CONVERSION TABLES

MASS

Metric

1 kilogram (kg.)	= 15,432 grains
	or 35·274 ounces
	or 2·2046 pounds
1 gramme (g.)	= 15·432 grains
1 milligram (mg.)	= 0·015432 grain

1 ton (2240 lb.)	= 1016 kilogrammes
1 hundredweight (112 lb.) (cwt.)	= 50·80 kilogrammes
1 stone (14 lb.) (st.)	= 6·35 kilogrammes
1 pound (avoirdupois) (lb.)	= 453·59 grammes
1 ounce (avoirdupois) (oz.)	= 28·35 grammes
1 grain (gr.)	= 64·799 milligrammes

CAPACITY

Metric

1 litre (l.)	= 1·7598 pints
1 millilitre (ml.)	= 16·894 minims

Imperial

1 gallon (160 fl. oz.) (gal.)	= 4·546 litres
1 pint (pt.)	= 568·25 millilitres
	or 0·56825 litre
1 fluid ounce (fl. oz.)	= 28·412 millilitres
1 fluid drachm (fl. dr.)	= 3·5515 millilitres
1 minim (min.)	= 0·059192 millilitres

LENGTH

Metric

1 kilometre (km.)	= 0·621 miles
1 metre (m.)	= 39·370 inches
1 decimetre (dm.)	= 3·9370 inches
1 centimetre (cm.)	= 0·39370 inch
1 millimetre (mm.)	= 0·039370 inch
1 micron (μ)	= 0·0039370 inch

Imperial

1 mile	= 1·609 kilometres
1 yard	= 0·914 metres
1 foot	= 30·48 centimetres
1 inch	= 2·54 centimetres
	or 25·40 millimetres

TEMPERATURE

Centigrade	Fahrenheit		Centigrade	Fahrenheit
110°	230°		38°	100·4°
100	212		37·5	99·5
95	203		37	98·6
90	194		36·5	97·7
85	185		36	96·8
80	176		35·5	95·9
75	167		35	95·0
70	158		34	93·2
65	149		33	91·4
60	140		32	89·6
55	131		31	87·8
50	122		30	86
45	113		25	77
44	111·2		20	68
43	109·4		15	59
42	107·6		10	50
41	105·8		+ 5	41
40·5	104·9		0	32
40	104·0		− 5	23
39·5	103·1		− 10	14
39	102·2		− 15	+ 5
38·5	101·3		− 20	− 4

To convert Fahrenheit into Centigrade, subtract 32, multiply the remainder by 5, and divide the result by 9.
To convert Centigrade into Fahrenheit, multiply by 9, divide by 5, and add 32.

VETERINARY MEDICINE

DEDICATED TO H.B. PARRY
AND TO THE MEMORY OF R.A. MACINTOSH
WHO BY THEIR CLINICAL TEACHING
LAID THE FOUNDATIONS
OF THIS BOOK

VETERINARY MEDICINE

FOURTH EDITION

D.C. Blood B.V.Sc., F.A.C.V.Sc.

Professor of Veterinary Medicine
Faculty of Veterinary Science, University of Melbourne

and

J.A. Henderson D.V.M., M.S.

Formerly Professor of Veterinary Medicine and Dean of the College of Veterinary Medicine
Washington State University, Pullman, Washington

THE WILLIAMS AND WILKINS COMPANY
BALTIMORE

BAILLIÈRE TINDALL
7 & 8 Henrietta Street, London WC2E 8QE

Cassell & Collier Macmillan Publishers Ltd, London
35 Red Lion Square, London WC1R 4SG
Sydney, Auckland, Toronto, Johannesburg

The Macmillan Publishing Company Inc.
New York

First published 1960
Fourth edition 1974
Reprinted 1975

ISBN 0 7020 0495 2

English Language Book Society Edition
Spanish Edition: *Editorial Interamericana, Mexico*
French Edition: *Vigot Frères, Paris*

Published in the United States of America by
The Williams and Wilkins Company, Baltimore.

Printed in Great Britain by William Clowes & Sons, Limited
London, Beccles and Colchester

Preface to the Fourth Edition

WHEN this book was first under discussion one of the major decisions to be made was whether there was a need for an omnibus-type book which dealt with the medical diseases of large animals. It was felt that species specialization and discipline specialization, and even specialization in body systems, were developing so rapidly that a textbook for generalists was unlikely to have a long life. In the intervening years specialization has developed in some degree but not to the extent that was anticipated. In clinical work, particularly with reference to food producing animals, specialization still tends to be a part-time occupation of individual veterinarians with practices providing a general service. Since this is a core book for large animal practitioners, and students with inclinations in that direction, we feel justified in writing this fourth edition in the same style as before, and with the same objectives.

The mass of published material which has appeared in recent years relating to the diseases of large animals is formidable and hard decisions were called for if the book was to remain of manageable size. Undoubtedly we have omitted items which should have been included and have included items which might well have been omitted. We claim no omniscience in these matters; given the constraints of time and distance we have done our best.

General Medicine is, as always, a relatively static section and we have made few changes; the sections on equine colic and diseases of the ruminant forestomach were exceptions and required significant additions. In Special Medicine there was much detail to add. So much had ensued in mastitis control since the last edition that the chapter had to be completely rewritten. Colibacillosis and salmonellosis were diseases on which much has been written recently and both sections required a good deal of modification. Vaccination against footrot in sheep, and the definition of the aetiology of swine dysentery were significant advances to be noted. Amongst the viral diseases there had been, as usual, a great deal of activity and almost every section required bringing up to date. The development of iso-immune haemolytic anaemia in calves after vaccination against protozoal diseases required a special note.

The descriptions of diseases caused by parasites have been updated, but there are special problems in the handling of parasitic diseases in a book of this type. Present-day advances in this field are related less to diagnosis and treatment than to those aspects of control which must be considered in formulating a preventive medicine or herd health programme. We point to this as an area which urgently requires its own literature, preferably in a herd health format. Amongst the nutritional deficiencies and metabolic diseases the most significant changes noted were in the 'metabolic profile' system of diagnosis and in vitamin E and selenium deficiencies. Again this group of diseases, currently designated as production diseases, needs to be considered within the framework of whole-farm economics.

A small beginning has been made in the section on Physical Agents on the matter of environmental pollution and its effect on animal health. Amongst chemical poisoning most advances have been made in the field of poison plants. The list of diseases caused by the inheritance of undesirable characters has had minor additions.

We fully expected that the chapter on diseases of unknown aetiology would be well reduced in length by the removal of finally identified aetiological entities such as 'hairy shaker' disease of lambs, and 'Manchester Wasting Disease'. But their places have been taken by the 'shaker foal' syndrome, trichomoniasis of horses, the 'mastitis–agalactia–metritis' syndrome of sows and gastric ulceration of pigs, most of which have been listed in previous editions but now have been given full status as diseases in their own right. The only really new addition in this chapter is the brief reference to the diseases of *Brunus edwardii*. Much of what is known about this area of animal disease is in the realm of folk-lore and we despair of ever being able to adapt it to present day methods of biochemical and biophysical evaluation. We include it as one reminder of what veterinary medicine was like before the cold analytical science of spectrophotometer, roentgen ray, oscilloscope, computer and standard deviation tipped the scales against the art of practice. To be sure we delight in the accuracy of science but we can still lament nostalgically for the obfuscation that the art of veterinary science made possible.

December 1973

D. C. Blood
J. A. Henderson

Contents

PART ONE   GENERAL MEDICINE

CONTENTS

PART TWO · SPECIAL MEDICINE

CONTENTS

List of Tables

PART ONE

GENERAL MEDICINE

1

Clinical Examination

In the investigation of any animal disease problem, whether involving a single animal or a group, the first and most important task is to carry out an accurate and complete clinical examination. The observations made should be recorded in detail. Clinical observations can and should be accurate although faulty interpretations, and hence faulty diagnoses, may occur because of inadequate knowledge.

The expression 'clinical examination' should not be misunderstood. It has three aspects: the animal, the history and the environment. Inadequate examination of any of these may lead to error. The examination of the affected animal represents only a part of the complete investigation. Careful questioning of the owner or attendant can yield information about the diet or the prior diet, about recent vaccination or surgery or about the introduction of animals into the group, that will provide the clues to a successful diagnosis. However, in certain instances, for example in arsenic poisoning, the most detailed examination of the animal and the most careful questioning of the owner may fail to elicit the evidence necessary for a correct diagnosis. Only a careful physical search for a source of arsenic can provide this information. Thus neglect of one aspect of the clinical examination can render valueless a great deal of work on the other aspects and lead to an error in diagnosis.

HISTORY-TAKING

In veterinary medicine history-taking is the most important of the three aspects of a clinical examination. The significance of the results obtained by examination of the patient and the environment are liable to be modified by a number of factors. Animals are unable to describe their symptoms and signs; they vary widely in their reaction to handling and examination and a wide range of normality must be permitted in the criteria used in a physical examination. These variations are much greater in some species than in others. Dogs, horses and cattle, because of their size and because they are accus-

tomed to human company, are relatively good subjects but sheep, goats and pigs are much more difficult. A satisfactory examination of the environment may prove difficult because of lack of knowledge of the factors concerned or because of the examiner's inability to assess their significance. Problems such as the measurement of the relative humidity of a barn and its importance as a predisposing factor in an outbreak of pneumonia or the determination of pH of the soil with reference to the spread of leptospirosis can present virtually insuperable difficulties to the veterinarian in the field. On the other hand a search for a specific factor such as a known poison may be relatively simple.

Nevertheless history-taking is the key to accurate diagnosis in veterinary medicine, and to be worth while it must be accurate and complete. Admittedly, human fallibility must be taken into consideration; there may be insufficient time, the importance of particular factors may not be appreciated, there may be misunderstanding. Although these are excusable to a point, failure to recognize the importance of the history can lead only to error. It is essential for the examiner to support and assess the accuracy of the history by careful examinations if he is not to be misled, but it is the inaccurate or incomplete history that can lead him furthest astray. For example, if the veterinarian rejects the possibility of erysipelatous endocarditis in a sow because there have never been cases of erysipelas on that particular farm, when in fact the patient has been purchased only 3 weeks previously, he is guilty of a cardinal error of omission.

The history should suggest not only the diagnostic possibilities but also the probabilities. A 1 year old heifer is unlikely to have clinical Johne's disease; an adult cow is more likely to have parturient paresis than a first-calf heifer, which in turn is more likely to have maternal obstetric paralysis than is the adult cow. The history may often indicate that special attention should be paid to the examination of a particular system in the animal, or a particular factor in the environment. For example in epilepsy, the animal may be seen when it is clinically normal and the only means of reaching a diagnosis is a consideration of the history.

History-taking Method

Successful history-taking involves certain intangibles which cannot be discussed here. However, a number of suggestions follow, which may prove helpful to the clinician. The owner or attendant must be handled with diplomacy and tact. The use of non-technical terms is essential since stockowners are likely to be confused by technical expressions or be reluctant to express themselves when confronted with terms they do not understand. Statements, particularly those concerned with time, should be tested for accuracy. Owners, and more especially herdsmen and agents, often attempt to disguise their neglect by condensing time or varying the chronology of events. It is amazing how many cattle can lose a hundred kilograms of body weight in a few hours! If a detailed cross-examination of the custodian seems likely to arouse his antagonism it is advisable for the veterinarian to forgo further questioning and be content with his own estimate of the dependability of the history. The clinician must try to separate the owner's observations from his interpretations. A statement that the horse had a bout of bladder trouble may, on closer examination, mean that the horse had an attack of abdominal pain in which it assumed a posture usually associated with urination. It is impossible to avoid the use of leading questions—'did the pigs scour?', 'was there any vomiting?'—but it is necessary to weigh the answers in accordance with the general veracity of the owner. Absence of a sign can only be determined by enquiring whether or not it occurred. Simply to ask for a complete history of what has happened almost invariably results in an incomplete history. The clinician must of course know the right questions to ask; this knowledge comes with experience and familiarity with disease. Laymen seldom describe symptoms and signs in their correct time sequence; part of the clinician's task is to establish the chronology of events.

For completeness and accuracy in history-taking the clinician should conform to a set routine. The system outlined below includes patient data, disease history and management history. The order in which these parts of the history are taken will vary. In general it is best to take the disease history first. The psychological effect is good: the owner appreciates the desire to get down to the facts about his animal's illness.

PATIENT DATA

If records are to be kept at all, even if only for financial purposes, accurate identification of the patient is essential. An animal's previous history can be referred to, the disease status of a herd can be examined, specimens for laboratory examination can be dispatched with the knowledge that the results can be related to the correct patient. And last but not least, financial statements will be sent, and to the correct owners, and will be correct in themselves. These points may have no bearing in establishing the diagnosis but they are of first importance in the maintenance of a successful practice. The relevant data include: the owner's name and initials, postal address and telephone number; the species, type, breed (or estimate of parentage in a crossbred), sex, age, name or number, body weight and, if necessary, a description including colour markings, polledness and other identifying marks of the patient. Such a list may appear formidable but many of the points, such as age, sex, breed, type (use made of animal, e.g. beef, dairy, mutton, wool), are often of importance in the diagnosis. A case history of a particular animal may suggest that further treatment is likely to be uneconomic because of age, or that a particular disease is assuming sufficient importance in a herd for different control measures to be warranted.

DISEASE HISTORY

History-taking will vary considerably depending on whether one animal or a group of animals is involved in the disease problem under examination. As a general rule in large animal work all disease states should be considered as herd problems until proved to be otherwise. It is often rewarding to examine the remainder of a group and find animals which are in the early stages of the disease.

Present Disease

Attempts should be made to elicit the details of the clinical abnormalities observed by the owner in the sequence in which they occurred. If more than one animal is affected, a typical case should be chosen and the variations in history in other cases should then be noted. Variations from the normal in the physiological functions such as intake of food or drink, milk production, growth, respiration, defaecation, urination, sweating, activity, gait, posture, voice and odour should be noted in all cases. There are many specific questions which need to be asked in each case but they are too numerous to list here and for the most part they are variations on the questions already suggested.

If a number of animals are affected information may be available from clinical pathological examinations carried out on living animals or necropsy examinations on fatal cases. The behaviour of animals before death and the period of time elapsing between the first observable signs and death or recovery are important items of information. Prior surgical or medical procedures such as castration, docking, shearing, or vaccination may be important factors in the production of disease.

Morbidity and Mortality Rates

The morbidity rate is usually expressed as the percentage of animals which are clinically affected compared with the total number of animals exposed to the same risks. The mortality rate, or percentage of affected animals which die, should also be estimated. These estimates may be important in diagnosis because of the wide variations in morbidity and mortality rates which occur in different diseases. An equally important figure is the proportion of animals at risk which are clinically normal but which show abnormality on the basis of laboratory or other tests.

Prior Treatment

The owner may have treated animals before calling for assistance. Exact details of the preparations used and doses given may be of value in eliminating some diagnostic possibilities. They will certainly be of importance when assessing the probable efficiency of the treatment, the significance of clinical pathological tests and in prescribing additional treatment.

Prophylactic and Control Measures

It should be ascertained if preventive or control procedures have already been attempted. There may have been clinical pathological tests, the introduction of artificial insemination to control venereal disease, vaccination, or changes in nutrition, management or hygiene. For example, in an outbreak of bovine mastitis careful questioning should be pursued regarding the method of disinfecting the cows' teats after each milking with particular reference to the type and concentration of the disinfectant used, and whether or not back-flushing of teat cups is practised. Spread of the disease may result from failure of the hygiene barrier at any one of a number of such points. When written reports are available they are more reliable than the memory of the owner. The history of the group relative to additions is of particular importance. Is the affected animal one of the group, or has it been

introduced, and how long ago? If the affected animal has been in the group for some time, have there been recent additions? Is the herd a 'closed herd' or are animals introduced at frequent intervals? Not all herd additions are potential carriers of disease. They may have come from herds where control measures are adequate, they may have been tested before or after sale or kept in quarantine for an adequate period after arrival; or they may have received suitable biological or antibiotic prophylaxes. They may come from areas where a particular disease does not occur, although a negative history of this type is less reliable than a positive history of derivation from an area where a particular disease is enzootic. The possibility of infection during transit is a very real danger and pre-sale certificates of health may be of little value if an animal has passed through a sale barn, a show or communal trucking yards while in transit. Highly infectious diseases may be transmitted via trucks, railway cars or other accommodation contaminated by previous inhabitants. Transient introductions, including animals brought in for work purposes, for mating or on temporary grazing, are often overlooked as possible vectors of disease. Other sources of infection are wild fauna which graze over the same area as domestic livestock, and inanimate objects such as human footwear, car tyres and feeding utensils.

A reverse situation may occur where imported stock has no resistance to enzootic infection in the home herd, or has not become adapted to environmental stresses such as high altitudes, high environmental temperatures and particular feeding methods or is not used to poisonous plants occurring in the new environment.

There may be considerable significance in the reasons for culling, and the number of animals disposed of for health reasons. Failure to grow well, poor productivity and short productive life will suggest the possible occurrence of a number of chronic diseases, including some caused by infectious agents, by nutritional deficiencies or by poisons.

Previous Disease

Information elicited by questioning on previous history of illness may be illuminating. If there is a history of previous illness enquiries should be made on the usual lines, including clinical observations, necropsy findings, morbidity and mortality rates, the treatments and control measures used and the results obtained. If necessary enquiries should be made about herds from which introduced animals have originated and also about herds to which other animals from the same source have been sent.

MANAGEMENT HISTORY

The management history includes nutrition, breeding policy and practice, housing, transport and general handling. It is most important to learn whether or not there has been any change in the prevailing practice prior to the appearance of disease. The fact that a disease has occurred when the affected animals have been receiving the same ration, deriving from the same source over a long period, suggests that the diet is not at fault, although errors in preparation of concentrate mixtures, particularly with the present-day practice of introducing additives to feeds, can cause variations which are not immediately apparent.

Nutrition

Livestock at pasture present a rather different problem from those being hand-fed in that they receive a diet which is less controlled and thus more difficult to assess. The risk of parasitic infestation, and, in some cases, infectious disease is much greater in grazing animals. Enquiries should be made as to the composition of the pasture, its probable nutritive value with particular reference to recent changes brought about by rain or drought, whether rotational grazing is practised, the fertilizer programme and whether or not minerals and trace elements are provided by top-dressing or mineral mixtures. The origin of mineral supplements, particularly phosphates which may contain excess fluorine, and home made mixtures which may contain excessive quantities of other ingredients should receive attention. Actual examination of the pasture area is usually more rewarding than a description of it. This facet of the examination will be dealt with in a later section.

Hand-fed animals are subjected to a more or less controlled food supply but because of human error they are frequently exposed to dietary mistakes. Types and amounts of foods fed should be determined. Young pigs may be stunted because they have not been kept on a starting ration for a sufficiently long period and the growing ration has not been introduced sufficiently gradually. Further examples of disease produced by inadequate handfed diets include osteodystrophia fibrosa in horses on diets containing excess grain, azoturia in the same species when heavy carbohydrate diets are fed during periods of rest, and lactic acid indigestion in cattle introduced to heavy grain diets too rapidly. The sources of the dietary ingredients may also be of importance. Grains from some areas are often much heavier and contain a much greater proportion of starch to husk than grains from other areas so that when feed is measured, rather than weighed, over- or under-feeding may occur. Exotic diseases may be imported in feed materials. Anthrax, foot-and-mouth disease and hog cholera are well-known examples. Variations in the preparation of ingredients of rations may produce variable diets. Overheating as in pelleting or the cooking of feeds can reduce their vitamin content; contamination with lubricating oil can result in poisoning by chlorinated naphthalene compounds; pressure extraction of linseed can leave considerable residues of hydrocyanic acid in the residual oil cake. Feeding practices may in themselves contribute to the production of disease. Pigs fed in large numbers with inadequate trough space or calves fed from communal troughs are likely to be affected by over-eating or inanition depending on their size and vigour. High-level feeding and consequent rapid growth may create deficiency states by increasing the requirement for specific nutrients.

In both hand-fed and grazing animals changes in diet should be carefully noted. Removal of animals from one field to another, from pasture to cereal grazing, from unimproved to improved pasture may all precipitate the appearance of disease. Periods of sudden dietary deficiency can occur as a result of bad weather, transportation or during change to unfamiliar feeds. Rapid changes are more important than gradual alterations, particularly in pregnant and lactating ruminants when metabolic diseases including those caused by hypocalcaemia, hypoglycaemia and hypomagnesaemia are likely to occur. The availability of drinking water must be determined; salt poisoning of swine occurs only when the supply of drinking water is inadequate.

Breeding

The breeding history may be of importance with regard to inherited disease. The existence of a relationship between sires and dams should be noted. Hybrid vigour in cross-bred animals should be considered when there is apparent variation in resistance to disease between groups maintained under similar environmental conditions. A general relationship between selection for high productivity and susceptibility to certain diseases is apparent in many breeds of animals and even in certain families. The possibility of genetotrophic disease, i.e. the inheritance of a greater requirement than normal of a specific nutrient, should be considered.

Breeding management may have some importance in the development of disease states; breeding early to avoid late calvings in the spring may result in calvings during cold weather when pasture is poor and in pasture-fed cattle this may lead to a high incidence of acetonaemia and hypomagnesaemic tetany. Similarly early beef calves born when the cows are confined may suffer losses from scours.

Climate

Many diseases are influenced by climate. Foot-rot in cattle and sheep reach their peak incidence in warm, wet summers and are relatively rare in dry seasons. Diseases spread by insects are encouraged when climatic conditions favour the propagation of the vector. Internal parasites are similarly influenced by climate. Cool, wet seasons favour the development of hypomagnesaemia in pastured cattle. Anhidrosis in horses is specifically a disease of hot, humid countries. The direction of prevailing winds is of importance in many disease outbreaks, particularly in relation to the contamination of pasture and drinking water by fumes from factories and mines and the spread of diseases carried by insects.

General Management

There are so many items in the proper management of livestock which if neglected can lead to the occurrence of disease that they cannot be related here; animal management in the prevention of disease is a subject in its own right. Some of the more important factors include hygiene, particularly in milking parlours and in parturition and rearing stalls; adequacy of housing in terms of space, ventilation, draining, situation and suitability of troughs; opportunity for exercise and the proper management of milking machines to avoid udder injury. The class of livestock under consideration is also of importance; for example, enterotoxaemia is most common in fattening lambs and pigs, parturient paresis in milking cows, obstructive urolithiasis in lambs and steers in feedlots and pregnancy toxaemia in ewes used for fat lamb production.

EXAMINATION OF THE ENVIRONMENT

A satisfactory examination of the environment necessitates an adequate knowledge of animal husbandry. Assessment of the various factors is often difficult but examination of the environment should never be neglected. It is often because of an observed relationship between environmental factors and the incidence of disease that suitable investigation of the disease can be undertaken. Even topography may be important. Flat, treeless plains offering no protection from wind predispose cattle to lactation tetany in inclement weather. Low marshy areas facilitate the spread of insect-borne diseases and soil-borne infections requiring damp conditions such as leptospirosis and Johne's disease, and diseases associated with liver fluke infestation are more prevalent in such areas. The soil type of a district may provide important clues to the detection of nutritional deficiencies; copper and cobalt deficiencies are most common on littoral sands and the copper deficiency/molybdenum excess complex usually occurs on peat soils. Predominant plant types, both natural and introduced, should be observed as they are often associated with soil types and may be the cause of actual disease; the high oestrogen content of some clovers, the occurrence of functional nervous diseases on pastures dominated by *Phalaris tuberosa* and perennial rye, liver damage on perennial rye grass pastures, the presence of selective absorbing 'converter' plants on copper- and selenium-rich soils are all examples of the importance of the dominant vegetation. The presence of specific poisonous plants, evidence of over-grazing, the existence of a bone-chewing or bark-chewing habit can be determined by an examination of the environment. Even in housed animals the presence of large quantities of bracken or spoiled sweet clover in the hay may go undetected if the actual feed is not examined. Vital clues in the investigation of poisoning in a herd may be the existence of rubbish heaps or ergotized grass or rye in the pasture, or the chewing of lead paint in the barn or careless handling of poisons in the feed area. In some cases the physical nature of the pasture plants may be important; old, bleached grass pasture can be seriously deficient in vitamin A, whereas lush young pasture can have rachitogenic potency because of its high carotene content or it may be capable of causing hypomagnesaemia if it is dominated by grasses. Lush legume pasture or heavy concentrate feeding with inadequate roughage can cause a serious bloat problem.

Drinking water may be an important factor in the production of disease. Deep artesian or subartesian waters may have a high fluorine content, shallow wells in rich organic soils may contain an excess of nitrate, water in ponds may be covered with algae containing neurotoxins or hepatoxic agents and flowing streams may carry effluent from nearby industrial plants.

EXAMINATION OF THE PATIENT

It is important that every patient receive a complete clinical examination. The omission of any part can lead to error in diagnosis and coincident diseases may be missed.

In this section a system for the examination of a patient is outlined. More detailed examination techniques are dealt with under the individual body systems. The examination of a patient consists of a general inspection carried out from a distance, followed by a physical examination in which the animal is examined at close quarters.

General Inspection

The importance of a general inspection of the animal cannot be over-emphasized, and yet it is often overlooked. Apart from the general impression gained from observation at a distance, there are some signs that can best be assessed before the animal is disturbed. The proximity of the examiner is particularly disturbing to animals that are unaccustomed to frequent handling.

GENERAL APPEARANCE

The general impression of the health of an animal obtained by an examination from a distance is difficult to analyse but the following points are important.

Demeanour

Separation of an animal from its group is often an indication of illness. The demeanour or bearing is also a reflection of the animal's health. If it responds normally to external stimuli such as sound and movement it is classified as bright. If the reactions are sluggish and the animal exhibits relative indifference to normal stimuli it is said to be dull or apathetic. A pronounced state of indifference in which the animal remains standing and is able to move but does not respond at all to external stimuli is usually referred to as the 'dummy' syndrome. This occurs in subacute lead poisoning, listeriosis and some cases of acetonaemia in cattle and encephalomyelitis and hepatic cirrhosis in the horse. The terminal stage of apathy or depression is coma in which the animal is unconscious and cannot be roused. Excitation states vary in severity. A state of anxiety or apprehension is the mildest form: here the animal is alert and looks about constantly but is normal in its movements. Such behaviour is usually expressive of moderate constant pain or other abnormal sensation as in early parturient paresis or in recent blindness. A more severe manifestation is that of restlessness in which the animal moves about a good deal, lies down and gets up and may go through other abnormal movements such as looking at its flanks, kicking at its belly and

rolling and bellowing. Again this demeanour is usually indicative of pain. More extreme degrees of excited demeanour include mania and frenzy. In mania the animal performs abnormal movements with vigour. Violent licking at its own body, licking or chewing inanimate objects, pressing forward with the head are typical examples. In frenzy, the actions are so wild and uncontrolled that the animals are a danger to anyone approaching them. In both mania and frenzy there is usually excitation of the brain as in rabies, acute lead poisoning and some cases of nervous acetonaemia.

Posture

Abnormal posture is not necessarily indicative of disease, but when associated with other signs it may indicate the site and severity of a disease process. One of the simplest examples is resting of a limb in painful conditions of the extremities: if a horse continually shifts its weight from limb to limb it may indicate the presence of laminitis or early osteodystrophia fibrosa. Arching of the back with the limbs under the body usually indicates mild abdominal pain; downward arching of the back and 'saw horse' straddling of the legs is characteristic of severe abdominal pain, usually spasmodic in occurrence; a 'dog-sitting' posture in the horse associated with rolling and kicking at the belly is usually associated with abdominal pain and pressure on the diaphragm such as occurs in acute gastric dilatation after engorgement on grain. In cattle this posture is commonly adopted by normal animals (4). Abduction of the elbows is usually synonymous with chest pain or difficulty in breathing. Elevation and rigidity of the tail, and rigidity of the ears and limbs are good indications of tetanus in animals. The carriage of the tail in pigs is a useful barometer of their state of health. Sheep that are blind, as in early pregnancy toxaemia, are immobile but stand with the head up and wear an expression of extreme alertness.

When the animal is recumbent there may also be abnormalities of posture. In cattle affected by dislocation of the hip or by sciatic nerve paralysis, the affected limb is not held flexed under the body but sticks straight out in an awkward position; unilateral pain in the chest may cause an animal to lie habitually on the other side, a weak hind leg may be kept under the animal. The head may be carried around towards the flank in parturient paresis in cows and in colic in horses. Sheep affected with hypocalcaemia, and cattle with bilateral hip dislocation, often lie in sternal recumbency with the hind legs extended behind in a frog-like attitude. Inability or lack of desire to rise are usually indicative of muscle weakness or of pain in the extremities as in enzootic muscular dystrophy or laminitis.

Gait

Movements of the limbs can be expressed in terms of rate, range, force and direction of movement. Abnormalities may occur in one or more of these categories. For example, in true cerebellar ataxia all qualities of limb movement are affected. In louping ill in sheep it is the range and force which are excessive giving a high-stepping gait and a bounding form of progression: in arthritis because of pain in the joints or in laminitis because of pain in the feet the range is diminished and the patient has a shuffling, stumbling walk. The direction of progress may be affected. Walking in circles is a common abnormality and is usually associated with rotation or deviation of the head; it may be a permanent state as in listeriosis or occur spasmodically as in acetonaemia and pregnancy toxaemia. Walking directly ahead regardless of obstructions is part of the 'dummy' syndrome mentioned earlier and is characteristic of encephalomyelitis and hepatic insufficiency in the horse.

Condition

The animal may be in normal bodily condition, obese, thin or emaciated. The difference between thinness and emaciation is one of degree; the latter is more severe but there are additional signs that are usually taken into consideration. In an emaciated (cachectic) animal the coat is poor, the skin is dry and leathery and work performance is reduced. Thin animals on the other hand are physiologically normal. The difference between fatness and obesity is of the same order. Most beef cattle prepared for the show-ring are obese.

Conformation

The assessment of conformation or shape is based on the symmetry and the shape and size of the different body regions relative to other regions. An abdomen which is very large relative to the chest and hindquarters can be classified as an abnormality of conformation. To avoid repetition points of conformation are included in the description of body regions.

Skin

Skin abnormalities can usually be seen at a distance. They include changes in the hair or wool, abnormal sweating, the presence of discrete or diffuse lesions, evidence of soiling by discharges and of itching. The normal lustre of the coat may be absent: it may be dry as in most chronic debilitating diseases or excessively greasy as in seborrhoeic dermatitis. In debilitated animals the long winter coat may be retained past the normal time. Alopecia may be evident: in hyperkeratosis it is diffuse; in ringworm it may be diffuse but more commonly occurs in discrete areas. Sweating may be diminished, as in anhidrosis of horses; patchy as in peripheral nerve lesions; or excessive as in acute abdominal pain. Hypertrophy and folding of the skin may be evident, hyperkeratosis being the typical example. Discrete skin lesions range in type from urticarial plaques, to the circumscribed scabs of ringworm, pox and impetigo. Diffuse lesions include the obvious enlargements due to subcutaneous oedema, haemorrhage and emphysema. Enlargements of lymph nodes and lymphatics are also evident when examining an animal from a distance.

BEHAVIOUR

Many aspects of the behaviour of the animal are of clinical importance.

Voice

Abnormality of the voice should be noted. It may be hoarse in rabies or weak in gut oedema: there may be continuous lowing in nervous acetonaemia or persistent bellowing indicative of acute pain. Soundless bellowing and yawning are commonly seen in rabid cattle and yawning is a common sign in animals affected with hepatic insufficiency.

Eating

In a patient which has retained its appetite there may be abnormality of prehension, mastication or swallowing and, in ruminants, of belching and regurgitation. Prehension may be marred by inability to approach feed, as in cerebellar ataxia, osteomyelitis of cervical vertebrae and other painful conditions of the neck. When there is pain in the mouth prehension may be abnormal and affected animals may be able to take only certain types of feed. Mastication may be slow, one-sided or incomplete when mouth structures, particularly teeth, are affected. Periodic cessation of chewing when food is still in the mouth occurs commonly in the 'dummy' syndrome, when there are space-occupying lesions of the cranium or an encephalomyelitis exists. Swallowing may be painful because of inflammation of the pharynx or oesophagus, as is found in strangles in the horse, in calf diphtheria, and where improper use of balling and drenching guns or bottles has caused laceration of the mucosa. Attempts at swallowing followed by coughing up of feed or regurgitation through the nostrils can also be the result of painful conditions but are most likely to be due to physical obstructions such as oesophageal diverticula or stenosis, a foreign body in the pharynx, or to paralysis of the pharynx. It is important to differentiate between material that has reached the stomach and ingesta regurgitated from an oesophageal site. Partial oesophageal obstruction resulting in difficult swallowing is usually manifested by repeated swallowing movements often with associated flexion of the neck and grunting.

In ruminants there may be abnormalities of rumination and belching. Absence of cudding occurs in many diseases of cattle and sheep; violent efforts at regurgitation with grunting suggest oesophageal or cardial obstruction. There may be inability to control the cud—'cud-dropping'—due to pharyngeal paralysis or painful conditions of the mouth. Failure to belch is usually manifested by the appearance of bloat.

Defaecation

In constipation and rectal paralysis or stenosis the act of defaecation may be difficult and be accompanied by much straining. When there is abdominal pain or laceration of the mucocutaneous junction at the anus defaecation may cause obvious pain. Involuntary defaecation occurs in severe diarrhoea and when there is paralysis of the anal sphincter. Consideration of frequency, volume and character of faeces is given later under the section on special examination of the digestive tract.

Urination

Micturition may be difficult when there is partial obstruction of the urinary tract, painful when there is inflammation of the bladder or urethra. In cystitis and urethritis there is increased frequency with the passage of small amounts of fluid and the animal remains in the urination posture for some time after the flow ceases. Incontinence, with constant dribbling of urine, is usually due to partial obstruction of the urethra or paralysis of its sphincter.

INSPECTION OF BODY REGIONS

As a general rule as much of a clinical examination as possible should be carried out before the animal is handled. This is partly to avoid unnecessary excitement of the patient but also because some abnormalities are better seen at a distance and in some cases cannot be discerned at close range. The general appearance of the animal should be noted and its behaviour assessed. Some time should also be devoted to an inspection of the various body regions.

Head

The facial expression may be abnormal, the rigidity of tetanus, the cunning leer or maniacal expression of rabies and acute lead poisoning are cases in point. The symmetry and configuration of the bony structure should be examined. Doming of the forehead occurs in some cases of congenital hydrocephalus and in chondrodysplastic dwarfs and in the latter there may be bilateral enlargement of the maxillae. Swelling of the maxillae and mandibles occurs in osteodystrophia fibrosa; in horses swelling of the facial bones is usually due to frontal sinusitis: in cattle enlargement of the maxilla or mandible is common in actinomycosis. Asymmetry of the soft structures may be evident and is most obvious in the carriage of the ears, degree of closure of the eyelids and situation of the muzzle and lower lip. Slackness of one side and drawing to the other are constant features in facial paralysis. Tetanus is accompanied by rigidity of the ears, prolapse of the third eyelid and dilation of the nostrils. The carriage of the head is most important; rotation is usually associated with defects of the vestibular apparatus on one side; deviation with unilateral involvement of the medulla and cervical cord; opisthotonus is an excitation phenomenon associated with tetanus, strychnine poisoning, acute lead poisoning, hypomagnesaemic tetany and encephalitis. The eyes merit attention: visible discharge should be noted, protrusion of the eyeball, as occurs in orbital lymphomatosis and retraction of the bulb as occurs commonly in dehydration are important findings: spasm of the eyelids and excessive blinking usually indicate pain or peripheral nerve involvement: prolapse of the nictitating membrane usually characterizes central nervous system derangement, generally tetanus. Dilation of the nostrils and nasal discharge suggest the advisability of closer examination of the nasal cavities at a later stage. Excessive salivation or frothing at the mouth denotes painful conditions of the mouth or pharynx or is associated with tremor of the jaw muscles due to nervous involvement. Swellings below the jaw may be inflammatory as in actinobacillosis and strangles, or oedematous as in acute anaemia, protein starvation or congestive heart failure. Unilateral or bilateral swelling of the cheeks in calves usually indicates necrotic stomatitis.

Neck

If there is enlargement of the throat this region should be more closely examined later to determine whether the cause is inflammatory and whether lymph nodes, salivary glands (or guttural pouches in the horse) or other soft tissues are involved. Goitre leads to local enlargement located further down the neck. A jugular pulse, jugular vein engorgement and oedema should be looked for and local enlargement due to oesophageal distension noted.

Thorax

The respiration should be examined from a distance, preferably with the animal in a standing position as recumbency is likely to modify it considerably. Allowance should be made for the effects of exercise, excitement, high environmental temperatures and fatness of the subject: obese show cattle may have respiratory rates two to three times that of normal animals. The rate, rhythm, depth and type of respiration should be noted.

Respiratory rate. In normal animals under average conditions the rate should fall within the following limits: horses 8 to 10, cattle 10 to 30, sheep and pigs 10 to 20 per minute. Increased respiratory rate is designated as polypnoea, decreased rate as oligopnoea and complete cessation as apnoea. The rate may be counted by observation of rib or nostril movements, by feeling the nasal air movements or by auscultation of the thorax or trachea. A significant rise in environmental temperature or humidity may double the normal respiratory rate (3).

Respiratory rhythm. The normal respiratory cycle consists of three phases of equal length; inspiration, expiration and pause; variation in the length of one or all phases constitutes an abnormality of rhythm. Prolongation of inspiration is usually due to obstruction of the upper respiratory tract, prolongation of the expiratory phase to failure of normal lung collapse as in emphysema. In most diseases of the lungs there is no pause and the rhythm consists of two beats instead of three. There may be variation between cycles: Cheyne-Stokes respiration, characteristic of advanced renal and cardiac disease, is a gradual increase and then a gradual decrease in the depth of respiration: Biot's breathing, which occurs in meningitis affecting the medullary region, is characterized by alternating periods of hypernoea and apnoea, the periods often being of unequal length.

Respiratory depth. The amplitude or depth of respiratory movements may be reduced in painful conditions of the chest or diaphragm, and increased in any form of anoxia. Moderate increase in depth is referred to as hypernoea and laboured breathing as dyspnoea. In dyspnoea the accessory respiratory movements are brought into play; there is extension of the head and neck, dilation of the nostrils, abduction of the elbows and breathing through the mouth plus increased movement of the thoracic and abdominal walls. Marked respiratory sounds, especially grunting, may also be heard.

Type of respiration. In normal respiration there is movement of the thorax and abdomen. In painful conditions of the chest, e.g. acute pleurisy, and in paralysis of the intercostal muscles there is fixation of the thorax and a marked increase in the movements of the abdominal wall; there is usually an associated pleuritic ridge caused by thoracic immobility with the chest expanded. This syndrome is usually referred to as an abdominal-type respiration. The reverse situation is thoracic type of respiration in which the movements are largely confined to the chest, as in peritonitis, particularly when there is diaphragmatic involvement.

Chest symmetry can also be gauged by inspection. Collapse or consolidation of one lung may lead to restriction of movements of the chest on the affected side. The 'rachitic rosary' of enlarged costochondral junctions is typical of rickets.

Respiratory noises or stridores include coughing due to irritation of the pharynx, trachea and bronchi, sneezing due to nasal irritation, wheezing due to stenosis of the nasal passages, snoring when there is pharyngeal obstruction as in tuberculous adenitis of the pharyngeal lymph nodes, roaring in paralysis of the vocal cords, and grunting, a forced expiration against a closed glottis, which happens in many types of painful and laboured breathing.

Abdomen

Variations in abdominal size are usually appreciated during the general inspection of the animal. An increase in size may be due to the presence of excess food, fluid, faeces, flatus or fat, the presence of a foetus or a neoplasm. Further differentiation is usually possible only on close examination, although foetal movements may be visible; in severe distension of the intestines with gas the loops of bowel may be visible in the flank. Gaseous distension is usually uniform whereas fluid tends to give an increased distension ventrally. The term 'gaunt' is often used to describe a decrease in abdominal size. It occurs most commonly in starvation, in severe diarrhoea and in many chronic diseases where appetite is reduced. Umbilical hernia or infection and dribbling from a pervious urachus may be apparent. Ventral oedema is commonly associated with approaching parturition, gangrenous mastitis, congestive heart failure, infectious equine anaemia, and rupture of the urethra due to obstructive urolithiasis. Ruminal movements are quite readily observed from a distance but are better examined at a later stage.

External Genitalia

Gross enlargements of the sheath or scrotum are usually inflammatory in origin but variocoele or tumours can also be responsible. Degenerative changes in the testicles may result in a small scrotum. Discharges of pus and blood from the vagina indicate infection of the genito-urinary tract.

Mammary Glands

Disproportionate size of the quarters of the udder suggests acute inflammation, atrophy or hypertrophy of a gland. These conditions can be differentiated only by palpation.

Limbs

Posture and gait have been described. Symmetry is important and comparison of pairs should be used when there is doubt of the significance of an apparent abnormality. Enlargement or distortion of bones, joints, tendons, sheaths and bursae should be noted and so should any enlargement of peripheral lymph nodes and lymphatic vessels.

Physical Examination

Some of the techniques used in making a physical examination are set out below.

Palpation

Direct palpation with the fingers or indirect palpation with a probe is aimed at determining the size, consistency, temperature and sensitiveness of a lesion or organ. Terms used to describe palpation findings include the following: doughy, when the structure pits on pressure as in oedema; firm, when the structure has the consistency of normal liver; hard, when the consistency is bone-like; fluctuating, when the structure is soft, elastic and undulates on pressure but does not retain the imprint of the fingers; emphysematous, when the structure is puffy and swollen, and moves and crackles under pressure because of the presence of gas in the tissue.

Percussion

In percussion the body surface is struck so as to set deep parts in vibration and cause them to emit audible sounds; the sounds vary with the density of the parts set in vibration. The sounds may be classified as follows: resonant, the sound emitted by organs containing air, e.g. normal lung; tympanitic, a drum-like note emitted by an organ containing gas under pressure such as a tympanitic rumen or caecum; dull, the sound emitted by solid organs such as heart and liver. The quality of the sound elicited is governed by a number of factors. The strength of the percussion blow must be kept constant as the sound volume increases with stronger percussion. Allowances must be made for the thickness and consistency of overlying tissues, the thinner the chest wall, the more resonant the lung; percussion on a rib must not be compared with percussion on an intercostal space; percussion in a fat animal may yield little information. The value of percussion as a diagnostic aid in large animals is limited. Man is the optimum size. Pigs and sheep are of a suitable size but the fatness of the pig and the wool coat of the sheep plus the unco-operative nature of both species make percussion impracticable. In cattle and horses the organs are too large and overlying tissue too thick for satisfactory outlining of organs or abnormal areas unless the observer is highly skilled.

Percussion can be carried out with the fingers using one hand as a plexor and one as a pleximeter. In large animals a pleximeter hammer may be used on a finger or a pleximeter disc. The use of the fingers is preferable as they produce little or no additional sound.

Tactile Percussion

By combining palpation and percussion it is possible to obtain information on the consistency and boundaries of organs not accessible by percussion alone. The technique consists essentially of an interrupted, firm, push stroke to push the organ away and allow it to rebound on to the finger-tips. Ballottement of a foetus is a typical example. A modification of the method is fluid percussion when a cavity containing fluid is percussed on one side and the fluid wave thus set up is palpated on the other.

Auscultation

Direct listening to the sounds produced by organ movement is performed by placing the ear to the body surface over the organ. Indirect auscultation by a stethoscope is much to be preferred. A considerable amount of work has been done to determine the most effective stethoscopic equipment including such things as the shape and proportions of bell chest pieces, the thickness of rubber tubes and the diameter and depth of phonendoscope chest pieces. A comparatively expensive unit from a reputable instrument firm is a wise investment. For large animal work a stethoscope with interchangeable 5 cm diameter phonendoscope and rubber (to reduce hair friction sounds) bell chest pieces is all that is required. The details of the sounds heard on auscultations of the various organs are described in their respective sections.

Combined Percussion and Auscultation

The fact that sounds are transmitted more efficiently through solid tissue than through tissue containing air can be utilized by combining percussion and auscultation. The stethoscope bell is placed over the area to be examined and a percussion sound produced by tapping on the trachea or on another part of the chest. Since the objective is to produce a sharp sound the tap should be short and forcible and be applied to tracheal cartilage or a prominent rib. An alternative method is to place one coin on the percussion site and strike it forcibly with the edge of another coin. When the tissue under examination is solid the percussion sound comes through sharply and loudly; when the tissue is air-filled it has an insulating effect and the sound produced is muffled and dull. The area of consolidation can be defined by comparing the sound with that heard in surrounding normal areas.

Succussion, or shaking of the body to detect the presence of fluid, is an adaptation of the above method. By careful auscultation while the body is shaken, free fluid in the chest or abdomen can be heard to rattle and an estimate of the fluid level can be made. One drawback of the technique is that fluid in the gut, especially when gas is present, will also rattle and may be confused with free fluid.

Miscellaneous special physical techniques including biopsy and paracentesis are described under special examination of the various systems to which they apply. With suitable equipment and technique one of the most valuable adjuncts to a physical examination is a roentgenological examination. The size, location and shape of soft tissue organs are often demonstrable in animals of up to moderate size.

EXAMINATION METHOD

The physical examination should be carried out as quietly and gently as possible to avoid disturbing the patient and thus upsetting the resting heart and respiratory rates. At a later stage it may be necessary to examine certain organs after exercise, but resting measurements should be carried out first. If possible the animal should be standing, as recumbency is likely to cause variation in pulse rate, respiration and other functions.

Temperature

Normally the temperature is taken per rectum. When this is impossible the thermometer should be inserted into the vagina. Ensure that the mercury column is shaken down, moisten the bulb to facilitate entry and if the anus is flaccid or the rectum full of hard faeces insert a finger also to ensure that the thermometer bulb is held against the mucosa. When the temperature is read immediately after defaecation, or if the thermometer is stuck into a ball of faeces or is left in the rectum for insufficient time, a false, low reading will result. As a general rule the thermometer should be left in place for 2 minutes. If there is doubt as to the accuracy of the reading, the temperature should again be taken. The normal temperature range for the various species at average environmental temperatures is as follows:

	Normal	Critical point
Horse	38·0 °C (100·5 °F)	39·0 °C (102·0 °F)
Cattle	38·5 °C (101·5 °F)	39·5 °C (103·0 °F)
Pig	39·0 °C (102·0 °F)	40·0 °C (103·5 °F)
Sheep	39·0 °C (102·5 °F)	40·0 °C (104·0 °F)

Temperature conversions are approximate.

These figures indicate the average resting temperature for the species and the critical temperature above which hyperthermia can be said to be present. Normal physiological variations occur in body temperature and are not an indication of disease: a diurnal variation of up to 1 °C (2 °F) may occur with the low point in the morning and the peak in the late afternoon. There may be a mild rise of about 0·6 °C (1 °F) in late pregnancy but the subnormal temperature quite often observed in bitches just before whelping is not constant in large animals. A precipitate but insignificant decline just before calving is not uncommon in cows and ewes (1) and lower temperatures than normal occur just before heat and at ovulation (2) but the degree of change (about 0·3 °C (0·6 °F)) is unlikely to attract clinical attention. High environmental humidity and temperature and exercise will cause elevation of the temperature; the deviation may be as much as 1·6 °C (3 °F) in the case of high environmental temperatures and as much as 2·5 °C (4·5 °F) after severe exercise: in horses, after racing, 2 hours may be required before the temperature returns to normal.

Marked temperature variations are an indication of a pathological process. *Hyperthermia* is simple elevation of the temperature past the critical point as in heat stroke. *Fever* or *pyrexia* is the state where hyperthermia is combined with toxaemia as in most infectious diseases. *Hypothermia*, subnormal body temperature, occurs in shock, circulatory collapse (as in parturient paresis and acute rumen impaction of cattle), hypothyroidism and just before death in most diseases.

Pulse

The pulse should be taken at the middle coccygeal or facial arteries in cattle, the facial artery in the horse and the femoral artery in sheep and goats. With careful palpation a number of characters may be determined, including rate, rhythm, amplitude, tone, maximum and minimum and pulse pressures and the form of the arterial pulse. Some of these characters are more properly included in special examination of the circulatory system and are dealt with under that heading.

Rate. The pulse rate is dependent on the heart alone and is not directly affected by changes in the peripheral vascular system. The pulse rate may or may not represent the heart rate; in cases with a pulse deficit where some heart-beats do not produce a pulse wave the rates will differ. Normal resting rates for the various species are:

Horses	30 to 40 per minute
Colts up to a year old	70 to 80 per minute
Cattle	60 to 80 per minute
Young calves	100 to 120 per minute
Sheep and goats	70 to 90 per minute

In newborn thoroughbred foals the pulse rate is 30 to 90 in the first 5 minutes, then 60 to 200 up to the first hour, and then 70 to 130 up to the first 48 hours after birth (6).

No pulse is palpable in the pig but the comparable heart rate is 60 to 100 per minute. *Bradycardia* or marked slowing of the heart-beat is unusual unless there is partial or complete heart block but it does occur in cases of space-occupying lesions of the cranium and in cases of diaphragmatic adhesions after traumatic reticulitis in cattle. *Tachycardia* or increased pulse rate is common, and occurs in most cases of septicaemia, toxaemia, circulatory failure and in animals affected by pain and excitement. Counting should be carried out over a period of at least 30 seconds.

Rhythm. The rhythm may be regular or irregular. All irregularities must be considered as abnormal except sinus arrhythmia, the phasic irregularity coinciding with the respiratory cycle. There are two components of the rhythm, namely the time between peaks of pulse waves and the amplitude of the waves. These are usually irregular at the one time, variations in diastolic filling of the heart causing variation in the subsequent stroke volume. Regular irregularities occur with constant periodicity and are usually associated with partial heart block. Irregular irregularities are due to ventricular extrasystoles or atrial fibrillation. Most of these irregularities, except that due to atrial fibrillation, disappear with exercise. Their significance lies chiefly in indicating the presence of myocardial disease.

Amplitude. The amplitude of the pulse is determined by the amount of digital pressure required to obliterate the pulse wave. It is largely a measure of cardiac stroke volume and may be considerably increased, as in the 'water hammer' pulse of aortic semilunar valve incompetence, or decreased as in most cases of myocardial weakness.

EXAMINATION OF BODY REGIONS

After the examination of the pulse, temperature and respiration the physical examination proceeds with an examination of the various body regions. This is best carried out in orderly fashion beginning at the head.

Head and Neck

Eyes. Any discharge from the eyes should be noted: it may be watery in obstruction of the lacrimal duct, serous in the early stages of inflammation and purulent in the later stages. Whether the discharge is unilateral or bilateral is of considerable importance; a unilateral discharge may be due to local inflammation, a bilateral discharge may denote a systemic disease. Abnormalities of the eyelids include abnormal movement, position and thickness. Movement may be excessive in painful eye conditions or in cases of nervous irritability including hypomagnesaemia, lead poisoning and encephalitis. The lids may be kept permanently closed when there is pain in the eye, or when the eyelids are swollen, as for instance in local oedema due to photosensitization or allergy. The membrana nictitans may be carried across the eye when there is pain in the orbit or in tetanus or encephalitis. There may be tumours on the eyelids.

Examination of the conjunctiva is important because it is a good indicator of the state of the peripheral vascular system. The pallor of anaemia and the yellow coloration of jaundice may be visible, although they are more readily observed on the oral or vaginal mucosae. Engorgement of the scleral vessels, petechial haemorrhages, oedema of the conjunctiva as in gut oedema of pigs or congestive heart failure, dryness due to acute pain or high fever are all readily observable abnormalities.

Corneal abnormalities include opacity varying from the faint cloudiness of early keratitis, to the solid white of advanced keratitis, often with associated vascularization, ulceration and scarring. Increased convexity of the cornea is usually due to increased pressure within the eyeball and may be due to glaucoma or hypopyon.

The size of the eyeball does not usually vary but

protrusion is relatively common and when unilateral is due in most cases to pressure from behind the orbit. Periorbital lymphoma in cattle, dislocation of the mandible and periorbital haemorrhage are common causes. Retraction of the eyeballs is a common manifestation of reduction in volume of periorbital tissues, for example in starvation when there is disappearance of fat and in dehydration when there is loss of fluids.

Abnormal eyeball movements occur in nystagmus due to anoxia or to lesions of the cerebellum or vestibular tracts. In nystagmus there is periodic, involuntary movement with a slow component in one direction and a quick return to the original position. The movement may be horizontal, vertical or rotatory. In paralysis of the motor nerves to the orbital muscles there is restriction of movement and abnormal position of the eyeball at rest.

Examination of the deep structures of the eye can be satisfactorily carried out only with an ophthalmoscope but gross abnormalities may be observed by direct vision. Pus in the anterior chamber, hypopyon, is usually manifested by yellow to white opacity often with a horizontal upper border obscuring the iris. The pupil may be of abnormal shape or abnormal in position due to adhesions to the cornea or other structures. An abnormal degree of dilation is an important sign, unilateral abnormality usually suggesting a lesion of the orbit. Bilateral excessive dilation (mydriasis) occurs in local lesions of the central nervous system affecting the oculomotor nucleus, or in diffuse lesions including encephalopathies, or in functional disorders such as botulism and anoxia. Peripheral blindness due to bilateral lesions of the orbits may have a similar effect. Excessive constriction of the pupils (miosis) is unusual unless there has been overdosage with organic phosphatic insecticides or parasympathetic drugs. Opacity of the lens is readily visible, especially in advanced cases.

Several tests of vision and of ocular reflexes are easily carried out, and when warranted should be done at this stage of the examination. Tests for blindness include a test for the eye preservation reflex and an obstacle test. In the former a blow at the eye is simulated, care being taken not to cause air currents. Reflex closure of the eyelids does not occur in peripheral or central blindness and in facial nerve paralysis there may be withdrawal of the head but no eyelid closure. An obstacle test in unfamiliar surroundings should be arranged and the animal's ability to avoid obstacles assessed. The results are often difficult to interpret if the animal is nervous. A similar test for night-blindness (nyctalopia) should be arranged in subdued light,

either at dusk or on a moonlit night. Nyctalopia is one of the earliest indications of avitaminosis A. Total blindness is called amaurosis, partial blindness is called amblyopia. The pupillary light reflex, closure and dilation of the iris in response to lightness and darkness, is best tested with a strong flashlight.

Nostrils. Particular attention should be paid to the odour of the nasal breath. There may be a sweet sickly smell of ketosis in cattle or a foetid odour which may originate from any of a number of sources including gangrenous pneumonia, necrosis in the nasal cavities or the accumulation of nasal exudate. Odours originating in the respiratory tract are usually constant with each breath and may be unilateral. The sour smell of alimentary tract disturbance is detectable only periodically coinciding with eructation. Odours originating in the mouth from bad teeth or from necrotic ulcers caused by *Sphaerophorus necrophorus* in calves may be smelled on the nasal breath but are stronger on the mouth breath.

In certain circumstances it may be important to note the volume of the breath expelled through the nostrils. It may be the only way of determining if the animal is breathing and in some cases of counting the respiratory rate. Variation in volume between nostrils, as felt on the hands, may indicate obstruction or stenosis of one nasal cavity. This can be examined further by closing off the nostrils one at a time; if obstruction is present in one nostril, closure of the other causes severe respiratory embarrassment.

Any nasal discharge that is present should receive special attention and its examination should be carried out at the same time as an inspection of the nasal mucosa. Discharges may be restricted to one nostril in a local infection, or be bilateral in systemic infection. The colour and consistency of the exudate will indicate its source. In the early stages of inflammation the discharge will be a clear, colourless fluid which later turns to a white to yellow exudate as leucocytes accumulate. In Channel Island cattle the colour may be a deep orange, especially in allergic rhinitis. A rust or prune juice colour indicates blood originating from the lower respiratory tract, as in pneumonia and in equine infectious anaemia in the horse. Blood clots derived from the upper respiratory tract or pharynx may be in large quantities or appear as small flecks. In general, blood from the upper respiratory tract is unevenly mixed with any discharge, whereas that from the lower tract comes through as an even colour. The consistency of the nasal discharge will vary from watery in the early stages of inflammation, through thick, to cheesy in long-standing cases. Bubbles or foam may be present. When the bubbles are coarse it signifies that the discharge originates in the pharynx or nasal cavities; fine bubbles originate in the lower respiratory tract. In all species vomiting or regurgitation caused by pharyngitis or oesophageal obstruction may be accompanied by the discharge of food material from the nose or the presence of food particles in the nostrils. In some cases the volume of nasal discharge varies from time to time, often increasing when the animal is feeding from the ground, suggesting infection of cranial sinuses.

Inflammation of the nasal mucosa varies from simple hyperaemia, as in allergic rhinitis, to diffuse necrosis, as in malignant head catarrh and mucosal disease, to deep ulceration as in glanders. In haemorrhagic diseases variations in mucosal colour can be observed and petechial haemorrhages may be present.

Mouth. Excessive salivation, with ropes of saliva hanging from the mouth and usually accompanied by chewing movements, occurs when a foreign body is present in the mouth and also in many forms of inflammation of the oral mucosa or of the tongue. Actinobacillosis of the tongue, foot-and-mouth disease and mucosal disease are typical examples. Identical signs appear in disease of the central nervous system when the salivary nucleus is involved, or where there is an encephalopathy as in acute lead poisoning in young cattle. Ingestion of a fungus sometimes found on red clover can induce excessive salivation, although the mechanism is unknown. Dryness of the mouth occurs in dehydration and poisoning with belladonna alkaloids or when high levels of urea are fed.

Abnormalities of the buccal mucosa include local lesions, haemorrhages in purpuric diseases, the discolorations of jaundice and cyanosis and the pallor of anaemia. Care must be taken to define the exact nature of lesions in the mouth, especially in cattle; differentiation between vesicles, erosive and ulcerative lesions is of diagnostic significance in the mucosal diseases of this species.

Examination of the teeth for individual defects is a surgical subject but a general examination of the dentition can yield useful medical information. Delayed eruption and uneven wear may signify mineral deficiency, especially calcium deficiency in sheep; excessive wear with mottling and pitting of the enamel is suggestive of chronic fluorosis.

The tongue may be swollen by local oedema or by inflammation as in actinobacillosis of cattle,

or shrunken and atrophied in post-inflammatory or nervous atrophy. Lesions of the lingual mucosa are part of the general buccal mucosal response to injury.

Examination of the pharyngeal region is difficult in large animals. In cattle it is usually performed with the hand using a mouth speculum. Foreign bodies, diffuse cellulitis and pharyngeal lymph node enlargement can be detected by this means. In horses, manual exploration can only be carried out under anaesthesia. Endoscopy is a useful method of examination in this species.

Submaxillary region. Abnormalities of the submaxillary region which should be noted include enlargement of lymph nodes due to local foci of infection, subcutaneous oedema as part of a general oedema, local cellulitis with swelling and pain, enlargement of salivary glands or guttural pouch distension in the horse. Thyroid gland enlargement is often missed or mistaken for other lesions, but its site, pulsation and surrounding oedema are characteristic.

Neck. Examination of the neck is confined mainly to the jugular furrow. Engorgement of the jugular vein may be due to obstruction of the veins by compression or constriction, or to failure of the right side of the heart. A jugular pulse of small magnitude is normal in most animals but it must be differentiated from a transmitted carotid pulse which is not obliterated by compression of the jugular vein at a lower level. Variations in size of the vein may occur synchronously with deep respiratory movements but bear no relation to the cardiac cycles. When the pulse is associated with each cardiac movement it should be determined whether it is negative or positive. The negative pulse is presystolic and due to atrial systole and is normal. The positive pulse is systolic and occurs simultaneously with the arterial pulse and the first heart sound; it is characteristic of an insufficient tricuspid valve.

Local or general enlargement of the oesophagus associated with vomiting or dysphagia occurs in oesophageal diverticulum, stenosis and paralysis, and in cardial obstructions. Passage of a stomach tube or probang can assist in the examination of oesophageal abnormalities.

Tracheal auscultation is often a worth-while procedure. Normally the sounds heard are soft and low but in upper respiratory tract disease they are purring or rattling when inflammatory exudate is present and whistling in the presence of stenosis. Tracheal auscultation is of particular value when there is doubt as to whether sounds heard over the chest are transmitted from the upper tract. If they are transmitted sounds they are audible only on inspiration.

Thorax

Examination of the thorax includes palpation, auscultation and percussion of the cardiac area (precordium) and the lung area.

Cardiac area. Palpation of the heart action has real value, the size of the cardiac impulses can be assessed and palpable thrills may on occasion be of more value than auscultation of murmurs. It is best carried out with the palm of the hand and should be performed on both sides. An increased cardiac impulse, the movements of the heart against the chest wall during systole, may be easily seen on close inspection of the left precordium and can be felt on both sides. It may be due to cardiac hypertrophy or dilation associated with cardiac insufficiency or anaemia or to distension of the pericardial sac with oedema or inflammatory fluid. Care should be taken not to confuse a readily palpable cardiac impulse due to cardiac enlargement with one due to contraction of lung tissue and increased exposure of the heart to the chest wall. Normally the heart movements can be felt as distinct systolic and diastolic thumps. These thumps are replaced by thrills when valvular insufficiencies or stenoses or congenital defects are present. When the defects are large the murmur heard on auscultation may not be very loud but the thrill is readily palpable. Early pericarditis may also produce a friction thrill. The cardiac impulse should be much stronger on the left than the right side and reversal of this situation indicates displacement of the heart to the right side. Caudal or anterior displacement can also occur.

Auscultation of the heart is aimed at determining the character of normal heart sounds and detecting the presence of abnormal sounds. Optimum auscultation sites are the fourth and fifth intercostal spaces, and, because of the heavy shoulder muscles which cover the anterior border of the heart, the use of a flat phonendoscope chest piece pushed under the triceps muscles is necessary. Extension of the forelimb may facilitate auscultation if the animal is quiet. Areas where the various sounds are heard with maximum intensity are not directly over the anatomical sites of the cardiac orifices because conduction of the sound through the fluid in the chamber gives optimum auscultation at the point where the fluid is closest to the chest wall. The first (systolic) sound is heard best over the cardiac apex, the tricuspid closure being most audible over the right apex, and mitral closure over the left apex. The second (diastolic) sound is heard best over the base of the heart, the aortic semilunar closure posteriorly and the pulmonary semilunar anteriorly, both on the left side.

In auscultation of the heart the points to be noted are the rate, rhythm, intensity and quality of sounds and whether abnormal sounds are present. Comparison of the heart and pulse rates will determine whether there is a pulse deficit due to weak heart contractions failing to cause palpable pulse waves: this is most likely to occur in irregular hearts. Normally the rhythm is in three time and can be described as LUBB-DUPP-pause, the first sound being dull, deep, long and loud and the second sound sharper and shorter. As the heart rate increases the cycle becomes shortened mainly at the expense of diastole and the rhythm assumes a two-time quality. More than two sounds per cycle is classified as a 'gallop' rhythm and may be due to reduplication of either the first or second sounds. Reduplication of the first sound is common in normal cattle and its significance in other species is discussed under diseases of the circulatory system. The rhythm between successive cycles should be regular except in the normal sinus arrhythmia associated with respiration. With irregularity there is usually variation in the time intervals between cycles and in the intensity of the sounds, louder sounds coming directly after prolonged pauses and softer than normal sounds after shortened intervals as in extrasystolic contractions. The intensity of the heart sounds may vary in two ways, absolutely or relatively; absolutely when the two sounds are louder than normal and relatively when one sound is increased compared to the other in the cycle. For example, there is increased absolute intensity in anaemia and in cardiac hypertrophy. The intensity of the first sound depends on the force of ventricular contraction and is thus increased in ventricular hypertrophy and decreased in myocardial asthenia. The intensity of the second sound depends upon the semilunar closure, that is on the arterial blood pressure and is, therefore, increased when the blood pressure is high and decreased when the pressure is low.

Abnormal sounds may replace one or both of the normal sounds or may accompany them. The heart sounds are muffled when the pericardial sac is distended with fluid. Sounds which are related to events in the cardiac cycle are murmurs or bruits and are caused mainly by endocardial lesions such as valvular vegetations or adhesions, insufficiency of closure of valves and to abnormal orifices such as a patent interventricular septum or ductus arteriosus. Interference with normal blood flow causes the development of turbulence with resultant eddying and the creation of murmurs. In attempting to determine the site and type of lesion it is necessary to identify its time of occurrence in the cardiac cycle; it may be presystolic, systolic or diastolic and it is usually necessary to palpate the arterial pulse and auscultate the heart simultaneously to determine accurately the time of occurrence. The site of maximum audibility may indicate the probable site of the lesion, but other observations including abnormalities of the arterial pulse wave should be taken into account. In many cases of advanced debility, anaemia and toxaemia soft murmurs which wax and wane with respiration (haemic murmurs) can be heard and are probably due to myocardial asthenia. In cases of local pressure on the heart by other organs, for example in diaphragmatic hernia in cattle, loud systolic murmurs may be heard, due probably to distortion of the valvular orifices.

Abnormal sounds not related to the cardiac cycle include pericardial friction rubs which occur with each heart cycle but are not specifically related to either systolic or diastolic sounds. They are more superficial, more distinctly heard than murmurs and have a to-and-fro character. Local pleuritic friction rubs may be confused with pericardial sounds especially if respiratory and cardiac rates are equal.

Percussion to determine the boundaries of the heart is of little value in large animal work because of the relatively large size of the heart and lungs and the depth of tissue involved. The area of cardiac dullness is increased in cardiac hypertrophy and dilation and decreased when the heart is covered by more than the usual amount of lung as in pulmonary emphysema. More detailed examination of the heart by electrocardiography, roentgenological examination, test puncture and blood pressure are described under diseases of the heart.

Lung area. Palpation, percussion and auscultation are again the methods available for examination of the lung area. Palpation may reveal the presence of a pleuritic thrill, bulging of the intercostal spaces when fluid is present in the thoracic cavity, or narrowed intercostal spaces and decreased rib movement over areas of collapsed lung.

Percussion may be by the usual direct means or indirectly by tracheal percussion when the trachea is tapped gently and the sound listened for over the lung area. With direct percussion the area of normal lung resonance can be defined and abnormal dullness or resonance detected. Increased dullness indicates the presence of underlying solid tissue, such as hepatized, oedematous or collapsed lung, or an accumulation of fluid. An overloud normal percussion note is obtained over tissue containing more air than usual, for example emphysematous lung. A definite tympanitic note can be elicited over pneumothorax or a gas-filled viscus penetrating through a diaphragmatic hernia. For percussion to be a satisfactory diagnostic aid affected areas need to be large with maximum abnormality, and the chest wall must be thin.

Auscultation. The lung area available for satisfactory auscultation is slightly larger than that available for percussion. The normal lung sound or vesicular murmur is heard over the bulk of lung tissue, particularly in the middle third anteriorly over the base of the lung and is a soft, sipping 'VEE-EFF', the latter, softer sound occurring at expiration. The sounds are caused by the movement of air in and out of alveoli and are heard with variable ease depending on the thickness of the chest wall and the amplitude of the respiratory excursion. In well-fleshed horses and fat beef-cattle the sounds may not be discernible at rest. Increased vesicular murmurs are heard in dyspnoea and in early pulmonary congestion and inflammation. The vesicular murmur may be diminished or absent when the alveoli and small bronchi are not filling with air, as in the later stages of pneumonia, pulmonary oedema and collapse. Bronchial tones are the sounds produced by the passage of air through the larger air passages and in normal animals are audible only at the base of the lung. If the lung is collapsed but there is no exudate in the bronchi, such as occurs in interstitial pneumonia, the area over which bronchial tones may be heard is much increased.

Abnormal sounds over the lung area include râles, friction rubs and peristaltic sounds. Râles may be moist when bronchioles are full of moist exudate and bubbling, gurgling sounds, easily moved by coughing are heard. Dry râles are whistling sounds caused by the presence of small amounts of tenacious exudate in the bronchioles and are most commonly heard in chronic pneumonia. Crepitant râles are fine, crackling sounds occurring when collapsed bronchi are dilated by the passage of air as in early pneumonia or emphysema. Pleuritic friction rubs are dry, crackling sounds caused by the rubbing together of dry inflamed pleural surfaces: they occur in emphysema and in early pleurisy, disappearing when the surfaces become separated by pleuritic effusion. Pleuritic friction rubs are likely to be confused with dry or crepitant râles but are more superficial, are not influenced by coughing and have a jerky character. They are heard equally well on inspiration and expiration whereas râles are most audible during inspiration.

Sounds of peristalsis are normally heard over the lung area on the left side in cattle and in horses. In cattle these sounds are due to reticular movement and in horses to movements of the colon. Their presence is not of much significance in these species unless there are other signs. In cattle, too, sounds of swallowing, belching and regurgitation may be confused with peristaltic sounds; ruminal movements and the oesophagus should be observed for the passage of gas or a bolus to identify these sounds. Other techniques for examination of the thorax are described under diseases of the respiratory system.

Abdomen

Palpation through abdominal wall. Palpation through the abdominal wall as is practised in small animals has very little place in large animal work. Palpation of an enlarged liver behind the right costal arch is sometimes possible in the cow. The focus of abdominal pain can sometimes be located by external palpation in horses and cattle. In pigs and sheep little can be accomplished by palpation since they are seldom sufficiently quiet and relaxed. In the detection of pain a firm even lift is required for deep-seated pain and a firm punch or jab for superficial pain. In cattle pain may be elicited over the right caudal ribs when there are liver lesions, over the hypogastrium in reticuloperitonitis or generally over the abdomen in diffuse peritonitis. If there is doubt as to whether pain is produced by the manipulation simultaneous auscultation of the trachea will detect a perceptible grunt when the affected area is reached. Percussion of the abdomen has little value in large animals. A distended rumen or caecum is usually discernible without the use of other aids. However, some clinicians derive a real advantage by percussing the abdomen of cattle for small acumulations of gas, such as occur with left abomasal displacement or obstruction of the duodenum. Percussion is carried out by a smart tap with a solid object such as a screwdriver, or by flicking with a fingernail, over the suspected area.

Rectal examination. Special care is necessary to avoid injuring the patient and causing it to strain. Suitable lubrication and avoidance of force are the two most important factors. Rectal examination enables observations to be made on the alimentary, urinary and genital tracts and on the vessels, peritoneum and pelvic structures. Palpable abnormalities of the digestive tract include paralysis and ballooning of the rectum, distension of the loops of the intestine with fluid or gas, the presence of hard

masses of ingesta as in caecal and colonic impactions in the horse, and intestinal obstruction due to volvulus, intussusception or strangulation. The detection of tight bands of mesentery leading to displaced segments may be a valuable guide. In cattle the caudal sacs of the rumen are readily palpable. When the rumen is distended as in bloat or vagus indigestion they may push well into the pelvis or be only just within reach when the rumen is empty. A distended abomasum may be felt in the right half of the abdomen in cases of abomasal torsion and occasionally in vagus indigestion. In normal animals there is little to feel because of the space occupied by normal intestines. Palpable objects should be carefully examined.

The left kidney in the cow can be felt in the midline and distinct lobulations are evident. In the horse the caudal pole of the left kidney can often be felt, but the right organ is out of reach. There may be abnormalities of size in pyelonephritis, hydronephrosis and amyloidosis, and pain on pressure in pyelonephritis. The ureters are not normally palpable nor is the empty bladder. A distended bladder or chronic cystitis with thickening of the wall can be felt in the midline at the anterior end of the pelvic cavity. Large calculi have a stone-like hardness and are occasionally observed in horses in the same position. Pain with spasmodic jerking of the penis on palpation of the urethra occurs in urinary obstruction due to small calculi, cystitis and urethritis. Enlarged, thickened ureters such as occur in pyelonephritis can be felt between the kidney and the bladder.

In the peritoneum and mesentery one may feel the small, grape-like lesions of tuberculosis, the large, irregular, hard masses of fat necrosis and the enlarged lymph nodes of lymphomatosis. The abdominal aorta is palpable, and in horses the anterior mesenteric artery and some of its branches can be felt. This may be an important examination if a verminous aneurysm is suspected, in which case the vessels are thickened but still pulsate, have an uneven rough surface and may be painful. In horses the caudal edge of the spleen is usually palpable in the left abdomen. There is an excellent description of rectal exploration in the horse (5).

Examination of the genital organs is usually carried out at this stage but is not discussed here because it is dealt with adequately in texts on diseases of the genital system.

Auscultation. Auscultation of the rumen in cattle and sheep is frequently a rewarding examination. In normal animals there are one to three movements per minute depending on the amount of time which has elapsed since feeding, and the type of feed consumed. The examination is made in the upper left flank and a normal sequence of sounds consists of a lift of the flank with a fluid gurgling sound, followed by a second more pronounced lift accompanied by a booming, gassy sound. Auscultation of the lower left ribs in these animals allows one to pick up the fainter fluid sounds of reticular contraction just prior to the contractions of the ventral ruminal sac and the dorsal ruminal sac described above. Reticular sounds have been described as being accompanied by a grunt in cases of traumatic reticulitis. Decrease in the loudness and frequency of these sounds occurs in many diseases and is discussed in detail under diseases of the ruminant stomachs.

Intestinal sounds are thin and faint in cattle and often masked by ruminal sounds. In horses the intestinal sounds are clearly audible. In the right flank and ventral abdomen one can hear the loud, booming borborygmi of the colon and caecum, and in the left flank the much fainter rushing fluid sounds of the small intestine. Increased sounds with a more fluid quality are heard in enteritis and spasmodic colic; there is a decrease or absence of sounds in impaction of the large intestine or verminous aneurysm. In intestinal stasis in the horse auscultation in the right flank often detects the tinkling sound of fluid dropping from the ileocaecal valve through gas into the body of the caecum.

A special form of auscultation in cattle is the auscultation of the left costal arch about one-third of the way up the rib for the fluid gurgling sounds of abomasal displacement. Special techniques for examination of the abdomen are described under that system.

DIAGNOSIS

The practice of medicine consists of two major facets, the making of a diagnosis and the provision of treatment and control measures. For treatment and control to be of optimum value the diagnosis must be accurate, so that diagnosis is the crux of all medical problems. In general there are two ways of making a diagnosis. The rote method is based on past experience and depends upon the recognition of a syndrome which is identical with one seen on a previous occasion. The second method is diagnosis by reasoning and is based on a rational summing up of the clinical findings and progression by logical steps to a final diagnosis. In a busy practice the first method is often used and as experience is enlarged becomes reasonably accurate in many cases. However, its weakness lies in the fact that so few cases

are identical and many will be seen that are sufficiently atypical to make the use of the method highly inaccurate. As a general rule diagnosis by reasoning is the method of choice and the following pattern provides a useful framework for its development.

Determination of the Abnormality of Function Present

Disease is abnormality of function which is harmful to the animal. The first step is to decide what abnormality of function is present. There may of course be more than one. Definition is usually in general terms such as paralysis, stasis of the alimentary tract, anoxia, respiratory failure, nervous shock and so on. These terms are largely clinical, referring to abnormalities of normal physiological functions, and their use requires a foreknowledge of normal physiology. It is at this point that the preclinical study of physiology merges into the clinical study of medicine.

The necessary familiarity with the normal, combined with observation of the case in hand, makes it possible to determine the physiological abnormality which may, for example, be anoxia. The next step is to determine the bodily system or systems involved in the production of the anoxia.

Determination of the System Involved

Having made a careful clinical examination and noted any abnormalities it is now possible to consider which bodily system is at fault. This may not be difficult with some systems: for example, anoxia must be due to failure of the circulatory or respiratory systems and examination of these systems is not difficult. However, special problems arise when one is attempting to examine the nervous system, the liver, kidney, spleen and haemopoietic systems. Routine physical examination by palpation, auscultation and percussion is not very rewarding. Ancillary methods of examination are necessary and are described under special examination methods for the various systems. As a guiding principle all functions of the organ under examination should be observed and any abnormalities noted. For example, if the integrity of the central nervous system is to be examined abnormality of muscle and sphincter tone including involuntary movement, abnormal posture, gait, mental state and defects of special senses should be looked for. Knowing the normal physiological functions of systems one looks for aberrations of them. When only simple physical examination is available it may be extremely difficult to choose between two or more systems as the possible seat of abnormality. For example, it may be difficult to decide between nervous and muscular origins of paralysis. If special diagnostic techniques are not available it is necessary to resort to probability as a guide. Paralysis due to muscle disease is unusual except in calves and lambs under special circumstances. If the patient is mature it is probable that the paralysis is of nervous origin. In some instances a secondary problem to be solved is the whereabouts within the system of the lesion. Dysentery or melaena may result from bleeding at various levels in the alimentary tract and the location of the site may be important in deciding the probable cause of the haemorrhage. This is particularly important when surgery is projected and only very careful examination and a detailed knowledge of localized function will answer the question accurately.

Determination of the Type of Lesion

The abnormality observed may be produced by lesions of different types. In general lesions can be divided into anatomical or physical lesions and functional disturbances. The physical lesions can be further subdivided into inflammatory, degenerative or space-occupying. These classifications are not mutually exclusive, a lesion may be both inflammatory and space-occupying; abscesses in the spinal cord or lung are typical examples. In these circumstances it is necessary to modify the diagnosis and say that such and such a lesion is space-occupying and may or may not be inflammatory.

The differentiation between functional disturbances and physical lesions is often extremely difficult because the abnormalities produced may be identical. For example, in a case of encephalopathy due to acute lead poisoning there is no physical lesion but the differentiation from the encephalitis of furious rabies may be impossible. As a rule, functional disturbances are transient, often recurrent or fluctuating and are readily reversible by treatment whereas structural lesions cause signs which are relatively static or at least change only gradually and are affected only gradually by treatment. This is by no means a regular rule; the acute abdominal pain of intestinal obstruction usually fluctuates but the lesion is a physical one whereas the paralysis of parturient paresis in cattle is static but the disturbance is functional only.

Differentiation between inflammatory, degenerative and space-occupying lesions is usually simpler. The latter produce signs characteristic of pressure on surrounding organs and can often be detected by physical means. Inflammatory lesions are characterized by heat, pain, swelling and a local or general leucocytosis and, in severe cases, a systemic toxaemia. Degenerative lesions produce the same loss or abnormality of function as lesions of the other types but are not usually accompanied by evidence of inflammation unless they are extensive. If the lesion is accessible biopsy should be considered as a means of determining its nature.

Determination of the Specific Cause of the Lesion

If the system involved, the nature of the abnormality and the type of lesion can be satisfactorily determined, it then remains to decide on the specific causative agent. If, for example, it could be said that a particular case of paralysis in a calf was caused by a degenerative lesion of the musculature only a few specific aetiological agents would have to be considered to make a final diagnosis. In many, if not most, cases it is impossible to go beyond this stage without additional techniques of examination, particularly laboratory examinations, and it is a general practice to make a diagnosis without this confirmatory evidence because of limitations of time or facilities.

It is at this stage that a careful history taking and examination of the environment show their real value. It is only by a detailed knowledge of specific disease entities, the conditions under which they occur, the epizootiology and the clinical niceties of each that this informed guess can be made with any degree of accuracy. If the diagnostic possibilities can be reduced to a small number, confirmation of the diagnosis by laboratory methods becomes so much easier because there are fewer examinations to be made and confirmation by response to treatment is easier to assess. If it is necessary to treat with a great many drugs serially, or in combination, to achieve a cure the expense is greater and the satisfaction of both the client and the veterinarian is diluted in proportion to the range of treatments. Accuracy in diagnosis means increased efficiency and this is the final criterion of veterinary practice.

REFERENCES

(1) Ewbank, R. (1969). *J. Reprod. Fertil.*, *19*, 569.
(2) Wrenn, T. R. (1958). *J. Dairy Sci.*, *41*, 1071.
(3) Taneja, G. C. (1960). *Indian J. vet. Sci.*, *30*, 107.
(4) Ewbank, R. (1964). *Vet. Rec.*, *76*, 388.
(5) Greatorex, J. C. (1968). *Equ. vet. J.*, *1*, 26.
(6) Rossdale, P. D. (1967). *Brit. vet. J.*, *123*, 521.

2

General Systemic States

THERE are several general systemic states which contribute to the effects of many diseases. Because they are common to so many diseases they are dealt with here as a group to avoid unnecessary repetition. Toxaemia, hyperthermia, fever and septicaemia are closely related in their effects on the body, and an appreciation of them is necessary if they are not to be overlooked in the efforts to eliminate the causative agent.

TOXAEMIA

Toxaemia is caused by the presence of toxins deriving from bacteria or produced by body cells. It does not include the diseases caused by toxic substances produced by plants or insects or ingested organic or inorganic poisons. Theoretically a diagnosis of toxaemia can be made only if toxins are demonstrable in the blood stream. Practically, toxaemia is often diagnosed when the syndrome described below is present. In most cases there is contributory evidence of a probable source of toxins which in many cases are virtually impossible to isolate or identify.

Aetiology

Toxins can be classified as antigenic and metabolic toxins. *Antigenic toxins* are produced by bacterial metabolism and probably to a less extent by helminth parasites. At least in the latter case there is the capacity to produce antigens resulting in the formation of antibodies. Bacterial toxins may be ingested preformed as in botulism, or be produced by excessive growth of alimentary tract flora, as occurs in enterotoxaemia caused by *Clostridium perfringens* Type D in lambs and calves. They may also arise from localized infection, as in metritis, mastitis and visceral abscesses including such specific diseases as necrotic hepatitis caused by *Cl. novyi* and bacillary haemoglobinuria caused by *Cl. haemolyticum*. *Metabolic toxins* may accumulate as a result of incomplete elimination of toxic materials normally produced by body metabolism, or by abnormal metabolism. Normally, toxic pro-

ducts produced in the alimentary tract or tissues are excreted in the urine and faeces or detoxified in the plasma and liver. When these normal mechanisms are disrupted, particularly in hepatic dysfunction, the toxins may accumulate beyond a critical point and the syndrome of toxaemia appears (3, 4). In obstruction of the lower alimentary tract there may be increased absorption of toxic phenols, cresols and amines which are normally excreted with the faeces, resulting in the development of the syndrome of auto-intoxication. In ordinary circumstances in monogastric animals these products of protein putrefaction are not absorbed by the mucosa of the large intestine but when regurgitation into the small intestine occurs there may be rapid absorption, apparently because of the absence of a protective barrier in the wall of the small intestine. In liver diseases many of the normal detoxification mechanisms, including oxidation, reduction, acetylation and conjugation with such substances as glycine, glucuronic acid, sulphuric acid and cysteine, are lost and substances not normally present in sufficient quantity to cause injury accumulate to the point where illness occurs. The production of toxins by abnormal metabolism is taken to include the production of histamine and histamine-like substances in damaged tissues. Ketonaemia due to a disproportionate fat metabolism, and lactic-acidaemia caused by acute ruminal impaction are two common examples of toxaemia caused by abnormal metabolism.

Pathogenesis

The effects of non-specific toxins on body functions are difficult to define. The more specific toxins, especially those of bacterial origin, have in many cases been isolated and their exact mode of action determined (1). For the most part the non-specific toxins exert their influence on carbohydrate metabolism (2): there is a fall in blood sugar level, the rate and degree varying with the severity of the toxaemia, a disappearance of liver glycogen and a decreased glucose tolerance of tissues so that administered glucose is not used rapidly. There is also an increase in protein breakdown and a rise in blood non-protein nitrogen levels. The means by which these metabolic changes are brought about are uncertain but two factors, damage to endocrine glands and interference with the normal activity of enzyme systems, appear to be logical means. Certainly lesions are present in endocrine glands, particularly the anterior pituitary and adrenal glands, in most toxaemias, and adrenocortical hormones do have protective and curative action in most toxaemic states. Damage to the liver and kidney parenchyma is also apparent.

The combined effects of the hypoglycaemia, interference with tissue enzymes and degenerative changes, reduce the functional activity of most tissues. The myocardium is weakened, the stroke volume decreases and the response to cardiac stimulants is diminished. There is dilatation and in some cases damage to capillary walls so that the effective circulating blood volume is decreased; this decrease, in combination with diminished cardiac output, leads to a fall in blood pressure and the development of circulatory failure. Respiration is little affected except in so far as it responds to the failing circulation. There is decreased liver function and the damage to renal tubules and glomeruli causes a rise in blood non-protein nitrogen and the appearance of albuminuria. The functional tone and motility of the alimentary tract is reduced and the appetite fails, digestion is impaired with constipation usually following. A similar loss of tone occurs in skeletal muscle and is manifested by weakness and terminally by prostration. Apart from the effects of specific toxins on the nervous system, such as those of *Cl. tetani* and *Cl. botulinum*, there is a general depression of function attended by dullness, depression and finally coma. Changes in the haemopoietic system include depression of haemopoiesis and an increase in the number of leucocytes, the type of cells which increase often varying with the type and severity of the toxaemia. Leucopenia may occur but is usually associated with aplasia of the leucopoietic tissue caused by viruses or specific exogenous substances such as radioactive materials.

Clinical Findings

The clinical picture in most non-specific toxaemias is approximately the same. It varies with the speed and severity of the toxic process but the variations in the syndrome are largely of degree. Depression, lethargy, separation from the group, anorexia, failure to grow or produce and emaciation are characteristic signs. Constipation is usual, the pulse is weak and rapid but regular and there

may be albuminuria. The heart rate is increased, the sounds reduced and a 'haemic' murmur may appear. There may or may not be fever; in most toxaemias due to bacterial infection or tissue destruction fever is present, but this is not so with metabolic toxins. Terminally there is muscular weakness to the point of collapse and death occurs in a coma or with convulsions.

Clinical Pathology

Isolation and identification of the toxin may be possible and the source of the toxic material may be found. A low blood sugar, high blood NPN (non-protein nitrogen), aplastic anaemia, leucocytosis and albuminuria can be anticipated. A glucose tolerance curve similar to that of diabetes mellitus in humans may be detectable in monogastric animals, and there is little response to insulin in correcting this deficiency. The importance of this factor in ruminants is unknown.

Necropsy Findings

Gross findings at necropsy are limited to those of the lesion which produces the toxin. Microscopically there is degeneration of the parenchyma of the liver, the glomeruli and tubules of the kidney and of the myocardium. There may also be degeneration or necrosis in the adrenal glands.

Diagnosis

A clinical diagnosis of toxaemia is frequently made and often with little more basis than the rather ill-defined syndrome described above. This is largely unavoidable because of the difficulties encountered in isolating a toxin or in determining its origin. It is easily confused with subacute poisoning by arsenic and other metals which have a general depressing effect on most body enzyme systems. In this instance an examination of the environment for a source of poison, characteristic signs of each poison and assays of food, gut contents and tissues are necessary to make a definite diagnosis. Toxaemia is a general symptom complex which forms part of many primary disease states, and it is largely in this secondary role that it requires recognition and adequate treatment. In all septicaemias, extensive inflammations and tissue degenerations it is a contributory mechanism in the production of sickness and death.

Treatment

If possible treatment should be directed at removal of the origin of the toxin, the provision of specific antitoxins and supportive treatment to counteract the effects of the toxaemia. Frequent provision of readily assimilable carbohydrate and protein is essential. If the appetite and digestion are impaired these substances should be provided by intravenous alimentation. Solutions containing glucose (2 to 10 ml. per kg. body weight of 5·5 per cent solution per day) and mixtures of amino-acids or protein hydrolysates are recommended. Insulin is unlikely to be of value, but concentrated vitamin preparations, particularly the B-complex group, may aid the utilization of glucose by supplementing impaired enzyme systems. Preparations containing sodium thiosulphate and methylene blue are in general use in veterinary practice for the treatment of non-specific toxaemias, but there seems to be little justification for their use except in specific poisonings caused by arsenic, hydrocyanic acid and nitrite.

REFERENCES

(1) Smith, H. (1969). *Brit. med. Bull.*, *25*, 288.
(2) Holmes, E. (1939). *Physiol. Rev.*, *19*, 439.
(3) Parke, D. V. & Williams, R. T. (1969). *Brit. med. Bull.*, *25*, 256.
(4) Judah, J. D. (1969). *Brit. med. Bull.*, *25*, 276.

HYPERTHERMIA, FEVER, HYPOTHERMIA

The symptom complexes characterized by significant changes in body temperature are dealt with together because they require some introduction in terms of the heat-regulating mechanisms of the body.

The body temperature is a reflection of the balance between heat gain (due to absorption from the environment and to metabolic activity) and heat loss. Absorption of heat from the environment occurs when the external temperature rises above that of the body. Most of the heat produced by the body derives from muscular movement and the maintenance of muscle tone. Heat losses occur by the standard physical phenomena of convection, conduction and radiation and the evaporation of moisture, including sweat, insensible perspiration and moisture vaporized by the respiratory tract. Losses by evaporation of moisture vary between species depending upon the development of the sweat gland system and are less important in animals than in man, beginning only at relatively high body temperatures. Horses sweat profusely, but in pigs, sheep and European cattle (1) sweating cannot be considered to be an effective mechanism of heat loss. In Zebu cattle the increased density of cutaneous sweat glands suggests that sweating may be more important (2). Profuse salivation and exag-

gerated respiration, including mouth breathing, are important mechanisms in the dissipation of excess body heat in animals. The tidal volume is decreased and the respiratory rate is increased so that heat is lost but alkalosis is avoided.

The balance between heat gain and heat loss is controlled by the heat-regulating functions of the hypothalamus. The afferent impulses derive from peripheral hot and cold receptors and the temperature of the blood flowing through the hypothalamus. The efferent impulses control respiratory centre activity, the calibre of skin blood-vessels, sweat gland activity and muscle tone. Heat storage occurs and the body temperature rises when there is a decrease in rate and depth of respiration, constriction of skin blood vessels, cessation of perspiration and increased muscle tone. Heat loss occurs when these functions are reversed. These physiological changes occur in, and are the basis of, the increment and decrement stages of fever.

An important development in recent years has been the investigation of variability between and within races and breeds of farm livestock in their susceptibility to high environmental temperatures (3). Interest in this subject has been aroused by the demands for classes of animals capable of high production in the developing countries of the tropical zone. As a result there has become available a sum of detailed information on the physiological effects of, and the mechanisms of adaptation to, high environmental temperatures (4, 5, 6, 7, 8).

As might have been expected these findings have also aroused interest in more temperate climates where the demand for more economic animal husbandry methods has led to investigation of all avenues by which productivity might be increased. Such subjects as the provision of shelter in hot weather, the use of tranquillizers to reduce activity and therefore heat increment, and the optimum temperature in enclosed pig houses are subjects of vital importance to farming economy but are not dealt with in this book because they appear to have little relation to the production of clinical illness.

The two clinical disorders of animals caused by exposure to high environmental temperatures are heat stroke, described below under hyperthermia, and anhidrosis described under diseases due to unknown causes. There appear to be no parallels to human prickly heat and heat syncope amongst animals. Heat exhaustion and anhidrotic asthenia, two well-recognized entities in human medicine (9), probably do occur in cattle and horses. The prominent features of these diseases in man are physical weakness, slight elevation of temperature, weight loss and dehydration, and these are seen often in large animals poorly adapted to tropical climates. Heat cramps have been described as a cause of equine colic after violent exercise and parenteral treatment with large volumes of normal saline solution has been recommended. Recently a form of hyperthermia in swine, manifested under certain forms of anaesthesia, has been described (10). Susceptible pigs exhibit temperatures as high as 45°C and death under anaesthesia is the usual result.

REFERENCES

(1) Brook, A. H. & Short, B. F. (1960). *Aust. J. agric. Res.*, *11*, 557.
(2) Taneja, G. C. (1960). *J. agric. Sci.*, *55*, 109.
(3) Robinson, D. W. (1969). *Brit. vet. J.*, *125*, 112.
(4) Yeates, N. T. M. (1955). *Aust. J. agric. Res.*, *6*, 891.
(5) Johnson, H. D. *et al.* (1958). *Res. Bull. Mo. agric. exp. Stn*, *683*, 31.
(6) McFarlane, W. V. *et al.* (1958). *Aust. J. agric. Res.*, *9*, 217 & 690.
(7) Dowling, D. F. (1959). *Aust. J. agric. Res.*, *10*, 736.
(8) Shrode, R. R. *et al.* (1960). *J. Dairy Sci.*, *43*, 1235, 1245, 1255, & 1263.
(9) Ladell, W. S. S. (1957). *Trans. roy. Soc. trop. Med. Hyg.*, *51*, 189.
(10) Jones, E. W. *et al.* (1972). *Anesthesiology*, *36*, 42.

Hyperthermia (Heat Stroke)

Hyperthermia is the elevation of body temperature due to excessive heat production or absorption, or to deficient heat loss when the causes of these abnormalities are purely physical. Heat stroke is the most commonly encountered clinical entity.

Aetiology

The major causes of hyperthermia are the physical ones of high environmental temperature and prolonged, severe muscular exertion especially when the humidity is high, the animals are fat, have a heavy hair coat, or are confined with inadequate ventilation, such as on board ship. The critical point in sheep with a light wool coat on board ship appears to be a temperature of 35°C (95°F) at a humidity of 33 to 39 mm. Hg vapour pressure (1). The original concept of sunstroke as being due to actinic irradiation of the medulla has now been discarded and all such cases are now classed as heat stroke.

The minor causes of hyperthermia include damage to the hypothalamus (neurogenic hyperthermia) and dehydration hyperthermia. Neurogenic hyperthermia is due usually to spontaneous haemorrhage, and although hyperthermia is the usual result, poikilothermia may also occur. In dehydration there is an insufficiency of tissue fluids to permit heat loss by evaporation.

It is of interest that hyperthermia has been shown to occur in sheep following the administration of tranquilizing drugs in hot weather (4). This points to the possibility of such drugs predisposing to heat stroke in some circumstances.

Pathogenesis

The means by which hyperthermia is induced have already been described. The physiological effects of hyperthermia are important and are outlined briefly here. Unless the body temperature reaches a critical point a short period of hyperthermia is advantageous in an infectious disease because phagocytosis and immune body production are facilitated and the viability of most invading organisms is impaired. These changes provide justification for the use of artificial fever to control bacterial disease. However, the metabolic rate may be increased by as much as 40 to 50 per cent, liver glycogen stores are rapidly depleted and extra energy is derived from increased endogenous metabolism of protein. If anorexia occurs because of respiratory embarrassment and dryness of the mouth, there will be considerable loss of body weight and lack of muscle strength accompanied by hypoglycaemia and a rise in blood non-protein nitrogen.

There is increased thirst due in part to dryness of the mouth. An increase in heart rate occurs due directly to the rise in blood temperature and indirectly to the fall in blood pressure resulting from peripheral vasodilatation. Respiration increases in rate and depth due directly to the effect of the high temperature on the respiratory centre. Urine secretion is decreased because of the reduced renal blood flow resulting from peripheral vasodilatation, and because of physicochemical changes in body cells which result in retention of water and chloride ions.

When the critical temperature is exceeded there is depression of nervous system activity, and depression of the respiratory centre usually causes death by respiratory failure. Circulatory failure also occurs due to myocardial weakness, the heart rate becoming fast and irregular. If the period of hyperthermia is unduly prolonged, rather than excessive in degree, the deleterious effects are those of increased endogenous metabolism and deficient food intake. There is often an extensive degenerative change in most body tissues but this is more likely to be due to metabolic changes than to the direct effects of elevation of the body temperature.

Clinical Findings

An elevation of body temperature is the primary requisite for a diagnosis of hyperthermia and in most species the first observable clinical reaction to hyperthermia occurs when the rectal temperature exceeds 39·5°C (103°F). An increase in heart and respiratory rates, with a weak pulse of large amplitude, sweating and salivation occur initially followed by a marked absence of sweating. The animal may be restless but soon becomes dull, stumbles while walking and tends to lie down. In the early stages there is increased thirst and the animal seeks cool places, often lying in water or attempting to splash itself. When the body temperature reaches 41°C (106°F) respiration is laboured and general distress is evident. Beyond this point the respirations become shallow and irregular, the pulse becomes very rapid and weak and these signs are usually accompanied by collapse, convulsions and terminal coma. Death occurs in most species when a temperature of 41·5 to 42·5°C (107 to 109°F) is attained. Abortion may occur if the period of hyperthermia is prolonged and a high incidence of embryonic mortality has been recorded in sheep which were 3 to 6 weeks pregnant (2). In cattle breeding efficiency is adversely affected by prolonged heat stress.

Clinical Pathology

No important clinico-pathological change is observed in simple hyperthermia.

Necropsy Findings

At necropsy there are only poorly defined gross changes. Peripheral vasodilatation may be evident, clotting of the blood is slow and incomplete, and rigor mortis and putrefaction occur early. There are no constant or specific histopathological changes.

Diagnosis

Simple hyperthermia must be differentiated from fever and septicaemia. Clinically there may be little to distinguish between them. The toxaemia which accompanies the latter conditions does not add much of significance to the clinical picture. In septicaemia petechial haemorrhages in the mucosae and skin may be present and blood cultures may be positive in bacterial infections. In most cases of hyperthermia examination of the environment reveals the causative factor.

Treatment

If treatment is necessary because of the severity or duration of the hyperthermia two methods are available. Cold applications, including immersion, spraying or cold packs are most effective if there is urgency. Drugs of the salicylate group increase heat loss by withdrawing fluid from the tissues into the vascular system and, by increasing the circulating blood volume, improve the efficiency of heat loss from the skin. Supportive treatment includes provision of adequate glucose and protein to compensate for increased utilization and in some cases deficient intake. The presence of adequate drinking water is essential and together with shade and air movement is of considerable assistance when animals are exposed to high air temperature. If animals have to be confined under conditions of high temperatures and humidity the use of tranquillizing drugs is recommended to reduce unnecessary activity. Chlorpromazine, for example, has been shown to increase significantly the survival rate of pigs exposed to heat and humidity stress (3).

REFERENCES

(1) Hamilton, F. J. *et al.* (1961). *Aust. vet. J.*, *37*, 297.
(2) Smith, I. D. *et al.* (1966). *Aust. vet. J.*, *42*, 468.
(3) Juszkiewicz, T. & Jones, L. M. (1961). *Amer. J. vet. Res.*, *22*, 553.
(4) Grosskopf, J. F. W. *et al.* (1969). *J. S. Afr. vet. med. Ass.*, *40*, 51.

Hypothermia

Hypothermia occurs when excess heat is lost or insufficient is produced so that the body temperature falls. It is of less importance than hyperthermia and occurs for the opposite reasons. Exposure to excessively cold air temperatures will cause heat loss if increased metabolic activity, muscle tone and peripheral vasoconstriction are unable to compensate. Decrease of muscle tone as in parturient paresis and acute ruminal impaction and during anaesthesia and sedation, peripheral vasodilatation in shock, and reduction of metabolic activity in the terminal stages of many diseases are common causes of hypothermia. In the latter case a sudden fall in temperature in a previously febrile animal, the so-called pre-mortal fall, is a bad prognostic sign.

Artificial hibernation or induced hypothermia has had experimental use as an anaesthetic for extensive surgical operations in humans, but it is necessary initially to overcome the normal thermostatic mechanisms by the use of an anaesthetic. In man consciousness fails at rectal temperature of 29·5 to 30·5°C (85 to 87°F) and fatal ventricular fibrillation is likely to occur at rectal temperatures of 25 to 26·6°C (77 to 80°F) (1). In dogs the body temperature can be reduced to as low as 5°C (41°F) permitting complete exsanguination for 45 minutes. Extensive reviews on hypothermia relative to surgery and to acclimation to cold environment are available (2, 3).

REFERENCES

(1) Pickering, G. (1958). *Lancet, 1*, 59.
(2) Drew, C. E. & Anderson, I. M. (1959). *Lancet, 276*, 745, 748 & 771.
(3) Edholm, O. G. *et al.* (1961). *Brit. med. Bull., 17*, 1–72.

Fever

Fever is the symptom complex in which hyperthermia and toxaemia are produced by substances circulating in the blood stream.

Aetiology

Fevers may be septic or aseptic, the septic type being the more commonly encountered.

Septic fevers result from infection with viruses, bacteria, fungi or protozoa. The infection may be localized in abscesses, in body cavities as empyemas, or be generalized with a bacteraemia or septicaemia. In septic fevers the hyperthermia is due to bacterial pyrogens, pyrexin (a complex of bacterial pyrogen and globulin), pyrogenic polysaccharides extractable from normal tissue, and leucocytic pyrogen liberated from functionally active leucocytes in inflammatory exudates (1, 2). The endogenous or leucocytic pyrogen is produced in many forms of inflammation other than those due to bacterial infection, including tuberculous sensitivity, virus infection and typhoid vaccination. It acts directly on the thermo-regulation centre and does not cause a leucopenia. The other pyrogens cause hyperthermia by indirect action on the hypothalamic centres and all cause a leucopenia.

Aseptic fevers include chemical fevers, caused by the injection of foreign protein or substances which cause tissue damage and a reaction to protein degradation products, and surgical fevers due to the breakdown of necrotic tissue and blood. Thus fever may occur in severe haemoglobinaemia or in extensive infarction or in necrosis of extensive tumours. The fever in such cases is usually slight. The toxaemia in all cases of fever is due to the deleterious effects of bacterial toxins or tissue breakdown products on functional body tissues.

Pathogenesis

The effect of bacterial and tissue pyrogens is exerted on the thermoregulatory centre of the hypothalamus so that the thermostatic level of the body is raised. The immediate response on the part of organs involved in heat regulation is the prevention of heat loss and the increased production of heat. This is the period of *increment* or chill which is manifested by cutaneous vasoconstriction, resulting coldness and dryness of the skin and an absence of sweating. Respiration is reduced and muscular shivering occurs while urine formation is minimal. Although the skin is cold the rectal temperature is elevated and the pulse rate increased. When the period of heat increment has raised the body temperature to the new thermostatic level the second period of fever, the *fastigium*, or period of constant temperature follows. In this stage the mechanisms of heat dissipation and production return to normal. Cutaneous vasodilatation causes flushing of the skin and mucosae, sweating occurs and may be severe and diuresis develops. During this period there is decreased ruminal motility (3), and metabolism is increased considerably to maintain the body temperature and tissue wasting may occur. There is also an inability to maintain a constant temperature when environmental temperatures vary.

When the effect of the pyrogenic substances is removed the stage of *decrement* or fever defervescence appears and the excess stored heat is dissipated. Vasodilatation, sweating and muscle flaccidity are marked and the body temperature falls. If the toxaemia accompanying the hyperthermia is sufficiently severe the ability of tissues to respond to heat production or conservation needs may be lost and as death approaches there is a precipitate fall in body temperature.

Clinical Findings

The effects of fever are the combined effects of toxaemia and hyperthermia. There is elevation of body temperature, an increase in pulse rate with a diminution of amplitude and strength, hyperpnoea, wasting, oliguria often with albuminuria, increased thirst, anorexia, constipation, depression and muscle weakness.

The form of the fever may vary. Thus the temperature rise may be *transient, continuous, remittent* when the diurnal variation is exaggerated, *intermittent* when fever peaks last for 2 to 3 days and are interspersed with normal periods and *atypical* when temperature variations are irregular. A biphasic fever consisting of an initial rise, a fall to normal and a secondary rise, occurs in some diseases, e.g. in strangles in the horse and in erysipelas in swine.

Clinical Pathology

There are no clinico-pathological findings characteristic of fever.

Necropsy Findings

The findings are a combination of those of hyperthermia, including vasodilatation, rapid onset of

rigor mortis and putrefaction, and those of toxaemia with microscopic evidence of degeneration in
parenchymatous organs.

Diagnosis

Differentiation from hyperthermia, where there
is no toxaemia and from septicaemia, which is
accompanied by infection of the blood stream, is
necessary.

Treatment

The general principles of treatment of fever are
to remove the source of the toxin and to treat the
toxaemia and the hyperthermia if the fever is excessive or prolonged. Stimulation of the circulation
and respiration may be necessary if these are failing. Removal of the toxin necessitates control of infections by antibacterial drugs and removal of necrotic material in aseptic fevers and local infections.
Specific antibodies and antitoxins find use in controlling infection and reducing the effects of bacterial toxins. Non-specific treatments include the
use of adrenocortical hormones to facilitate repair
processes and alleviate inflammation. These drugs
must be used with great caution and be supported
by large doses of broad-spectrum antibiotics. Inaccessible foci of infection may be benefited by the
systemic or local use of enzyme preparations.
Diuretics which have an important part to play in
the removal of transudates are unlikely to have any
effect on aggregations of inflammatory fluids.

REFERENCES

(1) Atkins, E. (1960). *Physiol. Rev.*, *40*, 580.
(2) van Miert, A. S. J. P. A. M. & Atmakusuma, A. (1971).
    J. comp. Path., *81*, 119.
(3) van Miert, A. S. J. P. A. M. (1968). *Vet. Rec.*, *82*, 632.

SEPTICAEMIA

Septicaemia is the disease state compounded of
toxaemia, hyperthermia and the presence of large
numbers of infectious micro-organisms, including
viruses, bacteria and protozoa in the blood stream.

Aetiology

Many infectious agents produce septicaemias.
The difference between septicaemia and bacteraemia is one of degree. In bacteraemia bacteria are
present in the blood stream for only transitory
periods and do not produce clinical signs. In septicaemia the causative agent is present throughout
the course of the disease and is directly responsible
for the signs which appear.

Pathogenesis

Two mechanisms operate in septicaemia. The
exotoxins or endotoxins produced by the infectious
agents produce a profound toxaemia and high fever
because of the rapidity with which they multiply
and their rapid spread to all body tissues. Also localization occurs in many organs and may produce
serious defects in animals which survive the
toxaemia. They also cause direct endothelial
damage and haemorrhages into tissue commonly
result. The same general principles apply to a
viraemia except that toxins are not produced by the
virus. It is more likely that the general signs which
occur are caused by the products of the tissue cells
killed by the multiplying virus (1).

Clinical Findings

The clinical findings in septicaemia are those of
toxaemia and hyperthermia and include fever and
submucosal and subepidermal haemorrhages,
usually petechial, or occasionally ecchymotic. The
haemorrhages are best seen under the conjunctiva
and in the mucosae of the mouth and vulva. Localizing signs may occur as the result of localization of
the infection in joints, heart valves, meninges, eyes
or other organs.

Clinical Pathology

Isolation of the causative bacteria from the blood
stream should be attempted by culture or animal
inoculation at the height of the fever. The presence
of leucopenia or leucocytosis is an aid in diagnosis
and the type and degree of leucocytic response may
be of prognostic significance.

Necropsy Findings

Apart from the changes caused by toxaemia and
hyperthermia there may be subserous and submucosal haemorrhages and embolic foci of infection in various organs but these are usually overshadowed by the lesions specific to the causative
agent.

Diagnosis

Only by the isolation of the causative agent from
the blood stream can a positive diagnosis of septicaemia be made. However, the presence of petechiae in mucosae and conjunctivae may suggest
septicaemia, and high environmental temperatures
suggest hyperthermia. Evidence of localization in
individual organs is contributory evidence that
septicaemia is present or has occurred.

Treatment

The same general recommendations for treatment apply here as in fever except that the need for treatment is more urgent and intravenous or parenteral treatment with antibacterial drugs or sera and antitoxins should be provided as soon as possible. Strict hygienic precautions to avoid spread of diseases may be necessary in many cases.

REFERENCE

(1) Downie, A. W. (1963). *Vet. Rec.*, *75*, 1125.

DISTURBANCES OF APPETITE, FOOD INTAKE AND NUTRITIONAL STATUS

Hunger is a purely local subjective sensation arising from gastric hypermotility caused in most cases by lack of distension by food. *Appetite* is a conditioned reflex depending on past associations and experience of palatable foods and is not dependent on hunger contractions of the stomach. The term appetite is used loosely with regard to animals and really expresses the degree of hunger as indicated by the food intake. When we speak of variations from normal appetite we mean variations from normal food intake, with the rare exception of the animal which demonstrates desire to eat but fails to do so because of a painful condition of the mouth or other disability. Variation in appetite includes increased, decreased or abnormal appetite.

Hyperorexia, or increased appetite, due to increased hunger contractions is manifested by *polyphagia* or increased food intake. Partial absence of appetite (*inappetence*) and complete absence of appetite (*anorexia*) are manifested by varying degrees of decreased food intake (*anophagia*). *Abnormal appetites* include cravings for substances, often normally offensive, other than usual foods. The abnormal appetite may be perverted, a temporary state, or depraved, the permanent or habit stage. Both are manifested by different forms of *pica* or *allotriophagia*.

Polyphagia

Starvation, functional diarrhoea, chronic gastritis and abnormalities of digestion, particularly pancreatic deficiency, may result in polyphagia. Metabolic diseases, including diabetes mellitus and hyperthyroidism, are rare in large animals but are causes of polyphagia in other species. Internal parasitism is often associated with poor growth response to more than adequate food intakes.

Although appetite is difficult to assess in animals it seems to be the only explanation for the behaviour of those which grossly over-eat on concentrates or other palatable feed. The syndromes associated with over-eating are dealt with under the diseases of the alimentary tract.

Anophagia or Aphagia

Decreased food intake may be due to physical factors such as painful conditions of the mouth and pharynx or to lack of desire to eat. Hyperthermia, toxaemia and fever all decrease hunger contractions of the stomach. In species with a simple alimentary tract a deficiency of thiamine in the diet will cause atony of the gut and reduction in food intake. In ruminants a deficiency of cobalt and a heavy infestation with trichostrongylid helminths are common causes of anophagia. In fact alimentary tract stasis due to any cause results in anophagia. Some sensations, including severe pain, excitement and fear may override hunger sensations and animals used to open range conditions may temporarily refuse to eat when confined in feeding lots or experimental units.

One of the important aims in veterinary medicine is to encourage an adequate food intake in sick and convalescent animals. Alimentary tract stimulants applied either locally or systemically are in common use but are of limited value unless the primary condition is corrected first. To administer strychnine orally or para-sympathomimetic drugs parenterally when there is digestive tract atony due to peritonitis is unlikely to increase food intake. If the primary cause of the lack of appetite is corrected but the animal still refuses to take food these drugs and thiamine are more likely to achieve a response. Rumen inoculation through cud transfers often produces excellent results. The provision of appetizing food is also of value. In nervous anophagia the injection of insulin in amounts sufficient to cause hypoglycaemia without causing convulsions is used in human practice, and in animals the use of tranquillizing drugs may achieve the same result. In ruminants the effects of blood glucose levels on food intake are debatable (1, 2) but it seems probable that neither blood glucose nor blood acetate levels are important factors in regulating the appetite (3, 4). Electrolytic lesions in the hypothalamic region can stimulate or depress food intake depending on the area affected (5). This indicates the probable importance of the hypothalamus in the overall control of appetite, a promising area for research in animal production.

REFERENCES

(1) Manning, R. *et al.* (1959). *Amer. J. vet. Res.*, *20*, 242.
(2) Vallenas, G. A. (1956). *Amer. J. vet. Res.*, *17*, 79.

(3) Bowen, J. M. (1962). *Amer. J. vet. Res.*, *23*, 948 & *24*, 73.
(4) Holder, J. M. (1963). *Nature, Lond.*, *200*, 1074.
(5) Baile, C. A. *et al.* (1968). *J. Dairy Sci.*, *51*, 1474.

Pica or Allotriophagia

Pica refers to the ingestion of materials other than normal food and varies from licking to actual eating. It is due in most cases to dietary deficiency, either of bulk or in some cases more specifically fibre, or of individual nutrients, particularly salt, cobalt or phosphorus. Boredom, in the case of animals closely confined, often results in the development of pica. Chronic abdominal pain due to peritonitis or gastritis and central nervous system disturbances including rabies and nervous acetonaemia are also causes of pica.

The type of pica may be defined as follows: *osteophagia* is the chewing of bones; *infantophagia* is the eating of young; *coprophagia* is the eating of faeces. Other types include wool eating in sheep, bark eating, the eating of carrion and cannibalism and salt hunger resulting in coat licking, leather chewing and the eating of earth. Cannibalism may become an important problem in housed animals, particularly swine, which bite one another's tails often resulting in severe local infections, and although some cases may be due to protein, iron or bulk deficiency in the diet many seem to be the result of boredom in animals given insufficient space for exercise. Provision of larger pens or a hanging object to play with, removal of incisor teeth and the avoidance of mixing animals of different sizes in the same pen are common control measures in pigs. In many instances only one pig in the pen has the habit and his removal may prevent further cases. One common measure which is guaranteed to be successful in terms of tail-biting is surgical removal of all tails with scissors during the first few days of life, when the needle teeth are removed. Unfortunately the cannibalistic tendency may then be transferred to ears. As in all picas the habit may survive the correction of the causative factor.

Infantophagia can be important in pigs in two circumstances. In intensively housed sows, especially young gilts, hysterical savaging of each pig as it is born can cause heavy losses. When sows are grazed and housed at high density on pasture it is not uncommon to find 'cannibal' sows who protect their own litters but attack the young pigs of other sows. This diagnosis should be considered when there are unexplained disappearances of young pigs.

Pica may have serious consequences. Cannibalism may be the cause of many deaths; poisonings, particularly lead poisoning and botulism are common sequelae; foreign bodies lodging in the alimentary tract or accumulations of wool, fibre or sand may cause obstruction; perforation of the oesophagus or stomach may result from the ingestion of sharp foreign bodies; grazing time is often reduced and livestock may wander away from normal grazing. In many cases the actual cause of the pica cannot be determined and corrective measures may have to be prescribed on a basis of trial and error.

Starvation

Complete deprivation of food causes rapid depletion of glycogen stores and a change-over in metabolism to fat and protein. In the early stages there is hunger, increase in muscle power and endurance, and a loss of body weight. In sheep there is often a depression of serum calcium levels sufficient to cause clinical hypocalcaemia. The development of ketosis and acidosis follows quickly on the heels of increased fat utilization. Muscular power and activity now decrease and the loss of body weight may reach as high as 50 to 60 per cent. The metabolic rate falls and is accompanied by a slowing of the heart and a reduction in stroke volume, amplitude of the pulse and blood pressure. In the final stages when fat stores are depleted massive protein mobilization occurs and a pre-mortal rise in total urinary nitrogen is observed whereas blood and urine ketones are likely to diminish from their previous high level. Great weakness of skeletal and cardiac musculature is also present in the terminal stages and death is due to circulatory failure. During the period of fat utilization there is a considerable reduction in the ability of tissues to utilize glucose and its administration in large amounts is followed by glycosuria. In such circumstances readily assimilable carbohydrates and proteins should be given in small quantities at frequent intervals but fatty foods may exacerbate the existing ketosis.

Inanition (Malnutrition)

Incomplete starvation, inanition or malnutrition is a more common field condition than complete starvation. The diet is insufficient in quantity and all essential nutrients are present but in suboptimal amounts. The condition is compatible with life and in general the same pattern of metabolic change occurs as in complete starvation but to a less degree. Thus ketosis, loss of body weight and muscular power and a fall in metabolic rate occur. In addition there is mental depression, lack of sexual desire and increased susceptibility to infection. The increased susceptibility to infection which occurs in some cases of malnutrition cannot be accepted as a general rule. In the present state of knowledge it can only be said that 'some nutritional influences affect resistance to some forms of infection' (1, 2). If there is a relative lack of dietary protein over a long period of time, anasarca occurs, particularly in the intermandibular space. Malnutrition makes a significant contribution to a number of quasi-specific diseases, 'weaner ill-thrift' and 'thin sow syndrome' among them, and these are dealt with elsewhere. Controlled malnutrition in the form of providing submaintenance diets to animals during periods of severe feed shortage is now a nutritional exercise with an extensive supporting literature. Animals fed on such diets undergo metabolic changes reflected in blood and tissue values as well as the more significant changes in weight (3). A deficiency of one or more specific dietary essentials is more appropriately described as partial starvation and is dealt with in Chapter 28.

REFERENCES

(1) Sprunt, D. H. & Flanigan, C. (1960). *Advances in Veterinary Science*, Vol. 6. New York: Academic Press.
(2) Hill, R. (1965). *Brit. vet. J.*, *121*, 402.
(3) Payne, E. *et al.* (1970). *Aust. J. exp. Agric. Anim. Husb.*, *10*, 256.

Thirst

Thirst is an increased desire for water manifested by excessive water intake (polydipsia). There are two important causes of thirst: dryness of the pharyngeal and oral mucosae increases the desire for water, irrespective of the water status of body tissues; in addition cellular dehydration due to a rise in blood osmotic pressure causes increased thirst. The latter occurs commonly in many cases of dehydration due to vomiting, diarrhoea, polyuria and excessive sweating. Increased thirst in early fever is due to changes in cell colloids leading to increased water retention. In humans several other factors appear to exert some effect on water intake; a deficiency of potassium and an excess of calcium in tissue fluid both increase thirst; an increased thirst also occurs in uraemia irrespective of the body's state of hydration. It has been suggested that these chemical factors may cause direct stimulation of the thirst centre in the hypothalamus (1). Clinically diabetes insipidus produces by far the most exaggerated polydipsia.

The clinical syndrome produced by water deprivation is not well defined. Animals supplied with saline water will drink it with reluctance and, if the salinity is sufficiently great, die of salt poisoning.

Cattle at pasture which are totally deprived of water usually become quite excited and are likely to knock down fences and destroy watering points in their frenzy. On examination they exhibit a hollow abdomen, sunken eyes and the other signs of dehydration. There is excitability with trembling and slight frothing at the mouth. The gait is stiff and uncoordinated and recumbency follows. Abortion of decomposed calves, with dystokia due to failure of the cervix to dilate, may occur for some time after thirst has been relieved and cause death in survivors. At necropsy there is extensive liquefaction of fat deposits, dehydration and early foetal death in pregnant cows (2).

REFERENCES

(1) Fourman, P. & Leeson, P. M. (1959). *Lancet*, *276*, 268.
(2) Knight, R. P. (1963–4). *Vict. vet. Proc.*, *22*, 45.

Hyperlipaemia

A disturbance of fat metabolism in ponies has achieved prominence largely because it is usually a prelude to death and because the primary disease of which it is a major secondary complication is not usually diagnosed (1, 2, 3). Affected ponies do not eat, lose body weight quickly and their serum is macroscopically hyperlipaemic. Most cases occur in pregnant mares. The mortality rate is decreased by supportive therapy including glucose saline infusion, vitamin mixtures and corticosteroids.

REFERENCES

(1) Schotman, A. J. H. & Wagenaar, J. (1969). *Ztbl. vet. Med.*, *16A*, 1.
(2) Wagenaar, G. *et al.* (1970). *T. Diergeneesk.*, *95*, 102.
(3) Schotman, A. J. H. & Kroneman, J. (1969). *Neth. J. vet. Sci.*, *2*, 60.

ALLERGY AND ANAPHYLAXIS

The importance of abnormal reactions between antigens and antibodies is to a large extent undetermined in veterinary medicine although it appears to be less than in human medicine. Allergy and anaphylaxis are the two major manifestations of hypersensitivity and they are closely allied in aetiology, the main difference being one of degree of reaction.

Anaphylaxis

Anaphylaxis is an acute disease caused by an antigen-antibody reaction with signs varying from species to species depending principally upon the degree of development of plain muscle in their various organs.

Aetiology

In general the reaction is due to sensitization to a protein substance entering the blood stream and a second exposure to the same substance. In veterinary practice such incidents are not uncommon although the sensitizing substance cannot always be isolated. Anaphylaxis can occur after repeated intravenous injections of glandular extracts and repeated blood transfusions from the same donor.

Although severe anaphylactic reactions occur usually after a second exposure to a sensitizing agent, reactions of similar severity can occur with no known prior exposure. In large-animal work this is most likely to occur after the injection of sera and bacterins, particularly heterologous sera and bacterins in which heterologous serum has been used in the culture medium. Occasional cases of anaphylaxis occur after the administration of conventional drugs such as penicillin and procaine. The occurrence of signs at the first injection is reminiscent of 'serum sickness' in man but, contrary to the usual delay in appearance of sickness in man, the reaction occurs usually within a few hours of exposure in animals. Because signs may occur at first exposure it is advisable to keep injected animals under close observation for some hours. There have been reports of the occurrence of anaphylaxis in calves after the injection of lyophilized Strain 19 *Brucella abortus* vaccine. In these circumstances it is probable that the animals have been unknowingly exposed to the antigen on a previous occasion.

Anaphylactic reactions to ingested protein occur in humans, and cases have been observed in animals, both at pasture and in the feed-lot. The fog fever syndrome in cattle characterized by pulmonary oedema and emphysema and occurring on improved pastures, hay aftermath and rape is usually described as allergic but may be anaphylactic in its severity. An anaphylactic reaction sometimes occurs in cows, especially Channel Island cattle, when they are dried off in preparation for calving. Severe urticaria and some respiratory distress occur 18 to 24 hours after milking is stopped (1).

Hypersensitivity reactions are sometimes observed at a higher incidence than normal in certain families and herds of cattle.

Pathogenesis

The manifestations of anaphylaxis are largely explainable in terms of the local liberation of histamine (3). Histamine is liberated in the affected tissues by the reaction between circulating antigen and fixed antibody. Depending upon the amount of plain muscle in the various organs and the situation of the tissues rich in histamine the reaction will vary between species. In the dog the reaction is chiefly in the liver, in cattle it is largely confined to the lungs and to a less extent the rumen. Sheep and pigs show largely a pulmonary reaction and horses manifest changes in the lungs, skin and feet.

Sensitization of a patient requires about 10 days after first exposure to the antigen, and persists for a very long time, months or years.

Clinical Findings

In cattle the initial signs include a very sudden and severe dyspnoea, muscle shivering, and anxiety. In some cases there is profuse salivation, in others moderate bloat and in others diarrhoea. After blood transfusions the first sign is often hiccough. Additional signs are urticaria, angioneurotic oedema and rhinitis. Muscle tremor may be severe and a rise in temperature of 40·5 °C (105 °F) may be observed. On auscultation of the chest there may be increased vesicular murmur, fluid bubbling sounds if oedema is present, and emphysema in the later stages if dyspnoea has been severe. In most surviving cases the signs have usually subsided within 24 hours, although dyspnoea may persist if emphysema has occurred.

Sheep and pigs show acute dyspnoea and horses (6) may do the same, although laminitis and angioneurotic oedema are also common signs in this species. Laminitis also occurs rarely in ruminants.

Clinical Pathology

Blood histamine levels may or may not be increased and little data are available on blood eosinophile counts. Tests for sensitivity to determine the specific sensitizing substance are rarely carried out for diagnostic purposes but their use as an investigation tool is warranted. Serological tests to determine the presence of antibodies to plant proteins in the diet have been used in this way (2).

Necropsy Findings

In acute anaphylaxis in young cattle and sheep the necropsy findings are confined to the lungs and are in the form of severe pulmonary oedema and vascular engorgement. In adult cattle there is oedema and emphysema without engorgement. In protracted anaphylaxis produced experimentally in young calves the most prominent lesions are hyperaemia and oedema of the abomasum and small intestines (5). In pigs and sheep pulmonary emphysema is evident and vascular engorgement of the lungs is pronounced in the latter. Pulmonary emphysema in the horse may be accompanied by subcutaneous oedema and the lesions of laminitis.

Diagnosis

A diagnosis of anaphylaxis can be made with confidence if a foreign protein substance has been injected within the preceding hour but should be made with reservation if the substance appears to have been ingested. Characteristic signs as described above should arouse suspicion and the response to treatment may be used as a test of the hypothesis. Acute pneumonia may be confused with anaphylaxis, but there is usually more toxaemia and the lung changes are more marked in the ventral parts of the lung; in anaphylaxis there is general involvement of the entire lung.

Treatment

Treatment should be administered immediately; a few minutes' delay may result in the death of the patient. Adrenaline administered intramuscularly (or one-fifth of the dose given intravenously) or antihistamine drugs are often immediately effective, the signs abating while the injection is being made. There is a good deal of variation between antihistamines in their efficiency in preventing anaphylaxis; atropine is of little value (4).

REFERENCES

(1) Campbell, S. G. (1970). *Cornell Vet.*, *60*, 654.
(2) Brownlee, A. & Baigent, C. L. (1964). *Vet. Rec.*, *76*, 1060.
(3) Aitken, M. M. & Sanford, J. (1967). *Proc. 18th int. vet. Congr.*, *2*, 823.
(4) Aitken, M. M. & Sanford, J. (1969). *Nature, Lond.*, *223*, 314.
(5) Wray, C. & Tomlinson, J. R. (1969). *J. Path.*, *98*, 61.
(6) Hidalgo, R. J. & Linrode, P. A. (1969). *Proc. 15th ann. Conv. Amer. Ass. equine Practnrs*, Dec. 1–3, p. 293.

Allergy

Allergy is a systemic state caused by an antigen-antibody reaction with signs varying depending upon the tissues involved. The signs are usually local and mild although more than one tissue may be involved, whereas in anaphylaxis the lesions are extensive and severe.

Aetiology

Exposure to any of the aetiological agents described under anaphylaxis may result in this milder form of hypersensitivity. Exposure may occur by injection, by ingestion, by inhalation or by contact with the skin.

Pathogenesis

As in anaphylaxis the lesions and signs can be taken to be the result of the liberation of histamine from tissues sensitized to the antigen.

Clinical Findings

In ruminants inhalation of a sensitizing antigen may cause the development of allergic rhinitis. On ingestion of the sensitizing agent there may be a sharp attack of diarrhoea and the appearance of urticaria or angioneurotic oedema; in ruminants mild bloat may occur. Contact allergy is usually manifested by eczema. In farm animals the eczematous lesion is commonly restricted to the skin of the lower limbs, particularly behind the pastern, and at the bulbs of the heels, or to the midline of the back if the allergy is due to insect bites. In many cases of allergic disease the signs are very transient and often disappear spontaneously within a few hours. Cases vary in severity from mild signs in a single system to a general illness resembling anaphylaxis. On the other hand cases of anaphylaxis may be accompanied by local allergic lesions.

Diagnosis

The transitory nature of allergic manifestations is often a good guide, as are the types of lesions and signs encountered. The response to antihistamine drugs is also a useful indicator. Skin test programmes as applied to man should be utilized when recurrent herd problems exist (1, 2). The differential diagnosis of allergy is discussed under the specific diseases listed above.

Treatment

As in anaphylaxis, adrenaline, antihistamines and corticosteroids are usually highly effective. Skin lesions other than oedema may require frequent local applications of lotions containing antihistamine substances. Continued exposure to the allergen may result in recurrence or persistence of the signs. Keeping the animals indoors for a week often avoids this, probably because the allergen occurs only transiently in the environment. Hyposensitization therapy, as it is practised in human allergy sufferers, may have a place in small animal practice but is unlikely to be practicable with farm animals.

REFERENCES

(1) Scherr, M. S. (1964). *J. Amer. vet. med. Ass.*, *145*, 798.
(2) Campbell, S. G. (1970). *Cornell Vet.*, *60*, 240.

AMYLOIDOSIS

Amyloidosis usually occurs in association with a chronic suppurative process elsewhere in the body. Extensive infiltration of various body organs with amyloid causes depression of function of the organs involved.

Aetiology

The aetiology is incompletely understood; most cases occur in animals injected frequently with antigenic substances for the commercial production of hyperimmune serum. Natural cases usually occur in animals suffering from long-standing suppurative processes (1, 2). In humans primary amyloidosis, in which no precipitating lesions can be found also occurs but such cases are rare in farm animals (3). The diseases are the same in other respects.

Pathogenesis

How amyloid is formed is uncertain but a hyperglobulinaemia is commonly present and this together with the circumstances under which it occurs suggest an abnormality of the antigen-antibody reaction. Extensive amyloid deposits may occur in the spleen, liver or kidneys and cause major enlargement of these organs and serious depression of their functions. In the latter case an extreme degree of proteinuria occurs. The amyloid material deposited in the tissues is a glycoprotein and has specific staining reactions.

Clinical Findings

Most cases of amyloidosis are detected incidentally at necropsy. Clinical cases are characterized by emaciation and enlargement of the spleen, liver or kidneys and involvement of the kidney causes proteinuria and is often accompanied by profuse, chronic diarrhoea, polydipsia and anasarca (4, 5). In man involvement of the heart causes a syndrome of congestive heart failure and involvement of the liver causes oedema, but these latter syndromes are not known to occur in animals.

Clinical Pathology

An extreme, persistent proteinuria should suggest the presence of amyloidosis. Electrophoretic studies of serum may be of value in determining the presence of hyperglobulinaemia. Alpha globulin levels are usually elevated and albumin levels depressed.

Necropsy

Affected organs are grossly enlarged and have a pale, waxy appearance. In the spleen, the deposits are circumscribed, in the liver and kidneys they are diffuse. Deposits of amyloid in tissues may be made visible by staining with aqueous iodine.

Diagnosis

Enlargement of parenchymatous organs associated with chronic suppurative processes should arouse suspicion of amyloidosis especially if there is emaciation and marked proteinuria. Pyelonephritis, non-specific nephritis and nephrosis bear a clinical similarity to amyloidosis.

Treatment

Treatment is of no value and affected animals should be discarded.

REFERENCES
(1) Rooney, J. R. (1956). Cornell Vet., 46, 369.
(2) Hadlow, W. J. & Jellison, W. L. (1962). J. Amer. vet. med. Ass., 141, 243.
(3) Radostits, O. M. & Palmer, N. (1965). Canad. vet. J., 6, 208.
(4) Grunder, H. D. & Trautwein, G. (1965). Dtsch. tierärztl. Wschr., 72, 442.
(5) Murray, M. et al. (1972). Vet. Rec., 90, 210.

The Alarm Reaction and the Adaptation Syndrome

The need to recognize these systemic states derives from the reactions of the animal body to conditions of strain or stress. They are also basic to the explanation of certain diseases of obscure aetiology particularly those described as collagen diseases in humans. The alarm reaction and the adaptation syndrome can be produced experimentally but there is some hesitation in accepting them as the basis for most diseases. The word 'stress' has come to include any noxious stimulus, whether in the internal or external environment. Such factors as toxaemia, infections, heat, cold, anoxia, trauma and physical exhaustion undoubtedly place the body under 'stress' and result in an increased secretion and utilization of adrenocortical steroids. The exact mechanisms by which secretion of these hormones is stimulated (other than the known stimulating effect of adrenocorticotrophic hormone of the anterior pituitary gland) and their rate of utilization increased, are unknown. At present it seems safe to assume that 'stress' of any nature is likely to promote increased adrenal cortical activity and if the stress is continued over a long enough period exhaustion of the gland may occur and resistance to further stress be seriously diminished. On the other hand, there is insufficient proof that hypersecretion of adrenocortical steroids during the period of resistance or 'adaptation' is the cause of such diseases as periarteritis nodosa and rheumatoid arthritis in humans. It appears likely that these diseases result from abnormality of the antigen-antibody reaction but whether adrenal cortical stimulation is the basic mechanism is not proven. The importance of existing knowledge about the 'alarm reaction-adaptation syndrome' to veterinary medicine appears to be very limited (1, 2).

REFERENCES

(1) Venzke, W. G. (1958). *Mod. vet. Pract.*, *39*, 52 (Oct. 1.)
(2) Veilleur, R. (1963). *Advances in Veterinary Science*, Vol. 8, p. 189. New York: Academic Press.

3

Diseases of the Newborn

BY AND LARGE morbidity and mortality rates are higher in new-born animals than in any other age group and the prevention of losses among them assumes special importance. This chapter deals with the general aspects of those diseases which are present at birth or occur within the first 2 weeks of life in animals born at term; the specific diseases are dealt with elsewhere as are the diseases causing abortion. In this discussion the diseases are grouped under two main headings, congenital defects, which may be inherited or due to other causes, and infections, acquired during uterine life or in the period immediately after birth. Many other defects and diseases of new-born animals occur sporadically in all species and are dealt with under the systems in which they occur. Neoplasms of the newborn are recorded rarely (1). There are many more causes of loss in new-born animals especially when they are on range, but most of such losses are caused by faults in management and cannot be considered as due to disease. Their omission does not in any way detract from their importance. Most work in this field has been done in lambs (2, 3, 4, 5).

CONGENITAL DEFECTS

When a noxious influence is applied to a pregnant female during the first third of pregnancy and after implantation, it may cause death of the dam, death with or without abortion of the embryo or congenital deformity of the embryo, depending upon the severity and nature of the influence. During the early part of pregnancy before implantation and before tissue differentiation commences the effect is likely to be that of embryonic death and resorption. If the insult occurs during the latter two-thirds of pregnancy injury to the foetus is unlikely unless the insult is sufficiently great to harm the dam, in which case approximately the same results will appear in the foetus; the end result is generally stillbirth or abortion. The resistance of the foetus in its later stage of development is due to the maturation of host defence factors (28). The embryo (first third of pregnancy) does not react to noxa in the same way as the foetus since no inflammation or leucocytosis develops. The reaction is one of abnormal development and it is often impossible to determine even histologically whether such an abnormality has been caused by infection or by heredity.

Although the type of noxious influence governs to a certain extent the type and severity of the defect which results, there is remarkable similarity between the defects observed after a wide range of insults (6). For example, the defects caused by vaccination of pregnant sows with attenuated hog cholera virus are similar to those caused by vitamin A deficiency in early pregnancy, and it seems therefore that the severity and time in gestation at which such influences are applied are of equal importance. The time during gestation is important in determining the organ which is affected; those organs which are developing rapidly at the time are most likely to be affected. There is a tendency for the range of abnormalities, and correspondingly the organs affected, to be increased by an increase in the duration and severity of the insult. This suggests the possibility that there may be a final common path through which all noxious influences exert their deleterious influence on actively differentiating embryonic tissues. In man most defects are attributed to defective blood supply to the foetus resulting from abnormal placentation, and in experimental animals anoxia produced by low atmospheric pressure causes a high incidence of embryonic defects (7). Anoxia may be the cause in individual cases but is unlikely to be the cause in all; however, by an extension of the same principle, it is possible that a deficiency of an essential metabolite or the presence of a cytopathic agent (viral or chemical) in an unimpaired circulation could have the same effect as anoxia by interfering with tissue metabolism at the same level. That is to say, the final common path may be the high rate of metabolism of rapidly dividing cells. On the other hand it is possible that increased activity of the adrenal cortex may be the final common path, the increased activity being due to deficiency of metabolites, anoxia or other stress factors.

One of the remarkable features of non-inherited congenital defects in animals and man is their tendency to occur in 'outbreaks'. This is understandable if known viral infections or nutritional deficiencies have a seasonal occurrence, but where the causative agent is not known the reason for the periodicity of the defect is obscure.

It is possible that many inherited defects, which need not be congenital, are due to inheritance of a higher requirement of a specific metabolite than normal, the so-called 'genetotrophic' diseases. Certainly some inherited defects including cleft palate can be reproduced by dietary deficiencies, the incidence of some inherited defects can be modified by dietary supplementation (8), and the effects of many noxious agents are modified by the genetic constitution of the animal (6).

The noxious influences which are known to produce congenital defects are listed below:

Inheritance

There are many examples among domestic animals (see Chapter 33).

Virus Infection

Rubella in humans produces defects of eyes, ears and heart (9); influenza (Asian flu) in human females causes defects of the central nervous system (10); vaccination of pregnant sows with modified hog cholera virus between the 15th and 25th day of pregnancy produces piglets with oedema, deformed noses and kidneys and causes many foetal resorptions (11); vaccinations of pregnant ewes with attenuated blue-tongue virus between the 35th and 45th days of pregnancy is reported to produce a high proportion of lambs with hydranencephaly (12) and similar defects are thought to occur after natural subclinical infections with the blue-tongue virus (13). The only well established examples of congenital defects in domestic animals as a result of naturally acquired virus infection during pregnancy are cerebellar hypoplasia in kittens, piglets and calves related to infection of the dam by panleucopenia virus, swine fever virus and mucosal disease virus, respectively. Arthrogryposis and cleft palate in calves have been suspected to occur after infection of the dam with mucosal disease virus.

Nutritional Deficiency

There are numbers of congenital defects in animals which are known to be caused by deficiencies of specific nutrients in the diet of the dam. Thus iodine deficiency causes goitre, copper deficiency causes enzootic ataxia in lambs, vitamin D deficiency causes neonatal rickets, and vitamin A deficiency causes eye defects, harelip and other abnormalities in piglets. Congenital defects suspected to be due to nutritional deficiency include paresis and paralysis in lambs and calves caused by vitamin E deficiency, and acorn calves thought to be due to a complex deficiency of unknown factors. The significance of experimentally produced congenital defects in laboratory animals for domestic animals is undetermined; deficiencies of choline, riboflavine, pantothenic acid, cobalamin and folic acid (14) and manganese and copper (15) have been used to produce a wide range of defects. Hypervitaminosis A produces defects in rats.

Simple inanition does not cause congenital defects but is a common cause of foetal resorption, stillbirths and weak offspring. A deficiency of protein may increase the abortion and stillbirth rates. The experimental production of congenital malformation by metabolic procedures has been reviewed (16).

Miscellaneous Causes

Exposure to a number of toxic substances including selenium, nitrogen mustards, tetanus toxin, sulphonamide drugs, physostigmine and radium or X-ray irradiation all result in an increased incidence of congenital defects (7). Exposure of rats to heliotrine, the pyrrolizidine alkaloid in plants of *Heliotropum* spp. to which domestic animals often have access, can cause foetal anomalies in rats (17). Ingestion of the plant *Veratrum californicum*, particularly around the 14th day of gestation, causes defects of the cranium and brain in lambs and prolonged gestation in their dams (25). The ingestion of locoweeds (*Astragalus* and *Oxytropis* spp.) and lupin (*Lupinus sericeus*) also causes limb contractures in calves and lambs (31) and the ingestion of tobacco plants has been suggested as a cause of limb deformities in young pigs (33). Considerable interest centres around the observation that cortisone administered early in pregnancy in mice and humans causes an increased incidence of cleft palate (18). The administration of oestrone and oestradiol to mice (12th to 16th day of pregnancy) causes a high incidence of cleft palate (19) and the feeding during early pregnancy of methallibure, a product used to suppress oestrus in sows, has resulted in limb and cranial deformities in pigs (24). Severe exposure to beta or gamma irradiation such as might occur after an atomic explosion can result in a high proportion of gross malformations in developing foetuses (20). Experimental radiation injury has caused the appearance of calves with defective limb development (21). Hyperthermia of the dam has been suggested as a cause of congenital brain defects (29). Bismuth (22) and apholate (23), an insect chemosterilant, are also suspected of causing multiple congenital defects in sheep.

Clinically a combination of defects is often seen in the one animal and care must be taken to ensure that all organs are examined. There are several defects which cannot be readily distinguished at birth and others which disappear subsequently. It is probably wise not to be too dogmatic in predicting the outcome in a patient with only a suspicion of a congenital defect or one in which the defect appears to be causing no apparent harm. A specific instance is the new-born foal with a cardiac murmur. Sporadic cases of congenital defects are usually impossible to define aetiologically, but when the number of affected animals increases it becomes necessary to attempt to determine the cause. The possibility of inheritance playing a part is most easily examined, but if there is no evidence suggesting heredity as a factor the occurrence of a virus disease or vaccination against a virus disease should be considered. Primary or secondary nutritional deficiencies are often most difficult to determine and this examination is usually left until last.

Although there is a great deal of variation between species in the prevalence of congenital defects the overall incidence is sufficient to attract attention. From available figures a prevalence of 5 to 6 per cent of new-born animals in all species are defective (26, 27).

REFERENCES

(1) Misdorp, W. (1965). *Path. vet.*, 2, 328.
(2) McFarlane, D. (1961). *Aust. vet. J.*, 37, 105.
(3) Watson, R. H. & Elder, E. M. (1961). *Aust. vet. J.*, 37, 283.
(4) Moule, G. R. (1960). *Aust. vet. J.*, 36, 154.
(5) Hughes, K. L. *et al.* (1964). *Proc. Aust. Soc. Anim. Prod.*, Sydney, 92, 100, 107 & 113.
(6) Fraser, F. C. & Fainstaat, T. D. (1951). *Amer. J. Dis. Child.*, 82, 593.
(7) Hogan, A. G. (1953). *Ann. Rev. Biochem.*, 22, 299.
(8) Gilman, J. P. W. (1956). *Cornell Vet.*, 46, 487.
(9) Annotation (1957). *Lancet*, 273, 1103.
(10) Coffey, V. P. & Jessop, W. J. E. (1959). *Lancet*, 277, 935.
(11) Young, G. A. *et al.* (1955). *J. Amer. vet. med. Ass.*, 126, 165.
(12) Shultz, G. & Delay, P. D. (1955). *J. Amer. vet. med. Ass.*, 127, 224.
(13) Griner, L. A. *et al.* (1964). *J. Amer. vet. med. Ass.*, 145, 1013.
(14) Giroud, A. (1954). *Biol. Rev.*, 29, 220.
(15) O'Dell, B. L. *et al.* (1961). *J. Nutr.*, 73, 151.
(16) Kalter, J. & Warkany, J. (1959). *Physiol. Rev.*, 39, 69.
(17) Queen, C. R. & Christie, C. S. (1961). *Brit. J. exp. Path.*, 62, 369.
(18) Harris, J. W. S. & Ross, I. P. (1956). *Lancet*, 270, 1045.
(19) Nishihara, G. (1958). *Proc. Soc. exp. Biol.*, 97, 809.
(20) Schjeide, O. A. (1957). *Nutr. Rev.*, 15, 225.
(21) Erickson, B. H. & Murphree, R. L. (1964). *J. Anim. Sci.*, 23, 1066.
(22) James, L. F. *et al.* (1966). *Amer. J. vet. Res.*, 27, 132.
(23) Younger, R. L. (1965). *Amer. J. vet. Res.*, 26, 991.
(24) King, G. J. (1969). *J. Reprod. Fertil.*, 20, 551.
(25) Binns, W. *et al.* (1965). *J. Amer. vet. med. Ass.*, 147, 839.
(26) Priester, W. A. *et al.* (1970). *Amer. J. vet. Res.*, 31, 1871.
(27) Gilmore, L. O. & Fechheimer, N. S. (1970). *Ohio agric. Res. Centre*, Res-Summary No. 45.
(28) Osburn, B. I. *et al.* (1970). *Fed. Proc.*, 29, 286.
(29) Edwards, M. J. (1969). *Aust. vet. J.*, 45, 189.
(30) Leipold, H. W. *et al.* (1970). *Amer. J. vet. Res.*, 31, 1367.
(31) James, L. F. *et al.* (1967). *Amer. J. vet. Res.*, 28, 1379.

NEONATAL INFECTION

Portal of Infection

Considerable interest centres about the question of whether some infections of the newborn are contracted before or after birth and in many instances this has not been determined. The point is of particular importance in foals where infections due to *Actinobacillus equuli*, *Escherichia coli*, *Salmonella abortivoequina* and *Streptococcus pyogenes equi* cause heavy mortality. The decision as to whether or not the disease is intra-uterine in origin may influence the control measures to be used. If it is intra-uterine the infection must gain entrance via the placenta and probably by means of a placentitis due to a blood-borne infection or an existing endometritis. In the latter case disinfection of the uterus before mating becomes an important hygienic precaution and disinfection of the environment may have little effect on the incidence of the disease. If the disease is post-natal the portal of entry of the infection may be through the navel or by ingestion. Contamination of the environment can arise from soiling of the udder or bedding by uterine discharges from the dam, or from previous parturitions, or from discharges from other affected new-born animals. The rapidity with which signs appear and death occurs is not a satisfactory criterion on which to judge whether an infection has occurred before or after birth, as the incubation period in a virulent infection in a new-born animal may be less than 24 hours. If the causative agent can be detected in the uterine exudate of the dam and in the foetus at birth and if signs are observed at birth the infection can be classed as intra-uterine. The presence of lesions in the foetus at birth, as in leptospiral abortion in pigs and *Act. equuli* infections in foals, is an additional proof that the infection gained entrance during intra-uterine life. Septicaemia in foals due to *Act. equuli* and *E. coli* can arise from infection *in utero*, and sporadic cases of tuberculosis occur in new-born animals, but by far the greatest proportion of neonatal infections occur after birth. Intra-uterine infections are more commonly associated with death of the dam or the foetus or with abortion.

Bacteria and viruses are frequently found in the foetus in domestic animals and in man. Whether or not a placentitis must develop first is undecided and experimental work on the permeability of the placenta to virus particles is equivocal (1). Because of the importance of viruses and possibly bacteria in the aetiology of congenital defects in man, sheep and pigs this situation needs to be clarified. It is possible that infection gains entrance to the exposed trophoblast before closure of the amniotic folds, infection coming from the uterine contents via an existing metritis or blood-borne infection (2).

Resistance to Infection

The new-born animal is particularly susceptible to infection. It is lacking in antibodies because of the failure of these substances to pass the placental barrier, it may lack certain protective minerals and vitamins and it has a poorly developed reticuloendothelial system and is therefore incapable of developing an active immunity or dealing satisfactorily with invading organisms. This neonatal susceptibility does not apply to all infectious agents. Thus there are specific diseases to which new-born animals are highly susceptible, e.g. lamb dysentery and enteritis due to *E. coli*, to which adults are relatively resistant (9). On the other hand some pathogens, e.g. *Brucella abortus*, are unable to survive in the tissues of the young.

Although information is incomplete, certain principles are well established and can be used as a working hypothesis when considering problems of immunity of the newborn. Transplacental transmission of antibodies does not occur in domestic animals, the passive immunity of the newborn coming from the ingestion of colostrum containing high concentrations of antibodies. Differing from the placental transmission of antibodies, absorption from colostrum through the intestinal wall is not markedly selective (3). This non-specificity extends as far as heterologous antibodies. For example, antibodies against *Salmonella cholerae suis* in horse serum are capable of passing through the intestinal wall of the new-born pig (4). On the other hand, antibodies of ovine origin are absorbed but less readily than those of equine or porcine origin (24). The antibody titre is much higher in colostrum than maternal serum but the titre falls as the colostrum gives way to normal milk. The concentration of antibodies reached in the suckling's serum depends on the concentration in the dam's colostrum

and the amount of colostrum taken. There is a great deal of variation in these factors between species, breeds and individuals (29). Persistence of the antibody titre in the suckling's serum and therefore its passive immunity also appears to depend upon the absolute amount of antibody absorbed from the gut. Absorption of antibodies from the gut occurs for only a short period after birth, the exact time varying with the species. In cattle absorption occurs for only 24 hours, for up to 4 days in goats and up to 12 days in dogs: absorption continues to somewhere between 29 and 48 hours in lambs (5), although it is greatly diminished at about 15 hours (23), and 24 to 36 hours in foals (6). In pigs cessation of absorption occurs somewhere between 12 and 27 hours (7, 8). The times at which absorption ceases are capable of a good deal of variation. One of the important factors determining the cut-off point is the time at which the first colostrum is ingested. If colostrum is withheld the capacity to absorb globulins is greatly prolonged (7, 9). The failure of antibodies to pass the placenta of domesticated animals prevents the occurrence of isoimmunization haemolytic anaemia until after the foetus is born.

The status of the new-born animal with regard to vitamins and minerals is dependent on the status of the dam, but in the case of vitamin A it is also dependent on placental permeability. Vitamin A in the alcohol form, as it occurs in the blood of the cow from the breakdown of carotene, does not pass the placental barrier but in the ester form, as it occurs in cod liver oil, it is transmissible. Thus a high green feed intake does not increase vitamin A storage in the foetus but does markedly increase the content in colostrum.

The importance of the colostrum is therefore largely related to its protective effects against infection due to its content of antibodies and to a less extent of vitamin A. Failure to obtain colostrum may be due to death of or agalactia in the dam, weakness of the offspring, premilking or removal of the new-born animal from the dam before it has sucked. Isolation of the newborn may be essential, for example in foals produced by incompatible matings and in such cases it is necessary to provide an alternative source of antibodies and vitamin A and prophylactic wide-range antibiotics.

It has been established that antibodies in the colostrum which reach the serum are found in the gamma globulin fraction, the major immunoglobulins, and are present as a member of immunochemically distinct entities. The immunoglobulins known to be present in bovine colostrum and to pass to the calf's serum after sucking are IgM and

IgG (30). The presence or absence of antibodies may not have much effect on the incidence of disease in a group of neonates but it is likely to markedly influence the mortality rate in the group (31).

The condition of agammaglobulinaemia as it occurs in man and which seems to be of some importance in that species in causing lowered neonatal resistance to infection is probably due to the small supply of colostrum and its low content of antibody. In domestic animals the elevation of blood globulins after the ingestion of colostrum is considerable and probably sufficient in most cases to provide immune substances until the developing reticulo-endothelial system is capable of reacting to infection. However, there is an increasing body of evidence which points to causes of hypogammaglobulinaemia in calves other than a deficient intake of colostrum (32). Some of the absorbed protein appears to be lost from the circulation in the urine. At least in the lamb there is a period of increased kidney permeability to protein which is concurrent with the period of intestinal permeability (5). There is a marked proteinuria and globulin and antibody are present in the urine. Agammaglobulinaemia may be the cause of chronic susceptibility to infection in young farm animals (10), and an incidence of hypogammaglobulinaemia up to a level of 4 per cent has been recorded in some cattle populations (11).

One of the corollaries of intestinal absorption of colostral antibodies is that sensitizing antibodies which cause isoimmunization haemolytic anaemia may be absorbed by the new-born animal. With a tuberculous dam sufficient antibodies may be absorbed to make the offspring sensitive to the tuberculin test for a considerable period. Another corollary is that the presence of excessive quantities of passively-acquired antibodies in the neonate's circulation may suppress the production of specific antibodies when the animal is exposed to the relevant antigen. The development of immunological competence after birth varies from antigen to antigen and from animal species to animal species, and this variation must obviously have a great deal of influence on the young animal's susceptibility to different infectious agents (12).

Environmental Factors

Two environmental factors which may predispose to infection, besides causing mortality themselves, are low environmental temperature (21) and deprivation of carbohydrate leading to hypoglycaemia (20). Piglets are particularly susceptible to both factors. Their thermo-regulation mechanism is highly inefficient during the first 9 days of life and is not working well until the 20th day (13). The preferred air temperature for neonatal pigs is 32°C (89·5°F) during the first day and 30°C (86°F) thereafter (22). Because of the importance of neonatal mortality in range lambs some observations have been made on their thermo-regulation efficiency (14, 15) and it is apparent that at high environmental temperatures it is not effective. Heat prostration and some deaths can occur when the environmental temperature is high especially if lambs have to perform prolonged physical exercise and if there is an absence of shade. Thermo-regulatory efficiency at low temperatures is moderately good in new-born lambs and is dependent on the presence of deposits of readily metabolizable 'brown fat' (25). There is little information on thermo-regulation in new-born foals but it is evident that healthy foals, within a normal environmental temperature range, are capable of a homeothermic response (26).

New-born lambs, calves and foals are much more capable of maintaining their blood glucose levels when starved than are piglets (16, 27) although occasional cases of hypoglycaemic coma may be seen in lambs. Piglets starved during the first week of life succumb quickly and manifest a specific syndrome known as neonatal hypoglycaemia or baby pig disease. Calves are also highly resistant to insulin-produced hypoglycaemia during the first 48 hours of life but are susceptible and respond convulsively to it at 7 days (17).

Nutrition of the dam is important in relation to resistance of the offspring (18), but it is impossible to be specific in recommending the ration to be used.

Methods of feeding the young may also be important in the production of disease. Pail-fed calves readily develop dietetic scours due to abnormal curd formation in the abomasum if they are fed large quantities of milk at long intervals. Housing is equally important, particularly in young pigs which are very sensitive to temperature variations. Hygiene is important especially when animals are confined to close quarters. Gross contamination of pens by pathogenic organisms and aerogenous spread in poorly ventilated, wet barns are two of the commonest environmental factors producing spread of disease in the newborn and requiring strict hygienic precautions. Movement of animals, either the dam just before parturition or the new-born animal during the first few days of life, presents a major environmental hazard. The dam may not have been exposed to and thus have no circulating antibodies against pathogens present in the new environment. A new-born animal may be in the same position both with regard to deficiency of antibodies and exposure to new infections.

Pre-milking of dairy cows to relieve udder congestion and improve post-parturient milk production has become a vogue in some areas. It may be advisable in certain circumstances but it has the deficiency of reducing the antibody content of colostrum and increasing the chances of infection in the calf.

Aetiology

Amongst domestic animals the common neonatal infections encountered are:

Cattle

Bacteraemia or septicaemia caused by *E. coli*, *Listeria monocytogenes*, *Pasteurella* spp., *Streptococci* or *Salmonella* spp.; enteritis caused by *Clostridium perfringens* types A, B and C, and pneumoenteritis due to a virus.

Pigs

Septicaemia with localization in joints, endocardium and meninges caused by *Streptococcus* spp.; bacteraemia, septicaemia and enteritis caused by *E. coli*; transmissible gastro-enteritis, swine pox and vomiting and wasting disease caused by viruses; enteritis caused by *Cl. perfringens*; arthritis and septicaemia caused by *E. insidiosa*; and septicaemia caused by *L. monocytogenes*.

Horses

Septicaemia with localization, particularly in joints, caused by *E. coli*, *Act. equuli*, *Sal. abortivoequina*, *Strep. pyogenes equi* and *Sal. typhimurium*: enteritis caused by *Cl. perfringens*; septicaemia caused by *L. monocytogenes*.

Sheep

Bacteraemia with localization in joints caused by streptococci, micrococci and *E. insidiosa*, gas gangrene of the navel caused by *Cl. septicum* and *Cl. oedematiens*; lamb dysentery caused by *Cl. perfringens* type B; septicaemia caused by *E. coli* and *L. monocytogenes*.

Non-specific infections caused by pyogenic organisms, including *Corynebacterium pyogenes*, *Sphaerophorus necrophorus*. *Streptococcus* and *Micrococcus* spp. and *Pasteurella* spp. occur in all species.

Pathogenesis of Neonatal Infection

The usual pattern of development in neonatal infections is a septicaemia, with a severe systemic reaction, or a bacteraemia with few or no systemic signs followed by localization in various organs. If the portal of entry is the navel local inflammation occurs—the so-called 'navel ill'—which can be easily overlooked if clinical examination is not thorough. From the local infection at the navel, extension may occur to the liver or via the urachus to the bladder and result in chronic ill-health, or systemically to produce septicaemia. In blood-borne infections localization is most common in the joints producing a suppurative or non-suppurative arthritis. Less commonly there is localization in the eye to produce a panophthalmitis, on the heart valves to cause valvular endocarditis or in the meninges to produce a meningitis. Most of these secondary lesions take some time to develop and signs usually appear at 1 to 2 weeks of age.

Dehydration and electrolyte imbalance can occur very quickly in new-born animals whether diarrhoea and vomiting are present or not. This is probably due to deprivation of fluid intake as much as to loss of fluid. The extreme depression observed in many cases is probably caused by biochemical changes in addition to the effects of bacterial toxins.

Principles of Treatment and Prevention in Neonatal Infections

In treatment, control of the infection must include the use of suitable antibiotics, preferably as indicated by bacteriological examination and sensitivity tests of cultures. Because of the poor immunological status of the new-born animal the provision of extra antibodies by transfusions of whole blood, infusion of serum or blood plasma or injections of specific antisera is often practised. When it is given by injection 2 to 4 ml. per lb. body weight of whole blood should be used, either by the intraperitoneal, intravenous or subcutaneous routes. Serum and plasma can be given similarly and at half the dose rate. If the animal is less than 24 hours old, the material may be fed but should be given at doses of four to five times the injection dose. If the dam is the only available source of a good antibody supply her blood may be used but as the titre is lower than normal, because of the drain of antibodies into colostrum, other animals in the group may be better donors. In the special case of foals likely to develop isoimmunization haemolytic anaemia, the dam's blood must not be used because of its high content of antibodies to which the foal is sensitized. When a particular infection is new to a group or when the antibody level is likely to be low in the adults such as in *E. coli* infections, vaccination of the dams before parturition to increase the colostral antibody content is highly recommended. When this is done the common practice is to give several injections of an autogenous vaccine at 1 to 2 months before parturition. Vaccination of the newborn before they are 2 months old is unlikely to be effective, but passive immunization by the injection of hyperimmune serum is often advisable. Passive immunization via the colostrum has also been attempted by intramammary vaccination of cows with *Salmonella dublin* antigen during the last month of pregnancy (28). The method has many obvious disadvantages and is not recommended. Vaccination *in utero* obviates many of these disadvantages and, should the procedure prove practicable, offers a more direct alternative (32).

Prophylactic measures should include removal of infection from the environment or removal of the animal from the infected environment, increasing the specific resistance of the new-born animal and suitable management to increase non-specific resistance. When attempting to remove the infection from the environment the problem of whether the infection derives from an intra- or extra-uterine source must receive consideration. Intra-uterine infection necessitates local uterine or systemic treatment of the dam to eliminate the infection from the uterus before conception occurs. Swabs of the uterine contents should be examined before and after treatment in suspected animals. Disinfection of maternity quarters is recommended. A rotation of fields should be used for animals at pasture. Increasing the specific resistance of the newborn can be carried out by vaccination of the dam in the latter part of pregnancy as described above or by the use of specific antisera immediately after birth.

An adequate supply of colostrum or alternatively blood transfusions should be provided to ensure non-specific resistance. It is a common field experience to encounter calves with very low serum globulin levels but with a history from the owner of having taken colostrum. Nevertheless, change of management to force feeding of colostrum may overcome the hypoglobulinaemia and the neonatal mortality. Partly to point up the occurrence of low serum globulin levels, and partly because of the need to detect them in purchased new-born calves, the measurement of serum globulin levels has become a standard laboratory procedure. Prophylactic action to be taken when affected animals are detected may include blood or serum transfusion, the administration of non-specific hyper-immune serum or purified gammaglobulin, usually freeze-dried. The latter is often too expensive for general use.

In special cases where infection is probable antibiotics or sulphonamides should be used prophy-

lactically, keeping in mind that adequate doses obviate the development of resistant strains of bacteria. Suitable management practices should be followed with particular reference to feeding methods when animals are reared artificially. An adequate supply of vitamins and other essential nutrients should also be provided for the dam and the newborn. Movement of heavily pregnant and newborn animals to new herds or flocks should be avoided. Disinfection of the navel at birth is a worth-while practice in all circumstances but is essential under conditions of heavy environmental contamination. Severance of the umbilical cord too quickly after the birth of thoroughbred foals has been suggested as a means by which the foals are deprived of large quantities of blood. This may result in the development of barkers and wanderers and predispose the foal to other diseases (19).

REFERENCES

(1) Biegeleisen, J. Z. & Scott, L. V. (1958). *Proc. Soc. exp. Biol.*, *97*, 411.
(2) Young, G. A. (1955). *Proc. 92nd ann. Meet. Amer. vet. med. Ass.*, 377–381.
(3) Brambell, F. W. R. (1961). *Proc. roy. Soc. Med.*, *54*, 992.
(4) Olsson, B. (1959). *Nord. Vet.-Med.*, *11*, 1.
(5) McCarthy, E. F. & McDougall, E. I. (1953). *Biochem. J.*, *55*, 177.
(6) Bruner, D. W. *et al.* (1950). *Amer. J. vet. Res.*, *11*, 22.
(7) Payne, L. C. & Marsh, C. L. (1962). *J. Nutr.*, *76*, 151.
(8) Asplund, J. M. *et al.* (1962). *J. Anim. Sci.*, *21*, 412.
(9) Lecce, J. G. & Morgan, D. D. (1962). *J. Nutr.*, *78*, 263.
(10) Perk, K. & Lobl, K. (1962). *Amer. J. vet. Res.*, *23*, 92.
(11) Cohen, R. & Trainin, Z. (1969). *Refuah vet.*, *26*, 18.
(12) Ingram, D. G. & Smith, A. N. (1965). *Canad. vet. J.*, *6*, 194 & 226.
(13) Holub, A. *et al.* (1957). *Nature, Lond.*, *180*, 858.
(14) Smith, I. D. (1961). *Aust. vet. J.*, *37*, 205.
(15) Alexander, G. (1962). *Aust. J. agric. Res.*, *13*, 82, 100, 122 & 144.
(16) Goodwin, R. F. W. (1957). *J. comp. Path.*, *67*, 289.
(17) Edwards, A. V. (1964). *J. Physiol.*, *171*, 46P.
(18) Wigglesworth, J. S. (1966). *Brit. med. Bull.*, *22*, 13.
(19) Rossdale, P. D. & Mahaffey, L. W. (1958). *Vet. Rec.*, *70*, 142.
(20) Shelley, H. J. & Neligan, G. A. (1966). *Brit. med. Bull.*, *22*, 34.
(21) Mount, L. E. (1966). *Brit. med. Bull.*, *22*, 34.
(22) Mount, L. E. (1963). *Nature, Lond.*, *199*, 1212.
(23) Lindqvist, K. (1963). *Proc. 9th Nordic vet. Congr., Copenhagen, 1962*, *1*, 283.
(24) Kaeberle, M. L. & Segre, D. (1964). *Amer. J. vet. Res.*, *25*, 1096 & 1103.
(25) Alexander, G. *et al.* (1970). *Biol. Neonate*, *15*, 198.
(26) Rossdale, P. D. (1968). *Brit. vet. J.*, *124*, 18.
(27) Dalton, R. G. (1967). *Brit. vet. J.*, *123*, 237.
(28) Butko, M. P. (1967). *Trudy vses. Inst. Vet. Sanit.*, *29*, 305.
(29) Kruse, V. (1970). *Anim. Prod.*, *12*, 619 & 627.
(30) Penhale, W. J. *et al.* (1970). *Brit. vet. J.*, *126*, 30.
(31) Hurvell, B. A. & Fey, H. (1970). *Acta vet. scand.*, *11*, 341.
(32) Gay, C. C. (1971). *Proc. 19th World vet. Congress*, Mexico, 1971, pp. 1004–5.
(33) Menges, R. W. *et al.* (1970). *Environ. Res.*, *3*, 285.

4

Diseases of the Alimentary Tract—I

INTRODUCTION

Principles of Alimentary Tract Dysfunction

THE primary functions of the alimentary tract are the prehension, digestion and absorption of food and water and the maintenance of the internal environment by modification of the amount and nature of the materials absorbed.

The primary functions can be divided into four major modes and, correspondingly, there are four major modes of alimentary dysfunction. There may be abnormality of motility, of secretion, of digestion or of absorption. The procedure in diagnosis should be to determine which mode or modes of function is or are disturbed before proceeding to the determination of the site and nature of the lesion and ultimately of the specific cause.

MOTOR FUNCTION

Hypermotility and Hypomotility

The most important facets of alimentary tract motility are the peristaltic movements which move ingesta and faeces from the oesophagus to the rectum, the segmentation movements which churn and mix the ingesta, and the tone of the sphincters. In ruminants these movements are of major importance in the forestomachs. Prehension, mastication and swallowing are other facets of alimentary tract motility which are essential for normal functioning of the tract.

Abnormal motor function may take the form of increased or decreased motility. Peristalsis and segmenting movements are usually affected equally and in the same manner. Motility depends upon stimulation via the sympathetic and parasympathetic nervous systems and is thus dependent on the activity of the central and peripheral parts of these systems, and upon the intestinal musculature and its intrinsic nervous plexuses. Autonomic imbalance, resulting in a relative dominance of one or other system, is manifested by hypermotility or hypomotility, and can arise as a result of stimulation or destruction of hypothalamic centres, the ganglia, or the efferent or afferent peripheral branches of the system. Debility, accompanied by weakness of the musculature, or severe inflammation, such as occurs in acute peritonitis or after trauma, result in atony of the gut wall. Less severe inflammation, such as occurs in mild gastritis and enteritis, causes an increase in muscular activity. Increased motility causes diarrhoea, decreased motility causes constipation, and both have deleterious effects on digestion and absorption.

Increased irritability at a particular segment increases its activity and disturbs the normal downward gradient of activity which ensures that the ingesta is passed from the oesophagus to the rectum. Not only is the gradient towards the rectum made steeper, thus increasing the rate of passage of ingesta in that direction, but the increased potential activity of an irritated segment may be sufficiently high to produce a reverse gradient to the oral segments so that the direction of the peristaltic waves is reversed, oral to the irritated segments. It is by this means that vomiting occurs and intestinal contents, even faeces, are returned to the stomach and vomited.

Distension

One of the major results of abnormality of motility is distension of the tract which occurs in a number of disturbances including the rapid accumulation or inefficient expulsion of gas, complete occlusion of the lumen by intestinal accident or pyloric or ileocaecal valve obstruction, and engorgement on solid or liquid foods. Fluids, and to a less extent gas, accumulate because of their failure to pass along the tract. Much of the accumulated fluid represents saliva and gastric and intestinal juices secreted during normal digestion. Distension causes pain and, reflexly, increased spasm and motility of adjoining gut segments. Distension also stimulates further secretion of fluid into the lumen of the gut and this exaggerates the distension. When the distension passes a critical point, the ability of the musculature of the wall to respond diminishes, the initial pain disappears, and a stage of paralytic ileus develops in which all muscle tone is lost.

Abdominal Pain

Visceral pain may arise in any organ but the mode of its development is always the same and it is discussed here because alimentary tract disease is the major cause of visceral, and more specifically, of abdominal pain. The most important mechanism is stretching of the wall of the organ which stimulates free pain endings of autonomic nerves in the wall. Contraction does not of itself cause pain but does so by causing direct and reflex distension of neighbouring segments. Thus spasm, an exaggerated segmenting contraction of one section of bowel, will result in distension of the immediately oral segment of bowel when a peristaltic wave arrives. When there is increased motility for any reason, excessive segmentation and peristalsis cause abdominal pain, and the frequent occurrence of intermittent bouts of pain depends upon the periodic increases in muscle tone which are typical of alimentary tract wall. Other factors which have some stimulating effect on the pain end-organs are oedema and failure of local blood supply such as occurs in local embolism or in intestinal accidents accompanied by twisting of the mesentery. A secondary mechanism in the production of abdominal pain is the stretching and inflammation of serous membranes.

Clinically abdominal pain can be detected by palpation and the elicitation of pain responses. The question arises as to whether the response elicited is due to involvement of underlying organs or to referred pain. It is difficult to decide whether referred pain occurs in animals. In humans it is largely a subjective sensation although often accompanied by local hyperalgesia. At least there are no known examples of referred pain which are of diagnostic importance in animals and a local pain response on palpation of the abdomen is accepted as evidence of pain in the serous membranes or viscera which underlie the point of palpation.

Dehydration and Shock

An immediate effect of distension of the stomach or small intestine by the accumulation of saliva and normal gastric and intestinal secretions is the stimulation of further secretion of fluid and electrolytes in the oral segments. The stimulation is self-perpetuating and creates a vicious cycle resulting in loss of fluid and electrolytes to the point where fatal dehydration can occur. The dehydration is accompanied by acidosis or alkalosis depending on whether the obstruction is in the intestine and accompanied by loss of alkali, or in the stomach and accompanied by heavy loss of acid radicals. The net effect is the same whether the fluid is lost by vomiting or is retained in the gut. The same cycle of events occurs in ruminants which gorge on grain but here the precipitating mechanism is not distension but a gross increase in osmotic pressure of the ingesta due to the accumulation of lactic acid. Dehydration is also of major importance in diarrhoea irrespective of the cause. An important additional factor in the production of shock, when there is distension of alimentary segments, is a marked reflex depression of vasomotor, cardiovascular and respiratory functions. In diarrhoea in calves in which there is no septicaemia nor toxaemia caused by bacteria, the end-point in the phase of dehydration can be cardiac failure due to severe metabolic acidosis. Renal ischaemia leading to uraemia may result from decreased circulating blood volume and also contribute to a fatal outcome.

SECRETORY FUNCTION

Diseases in which abnormalities of secretion occur are not generally recognized in farm animals. In humans, and to a less extent, in small animals, defects of gastric and pancreatic secretion produce syndromes which are readily recognized but, as they result in abnormal motility, they depend upon clinical pathological examination for diagnosis. If they do occur in farm animals, they have as yet been recognized only as aberrations of motility.

DIGESTIVE FUNCTION

The ability of the alimentary tract to digest food depends on its motor and secretory functions, and in herbivores, on the activity of the microflora which inhabit the forestomachs of ruminants, or caecum and colon of equidae. The flora of the forestomachs of ruminants are capable of digesting cellulose, of fermenting the end-products of other carbohydrates to volatile fatty acids, and converting nitrogenous substances to ammonia and protein. In a number of circumstances, the activity of the flora can be modified so that digestion is abnormal or ceases. Failure to provide the correct diet, prolonged starvation or inappetence, and hyperacidity as occurs in engorgement on grain all result in impairment of microbial digestion. The bacteria, yeasts and protozoa may also be adversely affected by the oral administration of antibiotic and sulphonamide drugs, or drugs which drastically alter the pH of the rumen contents.

ABSORPTIVE FUNCTIONS

Absorption of fluids and the dissolved end-products of digestion may be adversely affected by increased motility or by disease of the intestinal mucosa. In most instances, the two occur together but, occasionally, as with some helminth infestations, lesions occur in the intestinal wall without accompanying changes in motility.

AUTO-INTOXICATION

This mechanism is thought to operate when there is cessation of forward movement of ingesta. At one time it did enjoy a considerable vogue as a diagnosis in human medicine and was credited as the cause of many human ailments. It has largely been discarded as an important consequence of disease of the alimentary tract but, used in its widest sense, the term still retains an element of accuracy in that there are many clinical signs in these diseases which cannot be adequately explained or classified in any other way. The theory of auto-intoxication suggested that the toxic amines and phenols produced by putrefaction of protein in the large intestine but normally detoxified in the bowel wall could, if regurgitated into the small intestine, be absorbed and cause depression, anorexia and weakness. There seems to be some gross evidence at necropsy that protein putrefaction does occur in the rumen of the cow and in the stomach and large intestine of the horse when these animals overeat on protein-rich feeds, when there is prolonged ruminal stasis or starvation or when large quantities of antibiotics are administered orally. Clinically one is led to the viewpoint that some of the signs in these diseases are caused by auto-intoxication. The depression, anorexia and posterior paresis in constipated pigs seem unexplainable in other terms.

The common association of constipation with posterior paralysis in animals is difficult to explain. It is believed by some that paralysis is part of the syndrome of auto-intoxication. By others, the paralysis is thought to be due to pressure on the sciatic nerve, and by others, both constipation and paralysis are viewed as manifestations of a primary nervous dysfunction.

The Manifestations of Alimentary Tract Dysfunction

Inanition is the major physiological effect of alimentary dysfunction when the disease is a chronic one, dehydration is the major effect in acute diseases, and shock is the important physiological disturbance in hyperacute diseases. Some degree of abdominal pain is usual in most diseases of the alimentary tract, the severity varying with the nature of the lesion. Other manifestations include abnormalities of prehension, mastication and swallowing, and vomiting, diarrhoea, haemorrhage and constipation.

ABNORMALITIES OF PREHENSION, MASTICATION AND SWALLOWING

Prehension, including grazing and drinking, may be interfered with by paralysis of the muscles of the jaw or tongue, by deficiencies of the incisor teeth or by malapposition of the jaws in grazing animals. The latter is often an inherited condition in cattle and sheep but may also be a result of rickets. Pain in the mouth caused by stomatitis, foreign bodies or glossitis may also interfere with prehension. A particular example is inability to drink cold water in cattle affected by fluorosis. A simple examination of the mouth usually reveals the causative lesion. Paralysis is indicated by the behaviour of the animal as it attempts to ingest feed without success. In all cases, unless there is anorexia due to systemic disease, the animal is hungry and attempts to feed but cannot do so.

Mastication may be painful and this is manifested by slow jaw movements interrupted by pauses and expressions of pain if the cause is a bad tooth, but in a painful stomatitis there is usually complete refusal to chew. Incomplete mastication is evidenced by the dropping of food from the mouth while eating and the passage of large quantities of undigested material in the faeces.

Swallowing is a complex act governed by reflexes mediated through the glossopharyngeal, trigeminal, hypoglossal and vagal nerves. The mechanism of the act includes closure of all exits from the pharynx, the creation of pressure to force the bolus into the oesophagus, and involuntary movements of the musculature of the oesophageal wall to carry the bolus to the stomach. A defect in nervous control of the reflex or a narrowing of the lumen of the pharynx or oesophagus may interfere with swallowing and it is difficult to differentiate clinically between physical and functional causes of dysphagia (difficulty in eating).

Dysphagia is usually due to physical obstruction by a foreign body or tumour in the pharynx or oesophagus, although painful lesions or general inflammatory swelling insufficient in degree to completely prevent swallowing may have the same effect. A functional obstruction can also occur with oesophageal dilatation due to partial paralysis or to oesophageal diverticulum. Spasm or achalasia of the cardia of the stomach is a well-known entity in humans but it is not recognized in farm animals. Dysphagia is manifested by forceful attempts to swallow accompanied by extension of the head at first, followed by forceful flexion and violent contractions of the muscles of the neck and abdomen.

Inability to swallow is usually caused by the same lesions as dysphagia but in a greater degree. If the animal attempts to swallow, the results depend on the site of the obstruction. Lesions in the pharynx cause regurgitation through the nostrils or coughing up of the material. In the latter instance, there is danger that some of the material may be aspirated into the lungs and cause acute respiratory and cardiac failure or aspiration pneumonia. When the obstruction is at a low level in the oesophagus, a large amount of material may be swallowed and then regurgitated. It is necessary to differentiate between material regurgitated from the oesophagus and vomitus. The former is usually slightly alkaline, the latter acid.

DIARRHOEA AND CONSTIPATION

Abnormalities of peristalsis and segmentation usually occur together. With a general increase in activity caused by inflammation or autonomic imbalance, there is increased caudal flow resulting in a decrease in alimentary sojourn—diarrhoea. Because of lack of absorption of fluid, the faeces are usually softer than normal and increased in bulk. The frequency of defaecation is usually increased. The common causes of diarrhoea include enteritis, incomplete digestion with the passage of excess fibre or other feed constituents, and functional diarrhoea such as occurs in excitement. Increased venous pressure in the portal circuit caused by congestive heart failure or hepatic fibrosis also causes diarrhoea.

When the motility of the intestine is reduced, the alimentary sojourn is prolonged and constipation occurs. Because of the increased time afforded for fluid absorption, the faeces are dry, hard and of small bulk and are passed at infrequent intervals. The common causes of constipation include severe debility, deficient dietary bulk, dehydration, partial obstruction, painful conditions of the anus, and paralytic ileus. Grass sickness of horses is a specific disease in which severe constipation is accompanied by degenerative lesions in sympathetic ganglia. It is a common sign in chronic zinc poisoning in cattle.

VOMITING

Vomiting is the most complex of the motor disturbances of the alimentary tract. It is essentially a protective mechanism, in the nature of a reverse peristaltic movement, with the function of removing excessive quantities of ingesta or toxic materials from the stomach. It occurs in two forms. Projectile vomiting is based almost entirely on reverse peristalsis and is not accompanied by retching movements. Large amounts of fluid material are vomited with little effort. This is the common form of vomiting in horses and ruminants and occurs almost entirely as a result of overloading of the stomach or forestomachs with food or fluid. True vomiting is accompanied by retching movements including contraction of the abdominal wall and of the neck muscles and extension of the head. The movements are commonly prolonged and repeated and the vomitus is usually small in amount and of porridge-like or pasty consistency. It is most commonly a result of irritation of the gastric mucosa.

It is not proposed to deal extensively with vomiting here because it is not a common sign in farm animals. Examination of suspected vomitus to determine its site of origin should be undertaken. Vomiting is commonly designated as being either peripheral or central in origin depending on whether the stimulation arises centrally at the vomiting centre or peripherally by overloading of the stomach or inflammation of the gastric mucosa, or by the presence of foreign bodies in the pharynx, oesophagus or oesophageal groove. Central stimulation of vomiting by apomorphine and in nephritis and hepatitis are typical examples but vomiting occurs rarely, if at all, in these diseases in farm animals. In young pigs, vomiting is a common accompaniment of many systemic diseases.

Vomiting may have serious effects in that fluid and electrolytes may be lost in large quantities. In horses and cattle it may be followed by aspiration pneumonia or acute laryngeal obstruction. In these animals true vomiting is usually accepted as an ominous sign of grave involvement of the alimentary tract.

ALIMENTARY TRACT HAEMORRHAGE

Haemorrhage into the stomach or intestine may occur as a result of ulceration with erosion of blood vessels, acute vascular engorgement such as occurs in intestinal obstruction or thrombosis of mesenteric arteries and in acute gastritis or enteritis, especially when these are caused by helminths or protozoa which penetrate more deeply than most bacterial or viral infections. Haemorrhage into the stomach results in the formation of acid haematin which gives vomitus a dark brown colour like coffee grounds, and faeces a black or very dark brown, tarry appearance (melaena). The change in appearance of the faeces caused by haemorrhage into the bowel varies with the level at which the haemorrhage occurs. If the blood originates in the small intestine, the faeces may be brown-black but, if it originates in the colon or caecum, the blood is unchanged and gives the faeces an even red colour. Haemorrhage into the lower colon and rectum may cause the voiding of stools containing or consisting entirely of clots of whole blood.

Haemorrhage into the pharynx is unusual but when it occurs the blood may be swallowed and appear in the faeces or vomitus. If there is any doubt about the presence of blood in the faeces or vomitus, biochemical tests should be performed. The haemorrhage may be sufficiently severe to cause anaemia and, in more severe cases, acute peripheral circulatory failure.

ABDOMINAL PAIN

The pain associated with diseases of the abdominal viscera causes similar signs irrespective of the organ involved and careful clinical examination is necessary to locate the site of the lesion. The manifestations of abdominal pain vary with the species, horses being particularly sensitive, but comprise largely abnormalities of behaviour and posture.

When the abdominal pain is acute, affected horses are restless, paw violently with the front feet, kick at the belly, crouch with the hindlegs, go down heavily and roll and thrash with the legs. The pain is usually intermittent but attacks follow one another in rapid succession and the animal may soon bruise itself badly, particularly on the head and at the elbows and stifles. Abnormal postures, including sitting on the haunches, a straddling position as though the animal was about to urinate, accompanied in males by relaxation of the penis, and lying on the back with the legs in the air are common. The animal frequently turns its head to look at the flank. Patchy sweating, a marked increase in heart rate, usually to over 100 per minute, rapid, shallow, sobbing respiration, and injection of mucosal and conjunctival vessels are also present, particularly in cases of acute gastric dilatation, acute intestinal obstruction, or impaction of the ileocaecal valve. These signs are not so marked in intestinal hypermotility, impaction of the large intestine and obstruction of mesenteric vessels. Rectal examination and abdominal auscultation, are important aids to diagnosis. Renal and urethral colic are usually acute.

A similar but usually less severe syndrome is typical of acute abdominal pain in cattle due to the same acute causes but only subacute pain occurs in sheep and pigs.

Subacute pain in all species may be due to alimentary tract disease, particularly impaction of the large intestine in pigs and impaction of the forestomachs and abomasal obstruction in adult cattle, but it also occurs in acute hepatitis and peritonitis. Traumatic reticulo-peritonitis of cattle is the outstanding example; the emphasis is on immobility, the animal showing reluctance to move, arching of the back, grunting on walking or with each respiration, constipation, reluctance to urinate, rapid, shallow respiration and pain on abdominal percussion and palpation.

TENESMUS

Tenesmus, or severe straining, is a common sign of many diseases of the organs of the pelvic cavity including vaginitis and placental retention, in rabies and spinal cord abscess and in many cases in which the cause of straining cannot be determined. There appears to be an increased incidence in feed-lot cattle since stilboestrol feeding became widespread. Thus, although it is a common sign of intestinal disease especially when the colon is affected as in coccidiosis and intussusception, it is not a diagnostic sign of disease of the lower alimentary tract. Careful clinical examination is usually necessary to determine the system involved.

SHOCK AND DEHYDRATION

Acute rapid distension of the intestine or stomach causes reflex effects on heart, lungs and on blood vessels. The blood pressure falls abruptly, the temperature falls below normal and there is a marked increase in heart rate. In acute intestinal accidents in horses which terminate fatally in 6 to 12 hours, shock is probably the major cause of death. There appears to be some species difference in the susceptibility to shock because similar accidents in cattle rarely cause death in less than 3 to 4 days, although acute ruminal tympany may exert its effects in this way and cause death in a very short time. Less severe distension, vomiting and diarrhoea cause clinically recognizable dehydration.

ABNORMAL NUTRITION

Failure of normal motor, secretory, digestive or absorptive functions causes impairment of nutrient supply to body tissues. Inanition or partial starvation results and the animal fails to grow, loses body weight or shows other signs of specific nutritional deficiencies. Ancillary effects include decreased appetite when motility is decreased: in many cases where motility is increased and there is no toxaemia, the appetite is increased and may be voracious.

Special Examination

The greater part of the technique of the examination of the alimentary tract has been dealt with in the chapter on clinical examination but there are some special aspects which require discussion here.

Roentgenological examination is difficult in

horses and cattle and is little used in the examination of the alimentary tract of other species. It has been used extensively in the investigation of motor functions of the tract in sheep and can be used clinically in sheep, pigs, foals and calves if the expense is warranted.

External palpation of the abdomen is of limited value in farm animals and is replaced by the passage of a stomach tube, by rectal examination and by auscultation of the abdomen. Attempts to pass a stomach tube will detect complete or partial obstruction of the oesophagus. In gross distension of the stomach in the horse, there is an immediate rush of fluid contents as soon as the cardia is passed. Visual examination of the posterior fauces, pharynx and larynx of cattle is sometimes essential and general anaesthesia to permit the examination is often unsatisfactory. With patience and proper restraint the examination is possible if a mouth speculum is illuminated with a flashlight.

Examination of the faeces may provide valuable information on the digestive and motor functions of the tract. They should be examined for volume, consistency, form, colour, covering, odour and composition. Note should be made of the frequency and the time taken for material to pass through the tract. Laboratory examinations may be advisable to detect the presence of helminth eggs, occult blood, bile pigments, pathogenic bacteria or protozoa.

It is usually sufficient to say that the volume is scanty, normal or copious but, in special circumstances, it may be advisable to weigh or measure the daily output. Horses normally pass 30 to 40 lb. per day, cattle 50 to 90 lb., pigs 2 to 5 lb., and sheep and goats 1 to 3 lb. There is an increased bulk when much fibre is fed or during attacks of diarrhoea. The consistency and form of the faeces varies with each species and varies widely within a normal range, depending particularly on the nature of the food. Variations in consistency not explainable by changes in the character of the feed may indicate abnormalities of any of the functions of the tract. The consistency is more fluid in diarrhoea and less fluid than normal in constipation.

The colour of the faeces also varies widely with the colour of the food but faeces of a lighter colour than normal may be caused by an insufficient secretion of bile or by simple dilution of the pigments as occurs in diarrhoea. The effect of blood on the appearance of faeces has already been described. Discoloration by drugs should be considered when the animal is undergoing treatment.

Faecal odour also depends largely on the nature of the food eaten but in severe enteritis the odour is characteristically one of putrefaction. The composition of the faeces should be noted. In herbivorous animals, there is always a proportion of undigested fibre but excessive amounts suggest incomplete digestion due for example to bad teeth and faulty mastication. Excessively pasty faeces are usually associated with a prolonged sojourn in the tract such as occurs in vagal indigestion or abomasal displacement in cattle. Foreign material of diagnostic significance includes sand or gravel, wool, and shreds of mucosa. Mucus is a normal constituent but, in excessive amounts, indicates either chronic inflammation when it is associated with fluid, copious faeces, or constipation when the faeces are small in volume and hard. Mucosal shreds or casts always indicate inflammation.

Frequency of defaecation and the length of sojourn are usually closely allied, increased frequency and decreased sojourn occurring in diarrhoea and the reverse in constipation. Most animals defaecate 8 to 12 times a day but the sojourn varies widely with the species. Omnivores and carnivores with simple stomachs have an alimentary sojourn of 12 to 35 hours. In ruminants it is 2 to 4 days and in horses 1 to 4 days depending on the type of feed.

Observation of other acts associated with the functions of the alimentary tract may provide information of diagnostic value. Prehension, mastication, swallowing, vomiting and defaecation should be observed and an attempt made to analyse the behaviour of the animal when there is evidence of abdominal pain.

Principles of Treatment in Alimentary Tract Disease

Removal of the primary cause of the disease is essential but the major part of the treatment of diseases of the alimentary tract is supportive and symptomatic, and aimed at relieving pain, correcting the abnormality and repairing the damage done. The specific treatments are discussed elsewhere and include antibacterial, coccidiostatic and anti-fungal agents, surgical correction of accidents and displacements, the provision of specific antidotes for poisons, and treatment of helminth infestations.

Correction of abnormal motility. Either excessive or depressed motility should be corrected. When motility is increased, the administration of atropine or other spasmolytics is usually followed by disappearance of the abdominal pain and a diminution of fluid loss. An additional valuable measure when the hypermotility is caused by inflammation of the mucosa is the administration of oral astringent mixtures containing charcoal, alkalis and tannic acid derivatives.

When motility is decreased the usual practice is to administer parasympathomimetic drugs or purgatives, usually combined with an analgesic. The use of atropine may relieve the pain transiently in these circumstances but has no effect in removing the distending material.

Replacement of fluids and electrolytes. In gastric or intestinal obstruction, or when diarrhoea is severe, it may be necessary to replace lost fluids and electrolytes by the parenteral administration of large quantities of isotonic glucose-saline or other physiologically normal electrolyte solutions. The amount of fluid lost may be very large and fluids must be given in quantities of not less than 4 ml. and preferably up to 10 ml. per lb. of body weight daily, depending on severity. In young animals the need is much greater still and amounts of 50 ml. per lb. body weight given slowly intravenously, are probably not excessive. The treatment of shock is discussed elsewhere but should include the administration of fluids, plasma or blood and vaso-constrictor agents.

Relief of distension. This is one of the major principles of treatment in alimentary tract disease. It may be possible to relieve by medical means a distension caused by the accumulation of ingesta but surgical intervention is necessary in some cases. In purely functional distension, relief of the atony or spasm can be effected by the use of stimulants and spasmolytics respectively. Distension due to intestinal or gastric accidents usually requires surgical treatment.

Reconstitution of rumen flora and correction of acidity or alkalinity. When prolonged anorexia or acute indigestion occurs in ruminants, the rumen flora may be seriously reduced. In convalescence, the reconstitution of the flora can be hastened by the oral administration of a suspension of ruminal contents from a normal cow, or of dried ruminal contents which contain viable bacteria and yeasts and the substances necessary for growth of the organisms.

The pH of the rumen affects the growth of rumen organisms, and hyperacidity, such as occurs on overeating of grain, or hyperalkalinity, such as occurs on overeating of protein-rich feeds, should be corrected by the administration of alkalinizing or acidifying drugs as the case may be.

Relief of pain. The relief of pain is one of the major tasks in alimentary tract disease. No single drug is completely satisfactory and every effort should be made to correct the primary disease. Analgesics and narcotics are in general use and are discussed under the individual diseases.

Relief of tenesmus. This is a most difficult task. Commonly long-acting epidural anaesthesia and sedation are the aims and infusion of the rectum or vagina with a topical anaesthetic may be added but in many cases are partly or completely ineffective. A suggested treatment in cattle is the production of artificial pneumoperitoneum by the insufflation of air into the peritoneal cavity via a cannula inserted at the paralumbar fossa. Insufflation is continued until both fossae are vaulted to the height of the costal arch.

DISEASES OF THE BUCCAL CAVITY AND ASSOCIATED ORGANS

Stomatitis

Stomatitis is inflammation of the oral mucosa and includes glossitis (inflammation of the lingual mucosa), palatitis (lampas) and gingivitis (inflammation of the mucosa of the gums). Clinically it is characterized by partial or complete loss of appetite, by smacking of the lips and profuse salivation. It is commonly an accompaniment of systemic disease.

Aetiology

Stomatitis may be caused by physical, chemical or infectious agents, the latter being the largest group of causes. Under experimental conditions, stomatitis can be produced by some nutritional deficiencies but these are not known to cause clinical stomatitis under natural conditions.

Physical agents include trauma while dosing, foreign bodies, maloccluded teeth, sharp awns and spines on plants, and the eating of frozen food or drinking of hot water.

Chemical agents include irritant substances, particularly chloral hydrate administered in strong concentrations, acids, alkalis, and irritant drugs including mercury and cantharides preparations applied as counter-irritants and improperly covered so that animals can lick them. A moderate stomatitis may also occur in chronic mercury poisoning.

Bacterial stomatitis is usually necrotic and is manifested by ulceration and suppuration. The only common one is oral necrobacillosis caused by *Sphaerophorus necrophorus*. Mycotic dermatitis in cattle caused by *Nocardia dermatonomus* and ulcerative granuloma of pigs caused by *Borrelia suilla* may involve the lips and cheeks and spread to involve the labial mucosa. Actinobacillary (*Actinobacillus lignieresi*) lesions of the tongue in cattle may be accompanied by ulcerations on the dorsum and sides of the tongue and on the lips, and involvement of the gums may occur in actinomycosis.

Viral stomatitis assumes a number of forms, vesicular, erosive, ulcerative and proliferative, which are described in detail under clinical findings. Formation of vesicles is characteristic of foot-and-mouth disease, vesicular stomatitis and vesicular exanthema. Erosive and secondary ulcerative stomatitis occurs in rinderpest, bovine malignant catarrh, mucosal disease, muzzle disease, blue tongue and infectious ulcerative stomatitis and may occur in diseases which primarily involve the lips but which spread to involve the oral mucosa. Ulcerative dermatosis, sheep pox and contagious ecthyma are primarily skin diseases but may, in severe cases, involve the alimentary tract including the mouth. Proliferative lesions occur in proliferative stomatitis, papular stomatitis and in rare cases of papillomatosis.

Although the original lesions in these specific diseases are as described above, secondary bacterial invasion commonly follows and may convert them to suppurative and ulcerative lesions which resemble bacterial stomatitis. The lesions may spread extensively and produce a phlegmonous condition of the soft tissues of the face.

Mycotic stomatitis is in most cases caused by infections with *Monilia* spp. fungi.

Premature loss of teeth in sheep has aroused concern in some countries because of the number of animals which have to be discarded at an early age. Although some investigations have been initiated the cause of such losses has not been determined (3, 4). The ingestion of irritating materials such as particles of sand and spiny awns of grass seeds have been suggested but on many affected farms do not appear to be aetiological agents.

An unidentified ulceromembranous gingivitis has been recorded in sheep (1). Ulceration began at the gum-tooth margin and penetrated down into the alveoli causing expulsion of the teeth. Both incisors and molars were affected and spirochaetes and *Sphaerophorus necrophorus* were present on culture. Parenteral treatment with penicillin in the early stages resulted in rapid recovery but some deaths occurred in badly affected sheep. A comparable condition also recorded in New Zealand is a granulomatous periodontitis of adult sheep observed in certain limited geographical areas (2, 3).

Many other causes of stomatitis have been suggested but the relationship of these conditions to the specific diseases listed above is unknown. It is common to find stomatitides that cannot be defined as belonging to any of these aetiological groups. An example is necrotic glossitis reported in feeder steers in the U.S.A. (5, 6) in which the necrotic lesions are confined to the anterior part of the tongue.

Pathogenesis

The lesions of stomatitis are produced by the causative agents being applied directly to the mucosa, or gaining entrance to it by way of minor abrasions, or by localization in the mucosa from a viraemia. In the first two instances, the stomatitis is designated as primary. In the third, it is usually described as secondary because of the common occurrence of similar lesions in other organs or on other parts of the body, and the presence of a systemic disease. The clinical signs of stomatitis are caused by the inflammation or erosion of the mucosa and the signs vary in severity with the degree of inflammation.

Clinical Findings

There is partial or complete anorexia and slow, painful mastication. Chewing movements and smacking of the lips are accompanied by salivation, either frothy and in small amounts, or profuse and drooling if the animal does not swallow normally. The saliva may contain pus or shreds of epithelial tissue. A foetid odour is present on the breath only if bacterial invasion of the lesion has occurred. Enlargement of local lymph nodes may also occur if bacteria invade the lesions. Swelling of the face is observed only in cases where a cellulitis or phlegmon has extended to involve the soft tissues. An increased desire for water is apparent and the animal resents manipulation and examination of the mouth.

Toxaemia may be present when the stomatitis is secondary to a systemic disease or where tissue necrosis occurs. This is a feature of oral necrobacillosis and many of the systemic viraemias. In some of the specific diseases, lesions may be present on other parts of the body, especially at the coronets and mucocutaneous junctions.

The local lesions vary a great deal. Vesicular lesions are usually thin-walled vesicles 1 to 2 cm. in diameter, filled with clear serous fluid. The vesicles rupture readily to leave sharp-edged, shallow ulcers. Erosive lesions are shallow, usually discrete, areas of necrosis which are not readily seen in the early stages. They tend to occur most commonly on the lingual mucosa and at the commissures of the mouth. The necrotic tissue may remain *in situ* but is usually shed leaving a very shallow discontinuity of the mucosa with a dark-red base which is more readily seen. If recovery occurs, these lesions heal very quickly. Ulcerative lesions penetrate more deeply to the lamina propria.

Catarrhal stomatitis is manifested by a diffuse inflammation of the buccal mucosa and is commonly the result of direct injury by chemical or physical agents. Mycotic stomatitis usually takes the form of a heavy, white, velvety deposit with little obvious inflammation or damage to the mucosa.

Clinical Pathology

Material collected from lesions of stomatitis should be examined for the presence of pathogenic bacteria and fungi. Transmission experiments may be undertaken with filtrates of swabs or scrapings if the disease is thought to be due to a viral agent.

Necropsy Findings

The oral lesions are easily observed but complete necropsy examinations should be carried out on all fatally affected animals to determine whether the oral lesions are primary or are local manifestations of a systemic disease.

Diagnosis

Particularly in cattle, and to a less extent in sheep, the diagnosis of stomatitis is most important because of the occurrence of oral lesions in a number of highly infectious viral diseases. The diseases are listed under aetiology and their differentiation is described under their specific headings. Careful clinical and necropsy examinations are necessary to define the type and extent of the lesions if any attempt at field diagnosis is to be made. In cattle lymphoma of the ramus of the mandible may spread extensively through the submucosal tissues of the mouth causing marked swelling of the gums, spreading of the teeth, inability to close the mouth and profuse salivation. There is no discontinuity nor inflammation of the buccal mucosa but gross enlargement of the cranial lymph nodes is usual.

Treatment

Affected animals should be isolated and fed and watered from separate utensils if an infectious agent is suspected. Specific treatments are dealt with under the headings of the specific diseases. Non-specific treatment includes frequent application of a mild antiseptic collutory such as a 2 per cent solution of copper sulphate, a 2 per cent suspension of borax or a 1 per cent suspension of a sulphonamide in glycerin. Solutions containing 2 per cent potassium chlorate or alum serve a similar purpose. Indolent ulcers require more vigorous treatment and respond well to curettage or cauterization with a silver nitrate stick or tincture of iodine.

In stomatitis due to trauma, the teeth may need attention. In all cases, soft, appetizing food should be offered and feeding by stomach tube or intravenous alimentation resorted to in severe, prolonged cases. If the disease is infectious, care should be exercised to ensure that it is not transmitted by the hands or dosing implements.

REFERENCES

(1) Salisbury, R. M. *et al.* (1953). *N.Z. vet. J.*, *1*, 51.
(2) Porter, W. L. *et al.* (1970). *N.Z. vet. J.*, *18*, 21.
(3) McKinnon, M. M. (1959). *N.Z. vet. J.*, *7*, 18.
(4) Dalgarno, A. C. & Hill, R. (1961). *Res. vet. Sci.*, *2*, 107.
(5) Wake, W. L. (1961). *J. Amer. vet. med. Ass.*, *138*, 7.
(6) Hill, J. K. & Herrick, J. B. (1961). *Vet. Med.*, *56*, 190,

DISEASES OF THE PHARYNX AND OESOPHAGUS

Pharyngitis

Pharyngitis is inflammation of the pharynx and is characterized clinically by coughing, painful swallowing and lack of appetite. Regurgitation through the nostrils and drooling of saliva may occur in severe cases.

Aetiology

Pharyngitis in farm animals commonly occurs as part of some other primary disease. It is an important feature of strangles in horses, pharyngeal anthrax in pigs and horses and oral necrobacillosis. Granulomatous lesions may occur in the pharynx in actinobacillosis in addition to the more common involvement of the lymph nodes. Other specific diseases in which stomatitis occurs may have an associated pharyngitis and it is often present also in specific diseases which affect the upper respiratory tract. 'Pharyngeal phlegmon' or 'intermandibular cellulitis' in cattle is not a pharyngitis but has much in common with it except that it is almost always fatal. The cause is not known but *Sphaerophorus necrophorus* is commonly isolated from the swollen area.

Foreign bodies, particularly grass and cereal awns, and gelatin capsules may lodge in the pharynx, or in the suprapharyngeal diverticulum of pigs and cause local ulceration and irritation. The ingestion of irritant chemicals or hot or cold substances may cause stomatitis and pharyngitis.

Pathogenesis

Inflammation of the pharynx is attended by painful swallowing and disinclination to eat. If the swelling of the mucosa and wall is severe, there may be virtual obstruction of the pharynx.

Clinical Findings

The animal may refuse to eat or drink and, if it does so, swallows reluctantly and with evident pain. Opening of the jaws to examine the mouth is resented and manual compression of the throat from the exterior causes paroxysmal coughing. There may be a mucopurulent nasal discharge, sometimes containing blood, spontaneous cough and, in severe cases, regurgitation of fluid and food through the nostrils. Oral medication in such cases may be impossible. Affected animals often stand with the head extended, drool saliva and make frequent, tentative jaw movements. If the local swelling is severe, there may be obstruction to respiration and visible swelling of the throat. The retropharyngeal and parotid lymph nodes are commonly enlarged. In 'pharyngeal phlegmon' in cattle there is an acute onset with high fever (41 to 41·5°C, 106 to 107°F), rapid heart rate, profound depression and severe swelling of the soft tissues within and posterior to the mandible to the point where dyspnoea is pronounced. Death usually occurs 36 to 48 hours after the first signs of illness.

Palpation of the pharynx may be undertaken in large animals with the use of a gag if a foreign body is suspected, and endoscopic examination through the nostril may be undertaken in the horse. Most acute cases subside in 3 to 4 days but chronic cases may persist for many weeks especially if there is ulceration or a persistent foreign body. An occasional sequel is aspiration pneumonia when food is aspirated into the lungs. Severe toxaemia may accompany the local lesions especially in oral necrobacillosis and, to a less extent, in strangles. Empyema of the guttural pouches may occur in horses.

Clinical Pathology

Nasal discharge or swabs taken from accompanying oral lesions may assist in the identification of the causative agent.

Necropsy Findings

Deaths are rare in primary pharyngitis and necropsy examinations are usually undertaken only in those animals dying of specific diseases. In 'pharyngeal phlegmon' there is oedema, haemorrhage and abscessation of the affected area and on incision of the area a foul-smelling liquid and some gas usually escapes.

Diagnosis

The syndrome of pharyngitis is manifested by an acute onset and local pain. In pharyngeal paralysis and obstruction, the onset is usually slow except that obstruction by a foreign body may occur very acutely and cause severe distress and continuous, expulsive coughing but there are no systemic signs. Endoscopic examination of the pharyngeal mucous membranes is often of diagnostic value.

Treatment

The primary disease must be treated, usually parenterally, by the use of antibiotics or sulphonamides, although oral treatment with sulphonamides or iodides may be undertaken in chronic cases. In horses, drugs may be given mixed with syrup as an electuary or administered as a topical spray. Inhalations may also be of value in the recovery stages. Creolin, pine oil or turpentine (about 5 oz. per gallon of water) may be poured on to chopped hay in a nose bag or mixed into a hot bran mash. Electuaries containing sedative expectorants may be administered as an alternative. 'Pharyngeal phlegmon' is highly fatal and early treatment, repeated at frequent intervals, with a broad-spectrum antibiotic is necessary if there is to be any chance of recovery.

Pharyngeal Obstruction

Obstruction of the pharynx is accompanied by stertorous respiration, coughing and difficult swallowing.

Aetiology

Enlargement of the retropharyngeal lymph nodes may occur in tuberculosis, actinobacillosis and lymphomatosis, especially in cattle, and in strangles in horses. Large obstructive foreign bodies, including bones, corn cobs and pieces of wire may also cause obstruction. Occasional cases are caused by fibrous or mucoid polyps in cattle. These structures are usually pedunculated because of traction during swallowing and may cause intermittent signs of obstruction. Diffuse enlargement of lymphoid tissue in the pharyngeal wall and soft palate may also cause pharyngeal obstruction in cattle and pigs.

Pathogenesis

Reduction in calibre of the pharyngeal lumen interferes with swallowing and respiration.

Clinical Signs

There is difficulty in swallowing and animals may

be hungry enough to eat but, when they attempt to swallow, cannot do so and the food is coughed up through the mouth. Drinking is usually managed successfully. There is no dilatation of the oesophagus and usually little or no regurgitation through the nostrils. An obvious sign is a snoring inspiration, often loud enough to be heard some yards away. The inspiration is prolonged and accompanied by marked abdominal effort. Auscultation over the pharynx reveals loud inspiratory stertor. Manual examination of the pharynx is necessary if the nature of the lesion is to be determined. When the disease runs a long course, emaciation usually follows. Rupture of abscessed lymph nodes may occur when a nasal tube is passed and result in aspiration pneumonia.

Clinical Pathology

A tuberculin test may be advisable in bovine cases. Nasal swabs may contain *Streptococcus equi* when there is streptococcal lymphadenitis in horses.

Necropsy Findings

Death occurs rarely and in fatal cases the physical lesion is apparent.

Diagnosis

Signs of the primary disease may aid in the diagnosis in tuberculosis, actinobacillosis and strangles. Pharyngitis is accompanied by severe pain and commonly by systemic signs and there is usually stertor. It is of particular importance to differentiate between obstruction and pharyngeal paralysis when rabies occurs in the area. Oesophageal obstruction is also accompanied by the rejection of ingested food but there is no respiratory distress. Laryngeal stenosis may cause a comparable stertor but swallowing is not impeded. Nasal obstruction is manifested by noisy breathing but the volume of breath from one or both nostrils is reduced and the respiratory noise is more wheezing than snoring.

Treatment

Removal of a foreign body may be accomplished through the mouth. Treatment of actinobacillary lymphadenitis with iodides is usually successful and some reduction in size often occurs in tuberculous enlargement of the glands but complete recovery is unlikely to occur. Parenteral treatment of strangles abscesses with penicillin may effect a cure.

Pharyngeal Paralysis

Pharyngeal paralysis is manifested by inability to swallow and an absence of signs of pain and respiratory obstruction.

Aetiology

Pharyngeal paralysis accompanies several specific diseases including rabies and other encephalitides, botulism, and also occurs sporadically in cases of peripheral nerve damage caused by trauma, by a spreading suppurative process or pressure by tumour or abscess. In the horse pharyngeal paralysis may result from nerve damage resulting from the formation of diphtheritic membranes in the guttural pouch (1).

Pathogenesis

Inability to swallow and regurgitation are the major manifestations of the disease. The condition known as 'cud-dropping' in cattle may be a partial pharyngeal paralysis as there is difficulty in controlling the regurgitated bolus which is often dropped from the mouth. There may be an associated laryngeal paralysis accompanied by 'roaring'. In these circumstances, aspiration pneumonia is likely to develop.

Clinical Findings

The animal is usually hungry but, on prehension of food or water, attempts at swallowing are followed by dropping of the food from the mouth, coughing and the expulsion of food or regurgitation through the nostrils. Salivation occurs constantly and swallowing cannot be stimulated by external compression of the pharynx. The swallowing reflex is a complex one controlled by a number of nerves and the signs can be expected to vary greatly depending on which nerves are involved and to what degree. There is rapid loss of condition and dehydration. Clinical signs of the primary disease may be evident but, in cases of primary pharyngeal paralysis, there is no systemic reaction. Pneumonia may follow aspiration of food material into the lungs and produces loud gurgling sounds on auscultation.

In 'cud-dropping' in cows, the animal is normal except that regurgitated boluses are dropped from the mouth, usually in the form of flattened discs of fibrous food material. Affected animals may lose weight but the condition is usually transient, lasting for only a few days. On the other hand, complete pharyngeal paralysis is usually permanent and fatal.

Clinical Pathology

The use of clinico-pathological examinations is restricted to the identification of the primary specific diseases.

Necropsy Findings

If the primary lesion is physical, it may be detected on gross examination.

Diagnosis

In all species often the first impression gained is that there is a foreign body in the mouth or pharynx and this can only be determined by physical examination. Pharyngeal paralysis is a typical sign in rabies and botulism but there are other clinical findings which suggest the presence of these diseases. Absence of pain and respiratory obstruction are usually sufficient evidence to eliminate the possibility of pharyngitis or pharyngeal obstruction. Endoscopic examination of the guttural pouch is a useful diagnostic aid in the horse.

Treatment

Treatment is unlikely to have any effect. The local application of heat may be attempted. Feeding by nasal tube or intravenous alimentation may be tried if disappearance of the paralysis seems probable.

REFERENCE

(1) Cook, W. R. (1966). *Mod. vet. Pract.*, 47, 41.

Oesophagitis

Inflammation of the oesophagus is accompanied initially by signs of spasm and obstruction, pain on swallowing and palpation, and regurgitation of blood-stained, slimy material.

Aetiology

Primary oesophagitis caused by the ingestion of chemical or physical irritants is usually accompanied by stomatitis and pharyngitis. Laceration of the mucosa by a foreign body or too vigorous passing of a stomach tube or probang may cause oesophagitis unaccompanied by lesions elsewhere. Death of *Hypoderma lineata* larvae in the submucosa of the oesophagus of cattle may cause acute local inflammation and subsequent gangrene.

Inflammation of the oesophagus occurs commonly in many specific diseases, particularly those which cause stomatitis but the other clinical signs of these diseases overshadow those of oesophagitis.

Pathogenesis

The first reaction of the oesophagus to inflammation is an increase in muscle tone and involuntary movement and these, combined with local oedema and swelling, create a functional obstruction.

Clinical Signs

In the acute stages, there is salivation and attempts at swallowing which cause severe pain, particularly in horses. In some cases, swallowing is impossible and attempts to do so are followed by regurgitation and coughing, accompanied by pain, retching movements and vigorous contractions of the cervical and abdominal muscles. The regurgitus may contain much mucus and some fresh blood. If the oesophagitis is in the cervical region, palpation in the jugular furrow causes pain and the swollen oesophagus may be palpable. If perforation has occurred, there is local pain and swelling and often crepitus. Local cervical cellulitis may cause rupture to the exterior and development of an oesophageal fistula, or infiltration along fascial planes with resulting compression obstruction of the oesophagus, and toxaemia. Perforation of the thoracic oesophagus may lead to fatal pleurisy. Animals that recover from oesophagitis are commonly affected by chronic oesophageal stenosis with distension above the stenosis. Fistulae are usually persistent but spontaneous healing may occur (1). In the specific diseases such as mucosal disease and bovine malignant catarrh, there are no obvious clinical signs of oesophagitis, the lesions being mainly erosive.

Clinical Pathology and Necropsy Findings

Ante-mortem laboratory examinations and necropsy findings are restricted to those pertaining to the various specific diseases in which oesophagitis occurs. In traumatic lesions or those caused by irritant substances, there is gross oedema, inflammation and, in some cases, perforation.

Diagnosis

Oesophagitis may be mistaken for pharyngitis but, in the latter, the results of attempted swallowing are not so severe and coughing is more likely to occur. Local palpation may also help to localize the lesion. Pharyngitis and oesophagitis commonly occur together. When the injury is caused by a foreign body, it may still be in the oesophagus and, if suitable restraint and anaesthesia can be arranged, the passage of a nasal tube may locate it. Complete oesophageal obstruction is accompanied by bloat in ruminants, by palpable enlargement of the oesophagus and by less pain on swallowing than in oesophagitis although horses may show a great deal of discomfort.

In cattle perforation of the oesophagus is not uncommon. There is a persistent, moderate toxaemia, a moderate fever and a leucocytosis. Pus accumulates in surrounding fascial planes, but causes only slight physical enlargement which is easily missed on a physical examination.

Treatment

Food should be withheld for 2 to 3 days and the animal may need to be fed intravenously during this period. Parenteral antibacterial treatment should be administered, especially if laceration or perforation has occurred. If the animal can swallow, astringent and antibacterial electuaries should be given at frequent intervals.

REFERENCE

(1) Raker, C. W. & Sayers, A. (1958). *J. Amer. vet. med. Ass.*, *133*, 371.

Oesophageal Obstruction

Oesophageal obstruction may be acute or chronic and the clinical signs of inability to swallow, regurgitation of food and water, and bloat in ruminants are accompanied in acute cases by severe distress.

Aetiology

The commonest cause in cattle is obstruction by solid objects, particularly turnips, potatoes, oranges, apples and peaches, and in horses is incompletely masticated and ensalivated dry feed, particularly dried sugar beet pulp or bran. A particular occurrence has been recorded after dosing Shetland ponies with 0·5 oz. gelatin capsules (1). Chronic obstruction may result from stenosis after oesophagitis, external pressure by tuberculous or neoplastic lymph nodes in the mediastinum or at the base of the lung, by thymoma, by a persistent right aortic arch in new-born animals, or by cervical or mediastinal abscesses in adults. Other causes of chronic bloat in cattle are discussed elsewhere. Rarely there may be paralysis, or the presence of a diverticulum of the oesophagus. Cardial obstruction in horses may be caused by a carcinoma of the stomach (2), and in cattle, with intermittent bloat and vomiting, by oesophageal hiatus hernia (4).

Pathogenesis

There is physical inability to swallow and, in cattle, inability to belch with resulting bloat. In acute obstruction, there is initial spasm at the site of obstruction and forceful, painful peristalsis and swallowing movements.

Clinical Findings

Acute obstruction or choke. In cattle, the obstruction is usually in the cervical oesophagus just above the larynx or at the thoracic inlet. The animal suddenly stops eating and shows anxiety and restlessness. There are forceful attempts to swallow and regurgitate, salivation, coughing and continuous chewing movements. If obstruction is complete, bloating occurs rapidly and adds to the animal's discomfort. Ruminal movements are continuous and forceful and there may be a systolic murmur audible on auscultation of the heart.

The acute signs, other than bloat, usually disappear within a few hours. This is due to relaxation of the initial oesophageal spasm and may or may not be accompanied by onward passage of the obstruction. Many obstructions pass on spontaneously but others may persist for several days and up to a week. In these cases, there is inability to swallow, salivation and continued bloat. Passage of a nasal or stomach tube is impossible. Persistent obstruction causes pressure necrosis of the mucosa and may result in perforation or in subsequent stenosis due to fibrous tissue constriction.

In horses, the obstruction is often in the terminal part of the thoracic oesophagus and cannot be seen or palpated. The clinical signs are similar to those in the cow but are more severe and the horse's reaction may take the form of violent activity with very forceful attempts to swallow or retch. Persistent obstruction may also occur in the horse. Gelatin capsules are particularly liable to remain *in situ* for three or four days. Death may occur in either species from subsequent aspiration pneumonia or, when the obstruction persists, from dehydration.

Chronic obstruction. There is an absence of acute signs. In cattle, the earliest sign is chronic bloat which is usually of moderate severity and may persist for very long periods without the appearance of other signs. The rumen usually continues to move in an exaggerated manner for some weeks but, after prolonged distension, tone is usually depressed. In horses and in cattle in which the obstruction is sufficiently severe to interfere with swallowing, a characteristic syndrome develops. Swallowing movements are usually normal until the bolus reaches the obstruction when they are replaced by more forceful movements. Dilation of the oesophagus may cause a pronounced swelling at the base of the neck. The swallowed material either passes slowly through the stenotic area or accumulates and is then regurgitated. In the later stages, there may be no attempt made to eat solid food but fluids may be taken and swallowed satisfactorily.

When there is paralysis of the oesophagus, regurgitation does not occur but the oesophagus fills and overflows, and saliva drools from the mouth and nostrils. Aspiration into the lungs may follow. Passage of a stomach tube or probang is obstructed by stenosis but may be unimpeded by paralysis.

Clinical Pathology

Laboratory tests are not used in diagnosis although roentgenological examination is helpful to outline the site of stenosis, diverticulum or dilatation, even in animals as large as the horse (5).

Diagnosis

The clinical picture is typical but can be mistaken for that of oesophagitis in which local pain is more apparent and there is often an accompanying stomatitis and pharyngitis. Differentiation of the causes of chronic obstruction may be difficult. A history of previous oesophagitis or acute obstruction suggests cicatricial stenosis. Persistent right aortic arch is rare and confined to young animals. Mediastinal lymph node enlargement is usually accompanied by other signs of tuberculosis or lymphomatosis. Chronic ruminal tympany in cattle may be caused by ruminal atony in which case there is an absence of normal ruminal movements. Diaphragmatic hernia may also be a cause of chronic ruminal tympany in cattle and is sometimes accompanied by obstruction of the oesophagus with incompletely regurgitated ingesta. This condition and vagus indigestion, another cause of chronic tympany, are usually accompanied by a systolic cardiac murmur but passage of a stomach tube is unimpeded.

Treatment

In acute obstruction where there is marked distress, some attempt should be made to sedate the animal before proceeding with treatment. Administration of an ataractic drug or chloral hydrate may also help in relaxing the oesophageal spasm. Other means of relaxing the spasm include the subcutaneous administration of atropine sulphate (16 to 32 mg.) or the administration of fluid extract of belladonna (1 to 2 ml.) by stomach tube. The passage of the stomach tube or probang is usually necessary to locate obstructions low down in the oesophagus. Gentle attempts may be made to push the obstruction onward but care must be taken to avoid damage to the oesophageal mucosa.

Solid obstructions in the upper oesophagus of cattle may be reached by passing the hand into the pharynx through a speculum and having an assistant press the foreign body up towards the mouth. It is often difficult to grasp the obstruction sufficiently strongly to be able to extricate it from the spastic oesophagus. A long piece of strong wire bent into a loop may be passed over the object and an attempt made to pull it up into the pharynx. If both methods fail, it is advisable to leave the object *in situ* and use treatments aimed at relaxing the oesophagus. In such cases in cattle it is usually necessary to trocarize the rumen and leave the cannula in place until the obstruction is relieved.

Accumulations of particulate material such as those which are commonly found in the lower oesophagus of horses are more difficult to remove. Small quantities of warm saline should be introduced through a stomach tube passed to the point of obstruction and then pumped or siphoned out. This may be repeated a number of times until the fluid comes clear. If the obstruction is still present, fluid extract of belladonna should be administered before removal of the tube. Further attempts at irrigative removal should be attempted at short intervals. If the obstruction is palpable in the neck, vigorous squeezing from the exterior may break it up and aid in its removal. Two tubes may be used, one in each nostril, to make faster irrigation possible but care must be taken to avoid overflowing the oesophagus and causing aspiration into the lungs (3). This is a constant hazard whenever irrigative removal is attempted and the animal's head must always be kept low to avoid aspiration. Surgical removal by oesophagotomy may be necessary if other measures fail.

The animal must not be allowed access to water or food until the obstruction is removed. In chronic cases, especially those due to paralysis, repeated siphonage may be necessary to remove fluid accumulations. Treatment of chronic obstructions is usually unsuccessful.

REFERENCES

(1) Lundvall, R. L. & Kingrey, B. W. (1958). *J. Amer. vet. med. Ass.*, *133*, 75.
(2) Keown, G. H. (1956). *North Amer. Vet.*, *37*, 834.
(3) Baker, W. (1945). *Vet. Rec.*, *57*, 67.
(4) Kirkbride, C. A. & Noordsy, J. L. (1968). *J. Amer. vet. med. Ass.*, *152*, 996.
(5) Alexander, J. E. (1967). *J. Amer. vet. med. Ass.*, *151*, 47.

DISEASES OF THE STOMACH AND INTESTINES

Only those diseases which are accompanied by physical lesions or disturbances of motility are dealt with. Diseases caused by functional disturbances of secretion are not recognized in animals. In any case, disturbances of secretion are usually accompanied by disturbances of motility. Deficiencies of biliary secretion are dealt with in the chapter on diseases of the liver. Those diseases of the stomachs which are peculiar to ruminants are dealt with separately as they present rather special problems in diagnosis.

Equine Colic

Those diseases of the horse which cause abdominal pain, generally referred to as equine colic, are dealt with in the following sections. So that they may be readily identified a summary based on aetiology is set out in the table on p. 59. It has been drawn up on the assumption that the primary disturbance in all colics is distension of the stomach or intestines. The distension may be static when there is an accumulation of ingesta, gas or fluid, or transient when local, periodic distensions occur as the result of spasm and increased peristalsis of intestinal segments. The static accumulations are classified as physical colics, requiring physical treatments, the transient distensions as functional colics for which the rational treatment is the relief of both spasm and increased peristalsis. A secondary cause of abdominal pain, of most importance in acute intestinal accidents, is stretching of the peritoneum.

Clinical Signs of Colic

Restlessness is evident and is manifested by pawing or stamping or kicking at the belly, or by getting up and lying down frequently. Pain is manifested by looking at the flank, rolling, lying on the back, careful lying down and slowness in getting up, the horse often sitting like a dog for long periods. The posture is often abnormal, seen usually as a 'sawhorse' attitude. Geldings often protrude the penis without urinating.

The pain is usually intermittent, especially in the early stages, often to the point where recovery is incorrectly diagnosed. Bouts of pain may last for over 10 minutes with like periods of relaxation. In general the level of pain, which may be subacute or acute, is of about the same severity for the duration of the illness; impaction of the ileo-caecal valve is an exception. In the most severe cases the pain is almost continuous and although it has the same general pattern as above there may be in addition obvious signs of shock, profuse sweating, sobbing respiration and uncontrolled movements of such violence that the horse quickly does itself serious injury.

Diagnosis

Other diseases which have clinical signs reminiscent of colic are laminitis, hepatitis, lactation tetany, tetanus, urethral obstruction and peritonitis. In laminitis there is immobility rather than restlessness, the feet are held together and there is no evidence of abdominal pain, although the horse may be in great distress; the pain is obviously in the feet. In hepatitis the horse may look at the flank and show abdominal pain but the pain is dull and continuous and the horse does not adopt an abnormal posture or roll or stamp its feet. There may be compulsive walking and other evidence of delirium, and jaundice is common. Lactation tetany is rare but signs of tetany, incoordination and agitation in mares recently foaled or weaned, or in horses of any type after great excitement or fatigue, should arouse suspicions of hypocalcaemia. In tetanus, the extreme tetany, third eyelid prolapse and hypersensitivity are characteristic enough but if animals are down when they are first seen, the tetanic convulsions and gross sweating may suggest severe abdominal pain and lead to an incorrect diagnosis of colic. It is useful to remember that a horse with colic can always rise; a horse with tetanus that can rise has unmistakeable clinical signs. Casual observation of a gelding with obstructive urolithiasis may lead to an incorrect diagnosis of colic. A simple clinical examination will reveal the frequent attempts to urinate and the passage of a few drops of bloody urine. In most cases the distended bladder is easily palpated on rectal examination. Horses affected with subacute or acute peritonitis may be flank-watchers, but pain is evident on percussion or deep palpation. Fever is characteristic and also immobility, instead of the restlessness of colic.

Colic is one of the common disease complexes in the horse and its early recognition and accurate differentiation is very important (5). The clinical syndrome is described above. Having observed this it is then necessary to carry out a more complete examination. The following is suggested as a minimum.

The pulse rate should be less than 80 per minute for a favourable prognosis; a rate of over 100 will probably indicate an early demise. The temperature is rarely above the normal range, in fact a subnormal temperature is more usual. Too low a temperature indicates the development of shock; fever suggests some other cause of the signs observed. Auscultation of the abdomen, as discussed in Chapter 1, is essential. Continuous borborygmi suggest hypermotility; their absence indicates paralytic ileus. A rectal examination is the most important part of the procedure. Gas-filled loops of intestines indicate flatulent colic or, especially if accompanied by much fluid, intestinal obstruction. Long, unbroken columns of faeces are a sure indication of impaction. Isolated abnormal intestinal loops are often palpable in intussusception, strangulation, volvulus, verminous mesenteric arteritis. In fact these diseases can only be positively diagnosed in this way. Although the affected segment may be out of reach from the rectum it is usually possible to pick up the tight-stretched band of mesentery, or adhesion, that leads to it; it may be impossible to diagnose the nature of the lesion but it is often possible to predict its whereabouts, and this is most important in these highly fatal conditions because surgical intervention is the only means of salvage.

A complete clinical examination might also include the passage of a nasal tube to determine whether the stomach is grossly distended with fluid, and paracentesis to determine whether there is excess inflammatory exudate in the peritoneal cavity, or whether there is any evidence of intestinal or gastric rupture (6, 8).

The differentiation of the specific lesions which cause colic is necessary because the prognosis varies so greatly with each and the choice of treatment used depends on the nature of the lesion. In general the prognosis is excellent for diseases caused by hyper-motility, good for faecal impaction, and very bad in intestinal and vascular emergencies unless the diagnosis is accurate and surgery can be carried out immediately.

The more common colics are listed below:

Acute. Gastric dilatation, ileo-caecal valve impaction, intestinal emergency (intussusception, volvulus, strangulation, diaphragmatic hernia, enterolith or phytobezoar), enteritis especially that caused by sand, haemorrhage into the intestinal wall as in purpura haemorrhagica or anthrax or similar oedema and flatulent colic.

Subacute. Impaction of colon and/or caecum, spasmodic colic, retained meconium. These represent the bulk of colic cases and are seldom fatal (3).

Chronic or recurrent. Mesenteric verminous arteritis with vascular obstruction or constriction of gut by adhesions, peritonitis, grass sickness. The most common recurrent colic is simple impaction of caecum and colon due to poor condition of the molar teeth, indigestible coarse roughage, too frequent or heavy feeding, gluttonous feeders and debility due to disease or, more commonly, old age. The most recent introduction to the group is terminal ileal hypertrophy which is described elsewhere.

Clinical Pathology

Laboratory tests may not be of much use in determining the presence or location of colic but they are of very great assistance in making a prognosis and measuring progress (1, 6). A high packed cell volume, a marked leucopenia, high blood glucose, low blood chloride and pH suggest an unfavourable outcome (1). In terms of prognosis, the central venous pressure is the most helpful measurement in determining progress in severe cases (7, 8).

Treatment

The treatment of each case of colic depends upon the nature and situation of the lesion but the following principles apply. Analgesia is necessary to prevent self-inflicted injury without masking the signs necessary to determine the state of the disease. Pethidine (Meperidine) or chloral hydrate are satisfactory drugs for the purpose. Pethidine is subject to narcotics regulations and alternative analgesics would be advantageous. Pentazocine, a synthetic analgesic, is not a narcotic and has provided excellent pain relief in horses. Pethidine and pentazocine at the recommended dose of 1 mg. per lb. body weight give approximately the same effect. Dipyrone had no effect (4). Ataractics are not generally sufficiently analgesic and are to be avoided. In impaction with faecal material there is a choice between lubricants, e.g. mineral oil, and anthroquinone purgatives. The latter are much smaller in bulk and easier to carry but they are variable in efficiency and inclined to over-purgate. Parasympatheticomimetic drugs such as arecoline, physostigmine and a number of proprietary preparations have their place in the treatment of faecal impaction, but only as a follow-up or ancillary to a lubricant. The use of such drugs in horses whose colons are impacted by huge masses of very dry manure causes unnecessary pain. Antispasmodics, such as atropine, are to be avoided unless there is evidence of functional motility, when they are the drug of choice and are rapidly and dramatically effective. Because of this efficiency they tend to be over used.

In many cases of colic, especially when there is fluid loss into the gut lumen, there is a rapid and severe haemoconcentration and metabolic acidosis (1). In these cases the fluid and electrolyte status of the animals should be watched carefully, and the appropriate remedial measures, the parenteral administration of lactated Ringer's or Hartmann's solutions, commenced early. The dose rates required may be very high and can be determined only by reference to the central venous pressure. Very large doses of corticosteroids are currently fashionable in endotoxic shock and shock generally (7, 8).

Increasingly surgery is being undertaken for the relief of physical colic with best results being obtained in the longer-standing lesions (2). The very acute, major lesions such as torsion of the caecum

Aetiological Classification of Equine Colic

Classification	Primary Aetiological Agent	Pathogenesis	Cause of Distension
PHYSICAL COLICS	Lowgrade roughage Bad teeth Debility Exhaustion Excessive inspissation	Distension	Accumulation of ingesta (*Impaction of the large intestine*)
	Lush green feed *Clostridium perfringens* type A Secondary to acute obstruction	Distension	Accumulation of gas (*Flatulent colic. Intestinal tympany*)
	Engorgement with grain Engorgement with whey Pyloric obstruction	*Acute gastric dilatation*	Accumulation of fluid
	Impaction ileocaecal valve (finely ground roughage) Fibre-balls and enteroliths Acute intestinal accidents (volvulus, intussusception, strangulation, diaphragmatic hernia)	*Acute intestinal obstruction*	
	Verminous mesenteric arteritis (adhesions from) *Terminal ileal hypertrophy*	*Chronic intestinal obstruction*	
	Verminous mesenteric arteritis (Strongylosis) Peritonitis Grass sickness	Paralytic ileus	
FUNCTIONAL COLICS	Parasitism (Strongylosis) Bacteria (Salmonellosis, etc.) Viral (Equine viral arteritis) Physical (Sand colic) Chemical poison	*Enteritis*	Spasm and increased peristalsis
	Excitement Thunderstorms Cold drinks or chilling Reflex from other viscera Grass sickness *Verminous mesenteric arteritis*	Imbalance of autonomic nervous system (*Spasmodic colic*)	

or colon present two problems, that of counter-acting the severe shock and the difficulty of re-arranging these voluminous viscera in their natural positions. These challenges are being taken up by our intrepid surgical colleagues and will no doubt be conquered and reported at another time.

REFERENCES

(1) Kalsbeck, H. C. (1970). *T. Diergeneesk.*, 95, 429.
(2) Mason, T. A. *et al.* (1970). *Aust. vet. J.*, 46, 349.
(3) Korber, H. D. (1971). *Berl. Munch. tierärztl. Wshr.*, 84, 75.
(4) Low, J. E. (1969). *Proc. 15th ann. Conv. Amer. Ass. equine Practnrs*, Houston, Texas, p. 31.
(5) Koal, F. *et al.* (1966). *Proc. 12th ann. Conv. Amer. Ass. equine Practnrs*, Los Angeles, p. 263.
(6) Vaughan, J. T. (1970). *Proc. 16th ann. Conv. Amer. Ass. equine Practnrs*, Montreal, Quebec, p. 295.
(7) Gertsen, K. E. (1970). *Proc. 16th ann. Conv. Amer. Ass. equine Practnrs*, Montreal, Quebec, p. 309.
(8) Donawick, W. J. & Alexander, J. T. (1970). *Proc. 16th ann. Conv. Amer. Ass. equine Practnrs*, Montreal, Quebec, p. 343.

Gastric Dilatation

Dilatation of the stomach is accompanied by signs of abdominal pain and occasionally by projectile vomiting.

Aetiology

Theoretically acute gastric dilatation can be caused by sudden, complete obstruction of the pylorus by foreign body or achalasia, by gross overeating or the drinking of excessive quantities of fluid. This latter is particularly likely to occur in the horse where the anatomy of the stomach lends itself to occlusion of the cardia. The ingestion of large amounts of grain is the most common cause in horses but sporadic cases may also occur after drinking large quantities of whey or other palatable fluids. In the former circumstance, there may be the added effect of toxaemia from the putrefactive breakdown of protein in the food. In the pig, gastric distension is usually readily relieved by vomiting. Obstruction of the pylorus by foreign bodies is not common in farm animals, but obstruction by fibre balls occurs commonly in cattle in some areas, and obstruction by ingested objects occurs occasionally in calves. External compression of the pylorus by lipoma in horses or abdominal fat necrosis or lymphoma may occur in cattle.

Chronic dilatation may result from pyloric obstruction due to a tumour mass or cicatricial constriction, atony of the stomach wall in old or debilitated animals and those fed for long periods on coarse, indigestible roughage, and where ulceration causes pyloric spasm. The latter may occur in young calves about three months of age. Wind-sucking or crib-biting in horses may, in its advanced stages, cause chronic gastric dilatation.

Pathogenesis

Dilatation of the stomach stimulates vomition. In acute dilatation when vomition does not occur, the secretions accumulate and gastric motility is increased with powerful peristaltic waves passing towards the pylorus. The distension and hypermotility cause severe abdominal pain. Acute gastric dilatation is also accompanied by additional general effects. Reflex depression of the cardiac and peripheral vascular systems results in shock and there may be reflex depression of respiration. Excessive secretion and loss of fluid can result in fatal dehydration and alkalosis. Local damage to the gastric mucosa may cause additional shock and increase the permeability of the mucosa to toxic products produced by the abnormal digestion and putrefaction. Rupture of the stomach may occur especially if the wall is weakened by existing ulcers. In chronic dilatation, the stomach is atonic, the reflex spasm and motility are reduced, the pain less severe, and onward passage of fluid is not completely prevented but the prolonged gastric sojourn causes indigestion and interference with nutrition. A secondary gastritis may develop in these circumstances. The appetite is reduced because of the chronic fullness of the stomach and the absence of hunger contractions.

Engorgement on wheat in the horse results in the production of large quantities of lactic acid in all parts of the intestine. The increase in osmotic pressure of the bowel contents causes passage of much fluid into the lumen and severe dehydration may result. Absorption of lactic acid is minor and only a mild acidosis develops. These changes occur at intakes of wheat of 10 g. per kg. body weight and they are not necessarily accompanied by laminitis but, at intakes of 7 to 9 g. per kg. body weight, severe laminitis occurs without the production of much lactic acid (1).

Clinical Findings

Acute gastric dilatation may run a course of 2 to 3 days and the chronic condition may persist for a period of months. Vomiting is a cardinal sign in acute dilatation and may occur even in the horse. It is usually projectile in nature, manifested by the vomiting of large quantities of fluid with little effort. In the horse, much of the material is passed through the nostrils and it is usually a terminal event, sometimes accompanied by gastric rupture. If the cause of dilatation is engorgement on grain, most of the fluid is absorbed by the mass of food and vomiting does not occur. Abdominal pain is usually severe and, in horses, is manifested by sweating, rolling, kicking at the belly, sitting on the haunches, and an increase in pulse and respiratory rates. Dehydration is severe and there is looseness of the skin and sinking of the eyes. If alkalosis is severe, the clinical signs may include tetany, tremor and rapid respiration. Passage of a stomach tube usually results in the evacuation of large quantities of foul-smelling fluid, except in cases of grain engorgement where it is absorbed by large quantities of grain. The distension is not usually visible or palpable. Laminitis may be a sequel of grain engorgement in horses.

In chronic dilatation, there is anorexia, mild, continuous or recurrent pain, scanty faeces and gradual loss of body weight. Vomiting and bouts of pain may occur after feeding but they are not usually severe. Dehydration may be present but is usually only of moderate degree. In affected horses, the distended stomach may be palpable on rectal examination and the faeces are passed in small quantities and are usually of a soft, pasty consistency.

Clinical Pathology

The vomitus should be checked for acidity to determine that it has originated in the stomach. Reflux of intestinal fluid may cause secondary gastric dilatation but the vomitus will be alkaline. Roentgenological examination, with or without a barium meal, may be of diagnostic value in young animals.

Necropsy Findings

After grain engorgement in horses, the stomach is distended with a doughy, evil-smelling mass of food. In acute gastric dilatation due to other causes, the stomach is grossly distended with fluid and the wall shows patchy haemorrhages. Rupture may have occurred and the peritoneal cavity is then full of ingesta.

Diagnosis

The vomiting in gastric dilatation is more profuse and projectile than that of gastritis or enteritis but may be simulated by that of obstruction of the upper part of the small intestine. In both enteritis and intestinal obstruction, the vomitus may contain bile and is alkaline in reaction. A specific disease of horses, grass sickness, is characterized by an accumulation of fluid in the stomach and intestines.

When there is no history of overeating, and particularly in chronic cases, it is usually impossible to decide whether the pyloric obstruction is physical or functional but treatment with drugs likely to relax the pyloric sphincter may be of value in differentiating the two.

Treatment

Treatment is palliative only, except in cases of overeating in horses in which case an attempt should be made to empty the stomach by the passage of a tube or by the administration of purgatives. Gastric lavage is often unsuccessful in cases of grain engorgement because of the pastiness of the ingesta. As large a tube as possible should be used and 1 to 2 gallons of normal saline pumped in and then siphoned or pumped off. In many instances, the fluid cannot be recovered, or if it is recoverable, very little grain comes with it. The alternative is to administer mineral oil, preferably with a wetting agent, and follow this with a parasympathetic stimulant. There is danger that these latter drugs may cause rupture of an over-distended stomach.

Periodic removal of fluid by stomach tube in cases of obstruction relieves the discomfort and prolongs the animal's life provided the fluid and electrolyte loss is made good by the intravenous administration of electrolyte solutions. Relaxation of the pylorus by the repeated administration of belladonna preparations should be attempted in case the obstruction is functional. In human medicine, glyceryl trinitrate and atropine methonitrate (Eumydrin) are used with some success for this purpose.

Physical obstructions due to tumours or foreign bodies are uncommon in farm animals but gastrotomy is sometimes advisable in pigs and young calves when the history suggests that a foreign body may have been ingested. Chronic atony does not respond satisfactorily to treatment although stimulant strychnine preparations (14 ml. tincture of nux vomica twice daily to horses) are usually advocated. The provision of soft, palatable, concentrated food may reduce the frequence and severity of attacks of abdominal pain in these cases.

REFERENCE

(1) Commonwealth Scientific and Industrial Research Organization (1954). *C.S.I.R.O., Aust., 6th annual Rpt.*

Gastritis

Inflammation of the stomach causes disorders of motility and is manifested clinically by vomiting. It is commonly associated with enteritis in the syndrome of gastro-enteritis. Much of the discussion which follows, particularly on the subject of aetiology, might be better dealt with under a separate heading of dyspepsia. The pathogenesis, clinical findings and necropsy lesions are poorly defined and could very well be functional rather than based on structural changes.

Aetiology

Gastritis may be acute or chronic but both forms of the disease may be caused by the same aetiological agents acting with varying degrees of severity and for varying periods. The inflammation may be caused by physical, chemical, bacterial, viral or metazoan agents.

Physical agents. Gross over-feeding causing gastric dilatation is usually accompanied by some secondary gastritis. Frosted or frozen feeds, particularly roots, may cause a severe gastritis, although frozen roots in adult ruminants are more likely to cause severe indigestion accompanied by frothy bloat. The ingestion of coarse, fibrous feeds such as straw bedding may perpetuate a chronic gastritis, especially in pigs and calves, although it is probable that a primary gastro-enteritis causes the animal to develop a perverted appetite and eat the bedding in the first place. Bad teeth, leading to faulty mastication, may have the same effect as coarse roughage.

The feeding of damaged feeds, including mouldy and fermented hay and ensilage, commonly causes a moderate gastritis. Foreign bodies may also lacerate the gastric mucosa and cause gastritis. A particular example is traumatic reticuloperitonitis of cattle.

Chemical agents. A number of caustic and irritant poisons, including arsenic, lead, copper, mercury, phosphorus and nitrate cause severe gastro-enteritis and a number of poisonous plants have also been incriminated. Excess production of lactic acid in the rumen after engorgement on grain often leads to the development of acute rumenitis and subsequently gastro-enteritis.

Bacterial agents. A primary bacterial gastritis is uncommon in animals. It occurs in some cases of oral necrobacillosis, haemorrhagic enterotoxaemia and colibacillosis in calves, and in braxy. A gastritis perhaps better described as venous hyperaemia and infarction occurs in erysipelas, salmonellosis, vibrionic dysentery and acute colibacillosis of pigs past weaning age.

Viral agents. Transmissible gastro-enteritis of baby pigs is, as the name implies, a gastro-enteritis. The gastric lesions in hog cholera, African swine fever and swine influenza are of the nature described above under bacterial causes. The abomasal and, to a less extent, ruminal lesions which occur in rinderpest and the mucosal diseases in ruminants are accompanied by more extensive and obvious erosive lesions in the mouth, oesophagus and intestines.

Fungal agents. Fungi can produce diffuse or ulcerative gastritis in new-born animals, especially pigs. Mucormycosis and moniliasis are the two commonly recorded causes. In all species *Mucor* spp. and *Aspergillus* spp. fungi frequently complicate gastric ulcers caused by other agents.

Metazoan agents. Many nematodes cause abomasitis in cattle and sheep. *Trichostrongylus axei*, *Ostertagia* spp., and *Haemonchus* spp. are the most commonly encountered. Abomasitis may also be caused by heavy infestations with larval paramphistomes migrating to the rumen. In horses, the larvae of *Habronema megastomum* cause a granulomatous or ulcerative lesion of the stomach wall which may lead to perforation and the development of peritonitis. *H. muscae* and *H. microstoma* cause gastritis without the production of tumours. Massive infestation with larvae of the botfly (*Gasterophilus* spp.) may cause ulcerations which may have a variety of complications. In pigs, the red stomach worm (*Hyostrongylus rubidus*) and the thick stomach worms (*Ascarops stongylina* and *Physocephalus sexalatus*) inhabit the stomach and, although they are of low pathogenicity, cannot be disregarded as causes of gastritis in this species.

Pathogenesis

Gastritis is an anatomical concept and does not often occur in animals without involvement of other parts of the alimentary tract. Even in parasitic infestations where the nematodes are relatively selective in their habitat, infestation with one nematode is usually accompanied by infestation with others so that gastro-enteritis is produced. It is dealt with as a specific entity here because it may occur as such, and enteritis is common without gastric involvement. The net effects of gastroenteritis can be determined by a summation of the effects of gastritis and enteritis.

The reactions of the stomach to inflammation include increased motility and increased secretion. There is a particular increase in the secretion of mucus which does protect the mucosa to some extent but also delays digestion and permits putrefactive breakdown of the ingesta. This abnormal digestion may cause further inflammation and favours spread of the inflammation to the intestines. In acute gastritis, the major effect is on motility; in chronic gastritis, on secretion. In acute gastritis there is an increase in peristalsis causing abdominal pain and more rapid emptying of the stomach either by vomiting or via the pylorus in animals unable to vomit. In chronic gastritis, the emptying of the stomach is prolonged because of the delay in digestion caused by excessive secretion of mucus. This may reach the point where chronic gastric dilatation occurs. The motility is not necessarily diminished and there may be subacute abdominal pain or a depraved appetite due to increased stomach contractions equivalent to hunger pains.

Clinical Findings

Acute gastritis. When the inflammation is severe, pigs and sometimes horses and ruminants vomit. The vomitus contains much mucus, sometimes blood, and is small in amount, and vomiting is repeated with forceful retching movements. The appetite is always reduced, often absent, but thirst is usually excessive and pigs affected with gastroenteritis may stand continually lapping water or even licking cool objects. The breath usually has a rank smell and there may be abdominal pain. Diarrhoea is not marked unless there is an accompanying enteritis but the faeces are usually pasty and soft. Additional signs are usually evident when gastritis is part of a primary disease syndrome. Dehydration and alkalosis with tetany and rapid breathing may develop if vomiting is excessive.

Chronic gastritis. Here the syndrome is much less severe. The appetite is depressed or depraved and vomiting occurs only sporadically, usually after feeding. The vomitus contains much viscid mucus. Abdominal pain is minor and dehydration is unlikely to occur but the animal becomes emaciated due to lack of food intake and incomplete digestion.

Clinical Pathology

Specimens taken for laboratory examination are usually for the purpose of identifying the causative agent in specific diseases. Estimations of gastric acidity are not usually undertaken but samples of vomitus should be collected if a chemical poison is suspected.

Necropsy Findings

The signs of inflammation vary in severity from a diffuse catarrhal gastritis to severe haemorrhagic and ulcerative erosion of the mucosa. In the mucosal diseases, there are discrete erosive lesions. In parasitic gastritis, there is usually marked thickening and oedema of the wall if the process has been in existence for some time (1). Chemical inflammation is usually most marked on the tips of the rugae and in the pyloric region. In severe cases, the stomach contents may be haemorrhagic; in chronic cases the wall is thickened and the contents contain much mucus and have a rancid odour suggestive of a prolonged sojourn and putrefaction of the food.

It is important to differentiate between gastritis and the erythematous flush of normal gastric mucosa in animals which have died suddenly. Venous infarction in the stomach wall occurs in a number of bacterial and viral septicaemias of pigs and causes extensive submucosal haemorrhages which may easily be mistaken for haemorrhagic gastritis.

Diagnosis

Gastritis and gastric dilatation have many similarities but, in the latter, the vomitus is more profuse and vomiting is of a more projectile nature although this difference is not so marked in the horse in which any form of vomiting is severe. Gastritis in the horse is not usually accompanied by vomiting but gastric dilatation may be. In oesophageal obstruction, the vomitus is neutral in reaction and does not have the rancid odour of stomach contents. Intestinal obstruction may be accompanied by vomiting and, although the vomitus is alkaline and may contain bile or even faecal material, this may also be the case in gastritis when intestinal contents are regurgitated into the stomach. Vomiting of central origin is extremely rare in farm animals.

Determination of the cause of gastritis may be difficult but the presence of signs of the specific diseases and history of access to poisons or physical agents listed under aetiology above may provide the necessary clues. Analysis of vomitus or food materials may have diagnostic value if chemical poisoning is suggested.

Treatment

Treatment of the primary disease is the first principle and requires a specific diagnosis. Ancillary treatment includes the withholding of food, the use of gastric sedatives, the administration of electrolyte solutions to replace fluids and electrolytes lost by vomiting, and stimulation of normal stomach motility in the convalescent period.

In horses and pigs, gastric lavage may be attempted to remove irritant chemicals. Gastric sedatives usually contain insoluble magnesium hydroxide or carbonate, kaolin, pectin, or charcoal. Preparations rich in tannic acid, including catechu, are usually incorporated because of their astringent properties. Frequent dosing at intervals of 2 or 3 hours is advisable. If purgatives are used to empty the alimentary tract, they should be bland preparations such as mineral oil to avoid further irritation to the mucosa.

If vomiting is severe, large quantities of electrolyte solution should be administered parenterally. Details of the available solutions are given under the heading of dehydration. If the liquids can be given orally without vomiting occurring, this route of administration is satisfactory.

During convalescence, the animal should be offered only soft, palatable, highly nutritious foods. Bran mashes for cattle and horses and gruels for calves and pigs are most adequate and are relished by the animal. Alimentary tract stimulants, including ginger, strychnine preparations and ammonium carbonate are well tolerated and hasten return of normal gastric motility.

REFERENCE
(1) Martin, W. B. *et al.* (1957). *Vet. Rec., 69,* 736.

Gastric Ulcer

Ulceration of the gastric mucosa causes a syndrome including anorexia, abdominal discomfort, abnormal intestinal motility leading to constipation or diarrhoea, and in some cases gastric haemorrhage.

Aetiology

Gastric ulcers in farm animals are usually traumatic or associated with a primary erosive or ulcerative disease. Traumatic ulceration of the abomasum is relatively common in young calves about two to three months of age when they are weaned and begin to subsist largely on roughage. In most cases, they are symptomless but occasionally ulcers perforate (1). Similarly gastric ulcers in foals have been ascribed to irritation by rough feed (9). Shallow erosions occur in the abomasal mucosa of cattle in rinderpest, the mucosal diseases and bovine malignant catarrh. In occasional cases of the pox and vesicular diseases, lesions may also occur in the abomasum in sheep and cattle. Sporadic cases occur in cattle and these may rupture during times of stress, particularly in early lactation (2, 3, 4), or bleed intermittently. They may arise in association with abomasal displacement or torsion (12), lymphomatosis or vagus indigestion or apparently be unrelated to other disease. The latter are not un-common in adult bulls. An association between ulceration and grazing on pasture heavily fertilized with nitrogen has been suggested (13).

As a sequel to parasitic gastritis, ulcers may de-velop in horses infested with *Gasterophilus* spp., and *Habronema megastoma* larvae. Rupture of the ulcers may occur and cause local or diffuse peri-tonitis (5). Tumours of the mucosa may cause similar ulceration and perforation in this species.

In pigs, gastric ulceration with sudden death due to haemorrhage has become a disease of major proportions. It is dealt with separately under the heading of oesophago-gastric ulceration of swine. Ulcers have also been observed in association with hepatic dystrophy in vitamin E-deficient pigs. In many cases the fungus *Rhizopus microspora* is present in the ulcer. Fungal mycelia have also been observed in the abomasal ulcers of young calves described above but, in both calves and pigs, they are probably contaminants rather than pri-mary aetiological agents and are important only in that they delay healing (6).

Pathogenesis

The effects of gastric ulcer are largely reflex, causing spasm of the pylorus and increased gastric motility. The resulting syndrome is similar to that caused by chronic gastritis except that rupture of blood-vessels may lead to acute or chronic gastric haemorrhage or to perforation and fatal chronic peritonitis. In cattle, perforation is usually followed by the development of chronic peritonitis as the lesion is sealed off by the omentum. The same result is observed in horses except that secondary involve-ment of the spleen is more common.

Clinical Findings

Many gastric ulcers cause no apparent illness. In clinically affected animals the syndrome varies depending on whether ulceration is complicated by perforation, rupture of the stomach or haemor-rhage. In uncomplicated ulcers there are mild and intermittent signs of abdominal pain and anorexia and either constipation or diarrhoea. If haemor-rhage results there may be sudden death or melaena or a more chronic loss of blood in the faeces with a severe haemorrhagic anaemia developing in time. The faeces are very black and tarry, and usually pasty and of small volume because of the accom-panying pylorospasm. Perforation is usually fol-lowed by acute local peritonitis unless the stomach is overloaded and ruptures, when acute shock leads to death in a few hours (11). With acute local peri-tonitis, there is a chronic illness accompanied by a fluctuating fever, severe anorexia and intermittent diarrhoea. In cows, the milk yield is severely de-pressed, grinding of the teeth is common and rumi-nal movements and rumination are depressed or absent. Pain may be detectable on percussion of the abdomen (10). Rarely, death occurs rapidly from internal haemorrhage when the ulceration invades a blood-vessel which is of sufficient size (7).

Clinical Pathology

The dark brown to black colour of the faeces is usually sufficient proof of gastric haemorrhage but tests for blood may be necessary if pigmented pharmaceuticals are being used. When perforation has occurred, there is a sharp rise in total leucocytes and neutrophiles in the blood but these levels return to normal if the lesion is walled off. When splenitis develops in horses, they rise again to very high levels and are a diagnostic feature of the disease.

Necropsy Findings

Ulceration is most common at the pylorus al-though in cows ulcers are not infrequently found at the lowest point of the fundus area on the greater curvature (13). The ulcers are usually deep and well defined but may be filled with blood-clot or necrotic material and often contain fungal mycelia which may be of aetiological significance. Lesions of the primary disease may be evident.

Most cases of perforation in cattle are walled off by omentum with the formation of a large cavity 12 to 15 cm. in diameter in the peritoneal cavity which contains degenerated blood and necrotic debris. Material from this cavity may infiltrate widely through the omental fat. Adhesions may form between the ulcer and surrounding organs or abdominal wall (1). In horses, there is an area of local peritonitis, the stomach wall is adherent to the tip of the spleen and an extensive suppurative splenitis may be present. In some cases, especially when the stomach is very full at the time of perforation, a long tear develops in the wall and large quantities of ingesta spill into the peritoneal cavity.

Diagnosis

Gastric ulceration is not usually diagnosed antemortem unless haemorrhage occurs, because of the clinical resemblance of the disease to chronic gastritis and traumatic reticuloperitonitis. When haemorrhage occurs, melaena or haematemesis suggests the presence of ulcer but similar faecal discoloration occurs in abomasal torsion and acute intestinal obstruction.

Treatment

Protective and astringent preparations as are used in gastritis are recommended but need to be given over relatively long periods. If haemorrhage is severe, blood transfusions or haematinic drugs are necessary and parenteral coagulants are usually administered. Food containing harsh material which is likely to be physically irritating should be avoided. Surgical repair has been recorded in cows (4, 9, 10).

REFERENCES

(1) Rooney, J. R. et al. (1956). N. Amer. Vet., 37, 750.
(2) Pinsent, P. J. N. & Ritchie, H. E. (1955). Vet. Rec., 67, 769.
(3) Marr, A. & Jarrett, W. F. H. (1955). Vet. Rec., 67, 332.
(4) Tasker, J. B. et al. (1958). J. Amer. vet. med. Ass., 133, 365.
(5) Rainey, J. W. (1948). Aust. vet. J., 24, 116.
(6) Gitter, M. & Austwick, P. K. C. (1957). Vet. Rec., 69, 924.
(7) Bartlett, M. P. & Fincher, M. G. (1956). N. Amer. Vet., 37, 942.
(8) Tutt, J. B. et al. (1959). Vet. Rec., 71, 620.
(9) Rooney, J. R. (1964). Pathologia vet., 1, 497.
(10) Pinsent, P. J. N. (1968). Vet. Rev., 19, 50.
(11) Hemmingsen, I. (1967). Nord. Vet.-Med., 19, 17.
(12) Albert, T. F. & Ramey, D. B. (1967). J. Amer. vet. med. Ass., 150, 408.
(13) Aukema, J. J. (1971). Proefschrift. Faculteit Diergeneeskunde, Rijksuniversiteit, Utrecht.

Acute Intestinal Obstruction

Intestinal obstruction includes volvulus, intussusception and strangulation. The clinical signs typical of these conditions include acute abdominal pain, severe shock, absence of defaecation and often the passage of blood and mucus.

Aetiology

The commonest causes are the intestinal accidents, volvulus, intussusception and strangulation in which there is physical occlusion of the intestinal lumen. Functional obstructive lesions, such as those which occur with local or general paralytic ileus, can be considered with physical occlusions (11), but are dealt with separately here. In many cases, the causes of the obstruction are bizarre and not readily diagnosed. In horses torsion of the caecum or large colon may occur while rolling, especially if the rolling is violent and caused by a primary attack of impaction or spasmodic colic. Strangulation of an inguinal hernia is not uncommon in stallions, and strangulation of small intestine through the epiploic foramen (9), by bands of adhesions and by pedunculated lipomas has occurred. Impaction of the ileocaecal valve occurs in horses and is sometimes included in this category because of the acute nature of the syndrome. Intussusception is the commonest cause of intestinal obstruction in foals.

In calves, lambs and pigs, torsion of the mesentery is the commonest form. Intussusception is most common in adult cattle but herniation may occur through mesenteric tears or behind a ventral ligament of the urinary bladder (1, 2). Compression stenosis caused by organization of a blood clot after expression of a corpus luteum from an ovary has also been observed. Torsion of the caecum (3) and rotation of the coiled colon about its mesentery also occur. Dilatation of the caecum, caused probably by heavy feeding on grain, is considered to be an early stage of caecal torsion. Clinically the two stages are indistinguishable before laparotomy (13, 14, 15). The same comment applies to the colon which may suffer from a dilation without torsion. The response of the gut, in the form of dilation, to heavy feeding with carbohydrates has been shown to occur in pigs fed increasing amounts of lactose (18), and cattle fed on grain (24). Lipomas (6) and fat necrosis of the mesenteries and omenta are also causes of obstruction in cattle, and fibre balls (phytobezoars) may be a common cause in cattle and sheep, especially in areas where fibrous feed occurs extensively. For example a high incidence of intestinal obstruction has been recorded in an area infested by onion grass (Romulea bulbocodium), the disease appearing to occur most commonly in cows in late pregnancy or in the first 2 weeks after calving (10). A common history in cattle is of unusual activity such as occurs during oestrus prior to the onset of obstruction. A high incidence of intestinal rupture caused by phytotrichobezoars has been recorded in horses (19, 23).

Intestinal obstructions are not commonly recorded in sheep although heavy infestations of nodular worms (Oesophagostomum columbianum) are sometimes associated with obstruction due to adhesions or intussusception. A number of cases of ileal intussusception have been recorded in a group of travelling sheep in which nodular worms appeared to play no part (4).

Obstruction of the terminal small colon occurs in young piglets and may be caused by very hard faecal balls or by barley chaff used as bedding (5). Torsion of the coiled colon about its mesentery has also been observed in adult pigs. In all species, excessive trauma to the intestines during surgical operations, distension for periods of up to several days and acute diffuse peritonitis cause a functional stasis of the intestine which is similar in many respects to that produced by a physical obstruction. This syndrome of paralytic ileus also occurs in grass sickness in horses.

Pathogenesis

The effects of intestinal obstruction differ considerably between species, and within species depending on the site and type of obstruction. In general, obstructions high in the small intestine cause a more acute and severe syndrome than those in the large intestine but the difference may not be great. For example, obstructions of the small intestine or colon in horses usually kill within 24 hours while similar obstructions in cattle are not usually fatal in less than a week. This generalization is not without exceptions, due possibly to the presence or absence of toxigenic bacteria in isolated loops of intestine (10, 16). The type of lesion is important depending on whether the blood supply to a large section of intestine is cut off or whether circulatory effects are minimal. Obstructions caused by external pressure such as occurs in fat necrosis cause less acute signs than do torsion and intussusception.

There are several factors which are of importance in the production of clinical signs and in causing the death of the animals. Acute shock is the important factor in severe cases, particularly in the horse. Distension of the bowel causes reflex cardiovascular effects, and peripheral circulatory failure and collapse occur. In less severe cases, dehydration and loss of electrolytes are the important mechanisms as described under Principles of Alimentary Tract Dysfunction. The fluid and accompanying electrolytes are secreted into the lumen of the intestine in response to distension above the obstruction. It is this distension which is responsible for the abdominal pain observed. The greater severity of the disease in horses when obstruction occurs in the large intestine is probably due to the rapidity of the distension created by gas accumulation in this part of the alimentary tract. Distension is not a major factor in cattle or pigs unless there is occlusion of the lumen of the large intestine but, as compared to the horse, the syndrome produced is much less severe.

In the subacute cases which do not die from shock, there is the additional factor of interference with local blood supply when the vessels are occluded by twisting of the mesentery or by their passage into an intussusception. Because the veins are occluded most readily, there is usually considerable escape of fluid under pressure from the arteries into the intestinal wall and the peritoneal cavity. Gangrene of the intestinal wall occurs and the two factors of fluid loss and toxaemia add further insults.

Failure of ingesta to pass the obstruction and be absorbed is of little importance. Auto-intoxication may be a factor when faeces accumulate in obstruction of the large intestine but the importance of this factor is debatable.

Clinical Signs

In horses, there is a sudden onset of acute abdominal pain with rolling, pawing, sweating, an increase in rate and depth of respiration, an increase in heart rate (over 100 per minute), and weakness of the pulse. On rectal examination, there is an absence of faeces in the rectum and the intestines are distended with gas although there is no great external evidence of tympany. Intestinal sounds, other than occasional gurgles of gas moving, are absent. The mucosae and conjunctiva are usually congested. The body temperature falls, the horse becomes recumbent and may die within 12 hours and usually before 24 hours. On rectal examination one often finds the abdomen full of tightly-distended intestinal loops which make further examination difficult. In chronic cases of partial obstruction a great variety of abnormalities may be encountered. Chief among these are tight bands of adhesions and mesentery which usually lead to the obstructed loop of intestine. The findings in caecal displacement of the horse have been described (22).

In cattle, there is an initial attack of acute abdominal pain in which the animal kicks at its belly, treads uneasily with the hind feet, depresses the back and often groans or bellows with pain. The pain occurs spasmodically and at short, regular intervals and may occasionally be accompanied by rolling. This stage of acute pain usually passes off within a few (8 to 12) hours and during this time no food is taken and little or no faeces are passed. The temperature and respiratory rates are relatively unaffected and the pulse rate may be normal or elevated depending on whether or not blood-vessels are occluded. For example in caecal torsion the pulse rate may be normal (7). On rectal examination, the rectum is empty except for thick, tenacious mucus or a thick, dark-red, pasty material depending on whether blood has exuded into the lumen of the intestine. In some cases caused by obstruction by fibre-balls the faecal material is pasty, evil-smelling and yellow-grey in colour (10, 20). In cattle with intussusception there is a complete failure to defaecate; in other species the passage of abnormal faeces may continue. Signs of shock are evident but are not usually severe.

When the acute pain has subsided, the cow remains depressed, does not eat and passes no faeces. The circulation, temperature and respiration are normal but there is no ruminal or intestinal activity. Rectal examination is important at this stage. The rectum remains empty except for the mucous or tarry exudate described above and insertion of the arm usually causes pain and vigorous straining and peristalsis. Distension of loops of intestine is not nearly as obvious as in horses and may not occur unless the colon or caecum is involved.

The abdomen is slightly distended, and splashing sounds can be elicited by ballottement in the left and right flanks over the rumen and abomasum when the obstruction is in the upper part of the small intestine. In obstruction of the pylorus the sounds can be produced only on the right side, just behind the costal arch and approximately half way down its length. Regurgitation of fluid ingesta through the nose is common (10). When there is intussusception or torsion of the small intestine, the affected loop is usually felt in the lower right abdomen but the site varies with the nature of the obstruction. A careful examination must be carried out. In intussusception the affected loop is readily palpated as an oblong, sausage-shaped mass of firm consistency but in torsion the loop may be small, soft and mobile. In many cases, it is possible to follow a tightly-stretched mesenteric fold from the root of the mesentery to the loop. Palpation of the loop may cause distress especially in the early stages.

In torsion of the coiled colon, a number of distended loops can be palpated and these may be visible in the right flank. When there is torsion or dilation of the caecum, there is usually one grossly distended loop running horizontally across the abdomen just anterior to the pelvis and posteriorly or medially to the rumen. It may be possible to palpate the blind end of the caecum, and in cases which have been affected for several days the organ may be so distended with fluid and gas that it can be seen through the right flank or fluid sounds produced by ballottement (7, 8). Lipomas and fat necrosis are usually easily palpable as firm, lobulated masses which can be moved manually. They may encircle

the rectum. Affected cattle may remain in this state for 6 to 8 days but during this time there is a gradual development of a moderate, pendulous, abdominal enlargement, profound toxaemia and an increase in heart rate. The animal becomes recumbent and dies at the end of 8 to 10 days.

In pigs and sheep, distension of the abdomen, absence of faeces and complete anorexia are evident. The distension may be extreme in young pigs when the terminal colon is obstructed. Death usually occurs in from 3 to 6 days.

Clinical Pathology

Laboratory examinations are not used in the diagnosis of the disease but they may be of value in assessing the severity of the secondary disturbances and in giving an indication of the treatment required. When dehydration is advanced, there is haemoconcentration and oliguria and, when gangrene is developing, the blood NPN is high. Paracentesis of the abdomen may yield blood-stained serous fluid when there is extensive obstruction to vascular flow.

Necropsy Findings

The physical lesions are readily observed and are accompanied by varying degrees of gaseous and fluid distension of the oral segments of the intestine compared to aboral segments, and varying degrees of congestion, oedema, necrosis and gangrene of obstructed loops. In paralytic ileus, the same flaccidity of the gut and accumulation of fluid and gas occur but there is no physical obstruction.

Diagnosis

Acute intestinal obstruction must be differentiated from other causes of acute abdominal pain. These causes may be other diseases of the alimentary tract or diseases affecting other abdominal organs. Diseases affecting the alimentary tract include gastric dilatation caused by over-eating or pyloric obstruction, particularly abomasal obstruction in calves. Vomiting or the passage of large quantities of gas or fluid through a nasal tube, followed by relief of pain, are more common in this condition but, in obstruction of the upper part of the intestine, fluid may also fill the stomach. Complete absence of faeces and the passage of blood and mucus are more typical of intestinal obstruction and the obstructed segment of bowel can usually be felt on rectal examination in the cow and the horse. Abomasal torsion in cattle is a special case of gastric dilatation and may be accompanied by acute pain in the early stages.

In occasional cases of traumatic reticuloperitonitis in cattle there are early signs of acute abdominal pain but moderate fever, rumen stasis and abdominal tenderness are apparent and, although there may be constipation, some normal faeces are passed. Acute enteritis and intestinal hypermotility are accompanied by severe pain but increased peristaltic sounds can be heard and, in the former condition, there is diarrhoea. Intestinal hypermotility is transient and responds rapidly to treatment. Impaction of the ileocaecal valve is a disease restricted to horses, and may be distinguishable on palpation per rectum. It is rapidly fatal but affected horses usually survive for 48 hours compared to the course of 12 to 24 hours in acute obstruction.

Two of the most difficult diseases to differentiate from intestinal obstruction in horses are mesenteric vessel thrombosis and intestinal tympany because distension of the intestines with gas is typical of all three. Intestinal tympany is not usually accompanied by such severe pain and the shock of obstruction is not present. No obstructed intestinal loop can be palpated and, in most cases, flatus is passed per rectum. The syndrome in mesenteric vessel thrombosis is less acute and there may be passage of faeces containing blood rather than an absence of faeces. Careful rectal palpation may reveal the thickened, obstructed mesenteric vessels.

Renal and ureteric colic may simulate intestinal obstruction. Passage of a calculus down the ureter is not known to occur but transient bouts of pain in cattle are often ascribed to this cause. Acute involvement of individual renal papillae in pyelonephritis in cattle is also thought to cause some of these attacks of colic. In steers and wethers, urethral obstruction causes abdominal pain but there are additional signs of grunting, straining, distension of the urinary bladder and tenderness of the urethra. Defaecation is not impeded. Photosensitive dermatitis in cattle is also accompanied by kicking at the belly but the skin lesions are obvious and there are no other alimentary tract signs.

Treatment

Surgical removal of the obstruction is usually necessary. Resection of an intussusception may be followed by a period of intense and often painful peristalsis (21). Supportive treatment includes sedation in the early stages and the administration of antibiotics to control bacterial growth in the isolated section of gut, and of electrolyte solutions when dehydration has occurred (11). The administration of potassium by mouth is recommended to control the hypokalaemia which occurs, and which may be responsible for the severe muscular weakness which characterizes this disease (17). Restoration of normal motility after surgery is often difficult, and cases which have been in existence for four or five days may show persistent paralytic ileus even though the displacement is corrected surgically. Posterior pituitary extract is recommended (12) but mild stimulants including small doses of parasympathomimetic drugs or injectable cascara preparations are in more general use. Intestinal intubation, as it is practised in humans, has little practical value in large animal work, although some relief can be given to horses by draining the stomach when it has become filled with fluid regurgitated from the intestine.

Spontaneous correction of a displacement may occur especially if the animal is exercised vigorously or driven in a truck over a rough road. Immediate passage of large quantities of faeces heralds recovery. Spontaneous recovery has been recorded in intussusception when the gangrenous loop sloughs but subsequently fibrous constriction at the site may lead to a partial obstruction (21).

REFERENCES

(1) Bowen, R. W. (1946). *Aust. vet. J.*, *22*, 122.
(2) Wheat, J. D. (1947). *Cornell Vet.*, *37*, 254.
(3) Jones, E. W. et al. (1957). *J. Amer. vet. med. Ass.*, *130*, 167.
(4) Osborne, H. G. (1958). *Aust. vet. J.*, *34*, 42.
(5) Roneus, O. (1957). *Nord. Vet.-Med.*, *9*, 362.
(6) Edgson, F. A. (1952). *Vet. Rec.*, *64*, 449.
(7) Radostits, O. M. (1960). *Canad. vet. J.*, *1*, 405.
(8) Espersen, G. (1961). *Mod. vet. Pract.*, *42* (Aug. 15), 25.
(9) Lund, D. C. (1961). *Canad. vet. J.*, *2*, 265.
(10) Johnston, D. E. (1962). *Aust. vet. J.*, *38*, 294.
(11) Corker, E. & Dziuk, H. E. (1968). *Amer. J. vet. Res.*, *29*, 1429.
(12) Lowe, J. E. (1966). *Cornell Vet.*, *61*, 51.
(13) Sattler, H. G. (1963). *Wien. tierärztl. Mschr.*, *50*, 497.
(14) Pearson, H. (1963). *Vet. Rec.*, *75*, 961.
(15) Dirksen, G. (1962). *Dtsch. tierärztl. Wschr.*, *69*, 409.
(16) Weipers, W. L. (1963). *Bull. Off. int. Epiz.*, *59*, 1419.
(17) Hammond, P. B. et al. (1964). *J. comp. Path.*, *74*, 210.
(18) Shearer, I. J. & Dunkin, A. C. (1968). *N.Z.J. agric. Res.*, *11*, 923.
(19) Maconochie, J. R. et al. (1968). *Aust. vet. J.*, *44*, 81.
(20) Christie, B. A. (1967–68). *Vict. vet. Proc.*, *26*, 61.
(21) Pearson, H. (1971). *Vet. Rec.*, *89*, 426.
(22) Kalsbeck, H. G. (1971). *T. Diergeneesk.*, *96*, 472.
(23) Crook, I. G. (1967). *Aust. vet. J.*, *43*, 217.
(24) Svendsen, P. & Kristensen, B. (1970). *Nord. Vet.-Med.*, *22*, 578.
(25) Manahan, F. F. (1970). *Aust. vet. J.*, *46*, 231.

Enteritis

Inflammation of the intestinal mucosa causes increased motility of the gut, decreased absorption and increased secretion. Clinically it is manifested by abdominal pain, diarrhoea and sometimes dysentery. In many instances, it occurs coincidentally with gastritis.

Aetiology

There are very many causes of enteritis in farm animals and the disease varies a great deal in its severity depending upon the type and severity of the causative agent. The diseases listed below are those in which enteritis is a principal finding and there are many other diseases in which enteritis is a minor lesion. It should be borne in mind that there are influences exerted by the host which can play an important role in facilitating or suppressing the ability of a noxious agent to cause enteritis. Thus *Escherichia coli* may cause enteritis in new-born calves if their immunological status is reduced. Again in animals in the 2 to 4 weeks age group it may act as a secondary complication to hypermotility caused by a change in feed, and again in the post-weaning period due to a change in intestinal contents, because of lowered resistance after nutritional stress or because of a hypersensitivity reaction. For example it has been shown that the stimulus to *E. coli* proliferation lies in the host's response to intestinal irritation. In more exact terms the capacity of *E. coli* to colonize the intestine is directly related to the proportion of fluid in the faeces (6). Dietary indiscretions may cause significant increases in the fluid content of faeces and thus encourage the development of a bacterial enteritis.

Bacterial enteritis. Colibacillosis, salmonellosis, vibrionic dysentery, pasteurellosis and enterotoxaemia caused by *Clostridium perfringens* types B and C are all manifested by enteritis and occur in most species. Johne's disease is restricted to cattle and sheep and causes little clinical enteritis in the latter. Shigellosis in foals and baby pigs may be accompanied by diarrhoea, and occasional cases of anthrax show intestinal involvement.

Antibiotics administered by mouth to humans sometimes cause enteritis partly because of their irritant effect but largely because of the alteration of the intestinal flora which permits the overgrowth of bacteria (staphylococci, *Proteus* spp., and *Pseudomonas* spp.), and fungi (*Candida albicans*) which are normally kept under restraint (1). An identical occurrence has been described in foals with enteritis caused apparently by *Aspergillus fumigatus* (5), and in race horses in training (25), and a similar situation seems likely to occur in pigs and calves fed on antibiotics for long periods. Iron deficiency anaemia is a common predisposing cause of colibacillosis in pigs.

Viral enteritis. Cattle are the only species in which viral enteritides are common. Rinderpest, mucosal disease and bovine malignant catarrh are the important entities. Viral enteritis may be a significant cause of scours in calves. In pigs, transmissible gastro-enteritis is a disease of major importance. In horses some cases of equine viral arteritis develop enteritis.

Protozoan enteritis. Coccidiosis is of importance in all species of animals. Globidiosis may also be manifested by enteritis. An intestinal trichomoniasis has been reported in horses (14) but the significance of trichomonads in its aetiology has not been firmly established.

Enteritis caused by chemical agents. Poisoning by lead, arsenic, phosphorus, mercury, molybdenum, copper, sodium chloride, oxalates and nitrates causes enteritis when large doses are taken. Many poisonous plants commonly cause severe enteritis, and toadstools and unidentified fungi in mouldy feed occasionally do so. Overdosing with oral iron preparations may cause chemical enteritis in young pigs.

Enteritis caused by nutritional deficiency. Deficiency of nicotinic acid and other B vitamins may be of minor importance in the production of enteritis in pigs.

Parasitic enteritis. Enteritis caused by helminths is one of the commonest forms of the disease in animals. Massive infestations with stomach flukes (*Paramphistomum* spp.) may cause enteritis in ruminants (3) but in these animals infestations with *Strongyloides* spp., *Oesophagostomum* spp., *Trichostrongylus* spp., *Cooperia* spp., *Chabertia* spp. and *Nematodirus* spp. are more important. Hookworms (*Bunostomum* spp.) occasionally cause enteritis in calves, and heavy tapeworm (*Moniezia* spp.) infestations can cause enteritis in sheep. In horses, *Strongylus* spp. and *Trichonema* spp. are the common causes and *Ascaris* spp. to a much less extent. Pigs are not usually affected by parasitic enteritis although heavy infestations with *A. lumbricoides* may be accompanied by diarrhoea.

Enteritis caused by physical agents is uncommon in farm animals but the ingestion of large quantities of sand or soil either in feed contaminated during dust storms or when horses are grazed on sandy pasture and pull up plants by the roots causes an acute or chronic enteritis usually described as 'sand colic'. Acute enteritis may also occur as a result of lactic acid formation after engorgement on grain in ruminants and has been reported to occur following the feeding of grass silage with a high lactic acid content (15). The highly fatal diarrhoeic disease of horses known as 'colitis-X' has an uncertain aetiology but is probably an endotoxaemia (4).

Intestinal ulcers occur in animals only as a form of chronic enteritis and not, as far as is known, as a result of psychosomatic disease as they do in humans. Ulceration occurs in many specific erosive diseases listed above and in salmonellosis and hog cholera but the lesions are present in the terminal part of the ileum and more commonly in the caecum and colon.

Pathogenesis

Depending upon the causative agent, there may be a mild catarrhal inflammation, a severe haemorrhagic enteritis or an erosive or necrotic destruction of the intestinal mucosa, and the clinical signs vary accordingly. Apart from the direct toxigenic effects of bacteria on the intestinal epithelium, it is probable that the metabolic interaction between the bacteria and the substrate of intestinal contents has an effect on the mucosa (7). The primary reaction of the epithelium to inflammatory stimulation is to desquamate, and this is accompanied in most cases by an increase in motility. Absorption of fluids and digestion are impaired and the intestinal contents are passed along the lumen in a fluid state resulting in diarrhoea. Incomplete digestion, putrefaction of protein and carbohydrate fermentation are manifested by a foul odour. There is loss of fluid and electrolytes, and dehydration results. For example in calves the faecal excretion of water and nitrogenous substances may be 100 times normal (13). There may be also an extensive loss of protein (11), especially in parasitic enteritis and abomasitis, but the reasons for the loss are obscure. It may contribute to the loss of condition in chronic enteritis and to dehydration in the acute form of the disease.

In chronic enterocolitis there is often a serious loss of plasma proteins, possibly via an accompanying intestinal lymphangiectasia (12). In other cases lymphangiectasia may be the only lesion and probably contributes another cause of the so-called 'protein-losing enteropathies'.

When the enteritis is severe, there may be marked denudation of epithelium, permitting the absorption of toxic products and the entrance of pathogenic bacteria, and resulting in more acute loss of fluids and even whole blood so that shock and dysentery may occur. Shedding of large areas of mucosa may cause the appearance of shreds or casts of mucosa in the faeces.

In chronic enteritis, the intestinal wall becomes thickened and mucus secretion is stimulated, fluid absorption is decreased and the faeces are thin and watery and may contain much mucus.

Clinical Findings

Gastritis commonly accompanies enteritis and signs referable to inflammation of the gastric mucosa may be present also. In acute enteritis, there is abdominal pain which is most severe in the horse and is often sufficient in this species to cause rolling and kicking at the belly (2). This is unusual in cattle although it is seen occasionally in arsenic poisoning and salmonellosis in this species. In chronic enteritis, pain is seldom present, and when it is, is vague and intermittent.

Diarrhoea is the characteristic sign in acute enteritis. The faeces are soft and fluid and have an unpleasant odour. They may contain blood, shreds of mucosa and mucus. In chronic enteritis, the odour is not grossly abnormal, mucus may be present in large quantities, and there is an absence of systemic signs of shock and dehydration. The course is longer and the animal becomes emaciated. Anorexia is complete in acute enteritis but the appetite may be normal or even voracious in the chronic disease and thirst is usually increased. Straining may occur, especially in calves, and be followed by intussusception or rectal prolapse. Some indication of the nature of the enteritis may be obtained from the distribution of the diarrhoea on the animals' hind parts. Thus, in calves, the 'smudge pattern' may suggest both coccidiosis and the straining that commonly accompanies it when the faeces are smeared horizontally across the ischial tuberosities and the adjoining tail, or helminth infestation when there is little smearing on the pinbones but the tail and insides of the hocks are liberally coated (8).

Auscultation of the abdomen usually reveals sounds of increased motility and fluidity of intestinal contents. Pain may be evidenced on firm abdominal palpation in the smaller animals. Systemic signs vary with the severity of the inflammation. There may be shock and an increase in heart rate in severe cases. Rectal examination is negative except in 'sand colic' in horses when impacted loops of bowel can be palpated. Typical signs of the specific diseases will also be present. Acute cases may terminate within 24 hours, especially in young animals, but chronic enteritis may persist for several months.

Clinical Pathology

Examination of the faeces to determine the presence of causative bacteria, helminths, protozoa and chemical agents is dealt with under the specific diseases. It is most important that faecal specimens be taken as the differentiation of the aetiological groups depends largely on laboratory examinations.

With increasing sophistication in diagnostic laboratories it is now not uncommon to determine the plasma osmolality and the concentration of sodium, potassium, chlorine and bicarbonate ions, for purposes of prognosis and to determine the form that fluid and electrolyte therapy should take. Affected calves may show very markedly decreased plasma osmolality, and also marked reductions in total body water and extra- and intra-cellular fluids (10).

Necropsy Findings

Necropsy findings vary from a catarrhal enteritis manifested by swelling and reddening of the mucosa, the presence of submucosal oedema and petechial haemorrhages and offensive-smelling, soft intestinal contents, to acute haemorrhagic and necrotic enteritis. In the latter, there is obvious necrosis of the mucosa and the ingesta contains blood and epithelial shreds. The mesenteric lymph nodes show varying degrees of enlargement, oedema and congestion, and secondary involvement of spleen and liver is not unusual. In chronic enteritis, the epithelium may appear relatively normal but the wall is usually thickened and may be oedematous. In some of the specific diseases, there are lesions typical of the particular disease.

Diagnosis

A diagnosis of enteritis is usually not difficult to make because of the nature of the faeces. Diarrhoea occurs in peat scours and other forms of hypermotility but there is an absence of abnormal odour, excessive faecal mucus, and of a systemic reaction. Chronic enteritis due to Johne's disease and parasitism may also be accompanied by faeces of this type and can be differentiated only by laboratory examination.

Differentiation between the causes of enteritis may be facilitated by the presence of lesions or signs typical of one of the specific diseases listed under aetiology above or there may be evidence of exposure to a poisonous substance. In 'sand colic' in horses, the faeces usually contain large amounts of sand which can be estimated by mixing the faeces with water and washing off the organic matter.

Treatment

Primary treatment will depend on the nature of the causative agent, and identification of the agent is essential if specific treatment is to be administered. Ancillary treatment includes removal of the causative agent from the intestine, administration of astringent preparations and replacement of lost fluids and electrolytes.

Removal of toxic material from the intestine is always a difficult problem. The only feasible method is by hastening evacuation through the faeces but the administration of irritant purgatives can only cause an exacerbation of the enteritis and result in superpurgation. This is particularly likely to occur in the horse. In most instances, it is preferable to allow the supposed toxic material to be evacuated naturally or, at most, to use a bland oily purgative. Accumulations of sand or soil can be removed by repeated treatments with a bland preparation such as mineral oil if they are not too firmly compacted. Daily doses of about 1 to 2 pints may be necessary for a week or more in chronic cases. In acute cases, excellent results have been reported with the administration of 2 to 3 gallons of warm saline and $\frac{1}{8}$ grain arecoline at half-hour intervals for 8 hours (2). If the sand mass is firm and hard surgical intervention may be indicated (9).

Astringent and protective preparations, as described under the treatment of gastritis, have a definite place in the treatment of enteritis as they reduce fluid loss and ease discomfort. Sedatives and spasmolytic preparations are also useful in relieving pain, particularly if the animal is likely to injure itself by rolling, but they should be avoided if possible. Replacement of lost fluids and electrolytes can usually be effected only by parenteral administration. In young animals, this form of treatment is most important and is often the factor which decides the outcome of the case. Details of the preparations and dose rates are provided under the treatment of dehydration. Blood transfusions are not as effective as saline solutions unless antibodies are required in young animals.

The inclusion of bacteriostatic drugs in oral preparations for the treatment of enteritis is often justified on the basis that they may prevent bacterial invasion of devitalized epithelium. If they are used, it should be at therapeutic levels because of the danger of creating resistant strains of bacteria.

REFERENCES

(1) Binns, T. B. (1956). *Lancet*, *270*, 336.
(2) Bither, H. D. & Sullivan, E. M. (1954). *Cornell Vet.*, *44*, 294.
(3) Nobel, T. (1956). *Refuah. vet.*, *13*, 155, cited in (1957). *Vet. Bull.*, *27*, 472.
(4) Teigland, M. B. (1960). *Proc. 6th ann. Meet. Amer. Assoc. equine Practnrs*, pp. 81–92.
(5) Lundvall, R. L. & Romberg, P. F. (1960). *J. Amer. vet. med. Ass.*, *137*, 481.
(6) Kenworthy, R. & Allen, W. D. (1966). *J. comp. Path.*, *76*, 31.

(7) Kenworthy, R. & Allen, W. D. (1966). *J. comp. Path.*, *76*, 291.
(8) Fenwick, D. C. (1963–64). *Vict. vet. Proc.*, *22*, 48.
(9) Rines, M. P. (1963). *Mich. St. Univ. Vet.*, *24*, 19 (Fall).
(10) Fayet, J. C. (1971). *Brit. vet. J.*, *127*, 37.
(11) Marsh, C. N. *et al.* (1969). *Amer. J. vet. Res.*, *30*, 163.
(12) Nansen, P. & Nielsen, K. (1967). *Nord. Vet.-Med.*, *19*, 524.
(13) Michel, M. C. (1971). *Ann. Biol. anim.*, *11*, 303.
(14) Bennett, S. P. & Franco, D. A. (1969). *J. Amer. vet. med. Ass.*, *154*, 58.
(15) Tutt, J. B. (1972). *Vet. Rec.*, *90*, 91.

Intestinal Hypermotility

A functional increase in intestinal motility seems to be the basis of a number of diseases of animals. Clinically there is some abdominal pain and, on auscultation, an increase in alimentary tract sounds and, in some cases, diarrhoea. Affected animals do not usually die and necropsy lesions cannot be defined but it is probable that the classification as it is used here includes many of the diseases often referred to as catarrhal enteritis or indigestion.

The two major occurrences of intestinal hypermotility are spasmodic colic of the horse and dietary scours of the calf.

Other circumstances in which hypermotility and diarrhoea occur without evidence of enteritis include peat scours of cattle on pasture deficient in copper and containing an excess of molybdenum, allergic and anaphylactic states and a change of feed to very lush pasture.

Spasmodic Colic

Aetiology

Spasmodic colic occurs usually in horses which are predisposed to it by an excitable temperament. Precipitating causes include excitement, such as occurs during thunderstorms, preparations for showing or racing, and drinks of cold water when hot and sweating after work. Excitable cattle may suffer from transient attacks of diarrhoea during periods of excitement.

Pathogenesis

The hypermotility of spasmodic colic in horses is thought to arise by an increase in parasympathetic tone under the influence of the causative factors mentioned above. This explanation is not particularly satisfying but the condition is comparable to the vague intestinal upsets which occur in children and excitable adults.

In calves, there may be a similar element of autonomic imbalance, particularly in cases of colic which occur transiently in calves in the 3 to 6 months age group and more rarely in adult cattle.

Clinical Findings

Spasmodic colic of horses is characterized by short attacks of abdominal pain. The pain is intermittent, the horse rolling, pawing and kicking for a few minutes, then shaking itself and standing normally for a few minutes until the next bout of pain occurs. Intestinal sounds are often audible some distance from the horse and loud, rumbling borborygmi are heard on auscultation. The pulse is elevated moderately to about 60 per minute and there may be some patchy sweating but rectal findings are negative and there is no scouring. The signs usually disappear spontaneously within a few hours. A similar syndrome occurs in cows and in calves although intestinal sounds are not usually increased.

Clinical Pathology and Necropsy Findings

Laboratory examinations are not used in diagnosis and the disease is not fatal.

Diagnosis

Spasmodic colic may be confused with enteritis since both diseases are characterized by abdominal pain and increased intestinal sounds. Diarrhoea is usually present in enteritis although an exception to this rule is acute parasitic enteritis in the horse. Confusion may also occur in cattle and in horses between spasmodic colic and acute intestinal obstruction especially in cattle where rectal examination may be negative in early cases of obstruction, but the failure to pass faeces and the presence of blood and mucus in the rectum are typical of this condition. The disease has also been confused with obstructive urolithiasis because of the similar posture adopted by horses in both diseases.

Treatment

Acute hypermotility as manifested by spasmodic colic is best treated by a spasmolytic such as atropine. In horses, a standard treatment is 16 to 32 mg. of atropine sulphate given subcutaneously followed by $\frac{1}{2}$ gallon of mineral oil by nasal tube. Pethidine (Demerol, isonipecaine hydrochloride or meperidine hydrochloride) injected parenterally at a dose rate of 1·0 mg. per lb. body weight is an effective analgesic and spasmolytic. Novocain (0·05 g. per 100 lb. body weight) injected very slowly intravenously may produce immediate relief from pain which lasts for 15 to 20 minutes (1) but undesirable excitement is a common side-effect. Promazine derivatives have a tranquillizing and spasmolytic effect also, and, followed by a mild purgative, appear to be the treatment of choice in this form of colic. Analgesics are not usually required but, if they are administered, they can be used as described under impaction of the large intestine.

REFERENCE
(1) Brion, A. (1946). *J. Amer. vet. med. Ass.*, *108*, 254.

Dietetic Scours

Aetiology

In calves, scours can be caused by dietary abnormalities and this is commonly followed by secondary colibacillosis. Drinking too rapidly, feeding large quantities of cold milk, the feeding of milk high in fat and in solids-not-fat and a sudden change from whole milk to milk substitutes or meal may precipitate attacks (1). Calves fed on milk from cows grazing very lush, clover-dominant pastures may also develop a thin, watery diarrhoea (2). There is a similar occurrence of scours in young pigs 2 to 3 weeks old (3). It may be caused by over-eating when the sow is milking heavily or when the piglets eat too much creep feed. Occasional cases occur in foals and lambs when the dams have a profuse milk supply. While simple over-feeding on milk is commonly thought to cause scours in calves, this has not been borne out by experimental work (15). Field experience suggests that dietetic scours occurs much more frequently in neonates fed artificial milks or milk replacers than when they are left on their dams. This has been shown experimentally in pigs (16).

Pathogenesis

Most cases of dietary scours in younger calves up to 4 weeks of age are usually ascribed to physical causes. For example milk of a high casein content leads to the formation of a much denser abomasal curd than does milk of a low casein content. The milk of dairy cows has a much higher casein content than colostrum and failure to feed colostrum or the feeding of milk in large quantities at long intervals may lead to the formation of a large, indigestible curd which gradually enlarges as further concretions of curd are applied to it (4). A degree of abomasal dilatation and irritation occurs and milk tends to pass into the intestine in an undigested state leading to the development of scours (5). The speed of drinking is probably important also. Prolongation of drinking time results in dilution of the milk with saliva and the production of a frothy, easily-digested curd (6). Failure of the oesophageal reflex in pail-fed calves may also be important in the production of scours. The milk is deposited in the rumen where it undergoes putrefaction. Regurgitation of milk from the abomasum into the rumen may also occur when calves are fed large amounts of cold milk infrequently. Sudden changes of diet, such as occur at abrupt weaning, cause a temporary malabsorption of fat and carbohydrate resulting in an increase in the fluid content of faeces and the development of diarrhoea (12). Another factor which may influence the occurrence of dietetic scours is the sugar content of the milk. It has been shown in lambs that an increase in sugar content of the diet can cause diarrhoea (13).

Poor clotting of milk also leads to scours. Milk with a very low level of casein or calcium, or with a high level of sodium or high pH clots poorly and undigested milk passes into the intestine where protein putrefaction causes scouring and may lead to bacterial multiplication and the development of enteritis and systemic infection.

Clinical Findings

Dietetic scours of calves is manifested by the passage of soft, fluid faeces, varying from white to yellow to green in colour depending on the composition of the diet. Although the calves lose weight rapidly and have a gaunt appearance, the appetite is good, the demeanour bright and the temperature and pulse rate are normal. If the condition is prolonged, dehydration may become severe and abomasal dilatation may occur as an end result. Affected calves often show a depraved appetite and eat bedding and other indigestible materials which further exacerbate the condition.

Clinical Pathology

Laboratory examinations are of value only in so far as they help to eliminate other possible causes of scouring in the diagnosis of the disease in calves.

Necropsy Findings

Deaths do not usually occur in uncomplicated dietetic scours but secondary bacterial complications occur frequently in young animals and are highly fatal.

Diagnosis

Dietetic scours resembles enteritis and may in fact precede it but there is an absence of systemic signs and the faeces are bulky and pasty rather than watery. The animal continues to feed well and responds to simple palliative treatment if the cause is dietary abnormality.

Treatment

In calves affected with dietary scours, milk feeding should be stopped and the calf fed oral electrolyte solutions for 24 hours. Milk is then gradually reintroduced. Foals should be muzzled and allowed only limited access to the mare, which will require hand-stripping to relieve tension in the udder. Astringent and protective preparations are commonly administered and may be combined with prophylactic doses of antibacterial drugs. Severe cases may require intravenous alimentation. The feeding practices should be corrected so that the calves are fed at least three times a day and preferably on colostrum or milk of low fat content. The addition of lime water (1 part to 2 parts of milk) aids digestion and helps protect pail-fed calves. Pregastric esterase has some proponents as a treatment to aid digestion and allow the calf to remain on feed (14).

The use of slow-flowing nipples to feed young calves has been recommended to reduce scouring and the vice of sucking each other. Opinions vary as to the efficiency of nipple feeding in the prevention of scours (7, 8, 9) and the method has a number of disadvantages. The time required for feeding the calves is greatly prolonged, some calves may not drink their quota and minor bloating may occur. Calves fed on nurse-cows are much less affected by dietary scours than are pail-fed calves but cases may occur on very fast-milking cows and the incidence is higher in calves allowed to suckle only twice a day than in calves allowed to run with the cows.

Cud transfers or rumen transplants have been recommended as an aid to digestion in young calves (10) but, provided the feed is relatively digestible, no advantage appears to accrue (11).

One of the principal difficulties when attempting to make satisfactory recommendations about the prevention of dietetic scours, especially in calves, is the great lack of knowledge on normal digestion and nutritional requirements of neonates. The nutrition of the pre-ruminant calf has been reviewed recently (17).

REFERENCES

(1) Owen, F. G. et al. (1958). J. Dairy Sci., 41, 662.
(2) Shanks, P. L. (1950). Vet. Rec., 62, 315.
(3) Goodwin, R. F. (1957). Vet. Rec., 69, 1290.
(4) Sheehy, F. (1948). Agriculture, Lond., 55, 189.
(5) Blaxter, K. L. & Wood, W. A. (1953). Vet. Rec., 65, 889.
(6) Wise, G. H. et al. (1947). J. Dairy Sci., 30, 499.
(7) Geddes, H. J. (1950). Aust. vet. J., 26, 233.
(8) Hoyer, N. & Larkin, R. M. (1954). Queensland agric. J. (Aust.), 79, 46.
(9) Kesler, E. M. et al. (1956). J. Dairy Sci., 39, 542.
(10) Pounden, W. D. & Hibbs, J. W. (1949). J. Amer. vet. med. Ass., 114, 33.
(11) MacArthur, A. T. G. (1957). N.Z. J. Sci. Tech., Sec. A., 38, 696.
(12) Kenworthy, R. & Allen, W. D. (1966). J. comp. Path., 76, 31.
(13) Walker, D. M. & Faichney, G. J. (1964). Brit. J. Nutr., 18, 209.
(14) Campbell, M. R. et al. (1964). Vet. Med., 59, 610.
(15) Mylrea, P. J. (1966). Res. vet. Sci., 7, 417.
(16) White, F. et al. (1969). Brit. J. Nutr., 23, 847.
(17) Radostits, O. M. & Bell, J. M. (1970). Canad. J. Anim. Sci., 50, 405.

Impaction of the Ileocaecal Valve

Impaction of the ileocaecal valve occurs commonly only in horses, causing a syndrome of subacute abdominal pain followed by one of acute pain. It is commonly fatal and is comparable in severity to acute intestinal obstruction.

Aetiology

The common cause is feeding on low-grade, finely-chopped roughage (1).

Pathogenesis

The finely-chopped straw or poor hay passes through the stomach in an undigested form and collects in the terminal ileum at the ileocaecal valve. The obstruction is complete and the further pathogenesis is identical with that of acute intestinal obstruction except that the local vascular occlusion which occurs in the latter disease is not present and shock does not occur. For this reason, the course of the disease is more prolonged.

Clinical Findings

The syndrome develops in two stages (2). Initially there is a period of 8 to 12 hours in which subacute abdominal pain is evidenced, the horse doing some rolling and pawing and looking at the flank but there is no great increase in pulse rate or respiration. The intestinal sounds are increased in frequency and intensity. Rectal examination may reveal no abnormality although, with careful palpation, the enlarged, impacted ileum may be detectable in the upper right flank at the base of the caecum, although this is easily confused with an impaction of the small colon.

At the end of this phase, the pain increases in severity. There is severe depression, patchy sweating and coldness of the extremities and the animal stands with its head hung down, sits on its haunches and rolls and struggles violently. The abdominal pain becomes severe and continuous, the pulse rate rises to between 80 and 120 per minute and the pulse is weak. Respirations are increased to 30 to 40 per minute and the temperature up to 39·5 °C

(103°F). The abdominal sounds are almost entirely absent at this stage and passage of a nasal tube is followed by aspiration of sanguineous fluid, often in quantities up to several gallons. On rectal examination, the large intestine is small and contracted but the small intestine is so tightly distended with gas and fluid that proper examination of the viscera is impossible although tightly-stretched bands of mesentery may be palpable. Death usually occurs 36 to 48 hours after the onset of illness.

Clinical Pathology

Laboratory examinations are of no value in diagnosis.

Necropsy Findings

The distal 30 to 45 cm. in the ileum are firmly packed with finely-chopped fibrous material, and the small intestine and even the stomach are tightly distended with up to 90 to 135 litres of blood-stained fluid.

Diagnosis

In the early stages, the disease is easily mistaken for spasmodic colic or enteritis because of the moderate, acute pain and the increased intestinal sounds. The history of the diet and palpation of the impacted ileum are the principal differentiating features. In addition, the continuation of the illness suggests ileocaecal valve impaction. In the second phase, the disease resembles acute tympany of the intestine except that the small rather than the large intestine is obstructed, or acute intestinal obstruction where shock is more severe and again it is the large intestine which is usually affected. Horses which develop an acute obstruction while rolling due to the pain of spasmodic colic or impaction of the large intestine present a clinical syndrome almost identical with that of ileocaecal valve impaction. The characteristic features of ileocaecal valve impaction are the gross accumulation of fluid and the relatively long course.

Treatment

Removal of fluid from the stomach prolongs the animal's life and eases the discomfort but intravenous alimentation is necessary to replace the lost fluids. Sedatives must be administered because of the severe bruising usually incurred during bouts of violent struggling. Removal of the obstruction is necessary if the patient is to survive but often proves to be impossible. A large dose of mineral oil ($\frac{1}{2}$ to 1 gallon), preferably containing a wetting agent, should be followed in two or three hours by a parasympathetic stimulant. The increased intestinal motility causes a reappearance of severe pain and rupture of the intestine may occur. Enterotomy has been performed and the obstruction removed but the surgery is of an heroic order.

REFERENCES

(1) Hudson, J. (1936). *Vet. J.*, *92*, 50.
(2) Hutchins, D. R. (1952). *Aust. vet. J.*, *28*, 236.

Intestinal Tympany

Intestinal tympany causes distension of the abdomen and severe abdominal pain and is sometimes accompanied by the passage of much flatus.

Aetiology

Most cases of intestinal tympany occur in the horse and are secondary to obstruction of the intestinal lumen. All cases of tympany of the small intestine are caused by some form of intestinal obstruction. Tympany of the large intestine may be primary or secondary. Primary cases are caused by the ingestion of large quantities of highly fermentable green feed. Secondary cases are caused by acute intestinal obstruction or stenosis by constricting fibrous tissue bands after castration, or in association with verminous aneurysm. In pigs and ruminants, the tympany is always secondary, usually to acute intestinal obstruction.

Pathogenesis

The excessive production of gas or its retention in a segment of bowel causes distension and acute abdominal pain. In primary tympany, the distension is periodically reduced by the evacuation of some gas and the course is relatively long. In secondary tympany, the pathogenesis depends largely on the primary cause, the distension adding a further burden. Some interference with circulation and respiration occurs and may contribute to death in cases which terminate fatally.

Clinical Findings

Abdominal distension is evident in all species and the distended loops of intestine may be visible through the abdominal wall in thin animals. Pain is acute and affected horses may roll and paw violently. Peristaltic sounds are reduced but fluid may be heard moving in gas-filled, intestinal loops producing a tinkling, metallic sound. On rectal examination, gas-filled loops of intestine fill the abdominal cavity and make proper examination of its contents impossible. In primary tympanites much flatus is passed and the anus may be in a state of continuous dilatation.

Clinical Pathology

Laboratory examinations are of no value in diagnosis.

Necropsy Findings

In cases of secondary tympany, the causative obstruction is evident. In primary cases, the intestines are filled with gas and the faeces are usually pasty and loose.

Diagnosis

Primary tympany is always difficult to differentiate from secondary tympany and the presence of an intestinal obstruction may be difficult to determine as rectal examination is impeded. If flatus and faeces are passed and if there is a history of engorgement on lush, legume pasture, primary tympany is probably the cause. Intestinal obstructions usually cause death in a much shorter time and the distension is often restricted to short lengths of intestine whereas primary tympany usually involves most if not all of the tract.

Treatment

In severe primary cases, trocarization with a long, small-calibre, intestinal trocar and cannula may be necessary. This can be performed per rectum or through the upper right or left flank depending on the site of maximum distension. All cases should receive mineral oil ($\frac{1}{2}$ to 1 gallon) containing an antiferment such as oil of turpentine ($\frac{1}{2}$ to 1 oz.), formalin (1 oz.) or chloroform (1 oz.). It may be necessary to administer a sedative if pain is acute.

In secondary tympany, permanent relief can be obtained only by correction of the obstruction.

Verminous Mesenteric Arteritis

(Verminous Aneurysm)

Migration of the larvae of *Strongylus vulgaris* into the wall of the cranial mesenteric artery and its branches occurs commonly in horses and may cause restriction of the blood supply to the intestines. Cases may occur in foals as young as six months old. Chronic, low-grade impairment causes atony of segments of the large intestine. Pressure on sympathetic ganglia has been suggested as the cause of the recurrent attacks of spasmodic colic which occur in some cases (1). Recurrent attacks of colic also occur when a secondary bacterial infection, usually *Streptococcus equi*, *Actinobacillus equuli* or *Salmonella typhimurium*, becomes established in the aneurysm (6). The signs produced by mesenteric abscess are similar to those of verminous aneurysm but the temperature is usually elevated and rupture of the abscess may lead to the development of a diffuse peritonitis. This condition has been diagnosed by roentgenological examination after the production of pneumoperitoneum, but it is more likely that these are cases of recurrent mesenteric embolism. Complete vascular occlusion occurs in some cases and leads to necrosis and gangrene of sections of the large intestine. In these animals, there is moderately severe abdominal pain for three to four days with almost complete cessation of defaecation and absence of intestinal sounds due to stasis. On rectal examination, distended loops of intestines and tightly stretched mesentery may be felt, but the distension is neither severe nor general. If the horse is not too large, it is often possible to palpate the root of the cranial mesenteric artery as a fixed, firm swelling in the midline, level with the caudal pole of the left kidney. It will be much enlarged, have a rough, knobbly surface and it usually pulsates with each pulse wave. The colic and caecal arteries are usually thickened and enlarged to about a centimetre in diameter and have palpable lumps along them. These cases always terminate fatally, due either to peritonitis after rupture of the intestinal wall (7), or to toxaemia caused by gangrene of the intestinal wall. Occasional cases with extensive occlusion die quickly, in 12 to 24 hours, due probably to shock from the massive infarction (8). All forms of treatment, including parasympathetic stimulants, are ineffective but nitrites have been recommended to dilate the vessels (3).

At necropsy, the arteries are partially or completely occluded along a large part of their course and larvae are usually found in the walls or free in the lumen. In severe cases, large patches of gangrene are present in the wall of atonic loops of bowel. Secondary bacterial invasion of the aneurysm may occur and cause gross enlargement and local peritonitis with the development of adhesions and eventual constriction of the intestine. In these cases there is usually a history of intermittent or continuous low-grade abdominal pain over a period as long as several months. The clinical signs are very similar to those of terminal ileal hypertrophy (9) but the two conditions may be distinguishable on the basis of rectal findings. In both diseases confirmation of the diagnosis and treatment can only be effected via a laparotomy incision. Aberrant aneurysms have been found in the hepatic and middle caecal arteries (2) and the ascending aorta (4). Physical obstruction by compression of the caudal vena cava causing oedema of the hind legs has also been recorded (5).

Commonly the disease is not suspected until recurrent attacks of colic occur. Blood eosinophil counts and faecal examinations for worm eggs are of little value in diagnosis. Treatment with an anthelmintic such as thiabendazole (250 mg. per kg. per day), along with supportive treatment when indicated, is recommended (10).

REFERENCES

(1) Ottaway, C. W. & Bingham, M. L. (1946). *Vet. Rec.*, *58*, 155.
(2) Todd, A. C. *et al.* (1951). *J. Amer. vet. med. Ass.*, *118*, 102.
(3) Littlejohn, A. (1958). *J. S. Afr. vet. med. Ass.*, *29*, 67.
(4) Farrelly, B. T. (1954). *Vet. Rec.*, *66*, 53.
(5) Davis, R. W. & Epling, G. P. (1948). *J. Amer. vet. med. Ass.*, *113*, 339.
(6) Zeskov, B. *et al.* (1959). *Amer. J. vet. Res.*, *20*, 448.
(7) Curtis, R. A. (1964). *Canad. vet. J.*, *5*, 36.
(8) Nelson, A. W. *et al.* (1968). *Amer. J. vet. Res.*, *29*, 315.
(9) Mason, T. A. *et al.* (1970). *Aust. vet. J.*, *46*, 349.
(10) Coffman, J. R. & Carlson, K. L. (1971). *J. Amer. vet. med. Ass.*, *158*, 1358.

Impaction of the Large Intestine

Impaction of the large intestine causes moderate abdominal pain, constipation and a syndrome of general depression and anorexia.

Aetiology

In farm animals, the disease is common only in horses and pigs. A number of causative factors are implicated in horses. For the most part, they are dietary causes and include feeding on low-grade, indigestible roughage, particularly old hay and sorghum, defective teeth causing improper mastication of the roughage, and feeding at overlong intervals. Over-fed, fat horses and gross feeders are particularly susceptible to recurrent attacks of the disease. General debility is a predisposing cause in that the diminished intestinal muscle tone is incapable of moving the large bulk of ingesta. Interference with the local blood supply to the intestine, short of complete occlusion of vessels such as occurs in verminous mesenteric arteritis, has the same effect. Enteroliths and fibre-balls may also cause obstruction of the large intestine and usually result in recurrent attacks of colic. Recurrent attacks may also be caused by persistence of any of the causative factors listed above. Retention of the meconium in foals is a common and special occurrence of impaction of the large intestine (1). Colt foals are more commonly affected than fillies, and foals carried overtime and which have a narrow pelvis are most susceptible.

In cows and mares near parturition, an apparent rectal paralysis leading to constipation may occur. The cause is unknown but is considered to be the result of pressure by the foetus or foetuses on pelvic nerves. In pigs, impaction of the colon and rectum occurs sporadically, usually in adult sows which get little exercise and are fed wholly on grain. The disease also occurs in pigs which are overcrowded in sandy or gravelly outdoor yards. A special occurrence in young weaned pigs causes obstruction of the coiled colon. Rectal paralysis is also an occasional development in encephalitis of horses.

Pathogenesis

Continued overloading of the colon and caecum, either primarily, because of the nature of the food, or secondarily, because of poor intestinal motility, causes prolongation of the intestinal sojourn and excessive inspissation of faecal material so that movement of the mass by peristalsis is still further impaired. If the process is prolonged, the colon becomes insensitive to the stimuli caused by distension which normally provoke defaecation. Chronic constipation results.

In horses, the effects of impaction of the large intestine are more serious than in other animals because of the tremendous capacity of the organ. Accumulation of faecal material occurs gradually until sufficient distension is present to cause pain. Auto-intoxication may also play a part in the production of clinical signs. Although impaction of the caecum and colon usually occur together, it is not uncommon to find maximum impaction in one particular region. Thus impaction may be restricted to the caecum, the small colon or the pelvic flexure of the large colon.

In pigs, the effects appear to be due largely to auto-intoxication although the commonly occurring posterior paresis seems more likely to be due to pressure from inspissated faecal material.

Clinical Findings

Moderate abdominal pain is the typical sign in affected horses. This often continues for 3 to 4 days and sometimes for as long as 2 weeks. A very long course of more than 3 to 4 days is usually associated with caecal impaction. The horse is not violent and the bouts of pain are of moderate severity occurring at intervals of up to a half-hour. There is anorexia and constipation, and the faeces are passed in small amounts and are hard and covered with thick, sticky mucus. Intestinal sounds are absent or much decreased in intensity. Rectal palpation usually enables one to detect the cause of the trouble.

Impaction of the pelvic flexure of the large colon is the commonest site and the distended, solid loop of the intestine often extends to the pelvic brim or even to the right of the midline. Lying on the floor of the abdomen, it is easily palpated, the faecal mass can be indented with the fingers and the curvature and groove between the dorsal and ventral loops of the left colon can be easily discerned. Impaction of the caecum can be palpated in the right flank extending from high up and passing downwards and anteriorly. An impacted small colon may be felt dorsally to the right of the midline and almost at arm's length. Its diameter is much less than that of the other segments and it may be confused with an impacted terminal ileum.

The pulse rate may be moderately increased but does not usually rise above 50 per minute and the temperature and respiratory rates are unaffected. Although the animal does not eat, it may drink small quantities of water at frequent intervals, often standing by the water trough and sipping or lapping the water continuously. Most cases respond satisfactorily to treatment although impaction of the caecum is difficult to relieve and may cause a fatal termination. Recurrence of impaction of the large intestine is common and is usually due to failure to correct the cause. When deaths occur, they are due to rupture of the intestine or from exhaustion after a long course.

Retention of the meconium in foals causes continuous straining with elevation of the tail, humping of the back with the feet under the body and even walking backwards. There is no toxaemia and the colt continues to suck intermittently but is inclined to be restless and lie down for much of the time. Hard faecal balls can be palpated with the finger in the rectum.

In pigs, the syndrome has no specific signs. There is anorexia and dullness and the pig is recumbent much of the time. Faeces passed are scanty, very hard and covered with mucus. Weakness to the point of inability to rise occurs in some cases. Hard balls of faeces in the rectum are usually detected when a thermometer is inserted. In paralysis of the rectum, there is inability to defaecate and usually some straining. The anus and rectum are ballooned and manual removal of the faeces does not result in contraction of the rectum. Spontaneous recovery usually occurs three or four days after parturition.

Clinical Pathology

Laboratory examinations are not usually undertaken except for faecal examinations for nematode eggs.

Necropsy Findings

The large intestine is packed full of firm, dry faecal material and rupture may have occurred.

Diagnosis

Other causes of constipation such as peritonitis and dehydration must be considered when making a diagnosis of impaction of the large intestine.

Other forms of colic can be eliminated from consideration largely on the basis of rectal palpation, the absence of systemic signs and intestinal sounds. Acute gastric dilatation, acute intestinal obstruction and spasmodic colic are more severe and have a much shorter course. Palpation of the cranial mesenteric artery is necessary to make a diagnosis of verminous mesenteric arteritis. In foals, tympany of the large intestine occurs but is much more serious, with abdominal distension and acute abdominal pain the cardinal signs. Moderate straining, dullness and gradual distension of the abdomen are the main clinical features of rupture of the bladder in new-born foals and this can be mistaken for retention of the meconium.

Treatment

Many forms of treatment have been used in horses but the most satisfactory is the administration of $\frac{1}{2}$ to 1 gallon of mineral oil with $\frac{1}{2}$ to 1 oz. of chloral hydrate in 1 quart of water by nasal tube. A common alternative to the chloral is the parenteral administration of an ataractic drug. If the impaction is not relieved in 12 hours, the treatment is repeated, together with the subcutaneous injection of a parasympathetic stimulant. Parasympathetic stimulants should not be used without prior administration of oil to soften the faecal mass, or rupture of the over-distended intestine may result. Most cases respond to the first treatment but more severe cases may require a second treatment. Impactions of the caecum are the most intractable as soft faeces may be passed through the dorsal sac without emptying the ventral sac. For such cases the injection of 6 to 10 oz. of warm mineral oil directly into the caecal mass through the rectal or abdominal wall has been recommended (3). Linseed oil may be used instead of mineral oil but has no particular advantage. Detergents have been found to be of value when combined with mineral oil in severe constipation in humans (2) and are now used in the treatment of animals.

Other treatments include the use of more violent purgatives including the anthracene purgative aloes or its synthetic counterparts. These are quite effective and work more rapidly than mineral oil but have the disadvantage that the dose rate has to be carefully controlled to avoid overpurgation, and underdosing may result in failure to respond. Hot, soapy-water enemas used to be employed but are of debatable value. In constipated cows and sows mineral oil, Epsom or Glaubers salts or an anthracene purgative are usually used, but it has been suggested that non-irritant substances are to be preferred. Standardized senna is recommended for sows, particularly for those in late pregnancy (5).

Retention of the meconium in foals is treated by injecting mineral oil (2 to 3 oz.) or glycerin (1 oz.) or Coloxyl (dioctyl sodium sulphosuccinate) into the rectum with a 12 in. rubber tube. The enemas are repeated until soft faeces appear and the foal is comfortable. Oral doses of Coloxyl or 4 to 8 oz. of mineral oil are also advised. Affected foals should be treated regularly at 4-hour intervals until recovery. Some cases prove to be most obstinate and hard faecal masses continue to be passed for several days even though soft faecal material is being passed as well. Small doses of parasympathetic stimulants ($\frac{1}{8}$ to $\frac{1}{16}$ of the adult dose) may hasten recovery at this stage. In some cases, removal of the masses by traction with blunt forceps or by colostomy is necessary. Surgical removal is indicated when the foal has not sucked for more than 2 hours and its life is therefore endangered, or when the amount of meconium present is large, when the rectum has been damaged or is too small to permit of manipulation (4).

REFERENCES

(1) Leader, G. H. (1952). *Vet. Rec.*, *64*, 241.
(2) Annotation (1955). *Lancet*, *269*, 128.
(3) Nagorski, F. & Joszt, B. (1958). *Méd. Vét. Varsovie*, *14*, 470.
(4) Littlejohn, A. (1963). *Vet. Rec.*, *75*, 729.
(5) Sassoon, H. F. (1965). *Brit. vet. J.*, *121*, 171.

CONGENITAL DEFECTS OF THE ALIMENTARY TRACT

Congenital Atresia of the Salivary Ducts

Congenital atresia of salivary ducts usually results in distension of the gland followed by atrophy. Rarely the gland may continue secreting, resulting in a gross distension of the duct (5).

Agnathia and Micrognathia

These are variations of a developmental deficiency of the mandible, relatively common in sheep. The mandible and its associated structures is partially or completely absent (6).

Persistence of the Right Aortic Arch

Persistence of the right aortic arch as a fibrous band may occlude the oesophagus and cause signs of obstruction, particularly chronic bloat in young calves.

Terminal Ileitis

Terminal ileitis of pigs, horses and sheep occurs as a hyperplasia of the ileal musculature, sometimes with gross thickening of the intestinal wall and diverticulosis (2). Ulceration with perforation may lead to fatal peritonitis.

Congenital Atresia of the Colon and Anus

Atresia of the anus in pigs, the terminal colon in horses and the ileum and colon (3, 4) in cattle are thought to be inherited defects. Sporadic cases occur in the new-born animals of all species. The defect is obvious when the anus is absent but passage of a rectal tube may be necessary to detect atresia of the intestine (1).

REFERENCES

(1) Maclellan, M. & Martin, J. A. (1956). *Vet. Rec.*, *68*, 458.
(2) Cordes, D. O. & Dewes, H. F. (1971). *N.Z. vet. J.*, *19*, 108.
(3) Norrish, J. G. & Rennie, J. C. (1968). *J. Hered.*, *59*, 186.
(4) Osborne, J. C. & Legates, J. E. (1963). *J. Amer. vet. med. Ass.*, *142*, 1104.
(5) Fowler, M. E. (1965). *J. Amer. vet. med. Ass.*, *146*, 1403.
(6) Smith, I. D. (1968). *Aust. vet. J.*, *44*, 510.

NEOPLASMS OF THE ALIMENTARY TRACT

Neoplasms of the alimentary tract are uncommon in farm animals. Squamous-cell carcinomas occasionally develop in the mouth and stomach of horses and the rumen of cattle (1). In the mouth, the tumours usually arise from the gums and cause interference with mastication. They occur most commonly in aged animals and probably arise from alveolar epithelium after periodontitis has caused chronic hyperplasia. In the stomach of the horse, they occur in the cardiac portion and may cause obscure indigestion syndromes, including obstruction of the lower oesophagus, or ulcerate to permit perforation of the stomach wall and the development of peritonitis. Ruminal tumours may obstruct the cardia and cause chronic tympany. In lymphomatosis of cattle, there is frequently gross involvement in the abomasal wall causing persistent diarrhoea. Ulceration, haemorrhage and pyloric obstruction may also occur. Papillomas (2) sometimes involve the pharynx, oesophagus, oesophageal groove and reticulum and cause chronic ruminal tympany in cattle.

A high incidence of malignant neoplasia affecting the pharynx, oesophagus and rumen has been recorded in one area in South Africa (3, 4). The tumours were multicentric in origin and showed evidence of malignancy on histological examination. The clinical disease was chronic and confined to adult animals with persistent, moderate tympany of the rumen and progressive emaciation as typical signs.

REFERENCES

(1) Wood, C. *et al.* (1957). *Vet. Rec.*, 69, 1066.
(2) Ascott, E. W. (1946). *Vet. Rec.*, 58, 39.
(3) Plowright, W. (1955). *J. comp. Path.*, 65, 108.
(4) Plowright, W. *et al.* (1971). *Brit. J. Cancer*, 25, 72.

DISEASES OF THE PERITONEUM

Peritonitis

Inflammation of the peritoneum is accompanied by abdominal pain which varies in degree with the severity and extent of the peritonitis. Tenderness on palpation, rigidity of the abdominal wall, constipation and a systemic reaction are the typical manifestations.

Aetiology

In farm animals, the commonest causes of peritonitis are perforating lesions of the alimentary or genital tracts. Traumatic reticuloperitonitis in cattle and goats, perforation of an abomasal ulcer in cattle, perforation of ulcers in the ileum in regional ileitis in pigs, spread of infection from abscesses in the intestinal wall in oesophagostomiasis in sheep and from perforation of gastric ulcers caused by larvae of *Gasterophilus* spp. and *Habronema megastomum* in horses are among the common causes. Rupture of the stomach or intestine when acute dilatation or obstruction occurs is always followed by the development of acute peritonitis, although shock and internal haemorrhage are much more important as causes of death. Even before rupture in most obstructions, including abomasal torsion, a severe degree of peritonitis develops because of passage of infection through the devitalized and permeable wall of the obstructed portion. A similar picture is seen in acute rumenitis in cattle after overeating on grain.

Rupture of the vagina may occur when coitus is violent particularly when young heifers which are not properly in oestrus are served by young, active bulls. Spontaneous rupture of the uterus at parturition or during manual correction of dystocia is usually followed by shock and haemorrhage, although these may be remarkably slight in cattle, and peritonitis may not follow if the uterine contents are not contaminated. Failure of the uterus to heal or be repaired may be followed by peritonitis in several days. Sadistic rupture of the vagina is an occasional cause of peritonitis.

Traumatic perforation of the abdominal wall from the exterior by horn gores, stake wounds, trocarization to relieve ruminal or caecal tympany, faulty asepsis during laparotomy, and during intra-peritoneal injections are less common causes of peritonitis but are amongst the most difficult ones to treat because of the mixed bacterial flora which is usually present. Rupture of abscesses in the spleen, liver and umbilical vessels and in sub-peritoneal sites may also give rise to peritonitis. Less commonly, haematogenous infections localize in the peritoneum. Tuberculosis and actinomycosis may cause peritonitis in this way or be spread from local lesions in other organs. Spontaneous rupture of the rectum at calving has been recorded (1) and the possibility of sadistic rupture must always be borne in mind.

Peritonitis may also occur as part of several specific diseases, including Glasser's disease in pigs, in serositis-arthritis of sheep and goats and sporadic bovine encephalomyelitis in cattle, in all of which a serofibrinous inflammation occurs in all serous membranes.

Pathogenesis

At least four factors operate in the genesis of clinical signs in peritonitis. They are toxaemia or septicaemia, paralytic ileus, accumulation of fluid exudate, and the development of adhesions. Toxins produced by bacteria and by the breakdown of tissue are absorbed readily through the peritoneum. The resulting toxaemia is the most important factor in the production of clinical illness and its severity is usually governed by the size of the area of peritoneum involved. In acute diffuse peritonitis, the toxaemia is profound; in local inflammation, it is negligible. The type of infection present is obviously important because of variations between bacteria in their virulence and toxin production.

Paralytic ileus arises as a result of reflex inhibition of alimentary tract tone and movement in acute peritonitis. The net effect is one of functional obstruction of the intestine, and it is in many cases irreversible, playing a major part in causing a fatal outcome of the case. Initially there may be a temporary increase in motility, also mediated through extrinsic reflexes, but the resulting diarrhoea is usually transient and of minor degree.

In chronic peritonitis, the formation of adhesions is more important than either of the two preceding factors. Adhesions are an essential part of the healing process and are important in that they localize infection to a particular segment of the peritoneum. If this healing process is developing satisfactorily and the signs of peritonitis are diminishing, it is a common experience to find that vigorous exercise may cause breakdown of the adhesions, spread of the peritonitis and return of the clinical signs. Thus, a cow treated conservatively for traumatic reticuloperitonitis by immobilization on an incline may show an excellent recovery by the third day but, if allowed to go out to pasture at this time, may suffer an acute relapse. The secondary role of adhesions is to cause partial or complete obstruction of the intestine or stomach, or by fixation, to interfere with normal gut motility. Adhesions are of major importance in the production of vagus indigestion of cattle and may cause intestinal obstruction in horses as a sequel to mesenteric verminous arteritis or perforation of a gastric ulcer.

Accumulation of large quantities of inflammatory exudate in the peritoneal cavity may cause visible abdominal distension and interfere with respiration by obstruction of diaphragmatic movement. It is a comparatively rare occurrence but needs to be considered in the differential diagnosis of abdominal distension.

Abdominal pain is a variable sign in peritonitis. In acute, diffuse peritonitis, the toxaemia may be sufficiently severe to depress the response of the animal to the pain stimuli but, in less severe cases, the animal usually adopts an arched-back posture and shows evidence of pain on palpation of the abdominal wall. Inflammation of the serous surfaces of the peritoneum causes pain and a reflex effect is mediated through spinal cord reflex arcs to cause rigidity of the abdominal wall and the assumption of abnormal posture.

Clinical Findings

Acute diffuse peritonitis. The most constant signs, except in cases where the toxaemia is profound, are those of abdominal pain including arching of the back, lack of desire to move, and persistent standing. If the animal does lie down, it is usually with great care and after some preliminary fidgeting and grunting. Horses are probably more inclined to persistent recumbency than cattle but many of them do remain standing and lie down infrequently. Walking is usually only undertaken if the animal is forced and the gait is shuffling and cautious, the animal tending to keep its back arched and the trunk rigid. Grunting commonly occurs at each step, and when the animal defaecates or urinates. Affected animals are reluctant to pass urine and faeces and, when urination does occur, there are usually very large amounts voided. Sudden movements, including running and jumping, are always avoided and there is an absence of kicking or bellowing, and licking of the coat. There is usually complete anorexia.

The above clinical picture is observed in the most common syndrome of acute peritonitis. Less commonly, the early stages are accompanied by signs of acute abdominal pain, including kicking at the belly, rolling and restlessness. On physical examination in either case, there is an elevation of temperature which varies between 39·5 and 41·5 °C (103 and 107 °F), depending on severity, and a moderate increase in pulse and respiration rates, the latter caused by absence of abdominal movement. Alimentary tract sounds may be increased transiently in the early stages but disappear quickly and the abdomen is usually silent. Vomiting may occur at this stage in pigs. Evidence of pain can be elicited by percussion or palpation of the abdominal wall. It may be possible to elicit pain over the entire abdominal wall if the peritonitis is widespread, or over only a small area if it is localized. Tenseness of the abdominal wall produces the characteristic posture and apparent gauntness of the abdomen, but the rigidity cannot usually be detected clinically because in the normal animal the abdominal wall is tense. Rarely, inflammatory exudate accumulates in quantities sufficient to cause visible abdominal distension. Its presence can be confirmed by succussion and by paracentesis.

Constipation is usually present and the faeces are dark and often accompanied by large quantities of thick mucus and, in some cases, mucus only is voided. On rectal examination, no abnormality can be detected other than evidence of pain on palpation, and in long-standing cases adhesions may be present. Faeces are usually present in the rectum and, although the amount may be small, they are normal except for being dry and hard.

In those cases in which profound toxaemia occurs, especially in cows immediately after calving or when rupture of the alimentary tract occurs, the syndrome is quite different. There is severe weakness, depression and circulatory failure. The animal is recumbent and often unable to rise, depressed almost to the point of coma, has a subnormal temperature of 37 to 37·5 °C (99 to 100 °F), a high heart rate (100 to 120 per minute), and a very weak pulse. No abdominal pain is evidenced spontaneously or on palpation.

The outcome in cases of acute, diffuse peritonitis varies with the severity. Peracute cases accompanied by severe toxaemia usually die within 24 to 48 hours. The more common, less severe cases may be fatal in 4 to 7 days but adequate treatment may result in recovery in about the same length of time.

Acute local peritonitis. The clinical syndrome is similar to that of acute diffuse peritonitis but the signs are less severe. Arching of the back and disinclination to move occur but pain can be elicited over a small area only and the temperature and pulse rate are only moderately elevated. The outcome is more likely to be favourable unless adhesions are broken down and the peritonitis spreads.

Chronic peritonitis. The development of adhesions which interfere with normal alimentary tract movements, and gradual spread of infection as adhesions break down combine to produce a chronic syndrome of indigestion and toxaemia which is punctuated by short, recurrent attacks of more severe illness. The adhesions may be detectable on rectal examination but they are usually situated in the anterior abdomen and are impalpable. If partial intestinal obstruction occurs, the bouts of pain are usually accompanied by a marked increase in alimentary tract sounds and palpable distension of intestinal loops with gas and fluid. The course in chronic peritonitis may be as long as some months and the prognosis is not favourable because of the presence of physical lesions caused by scar tissue and adhesions.

In specific diseases in which peritonitis occurs secondarily, there are other signs which are usually more apparent clinically.

Clinical Pathology

Haematological observations are commonly used as an indicator of the presence and severity of peritonitis but do not usually add much to the clinical assessment of the case. In peracute cases, there is often a profound leucopenia (2000 to 3000 leucocytes per cmm.) but in most cases of acute diffuse peritonitis, there is an elevation of the leucocyte count to over 12,000 per cmm., and a marked neutrophilia and shift to the left. In acute local peritonitis, the neutrophilia and shift to the left occur but the total count may be within the normal range and, in chronic peritonitis, there is usually no detectable abnormality. Becteriological examination of fluid removed by paracentesis may be possible in some cases and may give some indication of the antibacterial treatment required. In cattle the abdomen is entered on the left of the midline and 3 to 4 cm. medial and 5 to 7 cm. cranial to the foramen for the left subcutaneous abdominal vein (2).

Necropsy Findings

In acute diffuse peritonitis, the entire peritoneum is involved but the most severe lesions are usually in the ventral abdomen. Gross haemorrhage into the subserosa, exudation and fibrin deposits in the peritoneal cavity and fresh adhesions which are easily broken down are present. In less acute cases, the exudate is purulent and may be less fluid, often forming a thick cheesy covering over most of the viscera. In cattle, *Sphaerophorus necrophorus* and *Corynebacterium pyogenes* are often present in large numbers and produce a typical, nauseating odour. Acute local peritonitis and chronic peritonitis are not usually fatal and the lesions are discovered only if the animal dies of intercurrent disease such as traumatic pericarditis or intestinal obstruction.

Diagnosis

The diagnosis of peritonitis is most difficult in cases accompanied by marked toxaemia and in severe chronic cases. In the former, the animal is in a state of collapse without localizing signs. In cattle, the syndrome is reminiscent of parturient paresis although the pulse rate is much more rapid in peritonitis and there is no response to calcium injections. Soon after the injection is commenced, the heart rate increases markedly and death due to acute heart failure may occur. Severe dehydration in acute ruminal impaction, in abomasal torsion or intestinal obstruction may be manifested by a similar syndrome in the terminal stage but there are usually clinical signs and items in the history which aid in the diagnosis.

The intermittent indigestion of chronic peritonitis may simulate that which occurs in lipomatosis or extensive fat necrosis of the mesentery and omentum, and in repeated overeating in horses. Vagus indigestion of cattle is a syndrome which has several characteristic features, including a continuous course, scanty faeces, abdominal distension and atony of the abomasum.

Differentiation of the cause of peritonitis is difficult if possible causes are not suggested by the history or by the presence of signs of primary, specific disease. Special diagnostic features are present in traumatic reticuloperitonitis, the commonest cause of peritonitis in cattle.

Treatment

The specific cause must be treated in each case and the treatments used are described under the specific diseases listed above. Non-specific treatment includes the administration of antibacterial drugs, including broad-spectrum antibiotics and sulphonamides, to control the infection, and the treatment of the toxaemia. Antibacterial drugs can be administered orally or parenterally but the best route is by intraperitoneal injection to give maximum concentration at the site of inflammation. The drug is usually administered in isotonic saline or electrolyte solutions, the quantity varying with the need to provide parenteral alimentation. If adhesions are likely to be present or the area of inflammation small, there is probably no advantage in the intraperitoneal route and, if the primary lesion is in the alimentary tract, there is probably an advantage in giving the drug by mouth provided the alimentary tract flora is not unfavourably depressed. If large quantities of exudate are present in the peritoneal cavity, surgical drainage is advisable to remove the source of toxins.

No attempt should be made to prevent the development of adhesions although, if they are extensive, they may cause inconvenience later. The treatment of toxaemia has been described elsewhere.

REFERENCES

(1) Kruiningen, H. J. van. *et al.* (1961). *Cornell Vet.*, *51*, 557.
(2) Oehme, F. W. & Noordsy, J. L. (1970). *Vet. Med.*, *65*, 55.

Lipomatosis

(*Abdominal Fat Necrosis*)

The hard masses of necrotic fat which occur relatively commonly in the peritoneal cavity of adult cattle, especially the Channel Island breeds and possibly Aberdeen-Angus, are commonly mistaken for a developing foetus and can cause intestinal obstruction (1). The latter usually develops slowly resulting in the appearance of attacks of moderate abdominal pain and the passage of small amounts of faeces. Many cases are detected during routine rectal examination of normal animals. One usually finds only sporadic cases but there is one report of a herd prevalence as high as 67 per cent (4). The cause is unknown but an inherited predisposition is suggested (2). An unusual form of the disease with many lesions in subcutaneous sites has been recorded in Holstein-Friesian cattle and is regarded as being inherited (3). There is no treatment and affected animals should be salvaged. A generalized steatitis has been reported in pony foals (5).

REFERENCES

(1) Edgson, F. A. (1952). *Vet. Rec.*, *64*, 449.
(2) Bridge, P. S. & Spratling, F. R. (1962). *Vet. Rec.*, *74*, 1357.
(3) Albright, J. L. (1960). *J. Hered.*, *51*, 231.
(4) Williams, D. J. *et al.* (1969). *J. Amer. vet. med. Ass.*, *154*, 1017.
(5) Platt, H. & Whitwell, K. E. (1971). *J. comp. Path.*, *81*, 499.

Diseases of the Alimentary Tract—II

DISEASES OF THE STOMACHS OF RUMINANTS

THE stomachs of ruminants are closely associated anatomically and functionally, and disease of one usually affects the others (1). The rumen is easily examined clinically and experimentally and it is usually used as an indicator of the state of the other stomachs. Bacterial digestion and fermentation, and physical maceration by contraction of the stomach walls are the two main functions of the forestomachs and the two are interdependent. Thus abnormality of one leads to abnormality of the other and of the two the motility is most readily examinable. Ruminal motility is therefore used as an index of digestive function in the ruminant.

The plain muscle of the forestomachs has no intrinsic contractile power and the movement of the walls of these organs depends upon the integrity of the afferent and efferent nerves and the reticulo-ruminal motor centre of the medulla. Both afferent and efferent fibres are carried in the vagus nerves and damage to one or other branches of the nerve causes interference with normal movements and produces the syndrome of vagus indigestion.

When food enters the forestomachs it normally divides into layers, an upper layer of free gas and a lower layer of fluid containing gas bubbles and suspended food particles. A layer of undigested fibre floats on top and heavy material such as grain sinks to the bottom, often in the reticulum. Much mixing of the contents of the rumen and reticulum takes place during ruminal movements which occur at the rate of 1 to 3 per minute, the more rapid rate occurring soon after feeding.

The movements occur in cycles commencing with a double reticular contraction, the second of which is accompanied by a strong contraction of the anterior dorsal sac of the rumen. These contractions pour the fluid reticular contents over the bulky food mass in the rumen. A contraction of the ventral sac follows and fluid is returned to the reticulum. The clinical evidence of this cycle of contractions has been dealt with in Chapter 1. During each reticular contraction fluid and food particles, particularly heavy grain, pass into the reticulo-omasal orifice and into the omasum and abomasum. It is this passage of heavy grain directly into the abomasum, without in many instances proper digestion in the rumen, which may lead to overloading of the abomasum and resultant displacement or torsion of this organ. It may also be important in the pathogenesis of enterotoxaemia caused by *Clostridium perfringens* Type D. If the floor of the reticulum is fixed to the ventral abdominal wall by adhesions it may be impossible for fluid to pass into the reticulo-omasal orifice. This may be a factor in the development of some forms of vagus indigestion.

Eructation contractions occur in the dorsal sacs, pass forward to the cardia of the oesophagus and in conjunction with a reticular relaxation depress the level of the reticular fluid. The cardia relaxes and gas is expelled. If the ruminal contents are frothy it may be impossible for the cardia to be cleared and eructation to occur; ruminal tympany follows. Eructation contractions are independent of mixing contractions, their rate depending upon the pressure of the gas in the rumen. They occur for the most part, immediately after the mixing contractions.

Rumination also depends upon additional ruminal contractions which are interposed before normal mixing movements of the rumen. These special contractions keep the area of the oesophageal cardia flooded with reticular fluid. A voluntary movement by the animal follows: an inspiratory effort is made with the glottis closed: the negative pressure in the thorax is greatly increased and the reticular fluid, carrying some floating ingesta, is carried up to the pharynx. Defects of regurgitation are usually due to inability to create the necessary negative pressure in the thorax; this may occur in chronic pulmonary emphysema. In these circumstances there are usually visible efforts at regurgitation, often accompanied by grunting. Regurgitation ceases as soon as ruminal atony occurs because of absence of the ruminal contractions necessary to keep the cardial region filled with fluid. However, regurgitation contractions play no part in the movement of the bolus up the oesophagus. Regurgitation also diminishes when regurgitation contractions are not stimulated by coarse fibre in the rumen. Cattle on pelleted or finely ground diets ruminate little or not at all. Rumination is also depressed by excitement and fear.

The factors which affect the motility of the rumen are discussed in the section on simple indigestion as are the principles of treatment in cases of ruminal atony.

REFERENCE

(1) Leek, B. F. (1969). *Vet. Rec.*, *84*, 238.

Simple Indigestion

Simple indigestion is caused by atony of the forestomachs and is characterized clinically by anorexia, lack of ruminal movement and constipation.

Aetiology

The disease is common in dairy cattle because of the variability in quality and the large amounts of the food consumed. It is not commonly observed in beef cattle or sheep probably because they are less heavily fed. The common causes are dietary abnormalities of minor degree including indigestible roughage, particularly when the protein intake is low, mouldy, over-heated and frosted feeds, and moderate excesses of grain and concentrate intake (10). Cases occur under excellent feeding régimes and are usually ascribed to over-feeding with grain. Although the difference between simple indigestion and acute impaction of the rumen is largely one of degree, their separation can be justified by the marked clinical difference between the two syndromes. Gross over-feeding usually occurs when cattle or sheep gain accidental access to large quantities of grain or are suddenly introduced to high grain diets in feed-lots. Indigestion is more common when heavily fed cows are fed a little more concentrate than they can digest properly. Sudden change to a new source of grain, especially from oats to wheat or barley may have the same effect.

Indigestible roughage may include straw, bedding or scrub fed during drought periods. It is probable that limitation of the available drinking water may contribute to the occurrence of the disease during dry seasons. Depraved appetite may also contribute to the ingestion of coarse indigestible material. Although good quality ensilage cannot be considered an indigestible roughage, cases of indigestion can occur in cattle which are allowed unlimited access to it. This is most likely to happen in heavy-producing cows running outside in cold weather and whose hay and grain rations are limited. It is not uncommon for big Holstein cows to eat 90 to 100 lb. of ensilage daily in such circumstances and the high intake of acetate and acetic acid (9) may be sufficient to depress their appetite. Prolonged or heavy oral dosing with sulphonamides or antibiotics may cause indigestion due to inhibition of the normal ruminal flora. Especially in Jersey cattle it is not uncommon to encounter ruminal atony which responds to parenteral treatment with calcium salts.

Pathogenesis

Primary atony caused by dietary abnormality is difficult to explain. Changes in the pH of its contents markedly affect the motility of the rumen and in cases caused by overeating on grain an increase in acidity is probably of importance. High protein diets including the feeding of excessively large quantities of legumes or urea, also depress motility because of the sharp increase in alkalinity which results (11). Atony which occurs after feeding on damaged feeds may have the same basis or be due to other unidentified agents in the food. The simple accumulation of indigestible food may physically impede ruminal activity. Putrefaction of protein may also play a part in the production of atony. The toxic amides and amines produced may include histamine which is known to cause ruminal atony when given intravenously and to be reversed by the administration of anti-histamine drugs (2, 3). Histamine is also probably responsible for the atony which occurs in allergy.

Affected cattle usually show a pronounced fall in milk yield caused probably by the sharp fall in volatile fatty acid production in the atonic rumen (1). Rumen contractions appear to play the same role as hunger contractions in simple stomachs and the decreased food intake is probably due to the ruminal atony.

Clinical Findings

A reduction in appetite is the first sign and is followed closely in milking cows by a slight drop in milk production. Both occur suddenly, the anorexia may be partial or complete but the fall in milk yield is relatively slight. The animal's posture is unaffected but there is mild depression and dullness. Rumination ceases and there is constipation with scanty, firm faeces in most cases although diarrhoea may occur on damaged feeds. Ruminal movements are depressed in frequency and force or are absent. There may be moderate tympany, especially with frozen and damaged feeds or in allergy but the usual finding is a firm, doughy, rumen without obvious distension.

There is no systemic reaction and the pulse, temperature and respiration rates are unaffected. Pain cannot be elicited by percussion of the abdominal wall. Most cases recover spontaneously or with simple treatments in about 48 hours.

Clinical Pathology

Examination of the urine for ketone bodies is usually necessary to differentiate indigestion from acetonaemia.

Two simple laboratory tests have been introduced to assess the activity of the ruminal microflora (6). The Sediment Activity Test is carried out on aspirated ruminal fluid strained to remove coarse particles. The strained fluid is allowed to stand in a glass vessel at body temperature and the time required for flotation of the particulate material recorded. The time in normal animals varies between 3 minutes, if the animal has just been fed, and 9 minutes if the last feeding has occurred some time previously. Settling of the particulate material indicates gross inactivity, less severe degrees being manifested by prolongation of the time required for flotation. The Cellulose Digestion Test is also performed on aspirated rumen fluid and depends upon the time required to digest a thread of cotton. A bead is tied to the end of the thread to indicate when separation occurs. Digestion times in excess of 30 hours indicate abnormality.

Necropsy Findings

The disease is not a fatal one.

Diagnosis

The major problem is to differentiate indigestion from acetonaemia and traumatic reticuloperitonitis. Acetonaemia occurs during the first two months after calving and is characterized by marked ketonuria. Traumatic reticuloperitonitis is manifested by a sharper fall in milk yield, a mild elevation of temperature, and pain on percussion of the ventral abdomen. Vagus indigestion is not usually accompanied by fever but runs a protracted course and may be accompanied by abdominal distension and hypermotility or hypomotility of the rumen. Abomasal displacement usually occurs immediately after parturition, is accompanied by ketonuria and abomasal sounds in the lower left flank, and runs a protracted course, often for months. The initial stages of some cases of abomasal torsion may be difficult to distinguish clinically from indigestion but they always terminate fatally. Acute ruminal impaction is a much more serious disease and is accompanied by signs of dehydration and nervous derangement. A history of engorgement on grain is usually forthcoming.

Secondary ruminal atony occurs in many diseases especially when septicaemia or toxaemia are present but there are usually additional clinical signs to indicate their presence. Parturient paresis of cattle and allergic and anaphylactic states are usually accompanied by ruminal stasis but do not cause a syndrome of indigestion, motility returning to normal as soon as the cause is corrected.

Treatment

Rational treatment is often difficult because of lack of knowledge of the aetiology, and for the most part treatment is symptomatic, consisting primarily of the use of rumenatoric drugs. Many drugs are used for this purpose. A number of these have little justification for their use (2, 3, 4) and their reputation depends to a large extent on the tendency of affected animals to recover spontaneously. Tartar emetic (10 to 12 g.) is effective when given orally but causes chemical reticulitis if given in concentrated form in a static rumen (5).

Parasympathetic stimulants are widely used as rumenatorics but have the disadvantage of creating undesirable side-effects and being very transitory in their action. Large doses depress rumen activity but small doses repeated at short intervals increase ruminal activity and promote violent emptying of the colon. Carbamylcholine chloride, physostigmine and neostigmine are most commonly used. The last is the most effective and should be given at a dose rate of 2·5 mg. per 100 lb. body weight (4). Carbamylcholine acts on the musculature only and causes uncoordinated and functionless movements (8). These drugs are not without danger, especially in very sick animals or those with peritonitis, and are specifically contraindicated during late pregnancy.

Epsom salt (1 to 2 pounds) and other magnesium salts are reasonably effective and have the merit of simplicity and cheapness (12). Anthraquinone purgatives in doses of 8 to 15 g. are commonly used with apparent good results, and strychnine preparations (containing up to 65 mg. of strychnine as a single dose for an adult cow) enjoy a good reputation.

More rational therapy should include the use of alkalis, such as magnesium hydroxide or carbonate when the rumen contents are excessively acid, or of an acid, such as acetic acid or vinegar, when the reaction is alkaline. A sample of rumen fluid can be readily obtained and the pH determined approximately by the use of reagent paper. If there is inspissation of ruminal contents 3 to 4 gallons of normal saline should be administered by stomach tube.

Cases of indigestion which have run a course of more than a few days, and animals suffering from prolonged anorexia due to any cause suffer an appreciable loss of ruminal microflora, especially if there have been marked changes in pH. Reconstitution of the flora by the use of rumen transplants is highly effective. An abattoir is the best source of material but it can be obtained from living animals by reaching into the mouth or kneeing the animal in the ribs as a bolus is regurgitated. Fluid may also be removed by siphoning or sucking with a special pump. Best results are obtained if 2 to 3 gallons of normal saline are pumped into the rumen and then withdrawn. The transplant material should be mixed with water, strained and administered as a drench or by stomach tube. Repeated dosing is advisable. The infusion will keep for several days at room temperature. Commercial products comprising dried rumen solids are available and provide some bacteria and substrate for their activity. They are of most value as adjuncts to transplants and have not been found to be highly effective in restoring gastric motility in lambs whose appetite has been reduced by oral administration of chloromycetin (7). To overcome the prevalence of indigestion on low roughage diets a number of commercial 'instant roughages' are available. These are administered once in a meat animal's lifetime and cause stimulation of rumenal activity (13).

When affected animals resume eating they are best tempted by good, stalky meadow or cereal hay. Good quality alfalfa or clover hay, green feed and concentrate may be added to the diet as the appetite improves.

REFERENCES

(1) Stone, E. C. (1949). *Amer. J. vet. Res.*, *10*, 26.
(2) Dougherty, R. W. (1942). *Cornell Vet.*, *32*, 269.
(3) Clark, R. (1950). *J. S. Afr. vet. med. Ass.*, *21*, 13 and 49.
(4) Clark, R. & Weiss, K. E. (1954). *Onderstepoort J. vet. Res.*, *26*, 485.
(5) Stevens, C. E. *et al.* (1959). *J. Amer. vet. med. Ass.*, *134*, 323.
(6) Nichols, R. E. & Penn, K. E. (1958). *J. Amer. vet. med. Ass.*, *133*, 275.
(7) Tucker, J. O. *et al.* (1956). *Amer. J. vet. Res.*, *17*, 498.
(8) Clark, R. (1956). *J. S. Afr. vet. med. Ass.*, *27*, 79.
(9) Dowden, D. R. & Jacobson, D. R. (1960). *Nature, Lond.*, *188*, 148.
(10) Hoflund, S. (1967). *Vet. Bull.*, *37*, 701.
(11) Forenbacher, S. *et al.* (1967). *Vet. Arh.* (*Zagreb*), *37*, 1.
(12) Lamberth, J. L. (1969). *Aust. vet. J.*, *45*, 223.
(13) Anon. (1971). *Vet. Rec. Info. Supp.* No. 76, p. 217.

Acute Impaction of the Rumen

(*Rumen Overload*)

The ingestion of large amounts of highly fermentable, carbohydrate feeds causes an acute illness due to the excess production of lactic acid in the rumen. Clinically the disease is manifested by severe toxaemia, dehydration, blindness, recumbency, complete ruminal stasis and a high mortality rate.

Aetiology

Accidental access to large quantities of whole or ground grain is the most common cause. Feeder cattle and lambs brought into feed-lots and fed on excessive amounts or allowed *ad lib.* access to self-feeders, without a prior period of adjustment to the feed are most commonly affected. Even in adjusted cattle the common practice of feeding to the limit of appetite maintains many animals on the brink of overload. The clinical disease is also recorded in goats (22). The commonly held view that freshly harvested grain is more toxic than old grain appears to have little foundation (17). Animals which break into fields of ripe, green corn, especially during dry seasons, will gorge themselves and develop acute ruminal impaction. Less common occurrences of the disease are after engorgement on apples, grapes (1), bread, bakers' dough, sugar beet, mangels, lush kikuyu grass (27) and sour, wet, brewers' grains (2, 16). Of the grains, oats and grain sorghum are the least dangerous but fatalities may occur when cattle accustomed to feed on the lighter grains are suddenly changed to wheat or barley (28). It is difficult to give an estimate of the amount of grain required to cause illness. Dairy cattle accustomed to heavy grain diets may consume 40 lb. of grain and develop only moderate illness while 20 lb. may be fatal in steers used to hay or pastures only. Intakes of 50 lb. are likely to be fatal but there is a great deal of unexplainable variation between animals (19). On all grain rations it has been suggested that lethal dose rates are 60 to 80 g. per kg. body weight for sheep and 20 g. per kg. for cattle (28).

Pathogenesis

The important factor in the production of the disease is the rapid fermentation of the carbohydrate in the feed by Gram positive cocci (usually *Streptococcus bovis*), with the formation of large quantities of lactic acid which may reach a concentration of 3 per cent (3, 4, 5). The disease can be produced experimentally by the oral administration of mineral acids or large quantities of glucose. As a result of the lactic acid production the osmotic pressure of the ruminal contents increases and fluid is drawn into the rumen from the vascular system and dehydration, haemoconcentration and anuria result. Rumen motility decreases as the pH falls, stasis being complete in a few hours, and the normal rumen microflora are largely destroyed (9) and replaced by lactobacilli and streptococci (20). The degree of acidity that develops governs the severity of the signs produced. In attempting to produce the disease experimentally in sheep, it has been found that signs do not appear if the pH remains above 5·0. In the pH range between 4·5 and 5·0 ruminal stasis occurs in some sheep; between 4·0 and 4·5 stasis occurs in most sheep and they are dejected and take no feed or water for 2 to 7 days. Ruminal movements are absent. Improvement occurs gradually over a period of about 4 days. There is severe depression of volatile fatty acid production due to the destruction of the ruminal bacteria and protozoa.

In sheep that die of the disease there are a number of factors which contribute to the fatality. Dehydration is probably most important but production of histamine and the absorption of lactic acid to produce acidosis also contribute. The acidosis is manifested by polypnoea and depression. When the disease is produced experimentally with mineral acids or glucose no laminitis is apparent but it may occur if wheat or mangels are used (3). This occurrence of laminitis is probably due to the formation of histamine in quantities which vary with the amount of protein in the feed and the degree to which putrefaction occurs. Levels of histamine greater than 70 μg. per ml. of rumen fluid are found in fatal cases (6) but only normal levels of histamine are found in cattle fed on heavy grain diets (23). Laminitis is not a common accompaniment of rumen overload and it is probable that when it does occur it is because the conditions in the affected animal are such as to encourage histamine formation.

Previous exposure to diets high in carbohydrates increases the ability of animals to deal with large amounts of lactic acid by the development of buffering mechanisms in the rumen. Cattle and sheep can become accustomed to intakes of grain which would be toxic at the beginning of the feeding period (7). Changes in the microbial population probably play a part in the adaptation mechanism.

Sufficient lactic acid is produced in most cases to cause a severe chemical rumenitis. This may be of little importance but bacterial or fungal invasion of the lesions may occur and give rise to a more serious rumenitis. Bacterial infections usually lead to the development of metastatic abscesses in the liver which may cause clinical hepatitis but more commonly are symptomless, resulting only in condemnation of the liver at slaughter. Because of the high prevalence of these hepatic lesions in cattle fed on barley some importance has been attributed to the barley awns as traumatic agents (24). Widespread necrosis and gangrene may affect as much as half of the forestomach walls and lead to the development of an acute diffuse peritonitis. The damage to the viscus causes complete atony and this, together with the toxaemia resulting from the gangrene, is usually sufficient to kill the animal.

Clinical Findings

The speed of onset of the illness varies with the nature of the feed, being faster with ground feed than whole grain. The severity of the illness increases with the amount of feed taken. In severe cases clinical illness is apparent within 12 hours of engorgement. In some cases the first sign may be abdominal pain with kicking at the belly. There is profound depression, with hanging of the head and disinclination to move. The respiration is usually increased in rate and may be accompanied by grunting. Anorexia is complete and affected animals usually do not drink much water. There may be moderate distension of the abdomen and slight ruminal tympany but these are never marked. The rumen contents palpated through the left paralumbar fossa are firm and doughy. The nose is dry and mucopurulent exudate accumulates in the nostrils. Grinding of the teeth is a common sign and there is usually diarrhoea with the passage of soft, light-coloured, smelly faeces. In very severe cases there may be profuse diarrhoea accompanied by the passage of much mucus and some blood. Overeating on grapes or apples may be suggested by the presence of large numbers of pips and skins in the faeces although an absence of faeces has been described in grape engorgement (1).

An increase in pulse rate up to 120 to 140 per minute is usual and the pulse is weak. The temperature is usually below normal, 37 to 38·5°C (99 to 101°F) but animals exposed to hot sun may have temperatures up to 41°C (106°F). Ruminal movements are completely absent although the gurgling sounds of gas rising through the large quantity of fluid which accumulates in the rumen may be heard on auscultation. Severely affected animals have a staggery, drunken gait and appear to be blind. They bump into objects and have no eye preservation reflex. The pupillary light reflex appears to be unimpaired. Laminitis may be present but it occurs more commonly as an independent disease in feed-lot cattle on full feed or in bulls being fattened for show.

Recumbency usually follows after about 48 hours but it may be present as an early sign. Affected animals lie quietly, often with the head turned into the flank, and their response to any stimulus is much decreased so that they resemble cases of parturient paresis very closely. Rapid development of acute signs, particularly recumbency, suggests an unfavourable prognosis and the necessity for urgent, radical treatment. Death occurs in 24 to 72 hours in most fatal cases and improvement during this time is best measured in terms of a fall in pulse rate, rise in temperature, return of ruminal movement and the passage of large amounts of soft faeces. Some animals appear to make a temporary improvement but become severely ill again on the third or fourth day. These are probably animals in which severe fungal rumenitis has occurred and death usually follows in 2 to 3 days due to acute diffuse peritonitis.

The syndrome described above is the commonest and most dramatic but when a number of animals have been exposed to over-feeding there are all degrees of severity from this to simple indigestion which responds readily to treatment. The prognosis varies with the severity. If the pulse rate is not increased simple medical treatment with purgatives is sufficient. Animals showing an increase in pulse rate but which remain standing require energetic medical treatment but usually recover. Those animals which stagger, are blind and recumbent, respond unfavourably to treatment and require rumenotomy for removal of the food material from the rumen.

Clinical Pathology

The severity of the disease can usually be determined by physical examination but field and laboratory tests are of some additional value. The degree of haemoconcentration, as indicated by haematocrit estimations, increases with the amount of fluid withdrawn from the tissues into the rumen. The haematocrit rises from a normal of 30 to 32 per cent up to 50 to 60 per cent in the terminal stages and is accompanied by a marked fall of blood pressure. The urine pH falls to about 5·0 and becomes progressively more concentrated and terminally there is complete anuria. Blood lactate and inorganic phosphate levels rise and blood pH and bicarbonate fall appreciably. In the terminal stages blood glucose and phosphate levels are usually greatly elevated (19).

The pH of the ruminal fluid falls and can be measured roughly by the use of indicator papers. A pH of between 4·5 and 5·0 suggests a moderate degree of abnormality but a pH of less than 4·5 suggests severe involvement and a need for energetic treatment. The predominantly gram-negative flora of the rumen is replaced by a gram-positive one and motile infusoria disappear from the ruminal fluid. The progress of the animal can be measured by a fall in haemoconcentration and a rise in pH of the ruminal contents. In experimental sheep affected with rumen overload a fall in pH of the urine was a very early sign. In sheep which were only moderately affected the pH fell from a normal of 8·0 to as low as 5·0 (12). A degree of proteinuria was also observed.

Necropsy Findings

In acute cases which die in 24 to 48 hours the contents of the rumen and reticulum are thin and porridge-like and have a typical odour suggestive of putrefaction. The cornified epithelium may be mushy and easily wiped off leaving a dark, haemorrhagic surface beneath. This change may be quite patchy, caused probably by the production of excess lactic acid in pockets where the grain collects, but is generally restricted to the ventral half of the sacs. Abomasitis and enteritis are also evident in many cases. There is a pronounced thickening and darkening of the blood and the visceral veins stand out prominently.

In cases which have persisted for 3 or 4 days the wall of the reticulum and rumen may be gangrenous. This change is again patchy but may be widespread. In affected areas the wall may be 3 or 4 times the normal thickness, show a soft black mucosal surface raised above surrounding normal areas and a dark red appearance visible through the serous surface. The thickened area is very friable and on cutting has a gelatinous appearance. Histological preparations show infiltration of the area by fungal mycelia and a severe, haemorrhagic necrosis. In the nervous system in cases of 72 hours or more duration demyelination has been reported (18). A terminal ischaemic nephrosis is present in varying degree in most fatal cases of more than several days standing.

If the post-mortem delay is less than an hour estimations of rumen pH may be of value in confirming the diagnosis. A secondary enteritis may be present in cases of long standing.

Diagnosis

A history of engorgement usually is sufficient to confirm the diagnosis but if this is not available the disease can be mistaken for parturient paresis, acute hepatic insufficiency, or poisoning, particularly with arsenic or lead. Parturient paresis is restricted to cows which have recently calved or ewes in late pregnancy or in early lactation. Other forms of hypocalcaemia are not so restricted but in these and in parturient paresis the faeces are hard and dry, there is no evidence of peripheral circulatory collapse and the heart rate is not greatly increased. Acute hepatic insufficiency may be accompanied by blindness and a staggering gait but there is usually jaundice and the heart rate is approximately normal. In arsenic poisoning the enteritis is usually more severe although scouring may not occur in animals which die quickly. Lead poisoning is manifested by more severe nervous signs. Assay of the ingesta, liver and kidney may be necessary if metallic poisons are suspected.

There may be confusion with primary disease of the nervous system but the low body temperature, gross increase in heart rate and complete ruminal stasis, typical of acute ruminal impaction are not manifestations of any of the common diseases. Enterotoxaemia caused by *Cl. perfringens* type D occurs in well-fed calves and lambs, and possibly in cattle up to 2 years of age, and can be diagnosed on the basis of the toxicity of bowel filtrates.

The syndrome of acute indigestion also resembles that of the early stages of traumatic reticuloperitonitis but there is no fever or grunt on abdominal percussion and no change in the white cell count.

Treatment

Mild cases can be treated with purgatives as described under indigestion. In severe cases treatment must be more vigorous. When only one or two animals are affected rumenotomy is advisable. For large numbers of animals the following procedures are recommended. Prevent access to further grain; exercise vigorously for $\frac{1}{2}$ hour three times daily; allow frequent access to water, preferably in limited amounts at a time (19); administer antihistamines, oral antibiotics and an alkaline purgative. More details of some of these procedures are provided below.

Oral treatment should include the use of an alkaline aperient. Magnesium hydroxide and magnesium carbonate are most commonly used and in cattle after an initial dose of $\frac{1}{2}$ to 1 pound additional 4 oz. doses should be given at 12 hour intervals. Orally administered antibiotics including penicillin and the tetracyclines are capable of restricting the growth of the bacteria which produce the lactic acid but the dose rates required have not been accurately estimated (5, 8). Doses of 0·5 to 1·0 million units of penicillin are effective in sheep and doses of 5 to 10 million units are recommended in cattle. Alternatively, doses of 8 to 10 g. of tetracycline are recommended in cattle. Acid production may occur

when the effect of the antibiotic wears off and repeated dosing at 12 hour intervals may be necessary.

Repair of the dehydration can be carried out by the parenteral administration of large quantities of isotonic fluids. At least 4 litres per day should be given and 8 to 10 litres may be barely sufficient in severe cases. A moderate transient improvement always occurs after the fluids are given and may last for 12 to 24 hours but even the most energetic treatment may serve only to prolong the life of the animal without avoiding a fatal outcome in severe cases. Attempts to control the acidaemia must be approached with caution. The intravenous injection of 500 ml. of a 2·5 per cent solution of sodium bicarbonate usually has a markedly beneficial but transient effect, and a fatal alkalosis with hyperpnoea and tetany may be produced if the injection is given too rapidly or repeated too frequently. Oral dosing with sodium bicarbonate (4 oz. twice daily in cattle) is less dangerous but severe alkalosis may occur, although its use is hard to justify in the light of the known pathogenesis of the disease. European reports indicate a favourable response following the intravenous injection of thiamine in doses of 2 to 4 g. Excellent results are claimed especially if the use of alkalinizing agents, both orally and parenterally, and calcium preparations are avoided (13, 20, 21). Methylene blue administered intravenously is recommended as a supportive treatment. For mild cases and as a follow-up to parenteral treatment with thiamine oral dosing with bakers' yeast (2 lb. daily) is recommended.

Ancillary treatments include particularly the use of antihistamines. There is controversy over the usefulness of these drugs but field experience suggests that they have value in the prevention of laminitis in cases of engorgement on grain. Calcium borogluconate in the dose rates used in the treatment of parturient paresis is used in recumbent animals and may cause sufficient improvement to permit the animal to rise.

Emergency rumenotomy should be performed in serious cases, the rumen emptied completely and even fluids siphoned off and the rumen washed out (10). The contents should be replaced by twists of hay, some water and if possible a rumen transplant although this can be given subsequently by drench. Because a large part of the ruminal microflora is destroyed by the acidity of the rumen in all cases which recover from grain engorgement, a rumen transplant is advisable as soon as clinical improvement commences. Rumen transplants should also be given to cattle treated with large doses of antibiotics by mouth. An alternative to rumenotomy is gastric lavage utilizing a large-bore stomach tube (14). Warm water is pumped in and sucked out repeatedly until most of the grain has been removed. The method has merit especially when fat steers are affected and surgery is undesirable but it is tedious and time consuming and not always satisfactory.

Prevention

The disease is so highly fatal and so unpredictable in its severity that all possible measures must be taken to prevent it especially in feeder cattle which are most commonly exposed. Commencement of feeding grain in a mixture of 25 per cent grain, 75 per cent roughage with gradual change over a month's time to a 75 per cent grain–25 per cent roughage mixture is a safe procedure especially if the grain and roughage are ground through the same machine (26). With present-day emphasis on more haste and less care, there is a strong demand to reduce the change-over period and it has been shown that adaptation to the new diet can be effected in 2 to 6 days (25) in some cases but 2 weeks has been insufficient in others (28). Also, modern beef cattle husbandry practice tends to aim towards greater utilization of grain in the ration, and rations consisting almost entirely of grain are now being fed. Although the results appear satisfactory (11), information is gradually accumulating on the high incidence of rumenitis and ruminal parakeratosis on high-concentrate rations.

Cattle fed very heavily on grain are often fed by self-feeders and if these are made available without suitable preparation many deaths may occur. The most satisfactory method of preparation is to feed gradually increasing amounts of grain until saturation is reached, the stage where the cattle do not clean up all the grain provided, and then move the self-feeders into the pen.

The addition of alkalinizing agents to the ration of beef cattle fed heavily on grain suggests itself as a preventive measure, and although it has not been recorded as preventing rumen overload under experimental conditions, supplementation of such rations to a level of 7·2 per cent with a mixture of ground limestone and sodium bicarbonate (15), or 7·5 per cent sodium bicarbonate (24), significantly increased feed consumption and improved gains and feed efficiency and the latter method reduced the incidence of rumenitis to negligible levels.

REFERENCES

(1) Portway, B. (1957). *Aust. vet. J., 33*, 210.
(2) Worden, A. N. *et al.* (1954). *Vet. Rec., 66*, 133.
(3) Scarisbrick, R. (1954). *Vet. Rec., 66*, 131.
(4) Mackenzie, D. D. S. (1967). *J. Dairy Sci., 50*, 1772.
(5) Bullen, J. J. & Battey, I. (1957). *Vet. Rec., 69*, 1268.
(6) Dain, J. A. *et al.* (1955). *J. Anim. Sci., 14*, 930.
(7) Reid, R. L. *et al.* (1957). *Aust. J. agric. Res., 8*, 691.
(8) Bullen, J. J. & Scarisbrick, R. (1957). *J. Path. Bact., 73*, 495.
(9) Hungate, R. E. *et al.* (1952). *Cornell Vet., 42*, 423.
(10) Fox, F. H. (1956). *Proc. 92nd. ann. gen. Mtg. Amer. vet. med. Ass.*, p. 43.
(11) Wise, M. B. *et al.* (1961). *J. Anim. Sci., 20*, 561.
(12) Krogh, N. (1961). *Acta vet. Scand., 2*, 103.
(13) Broberg, G. (1960). AB. Lovisa, Finland, Nya. Tryckeri, pp. 1–83.
(14) Pounden, W. D. (1954). *Vet. Med., 44*, 463.
(15) Nicholson, J. W. G. & Cunningham, H. M. (1961). *Canad. J. Anim. Sci.*, pp. 41–134.
(16) Owens, E. L. (1959). *N.Z. vet. J., 7*, 43.
(17) Bezeau, L. M. (1965). *Canad. vet. J., 6*, 205.
(18) Strafuss, A. C. & Monlux, W. S. (1966). *Cornell Vet., 56*, 128.
(19) Hyldgaard-Jensen, J. & Simesen, M. G. (1966). *Nord. Vet.-Med., 18*, 73.
(20) Krogh, N. (1963). *Acta vet. Scand., 4*, 27 and 41.
(21) Dirksen, G. (1965). *Vet. med. Rev., Leverkusen 2*, 98.
(22) Gnanaprakasam, V. (1970). *Indian vet. J., 47*, 904.
(23) Fell, B. F. *et al.* (1967). *Vet. Rec., 81*, 593.
(24) Kay, M. *et al.* (1969). *Res. vet. Sci., 10*, 181.
(25) Uhart, B. A. & Carroll, F. D. (1967). *J. Anim. Sci., 26*, 1195.
(26) Tremere, A. W. *et al.* (1968). *J. Dairy Sci., 51*, 1065.
(27) Cordes, D. O. *et al.* (1969). *N.Z. vet. J., 17*, 77.
(28) Morris, J. G. (1971). *Aust. vet. J., 47*, 129.

Traumatic Reticuloperitonitis and Allied Syndromes

Perforation of the wall of the reticulum by a sharp foreign body produces initially an acute local peritonitis which may spread to cause acute diffuse peritonitis or remain localized to cause subsequent damage including vagal indigestion and diaphragmatic hernia. The penetration of the foreign body may proceed beyond the peritoneum and cause involvement of other organs resulting in pericarditis, cardiac tamponade, pneumonia, pleurisy and mediastinitis, and hepatic, splenic or diaphragmatic abscess (27).

These sequelae of traumatic perforation of the reticular wall are set out diagrammatically in the table facing.

This complexity of development makes diagnosis and prognosis difficult, and the possibility that a number of syndromes may occur together further complicates the picture. All of these entities except endocarditis are dealt with together here, even though many of them are diseases of other systems.

TRAUMATIC RETICULOPERITONITIS

Perforation of the wall of the reticulum by a sharp foreign body produces initially an acute local peritonitis characterized clinically by sudden anorexia and fall in milk yield, mild fever, ruminal stasis and local pain in the abdomen. Rapid recovery may occur, or the disease may persist in a

Sequelae of Traumatic Perforation of the Reticular Wall

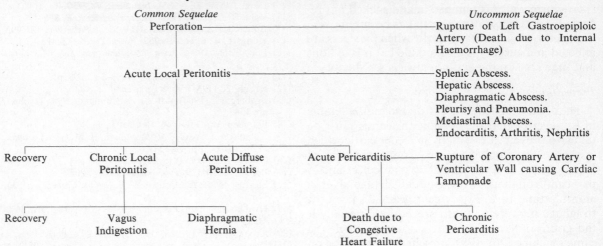

chronic form or spread widely to produce an acute, diffuse peritonitis.

Aetiology

Most cases are caused by the ingestion of foreign bodies in prepared feed. Baling or fencing wire which has passed through a chaff-cutter, feed chopper or forage harvester is the commonest cause of injury. In one series of 1400 necropsies, 58 per cent of lesions were caused by wire, 36 per cent by nails and 6 per cent by miscellaneous objects (1). The foreign bodies may be in the roughage or concentrate or may originate on the farm when repairs are effected to fences, yards and in the vicinity of feed troughs. Adult dairy cattle are most commonly affected because of their more frequent exposure but cases occur infrequently in yearlings, beef cattle, dairy bulls, sheep and goats. In the series of 1400 necropsies referred to 93 per cent were in cattle over two years old and 87 per cent were in dairy cattle.

The disease is of great economic importance because of the severe loss of production it causes and the high mortality rate. Many cases go unrecognized and many more make spontaneous recoveries. In one extensive series of examinations at abattoirs 70 per cent of dairy cows showed residual lesions caused by traumatic perforation of the reticulum (2). In a similar survey in sheep and goats there was one case in 17 goats examined and an incidence of 2 per cent in adult sheep and 0·1 per cent in lambs (20). The disease also occurs in camels, but only rarely, and presents a syndrome identical with that seen in cattle (25). The natural and experimental disease in goats is also identical with that seen in cattle (30).

Pathogenesis

Lack of oral discrimination in cattle leads to the ingestion of foreign bodies which would be rejected by other species. Swallowed foreign bodies may lodge in the upper oesophagus and cause obstruction, or in the oesophageal groove and cause vomiting but in most instances they pass to the reticulum. Many lie there without causing harm but the cell-like structure of the lining provides many spots for fixation of the foreign body and the vigorous contractions of the reticulum are sufficient to push a sharp-pointed object through the wall. Most perforations occur in the lower part of the anterior wall but some occur laterally in the direction of the spleen and medially towards the liver.

If the wall is injured without penetration to the serous surface no detectable illness occurs, and the foreign body may remain fixed in the site for long periods and gradually be corroded away. This applies particularly to wire but nails last much longer. The ease with which perforation occurs has been illustrated by the artificial production of the disease (3). Sharpened foreign bodies were given to 10 cows in gelatin capsules. Of 20 pieces of wire and 10 nails, 25 were found in the reticulum. Of the 20 pieces of wire 18 had perforated or were embedded in the wall or plicae. Only one of the nails was embedded. Complete perforations were caused by 13 foreign bodies and incomplete by 6. All cows suffered at least one perforation, showed clinical signs of acute local peritonitis, and recovered after surgical removal of the foreign bodies.

Many foreign bodies do not remain embedded and are found lying free in the reticulum if surgery is delayed until about 72 hours after illness commences (27). This is probably due to necrosis around the penetrating object and the returning reticular movements manipulating it from its position (4). Objects which are deeply embedded, have kinks or barbs, or have large diameters tend to remain *in situ* and cause persistent chronic peritonitis.

The initial reaction to perforation is one of acute local peritonitis, and in experimentally induced cases, clinical signs commence about 24 hours after penetration (3, 5). The peritonitis causes ruminal atony and abdominal pain. If the foreign body falls back into the reticulum spontaneous recovery may occur, although spread of the inflammation to affect most of the peritoneal cavity is likely to occur in cows which calve at the time of perforation, and in cattle which are forced to exercise. Immobility is a prominent sign of the disease and it serves as a protective mechanism in that adhesions are able to form and localize the peritonitis. Animals made to walk or transported long distances frequently suffer relapses when these adhesions are broken down during body movements.

During the initial penetration the foreign body may penetrate beyond the peritoneal cavity and into the pleural or pericardial sacs to set up inflammation there. It is often stated that foreign bodies which remain embedded in the reticular wall may be pushed further by the pressure of the calf during late pregnancy or the efforts of parturition. This may occur in some cases but the more common train of events is that in cows in advanced pregnancy the initial perforation is likely to extend further than in non-pregnant cows. At least it can be said that serious complications including pericarditis are more likely to occur in cows after the sixth month of pregnancy (4).

The pathogenesis of the more common complications are discussed under traumatic pericarditis, vagus indigestion, diaphragmatic hernia and traumatic abscess of the spleen and liver (pp. 99, 96, 98 and 101). Less common sequelae include rupture of the left gastro-epiploic artery causing sudden death due to internal haemorrhage (6) and the development of a diaphragmatic abscess which infiltrates tissues to the ventral abdominal wall at the xiphoid process, rupturing to the exterior and sometimes discharging the foreign body. Haematogenous spread of infection from a diaphragmatic abscess or chronic local peritonitis is one of the commonest causes of endocarditis and its attendant lesions of arthritis, nephritis and pulmonary abscess. Penetration into the pleural cavity causes development of an acute suppurative pleurisy and pneumonia. In rare cases the infection is localized chiefly to the mediastinum with the development of an extensive abscess which causes pressure on the pericardial sac and resulting cardiac embarrassment and congestive heart failure.

Clinical Findings

The onset is sudden with complete anorexia and a sharp fall in milk yield usually to about a third of the previous yield. These changes occur within a 12 hour period and their abrupt appearance is typical of this disease. There is subacute abdominal pain in all cases. The animal is reluctant to move and does so slowly. Walking, particularly downhill, is often accompanied by grunting. Most animals prefer to remain standing for long periods and lie down with great care; habitual recumbency is characteristic in others. Arching of the back is marked in about half of the cases but there is always rigidity of the back and of the abdominal muscles so that the animal appears gaunt or 'tucked-up'. Defaecation and urination cause pain and the acts are performed infrequently and usually with grunting. In rare cases an attack of acute abdominal pain with kicking at the belly, stretching and rolling is the earliest sign. In others there is recumbency and inability to rise.

A moderate systemic reaction occurs, the temperature rising usually to 39·5 to 40°C (103 to 104°F), rarely higher, the pulse rate to about 80 per minute and the respiratory rate to about 30 per minute. Temperatures above 40°C (104°F) accompanied by heart rates greater than 90 per minute should arouse suspicion of serious complications. The respirations are usually shallow and, if the pleural cavity has been penetrated, are painful and accompanied by an audible expiratory grunt. Rumination is suspended and ruminal movements are absent, or at least severely depressed to a rate of about 1 per 2 minutes with the sounds much reduced in intensity. The rumen may appear to be full because of the presence of mild tympany and in some cases there is moderate distension of the left flank. On palpation a typical cap of gas can be felt before the firm doughy ruminal contents are reached. The presence of this cap is caused by the separation of the gas from the solid and fluid contents and may occur in other forms of acute ruminal atony. Constipation is always present.

Pain can be elicited by vigorous palpation of the abdominal wall just behind the xiphoid process of the sternum. Pressure can be exerted by a short, sharp jab with the closed fist or knee. Pinching the withers to cause depression of the back or sharp elevation of a rail held under the abdomen are much less satisfactory. A positive response to any of these tests is a grunt of pain which may be audible some distance away but is best detected by auscultation of the trachea. Pain may also be manifested when the infrequent reticular contractions occur. Observation of pain or uneasiness coinciding with the primary ruminal movement or just prior to it is suggested as an aid to making a diagnosis (7).

The stage of acute local peritonitis is quite short and the signs described above are at their maximum on the first day and in most cases subside quickly thereafter so that they may be difficult to detect by the third day. The most constant sign is the abdominal pain which may require deep palpation for its demonstration. In cases which recover spontaneously or respond satisfactorily to conservative treatment there may be no detectable signs of illness by the fourth day. When chronic peritonitis persists the appetite and milk yield do not return completely to normal. Pain is not evident although the gait may be slow and careful, and grunting may occur during rumination, defaecation and urination. Rumination is depressed and chronic moderate bloat may be present although ruminal movements are usually normal.

The development of acute, diffuse peritonitis is manifested by the appearance of a profound toxaemia within a day or two of the onset of local peritonitis. Alimentary tract movements cease entirely, there is severe depression and the temperature may be higher than normal, or subnormal in fulminating cases, especially those which occur immediately after calving. The pulse rate rises to 100 to 120 per minute and pain can be elicited by palpation anywhere over the ventral abdominal wall. Usually this stage is followed by one of acute collapse and peripheral circulatory failure with all pain responses having disappeared. A terminal stage of recumbency and coma produces a clinical picture not unlike that of parturient paresis.

Metal detectors have come to be widely used in the diagnosis of traumatic reticuloperitonitis. The presence of ferrous, metallic foreign bodies and their whereabouts can be accurately determined through the body wall but the instruments are of limited usefulness because most normal dairy cows (about 80 per cent) give positive results. They do, however, lend themselves to the accumulation of a great deal of data (29).

Clinical Pathology

Haematological observations provide good diagnostic and prognostic data. In typical cases the total leucocyte count rises to between 8000 and 12,000 per cmm. on the first day and remains high for 12 to 24 hours, subsiding to slightly above normal on the third day. The neutrophil and unsegmented neutrophil counts show a similar curve, total neutrophils rising from a normal level of 30 to 35 per cent up to 50 to 70 per cent, and band forms showing a marked rise also (19). By the third day in uncomplicated cases the counts may approximate normal levels (3). In chronic cases the levels do not return completely to normal for long periods and a persistent elevation of the monocyte count to a level of 5 to 9 per cent is diagnostically significant (8). In acute diffuse peritonitis the total count often falls precipitously and most cases which are complicated by serious sequelae show a divergence from the usual downward curve either by this precipitate fall in total count or by an equally steep rise in total leucocyte and total neutrophil counts. The proportion of immature neutrophils present is of considerable importance.

Necropsy Findings

Neither acute local nor chronic local peritonitis is fatal. In acute diffuse peritonitis a fibrinous or suppurative inflammation affects the whole of the peritoneal surface. There is a characteristic smell and large quantities of fluid are usually present. The foreign body can usually be found perforating the anterior lower wall of the reticulum, although it may have fallen back into the reticulum leaving only the perforation site and its surrounding inflammation as evidence of the site of penetration.

Diagnosis

The diseases which are commonly confused with traumatic reticulo-peritonitis are ketosis, indigestion, rumen overload, abomasal displacement or torsion, impaction of the omasum, pyelonephritis and hepatic abscess or fascioliasis. Acute local peritonitis due to penetration of the uterine wall by a catheter or of the rectal wall by a foreign body thrust sadistically into the rectum may be difficult to differentiate unless the painful area of the peritoneum can be determined. Acute local peritonitis can be differentiated from indigestion, acute ruminal impaction and acetonaemia by the presence of fever, local abdominal pain and the abrupt fall in milk yield and appetite. Pyelonephritis can be distinguished by the presence of pus and blood in the urine and abomasal displacement by the presence of abomasal sounds in the left flank. Hepatic lesions may be distinguishable by the elicitation of pain over the posterior ribs on the right side and are not necessarily accompanied by ruminal stasis. Acute ruminal impaction is a much more serious disease and is usually accompanied by a marked increase in heart rate, staggering, recumbency, blindness and hypothermia. Acute diffuse peritonitis may present a similar clinical picture but there is no history of engorgement and no sign of haemo-concentration.

Traumatic reticuloperitonitis usually causes a secondary acetonaemia when it occurs during early lactation and the presence of ketonuria should not be used as the sole basis for differentiation of the diseases. Differentiation may be extremely difficult if the peritonitis is of 3 or 4 days duration and leucocyte counts and blood sugar estimations may be necessary in many cases. Response to treatment may also serve as a guide. The history is often helpful; the appetite and milk yield fall abruptly in traumatic reticuloperitonitis, but slowly over a period of several days, and not to the same degree in acetonaemia.

Continued high fever, high pulse rate and toxaemia suggest involvement of the pericardial sac, liver or spleen as traumatic pericarditis or traumatic splenitis and hepatitis. All are marked by high total leucocyte and neutrophil counts. Typical sounds are heard on auscultation of the heart in the former and signs of congestive heart failure are present. Pain responses can be elicited by deep palpation over the respective organs when hepatic or splenic involvement occur.

Traumatic reticuloperitonitis is clinically indistinguishable from ephemeral fever although there is a more marked tendency to recumbency in the latter. Peritonitis due to perforation of an abomasal ulcer is characterized by evidence of pain on palpation over a much larger area of the abdominal wall and in the early stages this is most marked on the right hand side (28). If, as is usual, the peritonitis becomes diffuse the syndrome cannot be distinguished clinically from that caused by traumatic reticuloperitonitis. Extension from a metritis to involve the peritoneum is suggested by other signs of the primary disease.

Treatment

Two methods of treatment are in general use, conservative treatment with or without the use of a magnet, and rumenotomy. Both have advantages and each case must be considered separately when deciding on the form of treatment to be used.

Conservative treatment comprises immobilization of the animal, administration of antibacterial drugs to control the infection and possibly the oral administration of a magnet to immobilize the foreign body. The cow is tied or stanchioned and not moved for 10 to 14 days. Milking, feeding and watering are carried out on the spot. The immobili-

zation facilitates the formation of adhesions and this, and removal of the foreign body, may be further aided by standing the animal on an inclined plane (9) made of a door or planks or by packing earth under the front feet of the cow. The front feet should be elevated about 9 in. above the floor. Feed, particularly the roughage, should be reduced to about half. The response is often so good that the farmer is tempted to turn the cow loose before the allotted time and relapses frequently occur.

Antibacterial treatment may be provided by the oral administration of a sulphonamide (1 g. per lb. body weight daily for 3 to 5 days) or parenteral injections of antibiotics, usually a combination of penicillin and streptomycin, for 3 days. Oral sulphonamides depress the activity of rumen bacteria (10) but give a high concentration of drug in the vicinity of the lesion. The general effect appears to be good and a high rate of recovery is recorded with this treatment combined with immobilization (3, 17) provided treatment is begun in the early stages of the disease. Cows past their sixth month of pregnancy are likely to show incomplete recovery or relapse.

Small cylindrical or bar magnets, 7·5 cm. long by 1·0 to 2·5 cm. diameter with rounded ends have been developed as a prophylactic measure against traumatic reticuloperitonitis (11, 12) but they have also come into fairly general use as an aid to treatment. It is unlikely that they will extract a firmly embedded foreign body from the wall of the reticulum but loosely embedded ones with long free ends may be returned to the reticulum and loose foreign bodies will be immobilized. Used prophylactically they reduce the incidence of the disease a great deal provided they lodge in the reticulum. However, many pass straight through into the rumen unless the amount of roughage fed is reduced for 24 hours beforehand (13). There have been no reports of physical harm to the wall of the reticulum being caused by the magnets and the incidence of traumatic reticuloperitonitis is very greatly reduced (24, 26).

A variation of the use of magnets has been the introduction of magnetic retrievers (14, 15, 16) which are passed into the reticulum through the mouth or through a small incision in the left flank. They can be used on their own or 24 to 48 hours after a small oral magnet has been administered. The latter technique avoids the necessity of an extensive search of the reticulum as the free magnet has had time to become attached to the metallic foreign bodies. The retriever instruments are designed to reduce the number of rumenotomies required but they have several disadvantages. Those designed for use by the mouth cause much discomfort and there is often great difficulty in restraining the animals. Vomiting with resulting aspiration pneumonia is not uncommon and many metallic foreign bodies are not removed. When they are used to retrieve a small oral magnet administered previously, the magnetic retrievers are much more effective (21). It is always difficult to determine where the retrieving magnet has reached and in many instances it passes on into the rumen and cannot be directed into the reticulum. The use of a metal detector in conjunction with a magnetic retriever is a better combination. The presence of a metallic foreign body in the reticulum can be detected beforehand, the arrival of the retrieving magnet in the reticulum can also be observed and the disappearance of all metal from the reticulum when the retriever is withdrawn indicates a successful operation.

Surgical removal of the foreign body through a rumenotomy incision is widely used as a primary treatment. It has the advantage of being both a satisfactory treatment and diagnostic procedure. The recovery rate varies, depending largely upon the time at which surgery is undertaken, but is approximately the same as that obtained with the conservative treatment described above. In both instances 80 to 90 per cent of animals recover compared with about 60 per cent in untreated animals (1, 3, 18, 22, 23). Failure to improve is usually due to involvement of other organs or to the development of diffuse peritonitis.

The choice of treatments is largely governed by economics and the facilities and time available for surgery. A rumenotomy, satisfactorily performed, is the best treatment but is unnecessary in many cases because of the tendency of the foreign body to fall back into the reticulum. The best general policy is to treat the animal conservatively for three days and if marked improvement has not occurred by that time to perform a rumenotomy. Cows in the last three months of pregnancy probably need a rumenotomy if serious sequelae are to be avoided. Movement of the cow during the early stages of the disease is most undesirable because of the risk of breaking down the adhesions which may localize the infection.

As a preventive measure all chopped feed should be passed over magnets to remove metallic material before being fed to cattle. The practice of tying bales of hay with string instead of wire has led to a major decrease in the incidence of the disease.

Cases of chronic traumatic reticuloperitonitis are best treated by rumenotomy because of the probability that the foreign body is still embedded in the wall. Acute diffuse peritonitis is highly fatal but if detected early vigorous treatment with broad-spectrum antibiotics results in recovery in a good proportion of cases. The best route of administration is in normal saline by intraperitoneal injection. Two to three grammes of oxytetracycline or tetracycline in 4 litres of saline or electrolyte solution provide needed fluids and good distribution of the antibiotic through the cavity. The treatment is repeated daily for 3 days.

REFERENCES

(1) Editorial, (1954). *J. Amer. vet. med. Ass.*, *125*, 331.
(2) Maddy, K. T. (1954). *J. Amer. vet. med. Ass.*, *124*, 113.
(3) Kingrey, B. W. (1955). *J. Amer. vet. med. Ass.*, *127*, 477.
(4) Blood, D. C. & Hutchins, D. R. (1955). *Aust. vet. J.*, *31*, 113.
(5) Dougherty, R. W. (1939). *J. Amer. vet. med. Ass.*, *94*, 357.
(6) Stinson, B. (1945). *Skand. vet. Tidskr.*, *35*, 622.
(7) Williams, E. I. (1955). *Vet. Rec.*, *67*, 907 & 922 & *68*, 835.
(8) Carroll, R. E. & Robinson, R. R. (1958). *J. Amer. vet. med. Ass.*, *132*, 248.
(9) Jensen, H. E. (1945). *N. Amer. Vet.*, *26*, 213.
(10) Oyaert, W. *et al.* (1951). *Onderstepoort J. vet. Sci.*, *25*, 59.
(11) Carroll, R. E. (1955). *J. Amer. vet. med. Ass.*, *127*, 311.
(12) Carroll, R. E. (1956). *J. Amer. vet. med. Ass.*, *129*, 376.
(13) Lundvall, R. L. (1957). *J. Amer. vet. med. Ass.*, *131*, 471.
(14) Schipper, I. A. & Eveleth, D. R. (1955). *N. Amer. Vet.*, *36*, 640.
(15) Nilsson, L. S. (1956). *Vet. Med.*, *51*, 565.
(16) Kettel, E. W. & Snook, M. D. (1957). *J. Amer. vet. med. Ass.*, *131*, 285.
(17) Muller, E. (1952). *Wien. tierärztl. Mschr.*, *39*, 299.
(18) Hansen, A. G. (1953). *J. Amer. vet. med. Ass.*, *122*, 290.
(19) Brown, J. M. *et al.* (1959). *Amer. J. vet. Res.*, *20*, 255.
(20) Maddy, K. T. (1954). *J. Amer. vet. med. Ass.*, *124*, 124.
(21) Rosenberger, G. & Strober, M. (1959). *Vet. Rec.*, *71*, 811.
(22) Hjerpe, C. A. (1961). *J. Amer. vet. med. Ass.*, *139*, 227, 230 & 233.
(23) Fraser, C. M. (1961). *Canad. vet. J.*, *2*, 65.
(24) Albright, J. L. *et al.* (1962). *J. Dairy Sci.*, *45*, 547.
(25) Said, A. H. (1963). *Vet. Rec.*, *75*, 966.
(26) Dunn, H. O. *et al.* (1965). *Cornell Vet.*, *55*, 204.
(27) Fuhrimann, H. (1966). *Schweiz. Arch. Tierheilk.*, *108*, 190.
(28) Pinsent, P. J. N. (1962). *Vet. Rec.*, *74*, 1282.
(29) Jagos, P. (1969). *Acta vet. Brno*, *38*, 401 & 545.
(30) Roztocil, V. *et al.* (1968). *Vet. Rec.*, *83*, 667.

VAGUS INDIGESTION

Lesions which involve the vagus nerve supply to the forestomachs and abomasum cause varying degrees of paralysis of the stomachs resulting in syndromes characterized by delayed passage of ingesta, distension, anorexia and the passage of soft pasty faeces in small quantities. It is a common disease in cattle and has recently been recorded in sheep.

Aetiology

In cattle, traumatic reticuloperitonitis is the commonest cause, the inflammatory and scar tissue lesions affecting the ventral branch of the vagus nerve as it ramifies over the anterior wall of the reticulum (1). Some cases have adhesions, for example between the rumen and abomasum, which do not appear to involve the vagus nerve (11). Induration of the medial reticular wall where vagal stretch receptors are located is sufficient to interfere with normal oesophageal groove reflexes (12). In most cases the lesions are situated on the right hand wall of the reticulum (13). Actinobacillosis of the rumen and reticulum is a less common cause (8). In sheep peritonitis caused by Sarcosporidia and *Cysticercus tenuicollis* has been found to be an apparent cause (10). Disturbances similar to those which occur under natural conditions have been produced by sectioning the vagus nerve. The possibility that naturally occurring lesions may exert their effects by physical impairment of stomach movement and interference with the functioning of the oesophageal groove rather than by actual involvement of the vagus nerve has also been suggested (2) but not received with enthusiasm (13).

Involvement of the vagus nerve in the thorax may occur as a result of enlargement of lymph nodes affected by tuberculosis or lymphomatosis. Similar disturbances may occur as a result of diaphragmatic hernia.

Pathogenesis

A number of syndromes develop depending upon the branches of the nerve which are involved and possibly upon the degree of immobilization caused by adhesion of the reticulum to the diaphragm. The major abnormality appears to be in the development of achalasia of the reticulo-omasal and the pyloric sphincters, although paralysis of the fore-stomach and abomasal walls also plays a part.

When there is achalasia of the reticulo-omasal sphincter, food material accumulates in the rumen. If the ruminal wall is atonic the food accumulates without bloat occurring; if it has normal motility the ruminal wall responds to the distension by increased motility and the production of frothy bloat. When there is achalasia of the pylorus there is blockage of food material at this point and a syndrome of pyloric obstruction develops, often accompanied by pyloric ulceration. Associated with pyloric achalasia there is in some cases an apparent failure of the oesophageal groove to permit the passage of food into the rumen, this organ containing only fluid. It is possible that the different syndromes represent stages in the development of the one disease but for satisfactory definition they are dealt with separately here. It is often difficult to reconcile the apparent defects in motility of the stomachs, as evidenced by clinical and necropsy findings with the effects of experimental vagotomy (5, 6, 7).

Clinical Findings

A number of syndromes have been described (4, 13) but the following arbitrary division into three is considered to be sufficiently descriptive.

Ruminal distension with hypermotility. The occurrence of this type is not related to pregnancy or parturition. The first obvious sign is moderate to severe ruminal tympany although the animal is usually in poor flesh and has not been eating well for some time. The abdomen is distended but the rumen is moving forcefully and almost continuously with the sounds much reduced in volume. The faeces are normal or pasty but scanty. There is no fever and the heart rate is usually slower than normal and the sounds are often accompanied by a systolic murmur which waxes and wanes with respiration, being loudest at the peak of inspiration. The murmur disappears when the tympany is relieved. Ruminal distension is apparent on rectal examination. Standard treatments for ruminal tympany and impaction have no effect on the course of the disease.

Ruminal distension with atony. This type occurs most commonly in late pregnancy and may persist after calving. The cow is clinically normal in all respects except that she will not eat, passes only small amounts of soft pasty faeces, has a distended abdomen and will not respond to treatment with purgatives, lubricants or parasympathetic stimulants. Ruminal movements are seriously reduced or absent and there may be persistent mild bloat. There is no fever or increase in heart rate and no pain on percussion of the abdomen. On rectal examination the only abnormality is gross distension of the rumen which may almost block the pelvic inlet. The animal loses weight rapidly, becomes very weak and eventually recumbent. At this stage the heart rate increases markedly. The animal dies slowly of inanition.

Pyloric obstruction. Most cases of this type also occur late in pregnancy and are manifested by anorexia and a reduced volume of pasty faeces. There is no abdominal distension and no systemic reaction until the late stages when the pulse rate rises rapidly. The distended abomasum may be palpable on the abdominal floor on rectal examination but this is impossible if the cow is pregnant. The abomasum is firm and not distended with gas or fluid. Rumen movements are usually completely absent. As in the first type death occurs slowly due to inanition.

Combinations of these types may occur; in particular, distension of the rumen with atony combined with abomasal obstruction is the most commonly observed syndrome (9).

Clinical Pathology

In most cases there are no abnormalities on haematological examination although a moderate neutrophilia, a shift to the left and a relative monocytosis may suggest the presence of chronic traumatic reticuloperitonitis.

Necropsy Findings

Cases of the disease in which there is ruminal hypermotility do not usually come to necropsy. In both of the other types there is impaction of the abomasum. The pyloric region contains a solid mass of sand or impacted, fine, partly digested fibre. The remainder of the organ is filled with coarse undigested material similar to that usually found in the rumen. Ulcers of the pyloric mucosa are a common accompaniment. When there is ruminal distension the contents are usually in an advanced state of digestion and may have undergone some putrefaction. Cases in which ruminal distension was absent before death have a contracted rumen containing thin clear fluid and a few particles of feed. In both types the intestines are relatively empty and the faeces have a thick, pasty consistency and are dark green in colour (3).

Lesions are usually present on the anterior wall of the reticulum which suggest that traumatic reticuloperitonitis occurred some time previously. The lesions comprise extensive adhesions, fibrous fistulae, sometimes containing a foreign body, or abscesses. The situation of these lesions is often such that physical involvement of the vagus nerve does not appear likely.

Diagnosis

Chronic intractable indigestion with constipation may also occur in cattle after calving when there is left abomasal displacement but there are usually audible abomasal sounds in the left lower flank and the abdomen is shrunken rather than distended. Ruminal movements too are usually normal even though the sounds are muffled and not absent or exaggerated as they are in vagus indigestion. Differentiation between vagus indigestion and chronic reticuloperitonitis is impossible without exploratory rumenotomy. Abomasal ulceration may present a similar clinical picture but is often part of the syndrome of vagus indigestion. In subacute abomasal torsion (right displacement) the distended abomasum can be readily palpated almost filling the right half of the abdominal cavity. Partial obstruction of the intestine by lipoma or fat necrosis can usually be detected by rectal palpation.

Treatment

Rumenotomy and emptying of the rumen is usually followed by slow recovery over a period of 7 to 10 days when there is ruminal hypermotility. Surgical interference, including abomasotomy, in the other types is usually unsatisfactory because the motility of the abomasum does not return (9, 13). Conservative medical treatment is not worth attempting because results are so poor. Mineral oil in doses of 1 quart daily repeated for 4 to 6 days may relieve the impacted abomasum. The administration of small doses of parasympathetic stimulants or parenteral cascara products may help when the oil has been administered for several days and the impacted mass softened. The most satisfactory procedure is to slaughter affected animals for meat.

REFERENCES

(1) Hoflund, S. (1940). *Svensk. veterinar. Tidskrift,* Supp. zum 45 Band.
(2) Hutchins, D. R. *et. al.* (1957). *Aust. vet. J.,* *33,* 77.
(3) Clark, C. H. (1953). *Vet. Med.,* *48,* 389.
(4) Kubin, G. (1955). *Wien. tierärztl. Mschr.,* *42,* 170.
(5) Habel, R. E. (1956). *Cornell Vet.,* *46,* 555.
(6) Titchen, D. A. (1958). *J. Physiol.,* *141,* 1.
(7) Stevens, C. E. & Sellers, A. F. (1956). *Amer. J. vet. Res.,* *17,* 588.
(8) Begg, H. (1950). *Vet. Rec.,* *62,* 797.
(9) Pope, D. C. (1961). *Vet. Rec.,* *73,* 1174.
(10) Naerland, D. G. & Helle, O. (1962). *Vet. Rec.,* *74,* 85.
(11) Jones, R. S. & Pirie, H. M. (1962). *Vet. Rec.,* *74,* 582.
(12) Leek, B. F. (1968). *Vet. Rec.,* *82,* 498.
(13) Neal, P. A. & Edwards, G. B. (1968). *Vet. Rec.,* *82,* 396.

DIAPHRAGMATIC HERNIA

Herniation of a portion of the reticulum through a diaphragmatic rupture causes chronic ruminal tympany, anorexia and displacement of the heart.

Aetiology

Most cases occur because of weakening of the diaphragm by lesions of traumatic reticuloperitonitis (1, 2, 3) but diaphragmatic rupture can occur independently of a foreign body (4, 5) and congenital defects of the diaphragm may be a cause in some animals (6, 8).

Pathogenesis

The usual syndrome produced is identical with that caused by vagus indigestion in which ruminal hypermotility is present. It seems probable that there is either achalasia of the reticulo-omasal sphincter due to involvement of the vagus nerve or impairment of function of the oesophageal groove caused by the fixation of the reticulum to the ventral diaphragm. The disturbance of function in the forestomachs suggests that food can get into the rumen but cannot pass from there to the abomasum. The hypermotility is thought to be due to over-distension of the rumen and be the cause of the frothy bloat.

There is usually no interference with respiration without major herniation but displacement and compression of the heart occur commonly.

Clinical Findings

There is a capricious appetite and loss of condition for several weeks before persistent moderate tympany of the rumen occurs. Grinding of the teeth may be conspicuous and the faeces are usually pasty and reduced in volume. Rumination does not occur but occasional animals vomit especially when a stomach tube is passed.

There is no fever and the pulse rate is usually slower than normal (40 to 60 per minute). Respiration is unaffected in most cases. A systolic murmur is usually audible on auscultation, and the intensity of the heart sounds may suggest displacement of the heart, usually anteriorly or to the left. Reticular sounds are audible just posterior to the cardiac area in many normal cows and they are not significantly increased in diaphragmatic hernia.

A more severe syndrome is recorded in cases where viscera other than a portion of the reticulum is herniated. Peristaltic sounds may be audible in the chest and there may be interference with respiration and signs of pain with each reticular contraction (5). Affected animals usually die from inanition in 3 or 4 weeks after the onset of bloat.

Clinical Pathology

Laboratory examinations are of no value in diagnosis.

Necropsy Findings

The majority of cases are sequelae to traumatic reticuloperitonitis and a fistulous tract is often found in the vicinity of the diaphragmatic rupture which is usually 15 to 20 cm. in diameter. A portion of the reticulum protrudes into the right pleural cavity to form a spherical distension usually 20·0 to 30 cm. in diameter, but more extensive in some cases. The reticulum is very tightly adherent to the hernial ring which is thickened by fibrous tissue. The omasum and abomasum are relatively empty but the rumen is over-filled with frothy, porridge-like material which contains very little fibre. Less common cases are those in which part of the reticulum, the omasum and part of the abomasum are herniated.

Diagnosis

Other causes of chronic bloat must be considered in the differential diagnosis, especially vagus indigestion with hypermotility which is also often accompanied by a systolic murmur. The two can only be differentiated by rumenotomy but there is the hazard that cases of diaphragmatic hernia are not relieved by the operation and tympany returns rapidly, sometimes necessitating a permanent ruminal fistula.

Passage of a stomach tube is usually necessary to determine whether or not a physical obstruction is present in the oesophagus. Vomiting is likely to occur in cases of diaphragmatic hernia and this occasionally causes blockage of the oesophagus with ingesta, simulating choke.

Treatment

Treatment should not be attempted and the animal should be sold for slaughter at the earliest opportunity. Most recorded attempts at surgical repair have been unsuccessful (6, 7). The ruminal contents are frothy and trocarization or passing a stomach tube has virtually no effect in reducing the tympany, nor do standard antifrothing agents. The tympany is usually not sufficiently severe to require emergency rumenotomy. The signs may be partly relieved by keeping the animal confined with the forequarters elevated.

REFERENCES

(1) Frost, J. N. & Danks, A. G. (1939). *Cornell Vet.*, *29*, 70.
(2) Roberts, S. J. (1946). *Cornell Vet.*, *36*, 92.
(3) Hutchins, D. R. *et al.* (1957). *Aust. vet. J.*, *33*, 77.
(4) Milne, F. J. (1951). *J. Amer. vet. med. Ass.*, *118*, 374.
(5) Robison, R. W. (1956). *N. Amer. Vet.*, *37*, 375.
(6) Jones, E. W. (1959). *Univ. Pennsylvania Bull.*, *Vet. Ext. Qtly*, *59*, 44.
(7) Dietz, O. (1961). *J. S. Afr. vet. med. Ass.*, *32*, 3.
(8) Trout, H. F. *et al.* (1967). *J. Amer. vet. med. Ass.*, *151*, 1421.

TRAUMATIC PERICARDITIS

Perforation of the pericardial sac by a sharp foreign body originating in the reticulum causes pericarditis with the development of toxaemia and congestive heart failure. Tachycardia, fever, engorgement of the jugular veins, anasarca, hydrothorax and ascites, and abnormalities of the heart sounds are the diagnostic features of the disease.

Aetiology

The aetiology has already been described. There is a greater tendency for perforation of the pericardial sac to occur during the last 3 months of pregnancy and at parturition than at other times. Approximately 8 per cent of all cases of traumatic reticuloperitonitis will develop pericarditis (1). Most affected animals die or suffer from chronic pericarditis and do not return to completely normal health.

Pathogenesis

The penetration of the pericardial sac may occur with the initial perforation of the reticular wall. On the other hand the animal may have a history of traumatic reticuloperitonitis some time previously, followed by a subsequent attack of pericarditis, usually during late pregnancy or at parturition. In this case it is probable that the foreign body remains in a sinus in the reticular wall after the initial perforation and penetrates the pericardial sac at a later date. Physical penetration of the sac is not essential to the development of pericarditis, infection sometimes penetrating through the pericardium from a traumatic mediastinitis. The introduction of a mixed bacterial infection from the reticulum causes a severe local inflammation, and persistence of the foreign body in the tissues is not essential for the further progress of the disease. The first effect of the inflammation is hyperaemia of the pericardial surfaces and the production of friction sounds synchronous with the heart beats. Two mechanisms then operate to produce signs, the toxaemia due to the infection and the pressure on the heart of the fluid which accumulates in the sac and produces congestive heart failure (5). In individual cases one or other of these two factors may be more important. Profound depression is characteristic of the first and oedema of the second. Thus an affected animal may be severely ill for several weeks with oedema developing only gradually, or extreme oedema may develop within 2 or 3 days. The rapid development of oedema usually indicates early death.

If chronic pericarditis persists there is embarrassment of the heart action due to adhesion of the pericardium to the heart. Chronic congestive heart failure results in most cases but some animals show a relatively good recovery. An uncommon sequel after perforation of the pericardial sac by a foreign body is rupture of a coronary artery or the ventricular wall. Death occurs almost immediately because of the cardiac tamponade.

Clinical Findings

There is profound depression, complete anorexia, habitual recumbency and rapid weight loss. Diarrhoea or constipation may be present and grinding of the teeth, salivation and nasal discharge are occasionally observed. The cow stands with the back arched and the elbows abducted. Respiratory movements are more obvious, being mainly abdominal, shallow, increased in rate to 40 to 50 per minute and often accompanied by grunting. Engorgement of the jugular vein, and oedema of the brisket and ventral abdominal wall occur and in severe cases there may even be oedema of the conjunctiva with grape-like masses of oedematous conjunctiva hanging over the eyelids. A prominent jugular pulse is usually visible and extends well up into the neck. Pyrexia (104 to 106 °F or 40 to 41 °C) is always present in the early stages and an increase in the pulse rate to the vicinity of 100 per minute and a diminution in the pulse amplitude are constant. Rumen movements are usually present but depressed. Pinching of the back and abdominal percussion produce a marked pain response. An even more pronounced grunt and an increased area of cardiac dullness can be detected by percussion over the precordial area, preferably with a pleximeter and hammer.

Auscultation of the chest reveals the diagnostic signs. In the early stages before effusion commences the heart sounds are normal but are accompanied by a pericardial friction rub which may wax and wane with respiratory movements. Care must be taken to differentiate this from a pleural friction rub due to inflammation of the mediastinum. In this case the rub is much louder and the heart rate will not be so high. Several days later when there is marked effusion the heart sounds are muffled and there may be gurgling, splashing or tinkling sounds. The cardiac impulse is increased in amplitude and is palpable over a larger area than usual. In all cases of suspected pericarditis careful auscultation of the entire precordium on both sides of the chest is essential as abnormal sounds may be audible only over restricted areas. This is especially so in chronic cases.

Most affected animals die within a period of 1 to 2 weeks although a small proportion persist with chronic pericarditis. The obvious clinical signs in the terminal stages are gross oedema, dyspnoea, severe watery diarrhoea, depression, recumbency and complete anorexia. Death is usually due to asphyxia and toxaemia.

Animals which have recovered from an initial pericarditis are usually affected by the chronic form of the disease (5). The animal is in poor condition and has a variable appetite although there is no systemic reaction and the demeanour is bright. Oedema of the brisket is usually not present but there is jugular engorgement. Auscultation reveals variable findings. The heart sounds are muffled and fluid splashing sounds may be heard over small discrete areas corresponding to the loculi of fluid in the sac, or there may be irregularity of the heart beat. The pulse rate is rapid (90 to 100 per minute) and the pulse is small in amplitude. These animals never do well and are unlikely to withstand the strain of another pregnancy or lactation.

Clinical Pathology

A pronounced leucocytosis with a total count of 16,000 to 30,000 cells per cmm. accompanied by a neutrophilia and eosinopenia is usual although less dramatic changes are recorded in one series of cases (4). When gross effusion is present the pericardial fluid may be sampled by paracentesis with a large bore bleeding needle over the site of maximum audibility of the heart sound, usually in the fourth or fifth intercostal space on the left side.

Necropsy Findings

In acute cases there is gross distension of the pericardial sac with foul-smelling, greyish fluid containing flakes of fibrin, and the serous surface of the sac carries very heavy deposits of newly formed fibrin. A cord-like, fibrous sinus tract usually connects the reticulum with the pericardium. Additional lesions of pleurisy and pneumonia are commonly present. In chronic cases the pericardial sac is grossly thickened and fused to the pericardium by strong fibrous adhesions surrounding loculi of varying size which contain pus or thin straw-coloured fluid.

Diagnosis

Endocarditis, lymphomatosis with cardiac involvement and congenital cardiac defects are all likely to be confused with traumatic pericarditis because of the similarity of the abnormal heart sounds. Endocarditis is usually associated with a suppurative process in another organ, particularly the uterus or udder, and although the abnormal heart sounds are typical bruits rather than pericardial friction sounds, this may be difficult to determine when extensive pericardial effusion has occurred (2). The diagnosis of lymphomatosis depends upon the detection of lymphomatous lesions in other organs or the presence of a marked leucocytosis and lymphocytosis. Congenital cardiac defects may not cause clinical abnormality until the first pregnancy but can be diagnosed by the presence of loud murmurs, a pronounced cardiac thrill and an absence of toxaemia. Sporadic bovine encephalomyelitis is accompanied by a severe fibrinous pericarditis and a pericardial friction rub but usually no signs of heart failure.

Less common causes of abnormal heart sounds include thoracic tumours and abscesses, diaphrag-matic hernia and chronic bloat which cause distortion of the atria and atrioventricular orifices. They are associated with other diagnostic signs, particularly displacement of the heart. In severely debilitated animals or those suffering from severe anaemia a haemic murmur which fluctuates with respiration may be audible. Occasional cases of haematogenous pericarditis are encountered and in some cases of pasteurellosis a fibrinous pericarditis may be present but there is usually serious involvement of other organs and the pericarditis is only secondary.

Treatment

The results of treatment are usually unsatisfactory but salvage of up to 50 per cent of cases can be achieved by long-term treatment with sulphonamides (1). The prognosis is much better in cases where toxaemia is the major factor, rapidly developing oedema presaging death in a short time. In these cases drainage of the pericardial sac may temporarily relieve the oedema and respiratory embarrassment but relapse is usually complete in about 24 hours. Selected cases of traumatic pericarditis have been treated satisfactorily by pericardiotomy (3).

REFERENCES

(1) Blood, D. C. & Hutchins, D. R. (1955). *Aust. vet. J.*, *31*, 229.
(2) Johns, F. V. (1947). *Vet. Rec.*, *59*, 214.
(3) Little, P. B. (1964). *J. Amer. vet. med. Ass.*, *144*, 374.
(4) Holmes, J. R. (1960). *Vet. Rec.*, *72*, 355.
(5) Fisher, E. W. & Pirie, H. M. (1965). *Brit. vet. J.*, *121*, 552.

TRAUMATIC SPLENITIS AND HEPATITIS

These conditions occur relatively uncommonly as sequelae to traumatic reticuloperitonitis and are manifested either by continuation of the illness caused by the initial perforation or by apparent recovery followed by relapse several weeks later (1). The prominent clinical signs include fever (103 to 105°F or 39·5 to 40·5°C), an increase in heart rate and a gradual fall in food intake and milk yield but ruminal movements are present and may be normal. Percussion of the abdomen over the site, usually used to detect the pain of traumatic reticuloperitonitis, gives a negative response although deep, forceful palpation may elicit a mild grunt. The diagnostic sign is pain on palpation with the thumb in the last two intercostal spaces halfway down the abdomen, on the right side when there is hepatic involvement, and on the left side when the spleen is affected.

Haematological examination is important, the total leucocyte count being greatly increased (above 12,000 per cmm.) and the differential count showing a marked neutrophilia and a shift to the left. Rumenotomy is not usually undertaken except for diagnostic purposes. Treatment with anti-bacterial drugs is effective if commenced sufficiently early. Oral treatment with sulphadimidine has been effective in some cases.

REFERENCE

(1) Blood, D. C. & Hutchins, D. R. (1955). *Aust. vet. J.*, *31*, 233.

Ruminal Tympany

(*Bloat*)

Ruminal tympany refers to over-distension of the rumen and reticulum with the gases of fermentation, either mixed with or separated from the fluid and solid ingesta. It occurs secondarily to a number of conditions in which the eructation of the gases is impeded but its major importance is as a primary disease in cattle under certain dietary regimens. Tympany causes heavy losses through death, severe loss of production, and the strict limitations placed on the use of some high-producing pastures for grazing. The incidence of the disease has increased markedly with the improvement of pastures by heavy applications of fertilizers and the use of high-producing leguminous pasture plants, and losses of cattle at times have reached enormous proportions. In New Zealand it is claimed that mortality due to bloat in cattle rose from 2·2 to 7·4 per 1000 cows per year in the period of 1942 to 1964 (2) and in the U.S.A. the annual losses due to the disease are reputed to be $50 million (3). Sheep can also be affected but appear to be much less susceptible than cattle.

Aetiology

Primary ruminal tympany. Many factors are known to have an influence on the occurrence of primary bloat and possibly to contribute to its causation (1, 37). These factors are conveniently divided into dietary and animal factors.

(a) *Dietary factors.* Of these, grazing on very succulent pasture, particularly young, rapidly growing legumes in the pre-bloom stage, is the biggest single cause of bloat in cattle, although the disease also occurs occasionally when cattle are grazed on cereal crops, rape, cabbages, leguminous vegetable crops including peas and beans, and young grass pasture with a high protein content. The common legumes have been classified in their tympany-producing potential in the order Alfalfa 108, Ladino 100, Red 83, White Dutch 64 and Crimson 7 (4). Ingestion of the more succulent parts of plants and avoidance of the more mature

portions can be a precipitating factor and tympany is less likely to occur if the crop is harvested and fed than if it is grazed. Restriction of the grazing area by forcing the cattle to eat the entire plants, has a similar effect. A high incidence is recorded when pasture is wet but this is probably due to the rapid growth of the plants during heavy rainfall periods rather than to physical wetness of the crop. Under experimental conditions the production of tympany is not influenced by the water content of clover or by wilting. Other plant factors which are known to be associated with an increased tendency to bloat are liberal administration of urea to the pasture, a high intake of glucose, calcium and magnesium and a high nitrogen intake (5).

Another common and economically important occurrence of primary ruminal tympany is in hand-fed animals confined in feed-lots and barns when insufficient roughage is fed or the feed is too finely ground.

(b) *Animal factors.* Cattle vary in their susceptibility to tympany and this individual idiosyncrasy may be inherited. Under experimental conditions the production of tympany is not influenced by the rate of intake, or the total intake of dry matter. Susceptibility increases with time when a tympany-producing diet is fed for a relatively short period (6). However, animals accustomed over very long periods to feeding on dangerous pastures may be less susceptible than other animals. Accordingly the mortality rate in young cattle is much higher than in mature animals.

Foaming of the ruminal contents. Foaming or frothiness of the ruminal contents is the vital factor in causing primary pasture bloat. This may be caused by any one of a number of factors and probably in many instances by a combination of these factors.

The cause of frothing in the rumen is a high viscosity or surface tension of the fluid in it. Several factors are thought to increase this viscosity including a number of plant constituents, particularly certain proteins, saponins and pectins and hemicelluloses (7). There are arguments for and against the importance of each (37). Of most significance appear to be the 18S series of proteins (39), although the concentration of pectin in the plant and the presence of the pectin methylesterase (PME) system, also in the plant, appear to be significant factors too. The PME is capable of converting pectin to pectic and polygalacturonic acids which have tremendous gelling properties and greatly increase the viscosity of the rumeno-reticular fluids (17, 18). One of the important features of froth formation by the 18S proteins is that their efficiency in this respect can be varied depending on the presence of cations such as nickel which bind the protein molecules to form a film. The pH of the rumen contents also plays an important part in the stability of the foam (maximum stability occurs at a pH of about 6·0) and the composition of the diet and the activity and composition of the rumen microflora are known to influence this factor. One of the major reasons for doubting the importance of saponins in naturally occurring cases of ruminal tympany is that they are inactivated at this pH.

The rate of flow and composition of the saliva has an effect on the tendency for tympany to occur. This effect may be exerted by means of the buffering effect of the saliva on the pH of the rumen contents or because of variations in its content of mucoproteins. Salivary mucin prevents the development of frothiness but mucinolytic bacteria in the rumen may destroy the mucin and permit bloating to develop in the presence of adequate saliva (8). The physical effects of dilution of ruminal ingesta by saliva may be important also; there is a negative correlation between the proportion of liquid present and the incidence of tympany, and feed of a low fibre and high water content depresses the volume of saliva secreted (9, 10). Also susceptible cows secrete significantly less saliva than non-susceptible cows (11).

Another factor remains to be considered in the development of frothiness in ruminal ingesta. This is the activity of the microflora (12, 13). An increase in slime-producing bacteria has been suggested as a predisposing cause of frothiness and there is some evidence to support this. The activity of these organisms and their rate of production of polysaccharides which encourage froth formation appear to be markedly affected by the amount of sucrose in the feed. Thus the increase in susceptibility to bloat with the length of the time the particular diet is fed could very well be due to a change in the predominant microbial flora of the rumen. It has also been suggested that the microflora may play an additional role by digesting plant lipids which would be expected to have an antifoaming effect (14).

In summary it is suggested that primary frothy bloat occurs when the ingesta contains foaming substances, the pH of the rumen is suitable for the growth of encapsulated bacteria which produce extracellular polysaccharides (slime) and mucinolytic bacteria which destroy salivary mucin, and salivation is insufficient either because of the failure of the diet to stimulate it or because of individual salivary paucity of the animal. In a particular set of circumstances one or more of these factors may be the critical one which triggers an outbreak of bloat.

Secondary ruminal tympany. Physical obstruction to eructation occurs in oesophageal obstruction caused by a foreign body, by stenosis or by pressure from enlargements outside the oesophagus or by obstruction of the cardia from the interior. Interference with oesophageal groove function in vagus indigestion and diaphragmatic hernia may cause chronic ruminal tympany and the condition also occurs in tetanus particularly in young animals due probably to spasm of oesophageal musculature. Carcinoma and papillomata of the oesophageal groove and reticulum are less common causes of obstructive bloat.

There may also be interference with the nerve pathways responsible for maintenance of the eructation reflex. The receptor organs in this reflex are situated in the dorsal pouch of the reticulum and are capable of discriminating between gas, foam and liquid. The afferent and efferent nerve fibres are contained in the vagus nerve but the location of the central coordinating mechanism has not been defined. Depression of this centre or lesions of the vagus nerve can interrupt the reflex which is essential for removal of gas from the rumen.

Normal tone and motility of the musculature of the rumen and recticulum are also necessary for eructation. In anaphylaxis, bloat occurs commonly because of muscle atony and is relieved by the administration of adrenaline or antihistamine drugs. A sudden marked change in pH of the rumen contents due either to acidity or alkalinity causes ruminal atony but the tympany which results is usually of a minor degree only, probably because the gas producing activity of the microflora is greatly reduced.

Chronic ruminal tympany occurs relatively frequently in calves up to six months of age without apparent cause. Persistence of an enlarged thymus, chronic ruminal atony caused by continued feeding on coarse indigestible roughage, and indigestion due to the accumulation of readily fermentable milk foods have all been suggested as causes but the condition usually disappears spontaneously in time and the cause in most cases is undetermined. Necropsy examination of a number of fatal cases has failed to detect any physical abnormality although a developmental defect appears to be likely because of the age at which it occurs. One case of chronic tympany in a calf has been recorded as caused by a partial rotation of the rumen about its long axis (15). Unusual postures, particularly lateral recumbency, are commonly characterized by secondary tympany.

Pathogenesis

Most interest centres around the pathogenesis of primary bloat on legume pasture. Two major groups of factors have received most attention—those factors which cause foaming of the ruminal contents and those which cause ruminal atony (16). Most cases of naturally occurring pasture or feed-lot bloat are not accompanied by ruminal atony; in fact in the early stages there is usually pronounced hypermotility. If atony were an important cause one would expect to find large quantities of gas free in the rumen but this does not occur. Almost without exception the great bulk of the gas is intimately mixed with the solid and fluid ruminal contents to form a dense froth. Some free gas is present but the amount which can be removed by a stomach tube or trocar and cannula does little to relieve the distension of the rumen. As a general rule it can be accepted that ruminal tympany characterized by the accumulation of free gas is due to oesophageal obstruction or ruminal atony.

If the eructation reflex can operate the experimental introduction of very large amounts of gas does not cause tympany since eructation removes the excess. Tympanogenetic feeds do not produce noticeably more gas than safe feeds and the simple production of excessive gas is known not to be a precipitating factor.

Frothiness of the ruminal contents causes physical obstruction of the cardia and inhibits the eructation reflex (10) and vomiting or eructation of the froth rarely occurs because the cranial sphincter of the oesophagus fails to open. Rumen movements are initially stimulated by the distension and the resulting hypermotility exacerbates the frothiness of the ruminal contents. Terminally there is a loss of muscle tone and ruminal motility.

The cause of death in bloat is obscure. The absorption of toxic gases, particularly hydrogen sulphide, or toxic amines, particularly histamine, has been suggested but is likely to be only a contributory factor. Distension probably plays an important part by reflexly depressing the cardiovascular and respiratory systems but experimental work shows a great deal of variation in the susceptibility of animals to ruminal distension (1).

Clinical Findings

In primary pasture bloat obvious distension of the rumen occurs suddenly, sometimes as soon as 15 minutes after going on to bloat-producing pasture. The distension is usually more obvious in the upper left flank but the whole of the abdomen is enlarged. There is discomfort and the animal may get up and lie down frequently, kick at the belly and even roll. Dyspnoea is marked and is accompanied by mouth breathing, protrusion of the tongue, salivation and extension of the head. The respiratory rate is increased up to 60 per minute. Occasionally projectile vomiting occurs and soft faeces may be expelled in a stream. Ruminal movements are usually much increased in the early stages and may be almost continuous but the sounds are reduced in volume because of the frothy nature of the ingesta. Later, when the distension is extreme, the movements are decreased and may be completely absent. The tympanic note produced by percussion is characteristic. Before clinical tympany occurs there is a temporary increase in eructation and rumination but both disappear in the acute stages. The course in ruminal tympany is short but death does not usually occur within three or four hours of the onset of clinical signs. Collapse and death almost without struggle occur quickly.

If animals are treated by trocarization or the passage of a stomach tube, only small amounts of gas are obtained before frothy material blocks the tube.

In a group of affected cattle there is usually a number of animals with clinical tympany and the remainder have mild to moderate distension of the abdomen. These animals are uncomfortable, graze for only short periods and suffer considerably in their milk production. This drop in production may be caused by depression of food intake or by failure of milk letdown.

In secondary bloat the excess gas is usually present as a free gas cap on top of the solid and fluid ruminal contents although frothy bloat may occur in vagus indigestion when there is increased ruminal motility. As in pasture bloat there is usually an increase in rate and force of ruminal movements in the early stages followed by atony. Passage of a stomach tube or trocarization results in the expulsion of large quantities of gas and subsidence of the ruminal distension. If an oesophageal obstruction is present it will be detected when the stomach tube is passed.

In both forms of bloat there is dyspnoea and a marked elevation of the heart rate up to 100 to 120 per minute in the acute stages. A systolic murmur is often audible, caused probably by distortion of the base of the heart by the forward displacement of the diaphragm. This murmur has been observed in ruminal tympany caused by tetanus, diaphragmatic hernia, vagus indigestion and oesophageal obstruction and disappears immediately if the tympany is relieved.

Clinical Pathology

Laboratory tests are not necessary in the diagnosis of ruminal tympany but a great deal of useful information about the pathogenesis of the disease can be obtained if estimations of ruminal pressure and examinations of ruminal microflora and the physical and chemical properties of rumen fluids are carried out.

Necropsy Findings

Animals that have died about an hour previously show protrusion and congestion of the tongue, marked congestion and haemorrhage of lymph nodes of the head and neck, epicardium and upper respiratory tract, friable kidneys and mucosal hyperaemia in the small intestine. The lungs are compressed, the cervical oesophagus shows congestion and haemorrhage, but the thoracic portion of the oesophagus is pale and blanched (41). In general congestion is marked in the front quarters and less marked or absent in the hind quarters. The rumen is distended but the contents are much less frothy than before death. A marked erythema is evident beneath the ruminal mucosa especially in the ventral sacs. The liver is pale due to expulsion of blood from the organ. Occasionally the rumen or diaphragm have ruptured. Animals that have been dead for some hours show subcutaneous emphysema, almost complete absence of froth in the rumen, and exfoliation of the cornified epithelium of the rumen with marked congestion of submucosal tissues (19).

Diagnosis

A diagnosis of ruminal tympany can be arrived at fairly easily and determination of the cause in primary bloat is in most cases a simple matter but in secondary bloat, particularly when it is chronic, this decision is often difficult to make. If the case is severe enough it is usually necessary to carry out emergency treatment without complete examination of the animal. Passage of a stomach tube will detect oesophageal obstruction or stenosis, both of which are accompanied by difficult swallowing, and in acute cases by violent attempts at vomiting. Vagus indigestion and diaphragmatic hernia have a prior history of traumatic reticuloperitonitis and partial anorexia. Tetanus is manifested by limb rigidity, prolapse of the third eyelid and hyperaesthesia. Carcinoma and papillomata of the oesophageal groove and reticulum and actinobacillosis of the reticulum cannot usually be diagnosed ante-mortem without exploratory rumenotomy.

One of the difficult situations encountered in veterinary practice is the post-mortem diagnosis of bloat, especially in animals found dead at pasture in warm weather (19). Blackleg, lightning stroke, anthrax and snakebite are common alternatives. A diagnosis of bloat must depend on an absence of local lesions characteristic of these diseases, the presence of marked ruminal tympany in the absence of other signs of post-mortem decomposition, the relative pallor of the liver and the other lesions described above.

Treatment

The treatment of secondary ruminal tympany depends on the removal of the cause. However, in any form of ruminal tympany it is often necessary to advise an owner to adopt first aid treatment until professional attention can be provided. Tying a stick in the mouth like a bit on a horse bridle, standing the cow with the front feet raised, smearing wood tar on the back of the tongue and careful drenching with a pint of any nontoxic vegetable or mineral oil are commonly advised. Veterinary treatment usually consists of the passage of a stomach tube or when this is not possible trocarization is performed. Alkaloidal extracts of the plants *Veratrum* spp. appear to show some promise as rumenatorics and in the treatment of non-frothy bloat (20).

The treatment of primary tympany is aimed at reducing the stability of the foam and this is best achieved by the oral administration of oils (21) or Poloxalene (25 to 50 g.) (44). The amount of oil needed is not great and 8 oz. is probably sufficient although it is more usual in practice to use 1 to 2 pints for cattle and 1 to 2 oz. for sheep. The type of oil is also unimportant, most vegetable and mineral oils and even cream being effective. An emulsified oil or one containing a detergent mixes with the ruminal contents more rapidly and gives consistently more rapid results than pure oil or fat (22). They are best administered by stomach tube to avoid aspiration and to remove free gas. If the case is urgent and trocarization is necessary the oil can be introduced through the cannula by a syringe with a long nozzle once gas has ceased to flow.

Of the older treatments turpentine (1 to 2 oz.) has remained in favour and owes its efficiency to its property of reducing the viscosity of ruminal foams. It is less satisfactory than bland oils because it is irritant and causes marked tainting of the milk. Other antifrothing agents, particularly silicones and detergents have been in general use but are less reliable than oils (1, 2, 3). It is general practice to administer a purgative with the oil to facilitate evacuation of the tympany-producing ingesta but this is unnecessary. Adrenaline and antihistamine compounds have been recommended in the treatment of allergic bloat but their use in frothy pasture bloat is dangerous (2).

Severe cases of frothy bloat which do not respond to medical treatment can be treated by rumenotomy but this should be avoided if possible because of the gross distension of the rumen and the ease with which it can be accidentally perforated causing soiling of the peritoneum.

Control

On pasture, prevention of frothy bloat is a difficult problem. In the past many husbandry practices have been recommended including the prior feeding of dry, scabrous hay, particularly Sudan grass, cereal hay and straw, restricting the grazing to 20 minutes at a time or until the first cow stops eating, cutting the crop and feeding it in troughs, and strip grazing to ensure that all available pasture is utilized each day. These methods have value when the pasture is only moderately dangerous but may be ineffective when the tympany-producing potential is high. In these circumstances the use of antibiotics to control the activity of the bacterial flora or of oils to reduce frothing is essential if dangerous pasture is to be used. One of the difficulties in bloat control is the cost of many currently recommended procedures.

Antibiotics have been used with limited success. Penicillin has been used to control bacterial activity in the rumen and to limit the amount of gas produced (16, 24, 25). Other single antibiotics have been used but have been less effective, but a rotation of antibiotics, using penicillin, erythromycin, tylosin, chloramphenicol, oxytetracycline and streptomycin each fed in grain for periods of a week, and a combination of streptomycin, tylosin, erythromycin and penicillin (STEP) is more effective. Both procedures have sufficient disadvantages to render them impractical in most circumstances (26). Antibiotics administered as slow release boluses have proved to be a satisfactory means of maintaining antibiotic levels in the rumen for periods of about 6 weeks but suffer from the expected deficiency of failing to control bloat within a relatively short period (3, 27). Potassium levopropylcillin reduces the incidence and severity of bloat for a substantially longer period than other antibiotics (27).

Oils and fats have achieved great success in the prevention of ruminal tympany and have been found to be 100 per cent effective by most workers provided they are administered regularly and in sufficient quantity (1). The major disadvantage is the difficulty of administering the prepara-

tions at least twice daily to cattle at pasture or in the feed-lot. The duration of the foam-preventing effect is short, lasting only a few hours and increasing the dose does not significantly lengthen the period of protection. If the oil or fat is emulsified with water it can then be sprayed on to a limited pasture area which provides part or all of the anticipated food requirements for the day. Backgrazing must be prevented and care is required during rainy periods when the oil is likely to be washed from the pasture. Two to 4 oz. of the oil per cow should be used each day. The method is ideal where strip-grazing is practised on irrigated pasture but is ineffective when grazing is uncontrolled. Under these conditions the oil can be administered at the rate of 4 oz. per head in concentrates fed before the cattle go on to the pasture or by addition to the drinking water to make a 2 per cent emulsion. The latter practice can be satisfactorily carried out by mixing a mineral oil with the water in all available troughs, turning off the water supply and refilling the troughs when they are emptied. A water-dispersible lard derivative gives good results in the prevention of bloat on alfalfa when used in the above manner (28). The serious disadvantage of this method is that the actual intake of the oil cannot be guaranteed and cattle which fail to drink after becoming accustomed to drinking the oil appear to be more susceptible than those which are not so accustomed (29). Climatic conditions also cause variations in the amount of water which is taken with consequent variation in the oil intake. It is probably safest to make provision for the daily intake of 8 to 10 ounces of oil per head during those periods when the pasture is at its most dangerous stage. Individual drenching is sometimes practised but because of the time and labour required the method is suitable only in emergency conditions. A recently introduced method of administering antifoaming agents is their application to the flanks of cows with a large paint brush as they go out of the milking shed. A preparation which is palatable to cattle and which encourages them to lick their flanks is preferred (2). As might be expected, failures with this technique are frequent.

Many oils have been used and all vegetable oils, mineral oil and emulsified tallow are effective. The choice of oil to be used depends on local availability and cost. If the oils are to be used over an extended period some consideration must be given to the effects of the oil on the animal. Continued administration of mineral oil causes restriction of carotene absorption and reduces the carotene and tocopherol content of the butter produced (30). Linseed oil, soya oil and whale oil have undesirable effects on the quality and flavour of the milk and butter (18). Peanut oil and tallow are the most satisfactory. In most areas the tympany-producing effect of pasture is short lived and may last for only 2 to 3 weeks. During this time the pasture can be grazed under the sheltering umbrella of oil administration until the bloat-producing period is passed.

Non-ionic surfactants (31, 32) especially poloxalene (polyoxyethylene polyoxypropylene block polymer) are highly effective, more so in cattle than sheep (43). In cattle daily intakes of poloxalene of 10 to 20 g. are recommended and daily dose rates of up to 40 g. are without deleterious effect. In very high risk situations it may be advisable to administer the drug at least twice daily. Poloxalene is rather unpalatable and its use in drinking water was not possible until the introduction of the pluronic L64 which is suitable for mixing with drinking water and is effective. It needs to be introduced to the cattle several weeks before the bloat season commences (38). It is in most general use as an additive to grain mixtures but it is also used in feed pellets and in mineral blocks (42).

Pectin methyl esterase inhibitors. In an attempt to inhibit PME and thus reduce the viscosity of ruminal fluids, a slow release granule in which sodium alkyl aryl sulphonate is impregnated onto vermiculite and coated with ethyl cellulose has been produced and found to be effective (33).

Sustained released capsules. These appliances have been under investigation in Australia and New Zealand for some time (40). A large capsule is administered into the rumen via a flexible large-bore tube. In the rumen the capsule opens exposing an antifoaming agent, which diffuses slowly from a matrix of ethyl-cellulose gel. The duration of effect is about 2 weeks.

Feedlot bloat is rather more resistant to the above mentioned procedures than pasture bloat (28) and continues to be a persistent problem in some feedlots. In some instances the addition of 2 oz. of mineral oil to the grain twice daily has given dramatic results and together with the addition of coarse roughage to the diet is strongly recommended. However, there are many reports of failure when comparatively large amounts are fed. In feedlot bloat vegetable oils and animal fats appear to be less effective than mineral oil, probably because of digestion of the former (35). Poloxalene at a dose rate of 10 g. daily appears to be efficient and has the advantage that it can be incorporated in a premix to be added to the grain ration (36). At a dose rate of 22·5 g. twice daily, a fairly expensive programme, this product did not completely prevent bloat (45).

Apart from the impressive reduction in clinical and fatal cases of ruminal tympany resulting from the prophylactic use of oils, there are the added advantages of being able to utilize dangerous pasture with impunity, and the reduction of subclinical bloat and its attendant lowering of food intake. Production may rise by as much as 25 per cent in 24 hours after the use of oil. Nevertheless these preventive methods should be considered as temporary measures only. The ultimate aim should be the development of a pasture of high net productivity where the maximum productivity is consistent with a low incidence of bloat and diarrhoea. At the moment a pasture comprising equal quantities of clovers and grasses comes closest to achieving this ideal but with available pasture plants and current methods of pasture management this clover/grass ratio is not easy to maintain. Two pasture management techniques are worthy of note. The usual 5 to 10 year period of clover dominance after a mixed pasture is established and the period of bloat susceptibility can be reduced to about 2 years by the administration of high levels of super phosphate (2 to 3 cwt. per acre per year). Also the use of high levels of nitrogen administration to pasture may reduce the risk of bloat during the development period of a pasture. One procedure which does have value is to concentrate on making dangerous pasture into hay and utilizing safer fields for grazing during dangerous periods.

REFERENCES

(1) Johns, A. T. (1956). *Vet. Rev. Ann.*, 2, 107.
(2) Clifford, H. J. *et al.* (1964). *Proc. Ruakura Fmrs Conf. N.Z.*, pp. 214–225.
(3) Anonymous (1965). *Mod. vet. Pract.*, 46, 47.
(4) Annotation (1957). *J. Amer. vet. med. Ass.*, 130, 49.
(5) Warner, D. *et al.* (1962). *J. Anim. Sci.*, 21, 757, 798.
(6) Lindahl, I. L. *et al.* (1957). *J. Anim. Sci.*, 16, 165.
(7) Head, M. J. (1959). *Nature, Lond.*, 183, 757.
(8) Bartley, E. E. & Yadava, I. S. (1961). *J. Anim. Sci.*, 20, 648 & 654.
(9) Weiss, K. E. (1953). *Onderstepoort. J. vet. Res.*, 26, 241.
(10) Meyer, R. M. *et al.* (1964). *J. Dairy Sci.*, 47, 1339.
(11) Mendel, V. E. & Boda, J. M. (1961). *J. Dairy Sci.*, 44, 1881.
(12) Bartley, E. E. *et al.* (1961). *J. Dairy Sci.*, 44, 553.
(13) Jacobson, D. R. *et al.* (1957). *J. Anim. Sci.*, 16, 515.
(14) Wright, D. E. & Frazer, J. G. (1961). *N.Z. J. agric. Res.*, 4, 203, 216, 224.
(15) Neal, P. A. & Edwards, G. B. (1963). *Vet. Rec.*, 75, 672.
(16) Johns, A. T. (1958). *Vet. Rev. Ann.*, 4, 17.
(17) Nichols, R. E. (1964). *Rep. 3rd intern. Meet. Dis. of Cattle, Copenhagen*, 2, 355.
(18) Nichols, R. E. (1968). *Amer. J. vet. Res.*, 29, 2005.
(19) Walker, D. (1960). *Aust. vet. J.*, 36, 17.
(20) Mullenax, C. H. *et al.* (1966). *Amer. J. vet. Res.*, 27, 211.
(21) Reid, C. S. W. & Johns, A. T. (1957). *N.Z. J. Sci. Tech., Sec. A.*, 38, 908.
(22) Johnson, R. H. *et al.* (1960). *J. Dairy Sci.*, 43, 1341.
(23) Johns, A. T. & McDowall, F. H. (1962). *N.Z. J. agric. Res.*, 4, 476 & 5, 1.

(24) Barrentine, B. F. *et al.* (1956). *J. Anim. Sci.*, *15*, 440.
(25) Johnson, R. H. *et al.* (1958). *J. Anim. Sci.*, *17*, 893.
(26) Van Horn, H. H. *et al.* (1963). *J. Anim. Sci.*, *22*, 399.
(27) Shellenberger, P. R. *et al.* (1964). *J. Anim. Sci.*, *23*, 196.
(28) Brown, L. R. *et al.* (1958). *J. Anim. Sci.*, *17*, 374.
(29) Southcott, W. H. & Hewetson, R. W. (1958). *Aust. vet. J.*, *34*, 136.
(30) McDowall, F. H. *et al.* (1957). *N.Z. J. Sci. Tech.*, *Sec. A.*, *38*, 839, 878, 1036, 1054.
(31) Helmer, L. H. *et al.* (1965). *J. Dairy Sci.*, *48*, 575, 799, 800.
(32) Bartley, E. E. (1965). *J. Amer. vet. med. Ass.*, *147*, 1397.
(33) Nichols, R. E. (1963). *J. Amer. vet. med. Ass.*, *143*, 998.
(34) Elam, C. J. *et al.* (1960). *J. Anim. Sci.*, *19*, 1089.
(35) Elam, C. J. & Davis, R. E. (1962). *J. Anim. Sci.*, *21*, 568.
(36) Shone, D. K. (1965). *J. S. Afr. vet. med. Ass.*, *36*, 373.
(37) Ayre-Smith, R. (1971). *Aust. vet. J.*, *47*, 162.
(38) Phillips, D. S. M. (1968). *N.Z. J. agric. Res.*, *11*, 85.
(39) Miltimore, J. E. *et al.* (1970). *Canad. J. Anim. Sci.*, *50*, 61.
(40) Gyles, A. (1970). *J. Agric. Vict. Dep. Agric.*, *68*, 156, 158.
(41) Mills, J. H. L. & Christian, R. G. (1970). *J. Amer. vet. med. Ass.*, *157*, 947.
(42) Foote, L. E. *et al.* (1968). *J. Dairy Sci.*, *51*, 584.
(43) Lippke, H. *et al.* (1969). *J. Anim. Sci.*, *28*, 819.
(44) Bartley, E. E. *et al.* (1967). *J. Amer. vet. med. Ass.*, *151*, 339.
(45) Bartley, E. E. & Meyer, R. M. (1967). *J. Anim. Sci.*, *26*, 913.

Ruminal Parakeratosis

Parakeratosis of the ruminal epithelium does not as far as is known cause clinical illness but opinions on its effects on weight gains and productivity vary. There is evidence that the development of parakeratosis increases and then reduces the absorption of volatile fatty acids from the rumen (5, 6) and that the addition of volatile fatty acids to a calf starter increases the incidence of the condition (7). The abnormality has been observed most commonly in cattle and sheep fed high-concentrate rations or alfalfa pellets which have been subjected to heat treatment and does not occur in cattle fed on rations containing normal quantities of unpelleted roughage (1, 5). The incidence of the disease does not appear to be related to the feeding of antibiotics or protein concentrates.

In affected rumens the papillae are enlarged, leathery, dark in colour and often adhered to form clumps. Histologically there is an increase in thickness of the cornified portion of the ruminal epithelium and a persistence of nuclei in the cornified cells (2). Some of the affected cells contain vacuoles. The aetiology and pathogenesis of the condition is obscure but it seems likely that the exciting factor is a chemical substance in the ruminal fluid. This is supported by the observation that parakeratosis of the stomach can be produced in rats fed ruminal fluid from affected cows (3), and by the greatest severity of lesions on the dorsal surface of the rumen about the level of the fluid ruminal contents. If such a chemical compound is present it may be produced from the feed constituents or accidentally added during processing of the feed. The incidence of affected animals in a group may be as high as 40 per cent (2, 4).

REFERENCES

(1) Harvey, R. W. *et al.* (1968). *J. Anim. Sci.*, *27*, 1438.
(2) Jensen, R. *et al.* (1958). *Amer. J. vet. Res.*, *19*, 277.
(3) Vidacs, G. *et al.* (1961). *J. Dairy Sci.*, *44*, 1178.
(4) Hopkins, H. A. *et al.* (1960). *J. Anim. Sci.*, *19*, 652.
(5) Harris, B. (1965). *Diss. Abstr.*, *26*, 1260.
(6) Hinders, R. F. & Owen, F. G. (1965). *J. Dairy Sci.*, *48*, 1069.
(7) Gilliland, R. L. *et al.* (1962). *J. Dairy Sci.*, *45*, 1211.

Impaction of the Omasum

Chronic omasal impaction as a clinical entity is difficult to define and is usually diagnosed at necropsy when the omasum is enlarged and excessively hard (2). It seems unlikely that it could cause death and is frequently observed in animals dying of other disease. It is reputed to occur when feed is tough and fibrous, particularly alfalfa stalks and loppings from fodder trees, or under drought feeding conditions in sheep which are fed on the ground. In the latter the impaction is due to the accumulation of soil in the omasum. Chronic recurrent bouts of indigestion occur and are manifested by normal rumen motility, infrequent and scanty faeces, refusal to eat grain and a negative ketone test (1). Pain may be elicited and the hard distended viscus palpated on deep pressure under the right costal arch or in the seventh to ninth intercostal spaces on the right side. Repeated dosing with mineral oil is recommended as treatment.

A more acute form of omasal atony in cattle is recorded in which the atony may be primary or secondary to other disease, particularly postparturient haemoglobinuria (5) and parturient paresis (3, 4). The omasum is grossly distended, the leaves and in some cases the wall of the organ show patches of necrosis and an associated peritonitis. Necrosis of the ruminal lining may also be present. Clinically the disease is manifested by complete anorexia, cessation of defaecation, an empty rectum and subacute abdominal pain with disinclination to move or lie down.

REFERENCES

(1) McDonald, J. S. & Witzel, D. A. (1968). *J. Amer. vet. med. Ass.*, *152*, 638.
(2) Hughes, W. A. & Cartwright, J. R. (1962). *Vet. Rec.*, *74*, 676.
(3) Blampied, P. H. *et al.* (1964). *Vet. Rec.*, *76*, 533.
(4) Albert, T. F. & Ramey, D. B. (1965). *J. Amer. vet. med. Ass.*, *147*, 617.
(5) Swarbrick, O. (1967). *Vet. Rec.*, *80*, 298.

Impaction of the Abomasum

(*Gastric Dyspepsia*)

The abomasum becomes impacted as part of the syndrome of vagus indigestion and in the unusual circumstance where cows are fed entirely on chopped straw. This is only likely to occur where husbandry is impoverished and where cattle are stimulated to eat large amounts because of very cold weather. It is probable that very little digestion of the straw occurs in the rumen and material which is fragmented by ruminal movements is carried over into the abomasum with rumen liquor but is unable to pass the pylorus. The clinical syndrome is very similar to that of vagus indigestion and, as in that disease, treatment even by abomasotomy is successful only rarely (1) although the prospects are improved if the cow is in good condition and there are no adhesions (3). Supplementation of the diet with a high-protein concentrate should encourage digestion of the straw and prevent impaction of the abomasum.

In young calves and lambs acute pyloric obstruction occurs after eating indigestible material including rags and shavings. Abomasal impaction in young animals also occurs as part of a syndrome of indigestion especially when calves are fed at infrequent intervals on over-large quantities of milk with a high content of casein (2, 4). An indigestible, rubbery curd develops in the abomasum which causes persistent scouring. If the feeding mismanagement continues the terminal stage of abomasal impaction develops. The calf becomes emaciated, has a pendulous, distended lower abdomen and fluid can be heard rattling in the abdomen when the animal is shaken. There is often a great deal of coarse straw and hair present in the abomasum but whether this is a primary cause of the impaction or is the result of a depraved appetite caused by indigestion is unknown. Abomasotomy is the only satisfactory treatment but atony of the stomach may persist even if the impacted material is removed.

REFERENCES

(1) Baker, G. T. & Lewis, M. R. W. (1964). *Vet. Rec.*, 76, 416.
(2) Hall, S. A. (1962). *Vet. Rec.*, 74, 814.
(3) Merritt, A. B. & Boucher, W. B. (1967). *J. Amer. vet. med. Ass.*, 150, 1115.
(4) Gray, J. D. L. (1968). *Vet. Rec.*, 82, 538.

Left Abomasal Displacement

In this disease the abomasum is displaced from its normal position on the abdominal floor either to the left or to the right or into an anterior position. In left displacement a sac of the abomasum comes to lie in a position behind the omasum and to the left of the rumen. The greater curvature passes under the rumen, is impounded between the rumen and the left abdominal wall and lies in the left lower flank. This form of the disease occurs most commonly at or soon after parturition and is characterized clinically by capricious appetite, reduced faecal volume and secondary ketosis. In anterior displacement the clinical picture is very similar to that of left displacement but the abomasum, or the major part of it, is displaced anteriorly and comes to lie between the reticulum and the diaphragm. In right displacement the abomasum is displaced to the right and is found lying between the liver and the right abdominal wall, and in severe cases may extend as far backwards as the pelvic brim. It is identical with the disease described by some authors as dilation of the abomasum and by others as subacute abomasal torsion. Because of the uncertainty as to nomenclature and its closer similarity to torsion than to left or anterior displacement it is described under the heading of dilatation in which there is usually some degree of torsion of the pylorus.

Aetiology

Left abomasal displacement has been observed in adult dairy cows with increasing frequency in recent years. This may be due to an increase in the surgical treatment of cases of chronic indigestion in cattle leading to more frequent observation of the displaced abomasum through laparotomy incisions. On the other hand there is a general impression that the disease has increased in incidence. This may be related to heavy feeding with grain in late pregnancy (1) since the highest incidence of abomasal displacement appears to be in those herds in which heavy grain or other concentrate feeding is practised. Opinions of research workers differ on the importance of heavy grain feeding as a causative factor (13, 14, 17) but the weight of evidence is that it does contribute to abomasal displacement. Occasional cases occur in calves and bulls but the disease rarely if ever occurs in beef cattle.

Parturition appears to be the most common precipitating factor (1, 2, 9). A few cases occur in late pregnancy and some dissociated from parturition but the condition is often so chronic that a history of the exact date of commencement may be difficult to obtain. It is probable that during pregnancy the rumen is lifted from the abdominal floor by the expanding uterus and the abomasum is pushed forward and to the left under the rumen. When parturition occurs the rumen subsides, trapping the abomasum, especially if it is atonic or distended with food as it is likely to be if the cow is fed heavily on grain. An additional, and probably highly important, factor is the diminution in size of the rumen which occurs on a minimal roughage diet and which would provide easy ventral access for the atonic abomasum (1). Unusual activity, including jumping on other cows during oestrus, is a common history in cases not associated with parturition. A marked predisposition to the disease is apparent in Channel Island cattle and most cases (up to 90 per cent) occur during the winter period (2). It is suggested that animals are predisposed to the disease by primary abomasal atony, possibly due to heavy grain feeding, and by inherited susceptibility, and that actual cases are precipitated by parturition, violent activity or misadventure. Dilation of the abomasum does not have the same relationship to pregnancy and cases occur in pregnant and non-pregnant animals in about equal numbers. An interesting difference is that of the incidence of these diseases in different countries. Left displacement is much the most common disease in the U.K. and North America but it is greatly overshadowed in numbers by abomasal dilation in Denmark.

Pathogenesis

There is a great deal of visceral displacement, the abomasum being displaced upward along the left abdominal wall, sometimes lateral to the spleen and sometimes between the spleen and the dorsal sac of the rumen. The omasum, reticulum, duodenum and liver are also displaced by rotation (10). Compression of the impounded part of the abomasum causes a great decrease in the volume of the organ and interference with normal movements. There is probably some interference with the function of the oesophageal groove due to slight rotation of all the stomachs in a clockwise direction and this impedes forward passage of ingesta. The obstruction of the displaced segment is incomplete and although it contains some gas and fluid, a certain amount is still able to escape and the distension rarely becomes severe. There is no interference with blood supply to the trapped portion so that the effects of the displacement are entirely those of interference with digestion and movement of the ingesta, leading to a state of chronic inanition.

Clinical Findings

In left displacement (3, 4, 5) there is initially a sudden decrease in appetite accompanied in occasional cases by signs of severe abdominal pain and abdominal distension. An obvious bulge caused by the distended abomasum may develop in the anterior part of the lower left paralumbar fossa and this may extend up behind the costal arch almost to the top of the fossa. The swelling is tympanitic and gives a resonant note on percussion. In most cases the medial displacement of the rumen results in a somewhat 'slab-sided' appearance. In acute cases the temperature may rise to 39·5 °C (103 °F) and the heart rate to 100 per minute but in the more common subacute cases the temperature and pulse rate are normal. The appetite returns but is intermittent and selective, the animal eating only certain feeds, particularly hay. The faeces are usually small in volume and pasty but periods of profuse diarrhoea may occur. Milk production decreases rapidly and the animal becomes thin with the abdomen greatly reduced in size.

Ruminal movements are present but may be decreased in frequency and are always decreased in intensity, often to the point where no sounds are heard. Auscultation of an area below a line from the centre of the left paralumbar fossa to just behind the left elbow reveals the presence of abnormal sounds of a much higher pitch and of a tinkling or splashing and more fluid nature than ruminal sounds. They often have a progressive peristaltic character. These are abomasal sounds and may occur frequently or as long as 15 minutes apart. They are not related in occurrence to ruminal movements and this can be ascertained by simultaneous auscultation of the left lower abdomen and palpation of the dorsal sac of the rumen. Auscultation in the tenth left intercostal space may reveal splashing sounds. Simultaneous ballottement and auscultation may stimulate typical sounds of abomasal displacement, and on simultaneous percussion of the last ribs and auscultation of the displaced organ a high pitched resonant note is heard (2, 4). Care must be taken not to mistake an atonic distended rumen for a displaced abomasum. This can best be done by carefully delimiting the area over which the characteristic resonant note can be heard on percussion. There may be transitory periods of improvement in appetite and disappearance of these sounds especially after transport or vigorous exercise.

On rectal examination a sense of negative pressure in the upper right abdomen may be appreciated. The rumen is small when the case is of several weeks' duration and the distended abomasum may be palpable to its left. In occasional cases there is chronic ruminal tympany and the rumen is distended. Untreated animals usually reach a certain level of inanition and then remain static for long periods. The disease is not usually fatal but affected animals are usually less than satis-factory production units. Occasional cases produce milk at normal levels (11).

In anterior displacement the clinical findings are very similar to those described above except that normal ruminal sounds can be heard in the usual position and gurgling sounds characteristic of a distended abomasum are heard just behind and above the heart and on both sides of the chest. If a rumenotomy is performed the distended aboma-sum can be felt between the reticulum and dia-phragm (15).

Clinical Pathology

There are no marked changes in the blood picture unless there is intercurrent disease, particularly traumatic reticuloperitonitis or abomasal ulcer. A moderate to severe ketonuria is always present (6) but the blood sugar level is normal. Paracentesis behind the costal arch, low down on the left side may permit the withdrawal of abomasal fluid which can be differentiated from ruminal fluid by the absence of motile protozoa and by its low pH (2 to 4 compared with 6 to 7·6 in ruminal fluid). Fluid is not always present in appreciable quantity in the abomasum and a negative result on puncture can-not be interpreted as eliminating the possibility of abomasal displacement.

Necropsy Findings

The disease is not usually fatal but carcases of affected animals are sometimes observed at abat-toirs. The displaced abomasum is trapped between the rumen and the ventral abdominal floor and contains variable amounts of fluid and gas. In occasional cases it is fixed in position by adhesions which usually arise from an abomasal ulcer.

Diagnosis

Most confusion occurs with primary ketosis or ketosis secondary to other diseases. The abomasal sounds audible on careful auscultation over the lower left flank are necessary to confirm the diag-nosis but the disease should be suspected in any case in which ketosis does not respond to treatment. The tinkling sounds of gas bubbles rising through fluid which can be heard in many cases of ruminal stasis may be confused with true abomasal sounds. Traumatic reticuloperitonitis is accompanied by ruminal stasis, mild fever and pain on abdominal percussion. Vagus indigestion is usually mani-fested by abdominal distension or palpable abo-masal enlargement and is more common before parturition. Diaphragmatic hernia is characterized by chronic ruminal tympany and abdominal en-largement. Exploratory laparotomy is necessary in many cases to confirm a diagnosis of abomasal dis-placement although peritoneoscopy has been used as an alternative.

Treatment

Rolling and manipulation have produced moder-ately good results for some workers (7). The cow is cast and laid on her back, then rolled vigorously to the right and the roll stopped abruptly in the hope that the abomasum will free itself. Chances of success are greatest in the advanced stages when the rumen is small. Starvation and restriction of fluid intake for several days beforehand may be advis-able. Violent exercise and transport over bumpy roads has on occasion caused spontaneous re-covery. Surgical relief of the displacement is now commonly practised and many techniques have been devised with emphasis on avoidance of re-currence of the displacement (6, 8, 12, 16). When coincident abomasal ulceration is suspected abo-masectomy may be necessary if perforation has occurred.

REFERENCES

(1) Neal, P. A. (1964). *Rep. 3rd int. Meet. Dis. Cattle, Copen-hagen*, 2, 361.
(2) Pinsent, P. J. N. *et al.* (1961). *Vet. Rec.*, 73, 729.
(3) Mason, T. A. (1967). *Vet. Rec.*, 80, 253.
(4) Richmond, D. H. (1964). *Canad. vet. J.*, 5, 5.
(5) Mather, M. F. & Dedrick, R. S. (1966). *Cornell Vet.*, 56, 323.
(6) Robertson, J. M. & Boucher, W. B. (1966). *J. Amer. vet. med. Ass.*, 149, 1423 & 1430.
(7) Cote, J. F. (1960). *Canad. vet. J.*, 1, 58.
(8) Gabel, A. A. & Heath, R. B. (1969). *J. Amer. vet. med. Ass.*, 155, 632.
(9) Robertson, J. McD. (1968). *Amer. J. vet. Res.*, 29, 421.
(10) Sack, W. O. (1968). *Amer. J. vet. Res.*, 29, 1567.
(11) Albert, T. F. & Ramey, D. B. (1968). *J. Amer. vet. med. Ass.*, 152, 1125.
(12) Weaver, A. D. (1970). *Brit. vet. J.*, 126, 194.
(13) Sack, W. O. & Svendsen, P. (1970). *Amer. J. vet. Res.*, 31, 1539.
(14) Svendsen, P. (1970). *Nord. Vet.-Med.*, 22, 571.
(15) Watering, C. C. v. d. *et al.* (1965). *T. Diergeneesk.*, 90, 1478.
(16) Lagerweij, E. & Numans, S. R. (1968). *Neth. J. vet. Sci.*, 1, 155.
(17) Svendsen, P. (1969). *Nord. Vet.-Med.*, 21, Suppl. 1, viii.

Dilation (Right Displacement) and Torsion of the Abomasum

Abomasal dilation, or right displacement as it is sometimes called, is a subacute disease character-ized by gradual distension of the right side of the abdomen due to fluid accumulation in the aboma-sum. It is probably a common, but not a necessary, precursor to abomasal torsion which is an acute obstruction of the alimentary tract and is manifested by severe abdominal pain, a short course and a high mortality rate.

Aetiology

Dilation and torsion of the abomasum are being observed in adult dairy cows with increasing frequency probably because of improvement in diagnostic techniques. Most cases of torsion occur in the period 3 to 6 weeks after calving (1, 2) but cases of dilation occur at any time. The cause is unknown, but the hypothesis for the aetiology of dilation is that a primary distension of the abomasum occurs either because of obstruction of the pylorus or primary atony of the abomasal musculature (3). Many cases have no apparent obstruction at the pylorus and atony of the abomasum seems to be a more likely cause but in Denmark the ingestion of large numbers of soil particles on unwashed roots is thought to be significant. This may be the reason for the higher incidence of the disease in the latter part of the winter (4). However attempts to reproduce the condition by feeding large quantities of sand have been unsuccessful (5). Because atony is often associated with vagus indigestion a relationship between the two has been suspected but there are usually no lesions affecting the reticulum or vagus nerves. Several cases have been recorded in calves (6, 7, 8, 9).

Pathogenesis

In torsion the twist is usually of the order of 180 to 270° and the syndrome is one of acute obstruction due to complete blockage. Fluid accumulates in the obstructed viscus and severe shock and dehydration follow. In subacute torsion the degree of rotation is less and although only small amounts of ingesta can pass there is no obstruction of the blood supply to the part. Alkalosis and dehydration develop but relatively slowly (10), the former because of increased secretion of hydrochloric acid. There are varying reports of the nature and direction of the torsion but most cases seem to fit into the following description (11). Torsion occurs in a vertical plane around a horizontal axis passing transversely across the body in the vicinity of the omaso-abomasal orifice; viewed from the right the torsion may be clockwise or anticlockwise.

Clinical Findings

In torsion (1, 12) there is a sudden onset of abdominal pain with kicking at the belly, depression of the back and crouching. The heart rate is increased to 100 to 120 per minute, the temperature is subnormal and ruminal movements are absent. The faeces are soft, and dark in colour and become blood-stained or melaenic in the ensuing 48 hours. They are usually passed in moderate quantity but there may be profuse diarrhoea. The abdomen is distended in the right flank and auscultation and percussion reveal tympany and the tinkling notes of a distended abomasum. Fluid movements may be heard on succussion. No food is taken but the animals are usually thirsty. Distension of the abomasum may be detectable on rectal examination but this is more usual in the subacute type. Death usually occurs in 48 to 96 hours from shock and dehydration.

In simple dilation (3, 12) the onset is more insidious and is marked by inappetence, slight ruminal tympany, a moderate increase in heart rate up to 90 per minute and a normal temperature. There is no acute abdominal pain. Ruminal movements are depressed but still present and the faeces are pasty and dark in colour. After 3 or 4 days the abdomen becomes obviously distended on the right side and the distended abomasum can be easily palpated on rectal examination. It may completely fill the right half of the abdomen and be of similar dimensions to the rumen. The wall is tense and the viscus is filled with gas and fluids which can be detected by auscultation, palpation and succussion of the area. In this form of the disease the course may be as long as 10 to 14 days. In both forms rupture of the abomasum may occur and cause the sudden death of the animal.

Clinical Pathology

Clinico-pathological examinations are not usually required for diagnosis. The blood picture is normal but haematological observations may be carried out in early subacute cases to rule out the presence of traumatic reticuloperitonitis. Because of the occurrence of the disease in the period after calving, tests for ketonuria are often performed and are usually moderately or markedly positive.

Necropsy Findings

In acute torsion the abomasum is grossly distended with brownish, sanguineous fluid and is twisted upon its long axis usually to the left, often with displacement of the omasum, reticulum and duodenum. In acute cases if the torsion is complete the wall of the abomasum is grossly haemorrhagic and gangrenous, and may have ruptured. In cases of dilation there may be impaction of the pylorus with particles of soil or an accompanying pyloric ulcer.

Diagnosis

Early subacute cases resemble traumatic reticulo-peritonitis but there is no pain on abdominal percussion and no abnormality of the leucocyte count. These cases may also be confused with primary acetonaemia and abomasal displacement but there is no response to treatment for acetonaemia and no abomasal sounds can be heard in the left flank. Differentiation between subacute cases of torsion and vagus indigestion with abomasal impaction is extremely difficult unless the abomasum can be palpated through a laparotomy incision or per rectum. In torsion the abomasum is tightly distended with gas and fluid; in impaction the contents are firm. Vagal indigestion usually develops much more slowly than torsion. In foetal hydrops, the two horns of the distended uterus are palpable and the organ is usually much tenser and more posterior. In caecal torsion the distended viscus is smaller in diameter, runs horizontally and its blind end may be palpable.

Acute cases resemble acute intestinal obstruction but there is no palpable loop of distended intestine, and the faeces are not so scanty nor heavily blood-stained until a later stage and are passed in greater quantity. The accumulation of fluid in the anterior part of the abdomen which can be heard on succussion is also indicative of abomasal torsion. Aspiration of this fluid by paracentesis may be of assistance in diagnosis. It is usually brown and sanguineous.

Treatment

In subacute cases laparotomy through the right flank with drainage of the abomasum and correction of the torsion has been carried out successfully but in many cases abomasal atony persists and the mortality rate is about 50 per cent (4, 11, 13). Rocking the cow on her back, followed by allowing her to get up from the right side, may sometimes be of value. In acute cases the treatment must be performed urgently as gangrene of the abomasal wall occurs quickly. Supportive treatment with large quantities of isotonic fluids is important to maintain the animal's fluid and electrolyte balance.

REFERENCES

(1) Bischoff, P. (1953). *Proc. 15th int. vet. Cong.*, Pt. 1, 2, 1040.
(2) Poelma, M. A. (1963). *Canad. vet. J.*, 4, 214.
(3) Jones, E. W. (1959). *Univ. Pennsylvania Bull., Vet. Ext. Qtly.*, 59, 44.
(4) Espersen, G. (1964). *Vet. Rec.*, 76, 1423.
(5) Svendsen, P. (1965). *Nord. Vet.-Med.*, 17, 500.
(6) Elam, C. J. *et al.* (1960). *J. Anim. Sci.*, 19, 1089.
(7) McNish, W. C. (1961). *Canad. vet. J.*, 2, 464.
(8) Macleod, N. S. M. (1964). *Vet. Rec.*, 76, 223.
(9) Martin, J. A. (1964). *Vet. Rec.*, 76, 297.
(10) Espersen, G. & Simesen, M. G. (1961). *Nord. Vet.-Med.*, 13, 147.
(11) Neal, P. A. & Pinsent, P. J. N. (1960). *Vet. Rec.*, 72, 175.
(12) Albert, T. F. & Ramey, D. B. (1964). *J. Amer. vet. med. Ass.*, 145, 553.
(13) Boucher, W. B. & Abt, D. (1968). *J. Amer. vet. med. Ass.*, 153, 76.

6

Diseases of the Liver

INTRODUCTION

PRIMARY DISEASES of the liver seldom occur in farm animals except as a result of poisonings. Secondary disease of the liver, arising as part of a generalized disease process or by spread from another organ, occurs more commonly. In primary hepatic disease the clinical manifestations are caused solely by the lesions in the liver while in secondary involvement the syndrome may include clinical signs unrelated to the hepatic lesions. This chapter is devoted to a consideration of primary diseases of the liver and to those aspects of other diseases in which manifestations of hepatic involvement occur.

The biliary system is not dealt with in detail because of its infrequent involvement in clinical disease. However, one does see occasional cases of cholangitis in cattle and horses. In horses a diffuse bacterial hepatitis, with signs of hepatic insufficiency, may be a sequel to cholangitis. In cattle concretions in the biliary system are usually a sequel to hepatic fascioliasis. Mild cases show temporary anorexia and pain on percussion over the liver. Severe cases are characterized by recurrent attacks of severe abdominal pain, alimentary tract stasis, and pain over the liver. Jaundice occurs only in the terminal stages of fatal cases and is accompanied by recumbency, depression and coma (1).

Principles of Hepatic Dysfunction

DIFFUSE AND FOCAL HEPATIC DISEASE

The liver has a very large reserve of function and approximately three-quarters of its parenchyma must be rendered inactive before clinical signs of hepatic dysfunction appear. Diffuse diseases of the liver are more commonly accompanied by signs of insufficiency than are focal diseases, which produce their effects either by the toxins formed in the lesions or by pressure on other organs, including the biliary system. The origin of a toxaemia is often difficult to localize to the liver because of the physical difficulty of examining the organ.

Diffuse diseases of the liver can be classified as hepatitis and hepatosis according to the pathological change which occurs, and the classification also corresponds roughly with the type of causative agent. Clinically the differences between these two diseases is not marked, although some assistance can be obtained from clinico-pathological examination.

HEPATIC DYSFUNCTION

There are no specific modes of hepatic dysfunction. The liver has a great many functions and any diffuse disease of the organ interferes with most or all of the functions to the same degree. Variations occur in the acuteness and severity of the damage but the effects are the same and the clinical manifestations vary in degree only. The major hepatic functions which, when disordered, are responsible for clinical signs include the maintenance of normal blood sugar levels by providing the source as glycogen, the formation of some of the plasma proteins, the formation and excretion of bile salts and the excretion of bile pigments, the formation of prothrombin, and the detoxification and excretion of many toxic substances including photodynamic agents. The clinical signs produced by interference with each of these functions are dealt with under manifestations of hepatic dysfunction. A rather special aspect is the role of the liver in the genesis of primary ketosis of cattle.

THE PORTAL CIRCULATION

The portal circulation and the liver are mutually interdependent, the liver depending upon the portal vein for its supply of nutrients and the portal flow depending upon the patency of the hepatic sinusoids. The portal flow is unusual in that blood from the gastrosplenic area and the lower part of the large intestine passes to the left half of the liver and the blood from the intestines to the right half, without mixing of the two streams in the portal vein. The restriction of toxipathic hepatitis to one half of the liver and the localization of metastatic abscesses and neoplasms in specific lobes results from the failure of portal vein blood from different gut segments to mix. The localization of toxipathic hepatitis may be because of selective distribution of the toxin or of protective metabolites. The passage of blood from the portal circuit through the liver to the caudal vena cava is dependent upon the patency of the hepatic vascular bed, and obstruction results in damming back of blood in the portal system, interference with digestion and absorption, and in the final stages the development of ascites.

Manifestations of Liver and Biliary Disease

JAUNDICE

Jaundice is a clinical sign which often arises in diseases of the liver and biliary system but also in diseases in which there are no lesions of these organs. It does not always occur and may be conspicuously absent in acute hepatitis. Although jaundice is a result of the accumulation of bilirubin, the staining is much more pronounced with direct bilirubin than with indirect bilirubin. Thus the jaundice is more intense in cases of obstructive and hepatocellular jaundice than in haemolytic jaundice. The levels of bilirubin in blood also affect the intensity of the jaundice, the obstructive form often being associated with levels of bilirubin which are ten times higher than those commonly seen in haemolytic anaemia. The staining of jaundice is due to staining of tissues, especially elastic tissue, and not to accumulation in tissue fluids so that it is best detected clinically in the sclera, and jaundice which may be detectable easily at necropsy may not be visible on clinical examination. Many classifications have been suggested but the simplest is that proposed by Popper and Schaffner (2) and illustrated diagrammatically in the table below.

The primary differentiation has to be made between jaundice with and without impairment of bile flow. Some indication of the type of jaundice can be derived from clinical examination. Thus jaundice is usually much more severe when impairment of flow occurs and when bile pigments are absent from the faeces. However, obstructive jaundice can occur with only partial occlusion of hepatic flow provided at least half of the bile flow is obstructed. In such cases jaundice may occur even though bile pigments are still present in the faeces. With lesser obstruction the portion of the liver and biliary tract which is functioning normally excretes the extra load of bile pigments. The only accurate basis for the differentiation between jaundice with impaired bile flow, and jaundice without impaired flow is the examination of the urine for the presence of bilirubin and urobilinogen and the determination of the relative amounts of direct and indirect bilirubin present in the serum. Indirect bilirubin which has not passed through hepatic cells is not excreted by the kidney, so that in haemolytic jaundice the indirect bilirubin content of serum is increased markedly and although the urine contains an increased amount of urobilinogen, no bilirubin is present. In those cases in which jaundice is caused by impairment of bile flow there is a marked increase in the serum level of direct bilirubin, and the bilirubin content of the urine is greatly increased. The amount of urobilinogen varies depending on whether any bilirubin reaches the intestine to be metabolized to urobilinogen and reabsorbed. In complete extrahepatic biliary obstruction urobilinogen is not present in the urine.

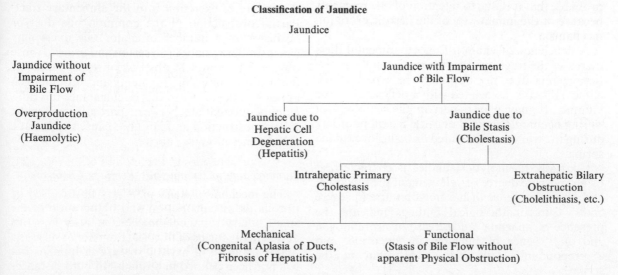

Classification of Jaundice

Jaundice

Jaundice without Impairment of Bile Flow

Jaundice with Impairment of Bile Flow

Overproduction Jaundice (Haemolytic)

Jaundice due to Hepatic Cell Degeneration (Hepatitis)

Jaundice due to Bile Stasis (Cholestasis)

Intrahepatic Primary Cholestasis

Extrahepatic Bilary Obstruction (Cholelithiasis, etc.)

Mechanical (Congenital Aplasia of Ducts, Fibrosis of Hepatitis)

Functional (Stasis of Bile Flow without apparent Physical Obstruction)

Adapted from Popper and Schaffner (2)

Overproduction or Haemolytic Jaundice

Haemolytic jaundice is common in animals and may be caused by bacterial toxins, invasion of erythrocytes by protozoa or viruses, inorganic and organic poisons and immunological reactions. Diseases in which bacterial toxins cause intravascular haemolysis are bacillary haemoglobinuria of cattle and leptospirosis although the mechanism by which haemolysis is produced in the latter disease does not seem to have been accurately determined. The common protozoan and viral diseases in which haemolysis occurs include babesiosis, anaplasmosis, eperythrozoonosis and equine infectious anaemia. Chronic copper poisoning, selenium poisoning in sheep (24), phenothiazine poisoning in horses, pasturing on rape and other cruciferous plants and bites by some snakes are other common causes. Post parturient haemoglobinuria has an uncertain aetiology but is usually attributed to a deficiency of phosphorus in the diet and the feeding of cruciferous plants. Iso-immunization haemolytic anaemia of the newborn is caused by an immunological reaction between the sensitized cells of the newborn and antibodies in the colostrum of the dam. The occurrence of acute haemolytic anaemia and jaundice in calves which drink large quantities of cold water may also be of the nature of an immunological response.

Neonatal jaundice is relatively common in babies and is regarded as a benign condition. It is rarely, if ever, observed clinically in new-born animals but may be noticeable at necropsy. Although it is generally stated that the jaundice is haemolytic and results from the destruction of excess erythrocytes when post-natal life begins, it appears more probable that it is due to retention of bile pigments because of the immaturity of the hepatic excretion mechanism.

A deficiency of vitamin E in experimental diets increases the fragility of erythrocytes but haemolytic anaemia does not appear to be a part of the clinical diseases associated with a deficiency of the vitamin. It may play a part in the aetiology of 'spring haemoglobinuria' of cattle fed on poor hay during the winter and pastured on lush clover in the spring.

Clinically haemolytic jaundice is characterized by a moderate degree of yellowing of the mucosae, and by the presence of haemoglobinuria in severe cases. Clinicopathological findings indicate the presence of anaemia, an increase in urobilinogen and an absence of bilirubin in the urine, and a preponderance of indirect bilirubin in the serum.

Jaundice due to Hepatic Cell Degeneration

The cause may be any of those diffuse diseases of the liver which cause degeneration of hepatic cells and which are listed under hepatitis. Because there is only partial obstruction of biliary excretion, the changes in serum and urine lie between those of haemolytic jaundice and extrahepatic biliary obstruction. Serum levels of total bilirubin are increased because of retention of direct bilirubin which also passes out in the urine, causing an elevation of urine levels. The urobilinogen levels in the urine also rise.

Extrahepatic Biliary Obstruction

Obstruction of the bile ducts or common bile duct by biliary calculi or compression by tumour masses is a rare occurrence in farm animals. Commonly listed causes are obstruction of the common duct by nematodes and inflammation of the bile ducts by extension from an enteritis or by infestation with trematodes.

A significant number of pigs die with biliary obstruction and purulent cholangitis secondary to invasion of the ducts by *Ascaris lumbricoides*. Parasitic cholangitis and cholecystitis also occur due to fascioliasis and infestation with *Dicrocoelium dendriticum*. In horses an ascending cholangitis may develop from a parasitic duodenal catarrh and cause signs of biliary obstruction.

Obstruction is usually complete and results in the disappearance of bile pigments from the faeces. Serum levels of direct bilirubin rise causing a marked elevation of total bilirubin in the serum. Excretion of the direct bilirubin in urine occurs on a large scale but there is no urobilinogen because of the failure of excretion into the alimentary tract. Partial obstruction of the common bile duct or occlusion of a number of major bile ducts may cause similar variations in serum and urine to those observed in complete obstruction except that the faeces do contain bile pigments and urobilinogen appears in the urine. In this circumstance it is difficult to differentiate between partial extrahepatic biliary obstruction and jaundice caused by hepatic cell degeneration (see above).

Jaundice due to Intrahepatic Primary Cholestasis

The mechanical stasis of biliary flow caused by fibrous tissue constriction and obliteration of the small biliary canaliculi may occur after hepatitis and in many forms of fibrosis. Functional stasis is a major problem in hepatic disease in humans but has not been defined in animals. In both instances the defect is the same as in extrahepatic biliary obstruction and the two diseases cannot be differentiated by laboratory tests. This poses a problem in the dog and man in that only extrahepatic biliary obstruction can be relieved by surgery.

NERVOUS SIGNS

Nervous signs including hyperexcitability, convulsions and coma, muscle tremor and weakness, psychic disturbances including dullness, compulsive walking, head-pressing, failure to respond to signals and, in some cases, mania, are common accompaniments of diffuse hepatic disease. The biochemical and anatomical basis for these signs has not been determined. Many factors including hypoglycaemia, and failure of normal hepatic detoxification mechanisms, leading to the accumulation of excess amino-acids and ammonia, or of acetylcholine, and the liberation of toxic breakdown products of liver parenchyma have all been suggested as causes and it is probable that more than one factor is involved.

One of the primary effects of severe, acute liver damage is a precipitate fall in blood sugar accompanied by nervous signs including hyperexcitability, convulsions and terminal coma. If the hepatic damage occurs more slowly the hypoglycaemia is less marked and less precipitous and is accompanied by inability to perform work, drowsiness, yawning and lethargy. With persistent hypoglycaemia structural changes may occur in the brain (hypoglycaemic encephalopathy) and these may be the basis for the chronically drowsy animals or dummies. However, hypoglycaemia does not always occur in acute hepatitis and cannot be considered to be the only or even the most important factor in producing the cerebral signs. Because of this it has been suggested that some unidentified hepatic principle is necessary for the utilization of glucose by neurones.

In many naturally occurring cases of hepatic insufficiency, in all species, degenerative changes in nervous tissue, identified as status spongiosus, have been identified. These changes have not been seen in normal sheep and appear to have a causal relationship to the nervous signs of chronic liver disease. Status spongiosus has been produced experimentally by the continuous infusion of ammonia into sheep who developed classical nervous signs (20).

OEDEMA AND EMACIATION

Failure of the liver to anabolize amino-acids and protein during hepatic insufficiency is manifested by tissue wasting and a fall in plasma protein. This may be sufficiently severe to cause oedema because of the lowered osmotic pressure of the plasma. Hepatic oedema is not usually very marked and is manifested most commonly in the intermandibular space (bottle jaw). If there is obstruction to the portal circulation, as may occur in hepatic fibrosis, the oedema is much more severe but is largely limited to the abdominal cavity.

DIARRHOEA AND CONSTIPATION

In hepatitis, hepatic fibrosis, and in obstruction or stasis of the biliary system the partial or complete absence of bile salts from the alimentary tract deprives it of the laxative and mildly disinfectant qualities of these salts. This, together with the reflex effects from the distended liver in acute hepatitis, produces an alimentary tract syndrome comprising anorexia, vomition in some species, and constipation punctuated by attacks of diarrhoea. The faeces are pale in colour and, if there is an appreciable amount of fat in the diet, there is steatorrhoea.

PHOTOSENSITIZATION

Most photosensitizing substances including phyllo-erythrin, the normal breakdown product of chlorophyll in the alimentary tract, are excreted in the bile. In hepatic or biliary insufficiency excretion of these substances is retarded and photosensitization occurs.

HAEMORRHAGIC DIATHESIS

In severe, diffuse diseases of the liver there is a deficiency in prothrombin formation and a consequent prolongation of the clotting time of the blood. Abnormality of the prothrombin complex is not the only defect, deficiencies of fibrinogen and thromboplastin occurring also. Prothrombin and other factors in the prothrombin complex depend upon the presence of vitamin K for their formation and an absence of bile salts from the intestine retards the absorption of this fat-soluble vitamin. Parenteral administration of vitamin K is advisable before surgery is undertaken in patients with severe hepatic dysfunction.

ABDOMINAL PAIN

Two mechanisms cause the pain in diseases of the liver; distension of the organ with increased tension of the capsule, and lesions of the capsule. Acute swelling of the liver occurs as a result of engorgement with blood in congestive heart failure and in acute inflammation. Inflammatory and neoplastic lesions of the capsule, or of the liver parenchyma just beneath the capsule, cause local irritation to its pain endorgans. The pain is usually subacute causing abnormal posture, particularly arching the back and disinclination to move. Tenseness of the abdominal wall and pain on deep palpation over the liver area may also be detected in the majority of cases.

ALTERATION IN SIZE OF THE LIVER

Great variation in the size of the liver is often seen at necropsy but clinical detection is not easy unless the liver is grossly enlarged. This is most likely to occur in advanced congestion of the liver due to congestive heart failure, in some plant poisonings in horses and when multiple abscesses or neoplastic metastases occur. In acute hepatitis the swelling is not sufficiently large to be detected clinically and in terminal fibrosis the liver is much smaller than normal.

DISPLACEMENT OF THE LIVER

The liver may be displaced from its normal position and protrude into the thoracic cavity through a diaphragmatic hernia causing respiratory distress and abnormal findings on percussion of the chest. Torsion of a lobe of the liver has been recorded in aged sows in the early part of lactation (3). Inappetence, uneasiness and unwillingness to suckle the young were followed by severe, prolonged vomiting, acute abdominal pain and dyspnoea. The twisted lobe was greatly increased in size and in one case the capsule was ruptured leading to severe internal haemorrhage.

RUPTURE OF THE LIVER

Rupture of the liver is an occasional accident in animals occurring usually as a result of trauma. In most instances rupture results in death from haemorrhage although small breaks in the capsule may heal. Horses used for the production of serum frequently develop hepatic amyloidosis, presumably as a reaction to repeated injection of foreign protein, and the death rate from rupture of the liver is relatively high in this group (19).

BLACK LIVERS OF SHEEP

Dark brown to black pigmentation of the liver and kidneys occurs commonly in sheep in certain parts of Australia. No illness is associated with the condition but the livers are not used for human consumption for aesthetic reasons and extensive financial loss may result. Commonly referred to as 'melanosis' the pigmentation has been determined to be the result of deposition of the pigment lipofuscin at various stages of oxidation (4). Areas in which the disease occurs carry many mulga trees (*Acacia aneura*) the leaves of which are fed to sheep in drought times.

The above condition should not be confused with the black livers found in a mutant strain of Corriedales in California (18). In these mutant sheep there is photosensitization following retention of phylloerythrin. The darkening of the liver is due to melanin.

Special Examination of the Liver

When disease of the liver is suspected after a general clinical examination, special techniques of palpation, biopsy and biochemical tests of function can be used to determine further the status of the liver.

PALPATION AND PERCUSSION

In farm animals the liver is well concealed by the rib cage on the right-hand side and its edge cannot be palpated. A general impression of the size of the liver can be obtained by percussion of the area of liver dullness but accurate definition is not usually attempted. Deep percussion or palpation to detect the presence of hepatic pain can be carried out over the area of liver dullness in the posterior thoracic region on the right-hand side. Percussion over the entire area is necessary as the pain of a discrete lesion may be quite localized.

If the liver is grossly enlarged its edge can be felt on deep palpation behind the costal arch and the edge is usually rounded and thickened in contradistinction to the sharp edge of the normal liver. This type of palpation is relatively easy in ruminants but is unrewarding in horses and pigs because of the thickness of the abdominal wall and the shortness of the flank.

BIOPSY OF THE LIVER

Biopsy of the liver has been used extensively as a diagnostic procedure in infectious equine anaemia, and poisoning by *Crotalaria* spp. and other species of plants, and in experimental work on copper and vitamin A deficiency. The technique requires some skill and anatomical knowledge. The most satisfactory instrument is a long, small calibre trocar and cannula to which is screwed a syringe capable of producing good negative pressure. The sharp point of the instrument is introduced in an intercostal space on the right-hand side, the number depending on the species, and advanced across the pleural cavity so that it will reach the diaphragm and diaphragmatic surface of the liver at an approximately vertical position. The point of insertion is made high up in the intercostal space so that the liver is punctured at the thickest part of its edge. The instrument is rotated until the edge of the cannula approximates the liver capsule; the trocar is then withdrawn, the syringe is attached and strong suction applied; the cannula is twisted vigorously and advanced until it reaches the visceral surface of the liver. If its edge is sufficiently sharp the cannula will now contain a core of liver parenchyma and if the instrument is withdrawn with the suction still applied a sample sufficient for histological examination and microassay of vitamin A, glycogen or other nutrient is obtained. Details of the technique for cattle (5, 6, 23), sheep (7) and horses (8, 9) are available.

The major deficiency of the method lies in the small sample which is obtained, and unless the liver change is diffuse the sample may not be representative. The procedure has been repeated many times on one animal without injury. The principal danger is that if the direction of the instrument is at fault it may approach the hilus and damage the large blood-vessels or bile ducts. If the liver is shrunken or the approach too caudal no sample is obtained. Fatal haemoperitoneum may result if a haemorrhagic tendency is present and peritonitis may occur if the liver lesion is an abscess containing viable bacteria. Biliary peritonitis results if a large bile duct is perforated.

ROENTGENOLOGICAL EXAMINATION

The application of roentgenology to examination of the liver and biliary system in large animals is limited to experimental work. Cholecystography after the oral administration of a halogenated phenolphthalein permits visualization of the gall-bladder but cholangiography can only be satisfactorily performed by direct injection of radio-opaque materials into the ducts after laparotomy.

BIOCHEMICAL TESTS OF HEPATIC FUNCTION

Laboratory tests of hepatic function are exacting and time consuming and are seldom undertaken at present in routine diagnostic work in farm animals. They find a place in the investigation of disease problems but in general insufficient work has been done with them to determine standards for normality and the relative usefulness of the different tests (10, 11). The tests in use in human medicine can be classified in three groups, those that measure the excretory rate of parenterally administered substances such as bromsulphalein; those that measure the metabolic activity of the organ by its capacity to metabolize such substances as galactose; and those which test detoxification

functions including the hippuric acid synthesis test and the glucuronic acid test. Apart from tests designed specifically for these particular functions, there is also a great deal of information to be gained from examination of body constituents which may however vary from causes which are not hepatic. These include serum bilirubin (direct and indirect), plasma protein, the albumin/globulin ratio and the non-specific serum-protein reactions on which the flocculation or turbidity tests are based. For full details of these tests and their comparative values up to date reviews should be consulted (5, 11).

In animals the bromsulphalein clearance test has been used in cattle (12), sheep (13), and horses (14) and although little information is available the test appears to have diagnostic value. It is time-consuming and care is needed with prepared solutions in open containers; anaphylactoid reactions have occurred after injection of solutions which are 10 days old (22). In carbon tetrachloride poisoning in cattle the Takata-ara test is the only one of the flocculation tests which appears to be of value and there is little variation in total or partitioned serum-protein levels. Significant variations occur in serum levels of alkaline phosphatase but the variations in normal cattle have such a wide range that results are difficult to interpret. Of the tests based on carbohydrate metabolism the galactose tolerance and adrenaline response tests appear to show some promise (11). Variations in urine bilirubin levels are not sufficiently great to indicate the presence or absence of hepatic disease in cattle unless the insufficiency is of extreme degree. An increase in the concentration of porphyrins (mainly coproporphyrin) in the urine also occurs and should not be mistaken for the porphyrins of inherited porphyria.

Determinations of serum levels of serum enzymes offers some promise in the detection of hepatic injury (17). The level of glutamic oxaloacetate transaminase is high in cardiac muscle and liver but the pyruvate transaminase is much higher in liver than in cardiac muscle in humans, and determination of respective serum levels of these substances may provide results of considerable diagnostic significance. Serum levels of glutamic oxaloacetate transaminase are greatly increased in hepatic damage in the horse, cow, pig and dog but the pyruvate transaminase is appreciably increased in hepatic damage only in the dog (15). In ruminants glutamate dehydrogenase occurs in high concentration in the liver and rises appreciably in serum when liver damage occurs (11). Serum levels of ornithine and carbamyl transferase (OCT) are also elevated even in chronic diseases (15), but only when there is active liver necrosis, not when the lesions are healing.

Measurement of the icteric index of plasma, by comparing its colour with a standard solution of potassium dichromate, cannot be considered to be a liver function test but it is used commonly as a measure of the degree of jaundice present. The colour of normal plasma varies widely between species depending upon the concentration of carotene. Horse, and to a less extent cattle, plasma is quite deeply coloured, but sheep plasma is normally very pale. The colour index needs to be corrected for this factor before the icteric index is computed.

In the early stages of hepatic dysfunction in cattle the serum enzyme tests, particularly glutamic oxalacetate transaminase, are efficient and sensitive tests. In the later stages when tests of biliary excretion are more applicable, estimations of serum bilirubin and phylloerythrin and the bromsulphalein test are indicated (16). In horses the estimation of sorbitol dehydrogenase is preferred (17). A satisfactory combination of tests for liver function is bromsulfalein clearance, OCT test and prothrombin time.

Principles of Treatment in Diseases of the Liver

In diffuse diseases of the liver no general treatment is satisfactory and the main aim should be to remove the source of the damaging agent. The most that can be attempted in acute hepatitis is to tide the animal over the danger period of acute hepatic insufficiency until the subsidence of the acute change and the normal regeneration of the liver restores its function. Death may occur during this stage because of hypoglycaemia, and the blood sugar level must be maintained by oral or intravenous injections of glucose. Because of the danger of guanidine intoxication an adequate calcium intake should be ensured by oral or parenteral administration of calcium salts.

There is some doubt as to whether protein intake should be maintained at a high level, as incomplete metabolism of the protein may result in toxic effects, particularly in the kidney. However, amino-acid mixtures, especially those containing methionine, are used with apparently good results. The same general recommendations apply in prevention as in the treatment of acute diffuse liver disease. Diets high in carbohydrate, calcium and protein of high biological value and a number of specific substances are known to have a protective effect against hepatoxic agents.

In chronic, diffuse, hepatic disease fibrous tissue replacement causes compression of the sinusoids and is irreversible except in the very early stages, when removal of fat from the liver by the administration of lipotrophic factors including choline, and maintenance on a diet low in fat and protein may reduce the compressive effects of fibrous tissue contraction. A high protein diet at this stage causes stimulation of the metabolic activity of the liver and an increased deposition of fat, further retarding hepatic function.

Local diseases of the liver require surgical or medical treatment depending upon the cause, and specific treatments are discussed under the respective diseases.

REFERENCES

(1) Stober, M. (1963). *Dtsch. tierärztl. Wschr.*, *68*, 608, 647.
(2) Popper, H. & Schaffner, F. (1957). *Liver: Structure and Function*, New York: McGraw-Hill.
(3) Gregersen, K. (1958). *Medlemsbl. danske Dyrlaegeforen*, *41*, 299.
(4) Winter, H. (1966). *Aust. vet. J.*, *42*, 40.
(5) Hoe, C. M. (1960). *Vet. Rev. Ann.*, *6*, 1.
(6) Holtenius, P. (1961). *Cornell Vet.*, *51*, 56.
(7) Dick, A. T. (1944). *Aust. vet. J.*, *20*, 298.
(8) Annotation (1944). *Vet. Rec.*, *56*, 278.
(9) Sova, Z. (1962). *Vet. Čas.*, *11*, 375.
(10) Harvey, D. G. (1958). *Vet. Rec.*, *70*, 616.
(11) Ford, E. J. H. (1965). *Vet. Rec.*, *77*, 1507.
(12) Cornelius, C. E. *et al.* (1958). *Amer. J. vet. Res.*, *19*, 560.
(13) Forbes, T. J. & Singleton, A. G. (1966). *Brit. vet. J.*, *122*, 55.
(14) Cornelius, C. E. & Wheat, J. D. (1957). *Amer. J. vet. Res.*, *18*, 369.
(15) Holtenius, P. & Jacobsson, S-O. (1964). *Rep. 3rd int. Meet. Dis. Cattle, Copenhagen, 1964*.
(16) Ford, E. J. H. & Boyd, J. W. (1962). *J. Path. Bact.*, *83*, 39.
(17) Freedland, R. A. & Kramer, J. W. (1970). *Adv. vet. Sci.*, *14*, 61.
(18) Arias, I. *et al.* (1964). *J. clin. Invest. 43*, 1249.
(19) Schützler, H. & Beyer, J. (1964). *Arch. exp. Vet.-Med.*, *18*, 1119.
(20) Hooper, P. T. (1972). *Vet. Rec.*, *90*, 37.
(21) Carper, H. A. (1967). *Amer. J. vet. clin. Path.*, *1*, 77.
(22) Morgan, H. C. *et al.* (1960). *Vet. Med.*, *55*, No. 8, 28.
(23) Thoonen, H. *et al.* (1967). *T. Diergeneesk.*, *36*, 3.
(24) De Boom, H. P. A. & Brown, J. M. M. (1968). *J. S. Afr. vet. med. Ass.*, *39*, 21.

Diffuse Diseases of the Liver

HEPATITIS

The differentiation of hepatic diseases into two groups of hepatitis and hepatosis has not achieved general acceptance and non-specific terms such as hepatic injury have been suggested to avoid the connotation of inflammation associated with the word hepatitis. To facilitate ease of reading, the word hepatitis is used throughout this chapter to include all diffuse, degenerative and inflammatory diseases which affect the liver. It is used here also to include the common pathological classification of cirrhosis. Clinically the syndrome caused by fibrosis of the liver is the same as that caused by hepatitis and the aetiology is the same, the only difference being that the onset of the disease is slower and less acute than in hepatitis.

Aetiology

Toxic hepatitis. The usual lesion is centrilobular and may be mild in degree and manifested by cloudy swelling, or be severe and accompanied by extensive necrosis. If the necrosis is severe enough or repeated a sufficient number of times fibrosis develops. The common causes of toxic hepatitis in farm animals are the inorganic poisons including phosphorus, arsenic and possibly selenium; organic chemicals, particularly carbon tetrachloride, hexachloroethane, gossypol from cottonseed, cresols from coal tar pitch, and chloroform (10); poisonous plants particularly *Senechio* spp., *Crotalaria* spp., *Heliotropum* spp., *Amsinckia* spp., lupins, Alsike clover (*Trifolium hybridum*), a number of fungi including *Pithomyces chartarum*, *Aspergillus flavus*, *Penicillium rubrum* and *Periconia* spp., and some algae. There are reports of an apparent toxic hepatitis in ruminants following the feeding of herring meal (8) and damaged alfalfa hay (9) but the toxic agent has not been identified. The relationship between chronic copper poisoning and hepatitis in sheep is discussed under toxaemic jaundice.

Moderate degrees of hepatitis occur in many bacterial infections irrespective of their location in the body and the hepatitis is usually classified as toxic, but whether the lesions are caused by bacterial toxins or by shock, anoxia or vascular insufficiency is unknown. The same position applies in hepatitis caused by extensive tissue damage occurring after burns, injury and infarction.

Infectious hepatitis. Diffuse hepatic lesions are rarely caused by infectious agents in farm animals. Infectious equine anaemia, salmonellosis, septicaemic listeriosis and leptospirosis are manifested by hepatic necrosis which is recognizable at necropsy but not by clinical signs of hepatic dysfunction. Some systemic mycoses are accompanied by multiple granulomatous lesions of the liver. Equine infectious arteritis causes hepatitis and may be accompanied by jaundice in severe cases, and in infectious equine rhinopneumonitis aborted foetuses show focal hepatic necroses. Foetal hepatopathy has been recorded in a viral epizootic abortion of cattle in California, U.S.A. (1) and a post-vaccinal hepatitis occurs in horses but the aetiological agent in the latter disease has not been determined.

Parasitic hepatitis. Massive liver fluke infestations and migration of larvae of *Ascaris* spp. are among the common causes of severe hepatitis in animals.

Nutritional hepatitis (trophopathic hepatitis). The cirrhosis of the liver caused by methionine deficiency, and acute hepatic necrosis caused by cystine deficiency in the diet of rats (2) are not known to have any importance in farm animals. The knowledge that vitamin E prevents acute hepatic necrosis in rats on cystine-deficient diets has led to the suggestion that the vitamin may be important in the prevention of dietary hepatic necrosis in pigs. There is an interesting relationship between the so called Factor 3, which contains selenium and protects against trophopathic hepatitis (4) and vitamin E, both agents protecting also against enzootic muscular dystrophy. Selenium and alpha-tocopherol have been shown capable of preventing dietary hepatic necrosis in pigs. A multiple dietary deficiency has also been suggested as the cause of a massive hepatic necrosis observed in lambs and adult sheep on trefoil pasture in California, U.S.A. (3).

Congestive hepatitis. Increased pressure in the sinusoids of the liver causes anoxia and compression of surrounding hepatic parenchyma. Congestive heart failure is the common cause and leads to centrilobular degeneration.

Inherited hepatic insufficiency in Southdown and Corriedale sheep is described later. It is not a hepatitis but a functional disease.

Pathogenesis

Hepatitis may be caused by a number of agents but the clinical effects are approximately the same in all instances as set out under manifestations of liver disease above. The usual lesion in toxipathic hepatitis is centrilobular and varies from cloudy swelling to acute necrosis with a terminal veno-occlusive lesion in some plant poisonings. In infectious hepatitis the lesions vary from necrosis of isolated cells to diffuse necrosis affecting all or most of the hepatic parenchyma. In parasitic hepatitis the changes depend upon the number and type of migrating parasites. In massive fluke infestations sufficient damage may occur to cause acute hepatic insufficiency, manifested particularly by submandibular oedema. In more chronic cases extension from a cholangitis may also cause chronic insufficiency. Trophopathic hepatitis in experimental animals is characterized by massive or submassive necrosis, and congestive hepatitis by dilatation of central veins and sinusoids with compression of the parenchymal cells. Hepatic fibrosis develops particularly if there is massive hepatic necrosis which destroys entire lobules. Degeneration is not possible as it is when the necrosis is zonal, and fibrous tissue replacement occurs. Thus fibrosis is a terminal stage of hepatitis which may have developed acutely or chronically and is manifested by the same clinical syndrome as that of hepatitis except that the signs develop more slowly. Fibrosis may also develop from a cholangitis. The term cirrhosis has been avoided because it carries connotations from human medicine which may be misleading when applied to animals.

Clinical Findings

The cardinal signs of hepatitis are anorexia, mental depression, with excitement in some cases, muscular weakness, jaundice and in the terminal stages somnolence, recumbency and coma with intermittent convulsions. Animals which survive the early acute stages may evidence photosensitization, a break in the wool or hair leading to shedding of the coat and susceptibility to metabolic strain for up to a year.

The initial anorexia is often accompanied by constipation and punctuated by attacks of diarrhoea. The faeces are lighter in colour than normal and if the diet contains much fat there may be steatorrhoea. Vomiting may occur in pigs. The nervous signs are often pronounced and vary from lethargy with yawning, or coma, to hyperexcitability with muscle tremor, mania and convulsions. A characteristic syndrome is the dummy syndrome in which affected animals push with the head, do not respond to normal stimuli and may be blind (7). There may be subacute abdominal pain usually manifested by arching of the back, and pain on palpation over the liver. The enlargement of the liver is usually not palpable.

Jaundice and oedema may or may not be present and are more commonly associated with the less acute stages of the disease. Photosensitization may also occur but only when the animals are on a diet containing green feed and are exposed to sunlight. A tendency to bleed more freely than usual may be observed. In chronic hepatic fibrosis the signs are similar to those of hepatitis but develop more slowly, and persist for longer periods, often months. Ascites and the dummy syndrome are more common than in hepatitis.

Clinical Pathology

Urine and blood samples and liver biopsy specimens may be submitted for laboratory examination as outlined under the discussion of jaundice and tests of hepatic dysfunction.

Necropsy Findings

The liver in hepatitis is usually enlarged and the edges swollen but the appearance of the hepatic surface and cross-section varies with the cause. In acute toxic and trophopathic hepatitis the lobulation is more pronounced and the liver is paler and redder in colour. The accentuation of the lobular appearance is caused by engorgement of the centrilobular vessels or centrilobular necrosis. There may be accompanying lesions of jaundice, oedema and photosensitization. In infectious hepatitis the lesions are inclined to be patchy and even focal in their distribution. Parasitic hepatitis is obviously traumatic with focal haemorrhages under the capsule and the necrosis and traumatic injury defineable as tracks. Congestive hepatitis is marked by the severe enlargement of the liver, a greatly increased content of blood, and marked accentuation of the lobular pattern caused by vascular engorgement and fatty infiltration of the parenchyma. In hepatic fibrosis the necropsy findings vary widely depending on the causative agent, the duration of its action and on its severity. The liver may be grossly enlarged or be much reduced in size with marked lobulation of the surface.

Diagnosis

Hepatitis is easily misdiagnosed as an encephalopathy unless jaundice or photosensitization is present. The nervous signs are suggestive of encephalomyelitis, encephalomalacia and cerebral oedema. Congestive hepatitis is usually not manifested by nervous signs, and being a secondary lesion in congestive heart failure, is usually accompanied by ascites and oedema in other regions and by signs of cardiac involvement. Hepatic fibrosis may produce ascites without evidence of cardiac disease.

Acute diseases affecting the alimentary tract, particularly engorgement on grain in cattle and horses, may be manifested by signs of nervous derangement resembling those of acute hepatic dysfunction but the history and clinical examination usually suggest a primary involvement of the alimentary tract.

Treatment

The principles of treatment of hepatitis have already been outlined. Results are seldom good (7). Protein and protein hydrolysates are probably best avoided because of the danger of ammonia intoxication. The diet should be high in carbohydrate and calcium, and low in protein and fat but affected animals are usually completely anoretic. Because of the failure of detoxification of ammonia and other nitrogenous substances by the damaged liver and their importance in the production of nervous signs, the oral administration of broad-spectrum antibiotics has been introduced in man to control protein digestion and putrefaction. The results have been excellent with neomycin and chlortetracyline (5, 6), the disappearance of hepatic coma coinciding with depression of blood ammonia levels. Purgation and enemas have also been used in combination with oral administration of antibiotics but mild purgation is recommended to avoid unnecessary fluid loss. Supplementation of the feed or periodic injections of the water soluble vitamins are desirable. Hepatic fibrosis is considered to be a final stage in hepatitis and treatment is not usually undertaken.

REFERENCES

(1) Howarth, J. A. *et al.* (1956). *J. Amer. vet. med. Ass., 128,* 441.
(2) Schwarz, L. (1954). *N.Y. Acad. Sci., 57,* 617.
(3) Cordy, D. R. & McGowan, B. (1956). *Cornell Vet., 46,* 422.
(4) Bunyan, J. *et al.* (1958). *Nature, Lond., 181,* 1801.
(5) Annotation (1957). *Lancet, 273,* 280.
(6) Dawson, A. M. *et al.* (1957). *Lancet, 273,* 1263.
(7) Fowler, M. E. (1965). *J. Amer. vet. med. Ass., 147,* 55.
(8) Koppang, N. (1964). *Nord. Vet.-Med., 16,* 305.
(9) Monlux, A. W. *et al.* (1963). *J. Amer. vet. med. Ass., 142,* 989.
(10) Wolff, A. A. *et al.* (1967). *Amer. J. vet. Res., 28,* 1363.
(11) Michel, R. L. *et al.* (1969). *J. Amer. vet. med. Ass., 155,* 50.

Focal Diseases of the Liver

HEPATIC ABSCESS

Local suppurative infections of the liver do not cause clinical signs of hepatic dysfunction unless they are particularly massive or extensively metastatic. They may, however, cause signs of toxaemia because of the destruction of hepatic tissue or the liberation of potent toxins. The toxaemia of traumatic hepatitis is usually due to toxins from *Corynebacterium pyogenes* and *Sphaerophorus necrophorus* which are implanted in the lesions by the perforating foreign body. Omphalophlebitis or rumenitis may also lead to hepatic invasions by *Sp. necrophorus* or other organisms and abscessed livers are common in cattle fed heavily on concentrates. Black disease is a profound toxaemia caused by the liberation of potent exotoxin from *Clostridium novyi*, and bacillary haemoglobinuria by a toxin from *Cl. haemolyticum* in focal hepatic necroses.

The clinical signs of these specific diseases are included under the discussion of each disease and the only finding common to all is local pain on palpation or percussion over the liver.

TUMOURS OF THE LIVER

Metastatic lesions of lymphomatosis in calves are the commonest neoplasms encountered in the liver of animals although primary adenoma, adenocarcinoma and metastases of other neoplasms in the area drained by the portal tract are not uncommon especially in ruminants. For the most part, they produce no signs of hepatic dysfunction but they may cause sufficient swelling to be palpable, and some abdominal pain by stretching of the liver capsule. Primary tumours of the gall-bladder also occur rarely and do not as a rule cause clinical signs (1).

REFERENCE

(1) Anderson, W. A. *et al.* (1958). *Amer. J. vet. Res. 19,* 58.

7

Diseases of the Cardiovascular System

INTRODUCTION

Principles of Circulatory Failure

THE primary function of the cardiovascular system is to maintain the circulation of the blood so that normal exchanges of fluid, electrolytes, oxygen, and other nutrient and excretory substances can be made between the vascular system and tissues. Failure of the circulation in any degree interferes with these exchanges and is the basis for circulatory failure, the primary concept in diseases of the cardiovascular system. The two functional units of the system are the heart and the blood-vessels and either may fail independently of the other, giving rise to two forms of circulatory failure—heart failure and peripheral failure. In heart failure the inadequacy is due to involvement of the heart itself; in peripheral circulatory failure the deficiency is in the vascular system which fails to return the blood to the heart.

HEART FAILURE

The two criteria used in assessing cardiac efficiency are the maintenance of circulatory equilibrium and the maintenance of the nutritional requirements of tissues. The maintenance of oxygen requirements is the most important, the nervous system in particular being very susceptible to deprivation of oxygen. Although both factors usually operate together, one of them is dominant in a particular case. It is therefore usual to subdivide heart failure into two types depending on which of the two factors is more important. However, a complete range of syndromes occurs and some of them do not fit neatly into one or other of the categories. Circulatory equilibrium is not maintained when the heart fails to eject all the blood returned by the venous system and the ventricular output does not equal the venous inflow. If this develops sufficiently slowly blood accumulates in the veins and congestive heart failure occurs. If on the other hand there is an acute reduction of cardiac output, as is caused by sudden cessation of the heart beat, the effect is to deprive tissues of their

oxygen supplies and the syndrome of acute heart failure develops.

PERIPHERAL CIRCULATORY FAILURE

In peripheral circulatory failure the effective blood volume is decreased because of loss of fluid from the vascular system or by pooling of blood in peripheral vessels. The failure of venous return results in incomplete filling of the heart and a reduction in its minute volume, although there is no primary defect in cardiac ejection. The effects are the same as those of congestive heart failure in that the supply of nutrients and oxygen to tissues is reduced but there is no cardiac failure and backward congestion of the venous system does not occur. Peripheral circulatory failure is unaccompanied by engorgement of any sort except in surgical shock in which there develops splanchnic vasodilatation and pooling of the blood in the visceral vessels.

CARDIAC RESERVE

The heart has considerable reserve with which to compensate for emergencies in circulatory dynamics. In normal circumstances this reserve is used to compensate for increased demands created by exercise and to a less extent by pregnancy, productivity—especially lactation—and by digestion. The compensatory mechanisms which operate in response to these demands are an increase in heart rate and an increase in stroke volume. The increased stroke volume results from increased diastolic filling of the ventricles due to dilatation and, in continued stress, by hypertrophy. This cardiac reserve is reduced by many pathological processes, and in many cases by the use of pharmacological agents. A stage of diminished cardiac reserve is the first step in heart disease and is manifested by inability of the animal to respond normally when called upon for extra effort. The compensatory mechanisms operate but not to the normal extent. The second stage in heart disease is one of decompensation when the heart is unable to maintain circulatory equilibrium at rest and all cardiac reserve is lost.

The estimation of cardiac reserve is important when a prognosis is to be made on an animal with heart disease. Some of the important criteria used in making this assessment include the heart rate, the intensity of its sounds, the size of the heart, the characters of the pulse, and the tolerance to exercise. A resting heart rate above normal indicates loss of cardiac reserve because the ability to raise the minute volume of the heart is thereby reduced. Heart rates above a certain limit (e.g. 100 to 120 per minute in adult horses and cattle) result in lesser diastolic filling and decreased minute volume. The absolute intensity of the heart sounds suggests the strength of the ventricular contraction, soft sounds suggesting weak contractions, and sounds which are louder than normal suggesting cardiac dilatation and possibly hypertrophy. The interpretation of variation in intensity must be modified by recognition of other factors, such as pericardial effusion, which interfere with audibility of the heart sounds. An increase in heart size may occur in dilatation or hypertrophy of the ventricles. Both of these are compensatory mechanisms and the presence of either suggests that the cardiac reserve is waning, but hypertrophy, when it is accompanied by a heart rate which is slower than normal, is an indication that reserve has been reinstated. Dilatation up to a critical point is a compensatory mechanism, but beyond this the contractile power of the myocardium is reduced and decompensation and congestive heart failure result.

Pulse characters are of value in determining the cardiac reserve but they are greatly affected by factors other than cardiac activity. An increased amplitude of the pulse occurs when the cardiac stroke volume is increased, but a decreased amplitude may result from reduced venous return as well as from reduced contractile power of cardiac muscle.

Exercise tolerance is a good guide to cardiac reserve. It is best measured by estimation of the maximum heart rate attained after a standard exercise test, and the speed with which the heart rate returns to normal. An increase in respiratory rate and depth is also a good guide but is modified by changes in the respiratory system as well as by changes in the cardiovascular system. Signs of congestive heart failure occur only when all cardiac reserve is lost. Other indications of cardiac disease, including cardiac irregularity, heart murmurs and the presence of pericarditis, are not signs of reduced cardiac reserve but it can usually be accepted that some loss of reserve must be present. A knowledge of the aetiology of the cardiac disease may be of value in prognosis in that a disease such as cardiac lymphomatosis, which is known to be progressive, must lead to further loss of reserve and eventually to congestive heart failure.

Manifestations of Circulatory Failure

The manifestations of circulatory failure depend on the manner and rapidity of its onset, and on its duration. They are best illustrated by a description of the three basic syndromes—congestive heart failure, acute heart failure or cardiac syncope, and peripheral circulatory failure. Some prior understanding of the abnormalities of cardiac rate and rhythm, and cardiac size, is necessary and these are dealt with first.

ABNORMALITIES OF CARDIAC RATE AND RHYTHM

Abnormalities of cardiac rhythm include tachycardia (increased rate), bradycardia (decreased rate), arrhythmia (irregularity) and gallop rhythms. Cardiac rhythm is influenced by the integrity of the neuromyocardium and abnormalities are of particular interest as an aid to diagnosis of myocardial disease. However, extrinsic factors also influence the rhythm and these need to be taken into account when the significance of abnormalities is being assessed.

Tachycardia

An increased heart rate results from an increased rate of discharge of impulses from the sino-atrial node which has its own intrinsic rate of discharge but which is also modified by external influences, particularly the vagus nerve. The term *simple tachycardia* is used to describe an increase in heart rate caused by detectable influences such as excitement, pain, hyperthermia, a fall in arterial blood pressure, an increase in venous pressure or the administration of adrenergic drugs.

Paroxysmal tachycardia is the term used to describe the temporary acquisition of a rapid heart rate without the apparent interference of any of the known influences described above. It occurs comparatively rarely in animals but may be encountered in horses. Attacks usually last for an hour or two and begin and end abruptly. The rhythm is quite regular and the rate is not appreciably influenced by exercise or fear and is usually more than double the normal rate for the particular animal. The pulse is small in amplitude but the absolute intensity of the heart sounds is usually greatly increased. Attention is drawn to the defect because of poor exercise tolerance but attacks may be sufficiently severe to cause acute heart failure. Less severe attacks may be followed by congestive heart failure if they are of sufficient duration.

Paroxysmal tachycardia is usually an indication of the presence of myocardial disease and its occurrence has prognostic significance in that affected animals may die suddenly of acute heart failure or, less commonly, of congestive heart failure. Digitalis, acetyl beta-methylcholine (which has effects similar to those of acetylcholine) and quinidine are used to terminate dangerous attacks of paroxysmal tachycardia in man.

Atrial flutter is also an intrinsic cardiac fault in which the atrium beats at a very rapid rate (e.g. 200 to 400 per minute in adult large animals) and the ventricular rate is also fast (100 to 200 per minute) but is less than the atrial rate because of a partial heart block. The rhythm is regular and the rate is not influenced by exercise or fear but distinct from paroxysmal tachycardia is the fact that the abnormality is continuous and does not occur in short attacks. The two can be differentiated by electrocardiographic examination. Atrial flutter is an indication of the presence of myocardial disease and may lead to congestive heart failure. Sudden assumption of the full atrial rate by the ventricles is always followed by the development of acute heart failure. Treatment with digitalis is usually effective.

Atrial fibrillation in which the atrium contracts at a very rapid rate is a more severe defect of atrial activity than flutter. The ventricular rhythm is grossly irregular and usually much faster than normal. The irregularity persists even when the heart rate is elevated by exercise, a point of differentiation from most other irregularities which tend to disappear with exercise (1). Ectopic heart beats tend to become worse with exercise. Gross irregularity in time and amplitude of the pulse is characteristic and a pulse deficit is common, not all ventricular contractions being sufficiently forceful to cause a pulse wave. Atrial fibrillation occurs usually in the presence of severe myocardial disease and is then accompanied by congestive heart failure. The condition is usually permanent and only palliative treatment is available. It is most common in large aged horses. Quinidine has proved to be an at least temporarily effective treatment (2) provided there is no toxaemia or congestive heart failure, when digitalis is preferred (3). A high proportion of successful treatments has been recorded in horses (34) when a regimen of premedication with digitalis is followed by quinidine until normal rhythm is established and a continuous maintenance with digitalis is instituted. Although spontaneous recovery has occurred and affected animals may perform normally, horses with atrial fibrillation must be considered to have a dubious future and death may occur at any time (4).

Ventricular fibrillation is not usually observed clinically because the incoordinated twitching of the myocardium does not result in ventricular ejection and the patient dies very quickly. Ventricular fibrillation occurs in the terminal stages of most suddenly fatal diseases including lightning stroke, overdosage with chloroform, severe toxaemia and acute anoxia of the myocardium. There is complete absence of the pulse and heart sounds, the blood pressure falls rapidly and the animal dies within a minute or two of acute heart failure. Treatment is usually impractical although deaths during anaesthesia may be prevented by cardiac massage or electrical defibrillation. Intracardiac injections of adrenaline are often used in acute cardiac arrest but do not correct fibrillation and are of little value.

Bradycardia

Simple bradycardia is a normal heart action at a reduced rate due to a decreased rate of discharge of stimuli from the sino-atrial node. Most simple bradycardias have an extracardiac origin and are caused by an increase in blood pressure, a highly efficient myocardium, space-occupying lesions of the cranium and increased intracranial pressure. Bradycardia is sometimes associated with vagus indigestion and diaphragmatic hernia in cattle but the mechanism is not obvious.

Heart block is caused by failure of transmission of the wave of impulse through the heart. The block may occur at the S-A node (S-A block), or at the A-V node (A-V block). S-A block is less common and is characterized by absence of an atrial sound, irregular irregularity and absence of complete complexes from the electrocardiogram. It has been observed in the horse (5).

A-V block occurs when the ventricle does not contract in response to atrial contraction because of interference with conduction through the atrioventricular bundle. Although partial A-V block may be associated with cardiac disease, in horses it occurs in otherwise normal animals especially when they are quiet and resting. The irregularity disappears with exercise and an increase in heart rate. In this species it must be considered to have no diagnostic significance unless it is accompanied by other signs of cardiac disease (6). The opposite situation of lack of exercise tolerance coupled with a normal resting but irregular post-exercise cardiac rhythm is probably indicative of serious cardiac disease (32).

In some cases there are no detectable myocardial changes (30) but when A-V block is a manifestation of pathological change it is because lesions develop in the A-V bundle, usually as a result of local inflammation in the myocardium. Overdosing with calcium salts or digitalis, poisoning with the toxin of *Clostridium perfringens* Type D and early asphyxia are other causes of heart block.

Heart block may be partial or complete. When it is partial the pulse may be regular or irregular depending on whether the ventricle responds to every second or other beat. The heart rate is slow but quickly speeds up and becomes regular on exercise or after administration of atropine, reverting suddenly to the prior rate when the stimulus is removed. When heart block is complete (32) the ventricle beats with its own inherent, regular, slow rhythm, the pulse is regular and slow and does not vary with exercise or after the administration of atropine. In A-V block in horses careful auscultation of the heart may reveal faint atrial sounds coincident with small pulses in the jugular veins in the intervals between ventricular sounds. With complete block in horses the ventricular rhythm may be so slow that cerebral anoxia and syncope ensue. In one such case an internal pacemaker has been used to improve cardiac function (33).

Bradycardia is important as an indication of heart disease if heart block is present. Congestive heart failure may be present because of the accompanying myocardial asthenia. Acute heart failure may occur in animals with heart block especially if violent exercise is undertaken. With the exception of partial A-V block in the horse in which it appears to be a normal occurrence, the prognosis is grave if heart block is present in any degree, because treatment is usually ineffective unless the primary cause can be eliminated. Affected animals should not be allowed to exert themselves and it will be necessary to treat congestive heart failure if it is present.

Arrhythmia

The arrhythmias of heart block and atrial fibrillation have already been described. There still remain the arrhythmias which are not characterized by tachycardia or bradycardia.

Sinus arrhythmia is a rhythmical variation in heart rate, occurring synchronously with respiration, the rate increasing with inspiration and decreasing with expiration. As far as is known it has no diagnostic significance, occurring in normal animals especially when respiration is slow and deep. It is distinguished from other arrhythmias by its close relation to respiratory movements. The arrhythmia disappears when the heart rate increases due to exercise or the administration of atropine.

Atrial and ventricular extrasystoles occur when impulses capable of stimulating myocardial contraction arise at points in the heart muscle away from the S-A node. The impulses usually arise from foci of damaged myocardium although they may occur in a number of intoxications including digitalis and chloroform. Different patterns of irregularity of the heart beat occur depending on whether the focus of irritation is in the atrium or the ventricles, but the irregular contractions may not be reflected in the pulse as the ventricular contractions which arise ectopically may not be sufficiently strong to cause a pulse wave. The characteristic features of extrasystolic contractions are regular irregularity of the heart, a pulse deficit at normal rates and a tendency for these abnormalities to become more severe with exercise (1). Clinically they can be differentiated from heart block by the presence of a pulse deficit but faint atrial sounds in the horse may have to be distinguished from ventricular sounds. The importance of extrasystoles is the same as for the other irregularities in that they indicate the presence of myocardial damage which may lead to the development of congestive heart failure. The condition is thought to be rare but has been observed in 1·5 per cent of a series of 270 horses (7). No specific treatment is available but treatment of a coincident congestive heart failure may be necessary.

Differentiation of the various arrhythmias is most accurately carried out by electrocardiographic examination, but accurate identification is of no great value in farm animals because single entities do not have particular prognostic significance. Some indication of the type of the irregularity can be gained by careful auscultation, checking for the presence of a pulse deficit, and determining the effects of exercise on the irregularity. Most irregularities disappear with exercise except atrial fibrillation which becomes much worse.

Gallop Rhythms

Reduplication of the first or second sound to give a triple instead of a double heart sound is described as a gallop rhythm and is usually associated with severe myocardial disease in man. In animals it occurs quite commonly in dairy cows, especially when the heart rate is slow and does not appear to have any prognostic significance. The first sound is usually reduplicated in these animals and is probably caused by asynchronous closure of the atrioventricular valves. In horses careful auscultation often reveals four heart sounds in normal animals. The 'fourth' heart sound is caused by atrial systole and occurs just prior to the standard first heart sound caused by ventricular systole. The 'third' heart sound is caused by rapid filling of the ventricles and occurs just after the standard second sound caused by closure of the semilunar valves (8, 9).

CARDIAC ENLARGEMENT

Enlargement of the heart is a compensatory response to an increased load on ventricular ejection. It may occur as a result of increased demand during hard labour but is usually significant only when there are valvular lesions or inefficient myocardial contractions. The two components of cardiac enlargement are hypertrophy of the wall and dilatation of the ventricular cavities. When an increased load is applied the initial response is usually dilatation and if the myocardium is healthy and nutrition is good hypertrophy follows. If hypertrophy does not occur and dilatation develops beyond a critical point ventricular contractions do not empty the ventricles, circulatory equilibrium is not maintained and other mechanisms, particularly an increase in rate, come into play. If these cannot compensate for the increased load congestive heart failure develops.

The significance of cardiac enlargement is that it indicates the presence of myocardial disease or increased resistance to blood flow in the pulmonary or aortic circuits and a diminution in cardiac reserve. The degree of enlargement is a good indication of the degree of cardiac embarrassment but accurate measurement is not usually undertaken in farm animals. Detection of cardiac enlargement is aided by careful auscultation of the heart and palpation of the apex beat. A palpable and audible increase in the apex beat and area of audibility, backward displacement of the apex beat, and increased visibility of the cardiac impulse at the base of the neck and behind the elbow are all indications of cardiac enlargement. Care must be taken that the abnormalities observed are not due to displacement of the heart by a space-occupying lesion of the thorax, or to collapse of the ventral parts of the lung and withdrawal of lung tissue from the costal aspects of the heart. Careful percussion may also be of value but enlargement is only detectable by this method when it is extreme because of the situation of the heart behind the heavy shoulder muscles. Roentgenological examination is the most satisfactory method of measurement if the animal's size permits it. Treatment of cardiac enlargement depends upon the treatment of the primary condition.

Congestive Heart Failure

In congestive heart failure, the heart, due to some intrinsic defect, is unable to maintain circulatory equilibrium at rest and congestion of the venous circuit occurs, accompanied by dilatation of vessels, oedema of the lungs or periphery, enlargement of the heart and an increase in heart rate.

Aetiology

Disease of the myocardium, endocardium and pericardium, diseases which primarily interfere with the flow of blood away from the heart (flow load) and diseases which impede heart action may all result in congestive heart failure. Diseases of the myocardium may be manifested by weakness of the myocardial contractions or, if the neuromyocardium is involved, by irregularity. In both cases the minute volume of the heart is reduced.

Myocarditis, myocardial dystrophy and neoplasms of the heart are the common causes of myocardial asthenia and irregularity. Endocardial diseases are largely inflammatory although congenital defects, including fibro-elastosis, also occur. Pericardial diseases comprise pericarditis, cardiac tamponade and hydropericardium. Diseases in which there is an increased flow load include congenital defects of the heart and large vessels, pulmonary emphysema, pneumothorax and pneumonia. Hypertension is one of the commonest diseases in man in which an increased flow load occurs but its occurrence in animals has not been determined.

Anoxia and toxaemia cause myocardial asthenia and these syndromes are accompanied by some signs of reduced cardiac reserve but congestive heart failure does not occur. Brisket disease is a possible exception, the main cause appearing to be continued exposure to low atmospheric pressures at high altitudes. If the cardiac reserve is already diminished by a prior lesion these factors may precipitate an acute cardiac insufficiency.

Pathogenesis

When an increased load is placed upon ejection of the blood from the heart, or the contractile power of the myocardium is reduced, compensatory mechanisms including increased heart rate, dilatation and hypertrophy, come into play to maintain circulatory equilibrium. However, cardiac reserve is reduced and the animal is not able to cope with circulatory emergencies as well as a normal animal. This is the stage of waning cardiac reserve in which the animal is comparatively normal at rest but is incapable of performing exercise, the phase of poor exercise tolerance. When these compensatory mechanisms reach their physiological limit and the heart is unable to cope with the circulatory requirements at rest, congestive heart failure develops. Many of the signs which appear can be explained by the increased hydrostatic pressure in the venous system, but the decreased forward output of blood from the heart also contributes to the clinical signs by the production of a degree of anoxia. Thus oedema is due largely to increased hydrostatic pressure in vessels but damage caused to the capillaries by anoxia facilitates the passage of plasma protein into tissues and further exacerbates the oedema. Hepatic injury, and a retention of salt and water due to the reduction in circulating blood volume also probably contribute to the oedema.

In animals congestive heart failure may occur in either the right or left ventricles or in both together. With failure of the right side venous congestion is manifested only in the greater circulation, and with failure of the left side the resulting engorgement and oedema are restricted to the lesser pulmonary circulation. Right-sided failure causes involvement of the liver and kidneys and reduces their normal function. In the kidneys the increase in hydrostatic pressure is off-set by the reduced flow of blood through the kidney and urine output is reduced. Anoxic damage to the glomeruli causes increased permeability and escape of plasma protein into the urine. Venous congestion in the portal system is an inevitable sequel of hepatic congestion and is accompanied by impaired digestion and absorption and eventually by transudation into the intestinal lumen and diarrhoea.

Clinical Findings

In the very early stages when cardiac reserve is reduced but decompensation has not yet occurred there is respiratory distress on light exertion. The time required for return to the normal respiratory and pulse rates is prolonged. In affected animals there may be evidence of cardiac enlargement and the resting heart rate is moderately increased.

Congestive heart failure referable to failure of the left side is manifested by an increase in the rate and depth of respiration at rest, cough, the presence of moist râles at the base of the lungs and increased dullness on percussion of the ventral borders of the lungs. Terminally there is severe dyspnoea and cyanosis. The heart rate is increased and there may be a murmur referable to the left atrioventricular or aortic semilunar valves.

In congestive heart failure of the right side the heart rate is increased and there is oedema, usually anasarca, ascites, hydrothorax and hydropericardium. The anasarca is characteristically limited to the ventral surface of the body, the neck and the jaw. If the congestion is sufficiently severe the liver is palpably enlarged, protruding beyond the right costal arch and the edge is thickened and rounded. The respiration is deeper than normal and the rate may be slightly increased. Urine flow is usually reduced and the urine is concentrated and contains a small amount of albumen. The faeces are usually normal at first but in the late stages diarrhoea may be profuse. Body weight may increase because of oedema but the appetite is poor and condition is lost rapidly. The superficial veins are dilated, particularly the jugular vein, and the normal jugular pulse is more visible and its maximum movement occurs higher up the neck than usual. Epistaxis may occur in the horse but is rare in other species. The attitude and behaviour of the animal is one of listlessness and depression, exercise is undertaken reluctantly, and the gait is shuffling and staggery due to weakness.

The prognosis in congestive heart failure varies to a certain extent with the cause but in most cases in large animals it is unfavourable. With a defect of the neuromyocardium the possibility of recovery exists but when the myocardium or endocardium are involved complete recovery rarely if ever occurs, although the animal may survive with a permanently reduced cardiac reserve. Uncomplicated defects of rhythm occur commonly only in the horse and these defects are more compatible with life than are extensive anatomical lesions.

Clinical Pathology

Clinico-pathological examinations are usually of value only in differentiating the causes of congestive heart failure. Venous pressure is increased and on venepuncture the pressure of blood from the needle is much greater than normal although it is not usually measured. Aspiration of fluid from accumulations in any of the cavities may be thought necessary if the origin of the fluid is in doubt. Classically the fluid is described as an oedematous transudate containing no protein but in most cases protein is present in large amounts due to leakage of plasma from damaged capillary walls. Proteinuria is often present for the same reason.

Necropsy Findings

Lesions characteristic of the specific cause are present and may comprise abnormalities of the endocardium, myocardium, lungs or large vessels. Space-occupying lesions of the thorax may also exert pressure on the heart and interfere with its function. The lesions which occur in all cases of congestive heart failure, irrespective of cause, are pulmonary congestion and oedema if the failure is left-sided, and anasarca, ascites, hydrothorax and hydropericardium, and enlargement and engorgement of the liver if the failure is right-sided.

Diagnosis

Accumulations of free fluid in the abdomen may also occur in peritonitis, rupture of the bladder and hepatic fibrosis. In chronic peritonitis fluid removed by paracentesis contains bacteria and many leucocytes and there is an absence of signs of cardiac involvement. A normal heart is characteristic of the other two conditions also and when the bladder is ruptured no urine is passed, the blood urea nitrogen is grossly elevated and there is usually a history of abdominal pain and straining to urinate. Fibrosis of the liver is usually accompanied by other signs of hepatic insufficiency including jaundice and photosensitization.

Oedema may occur without cardiac insufficiency in mares and cows near the end of pregnancy but it characteristically commences at the udder and reaches its maximum degree in this region. It may be sufficiently severe to extend to the brisket but there is no engorgement of the jugular veins and no evidence of cardiac involvement. Other causes of generalized oedema include particularly hypoproteinaemia, as it occurs in parasitism, but the oedema is not usually severe, is most apparent in the intermandibular space, and is usually accompanied by anaemia. Bottle-jaw, as it is called, is most noticeable in grazing animals and it may disappear when the animal is fed from a trough, the dependence of the part being reduced.

Dyspnoea has many causes but when it is accompanied by pulmonary oedema it is usually due either to left-sided congestive heart failure or to acute pulmonary oedema as it occurs in fog fever of cattle or other allergic and anaphylactic states. Poisoning with organic phosphates may have the same effect. It may be difficult to differentiate acute pulmonary emphysema from pulmonary oedema, especially since emphysema often occurs as a complication of oedema.

Treatment

The primary cause may be amenable to specific treatment. Non-specific treatment of congestive heart failure is applicable in most cases irrespective of the cause. Rest, or at least avoidance of violent exercise, is the primary consideration. If oedema is present the salt intake should be reduced to as low as possible and the water intake limited. Diuretics, either mercurials, acetazolamide, chlorothiazide or frusemide, may reduce the embarrassment caused by large accumulations of fluid in body cavities.

Venesection can be used as an emergency treatment and 2 to 4 ml. of blood per lb. body weight may be withdrawn at a time. The immediate embarrassment of respiration is removed but the hydrostatic pressure usually returns to pre-treatment levels within 24 hours. The same applies to drainage of the serous cavities by paracentesis, and the fluid loss should not be permitted to reach the point where dehydration occurs. If venesection is required at intervals of less than 7 days it is probably inadvisable to persist.

The use of drugs which increase the contractile power of the myocardium, e.g. digitalis and ouabain, has not received much attention in large animals. Oral administration in ruminants is probably of little value because of digestion of the glucosides. Intramuscular administration of purified extracts gives erratic results and intravenous injections must be given cautiously because of the danger of acute toxicity. The use of these drugs is also dangerous when there is severe infection, toxic myocarditis, or vegetative lesions of the valves and since these constitute the majority of conditions in which congestive heart failure occurs in farm animals the drugs do not find wide application. If they are used it is essential that the dosage be arranged in accordance with the principle of digitalization in which large, loading doses are given initially to obtain maximum improvement in cardiac output in a short time, followed by small maintenance doses to avoid intoxication. Unless myocardial damage is transient administration of the drug will probably have to be continued for life and this is unlikely to be a practicable procedure.

Acute Heart Failure

In acute heart failure there is sudden loss of consciousness, falling with or without convulsions, severe pallor of the mucosae and either death or complete recovery from the episode.

Aetiology

Acute heart failure may occur as the result of cardiac tamponade in which the pericardial sac is suddenly filled with fluid, in excessive tachycardia or ventricular fibrillation, such as occurs in falling disease of cattle and enzootic muscular dystrophy. Sporadic cases occur when intravenous injections are given too quickly, in lightning stroke and electrocution, and in excessive bradycardia. Bradycardia may be caused by heart block when there is disease of the myocardium or may occur during the intravenous injection of calcium preparations during the treatment of parturient paresis. Bradycardia caused by hypersensitivity of the carotid sinus is a specific syndrome in man but there appears to be no parallel in animals. Occlusion of a coronary vessel is another common cause of acute heart failure in man which is recorded rarely in animals. Complete cardiac asystole is most likely to occur during anaesthesia and is the result of myocardial anoxia combined with reflex vagal inhibition.

Pathogenesis

With excessive tachycardia the diastolic period is so short that filling of the ventricles is impossible and cardiac output is grossly reduced. In ventricular fibrillation no coordinated contractions occur and no blood is ejected from the heart. The cardiac output is also seriously reduced when the heart rate slows to beyond a critical point. In all of these circumstances there is a precipitate fall in minute volume of the heart and a severe degree of tissue anoxia. In peracute cases the most sensitive organ, the brain, is affected first and the clinical signs are principally nervous in type. Pallor is also a prominent sign in these cases because of the reduction in arterial blood flow.

In less acute cases respiratory distress is more obvious because of pulmonary oedema and although these can be classified as acute heart failure they are more accurately described as acute congestive heart failure.

Clinical Findings

The animal usually shows dyspnoea, staggering and falling, and death often follows within seconds or minutes of the first appearance of signs. There is marked pallor of the mucosae. Although clonic convulsions may occur they are never severe and consist mainly of sporadic incoordinated movements of the limbs. Death usually is accompanied by deep, asphyxial gasps. If there is time for physical examination, absence of a palpable pulse and bradycardia, tachycardia or absence of the heart sounds are observed.

In less acute cases, such as those which occur in enzootic muscular dystrophy in calves, the course may be as long as 12 to 24 hours, and dyspnoea and pulmonary oedema are prominent signs. These animals present a syndrome which has some of the characteristics of congestive heart failure.

Transient attacks of acute heart failure, manifested as cardiac syncope or vasovagal syncope occur in man but do not occur in animals, possibly because of their psychic origin.

Clinical Pathology

Insufficient time is available in which to conduct laboratory tests.

Necropsy Findings

In typical acute cases engorgement of visceral veins may be present if the attack has lasted for a few minutes but there are none of the lesions characteristic of congestive failure. There is insufficient time for the development of oedema, or hepatic enlargement. The primary cause may be evidenced by macroscopic or microscopic lesions of the myocardium.

Diagnosis

Acute heart failure may be mistaken for primary disease of the nervous system but is characterized by excessive bradycardia or tachycardia, pallor of mucosae, absence of the pulse, and the mildness of the convulsions. Epilepsy is usually transient and repetitive and has a characteristic pattern of development.

Treatment

Treatment of acute heart failure is not usually practicable in large animals because of the short course of the disease. Deaths due to sudden cardiac arrest or ventricular fibrillation while under anaesthesia can be avoided to a limited extent in animals (10) and humans by direct cardiac massage or electrical stimulation but these techniques are generally restricted to the more sophisticated institutional surgical units. Intracardiac injections of very small doses of adrenaline are used but are likely to do as much harm as good, especially if ventricular fibrillation is present (10).

Peripheral Circulatory Failure

Peripheral circulatory failure occurs when the cardiac output is reduced because of a failure of venous return to the heart. The decreased blood flow to tissues and the resulting anoxia causes depression of tissue function. Clinical manifestations include muscle weakness, subnormal temperature, increased respiratory and heart rates, and depression, coma, and in some cases mild clonic convulsions.

Aetiology

Failure of venous return occurs when there is peripheral vasodilatation and pooling of blood in the vessels, and when there is a reduction in circulating blood volume. When the defect is vascular the failure is termed vasogenic and when due to reduced blood volume it is termed haematogenic.

Vasogenic failure occurs principally in shock when the blood collects in dilated splanchnic vessels. In the initial stages the total blood volume is normal but the circulating blood volume is greatly reduced. In later stages there is reduction of total blood volume and irreversible shock develops as the peripheral circulatory failure progresses to the haematogenic type. Parturient paresis is a classical example of a vasogenic failure syndrome.

Haematogenic failure is manifested by a decrease in total and circulating blood volumes and occurs in haemorrhage, the terminal stages of shock, and in dehydration.

Pathogenesis

Compensatory mechanisms, including peripheral vasoconstriction and evacuation of blood stored in the spleen and other organs, can maintain the circulating blood volume up to a critical point but beyond this peripheral circulatory failure develops. The cardiac output falls and anoxia of tissues begins. If the circulating blood volume can be restored to normal by treatment before permanent damage to capillaries occurs recovery may be complete. Severe anoxia may cause permanent damage to the central nervous system and the renal parenchyma but this is not a common occurrence.

The speed with which fluid loss or splanchnic vasodilatation occurs has some bearing on the severity of the illness, as the compensatory mechanisms are capable of a continued response and are more readily overcome by acute than chronic stress. It is in circumstances where the failure is acute that damage to the central nervous system is most likely to occur. The major response to decreased venous return is observable clinically in the circulatory system where there is a fall in blood pressure and an increase in heart rate. Failure of the circulation also stimulates respiratory activity.

Clinical Findings

A general depression, weakness and listlessness are accompanied by a fall in temperature to below normal, an increase in heart rate with abnormalities of the pulse including small amplitude, weak pressures and an increased vessel tone, although this latter is decreased in the terminal stages. The absolute intensity of the heart sounds may also be reduced because of the fall in blood pressure. The skin is cold and the mucosae pale. The respiratory rate is increased and respirations are usually shallow. Anorexia is usual but thirst may be evident. Nervous signs include depression and listlessness, and coma in the terminal stages. Clonic convulsions may occur but they are not a prominent part of the syndrome. Acute vasogenic failure, as it occurs in vasovagal syncope in man, is manifested by fainting and falling but this syndrome does not appear to occur in animals except possibly as a cause of death when vomitus is aspirated during anaesthesia.

Clinical Pathology

Clinico-pathological examinations to determine the severity of a haemorrhagic anaemia, or the degree of haemoconcentration in cases of shock or dehydration, give an excellent estimate of the severity of the primary condition.

Necropsy Findings

The findings at necropsy examination vary with the cause and there are no lesions which are characteristic of peripheral circulatory failure.

Diagnosis

Peripheral circulatory failure can be diagnosed when there is evidence of circulatory failure but no detectable cardiac abnormality, and when a primary cause, such as haemorrhage, shock or dehydration, is known to be present. It is only by inclusion of the latter proviso that peripheral failure can be differentiated from severe toxaemia. Differentiation of the causes of peripheral failure depends upon ability to recognize the existence of shock, dehydration and haemorrhage and these subjects are discussed elsewhere.

Treatment

The main principle of treatment in peripheral circulatory failure is to restore the circulating blood volume to normal and maintain it so that tissue anoxia is avoided. The method of doing this varies with the cause. In vasogenic failure it is necessary to combat the peripheral vasodilatation by the administration of vasoconstrictor drugs such as adrenaline and pitressin. In haematogenic failure lost fluids should be replaced, the type of replacement depending on how the loss has occurred; in shock plasma is required; in dehydration, isotonic fluids; and in haemorrhage, whole blood. The preparations used and the methods of administration are discussed in more detail under the headings of these specific forms of fluid loss. In all cases there is a critical point at which recovery cannot occur because of capillary damage, particularly in the kidneys, but this can be detected only by the response to treatment.

Cardiac stimulants are of no value in peripheral circulatory failure because of the absence of any cardiac deficiency. In haematogenic failure vaso-constrictor drugs should be avoided as they further restrict blood flow.

Special Examination of the Cardiovascular System

The more commonly used techniques of examination of the heart and pulse are described in Chapter 1 but special techniques are available which may be of value in some cases and in investigational work. The use of some of these techniques is limited in many instances by the value of the animal and by its size.

Electrocardiography

It is not proposed to deal with this subject in detail here but extensive data are available on horses (11, 12, 13) and some on cattle (14, 15), goats (16) and lambs (17). Some information is also available for elephants (18) and camels (19). Foetal electrocardiography is practised in horses and is valuable as a diagnostic tool and also for determining that foetuses are viable (31). The recording of ECG signals from horses (20) and cattle (21) in motion has been satisfactorily achieved by the use of radiotelemetry.

Of particular importance in the assessment of electrocardiograms are the shape and duration of the various waves and their positive or negative polarity. These characters vary considerably with the leads used and care must be taken in comparing results that comparisons are made between identical leads.

Abnormalities of the P wave include a number of small waves in atrial flutter and the absence of P waves in atrial fibrillation. Prolongation of the PR interval indicates the presence of heart block and there will be an associated absence of QRS complexes. Complete independence of P wave and QRS complex rhythmicity is observed in complete heart block. Involvement of one or other of the branches of the bundle of His may be detectable by comparing the PR intervals obtained by the different leads. Varying degrees of heart block occur commonly in horses and details of electrocardiographic changes caused by atrial fibrillation (1) and ventricular pre-excitation (22) have been recorded in this species.

Using the standard leads I (left fore and right fore limbs), II (right fore and left hind) and III (left hind and right hind) in horses the P wave is usually positive, sometimes biphasic, the QRS complex usually small in amplitude and variable in form. The normal range of times for the standard measurements are P wave, 0·085 to 0·115 sec.; PR interval, 0·187 to 0·382 sec.; QRS complex, 0·074 to 0·140 sec.; and QT interval, 0·339 and 0·575 sec. (7).

In cattle the times are PR interval, 0·19 sec.; QRS complex, 0·09 sec.; QT interval, 0·39 sec. (23). The P and T waves are often biphasic and the QRS complex is variable in form.

In all species electrocardiographic studies are of value in determining the presence of myocardial disease and in many instances in giving some indication of the location of the lesion and the type of defect. Electrocardiograms taken before and immediately after exercise are of value in determining the type of abnormality because of the tendency for some arrhythmias to disappear when the heart rate increases.

Tests of Circulation Time and Cardiac Output

Estimation of the time required for blood to complete a circuit of the circulation is of value in determining the efficiency of the circulation. None of the tests used in man are suitable for general clinical use in large animals but similar tests have been used to measure cardiac output. In cattle and horses the cardiac output has been measured by the use of the dye Evans Blue (T–1824) (24) and in sheep by using indocyanine green (25). Cardiac output is also measurable by techniques utilizing cardiac catheterization (26). The circulation time will be decreased and the cardiac output increased under the same conditions, such as after exercise, during fever and in cases of anaemia. Increase of the circulation time and decrease in cardiac output occur in congestive heart failure.

Roentgenological Examination

Although standard data are not available for heart size as estimated on roentgenological examination, significant enlargement of the heart as a whole or of one or other of the ventricles or displacement can be detected by this means.

Special Examination of the Pulse

The more commonly used criteria for examination of the pulse have been described in Chapter 1. Additional information on blood pressure may be obtained by careful palpation. An estimate of the systolic pressure can be made by determining the amount of pressure that has to be exerted with a proximal finger to obliterate the pulse felt by a distal finger. Care must be taken that sufficient pressure is exerted with the distal finger to obtain maximum amplitude.

An estimate of the diastolic pressure can be obtained by gradually increasing pressure with one finger and determining the amount of pressure required to obtain the maximum amplitude of the pulse wave. An artery with a low diastolic pressure is flattened by light pressure between pulse waves and the maximum amplitude is felt with little digital pressure. Conversely a high diastolic pressure in an artery requires much pressure to flatten it and the maximum amplitude is only obtained by the exertion of considerable digital pressure.

The form of the pulse wave may have significance. A rapid rise and fall in the wave and a large amplitude are usually associated with aortic semilunar insufficiency and patent ductus arteriosus. In such cases there may be visible pulsation of small arteries. Low blood pressure, arteriovenous fistulae and anaemia are also accompanied by a rapid rise and fall of the pulse wave and an increased amplitude of the pulse. A slow-rising pulse is characteristic of stenosis of the aortic semilunar valves.

Special examinations of the arterial pulse include palpation of the external iliac and volar digital arteries in iliac thrombosis of horses, of the middle uterine arteries in pregnancy diagnosis of cattle, and the cranial mesenteric arteries of horses affected by verminous arteritis.

Examination of the Arteriolar-Capillary Circulation

The warmth and colour of the skin, mucosae and conjunctivae give some information on the state of the circulation in the smaller vessels. The colour of these surfaces depends upon the amount of blood present in the capillaries, pallor indicating emptiness of the capillaries, reddening indicating engorgement. Temperature of the skin depends largely upon the degree of arteriolar flow, warmth indicating good arteriolar flow, coldness suggesting poor flow.

In man fragility of capillary walls can be measured by the amount of negative pressure, applied through a suction cup, required to cause petechiation in the underlying skin. Standard data are not available for such tests in animals. The spontaneous occurrence of petechiae usually indicates increased capillary fragility but defects in the clotting mechanisms may also cause apparently spontaneous haemorrhages of varying sizes.

Ophthalmoscopic examination may reveal the presence of haemorrhages in the retina and, provided trauma to the orbit has not occurred, these may suggest increased vascular fragility. The haemorrhages may appear as red patches of various size which become brown to orange with increasing age. Discontinuities of vessels or lack of definition of their walls may also suggest vascular disease. Gross haemorrhage into the anterior chamber may also occur and is usually visible on direct examination of the eye.

Estimation of Arterial Blood Pressure

Direct estimation of arterial blood pressure is impractical clinically and indirect measurements have not been satisfactorily applied to farm animals because of their failure to relax during examination and the difficulty of applying standardized human equipment. A modified Baumanometer cuff, adapted to fit the foreleg of the horse, has been used to determine the blood pressure in the dorsal interosseous artery (27). The systolic and diastolic pressures recorded were 144 to 194 and 105 to 150 respectively.

Exercise Tolerance Tests

Tests used in man to determine cardiac sufficiency and reserve are not generally used as an aid to the diagnosis of heart disease in animals. However, because of the need to predict physical fitness for endurance tests on horses, some data have become available on the effects of exercise on heart and respiratory rates and these are of value in assessing ability to carry out prolonged, arduous exercise (28, 35). Standardized exercise tolerance tests have not been developed for animals but in horses most attention is given to the rapidity of the heart rate after exercise and the time at which the heart rate returns to normal. This time should be of the order of 6 to 8 minutes in horses accustomed to exercise and which are given moderate work for 10 to 15 minutes. After racing the heart rate diminishes little in the first 10 minutes, precipitately in the second 10 minutes, followed by a gradual return to normal over several hours (29).

Principles of Treatment of Circulatory Failure

The aim of treatment in congestive heart failure is to increase the efficiency of cardiac ejection and thus restore circulatory equilibrium. If oedema is incapacitating the use of diuretics is indicated, although improvement of cardiac function will have the same effect in time. In severe cases the combined use of digitalis and a diuretic provide the greatest chances of rapid response. In acute heart failure the aim is to restore normal cardiac rhythm. Complete arrest can only be satisfactorily reversed by electrical stimulation or physical massage.

Peripheral circulatory failure can be corrected, if only temporarily, by the provision of fluids or whole blood if the failure is haematogenic, or by the administration of vasoconstrictor drugs if the failure is primarily vasogenic. If capillary damage has occurred to the point that plasma protein is leaking into tissue spaces and the urine, the failure of the peripheral circulation is probably irreversible.

In all types of circulatory failure the basic defect is tissue anoxia, either stagnant or anaemic in type, and the provision of extra oxygen to ensure saturation of available haemoglobin may serve temporarily to counteract this defect. Oxygen is not usually available in large animal practice but it may be advantageous to supply it in individual cases where the primary cause of the failure can be corrected.

REFERENCES

(1) Holmes, J. R. & Alps, B. J. (1966). *Vet. Rec.*, 78, 672.
(2) Glendinning, S. A. (1965). *Vet. Rec.*, 77, 951.
(3) Detweiler, D. K. (1955). *J. Amer. vet. med. Ass.*, 126, 47.
(4) Glazier, D. B. *et al.* (1959). *Irish vet. J.*, 13, 47.
(5) Nicholson, J. A. *et al.* (1959). *Irish vet. J.*, 13, 168.
(6) Holmes, J. R. & Alps, B. J. (1966). *Canad. vet. J.*, 7, 280.
(7) Glazier, D. B. & Nicholson, J. A. (1959). *Irish vet. J.*, 13, 82.
(8) Patterson, D. F. *et al.* (1965). *Ann. N.Y. Acad. Sci.*, 127, 242 & 306.
(9) Smetzer, D. L. & Smith, D. R. (1965). *J. Amer. vet. med. Ass.*, 146, 937.
(10) Walker, R. G. & Rex, M. A. E. (1958). *Vet. Rec.*, 70, 667.
(11) Kroneman, J. (1966). *T. Diergeneesk.*, 91, 341.
(12) Steel, J. D. (1963). *Studies on the Electrocardiogram of the Racehorse*, Sydney: Australian Medical Publishing Co.
(13) Detweiler, D. K. (1958). *Univ. Pennsylvania Bull., Vet. Ext. Qtly.*, 59, 4.
(14) Lank, R. B. & Kingrey, B. W. (1959). *Amer. J. vet. Res.*, 20, 273.
(15) Sellers, A. F. *et al.* (1958). *Amer. J. vet. Res.*, 19, 620.
(16) Szabuniewiez, M. & Clark, D. R. (1967). *Amer. J. vet. Res.*, 28, 511.
(17) Hilmy, M. I. *et al.* (1960). *Amer. J. vet. Res.*, 21, 1001.
(18) Jayasinghe, J. B. *et al.* (1963). *Brit. vet. J.*, 119, 559.
(19) Jayasinghe, J. B. *et al.* (1963). *Amer. J. vet. Res.*, 24, 883.
(20) Holmes, J. R. *et al.* (1966). *Vet. Rec.*, 79, 90.
(21) Dracy, A. E. & Jahn, J. R. (1964). *J. Dairy Sci.*, 47, 561.
(22) Cooper, S. A. (1962). *Vet. Rec.*, 74, 527.
(23) Alfredson, B. V. & Sykes, J. F. (1943). *J. agric. Res.*, 65, 61.
(24) Fisher, E. W. & Dalton, R. G. (1961). *Brit. vet. J.*, 117, 143.
(25) Hamlin, R. L. & Smith, C. R. (1962). *Amer. J. vet. Res.*, 23, 711.
(26) Reeves, J. H. (1962). *Circulat. Res.*, 10, 166.
(27) Chowdhury, A. K. & Banerjee, A. K. (1960). *Indian vet. J.*, 37, 341.
(28) Cardinet, G. H. *et al.* (1963). *J. Amer. vet. med. Ass.*, 143, 1303.
(29) Witherington, D. H. (1971). *Equ. vet. J.*, 3, 99.
(30) Smetzer, D. L. *et al.* (1969). *Amer. J. vet. Res.*, 30, 337.
(31) Holmes, J. R. (1968). *Vet. Rec.*, 82, 651.
(32) Fisher, E. W. *et al.* (1970). *Vet. Rec.*, 86, 499.
(33) Taylor, D. H. & Mero, M. A. (1967). *J. Amer. vet. med. Ass.*, 151, 1172.
(34) Kroneman, J. & Breukink, H. J. (1966). *T. Diergeneesk.*, 91, 223.
(35) Holmes, J. R. (1968). *Equ. vet. J.*, 1, 10.

DISEASES OF THE HEART

Myocardial Asthenia

Myocardial asthenia or weakness is manifested by decreased power of contraction resulting in reduction of cardiac reserve and, in severe cases, in congestive heart failure or acute heart failure.

Aetiology

Myocarditis of clinical importance occurs rarely in farm animals although some animals affected with blackleg, foot-and-mouth disease and equine infectious anaemia (8) develop severe lesions. A gross myocarditis has been observed as a characteristic lesion in a viral disease of pigs in North America (6). Sporadic cases may occur after localization from bacteraemia in navel ill and strangles and by extension from pericarditis and endocarditis. A focal suppurative myocarditis may be a common finding in neonatal lambs infected with *Staphylococcus aureus* (7). Parasitic myocarditis also occurs sporadically especially in horses and is caused in most cases by migrating larvae of *Strongylus* spp. and the cystic stage of a number of cestodes may become implanted in the myocardium. Eosinophilic myocarditis also occurs occasionally but the primary cause is unknown.

Myocardial infarction due to occlusion of coronary arteries is recorded in horses and is usually due to parasitic arteritis or to bacterial emboli (1, 2).

Degenerative lesions of the myocardium are more common and occur in a number of specific diseases of farm animals. Myocardial dystrophy is a major lesion in avitaminosis E in calves and to a lesser extent in sheep. The so called 'herztod' of pigs is an acute myocardial degeneration. Severe chronic copper deficiency in cattle may lead to myocardial degeneration and fibrosis culminating in falling disease, and iron deficiency anaemia of young pigs is often accompanied by severe myocardial degeneration. Similar lesions occur in a number of poisonings, particularly selenium and gossypol and to a lesser extent arsenic, mercury and phosphorus. With the last-mentioned poisons and in many septicaemias there is a reduction in cardiac output due to physical or functional disturbances of the myocardium and the resulting cardiac embarrassment contributes to the illness or to death but in most cases does not produce a syndrome characteristic of acute or congestive heart failure. Ossification of the right atrium occurs sporadically in horses but is usually observed only at necropsy (3). It is often associated with tuberculosis. In adult cattle lymphomatosis commonly affects the right atrium and causes impairment of blood flow and congestive heart failure.

An important recent observation has been that of vascular damage and myocardial injury in horses caused by the intravenous injection of succinyl choline chloride. The drug has been used extensively to procure muscular relaxation for castration and other short term surgical procedures but there have been a disturbing number of reports of reduction in racing performance or sudden death. A high proportion of horses treated with the drug show electrocardiographic evidence of myocardial injury and at necropsy have macroscopic petechial and ecchymotic haemorrhages, particularly in the right ventricular myocardium (5).

Pathogenesis

The primary effect of any myocardial lesion is to reduce cardiac reserve and restrict compensation in circulatory emergencies. Many of the manifestations of heart disease described earlier, including cardiac enlargement, arrhythmia, or abnormalities of rate may occur and in the terminal stages a syndrome of congestive heart failure or acute heart failure develops depending upon the rate at which failure occurs. For example, in a collection of 63 cases of atrial fibrillation in horses, 4 horses showed dependent oedema, many had gross valvular lesions manifested by murmurs, largely systolic, and in 80 per cent of the animals there were gross and microscopic lesions of myocarditis (10).

Clinical Findings

In early cases there is decreased exercise tolerance. This is usually accompanied by an increase in heart rate and heart size although the latter may not be detectable. If the neuromyocardium is involved there may be clinically recognizable abnormalities of rate or rhythm, particularly bradycardia due to heart block and irregularity due to atrial flutter or fibrillation. The characters of the pulse and heart sounds are also changed but these changes can also occur due to extracardiac influences.

In the late stages there may be sudden death or attacks of cardiac syncope due to acute heart failure, or severe dyspnoea or general oedema due to congestive heart failure. Myocardial weakness is frequently accompanied by a haemic murmur which occurs with the first heart sound and reaches maximum intensity at the peak of inspiration and diminishes or disappears with expiration.

Clinical Pathology

Electrocardiography should be carried out when possible as it gives a good indication of the status of the myocardium even though the type of lesion cannot be diagnosed. Other tests as outlined in special examination of the cardiovascular system (p. 132) are not generally practicable. The release of transaminases into the bloodstream after acute myocardial infarction in man (4) and cattle has aroused much interest as a diagnostic test for this disease.

Necropsy Findings

Bacterial infections may cause discrete abscesses in the myocardium but viral infections and degenerations due to nutritional deficiencies and poisonings usually produce a visible pallor of the muscle which may be uniform or present as streaks between apparently normal bundles of muscle. The degenerated muscle may also be present in only the inner layers of the wall, leaving the external layers with a normal appearance. In coronary thrombosis infarction of a large area of the wall may have occurred but this is not visible unless the animal survives for at least 24 hours afterwards. Careful examination of the coronary arteries is usually necessary to detect the causative embolus. In horses infarction occurs most commonly in the right atrium.

The terminal stage of myocardial degeneration or myocarditis is often fibrous tissue replacement of the damaged tissue. The heart is flabby and thin walled and shows patches of shrunken, tough fibrous tissue. Rupture of the atrial walls may result, with sudden death occurring due to the pressure of blood in the pericardial sac. The lesions of lymphomatosis are characteristic of this disease: large, uneven masses of pale, firm, undifferentiated tissue with the consistency of lymphoid tissue.

Diagnosis

A diagnosis of myocardial asthenia is usually made when decreased exercise tolerance or acute or congestive heart failure occur without an associated distinctive cardiac abnormality. Endocardial lesions and congenital defects of the heart or large vessels are usually accompanied by an audible murmur, and in some cases a palpable cardiac thrill, and abnormalities of the pulse. Pericarditis causes muffling of the heart sounds and is accompanied in the early stages by a pericardial friction rub and in the later stages by fluid sounds on auscultation. Hydropericardium is also accompanied by muffling of the heart beat and adventitious fluid sounds. Cardiac rupture and tamponade may cause acute heart failure but affected animals die so quickly that clinical examination is usually not possible.

The cardiac dilatation of myocardial asthenia needs to be differentiated from increased audibility of heart sounds caused by retraction of the lung, and decreased audibility of the sounds from muffling by expanded lungs in pulmonary emphysema. Space-occupying lesions of the chest, including diaphragmatic hernia, mediastinal abscess and tumour, may also cause a degree of congestive heart failure and displacement of the heart, and are probably the commonest causes of error in the diagnosis of myocardial disease. They can be diagnosed only by careful auscultation and percussion.

Treatment

The primary cause must be treated and details are given under the specific diseases listed above. Supportive treatment is usually ineffective in acute heart failure and is not practicable in congestive heart failure.

REFERENCES
(1) Farrelly, B. T. (1954). *Vet. Rec.*, *66*, 53.
(2) Cronin, M. T. I. & Leader, G. H. (1952). *Vet. Rec.*, *64*, 8.
(3) Detweiler, D. K. (1958). *Univ. Pennsylvania Bull.*, *Vet. Ext. Qtly*, *59*, 4.
(4) Keele, K. D. *et al.* (1958). *Lancet*, *2*, 1187.
(5) Larsen, L. H. *et al.* (1959). *Aust. vet. J.*, *35*, 269.
(6) Gainer, J. H. (1967). *J. Amer. vet. med. Ass.*, *151*, 421.
(7) Dennis, S. M. (1966). *Vet. Rec.*, *79*, 38.
(8) Dobin, M. A. & Epschtein, J. F. (1968). *Mh. Vet.-Med.*, *23*, 627.
(9) Bishop, S. P. *et al.* (1966). *Lab. Invest.*, *15*, 1124.
(10) Else, R. W. & Holmes, J. R. (1971). *Equ. vet. J.*, *3*, 56.

Rupture of the Heart

Rupture of the heart occurs rarely in animals. It is recorded in cattle where a foreign body penetrating from the reticulum perforates the ventricular wall and as a spontaneous occurrence in horses. Rupture of the base of the aorta is not uncommon in horses and has the same effect as cardiac rupture. The pericardial sac immediately fills with blood and the animal dies of acute heart failure. A similar cardiac tamponade occurs when reticular foreign bodies lacerate a coronary artery or when foals suffer severe laceration of the epicardium during a difficult parturition.

When the aorta ruptures it may do so through its wall just above the aortic valves. The wall may have been weakened previously by verminous arteritis or by the development of medionecrosis. Another form of rupture occurs through the aortic ring (1). Death occurs very suddenly; all 8 cases reported by one author affected stallions and coincided with the time of breeding. Cardiac tamponade may occur but the common finding is a dissecting aneurysm into the ventricular myocardium.

REFERENCE
(1) Rooney, J. R. *et al.* (1967). *Path. vet.*, *4*, 268.

Valvular Disease

Disease of the heart valves interferes with the normal flow of blood through the cardiac orifices, causing murmurs and, in severe cases, congestive heart failure.

Aetiology

Endocarditis, in its acute or chronic form, is the commonest cause of valvular disease in animals and is described in detail below. Laceration or detachment of valves during severe exercise may occur but probably only when there is prior disease of the endocardium. Fenestration of the aortic and pulmonary semilunar valves has been observed commonly in horses. The cause of the lesions is unknown although their presence in very young animals, including newborn foals, suggests that some may be congenital defects (1). The importance of these lesions as causes of valvular insufficiency is doubtful although they may cause valvular murmurs if they are present close to the attachments of the cusps. A systolic murmur most audible on the left side behind the shoulder joint is common in normal newborn foals and is caused by patency of the ductus arteriosus. The persistence of this murmur to the fifth day suggests the presence of a congenital defect (9). Excessive cardiac dilatation in any form of myocardial asthenia or when there is excessive overloading of the arterial flow may result in dilatation of the orifices and functional insufficiency of the valves. Careful examination of the heart sounds is most commonly performed in the horse but the incidence of significant valvular lesions is remarkably low. Verrucose endocarditis of the atrioventricular valves occurs occasionally (2) and degenerative lesions of the aortic valves resulting in insufficiency have been observed in this species (7).

Cardiac murmurs are common in old horses, as they are in newborn foals, and it is often difficult to know how much importance one should attach to them. The commonest murmur is a diastolic murmur loudest over the aortic valve area and in most cases there is some evidence of aortic valvular insufficiency (9).

Pathogenesis

The presence of valvular lesions and murmurs may mean little except that some degree of cardiac reserve is lost. This may be small in degree, and moderate stenosis or incompetence can be compensated and supported for long periods provided myocardial asthenia does not develop. The importance of valvular lesions lies in their possible contribution to disease in other organs by the liberation of emboli, and the necessity for close examination of the heart when they are present. The purpose for which the animal is maintained also has some bearing on the significance of a murmur. Valvular lesions are of much greater importance in racing animals than in those kept for breeding purposes.

The important clinical indications of valvular disease are audible murmurs and palpable thrills. Both are caused by the eddying and turbulence created by the flow of blood through valvular leaks. In general the loudest murmurs are produced by leaks of only moderate size but a cardiac thrill always indicates the presence of a large leak. The turbulence may occur when the valves do not close properly (insufficiency) and blood is forced through atrioventricular orifices during ventricular systole, or through semilunar orifices during ventricular diastole. Turbulence may also occur when the valves do not open completely (stenosis) and blood enters the ventricle through a narrow atrioventricular orifice during its diastolic phase or is forced through a stenotic semilunar orifice during ventricular systole. Simple stenosis or insufficiency may occur independently but in many cases in animals, especially those in which there are vegetative lesions, insufficiency and stenosis of the one group of valves occur at the same time.

Impediment of blood flow through an orifice induces compensatory responses by the myocardium. If the stroke volume has to be increased to maintain the minute volume there is an accompanying dilatation. This is the case when the valves are insufficient, much of the ejecting force being wasted in the leakage of blood back through the incompetent valves. If the valves on the left side of the heart are affected the changes in ejection of blood from the ventricle produce changes in the character of the peripheral pulse.

Clinical Findings

Only the clinical findings referable to valvular disease are discussed here. The clinical findings in congestive heart failure, which may coexist, are discussed elsewhere. There is an obvious need for very careful auscultation if accurate observations are to be made. The need is perhaps greatest in the horse in which minimal lesions may be of great importance. Good equipment and a knowledge of the optimum areas of auscultation and the significance of the murmurs encountered are essential (6).

Stenosis of the aortic semilunar valves (8). There is a harsh systolic murmur, most audible high up over the base of the heart on the left side and posteriorly. The murmur replaces or modifies the first heart sound. A systolic thrill may be palpable over the base of the heart and the cardiac impulse is increased due to ventricular hypertrophy. The stenosis has no functional significance unless the pulse is abnormal, with a small amplitude rising slowly to a delayed peak. There may be signs of left-sided heart failure.

Insufficiency of the aortic semilunar valves. There is a loud diastolic murmur displacing or modifying the second heart sound and caused by the reflux of blood from the aorta into the left ventricle during ventricular diastole. The murmur is heard best over the base of the heart on the left side and posteriorly. There is no thrill but the apex beat is markedly increased because of the cardiac dilatation and the great increase in stroke volume. Valvular insufficiency of sufficient degree to have functional significance is accompanied by a pulse of very large amplitude and high systolic and low diastolic blood pressures. The pulse wave may be great enough to cause a visible pulse in small vessels and even in capillaries.

Stenosis and insufficiency of the pulmonary semilunar valves. The signs are the same as for aortic valve lesions except that there are no abnormalities of the pulse. Differentiation may be difficult when aortic valve lesions are small and produce no pulse signs. Pulmonary valve lesions are more audible anteriorly than aortic valve lesions and heart failure, if it occurs, is right-sided.

Stenosis of the left atrioventricular valves. There is a diastolic murmur caused by passage of blood into the left ventricle through a stenosed valve during diastolic filling. The severity of the stenosis governs the duration of the murmur rather than its intensity. In severe stenosis the murmur can be heard right through from the second to the first sound in each cardiac cycle. The murmur is most audible at the apex of the heart on the left side. A diastolic thrill may be palpable but the pulse characters are unchanged unless left-sided congestive heart failure is present due to incomplete filling of the ventricle.

Insufficiency of the left atrioventricular valve.
There is a systolic murmur, most audible at the apex of the heart on the left side, caused by leakage of blood through the valve during systole. The pulse characters, as in stenosis of this valve, are unchanged.

Stenosis and insufficiency of the right atrioventricular valves. The murmurs are the same as those of stenosis and insufficiency of the left A-V valves except that they are most audible over the right apex. Insufficiency of these valves is usually accompanied by an exaggeration of the jugular pulse. Congestive heart failure, if it occurs, will be manifested in the greater circulation.

Clinical Pathology

Clinico-pathological findings will reflect the changes caused by the primary disease and are significant only when there is endocarditis.

Necropsy Findings

Care is needed when the heart is opened to ensure that the valves can be viewed properly from both upper and lower aspects. Lesions of endocarditis may be visible or there may be perforations, distortion or thickening of the valves or breakage of the chordae tendinae. The lesions of congestive heart failure may also be present.

Diagnosis

Diagnosis of valvular disease depends largely on recognition of an endocardial murmur. Murmurs must be differentiated from pericardial and pleural friction sounds and from murmurs due to congenital defects. Valvular murmurs always accompany or replace the normal heart sounds and although a systolic and a diastolic murmur may be present in the one animal there is a strict relation to the cardiac cycle. Pleural friction rubs may be localized to the cardiac area but can be distinguished by their occurrence with each respiratory cycle. Pericardial friction sounds are more clearly audible and are present throughout the cardiac cycle, waxing and waning in intensity during diastole and systole. Murmurs caused by congenital defects are usually very loud, do not displace the normal heart sounds and can be heard in specific sites. A thrill is more commonly felt in congenital defects but may occur in valvular disease.

Special attention should be given to the differentiation of functional haemic murmurs and those due to structural lesions of the valves. Haemic murmurs can be expected in animals suffering from anaemia and in emaciated and debilitated animals.

The murmur is soft and usually only discernible by careful auscultation and characteristically waxes and wanes with each respiratory cycle, reaching maximum intensity at the height of inspiration.

Murmurs of endocardial origin are commonly encountered in otherwise normal animals, especially horses and pigs, and too much attention should not be paid to them unless there is supporting evidence of cardiac disease (3, 6). The murmurs are most commonly encountered in newborn animals and in those examined in sternal or lateral recumbency. A common murmur encountered in 2 to 3 year old normal horses is a short, high pitched squeak, most audible over the apex of the left side, and occurring midway between the second and first sounds and without being associated with either sound (4). In newborn pigs a continuous murmur may be heard and this is often replaced by an early systolic murmur audible for the first week of life. The murmur is thought to be caused by patency of the ductus arteriosus which subsequently disappears (5).

Treatment

There is no specific treatment for valvular disease. Methods for the treatment of congestive heart failure and endocarditis are discussed under those headings.

REFERENCES

(1) Mahaffey, L. W. (1958). *Vet. Rec.*, *70*, 415.
(2) Miller, W. C. (1962). *Vet. Rec.*, *74*, 825.
(3) Castle, R. F. (1961). *J. Amer. Med. Ass.*, *177*, 1.
(4) Glendinning, S. A. (1964). *Vet. Rec.*, *76*, 341.
(5) Evans, J. R. *et al.* (1963). *Circulat. Res.*, *12*, 85.
(6) Littlewort, M. C. G. (1962). *Vet. Rec.*, *74*, 1247.
(7) Bishop, S. P. *et al.* (1966). *Path. vet.*, *3*, 137.
(8) Fisher, E. W. (1968). *Vet. Rec.*, *82*, 618.
(9) Rossdale, P. D. (1967). *Brit. vet. J.*, *123*, 521.

Endocarditis

Inflammation of the endocardium may interfere with the ejection of blood from the heart by causing insufficiency or stenosis of the valves. Murmurs associated with the heart sounds are the major clinical manifestation and, if interference with blood flow is sufficiently severe, congestive heart failure develops.

Aetiology

Most cases of endocarditis in farm animals are caused by bacterial infection but whether the infection gains entrance by direct adhesion to undamaged endothelium, or through minor discontinuities of the valvular surfaces, or by haematogenous spread through the capillaries at the base of the valve is uncertain. The common infectious causes of endocarditis in animals are listed below. In cattle alpha-haemolytic streptococci and *Corynebacterium pyogenes* are the commonest bacteria found in valvular endocarditis (1, 2, 6). The infection may be embolic from suppurative lesions in other sites, especially traumatic reticulitis, metritis and mastitis, but many appear to be primary. Endocarditis is not uncommon in blackleg and has also been recorded in young calves vaccinated with viable *Mycoplasma mycoides*. In horses *Actinobacillus equuli* has been recorded as a cause (3), *Streptococcus equi* is frequently encountered and *Meningococcus* spp. are recorded as a cause in animals undergoing hyperimmunization with meningococci (4). Endocarditis in horses may also be caused by migrating *Strongylus* spp. larvae. In pigs *Streptococcus* spp. and *Erysipelothrix insidiosa* and in lambs *Streptococcus* spp and *E. coli* are common causes.

Pathogenesis

Vegetative or ulcerative lesions may develop and interfere with the normal passage of blood through the cardiac orifices, resulting in congestive heart failure. Fragments of vegetative lesions may become detached and cause embolic endarteritis, with the production of miliary pulmonary abscesses, or abscesses in other organs including myocardium, kidneys and joints.

Chronic lesions are less crumbly and less likely to release emboli but adhesions between cusps develop and retraction of scar tissue causes shrinking, distortion, and thickening of the valve cusps. At this stage interference with blood flow is severe and congestive heart failure almost always follows.

In cattle valvular lesions occur most commonly on the right AV valve and venous congestion is most marked in the general systemic vessels but bilateral or left-sided involvement of the AV valves is not uncommon (7). In horses the aortic semilunar valves are most commonly affected although the left AV valves may also be involved (5).

Clinical Findings

The important finding is a murmur on auscultation or a thrill on palpation of the cardiac area. The maximum intensity of the murmur varies with the situation of the affected valves (7) and this also governs whether or not there are abnormalities of the amplitude and pressure of the pulse, lesions of the left AV or aortic semilunar valves causing detectable abnormalities.

In compensated cases there may be poor exercise tolerance. In advanced cases, particularly where a concurrent myocardial asthenia reduces cardiac compensation, congestive failure develops. At all stages a moderate, fluctuating fever is common and secondary involvement of other organs may cause the appearance of signs of peripheral lymphadenitis, embolic pneumonia, nephritis, arthritis, tenosynovitis or myocarditis. There is usually much loss of condition, pallor of mucosae and an increase in heart rate. In cattle additional signs observed include a grunting respiration as though the animal was in pain, moderate ruminal tympany, scouring or constipation, blindness, facial paralysis, muscle weakness to the point of tremor or recumbency, jaundice and sudden death (2). Distension of the jugular vein, general oedema and a systolic or diastolic murmur are also present in many cases. In horses oedema occurs rarely and jugular engorgement is not a marked sign until the terminal stages.

The course in endocarditis may be as long as several weeks or months, or animals may drop dead without premonitory signs. In sows it is common for agalactia to develop in the first two or three weeks after farrowing, followed by a loss of weight, intolerance to exercise and dyspnoea at rest.

Clinical Pathology

A marked leucocytosis and a shift to the left occurs in acute cases (8). A significant increase in monocytes and macrophages and a severe anaemia have been observed in cattle at this time (1). In chronic cases where the lesions are due largely to scarring of the valves haematological findings are usually normal. Blood cultures should be attempted at the peaks of the fever but may have to be repeated on a number of occasions. Determination of the sensitivity of the organism to antibacterial drugs may aid in treatment. Repeated examination of the urine may reveal transient episodes of proteinuria and the shedding of bacteria.

Necropsy Findings

The lesions are termed vegetative when they are large and cauliflower-like and verrucose when they are small and wart-like. The former are present on the valves in most fatal cases. In the later stages the valves are shrunken, distorted and often thickened along the edges. This stage of recovery is rare in farm animals but may be observed in the semilunar valves in horses. Spontaneous healing is rare and in most cases treatment is commenced at too late a stage.

Embolic lesions may be present in any other organ. Culture of the valvular lesions should be undertaken but in many cases no growth is obtained. The causative bacteria may be dead or not cultivable and the examination of direct smears should always be undertaken.

Diagnosis

The differentiation of valvular disease from other conditions in which heart murmurs occur has already been discussed. Failure to observe a valvular murmur may result in confusion between endocarditis and pericarditis or other causes of congestive heart failure. The commonest error in cattle is in differentiation of the disease from lymphomatosis. The only satisfactory differential feature is the failure of lymphomatosis to respond to treatment with penicillin.

Treatment

Treatment is not highly successful because of the difficulty encountered in completely controlling the infection. The thickness of the lesions prevents adequate penetration of the drugs and unless the sensitivity of the causative organism is known a range of antibacterial drugs may have to be tried. The streptococci which cause endocarditis in cattle are reported to be often resistant to all antibiotics (1) but the parenteral administration of penicillin is usually effective. Large doses (4 to 6 million units daily for a cow weighing 1200 lb.) should be given for 3 days. If relapse occurs a 7 to 10 day course is recommended in valuable animals. If treatment is attempted a fall in temperature can be taken as an indication that the infection is being brought under control but treatment should be continued for at least a week.

The sequelae of embolic lesions in other organs and permanent distortion of valves resulting in valvular insufficiency also militate against a satisfactory outcome. The use of parenteral anticoagulants, as used in man to prevent further deposition of material on vegetative lesions, has not been found to be practicable in animals.

REFERENCES

(1) Rees Evans, E. T. (1957). *Vet. Rec.*, *69*, 1190.
(2) John, F. V. (1947). *Vet. Rec.*, *59*, 214.
(3) Innes, J. R. M. *et al.* (1950). *Brit. vet. J.*, *106*, 245.
(4) Miller, J. K. (1944). *Amer. J. Path.*, *20*, 269.
(5) Detweiler, D. K. (1958). *Univ. Pennsylvania Bull.*, *Vet. Ext. Qtly*, *59*, 4.
(6) Larsen, H. E. *et al.* (1963). *Nord. Vet.-Med.*, *15*, 645, 668 & 691.
(7) Wagenaar, G. (1963). *T. Diergeneesk.*, *88*, 1760.
(8) Kroneman, J. (1970). *T. Diergeneesk.*, *95*, 862.

Pericarditis

Inflammation of the pericardial sac causes an audible friction rub initially, followed by muffling of the heart sounds and congestive heart failure as fluid accumulates in the sac, or the exudate organizes to form obliterating and restrictive adhesions.

Aetiology

Perforation of the pericardial sac by an infected foreign body occurs commonly only in cattle. The resulting syndrome of traumatic pericarditis has already been discussed. Localization of a blood-borne infection occurs sporadically in many diseases including strangles and tuberculosis in horses. A generalized infection in horses has been observed in which pericarditis is accompanied by arthritis, pleurisy and peritonitis (1, 2) and *Strep. faecalis* has been isolated from the pericardial sac. Pericarditis occurs in cattle in sporadic bovine encephalomyelitis, tuberculosis and pasteurellosis. In sheep pericarditis may occur in pasteurellosis, and in pigs in pasteurellosis, pneumonia caused by *Mycoplasma* sp., salmonellosis, streptococcal infections and in Glasser's disease. Direct extension of infection from pleurisy or myocarditis may also occur in all animals but the clinical signs of pericarditis in such cases are usually dominated by those of the primary disease. A sporadic pericarditis from which no infectious agent can be isolated occurs in adult dairy cows. An homogeneous turbid fluid can be drawn off in large quantities by paracentesis and recovery is usual.

Pathogenesis

In the early stages inflammation of the pericardium is accompanied by hyperaemia and the deposition of fibrinous exudate which produces a friction rub when the pericardium and epicardium rub together during cardiac movement. As effusion develops the inflamed surfaces are separated, the friction rub is replaced by muffling of the heart sounds, and the accumulated fluid compresses the atria and right ventricle, preventing their complete filling. Congestive heart failure follows. A severe toxaemia is usually present in suppurative pericarditis because of the toxins produced by the bacteria in the pericardial sac.

In the recovery stage of non-suppurative pericarditis the fluid is resorbed, and adhesions form between the pericardium and epicardium to cause an adhesive pericarditis but the adhesions are usually not sufficiently strong to impair cardiac movement. In suppurative pericarditis the adhesions which form become organized and may cause complete attachment of the pericardium to the epicardium, or this may occur only patchily to leave some loculi which are filled with serous fluid.

In either case restriction of cardiac movement will probably be followed by the appearance of congestive heart failure.

Clinical Findings

In the early stages there is pain, avoidance of movement, abduction of the elbows, arching of the back and shallow, abdominal respiration. Pain is evidenced on percussion or firm palpation over the cardiac area of the chest wall, and the animal lies down carefully. A pericardial friction sound is detectable on auscultation of the cardiac area. The temperature is elevated to 39·5 to 41 °C (103 to 106 °F) and the pulse rate is increased. Associated signs of pleurisy, pneumonia and peritonitis may be present.

In most cases of pericarditis caused by traumatic reticuloperitonitis, haematogenous infection, or spread from pleurisy, the second stage of effusion is manifested by muffling of the heart sounds, decreased palpability of the apex beat and an increase in the area of cardiac dullness. If gas is present in the pericardial sac each cardiac cycle may be accompanied by splashing sounds. Signs of congestive heart failure become evident. Fever is present, the heart rate is markedly increased and toxaemia is severe, although this varies with the types of bacteria present. This is the most dangerous period and affected animals usually die of congestive heart failure, or of toxaemia, in 1 to 3 weeks. Those that survive pass through a long period of chronic ill health during which the toxaemia subsides relatively quickly but congestive heart failure diminishes slowly. In this stage of chronic pericarditis additional signs of myocarditis, particularly irregularity, may appear. The heart sounds become less muffled and fluid sounds disappear altogether or persist in restricted areas. Complete recovery is not common but with suitable antibacterial treatment relative normality may be regained.

Clinical Pathology

A marked leucocytosis and shift to the left is detectable on haematological examination in traumatic pericarditis. In the other forms of pericarditis changes in the blood depend upon the other lesions present and on the causative agent. In the stage in which effusion occurs a sample of fluid may be aspirated from the pericardial sac and submitted for bacteriological examination. The technique is not without danger as infection may be spread to the pleural cavity.

Necropsy Findings

In the early stages there is hyperaemia of the pericardial lining and a deposit of fibrin. When effusion occurs there is an accumulation of turbid fluid and tags of fibrin are present on the greatly thickened epicardium and pericardium. Gas may also be present and the fluid may have a putrid odour if *Sphaerophorus necrophorus* or *Corynebacterium pyogenes* are present. When the pericarditis has reached a chronic stage the pericardium is adherent to the epicardium over a greater or lesser part of the cardiac surface. Loculi containing serous fluid often remain. Embolic abscesses may be present in other organs. Lesions typical of the specific causative diseases listed above are described under their specific headings.

Diagnosis

Pericardial friction sounds may be mistaken for the friction sounds of early pleurisy. Synchronization of friction sounds with respiratory cycles indicates that the sounds are pleural in origin. Cardiac movement may produce friction sounds when pleurisy is localized to the pleural surface of the pericardial sac but there is an absence of other signs of pericardial involvement. Pericardial sounds may also be confused with valvular murmurs, or murmurs caused by congenital defects, but pericardial sounds are usually present throughout the cardiac cycle rather than accompanying or displacing one or other of the heart sounds.

Muffling of the heart sounds may also occur in pleurisy with effusion and in pulmonary emphysema but there are prominent signs of respiratory involvement. Hydropericardium is usually found in association with oedema and an increase in the cardiac impulse. It occurs commonly in congestive heart failure, in mulberry heart disease of pigs, in herztod of pigs, gossypol poisoning, clostridial intoxications of sheep and in lymphomatosis. Mediastinal abscess may also cause signs of congestive heart failure and local pleurisy.

Treatment

Antibacterial treatment of the specific infection should be undertaken if possible. Non-specific treatment should include broad spectrum antibiotics or sulphonamides. Intravenous alimentation is usually not indicated because of the long course. Repeated paracentesis to relieve the fluid pressure in the pericardial sac affords only temporary relief of the cardiac embarrassment, the fluid returning quickly. If the infection can be brought under control paracentesis of the pericardial sac followed by the administration of diuretics is recommended, but digitalization is usually not very effective and is dangerous if infection is still present. Surgical treatment, to provide continuous drainage of the sac, has been used, but is not usually successful (3).

REFERENCES
(1) Rainey, J. W. (1944). *Aust. vet. J.*, *20*, 204.
(2) Ryan, A. F. & Rainey, J. W. (1945). *Aust. vet. J.*, *21*, 146.
(3) Horney, F. D. (1960). *Canad. vet. J.*, *1*, 363.

Congenital Cardiac Defects

Some of the defects described in this section are actually defects of the peripheral vascular system but are described here for convenience. The defects often produce clinical signs at birth and cause severe illness or death in the first few weeks of life but in a number of cases adequate compensation occurs and the defect may not be observed until a comparatively late age. It is probably wise to avoid giving a too unfavourable prognosis in newborn animals which have a cardiac murmur, especially in foals and baby pigs and when the murmur is minimal. It is possible that in many such cases there is no structural defect and the murmur is innocent and functional and will disappear early in life. This is a common finding in human infants (6). In one extensive survey 48 per cent of all infants with systolic murmurs at birth were normal one year later.

The important factor in the pathogenesis of most congenital cardiac defects is the mixing of oxygenated and reduced blood through an anastomosis between the pulmonary and systemic circuits. The blood leaving the left ventricle or aorta therefore includes some oxygenated and some reduced blood. The resulting anoxic anoxia causes severe dyspnoea, and cyanosis may be marked if the proportion of unsaturated blood is high. This is most likely to occur when there is obstruction of the pulmonary artery. There is a notable absence of fever and toxaemia if intercurrent disease does not develop. Cardiac enlargement is usually detectable.

In animals which survive to maturity, sudden death due to acute heart failure or congestive heart failure are likely to occur when the animals are subjected to a physical stress such as the first pregnancy. The primary appearance of signs of cardiac disease when an animal is 2 or 3 years of age should not eliminate congenital defects from consideration. One of the major difficulties in clinical cardiology is to distinguish between the congenital anomalies themselves. Unless cardiac catheterization can be carried out (16) and pressure gradients and CO_2 and O_2 pressure gradients between the two sides of the heart determined an accurate pre-surgical diagnosis is impossible.

Congenital cardiac anomalies occur in all species (13) but are not common in any one of them. The greatest frequency is probably in cattle (9). The incidence is low in horses (10). In a large series of necropsy examinations of lambs 1·3 per cent were found to have cardiac, mostly septal, defects (19). The more common defects are set out below.

Ectopia cordis. An abnormal position of the heart outside the thoracic cavity is most common in cattle, the displacement usually being to the lower cervical region (11). The heart is easily seen and palpated and there is an accompanying divergence of the first ribs and a ventrodorsal compression of the sternum giving the appearance of absence of the brisket. Affected animals may survive for periods of years, as they also may with an abdominal displacement, but those with a displacement through a defective sternum or ribs rarely survive for more than a few days

Patent interventricular septum (subaortal septal defect). This defect occurs in all species and may be manifested by clinical signs in the first few days of life or by failure to grow well when young (8), or permit an apparently normal existence until maturity (1, 7, 15). There is a loud, blowing murmur audible over the base of the heart on both sides of the chest, the murmur being characteristically most audible over a circumscribed area but it can be heard faintly over a much larger area (2). The murmur in this defect is one of the loudest and most obvious murmurs encountered. It is systolic in time but the normal heart sounds can also be heard and these are increased in intensity. A pronounced cardiac thrill is palpable. Attention is usually drawn to the animal by the clinical appearance of severe dyspnoea at rest or after mild exercise. The size of the defect varies from a small orifice high up under the aorta to almost complete absence of the septum and governs the severity of the clinical signs. In most cases the cause of the defect is unexplained but in one reported occurrence of 3 cases in a herd of Hereford cattle, it may have been conditioned by inheritance (8).

A special variant of the condition is the tetralogy of Fallot in which the aorta overrides both ventricles and there is almost complete absence of the interventricular septum (18, 21). Stenosis of the pulmonary artery is also present. The functional defect is severe and cyanosis is usually marked because of the large amounts of unoxygenated blood which pass into the left ventricle. A similar variant, the Eisenmenger Complex, has been recorded in cattle (12, 17). It differs from the previous defect in that there is no stenosis of the pulmonary artery but there may be hypoplasia of the aorta. The clinical signs associated with this defect are similar to those seen in cases with tetralogy of Fallot except that cyanosis is not evident although exercise tolerance is low. The heart sounds may also be normal (12, 15).

Patent foramen ovale. This defect of the atrial septum usually causes no clinical signs and is detected only at necropsy.

Patent ductus arteriosus. The clinical signs are comparable to those of insufficiency of the aortic semilunar valves. The pulse is large in amplitude but has a low diastolic pressure. A murmur is audible high up over the base of the heart and is both systolic and diastolic in time, blood passing through the anastomosis during systole and diastole. The intensity of the murmur waxes and wanes giving rise to the name of 'machinery murmur'.

Coarctation of the aorta. Constriction of the aorta at the site of entrance of the ductus arteriosus causes a syndrome similar to that of stenosis of the aortic semilunar valves; there is a systolic murmur and a slow-rising pulse of small amplitude.

Persistence of the right aortic arch. Persistence of the right aortic arch causes constriction of the oesophagus, dysphagia and regurgitation (3). Clinical signs are evident soon after birth but survival until five years of age has been recorded in a bull which manifested chronic bloat and visible oesophageal dilatation (4). The aorta is situated to the right of the oesophagus and trachea and is connected by a ligamentum arteriosum to the left pulmonary artery, the oesophagus and trachea being contained in the triangle.

Fibro-elastosis. Congenital fibro-elastosis has been observed in calves and pigs. The endocardium is converted into a thick fibro-elastic coat, and although the wall of the left ventricle is hypertrophied the capacity of the ventricle is reduced. The aortic valves may be thickened and irregular and obviously stenosed. A similar condition occurs in humans but the cause in all species is unknown. The syndrome is one of congestive heart failure but there are no signs which indicate the presence of specific lesions of the myocardium, endocardium or pericardium. The defect may cause no clinical abnormality until the animal is mature.

Subvalvular aortic stenosis. Stenosis of the aorta at or just below the point of attachment of the aortic semilunar valves has been recorded as a common defect in pigs (5) but its differentiation from other causes of heart failure is difficult and the significance of the stenosis is open to doubt.

Clinically affected animals may die suddenly with asphyxia, dyspnoea and foaming at the mouth and nostrils, or after a long period of ill-health with recurrent attacks of dyspnoea. In the acute form death may occur after exercise or be unassociated with exertion.

Anomalous origin of carotid arteries. Either or both carotid arteries may originate from the pulmonary artery instead of the aorta. The resulting anoxia causes myocardial weakness in the ventricle of the affected side. Congestive heart failure usually follows. The defect has been recorded in cattle (14) and dogs.

REFERENCES

(1) Meyerowitz, B. (1942). *Amer. J. vet. Res., 3,* 368.
(2) Blood, D. C. & Steel, J. D. (1946). *Aust. vet. J., 22,* 22.
(3) Rooney, J. R. & Watson, D. F. (1956), *J. Amer. vet. med. Ass., 129,* 5.
(4) Roberts, S. J. *et al.* (1953). *Cornell Vet., 43,* 537.
(5) Emsbo, P. (1956). *Nord. Vet.-Med., 8,* 261.
(6) Benson, P. F. *et al.* (1961). *Lancet, 280,* 627.
(7) Blood, D. C. (1960). *Canad. vet. J., 1,* 104.
(8) Belling, T. H. (1961). *J. Amer. vet. med. Ass., 138,* 595.
(9) Schmidt, P. & von Mickwitz, C. U. (1964). *Mh. Vet.-Med., 19,* 541.
(10) Rooney, J. R. & Franks, W. C. (1964). *Path. vet., 1,* 454.
(11) Bowen, J. M. & Adrian, R. W. (1962). *J. Amer. vet. med. Ass., 141,* 1162.
(12) Fisher, E. W. *et al.* (1962). *Vet. Rec., 74,* 447.
(13) Godglück, G. (1962). *Dtsch. tierärztl. Wschr., 69,* 98.
(14) Botts, R. P. & Kintner, L. D. (1964). *Canad. J. comp. Med., 28,* 169.
(15) Fisher, E. W. & Pirie, H. M. (1964). *Brit. vet. J., 120,* 253.
(16) Buergelt, C. D. *et al.* (1970). *J. Amer. vet. med. Ass., 157,* 313.
(17) Säss, B. & Albert, T. F. (1970). *Cornell Vet., 60,* 61.
(18) Dear, M. G. & Price, E. K. (1970). *Vet. Rec., 86,* 219.
(19) Dennis, S. M. & Leipold, H. W. (1968). *Amer. J. vet. Res., 29,* 2337.
(20) Milledge, R. D. *et al.* (1968). *J. Amer. vet. med. Ass., 152,* 161.
(21) Breukink, H. J. *et al.* (1965). *T. Diergeneesk., 90,* 1164.

DISEASES OF THE BLOOD VESSELS

Arterial Thrombosis and Embolism

Arteritis leading to thrombus formation causes ischaemia of the tissues supplied by the affected artery. Clinical signs of reduced function or ischaemic necrosis vary with the site of the obstruction.

Aetiology

Parasitic arteritis is the most common form of arterial disease in farm animals. The migrating larvae of *Strongylus vulgaris* cause arteritis of the anterior mesenteric artery, the iliac arteries, the base of the aorta and less commonly the cerebral, renal and coronary arteries in horses. Onchocerciasis in cattle and elaeophoriasis in sheep are also accompanied by arteritis. Arteritis and arteriolar spasm are characteristic of ergotism and lead to gangrene of the extremities. Exposure to extreme cold has the same effect.

Arteritis is also the primary lesion in bovine malignant catarrh and equine viral arteritis. Periarteritis nodosa occurs occasionally in animals but the cause is not known (1, 2). Embolic endarteritis is also an occasional finding at necropsy in animals with suppurative lesions, or in cases of vegetative endocarditis or arterial thrombosis in other sites. Non-infected arterial embolism may occur when globules of fat enter vessels during surgery. Similar embolism in the pulmonary arteries is thought to occur in horses after castration in the cast position.

Pathogenesis

In parasitic arteritis inflammation and thickening of the arterial wall result in the formation of thrombi which may partially or completely occlude the artery. The common site is in the anterior mesenteric artery, obstruction of the vessel causing recurrent colic or fatal ischaemic necrosis of a segment of the intestine. Less common sites include the origin of the iliac artery at the abdominal aorta causing iliac thrombosis, the base of the aorta leading to rupture and haemopericardium, and the coronary arteries causing myocardial infarction. Occlusion of the arteries to the extremities in frostbite and ergotism causes local ischaemic necrosis. Sporadic cases of dry gangrene of the extremities are seen in calves which resemble the lesions seen in ergotism but in situations where contact with the fungus is not possible. The calves are usually chronically affected with diarrhoea and infection with *Salmonella* sp. has been suggested as a cause of the gangrene (12). Periarteritis nodosa and embolic endarteritis cause a variety of syndromes depending on the localization of the lesions. Large emboli which lodge in the pulmonary arteries cause anoxic anoxia, and emboli arising from the pulmonary veins may lodge in any organ particularly the brain and kidneys. Embolism in the renal artery causes acute cortical necrosis and gross haematuria. An aneurysm of the abdominal aorta which involved a ureter in a horse caused recurrent haemorrhage into the urinary tract (6).

Clinical Findings

The clinical findings in mesenteric verminous arteritis of horses and renal and myocardial infarction have been described elsewhere.

Iliac thrombosis in the horse. The clinical signs in thrombosis of the iliac artery comprise two common syndromes, a mild and an acute form of ischaemia of a hind limb. In the mild form there is lameness only on exercise, the animal returning to normal after a short rest. If the horse is forced to work when lameness develops the signs may increase to resemble those of the acute form. The lameness takes the form of weakness, usually of one hind limb which tends to give way especially when the animal turns on it.

In the acute form there is great pain and anxiety and the pulse and respiration rates are markedly increased. Profuse sweating may be evident, but the affected limb is usually dry and may be cooler than the rest of the body. The amplitude of the pulse in the common digital artery may be less in the affected than in the normal limb, and the thickening and irregularity of the arterial wall are palpable on rectal examination. The pain is often sufficiently severe to cause the animal to go down and refuse to get up. Recovery by the development of a collateral circulation or shrinkage of the thrombus is unlikely to occur.

Pulmonary embolism. Severe dyspnoea develops suddenly and is accompanied by profuse sweating and anxiety. The temperature and pulse rate are elevated but the lungs are normal on auscultation. In horses the signs usually pass off gradually in 12 to 24 hours but in cattle the anoxia may be more severe and cause persistent blindness and imbecility.

Clinical Pathology

Extensive thrombus formation is usually associated with a leucocytosis and a shift to the left.

Necropsy Findings

Obstruction of the affected artery is easily seen when it is opened. The thrombus or embolus is adherent to the intima and is usually laminated. Local or diffuse ischaemia or infarction may be evident if the embolus has been present for some time and may have progressed to the point of abscess formation.

Diagnosis

Iliac thrombosis in its acute form may be confused with azoturia but the muscles of the thigh and rump are not hard, there is no myoglobinuria and usually no history of working after a period of rest on full rations. In the less acute form it resembles a number of non-specific lamenesses and enzootic incoordination of horses. The fact that it commonly affects only one limb may be of assistance in identifying the vascular lesion. Pulmonary embolism may be confused with pneumonia but the onset is more sudden, and with acute emphysema although this disease is accompanied by characteristic pulmonary signs.

Causes of arterial rupture other than verminous arteritis include a possibly inherited tendency to aneurysm of the abdominal aorta in cattle (5), and copper deficiency in pigs causing rupture of major blood vessels and the heart wall (7).

Although clinical atherosclerosis occurs rarely in farm animals, it has been recorded in a horse in which sufficient vascular obstruction occurred to cause severe central nervous signs and a fatal outcome (3). Spontaneous atherosclerosis is a common necropsy finding in swine, cattle and wild animals but its relationship to disease has not been established (8, 9, 10). Arteriosclerosis is a major necropsy finding in Manchester Wasting Disease.

Treatment

Treatment with parenteral anticoagulants or enzymes is carried out only rarely. There are several records of good results in iliac thrombosis in horses after the intravenous injection of sodium gluconate (4, 11). The use of antibiotics has merit if a bacterial arteritis or endocarditis is suspected.

REFERENCES

(1) Helmboldt, C. F. *et al.* (1959). *J. Amer. vet. med. Ass., 134,* 556.
(2) Wickware, A. B. (1944). *Canad. J. comp. Med., 8,* 303.
(3) Rothenbacher, H. J. & Tufts, S. (1964). *J. Amer. vet. med. Ass., 145,* 132.
(4) Tillotson, P. J. & Kopper, P. H. (1966). *J. Amer. vet. med. Ass., 149,* 766.
(5) Schuiringa-Sybesma, A. M. (1961). *T. Diergeneesk., 86,* 1192.
(6) Nolan, V. J. & Henigan, M. J. (1964). *Vet. Rec., 76,* 298.
(7) Anonymous, (1962). *N.Z. J. agric., 105,* 261.
(8) Skold, B. *et al.* (1966). *Amer. J. vet. Res., 27,* 257.
(9) French, J. E. *et al.* (1965). *Ann. N.Y. Acad. Sci., 127,* 780.
(10) McKinney, B. (1962). *Lancet, 2,* 281.
(11) Branscomb, B. L. (1968). *J. Amer. vet. med. Ass., 152,* 1643.
(12) Mouwen, J. M. V. M. (1967). *T. Diergeneesk., 92,* 1282.

Venous Thrombosis

The development of thrombi in veins may result in local obstruction to venous drainage or in liberation of emboli which lodge in the lungs, liver or other organs.

Phlebitis is the common origin of thrombi and may be caused by localization of a blood borne infection, by extension of infection from surrounding diseased tissues, by infection of the umbilical veins in the newborn, and by irritant injections into the major veins. Venous thrombi are relatively common in strangles in the horse, and may affect the jugular veins or the caudal vena cava. Thrombosis of the caudal vena cava is recorded in cows (1, 2). Clinically it may be manifested by hepatic abscess, ascites, proteinuria and a marked left shift in the haemogram. Less common examples of venous thrombosis are those occurring in the cerebral sinuses either by drainage of an infection from the face or those caused by the migration of parasite larvae. Purpling and later sloughing of the ears which occur in many septicaemias in pigs are also caused by phlebitis and venous thrombosis.

Engorgement of the vein, pain on palpation and local oedema are the important signs. In unsupported tissues rupture may occur and lead to fatal internal or external haemorrhage. There are no typical findings on clinico-pathological examination and at necropsy the obstructed vessel and thrombus are usually easily located by the situation of the oedema and local haemorrhage.

The diagnosis depends on the presence of signs of local venous obstruction in the absence of obvious external pressure by tumour, enlarged lymph nodes, haematomas or fibrous tissue constriction. Pressure of a foetus may cause oedema of the perineum, udder and ventral abdominal wall during late pregnancy. Local oedema due to infective processes such as blackleg, malignant oedema and peracute staphylococcal mastitis are accompanied by fever, severe toxaemia, acute local inflammation and necrosis.

Parenteral treatment with antibacterial drugs and surgical measures, such as hot fomentations to external veins, are usually instituted to remove the obstruction or allay the swelling.

REFERENCES

(1) Wagenaar, G. (1965). *T. Diergeneesk., 90,* 873.
(2) Stober, V. M. (1966). *Schweiz. Archiv. Tierheilk., 108,* 613.

Haemorrhagic Disease

Spontaneous haemorrhage or excessive bleeding after minor injury may result from increased capillary fragility or from defects in the coagulation mechanism of the blood. The latter would be more properly considered in the next chapter but for convenience it is dealt with here.

Defects in the vascular wall occur in purpura haemorrhagica and in septicaemia. In septicaemia (or viraemia) the haemorrhages are petechial or ecchymotic. In purpura haemorrhagica they may also occur as large extravasations into tissues. In all cases there is an increase in capillary permeability caused by endothelial damage which results from bacterial or viral infection, from allergy or from some forms of poisoning.

Purpura haemorrhagica is a common haemorrhagic disease and has an allergic basis. Bracken fern poisoning in cattle, poisoning caused by trichloroethylene-extracted soyabean meal and radiation injury are also manifested by spontaneous haemorrhage due to bacteraemia facilitated by severe leucopenia. In viral epizootic haemorrhagic disease of deer there are both degenerative changes in the vessel walls and a platelet deficiency (6).

In septicaemia, haemorrhages are only a manifestation of the primary disease and contribute little to its pathogenesis. In purpura haemorrhagica the haemorrhage and exudation of serum may cause severe anaemia and depression of the circulating blood volume. Haemorrhagic diseases may be confused with those in which there is a defect of the clotting mechanism and differentiation depends upon accurate measurements of the clotting and prothrombin times in the laboratory. Tests for the measurement of capillary fragility are not used in veterinary medicine.

Treatment other than that of the primary condition is largely empirical. Antihistamines are used when allergy appears to be an important mechanism but response is poor when the extravasations have already occurred. Adrenaline applied locally on a pad may be of assistance when bleeding occurs from the nostrils. Agents which enhance coagulability of the blood are extensively used when the clotting mechanism is at fault but effect little response when endothelial damage has occurred.

Coagulation defects occur as a result of a deficiency of platelets (thrombocytopenic purpura), a thromboplastin deficiency as in haemophilia (3, 4, 5), a deficiency of prothrombin as in coumarol poisoning or vitamin K deficiency, or of poisoning by biological anticoagulants such as snake venoms. Thrombocytopenic purpura is rarely diagnosed in farm animals but has been observed in newborn pigs, apparently due to maternal auto-immunization (1, 2, 7, 8). Piglets are normal at birth but become thrombocytopenic after sucking. There is a heavy mortality rate, death being preceded by a generalized development of submucosal and subcutaneous haemorrhages, drowsiness, weakness and pallor. The treatment of coagulation defects can only be effected rationally if the missing factor can be defined.

REFERENCES

(1) Stomorken, H. *et al.* (1963). *Nature, Lond.*, *198*, 1116.
(2) Saunders, C. N. *et al.* (1966). *Vet. Rec.*, *79*, 549.
(3) Archer, R. K. (1961). *Vet. Rec.*, *73*, 338.
(4) Hutchins, D. R. *et al.* (1967). *Aust. vet. J.*, *43*, 83.
(5) Sanger, V. L. *et al.* (1964). *J. Amer. vet. med. Ass.*, *144*, 259.
(6) Fletch, A. L. & Karstad, L. H. (1971). *Canad. J. comp. Med.*, *35*, 224.
(7) Lie, H. (1968). *Acta vet. scand.*, *9*, 285.
(8) Nansen, P. *et al.* (1970). *Nord. Vet.-Med.*, *22*, 1.

8

Diseases of the Blood and Blood-forming Organs

INTERFERENCE with the normal functions of the blood can occur in a number of ways. There may be a decrease in the circulating blood volume, abnormalities of the cellular constituents, and abnormalities of the non-cellular constituents including protein, electrolytes and the buffering systems. In all of these dysfunctions there is a failure of one or more of the transportation mechanisms of the blood and the tissues are deprived of their essential nutrients or are not relieved of their excretory products. Because of the multiplicity of the modes of dysfunction which can occur it is not possible to summarize the physiological basis and major manifestations of diseases of the blood and these aspects are dealt with in the discussion of the individual diseases.

Diseases Characterized by Abnormalities of Blood Fluids

DEHYDRATION

A disturbance of body water balance in which more fluid is lost from the body than is absorbed results in reduction in the circulating volume of the blood and in dehydration of tissues.

Aetiology

Dehydration occurs when there is deprivation of drinking water but the more common occurrence is when excessive fluid is lost. Diarrhoea is the most common cause although vomiting, polyuria, loss of fluid from extensive skin wounds or by copious sweating may be important in sporadic cases. Severe dehydration also occurs in acute ruminal impaction, acute intestinal obstruction and torsion of the abomasum. In most forms of dehydration, deprivation of drinking water being an exception, the serious loss, and the one that most needs repair, is not the fluid but the electrolytes.

The ability to survive for long periods without water in hot climates represents a form of animal adaptation which is of some economic importance. This adaptation has been examined in camels and in Merino sheep. In the latter the ability to survive

in these dry, arid conditions depends on a number of factors including insulation, the ability to carry water reserves in the rumen and extracellular fluid space, the ability to adjust electrolyte concentrations in the several fluid locations, the ability of the kidney to conserve water and the ability to maintain the circulation with a lower plasma volume (1).

Pathogenesis

There are two factors involved in the pathogenesis of dehydration, the depression of tissue fluid levels with resulting interference in tissue metabolism, and anhydraemia with reduction in the fluid content of the blood. The initial response to negative water balance is the withdrawal of fluid from the tissues and the maintenance of normal blood volume. The fluid is drained first from tissue spaces (extracellular fluid) and then from the cells (intracellular fluid). Essential organs including the central nervous system, heart and skeleton contribute little and the major loss occurs from connective tissue, muscle and skin. In the goat, total body water may be reduced as much as 44 per cent before death occurs (3).

The secondary response is a reduction in the fluid content of the blood causing reduction in circulating blood volume (oligaemia) and an increase in the concentration of the blood (haemoconcentration). Because of the haemoconcentration there is an increase in the viscosity of the blood which impedes blood flow and further exacerbates the peripheral circulatory failure.

Dehydration exerts some important effects on tissue metabolism. There is an increase in breakdown of fat, then carbohydrate and finally protein to produce water of metabolism. The increased endogenous metabolism under relatively anaerobic conditions results in the formation of acid metabolites and the development of acidosis. Urine formation decreases because of the restriction of blood flow and this, together with the increased endogenous metabolism, causes a moderate increase in blood levels of non-protein nitrogen. The body temperature rises slightly—dehydration hyperthermia—because of insufficient fluid to maintain the loss of heat by evaporation. The onset of sweating in steers after exposure to high environmental temperatures has been shown to be delayed by dehydration (2).

Dehydration may cause death especially in acute intestinal obstruction, vomiting and diarrhoea, but it is chiefly a contributory cause of death when combined with other systemic states, particularly toxaemia and septicaemia.

Clinical Findings

The first and most important sign in dehydration is dryness and wrinkling of the skin giving the body and face a shrunken appearance. The eyeballs recede into the sockets and the skin subsides slowly after being picked up into a fold. Loss of body weight occurs rapidly, there is muscular weakness, lack of appetite and increased thirst. Urine excretion decreases and the urine becomes progressively more concentrated. The respiratory rate increases due to acidosis, the temperature rises, the heart rate increases and the pulse has a small amplitude and low pressure. Terminally there is profound depression and coma. Investigations in the dog indicate that dry mouth, doughy skin and congestion of conjunctival vessels occur at about 5 per cent body weight loss due to dehydration, at 7 per cent loss there is reduced skin elasticity, dry sunken eyes, and high concentration, small volume urine (4) and beyond 10 to 12 per cent loss of body weight there is circulatory collapse and muscle tremor.

Clinical Pathology

On haematological examination there is polycythaemia, and an increase in specific gravity, haematocrit, plasma protein concentration and viscosity. There is a rise in plasma non-protein nitrogen and a decrease in carbon dioxide combining power.

Necropsy Findings

At necropsy there is a general appearance of dehydration of tissues but gross lesions are confined to those of the primary disease.

Diagnosis

There is usually little difficulty in determining that dehydration is present because of the obvious loss of fluid by vomiting, diarrhoea or in increased urine flow, and the characteristic clinical signs. The difficulty usually is to determine the degree of loss so that adequate treatment can be instituted in the early stages and optimum amounts of fluid provided.

Treatment

The rational treatment of dehydration comprises the administration of adequate quantities of isotonic fluids containing the appropriate electrolytes, particularly sodium, to ensure that the fluid is retained. Oral administration is as effective as parenteral administration provided that absorption is normal. Most cases of dehydration in large animals are caused by diseases of the alimentary tract and oral administration is unsatisfactory. The volumes of fluid required are usually sufficiently large to preclude subcutaneous injection as a method of administration and intravenous or intraperitoneal routes are usually used. The latter route has the advantage that the rate of flow is immaterial (5) but the risk of perforating a viscus or major blood vessel is sufficient deterrent to make this an uncommon technique. Care must be exercised in intravenous injection as too rapid a flow may cause cardiac embarrassment, especially if there is already some loss of cardiac reserve due to toxaemia, or some diminution of the pulmonary capillary bed. Provided isotonic solutions are used this seems to be a theoretical rather than a practical danger in cardiac disease but caution is necessary in cases of pneumonia and pulmonary oedema. It is a common practice to administer 4 litres of isotonic solution intravenously in 30 minutes to a cow and cardiac embarrassment rarely occurs. Hypertonic solutions appear to be more dangerous and their use should be avoided in dehydration, especially as they cause further dehydration of tissues by withdrawal of fluid into the circulation.

A number of preparations are routinely used to combat dehydration. An isotonic solution of sodium chloride (0·95 per cent) is adequate and is preferred to an isotonic solution of glucose (5·5 per cent) because of the rapid metabolism of glucose and the subsequent loss of the water. Physiologically more complete solutions are provided by lactate-Ringer solution (0·6 per cent sodium chloride, 0·27 per cent sodium lactate, 0·04 per cent potassium chloride and 0·02 per cent calcium chloride). Darrow's solution contains sodium bicarbonate instead of lactate but is difficult to prepare because the bicarbonate loses carbon dioxide on heating and the solution cannot be sterilized by boiling, although autoclaving is satisfactory. Both solutions satisfactorily combat acidosis, the lactate being metabolized to bicarbonate in the body. The use of potassium salts has the advantage that intracellular fluid is more readily restored, sodium being restricted in its distribution to extracellular sites. The intracellular fluid of all body tissues is the last to be lost in dehydration but is much larger in volume than extracellular and intravascular fluid volumes and is correspondingly more important. The use of a solution containing glucose has several advantages: it provides a source of energy when alimentary absorption is poor and it aids in the reversal of ketosis and thus reduces acidosis.

Solutions containing protein hydrolysates and glucose (usually 5 per cent of each) are an advantage if there is an accompanying toxaemia or fever of long duration but the preparations are usually too expensive to use routinely. Although it is important to attempt to provide fluids and electrolytes to replace those which are deficient it is usually not possible to determine the exact requirements, and the standard electrolyte solutions described above are usually used.

The dose rate of fluids administered to animals is in many instances too low for maximum efficiency. If dehydration is severe a minimum of 12 ml. of solution per lb. body weight per day should be given, preferably in three divided doses. In calves some suggested effective levels are available (6, 7) and in severe dehydration dose rates of the order of 50 ml. for lb. body weight seem necessary.

For the efficient management of patients with dehydration the amount and type of electrolyte solution administered should be determined by frequent monitoring of serum electrolyte, usually Na, and to a less extent, K, Cl. There is a need to be cautious in interpreting the results of clinico-pathological tests to determine 'hydration status'. The fluid electrolyte balance is always a dynamic one and at times of acute illness the movement of blood, fluid and electrolytes may be extreme and independent of each other. Thus serial observations are almost imperative, and the laboratory findings must be considered in the light of the clinical history and status of the patient.

REFERENCES

(1) Macfarlane, W. V. et al. (1961). Aust. J. agric. Res., 12, 889.
(2) Bianca, W. (1965). Res. vet. Sci., 6, 33, 38.
(3) Ohya, M. (1965). Jap. J. vet. Sci., 27, 41.
(4) Michell, A. R. (1967). Vet. Rec., 81, 2.
(5) Ketchell, R. J. et al. (1964). Canad. vet. J., 5, 199.
(6) Watt, J. G. (1967). J. Amer. vet. med. Ass., 150, 742.
(7) Radostits, O. M. (1965). J. Amer. vet. med. Ass., 147, 1367.

HAEMORRHAGE

The rapid loss of whole blood from the vascular system causes peripheral circulatory failure and anaemia.

Aetiology

Spontaneous rupture or traumatic injury to large blood vessels are the common causes of severe haemorrhage but rapid blood loss may occur by bleeding from the mucous surfaces or by massive infestation by blood-sucking nematodes. Severe haemorrhage can thus occur in coccidiosis and salmonellosis. An important occurrence of nasal haemorrhage is in horses while racing.

Extensive blood loss into tissues may also occur when there are defects of vessel walls or the clotting mechanism as described under the heading of haemorrhagic diseases. For example a congenital multiple defect in the coagulation mechanism has caused fatal haemorrhage in Holstein calves (4). Authentic cases of haemophilia (5, 6, 7) and one case of idiopathic hypoplastic anaemia (8) have been described in foals.

Pathogenesis

The major effects of haemorrhage are loss of blood volume, loss of plasma protein and loss of erythrocytes. If the rate of blood loss is rapid the loss of circulating blood volume results in peripheral circulatory failure and anaemic anoxia results from the loss of erythrocytes. The combination of these two factors is often fatal. If the rate of blood loss is less rapid the normal compensatory mechanisms, including evacuation of blood stored in the spleen and liver and the withdrawal of fluid from the tissue spaces may maintain a sufficient circulating blood volume but the anaemia is not relieved and the osmotic pressure of the blood is reduced by dilution of residual plasma protein. The resulting anaemia and oedema are repaired with time provided the blood loss is halted.

Clinical Findings

Pallor of the mucosae is the outstanding sign but there is in addition, weakness, staggering and recumbency, a rapid heart rate and a subnormal temperature. The respirations are deep but not dyspnoeic. There is listlessness and dullness and in fatal cases the animal dies in a coma in lateral recumbency.

Clinical Pathology

Examination of the blood for haemoglobin and haematocrit levels, and the erythrocyte count are of value in indicating the severity of the blood loss and provide an index to the progress of the disease. Estimation of clotting and prothrombin times should be undertaken in cases in which unexplained spontaneous haemorrhages occur.

Necropsy Findings

Extreme pallor of all tissues and a thin watery appearance of the blood may be accompanied by large extravasations of blood if the haemorrhage has been internal. Where the haemorrhage has been chronic anaemia and oedema are characteristic findings.

Diagnosis

Other forms of peripheral circulatory failure include shock and dehydration but they can usually be differentiated on history alone. Anaemia due to other causes is not accompanied by signs of peripheral circulatory failure.

Treatment

All elements of the blood should be replaced and in severe cases blood transfusion is the most satisfactory treatment (1, 2, 3, 9). In large animal practice donors are usually readily available and the need for storing blood does not arise.

Blood can be collected into an anticoagulant solution in an open-mouthed vessel. Venepuncture into the jugular vein is the method of choice, using a 12- or 14-gauge needle or a small diameter trocar and cannula. A choke-rope to increase the venous blood pressure facilitates collection in cattle. Bottles from which air has been evacuated reduce the collection time and avoid clotting in the needle, which usually occurs after about a litre has been collected by the open method. An excellent method is to use a milking machine to create a negative pressure in the flask which is fitted up so that the blood passes through the anticoagulant solution as it flows into the flask. In dairy cattle a gallon of blood can be collected in 10 to 15 minutes by this method. Sodium citrate (10 ml. of a 3·85 per cent solution to each 100 ml. of blood collected) is the standard anticoagulant used. There is usually little risk to the donor if it is in good health and 4 to 7 ml. of blood per lb. body weight can be drawn off at one time without danger.

Blood is usually administered intravenously but there are occasions when this is very difficult to do, especially in shocked or unco-operative animals, and intraperitoneal injections are then used. The only criticism of this method is that absorption is delayed. However, in dogs 48 per cent of the cells are absorbed in 24 hours, 65 per cent in 48 hours and 82 per cent in 1 to 2 weeks (10), but the erythrocytes are taken up by the blood stream in an unaltered state. From our own observations the absorption of erythrocytes from the bovine peritoneal cavity appears to be rapid and complete. The method has particular advantages for newborn calves and baby pigs with iso-immune haemolytic anaemia. It is used extensively in human infants and is considered to be safe and effective (11). Its use is contra-indicated when the animal is in a state of oligaemic shock, when intravenous transfusion is obligatory. It is not recommended in cases with ascites, peritonitis, abdominal distension, peritoneal adhesions, recent abdominal surgery or abdominal distension due to any cause

If the blood is properly mixed with anticoagulant during collection there is little need to filter it and the urgency in most cases precludes this. Clotted blood inevitably blocks the needle and the blood has to be discarded. Cross matching of bloods to determine compatibility is not often practised in animals other than the horse, although repeated transfusions from one donor may provoke anaphylactic shock. Even in horses an initial transfusion from any donor can be made without much risk (12) except in the special case of iso-immunization haemolytic anaemia. To avoid any possibility of producing an agglutination-haemolysis reaction a matching test should be carried out by mixing the serum of the recipient with the cells of the donor. Two drops of donor blood are mixed in 2 ml. of a 3·85 per cent citrate solution and 2 drops of the mixture are added to 2 drops of the recipient's serum on a glass slide, which is then gently rocked. Agglutination between incompatible samples is readily seen. A reasonably satisfactory alternative is to inject a small amount of blood (200 ml. in an adult cow) and wait for 10 minutes. If no transfusion reaction occurs, the remainder of the blood can then be injected without risk. In an emergency interspecies transfusion may be used but is limited in value because of the poor longevity of the transfused erythrocytes particularly when the horse is used as a donor. Transfusion reactions are unlikely except with horse blood transfused into other species (13). In cattle the incidence of transfusion reactions is greatest in young animals (14 per cent incidence but sufficiently severe to require treatment in only 6 per cent) and in pregnant cattle (41 per cent incidence with a high proportion of cows aborting within 8 days). There is no individual blood group factor in cattle which is more important than others in transfusion reaction (17).

Anaphylactic reactions occur more commonly and are more severe when repeated transfusions from one donor are given more than a week after the initial transfusion (14). Sensitization to the blood of a particular donor may persist for more than a year. At the third transfusion almost 50 per cent of cattle will show a moderate to severe reaction. Signs may appear while the transfusion is in progress or within a few minutes afterwards. Hiccough usually occurs first, followed by dyspnoea, muscle tremor, salivation, frequent coughing, lacrimation, fever (40 to 40·5°C or 104 to 105°F) and in some cases ruminal tympany. Haemoglobinuria and abortion may also occur. The illness is usually mild and responds within a few minutes to the administration of adrenaline hydrochloride (4 to 5 ml. of 1:1,000 solution injected intramuscularly or 0·2 to 0·5 ml. intravenously in large animals). Intramuscular injection is safest and produces an effect within 3 to 4 minutes. Necropsy findings in animals dying of transfusion reaction are similar to those seen in acute anaphylaxis and include pulmonary oedema and subserosal petechiation.

A third reaction to transfusion, the pyrogenic reaction, occurs in man and in small animals but has not been recorded in farm animals. Administration of the blood at too rapid a rate may cause overloading of the circulation and acute heart failure. This is most likely to occur if blood is administered when there is myocardial asthenia due to toxaemia. The heart rate increases rapidly and weakness and dyspnoea precede collapse. A gallon (4·5 litres) of blood usually requires an hour to administer to a cow and comparable rates in the smaller species are advisable. Four to 7 ml. of blood per lb. body weight is an average figure worth remembering but in severe cases it is probably better to continue transfusion until improvement is apparent. In the event of cardiac failure during transfusion the blood flow should be stopped immediately and atropine administered.

The most common causes of failure in treatment by blood transfusion are failure to administer sufficient blood, and the irreversible changes which may have occurred in the patient before treatment commences. Citrate poisoning has also been blamed as a cause of failure in humans (8), the citrate causing constriction of the pulmonary capillary bed and myocardial embarrassment. The administration of 10 ml. of 10 per cent calcium gluconate at the beginning of the transfusion and after each 100 ml. of blood has been recommended to overcome this difficulty but the importance of this precaution in animals is unknown.

Alternatives to blood transfusion include the infusion of blood plasma, or plasma extenders such as acacia (6 per cent solution in 0·9 per cent saline), gelatin (6 per cent solution of special gelatin of known molecular size and capable of being retained in the circulation, in a solution of 0·85 per cent saline) or dextran, a neutral polysaccharide. These preparations find little place in large animal work because of the ready availability of whole blood and the possible toxicity of dextran in the horse (15). Intravenous injections of those fluids used in the treatment of dehydration have some value in that they help to restore the circulating blood volume but the important deficit of haemoglobin is not made good.

Cardiac stimulants are of no value because the efficiency of the heart is unimpaired. Vasoconstrictor drugs should not be used as they tend to further aggravate the existing anoxia. Parenterally administered coagulants have found favour in recent years and many proprietary preparations are available. Their value is open to doubt (16) but they are in general use because in most cases the situation is sufficiently serious to encourage the use of all available forms of treatment.

REFERENCES

(1) Ferguson, L. C. (1947). *J. Amer. vet. med. Ass., 111,* 466.
(2) Metcalf, F. L. & Stahl, W. E. (1942). *J. Amer. vet. med. Ass., 101,* 265.
(3) Williams, R. E. (1947). *Vet. Rec., 59,* 637.
(4) Bentinck-Smith J. *et al.* (1960). *Cornell Vet., 50,* 15.
(5) Archer, R. K. (1961). *Vet. Rec., 73,* 338.
(6) Hutchins, D. R. *et al.* (1967). *Aust. vet. J., 43,* 83.
(7) Sanger, V. L. *et al.* (1964). *J. Amer. vet. med. Ass., 144,* 259.
(8) Firt, P. & Hejhal, L. (1957). *Lancet, 273,* 1132.
(9) Holmes, J. W. H. (1949). *Vet. Rec., 61,* 551.
(10) Clark, C. H. & Woodley, C. H. (1959). *Amer. J. vet. Res., 20,* 1062.
(11) Scopes, J. W. (1963). *Lancet, 1,* 1027.
(12) Ferguson, L. C. (1955). The Blood Groups of Animals. In *Advances in Veterinary Science,* Vol. 2, pp. 106–137. New York: Academic Press.
(13) Clark, C. H. & Kiesel, G. K. (1963). *J. Amer. vet. med. Ass., 143,* 400.
(14) Humble, R. J. (1957). *Canad. J. comp. Med., 21,* 296.
(15) Archer, R. K. & Franks, D. (1961). *Vet. Rec., 73,* 657.
(16) Archer, R. K. (1957). *Vet. Rec., 69,* 56.
(17) Walt, K. V. D. & Osterhoff, D. R. (1969). *J. S. Afr. vet. med. Ass., 40,* 107.

SHOCK

Secondary or surgical shock occurs some hours after trauma and is manifested by peripheral circulatory failure without evidence of fluid or blood loss.

Aetiology

Shock follows severe injury to tissues caused by accidental trauma, surgery, especially when the abdominal viscera are roughly handled, and occurs also after prolapse of the uterus, and when large quantities of fluid are released from body cavities. Acute infections including particularly septicaemias and peritonitis may have a similar effect.

Pathogenesis

Although there need be no actual blood loss there is an appreciable fall in circulating blood volume (CBV) and peripheral circulatory failure is manifested. The reason for this depression of CBV is the subject of many hypotheses. Exhaustion of adrenal cortical activity, liberation of histamine from damaged tissues resulting in peripheral vasodilatation, and overstimulation of the adrenal-sympathetic system have all been advanced as causes of traumatic shock but complete evidence is lacking to support any of them as other than contributory factors. The current view is that sufficient fluid is lost from the circulation into the tissue spaces of the damaged part to account for the peripheral circulatory failure that occurs. One of the salient features of shock is the short period during which it is reversible. This is in contrast to peripheral circulatory failure caused by haemorrhage which is reversible by transfusion for long periods and until anoxic damage to capillaries causes irreversible continuing loss of plasma.

Clinical Findings

Coldness of the skin, a subnormal temperature, rapid, shallow breathing, and a rapid heart rate accompanied by a weak pulse of small amplitude and low pressures are characteristic of shock. Venous blood pressure is greatly reduced and the veins are difficult to raise. The mucosae are pale but not to the severe degree of blanching observed in haemorrhage. The animal is dull, weak, often recumbent and if the condition is fatal, dies in a coma.

Clinical Pathology

Measurement of the CBV is possible by the use of dyes or radioactive substances but the techniques are unlikely to be used in clinical practice. Haemoconcentration may or may not occur depending on whether the fluid loss is in the form of plasma or whole blood, but measurement of the haematocrit may be of value in individual cases to determine the progress of the disease. A high eosinophil count may suggest that adrenal cortical dysfunction has occurred and that treatment with adrenocorticotropic hormones or adrenal corticosteroids may be necessary.

Necropsy Findings

There may be evidence of trauma and the capillaries and small vessels of the splanchnic area may be congested.

Diagnosis

Shock is usually anticipated when severe trauma occurs, and is diagnosed when peripheral circulatory failure is present without evidence of haemorrhage or dehydration.

Treatment

The primary aim in the treatment of shock is to restore the circulating blood volume, preferably by blood transfusion although the use of plasma or plasma expanders is of much greater value than in severe blood loss. The use of peripheral vasoconstrictors is also of value to increase the effective blood volume. Pitressin is preferred to adrenaline for this purpose because of the transience of the reaction with the latter drug. Although the animal should be kept warm, overheating should be avoided because it causes peripheral vasodilatation and a further decrease in circulating blood volume.

The important principle in shock is to anticipate its occurrence and treat the animal prophylactically before the irreversible stage is reached. Blood transfusions and the administration of pitressin can, in many cases, prevent the irreversible anoxic damage to capillaries. Even when this has occurred there may still be a transient response but the animal soon reverts to its prior state of peripheral circulatory failure.

WATER INTOXICATION

The ingestion of excessive quantities of water when animals are very thirsty may result in water intoxication, especially if there has been much loss of salt due to severe exercise or high environmental temperatures (1). Experimentally the condition is difficult to reproduce unless the antidiuretic principle of the pituitary gland is administered, since the normal excretory mechanisms remove the bulk of the administered fluid. Under field conditions calves are most commonly affected (2, 3).

Cellular hydration occurs and in organized tissues the cells increase in turgor. This is particularly noticeable in the brain where a condition analogous to cerebral oedema occurs and causes nervous signs including muscle weakness and tremor, restlessness, ataxia, tonic and clonic convulsions and terminal coma. In unorganized tissues, particularly the erythrocytes, lysis occurs and the resulting haemolysis may cause severe haemolytic anaemia and haemoglobinuria. Additional signs include hypothermia and salivation.

Water intoxication does not occur commonly and can be avoided by allowing thirsty animals to have limited access to water. Treatment of affected animals should include sedation, the administration of diuretics and in severe cases the intravenous injection of hypertonic solutions.

REFERENCES

(1) Lawrence, J. A. (1965). *J. S. Afr. vet. med. Ass.*, 36, 277.
(2) Hannan, J. (1965). *Irish vet. J.*, 19, 211.
(3) Kirkbride, C. A. & Frey, R. A. (1967). *J. Amer. vet. med. Ass.*, 151, 742.

OEDEMA

Oedema is the excessive accumulation of fluid in tissue spaces caused by a disturbance in the mechanism of fluid interchange between capillaries, the tissue spaces and the lymphatic vessels.

Aetiology

Oedema results mainly from an increase in hydrostatic pressure in the capillaries, from a fall in osmotic pressure of the blood, from obstruction to lymphatic drainage or from damage to capillary walls. Increased hydrostatic pressure occurs mainly as a result of congestive heart failure but it may also occur in more limited regions such as in the portal circuit when there is hepatic fibrosis. Oedema of the udder and ventral abdominal wall occurs commonly in late pregnancy in cows and to a less extent in mares and is caused largely by foetal compression of venous drainage, although hypoproteinaemia is also thought to play a part in this form of oedema.

Decreased plasma osmotic pressure is caused in most instances by a reduction in the concentration of plasma protein. Continuous haemorrhage, especially in heavy parasitic infestations, often leads to oedema, not because of the loss of erythrocytes, but because of the loss of plasma protein. Continued loss of protein may also occur in renal disease but nephritic oedema rarely occurs in animals. Another cause of serious plasma protein loss is protein-losing enteropathy, sometimes associated with enterocolitis (2), sometimes not. Liver damage causes failure of synthesis of plasma proteins and the hepatic fibrosis of congestive heart failure may contribute to the development of oedema in this condition. Malnutrition may also be a factor. Animals on rations which are low in protein commonly develop anasarca because of hypoproteinaemia. This is most likely to occur in cattle and sheep at range during periods of prolonged drought although it has occurred in ruminants in feedlots. The occurrence of anasarca in cattle on vitamin A deficient diets has also been recorded. Oedema of newborn pigs is also thought to be caused by protein deprivation resulting from inadequate nutrition of the sow (1).

Obstruction of lymphatic flow plays a part in the production of most local oedemas caused by tumours and inflammatory swellings. Congenital lymphatic obstruction of calves and pigs and sporadic lymphangitis of horses are typical examples of obstructive oedema. Allergic oedema, manifested by urticaria, angioneurotic oedema and purpura haemorrhagica occur as a result of capillary dilation and damage caused by the local or general liberation of histamine. Fog fever probably has a similar basis. Damage to small vessels by toxins or infectious agents may also result in oedema. The oedema of septicaemic pasteurellosis of cattle, anthrax, blackleg, malignant oedema, gut oedema and mulberry heart disease of pigs and of infectious equine rhinopneumonitis, equine viral arteritis and infectious equine anaemia originates in this way.

Pathogenesis

At the arterial end of the capillaries the hydrostatic pressure of the blood is sufficient to overcome its osmotic pressure and fluid tends to pass into the tissue spaces. At the venous end of the capillaries the position is reversed and fluid tends to return to the vascular system. The pressure differences are not great and a small increase in hydrostatic pressure or decrease in osmotic pressure leads to failure of the fluid to return to the capillaries. The resulting accumulation of fluid in the tissue spaces, or by escape into serous cavities, constitutes oedema.

Clinical Findings

Accumulations of oedematous transudate in subcutaneous tissues are referred to as anasarca, in the peritoneal cavity as ascites, in the pleural cavities as hydrothorax and in the pericardial sac as hydropericardium. Anasarca in large animals is usually confined to the ventral wall of the abdomen and thorax, the brisket and, if the animal is grazing, the intermandibular space. Intermandibular oedema may be less evident in animals which do not have to lower their heads to graze. Oedema of the limbs is uncommon in cattle, sheep and pigs but occurs in horses quite commonly when the venous return is obstructed or there is a lack of muscular movement.

Oedematous swellings are soft, painless and pit on pressure. In ascites there is distension of the abdomen and the fluid can be detected by a fluid thrill on tactile percussion, fluid sounds on succussion and by paracentesis. A level top line of fluid may be detectable by any of these means. In the pleural cavities and pericardial sac the clinical signs produced by the fluid accumulation include restriction of cardiac movements, embarrassment of respiration and collapse of the ventral parts of the lungs. The heart sounds and respiratory sounds are muffled and the presence of fluid may be ascertained by percussion, succussion and paracentesis.

More localized oedemas cause more localized signs; pulmonary oedema is accompanied by respiratory distress, moist r

âles and in some cases by an out-pouring of froth from the nose; cerebral oedema is manifested by severe nervous signs. A not uncommon entity is a large oedematous plaque around the umbilicus in yearling horses. The plaque develops rapidly, causes no apparent illness and subsides spontaneously after about 7 days.

Clinical Pathology

Examination of a sample of fluid reveals an absence of signs of inflammation. In some instances the transudate is free of protein but in advanced cases much protein may be present because of the capillary damage which has occurred. The fluid may clot, have a high specific gravity and even contain free blood, particularly if the oedema is caused by increased hydrostatic pressure.

Necropsy Findings

The cause of the accumulation of fluid is obvious in many cases but estimations of the concentration of protein in the plasma may be necessary if hypoproteinaemia is thought to be the cause. If the primary cause is endothelial damage this will probably be detectable only on histological examination.

Diagnosis

Differentiation of the specific causes of oedema listed in aetiology above depends upon identification of the primary disease. Subcutaneous and peritoneal accumulations of urine occur when the urethra or bladder ruptures after urethral obstruction by calculi. Peritonitis, pleurisy and pericarditis are also characterized by local accumulations of fluid but toxaemia and other signs of inflammation are usually present.

Treatment

The treatment of oedema should be aimed at correcting the primary disease. Myocardial asthenia should be relieved by the use of digitalis, pericarditis by drainage of the sac, and hypoproteinaemia by the administration of plasma or plasma substitutes and the feeding of high quality protein. Ancillary measures include restriction of water intake and the amount of salt in the diet, the use of diuretics and aspiration of fluid. Diuretics may relieve the effects of pressure temporarily but are of little value if the transudate has a high content of protein. Aspiration of fluid must be carried out slowly to avoid acute dilatation of splanchnic vessels and subsequent peripheral circulatory failure. The technique usually gives only temporary relief because the fluid rapidly accumulates again causing further withdrawal of fluids from tissues.

REFERENCES

(1) Edwards, B. L. (1961). *Vet. Rec.*, *73*, 540.
(2) Nansen, P. & Nielsen, K. (1967). *Nord. Vet.-Med.*, *19*, 524.

Diseases Characterized by Abnormalities of the Cellular Elements of the Blood

ANAEMIA

Anaemia is defined as a deficiency of erythrocytes, or haemoglobin, per unit volume of blood. It is manifested by pallor of the mucosae, an increase in the rate and force of the heart beat and by muscle weakness. Dyspnoea at rest is not a common sign, a feature which helps to distinguish it from uncompensated heart failure.

Aetiology

Anaemia may be caused by excessive loss of blood by haemorrhage, or by increased destruction or the inefficient production of erythrocytes. Anaemias are therefore usually classified as haemorrhagic or haemolytic anaemia, or anaemia due to decreased production of erythrocytes.

Haemorrhagic anaemia may occur after acute haemorrhage or with chronic blood loss as it occurs in parasitism, particularly haemonchosis in ruminants (1) and strongylosis in horses (2). Enzootic haematuria, coccidiosis and poisoning by sweet clover, Warfarin and bracken fern are less common causes in cattle. Heavy infestation with ticks (3) and sucking lice may also cause an appreciable anaemia. Sporadic cases occur due to ulceration in the alimentary tract, particularly in cases of abomasal ulcer in cattle and gastric haemorrhage in swine. Multiple defects of coagulation, causing a severe bleeding tendency, have been observed in newborn Holstein calves which bleed excessively from the navel, nostrils and into the abdominal cavity soon after birth (6). The cause is unknown and the disease closely resembles sweet clover poisoning of newborn calves.

Haemolytic anaemia is a manifestation of many infectious and non-infectious diseases. Protozoan diseases in which haemolytic anaemia occurs include babesiasis which occurs in all species, anaplasmosis of ruminants and eperythrozoonosis of swine and ruminants. In cattle other common causes are leptospirosis, bacillary haemoglobin-uria, poisoning by onions or by rape and other cruciferous plants and postparturient haemo-globinuria. Calves which drink large quantities of cold water may also suffer an acute haemolytic epi-sode and this may also occur as part of a transfusion reaction. In horses equine infectious anaemia, phenothiazine poisoning and iso-immunization haemolytic anaemia of foals are the common causes. Although uncommon, haemolytic disease of the newborn occurs also in pigs and cattle. Chronic copper poisoning in sheep causes severe haemolytic anaemia and is a major factor in the production of the clinical signs of toxaemic jaun-dice in this species. The same effect may be pro-duced in cattle. Sheep are also susceptible to the haemolytic agent which is present in rape and other cruciferous plants. Haemolytic anaemia is rare in pigs but occurs in eperythrozoonosis. An acute haemolytic anaemia has been observed in associa-tion with acute pneumonia in beef calves housed in barns during the winter months. The cause is un-known and although multiple petechiae are present at necropsy, no specific bacterial agent has been identified. An acute haemolytic anaemia has also been recorded in association with primary atypical pneumonia in humans (4) and there may be some association between the two conditions. Some snake venoms also cause acute intravascular haemolysis.

Anaemia due to decreased production of erythro-cytes or haemoglobin. These comprise the bulk of the naturally occurring anaemias of animals and are due in most cases to nutritional deficiency, although toxic depression of the erythropoietic activity of bone marrow may also be a cause. Nutritional deficiencies of cobalt and copper cause anaemia in ruminants and although these elements are probably necessary for erythropoiesis in other species, the requirement of them does not seem to be so great and clinical anaemia does not occur under natural conditions. A deficiency of iron in the diet causes anaemia in piglets but under natural conditions does not appear to be of major impor-tance in the other species. Anaemia in racing horses attracts a good deal of interest and many deficiency diseases are postulated. One with some supporting data is the possible response of stabled horses, particularly pregnant mares who have no access to grass, to folic acid administration (10). A sudden change to a high altitude may be followed by a degree of anaemia lasting several weeks (13).

Chronic suppurative processes often cause marked depression of the activity of bone marrow and result in severe anaemia. Radiation disease is accompanied by depression of all erythropoietic and leucopoietic function. Poisoning by bracken fern, trichloroethylene-extracted soyabean meal and arsenic may also cause aplastic anaemia. An idiopathic hypoplastic anaemia has been described in a foal (8).

Myelophthisic anaemias, in which the bone marrow cavities are occupied by other, usually neo-plastic, tissues, are rare in farm animals. Plasma cell myelomatosis has been observed as a cause of such anaemia in pigs, calves and a horse (7). Clinical signs, other than of the anaemia, which is macro-cytic and normochromic, include skeletal pain, pathological fractures and paresis due to the osteolytic lesions produced by the invading neo-plasm. Cavitation of the bone may be detected on roentgenological examination.

Pathogenesis

Irrespective of the cause of anaemia the primary abnormality of function is the anaemic anoxia which follows. In acute haemorrhagic anaemia there is in addition a loss of circulating blood volume and plasma proteins. The fluid loss is quickly repaired by equilibration with tissue fluids and by absorption and, provided haemorrhage does not continue, the plasma proteins are quickly re-stored to normal by synthesis in the liver. However erythropoiesis requires a longer time interval to alleviate the anaemia. Haemolytic anaemia is often sufficiently severe to cause haemoglobinuria and may result in haemoglobinuric nephrosis and de-pression of renal function. Aplastic anaemia caused by toxins from a suppurative process is a secondary manifestation and is relieved by removal of the cause, and anaemia due to nutritional deficiency is similarly reversible.

The primary responses to tissue anoxia caused by anaemia are an increase in cardiac output due to increases in stroke volume and heart rate, and a decrease in circulation time. A diversion of blood from the peripheral to the splanchnic circulation also occurs. In the terminal stages when the tissue anoxia is sufficiently severe there may be a moder-ate increase in respiratory activity. Provided the activity of the bone marrow is not reduced ery-thropoiesis is stimulated by lowering of the tissue oxygen tension.

Clinical Findings

Pallor of the mucosae is the outstanding clinical sign but appreciable degrees of anaemia can occur without clinically visible change in mucosal or skin colour. These degrees of anaemia are usually not sufficient to cause signs of illness but they may interfere with performance, particularly in race-horses, and this aspect of equine medicine has come into prominence in recent years (5). Many horses suffer from moderate anaemia, due probably in most cases to strongylosis, and respond spectacularly to treatment with haematinic drugs.

In clinical cases of anaemia there are signs of pallor, muscular weakness, depression and anorexia. The heart rate is increased, the pulse has a large amplitude and the absolute intensity of the heart sounds is markedly increased. Terminally the moderate tachycardia of the compensatory phase is replaced by a severe tachycardia, a decrease in the intensity of the heart sounds and a weak pulse. The initial increase in intensity of heart sounds is caused by cardiac dilatation and an increase in blood pressure. If the dilatation is sufficiently severe the atrioventricular orifices become dilated causing relative insufficiency of the valves and a haemic systolic murmur which waxes and wanes with each respiratory cycle, reaching its maximum at the peak of inspiration. This type of murmur is not pathognomonic of anaemia and may be present in any form of myocardial asthenia or when the viscosity of the blood is reduced for any other reason.

Dyspnoea is not pronounced in anaemia, the most severe degree of respiratory distress appearing as an increase in depth of respiration without much increase in rate. Laboured breathing occurs only in the terminal stages. Additional signs which often accompany anaemia but are not essential parts of the syndrome are oedema, jaundice and haemoglobinuria. Cyanosis does not occur because of the relative deficiency of haemoglobin.

Clinical Pathology

Clinical signs do not appear until the haemoglobin level of the blood falls below about 50 per cent of normal. The erythrocyte count and the haematocrit are usually depressed. In haemorrhagic and haemolytic anaemias there is an increase in the number of immature red cells in the blood. The characteristic finding in anaemia caused by a deficiency of iron is hypochromasia caused by a reduction in mean corpuscular haemoglobin concentration; the haemoglobin level is low but the erythrocyte count may be normal.

Necropsy Findings

Necropsy findings include those specific to the primary cause. Findings indicative of anaemia include pallor of tissues, thin, watery blood and contraction of the spleen. Centrilobular hepatic necrosis is commonly present in cattle, and probably in other animals, if the anaemia has existed for some time (9).

Diagnosis

A diagnosis of anaemia is usually suggested by the obvious clinical signs. Differentiation between haemorrhagic and haemolytic anaemias and those caused by deficient production of erythrocytes or haemoglobin depends upon the history of haemorrhage, haemoglobinuria, jaundice, or diet, and upon clinical evidence of these signs. The clinico-pathological findings may also suggest the origin of the anaemia. Haemorrhagic and haemolytic anaemias are manifested by the presence of immature erythrocytes in the blood; deficiency anaemias by hypochromasia; and aplastic anaemia caused by toxins is manifested by low erythrocyte counts without evidence of regeneration. These generalizations are often not of much assistance in urgent situations where an animal is seriously ill, as so often happens with anaemia, or a number are affected. More accurate methods of determining the classification of the anaemia would be an advantage. The estimation of haptoglobins as a measure of haemolysis (11) and the measurement of lactic dehydrogenase, cholinesterase and protein profiles (12) are of assistance in this respect.

Treatment

Treatment of the primary cause of the anaemia is essential. Non-specific treatment includes blood transfusion in acute haemorrhage and even in chronic anaemia of severe degree. Haematinic preparations are used in less severe cases and as supportive treatment after transfusion. Iron administered by mouth or parenterally is in common use. Preparations injected intravenously give a rapid response and intramuscular injections of organic-iron preparations give less rapid but more prolonged results. Vitamin B_{12} is widely used as a non-specific haematinic, particularly in horses. In extreme cases of anaemia irreversible changes caused by anoxia of kidneys and heart muscle may prevent complete recovery in spite of adequate treatment.

REFERENCES

(1) Shumard, R. F. et al. (1957). Amer. J. vet. Res., 18, 330.
(2) Archer, R. K. & Poynter, D. (1957). J. comp. Path., 67, 196.
(3) Riek, R. F. (1957). Aust. J. agric. Res., 8, 209.
(4) Stewart, J. W. & Friedlander, P. H. (1957). Lancet, 273, 774.
(5) Brenon, H. C. (1956). J. Amer. vet. med. Ass., 128, 343.
(6) Bentinck-Smith, J. et al. (1960). Cornell Vet., 50, 15.
(7) Cornelius, C. E. et al. (1959). Cornell Vet., 49, 478.
(8) Archer, R. K. & Miller, W. C. (1965). Vet. Rec., 77, 538.

(9) Urbaneck, D. & Rossow, N. (1962). *Mh. Vet.-Med.*, *17*, 941.
(10) Seekington, I. M. *et al.* (1967). *Vet. Rec.*, *81*, 158.
(11) Allen, B. & Archer, R. K. (1971). *Vet. Rec.*, *89*, 106.
(12) Osbaldiston, G. W. *et al.* (1970). *J. Amer. vet. med. Ass.*, *157*, 322.
(13) Collins, J. D. *et al.* (1969). *Irish. vet. J.*, *23*, 42.

LEUKAEMIA

Leukaemia is manifested by abnormal proliferation of myelogenous or lymphatic tissues causing a marked increase in the number of circulating leucocytes. The disease is probably neoplastic in origin and is usually accompanied by enlargement of the spleen, lymph nodes and bone marrow, singly or in combination. There is sufficient evidence that some leukaemias are transmissible by means of viruses to suggest that some of those which occur commonly in livestock have a similar cause. There is as yet no concrete evidence that this is so.

In leukaemic leukaemia immature leucocytes appear in the blood, in aleukaemic leukaemia the total leucocyte count may or may not be increased. In leukaemia the differential leucocyte count may be distorted, a preponderance of immature granulocytes occurring in myelogenous leukaemia and a relative increase in lymphocytes occurring in lymphatic leukaemia. There may be an accompanying aplastic anaemia if erythropoiesis is depressed by expansion of myeloid tissue in the bone marrow—a myelophthisic anaemia. Examination of smears of bone marrow has become commonplace in cases of leukaemia in large animals. Samples of bone marrow contents are easily obtained from the sternum of animals in the standing position. In the horse specimens can be readily obtained from the ilium, entrance being made through the tuber coxae (1). Bone marrow biopsy techniques have also been described for cows (3, 4) and goats (5).

In farm animals the only common form of leukaemia is lymphomatosis. Myelogenous leukaemia is rare but has been recorded in all species. Erythroblastic and plasma cell tumours and monocytic leukaemia are still less frequent. Information on haemopoietic tissue tumours has been reviewed recently (2) and is not recapitulated here. When the leukaemia is leukaemic there is usually no difficulty in making a diagnosis because of the very high total white cell count, the distortion of the differential count, and the presence of immature cells. Most cases of lymphomatosis in farm animals are subleukaemic, at least when the disease is clinically recognizable, and the differentiation from lymphadenitis may be difficult. In lymphadenitis enlargement of the nodes usually occurs rapidly and asymmetrically and the enlargement may fluctuate or completely regress.

The leucocytosis associated with local or generalized infections is usually less severe in degree than that of leukaemic leukaemia and the distortion of the differential count is not so marked, following a standard pattern. There is a neutrophilia with a relative increase in band forms in acute generalized or local inflammatory processes, and a lymphocytosis or monocytosis in chronic suppurative infections.

A number of leucopenia-producing drugs, including nitrogen and sulphur mustards, urethane and antifolic acid compounds have been used in the treatment of leukaemia in human and small animal practice but the poor results obtained do not justify their use in farm animals.

REFERENCES

(1) Archer, R. K. (1964). *Vet. Rec.*, *76*, 465.
(2) Squire, R. A. (1964). *Cornell Vet.*, *54*, 97.
(3) Lawrence, W. C. *et al.* (1962). *Cornell Vet.*, *52*, 297.
(4) Wilde, J. K. H. (1961). *Res. vet. Sci.*, *2*, 315.
(5) Wilkins, J. H. (1961). *Vet. Rec.*, *74*, 244.

LEUCOPENIA

Leucopenia does not occur as a specific disease entity but is a common manifestation of a number of diseases. Virus diseases, particularly hog cholera, are frequently accompanied by a panleucopenia in the early acute stages. Leucopenia has also been observed in leptospirosis in cattle although bacterial infections are usually accompanied by a leucocytosis. Acute local inflammations may cause a transient fall in the leucocyte count because of withdrawal of the circulating cells to the septic focus.

Leucopenia may also occur as part of a pancytopenia in which all cellular elements of the blood are depressed. Agents which depress the activity of the bone marrow, spleen and lymph nodes and result in pancytopenia occur in trichloroethylene-extracted soya bean meal and bracken fern. Pancytopenia occurs also in radiation disease. Chronic arsenical poisoning, and poisoning by sulphonamides, chlorpromazine and chloramphenicol cause similar blood dyscrasias in man but do not appear to have this effect in animals.

The importance of leucopenia is that it reduces the resistance of the animal to bacterial infection and may be followed by a highly fatal, fulminating septicaemia. Treatment of the condition should include the administration of broad spectrum antibiotics to prevent bacterial invasion. Drugs, including pentnucleotide, which have been used to stimulate leucopoietic activity, have not been shown to materially affect most leucopenias.

Diseases Characterized by Abnormalities of Blood Chemistry

ABNORMALITIES OF ACID–BASE BALANCE

The pH of the blood is maintained at the normal level of 7·4 by its buffer systems, of which the bicarbonate system is most important. The addition of relatively large amounts of acid or alkali to the blood is necessary before its buffering capacity is exhausted and its pH changed. The proportions of the dissolved carbon dioxide and the bicarbonate ion, which form the components of the buffer system, are maintained at a constant level by either increased pulmonary ventilation and discharge of carbon dioxide, or by increased urinary excretion of the bicarbonate radical.

Changes from normal acid–base balance, towards either alkalosis or acidosis, make significant contributions to ill-health and to clinical signs observed. Some information on acid–base balance is available for horses (1) and for cattle (2).

Acidosis

In acidosis there is a tendency for the pH of the blood to change towards acidity but clinical signs can occur without detectable change of pH. The alkali reserve (bicarbonate) of the blood may be reduced in severe diarrhoea, or in persistent vomiting in which regurgitation of alkaline intestinal secretion occurs. Metabolic acidosis is understandably a very significant factor contributing to the clinical syndrome in enteric colibacillosis in calves and in acute intestinal obstruction in the horse. It has also been linked with the convulsive respiratory distress 'neonatal maladjustment syndrome' of foals (3). An increased excretion of base in the urine may also occur when fixed acids are absorbed from the alimentary tract. This may occur when acid-producing salts are fed or when ruminants ingest excessive amounts of grain. Ketosis may also result in a depletion of plasma bicarbonate. Acidosis also occurs when there is retention of carbon dioxide in the blood due to interference with normal respiratory exchange. Thus pneumonia, severe pulmonary emphysema, depression of the respiratory centre and congestive heart failure may all be accompanied by acidosis.

The clinically observable effects of acidosis are related chiefly to the respiratory system. The increased carbon dioxide tension of the blood and depletion of alkali reserve cause an increase in the depth and rate of respiration by stimulation of the respiratory centre. Hyperpnoea and dyspnoea appear when the alkali reserve is diminished to about 50 per cent of normal. The increased urinary excretion of fixed acids causes polyuria which may be sufficiently severe to cause dehydration. Anorexia, weakness, lassitude and terminal coma are other clinical signs. Vomiting may occur in pigs.

Treatment is directed towards replacement of the lost base and is usually effected by the oral administration of sodium bicarbonate in doses of 4 g. for sheep and 15 to 30 g. for large animals. It is often necessary to replace fluids at the same time and it is common practice to give intravenous injections of electrolyte solutions containing sodium bicarbonate or sodium lactate such as those recommended for the treatment of dehydration (p. 149).

Alkalosis

Alkalosis can be caused by an increased absorption of alkali, excessive loss of acid or a deficit of carbon dioxide. Overdosing with sodium bicarbonate or other alkali, prolonged vomiting in monogastric animals leading to continued loss of acid gastric juice, and hyperpnoea due to fever which may cause excessive loss of carbon dioxide, are the commonest causes of alkalosis.

Vomiting, lassitude, weakness, anorexia and polyuria develop as in acidosis but the hyperpnoeic stage is accompanied by muscle tremor and tetany with tonic and clonic convulsions rather than flaccidity and coma. The tetany is caused by depression of the ionized fraction of the serum calcium and can be relieved by the intravenous administration of calcium salts. Oral administration of acidifying salts, including ammonium chloride, chlorethamine or calcium chloride, correct the alkalosis. The provision of fluids and electrolytes by parenteral injection may be necessary if vomiting and fluid loss are severe.

REFERENCES

(1) Littlejohn, A. & Mitchell, B. (1969). *Res. vet. Sci.*, *10*, 260, 263.
(2) Schotman, A. J. H. (1970). *T. Diergeneesk.*, *95*, 331.
(3) Rossdale, P. D. (1969). *Res. vet. Sci.*, *10*, 279.

Diseases of the Spleen and Lymph Nodes

SPLENOMEGALY

Diffuse diseases of the spleen which result in enlargement are usually secondary to diseases in other organs. Splenomegaly with complete destruction of splenic function is virtually symptomless, especially if the involvement occurs gradually, and in most cases clinical signs are restricted to those caused by involvement of other organs. An enlarged spleen may be palpable on rectal examination in the horse and careful percussion may detect enlargement of the spleen in cattle but in most instances involvement of the organ is not diagnosed at antemortem examination unless laparotomy is performed. Rupture of a grossly enlarged spleen may cause sudden death due to internal haemorrhage.

Moderate degrees of splenomegaly occur in many infectious diseases, especially salmonellosis, anthrax and babesiasis. Animals which die suddenly because of lightning stroke, electrocution and euthanasia may also show a moderate degree of splenomegaly but the enlargement is minor compared to that observed in congestive heart failure, portal obstruction or neoplastic change. Neoplasms of the spleen are not common in large animals but may include lymphosarcoma, myelocytic leukaemia or malignant melanoma.

SPLENIC ABSCESS

Splenic abscess may result when a septic embolus lodges in the spleen, but is more commonly caused by extension of infection from a neighbouring organ. Perforation by a foreign body in the reticulum of cattle is the commonest cause of the disease in large animals and penetrations by sharp metal have caused splenitis in the horse (1). Perforation of a gastric ulcer in the horse may cause a similar clinical syndrome.

If the abscess is extensive and acute there are systemic signs of fever, anorexia and increased heart rate. Pain is evidenced on palpation over the area of the spleen and haematological examination reveals a marked increase in the total white cell count and a distinct shift to the left in the differential count. Peritonitis is often co-existent and produces signs of mild abdominal pain with arching of the back and disinclination to move. Mild recurrent colic may also occur. Anaemia, with marked pallor of mucosae, and terminal ventral oedema are also recorded (1).

Treatment of splenic abscess is often unrewarding because of the extensive nature of the lesion before clinical signs appear. The systemic signs can usually be brought under control by treatment with sulphonamides or antibiotics over a period of about 7 days but relapses are common and death is the almost certain outcome. Splenectomy is recommended if adhesions and associated peritonitis are absent.

REFERENCE

(1) Swan, R. A. (1968). *Aust. vet. J.*, *44*, 459.

ENLARGEMENT OF THE LYMPH NODES

Enlargement of the lymph nodes may occur as a result of infection or of neoplastic invasion. Metastases may develop as a result of spread from neoplasms in surrounding tissues. Primary neoplasms involving lymph nodes include lymphomatosis and myeloid leukaemia. In both of these diseases and in bacterial endocarditis simultaneous enlargement of a number of lymph nodes is characteristic.

Lymphadenitis accompanies other signs in many specific diseases including strangles, bovine malignant catarrh, sporadic bovine encephalomyelitis, glanders, enzootic lymphangitis and ephemeral fever, but as a sole presenting sign it occurs commonly in tuberculosis, caseous lymphadenitis of sheep and in some cases of actinobacillosis. In acute lymphadenitis there may be pain and heat on palpation but the nodes are for the most part painless.

Enlargement of peripheral nodes causes visible and palpable swellings and in some cases obstruction to lymphatic drainage and subsequent local oedema as in sporadic lymphangitis of horses. Enlargement of internal nodes may cause obstruction of the oesophagus or pharynx, trachea, or bronchi. Differentiation between lymphadenitis and neoplastic enlargement may require examination of a biopsy specimen.

9

Diseases of the Respiratory System

INTRODUCTION

Principles of Respiratory Insufficiency

THE functional efficiency of the respiratory system depends on its ability to oxygenate and to remove carbon dioxide from the blood in the respiratory circulation. Interference with these functions can occur in a number of ways but the underlying defect in all instances is lack of adequate oxygen supply to tissues. The anoxia (or more correctly hypoxia) of respiratory insufficiency is responsible for most of the clinical signs of respiratory disease and for respiratory failure, the terminal event of fatal cases. An understanding of anoxia and respiratory failure is essential to the study of clinical respiratory disease.

Anoxia

Failure of the tissues to receive an adequate supply of oxygen occurs in a number of ways. *Anoxic anoxia* occurs when there is defective oxygenation of blood in the pulmonary circuit and is usually caused by primary disease of the respiratory tract. *Anaemic anoxia* occurs when there is a deficiency of haemoglobin per unit volume of blood. The percentage saturation of the available haemoglobin and the oxygen tension are normal but the oxygen-carrying capacity of the blood is reduced. Anaemia due to any cause has these characteristics. Alteration of haemoglobin to pigments which are not capable of carrying oxygen has the same effect. Thus in poisoning caused by nitrite, in which haemoglobin is converted to methaemoglobin, and that due to carbon monoxide, when the haemoglobin is converted to carboxyhaemoglobin, there is an anaemic anoxia. *Stagnant anoxia* is the state in which the rate of blood flow through the capillaries is reduced. The oxygen saturation of arterial blood, the total oxygen load and the oxygen tension of arterial blood are normal, but because of the prolonged sojourn in the tissues the oxygen tension there falls to a very low level, reducing the rate of oxygen exchange. A relative anoxia of tissues results. Stagnant anoxia is the basic defect in conges-tive heart failure, peripheral circulatory failure and local venous obstruction. *Histotoxic anoxia* occurs when the blood is fully oxygenated but because of failure of tissue oxidation systems the tissues cannot take up oxygen. Cyanide poisoning is the only common cause of this form of anoxia.

Anoxic anoxia may occur when the oxygen tension in the inspired air is too low to oxygenate the pulmonary blood efficiently, but the common causes in animal disease are lesions or dysfunctions of the respiratory tract which reduce the supply of alveolar air. Abnormalities of the alveolar epithelium such as occur in pneumonia, decreased vital capacity as it occurs in pulmonary atelectasis, pneumonia, pneumothorax, pulmonary oedema and congestion, and decreased amplitude of chest movement due to pain of the chest wall all reduce the oxygen tension of the blood leaving the lungs. Obstruction of the air passages by the accumulation of exudate, and depression of the respiratory centre by drugs or toxins have the same effect. Anoxic anoxia is also the basic defect in congenital defects of the heart and large blood vessels when mixing of arterial and venous blood occurs through shunts between the two circulations. Anoxic anoxia also occurs when there is paralysis of the respiratory muscles in tick paralysis, botulism, tetanus and strychnine poisoning.

If the development of anoxia is sufficiently slow several compensatory mechanisms operate. An increase in depth of the respiratory movements (hyperpnoea) occurs as a result of the anoxia and is mediated by the chemoreceptors of the carotid and aortic bodies. Stimulation of splenic contraction and erythropoiesis in the bone marrow are produced by the anoxia and may result in polycythaemia. An increase in heart rate and stroke volume results in an increased minute volume of the heart. If these compensatory mechanisms are insufficient to maintain an adequate supply of oxygen to tissues, signs of dysfunction appear in the various organs. The central nervous system is most susceptible to anoxia and signs referable to cerebral anoxia are usually the first to appear.

Myocardial asthenia, renal and hepatic dysfunction and reduction of motility and secretory activity of the alimentary tract also occur.

Carbon Dioxide Retention (Hypercapnia)

Respiratory insufficiency results in faulty elimination of carbon dioxide and its accumulation in blood and tissues. This appears to have little effect other than to stimulate an increase in respiratory effort by its action on the respiratory centre.

Respiratory Failure

Respiratory movements are involuntary and are stimulated and modified by the respiratory centres in the medulla. The centres appear, at least in some species, to have spontaneous activity which is modified by afferent impulses from higher centres including cerebral cortex and the heat regulating centre in the hypothalamus, from the stretch receptors in the lungs via the pulmonary vagus nerves, and from the chemoreceptors in the carotid bodies. The activity of the centre is also regulated directly by the pH and oxygen and carbon dioxide tensions of the cranial arterial blood supply. Stimulation of almost all afferent nerves may also cause reflex change in respiration, stimulation of pain fibres being particularly effective.

Respiratory failure is the terminal stage of respiratory insufficiency in which the activity of the respiratory centres diminishes to the point where movements of respiratory muscles cease. Respiratory failure can be paralytic, dyspnoeic or asphyxial, or tachypnoeic, depending on the primary disease. In asphyxial failure, which occurs in pneumonia, pulmonary oedema, and upper respiratory tract obstruction there is hypercapnia and anoxia. The hypercapnia stimulates the respiratory centre, and the anoxia the chemoreceptors of the carotid body so that respiratory movements are dyspnoeic, followed by alternating periods of gasping and apnoea just before death. Paralytic respiratory failure is caused by poisoning with respiratory centre depressants or by nervous shock. Acute heart failure or haemorrhage may cause paralytic respiratory failure but there is usually a variable degree of dyspnoea and gasping, although not usually as severe as in typical asphyxial failure. In typical paralytic failure the respiratory centres are paralysed so that the respirations rapidly become more shallow and less frequent and then cease altogether without the appearance of dyspnoea or gasping.

Tachypnoeic respiratory failure is the least common form and arises when pulmonary ventilation is increased as in hyperthermia so that there is hypoxia but no carbon dioxide retention (acapnia). Because of the lack of carbon dioxide to stimulate the respiratory movements they are rapid and shallow—tachypnoea. The differentiation of these types of failure is of some importance in determining the type of treatment which is necessary. In the paralytic form a respiratory centre stimulant is required, in the asphyxial form oxygen is the rational treatment, and in the tachypnoeic form oxygen and carbon dioxide should be provided.

Principal Manifestations of Respiratory Insufficiency

The principal manifestations of respiratory dysfunction are those which derive from anoxia but in infectious diseases or where tissue destruction is extensive there is the added effect of toxaemia, the manifestations of which have been discussed elsewhere.

Hyperpnoea and Dyspnoea

Hyperpnoea is defined as increased pulmonary ventilation. Dyspnoea has a subjective element in that it is defined as the consciousness of the necessity for increased respiratory effort, and is loosely applied to animals to include increased respiratory movement which appears to cause distress to the animal. Hyperpnoea becomes dyspnoea at an arbitrary dyspnoeic point and the two are discussed together.

Dyspnoea is a physiological occurrence after strenuous exercise and is abnormal only when it occurs at rest or with little exercise. It is usually caused by anoxia and hypercapnia arising most commonly from diseases of the respiratory tract. In pulmonary dyspnoea one other factor may be of contributory importance; there may be an abnormally sensitive Hering-Breuer reflex. This is most likely to occur when there is inflammation or congestion of the lungs or pleura. Rapid, shallow breathing results. The dyspnoea of pulmonary emphysema is characteristically expiratory in form and is caused by anoxic anoxia and the need for forced expiration to achieve successful expulsion of the tidal air.

Cardiac dyspnoea results from backward failure of the left ventricle with congestion and oedema of the lungs. Stagnant anoxia plays some part in the production of this form of dyspnoea but diminished ability of the lungs to distend, with increased sensitivity of the Hering-Breuer reflex, and the effect of increased venous pressure on the respiratory centre are probably more important.

Dyspnoea is never marked in anaemic anoxia

when the patient is at rest because of the absence of hypercapnia. In acidosis the liberation of carbon dioxide stimulates the respiratory centre and dyspnoea may occur, and in some cases of encephalitis or space occupying lesions of the cranial cavity stimulation of the centre may cause neurogenic dyspnoea.

Other less common and important respiratory signs indicative of respiratory disease include abnormalities of the respiratory cycle such as prolongation of expiration or inspiration, disproportionate movements of the two sides of the chest, respiratory stridor and evidence of pain with respiratory movements. These have been discussed under examination of the thorax in Chapter 1.

Cyanosis

Cyanosis is a bluish discolouration of the skin, conjunctivae and visible mucosae caused by an increase in the absolute amount of reduced haemoglobin in the blood. It can occur only when the haemoglobin concentration of the blood is normal or nearly so, and when there is incomplete oxygenation of the haemoglobin. It can occur in all types of anoxic anoxia and in stagnant anoxia but not in anaemic patients because there is insufficient haemoglobin present. On the other hand polycythaemia predisposes to cyanosis. To satisfy all criteria of cyanosis the bluish discolouration should disappear when pressure is exerted on the skin or mucosa and blood flow is stopped temporarily. Methaemoglobinaemia is accompanied by discolouration of the skin and mucosae but the colour is more brown than blue and cannot be accurately described as cyanosis. The most marked cyanosis occurs in congenital cardiac defects and is never marked in acquired heart disease. It is not usually marked in pulmonary disease unless the degree of pulmonary collapse is severe without the circulation being impeded so that blood flows through large sections of lung without being oxygenated.

Cough

Coughing is a reflex act initiated by irritation of the respiratory mucosa of the air passages. It has a primary expulsive function but material of low viscosity may be spread further back into smaller bronchial passages and to other parts of the lung. It is a sign of importance in that it indicates the presence of primary or secondary disease of the respiratory system.

Nasal Discharge

Excessive or abnormal nasal discharge is usually an indication of respiratory tract disease. When the discharge is mucoid or purulent it usually indicates the presence of inflammation in the nasal cavities or paranasal sinuses but sanguineous or frothy exudate may suggest the presence of pulmonary congestion or oedema.

Epistaxis or nosebleed is in most instances a result of disease of the mucosae of the upper respiratory tract.

Small amounts of serosanguineous fluid in the nostrils as occurs in equine infectious anaemia and infectious equine pneumonia, does not represent epistaxis which must also be differentiated from the passage of blood-stained froth caused by acute pulmonary oedema. In this instance the bubbles in the froth are very small in size and passage of the froth is accompanied by severe dyspnoea, coughing and auscultatory evidence of pulmonary oedema.

In epistaxis blood may flow from one or both nostrils in drops or as a stream if the site of origin is in the nasal cavities. When the blood originates from a pharyngeal lesion there are frequent swallowing movements and a short, explosive cough which may be accompanied by the spitting-out of blood clots from the mouth. Unless bleeding is extremely profuse and causes death from haemorrhagic anaemia within a few hours, it usually stops spontaneously. The application of cold packs and the insertion of tampons soaked in adrenaline are often recommended as treatment for epistaxis but the tampons are difficult to insert and treatment is best directed towards stopping the haemorrhage by the administration of parenteral coagulants. Blood transfusion is sometimes necessary when large amounts of blood have been lost.

Special Examination of the Respiratory System

Opportunities for examination of the respiratory system by special techniques do not often arise and are not often used because of the need for expensive facilities. Nevertheless, special examinations may be carried out on valuable young farm animals and in the smaller species. For example methods are available for measuring tidal and minute respiratory volumes in foals as an aid to the assessment of pulmonary efficiency (2).

Roentgenological examination of the chest is a practicable procedure in calves, sheep, goats and pigs and may aid in the diagnosis of tumour, pneumonia and atelectasis. Bronchography, utilizing contrast agents, is of value in determining the patency of the trachea and bronchi but general anaesthesia is required to overcome the coughing stimulated by the passage of the tracheal catheter. Using a fluoroscope to determine the situation of the catheter tip, the contrast agent can be deposited in each dependent lobe in turn.

When an infectious process is suspected in the respiratory system it is customary to collect samples for examination. A direct swab from the nasal passages is the simplest but least satisfactory test. The resulting bacteriological examination usually reveals a large population of normal flora. Nevertheless, the method is not without value. For example, using a special nasal swab frequent isolations of *Pasteurella haemolytica* in young bulls were associated with frequent cases of bacterial pneumonia, but the isolation was not related to the development of pneumonia in the individual calf (3). For virological purposes nasal washings are usually collected, the simplest technique being irrigation of the nasal cavities and collection into an open dish. For more reliable results swabs of the laryngeal–pharyngeal area are collected. A swab in a long covering sheath, of the type used for collecting cervical swabs from mares, is easily passed up the nostril and provides a suitable sampling method.

A sputum cup is sometimes of value in obtaining a sample of tracheal mucus for bacteriological examination. The technique is practicable in cattle but good restraint and a heavy dose of an ataractic drug are necessary so that the tongue can be fully drawn and the laryngeal orifice brought into view. Paracentesis of the pleural cavity is of value when the presence of fluid in the sac is suspected. The needle should be introduced in the sixth or seventh intercostal space, below the anticipated level of fluid, and aspiration effected with a syringe. Care must be taken to avoid the pericardial sac. Needle puncture of a suspected lung abscess to determine the species of bacteria present is sometimes practised but there is the risk that infection will be spread to the pleura by this technique.

The techniques of auscultation and percussion used in examination of the chest are discussed in Chapter 1.

Principles of Treatment of Respiratory Tract Disease

If the disease is caused by bacterial or fungal infection, suitable treatment to control the causative agent should be provided. Obstruction of the upper respiratory tract by inflammatory or non-inflammatory lesions may necessitate tracheotomy to permit respiratory exchange until such time as the lesions are effectively treated. The principal ancillary treatment in diseases of the lungs should be the administration of oxygen. This method is not often adopted in large animal work but the use of a portable oxygen cylinder may find a place in tiding animals over a period of critical anoxia until inflammatory lesions of the lung subside. The disadvantages of oxygen therapy are that it must be given continuously, requiring constant attendance on the animal and suitable apparatus is required or much oxygen is wasted. The use of an oxygen tent is impractical and a mask must be used or a tube introduced into the pharynx via the nostril. Tracheal catheterization is practicable only in anaesthetized animals. For greatest efficiency the gas should be warmed and moistened as it is discharged and not permitted to impinge directly on mucosa. As a practical emergency measure these refinements may have to be disregarded.

In cattle the nasal tube must be inserted to the correct point because passage short of this causes excessive waste of oxygen and beyond this much is swallowed (1). The length of tube inserted should equal the distance from the nostril to a point one-third of the way from the lateral canthus of the eye to the base of the ear. Insertion of a nebulizer in the system permits the simultaneous administration of antibiotics and moisture to prevent drying of the pharyngeal mucosa. The volume of oxygen used should be about 4 to 8 litres per minute for an animal of 200 lb. weight.

Oxygen therapy is of value only when anoxic anoxia is present and oxygen saturation of the available haemoglobin is incomplete. Cases of pneumonia, pleurisy, and oedema and congestion of the lungs are the ones most likely to benefit. Relief may also be obtained in emphysema but the disease is incurable and no real advantage is gained. Anaemic and histotoxic anoxia are unlikely to respond and the response in stagnant anoxia is small because, although the degree of saturation of haemoglobin may be increased, the rate of blood flow through capillaries is slow and the rate of oxygen transfer to tissues is not greatly increased.

When depression of the respiratory centre occurs the use of respiratory stimulants is advisable but these drugs are unlikely to effect any improvement in animals in which the respiration is already deep. The most effective respiratory stimulant is carbon dioxide and this can be administered most efficiently as a mixture with oxygen containing 5 to 10 per cent of carbon dioxide. Increase in the depth of respiration results and improves the intake of oxygen. Improvement in the pulmonary circulation also occurs and the chances of pulmonary congestion in recumbent animals are correspondingly reduced. The impracticability of carrying gas cylinders and supervising continuous administration of the gas reduces the suitability of the technique in large animal work and parenterally administered stimulants are generally used. Picrotoxin, Metrazol, Coramine, caffeine and amphetamine sulphate are widely used for this purpose. Artificial respiration should not be neglected in acute cases and should be performed until respiration recommences or until failure to respond to the administration of a parenteral stimulant is apparent.

Removal of physical lesions which obstruct expansion of the lungs is usually practicable only when the obstruction is in the form of an accumulation of fluid in the pleural sac.

Expectorants are commonly used in farm animals, especially horses, and the choice of the most suitable drug for each case may improve the response obtained. Knowledge of the nature of the lesion, the character of the bronchial exudate and the type of cough are necessary before the choice can be made. When the cough is painful and exhausting and the secretion tenacious sedative expectorants, such as ammonium or potassium salts, stimulate secretion of protective mucus and lessen the coughing. In chronic bronchitis when the cough is soft and the bronchial exudate voluminous a stimulant expectorant such as creosote, turpentine, guaiacol or eucalyptus is more valuable. These drugs cause slight irritation and hyperaemia of the respiratory mucosa and tend to stimulate healing and diminish bronchial secretions. When the cough is exhausting and interferes with activity but there is little exudation an anodyne expectorant such as morphine, codeine or heroin, or belladonna is indicated. This situation is most commonly encountered in infectious equine bronchitis.

REFERENCES

(1) Kowalczyk, T. (1957). *J. Amer. vet. med. Ass.*, *131*, 333.
(2) Rossdale, P. D. (1969). *Brit. vet. J.*, *125*, 157.
(3) Magwood, S. F. *et al.* (1969). *Canad. J. comp. Med.*, *33*, 237.

DISEASES OF THE LUNGS

Pulmonary Congestion and Oedema

Pulmonary congestion is caused by an increase in the amount of blood in the lungs due to engorgement of the pulmonary vascular bed. It is sometimes followed by pulmonary oedema when intravascular fluid escapes into the parenchyma and alveoli. The various stages of the vascular disturbance are characterized by respiratory embarrassment, the degree depending upon the amount of alveolar air space which is lost.

Aetiology

Pulmonary congestion and oedema is a common terminal event in a great many diseases but is frequently overshadowed by other disturbances. Congestion which is clinically apparent may be primary when the basic lesion is in the lungs or secondary when it is in some other organ, most commonly the heart. Primary congestion is the first stage in most cases of pneumonia, after the inhalation of smoke and irritant fumes, and in anaphylactic reactions. It also occurs as hypostatic congestion in recumbent animals. Secondary congestion is usually a manifestation of congestive heart failure affecting the left ventricle in which the flow of blood through the lungs is impeded by increased pressure in the pulmonary veins.

Severe over-exertion in horses not accustomed to hard work is characterized by pulmonary congestion and, in this instance, it is probably partly primary and partly secondary due to acute myocardial asthenia. In man 'heart-strain' due to over-exertion is considered to be an unlikely development, muscular activity failing when the circulation is over-taxed, but horses which are forcibly driven appear to develop this syndrome.

Pulmonary oedema occurs most commonly as a sequel to congestion in acute anaphylaxis, in fog fever, and in congestive heart failure. It also occurs after the inhalation of smoke and in some toxaemias including mulberry heart disease of swine and poisoning with organic phosphorus compounds. Poisoning by alphanaphthyl thiourea (ANTU) causes pulmonary oedema in rodents and this may occur in farm animals.

Pathogenesis

In pulmonary congestion much of the effective alveolar air space is lost because of engorgement of the pulmonary capillaries. The vital capacity is reduced and oxygenation of the blood is impaired. Oxygenation is further reduced by the decreased rate of blood flow through the pulmonary vascular bed. Anoxic anoxia develops and is the cause of most of the clinical signs that appear.

The vital capacity is still further reduced when oedema, the secondary stage, occurs. The oedema is caused by damage to the capillary walls by toxins or anoxia or by transudation of fluid due to increased hydrostatic pressure in the capillaries. Filling of the alveoli, and in severe cases the bronchi, effectively prevents gaseous exchange.

Clinical Findings

All degrees of severity occur and only the most severe form is described here. The depth of respiration is increased to the point of extreme dyspnoea with the head extended, the nostrils flared and mouth-breathing. The respiratory movements are greatly exaggerated and can be best described as heaving; there is marked abdominal and thoracic movement during inspiration and expiration. A typical stance is usually adopted, with the front legs spread wide apart, the elbows abducted and the head hung low. The respiratory rate is usually increased especially if there is hyperthermia which occurs in acute anaphylaxis and after violent exercise as well as in the early stages of pneumonia. The pulse rate is usually elevated (up to 100 per minute) and the nasal mucosa is bright red. In acute congestion there is a harsh vesicular murmur but no râles are present on auscultation. When oedema develops there may be little air entry so that bronchial tones and fluid râles are the only audible sounds, particularly in the ventral parts of the lungs. In cases of long standing there may be emphysema of the dorsal parts of the lungs, especially if the lesion is caused by allergy. Percussion sounds vary from normal in early congestion to dullness when there is oedema.

Cough is usually present but it is soft and moist and appears to cause little discomfort. A slight to moderate serous nasal discharge occurs in the early stage of congestion but in severe pulmonary oedema this increases to a voluminous, frothy nasal discharge which is often blood-tinged.

The main importance of pulmonary congestion is as an indicator of early pathological changes in the lung or heart. Spontaneous recovery occurs quickly unless there is damage to alveolar epithelium or myocardial asthenia develops. Severe pulmonary oedema has much greater significance and usually indicates a stage of irreversibility. Death in cases of pulmonary oedema is accompanied by asphyxial respiratory failure.

Clinical Pathology

Laboratory examinations are of value only in differentiating the causes of the congestion or oedema. Bacteriological examination of nasal swabs and a complete haematological examination, looking particularly for the presence of eosinophilia are the standard examinations which are carried out.

Necropsy Findings

In acute pulmonary congestion the lungs are dark red in colour. Excessive quantities of venous blood exude from the cut surface. Similar but less marked changes occur in milder forms of congestion but are only seen in those animals which die from intercurrent disease. Histologically the pulmonary capillaries are markedly engorged and some transudation and haemorrhage into alveoli is evident.

Macroscopic findings in pulmonary oedema include swelling and loss of elasticity of the lungs which pit on pressure. They are usually paler than normal. Excessive quantities of serous fluid exude from the cut surface of the lung. Histologically there are accumulations of fluid in the alveoli and parenchyma.

Diagnosis

The diagnosis of pulmonary congestion and oedema is always difficult unless there is a history of a precipitating cause such as over-exertion or inhalation of smoke or fumes. Pneumonia usually presents itself as an alternative diagnosis and a decision cannot be based entirely on the presence or absence of hyperthermia. The best indication is usually the presence of toxaemia but this again is not entirely dependable. Bacterial pneumonia is usually accompanied by some toxaemia but cases of viral pneumonia are often free of it. Response to antibacterial treatment is one of the best indications, the only variable being the tendency for congestion and oedema of allergic origin to recover spontaneously. In many instances there will be doubt and it is then advisable to treat the animal for both conditions.

Treatment

The treatment of pulmonary congestion and oedema must first be directed at correction of the primary cause as listed under aetiology. Affected animals should be confined at rest in a clean, dry environment and exercise avoided. Venesection with the removal of 4 ml. of blood per lb. body weight is recommended in severe congestion. Oxygen therapy may effectively reduce the anoxia but administration of carbon dioxide or parenteral respiratory stimulants is unlikely to have any beneficial effect.

When oedema is severe prompt administration of atropine may reduce fluid transudation. In these cases the animal is in considerable danger and repeated injections may be necessary. Details of the recommended treatment régime are given in the section on treatment of poisoning by organic phosphorus compounds. Nebulized solutions are administered as inhalants in acute pulmonary oedema accompanied by froth in the air passages in humans; ethyl alcohol (95 per cent), and a mixture of silicones and polyhydric alcohols similar to those used in the treatment of frothy bloat in ruminants, are recommended to break down the froth (1).

REFERENCE

(1) Balagot, R. C. *et al.* (1957). *J. Amer. vet. med. Ass.*, *163*, 630.

Pulmonary Emphysema

(*Heaves*)

Abnormal distension of the lung caused by rupture of alveolar walls with or without escape of air into the interstitial tissue causes reduction in air space and embarrassment of respiration. Failure of the elastic recoil of the lungs results in forced expiration.

Aetiology

In cattle emphysema is an important lesion in atypical pneumonia, parasitic pneumonia and anaphylaxis. The most common form in animals is chronic alveolar emphysema or 'heaves' in horses (7). The cause of this condition is not known but the highest incidence is in adult horses and is usually associated with prolonged feeding on poor grade roughage and especially when the feed is dusty. It is most common where horses are housed in barns for long periods and is virtually unknown where horses are run at pasture all year round. Chronic bronchitis accompanied by bronchial stenosis, paroxysmal or chronic coughing, and excessive expiratory movement due to over-exertion are often quoted as precipitating causes but many cases occur in the apparent absence of these conditions. A similar clinical syndrome has been produced by the intravenous injection of histamine and there is increasing support for the hypothesis that the typical condition is an allergic phenomenon, possibly of mycotic origin (5, 6).

Sporadic cases of acute emphysema occur due to perforation of the lung by foreign bodies as in traumatic reticuloperitonitis, or pulmonary abscess. Local or perifocal emphysema is a common necropsy finding around local pulmonary lesions, especially atelectasis, and may cause little or no respiratory dysfunction, although in calves and pigs the emphysema is sometimes sufficiently extensive to kill the animal.

Pathogenesis

Excessive dilatation of alveoli can only occur by over-stretching of the supporting and elastic tissue of the pulmonary parenchyma. There are in the main two schools of thought on the pathogenesis of pulmonary emphysema. One proposes that there is a primary deficiency in the strength of the suppor-

tive tissues which are thus unable to support the alveolar walls during coughing or exertion. The other hypothesis is that chronic bronchitis and bronchiolitis or bronchial spasm due to allergy cause obstruction of the air passages but air still enters the alveoli through the communications between them. This air accumulates, causes overdistension and finally rupture of the alveoli (1). In either case an initial lesion probably leads to an area of weakness from which emphysema spreads during coughing or exertion. In interstitial emphysema there is the additional factor of distension of the connective tissue with air and compression collapse of the alveoli. The development of interstitial emphysema depends largely upon the amount of interstitial tissue which is present and is most common in cattle and pigs. In horses the emphysema is usually purely alveolar.

Emphysema which develops in association with another lesion such as atelectasis or oedema is often spoken of as compensatory, as though overdistension of residual lung causes alveolar dilatation. This may be the case but it seems probable that an agent which causes the primary lesion may also reduce the strength of the surrounding, supporting tissue and cause obstruction of neighbouring bronchioles with emphysema developing in the usual way as set out above.

The pathologic physiology of emphysema depends upon the inefficiency of evacuation of pulmonary air-space and failure of normal gaseous exchange in the lungs. The elastic recoil of the tissue is diminished and when the chest subsides during expiration incomplete evacuation occurs. Because of the increase in residual volume the tidal volume must be increased to maintain normal gaseous exchange. Retention of carbon dioxide stimulates an increase in the depth of respiration but maximum respiratory effort necessitated by exercise cannot be achieved. Anoxia develops and metabolism of all body tissues is reduced (2). The characteristic effect of emphysema is to produce an increase in expiratory effort necessitated by the failure of normal elastic recoil.

Interference with the pulmonary circulation results from collapse of much of the alveolar wall area and a consequent diminution of the capillary bed. The decreased negative pressure in the chest and the abnormally wide respiratory excursion also cause a general restriction of the rate of blood flow into the thorax. The combined effect of these factors may be sufficient to cause failure of the right ventricle especially if there is a primary defect of the myocardium. Acidosis may also result because of the retention of carbon dioxide.

Clinical Findings

In acute emphysema the onset is sudden and severe signs are present at rest. In general the signs are similar to those of chronic emphysema but the dyspnoea is much more severe and on auscultation the breath sounds may not be grossly abnormal.

In the chronic disease the signs appear gradually and in the early stages are evident only during exercise. Prolongation and exaggeration of the expiratory phase of each respiratory cycle is the major manifestation. Respiration is increased in depth and during expiration there is normal collapse of the rib cage followed by an expiratory uplift of the abdominal wall. In time the size of the chest increases so that the animal develops a barrel chested appearance with obvious protrusion of the costal arch. Subcutaneous emphysema may develop from an interstitial emphysema in cattle, or in other species when there is perforation of the pleura. In cattle the emphysema spreads from the interstitial tissue to beneath the pleura and from there to the hilus of the lung, through the mediastinum and fascial planes to the subcutaneous tissue.

A short, weak cough is characteristic and becomes more pronounced and wheezing with exercise. Exercise tolerance is poor and clinically affected horses are of little use for work. In advanced cases auscultation reveals the presence of loud crepitant râles accompanied by sibilant, whistling sounds and a pleuritic friction rub over most of the lung area. These sounds are most obvious in cattle, and although they may be present in horses, it is also common to find comparatively normal breath sounds in this species probably because of the absence of interstitial emphysema. On percussion the chest is hyperresonant and the area of cardiac dullness and the apex beat are diminished. The heart sounds are usually muffled by the expansion of the lung over the heart. Terminally congestive heart failure may develop but the usual course in horses is the gradual development of the emphysema until the horse is disposed of because of incapacity (4).

Clinical Pathology

The retention of carbon dioxide may cause an increase in alkali reserve, and a compensatory polycythaemia may develop.

Necropsy Findings

The lungs are distended and pale in colour and may bear imprints of the ribs. In interstitial emphysema the interalveolar septae are distended with air which may spread to beneath the pleura, to the mediastinum and under the parietal pleura. There may be evidence of congestive heart failure. On histopathological examination a bronchiolitis is present in most cases. This may be diffuse and apparently primary or originate by spread from a nearby pneumonia.

Diagnosis

Chronic emphysema of horses is characterized by a pattern of development and pathognomonic signs which are not readily mistaken for those of other diseases. Acute emphysema in cattle and horses is often accompanied by pulmonary oedema with the presence of consolidation and fluid râles in the ventral parts of the lungs. It may be confused with acute pulmonary congestion and oedema caused by anaphylaxis but forced expiration is not a characteristic of these latter conditions. Pneumonia is characterized by fever and localization of abnormal respiratory sounds which are not as marked nor as widely distributed as those of emphysema. Crepitant and sibilant râles may occur in chronic pneumonia but are evident only at the periphery of areas of consolidation. Pneumothorax is accompanied by forced inspiration and an absence of normal breath sounds.

Treatment

In acute emphysema rest is essential and the animal should be housed where respiration will not be impeded by humidity, high environmental temperatures or foul air. Oxygen therapy is indicated and should be provided if possible (2). Atropine usually produces temporary relief from the dyspnoea, as do corticosteroids, especially if oedema is present. Antihistamine drugs are a standard treatment in acute alveolar emphysema in cattle and may be of value in chronic emphysema in horses because it is known that histamines cause broncho-constriction in these animals (3, 5).

In all cases attempts should be made to treat any predisposing or precipitating cause and the animal should be protected from exposure to inclement weather, respiratory infection and dusty atmospheres. The elimination of dust is particularly important and this may require the dampening or soaking of both hay and grain. Pelleted rations are convenient and have been recommended along with beet pulp and molasses for acutely affected horses. Complete recovery is rare but in many cases useful work can be performed under careful feeding and management.

REFERENCES

(1) Lister, W. A. (1958). *Lancet*, *276*, 66.
(2) Simpson, T. (1955). *Lancet*, *273*, 105.

(3) Obel, N. J. & Schmiterlow, C. G. (1948). *Acta pharmacol.*, *4*, 71.

(4) Cook, W. R. (1965). *Vet. Rec.*, *77*, 516.

(5) Cook, W. R. & Rossdale, P. D. (1963). *Proc. R. Soc. Med.*, *56*, 972.

(6) Eyre, P. (1972). *Vet. Rec.*, *91*, 134.

(7) Gillespie, J. R. & Tyler, W. S. (1969). *Adv. vet. Sci. comp. Med.*, *13*, 59.

Pneumonia

Pneumonia is inflammation of the pulmonary parenchyma usually accompanied by inflammation of the bronchioles and often by pleurisy. It is manifested clinically by an increase in respiratory rate, cough, abnormal breath sounds on auscultation and, in most bacterial pneumonias, by evidence of toxaemia.

Aetiology

Pneumonia is often classified into primary and secondary categories but differentiation is becoming increasingly difficult because of the uncertain role of viruses in many bacterial pneumonias of animals. The importance of primary viral infection has become apparent only in recent years when techniques for their isolation, cultivation and identification have come into general use. The classification set out below is based on the generally accepted aetiology of each disease. Atypical interstitial pneumonia, which occurs in sheep and is common in cattle, is dealt with under that heading. Pulmonary abscess and aspiration pneumonia are dealt with elsewhere (p. 172).

Viral pneumonia. Virus pneumonia of pigs, virus pneumonia of calves and virus pneumonia of lambs are recognized as specific pneumonias. Infectious equine pneumonia probably commences as a viral infection, and equine viral rhinopneumonitis and equine viral arteritis are specific viral diseases of horses which cause some pulmonary inflammation. Maedi and jaagsiekte of sheep are chronic pneumonias caused by viruses.

Bacterial pneumonia. Contagious bovine pleuropneumonia (*Mycoplasma mycoides*) of cattle, and pleuropneumonia (*Mycoplasma mycoides*) of sheep and goats are important diseases in some countries. Pneumonia caused by *Pasteurella multocida* and *P. haemolytica* is an important disease in ruminants and swine possibly as a complication of a primary viral pneumonia. Pneumonia caused by *Klebsiella pneumoniae* has been recorded in calves in association with mastitis caused by this organism in cows, and pneumonia in lambs caused by *P. multocida* may have the same association.

Bacterial pneumonia may also occur as part of a systemic disease. Salmonellosis in pigs, tuberculosis and oral necrobacillosis in cattle, glanders and strangles in horses and melioidosis in sheep are often accompanied by severe pneumonia. Many other bacteria including *Streptococcus* spp., *Corynebacterium* spp., *Haemophilus* spp., *Bordetella bronchisepticus*, *Dermatophilus* spp. and pleuro-pneumonia-like organisms are found in sporadic outbreaks or cases of pneumonia in farm animals, especially in calves.

Pneumonia caused by fungi. Some of the systemic mycoses are accompanied by pulmonary involvement but the lesions are granulomatous and tend to be focal.

Pneumonia caused by metazoan parasites. Verminous pneumonia occurs in all species and invasion of the lungs of pigs and atypical hosts by the larvae of *Ascaris lumbricoides* var. *suum* may also cause pneumonia.

Pneumonia caused by physical and chemical agents. Aspiration pneumonia is dealt with as a separate entity and other physical and chemical pneumonias are rare in animals. Inhalation of nitrogen dioxide gas has been suggested as a cause of atypical pneumonia of cattle and a poisonous plant, Crofton weed, has been suggested as a cause of pneumonia in horses.

Pathogenesis

The process by which pneumonia develops varies with the causative agent and its virulence and with the portal by which it is introduced into the lung. Bacteria are introduced largely by way of the respiratory passages and cause a primary bronchiolitis which spreads to involve surrounding pulmonary parenchyma. The reaction of the lung tissue may be in the form of an acute fibrinous process as in pasteurellosis and contagious bovine pleuropneumonia, a necrotizing lesion as in infection with *Sphaerophorus necrophorus*, or as a more chronic caseous or granulomatous lesion in mycobacterial or mycotic infections. Spread of the lesion through the lung occurs by extension but also by passage of infective material along bronchioles and lymphatics. Spread along the air passages is facilitated by the normal movements of the bronchiolar epithelium and by coughing. Haematogenous infection by bacteria results in a varying number of septic foci which may enlarge to form lung abscesses. Pneumonia occurs when these abscesses rupture into air passages and spread as a secondary bronchopneumonia.

Viral infections are also introduced chiefly by inhalation and cause a primary bronchiolitis but there is an absence of the acute inflammatory reaction which occurs in bacterial pneumonia.

Spread to the alveoli causes enlargement and proliferation of the alveolar epithelial cells and the development of alveolar oedema. Consolidation of the affected tissue results but again there is an absence of acute inflammation and tissue necrosis so that toxaemia is not a characteristic development. Histologically the reaction is manifested by enlargement and proliferation of the alveolar epithelium, alveolar oedema, thickening of the interstitial tissue and lymphocytic aggregations around the alveoli, blood vessels and bronchioles. This interstitial type of reaction is characteristic of viral pneumonias.

Irrespective of the way in which lesions develop, the pathologic physiology of all pneumonias is based upon interference with gaseous exchange between the alveolar air and the blood. Anoxia and hypercapnia develop. In bacterial pneumonias there is the added effect of toxins produced by the bacteria and necrotic tissue, and the accumulation of inflammatory exudate in the bronchi is manifested by moist râles on auscultation. Interstitial pneumonia results in consolidation of pulmonary parenchyma without involvement of the bronchi and on auscultation loud bronchial tones are heard. These are caused by the passage of air through unobstructed bronchioles and are made more audible by the consolidation of the surrounding tissue. The presence of pleurisy is not necessarily indicative of either form of pneumonia. It occurs in both and its development depends more on the aetiological agent than on the mode of development of the lesion.

Restriction of gaseous exchange occurs because of the obliteration of alveolar spaces and obstruction of air passages. In the stage before blood flow through the affected part ceases, the reduction in oxygenation of the blood is made more severe by failure of part of the circulating blood to come into contact with oxygen. Cyanosis is most likely to develop at this stage and be less pronounced when hepatization is complete and blood flow through the part ceases. An additional factor in the production of anoxia is the shallow breathing which occurs. Pleuritic pain causes reduction in the respiratory excursion of the chest wall but when no pleurisy is present the explanation of the shallow breathing probably lies in the increased sensitivity of the Hering-Breuer reflex. Retention of carbon dioxide with resulting acidosis, is most likely to occur in the early stages of pneumonia because of this shallow breathing.

Clinical Findings

Rapid, shallow respiration is the cardinal sign of early pneumonia, dyspnoea occurring in the later stages when much of the lung tissue is non-functional. Polypnoea may be quite marked with only minor pneumonic lesions and the rapidity of the respiration is an inaccurate guide to the degree of pulmonary involvement. Cough is another important sign, the type of cough varying with the nature of the lesion. Bronchopneumonia is usually accompanied by a moist, painful cough, interstitial pneumonia by frequent, dry, hacking coughs, often in paroxysms. Auscultation of the chest before and after coughing may detect exudate in the air passages. Cyanosis is not a common sign and occurs only when large areas of the lung are affected. A nasal discharge may or may not be present, depending upon the amount of exudate present in the bronchioles and whether or not there is accompanying inflammation of the upper respiratory tract. The odour of the breath may be informative. It may have an odour of decay when there is a large accumulation of inspissated pus present in the air passages, or be putrid, especially in horses, when pulmonary gangrene is present.

Auscultation is a valuable aid to diagnosis. The stage of development and the nature of the lesion can be determined and the area of lung tissue affected can be outlined. In the early congestive stages of bronchopneumonia and interstitial pneumonia the vesicular murmur is increased. Moist râles develop in bronchopneumonia as bronchiolar exudation increases but in uncomplicated interstitial pneumonia clear, harsh, bronchial tones are audible. When complete consolidation occurs in either form bronchial tones are the only sounds audible over the affected lung but moist or crepitant râles can be heard at the periphery of the affected area in bronchopneumonia. Consolidation also causes increased audibility of the heart sounds. When pleurisy is also present it causes a pleuritic friction rub in the early stages and muffling of the pulmonary sounds in the late exudative stages. Consolidation can be detected also by percussion of the thorax or by tracheal percussion.

There may be an observable difference in the amount of movement in the two sides of the chest if the degree of consolidation is much greater in one lung. Additional signs evident in pneumonia include fever of variable severity, anorexia, depression, an increase in pulse rate and a reluctance to lie down. In the terminal stages mania and a tendency to attack are not uncommon, especially in cattle.

With adequate treatment in the early stages, bacterial pneumonia usually responds quickly and completely but viral pneumonia may not respond at all or may relapse after an initial response. The transient response is probably due to control of secondary bacterial invaders. In some bacterial pneumonias the same course is apparent due either to reinfection or to persistence of the infection in necrotic foci out of reach of usual therapeutic measures. The final outcome depends on the susceptibility of the causative agent to the treatments available and the severity of the lesions when treatment is undertaken. Although pleurisy is a common accompaniment of pneumonia and rarely occurs independently of it, it has been dealt with separately to facilitate the description of the two conditions.

Clinical Pathology

Ante-mortem laboratory examinations consist largely of cultural examinations of nasal swabs or tracheal sputum and determination of the sensitivity of isolated bacteria to antibacterial agents. Roentgenological examination is undertaken only in animals of suitable size when pulmonary abscess is suspected. Haematological observations usually reveal a leucocytosis and a shift to the left in bacterial pneumonias.

Necropsy Findings

Gross lesions are usually observed in the anterior and dependent parts of the lobes, and even in fatal cases where much of the lung is destroyed, the dorsal parts of the lobes may be unaffected. The gross lesions vary a great deal depending upon the type of pneumonia present. Bronchopneumonia is characterized by the presence of serofibrinous or purulent exudate in the bronchioles, and lobular congestion or hepatization. In the more severe, fibrinous forms of pneumonia there is gelatinous exudation in the interlobular septae and an acute pleurisy, with shreds of fibrin present between the lobes. In interstitial pneumonia the bronchioles are clean and the affected lung is sunken, dark red in colour and has a granular appearance under the pleura and on the cut surface. There is often an apparent, firm thickening of the interlobular septae. These differences are readily detected on histological examination. Lesions typical of the specific infections listed under aetiology are described under the headings of the specific diseases.

Diagnosis

Respiratory distress may result from involvement of other systems. Congestive heart failure, the terminal stages of anaemia, poisoning by histotoxic agents such as hydrocyanic acid, hyperthermia and acidosis are accompanied by respiratory embarrassment but not by the auscultation sounds typical of pulmonary involvement. Pulmonary oedema, congestion, embolism of the pulmonary artery and emphysema are often mistaken for pneumonia but can usually be differentiated by the absence of fever and toxaemia, on the basis of the history and on the auscultation findings. Pleurisy, pneumothorax and hydrothorax may be more difficult to distinguish because of obliteration of pulmonary sounds by a pleuritic friction rub, collapse or fluid accumulation.

Upper respiratory disease may also be accompanied by respiratory embarrassment, cough and abnormal sounds on auscultation but the sounds are most marked on inspiration; in pneumonia they occur in both parts of the cycle. Laryngitis, laryngeal oedema and tracheobronchitis are common upper respiratory diseases but they are usually accompanied by a more frequent cough, the cough being readily stimulated by squeezing the larynx or trachea. The degree of toxaemia in these diseases is usually less severe than in pneumonia.

Treatment

In specific infections as listed above, isolation of affected animals and careful surveillance of the remainder of the group to detect cases in the early stages should accompany the administration of specific antibacterial drugs or biological preparations to affected animals. Supportive treatment may include the provision of oxygen if it is available, especially in the critical stages when anoxia is severe. Respiratory stimulants serve no useful purpose in pneumonia but expectorants have value in chronic cases and during convalescence. Treatment with enzymes administered parenterally may be of value in chronic bronchopneumonia, especially in cases where relapses occur because of the persistence of foci of necrosis or accumulations of bronchial exudate. Prior treatment with antibacterial drugs is recommended to avoid spread of the infection via the air passages when the exudate becomes more fluid.

Steam inhalations and hot or stimulant applications to the chest wall have limited value although the latter may ease discomfort if pleurisy is present. Affected animals should be housed in warm, well ventilated, draught-free accommodation, provided with ample fresh water, and light nourishing food. During convalescence premature return to work or exposure to inclement weather should be avoided. If the animal does not eat, oral or parenteral forcefeeding should be instituted. If fluids are given intravenously care should be exercised in the speed with which they are administered. Injection at too rapid a rate may cause over-loading of the right ventricle and death due to acute heart failure.

Aspiration Pneumonia

Aspiration or inhalation pneumonia is a common and serious disease of farm animals. Most cases occur after careless drenching or passage of a stomach tube during treatment for other illness. Even when care is taken these procedures are not without risk. Other causes include the feeding of calves and pigs on fluid feeds in inadequate troughing, inhalation occurring in the struggle for food. Dipping of sheep and cattle when they are weak, or by keeping their heads under for too long, also results in inhalation of fluid. Vomiting in ruminants and horses may be followed by aspiration especially in cattle with parturient paresis or during the passage of a stomach tube if the head is held high. Rupture of a pharyngeal abscess during palpation of the pharynx or passage of a nasal tube may cause sudden aspiration of infective material. Animals suffering from paralysis or obstruction of the larynx, pharynx or oesophagus may aspirate food or water when attempting to swallow.

Although farm animals fed on dusty feeds inhale many dust particles and bacteria which can be readily isolated from the lung, this form of infection rarely results in the development of pneumonia. Much of the dust is filtered out in the bronchial tree and does not reach the alveoli. However, this may be of importance in the production of the primary bronchiolitis which so often precedes alveolar emphysema in horses. Liquids and droplets penetrate to the depths of the alveoli and run freely into the dependent portions, and aspiration pneumonia often results. An uncommon but important effect of aspiration with lodgement of food at the glottis is the production of asphyxia or sudden death due to vagal inhibition and cessation of respiration and circulation.

If large quantities of fluid are aspirated after passage of a stomach tube into the trachea death may be almost instantaneous, but with smaller quantities the outcome may depend on the composition of the aspirated material. Absorption from the lungs is very rapid and soluble substances such as chloral hydrate and magnesium sulphate exert their systemic pharmacological effects very rapidly. With insoluble substances and vomitus the more common occurrence is the development of a pneumonia with profound toxaemia which is usually fatal in 48 to 72 hours. Signs of pneumonia, including polypnoea, cough and the presence of râles, consolidation and an associated pleuritic friction rub, are present but the latter may be localized. The severity of aspiration pneumonia depends largely upon the bacteria which are introduced although in animals the infection is usually mixed, causing in many cases an acute gangrenous pneumonia which may be manifested by a putrid odour on the breath, or extensive pulmonary suppuration. Occasionally animals survive the acute stages but persist in a state of chronic ill-health due to the presence of pulmonary abscess.

If the lesion is well advanced treatment is not often effective but treatment with a broad spectrum antibiotic or sulphonamide may prevent development of the disease if administered soon after aspiration occurs.

Pulmonary Abscess

The development of single or multiple abscesses in the lung causes a syndrome of chronic toxaemia, cough and emaciation. Suppurative bronchopneumonia may follow.

Aetiology

Infected emboli originating in other organs and localizing in the pulmonary capillaries are the most common cause of pulmonary abscess. Endocarditis, metritis, mastitis and omphalophlebitis are common primary lesions often associated with pulmonary embolism. In tuberculosis and occasionally in actinomycosis granulomatous lesions develop in the lung and simulate pulmonary abscess. Systemic mycoses may also be accompanied by pulmonary lesions but these are probably aerogenous infections. Aspiration pneumonia or penetration of the lung by a foreign body from the reticulum in cattle may also be followed by the development of pulmonary abscesses. Many bacterial pneumonias, especially contagious bovine pleuropneumonia, may be followed by sequestration in the lung.

Pathogenesis

Pulmonary abscesses may be present in many cases of pneumonia and are not recognizable clinically. In the absence of pneumonia pulmonary abscess is usually a chronic disease, clinical signs being produced by toxaemia rather than by interference with respiration. However, when the spread is haematogenous and large numbers of small abscesses develop simultaneously, polypnoea and hyperpnoea appear, caused probably by stimulation of stretch receptors in the alveolar walls or by the sudden development of extensive embolic endarteritis. In these animals the respiratory embarrassment cannot be explained by the reduction in vital capacity of the lung. However, in more chronic cases the abscesses may reach a tremendous size and cause respiratory difficulty by obliteration of large areas of lung tissue.

In many cases there is a period of chronic illness of varying degree when the necrotic focus is walled off by connective tissue. Exposure to environmental stress or other infection may result in a sudden extension from the abscess to produce a fatal, suppurative bronchopneumonia, pleurisy or empyema.

Clinical Findings

In typical cases there is dullness, anorexia, emaciation and a fall in milk yield in cattle. The temperature is usually moderately elevated and fluctuating. Coughing is marked. The cough is short and harsh and usually not accompanied by signs of pain. Respiratory signs are variable depending on the size of the lesions, and although there is usually some increase in the rate and depth this may be so slight as to escape notice. Careful auscultation and percussion will reveal the presence of a circumscribed area of dullness in which no breath sounds can be heard. Crepitant râles are often audible at the periphery of the lesion.

Multiple small abscesses may not be detectable on physical examination but the dyspnoea is usually more pronounced. There may be a purulent nasal discharge and foetid breath but these are unusual unless bronchopneumonia has developed from extension of the abscess.

Most cases progress slowly and many affected animals have to be discarded because of chronic ill health; others terminate as a bronchopneumonia or emphysema. A rare sequel is the development of hypertrophic pulmonary osteoarthropathy.

Clinical Pathology

Examination of nasal or tracheal mucus may determine the causative bacteria but the infection is usually mixed and interpretation of the bacteriological findings is difficult. Roentgenological examination in young animals can be used to detect the presence of the abscess and give some information on its size and location. Haematological examination may give an indication of the severity of the inflammatory process but the usual leucocytosis and shift to the left may not be present when the lesion is well encapsulated.

Necropsy Findings

An accumulation of necrotic material in a thick-walled, fibrous capsule is usually present in the ventral border of a lung, surrounded by a zone of bronchopneumonia or pressure atelectasis. In sheep there is often an associated emphysema. In rare cases the abscess may be sufficiently large to virtually obliterate the lung. A well encapsulated lesion may show evidence of recent rupture of the capsule and extension as an acute bronchopneumonia. Multiple small abscesses may be present when haematogenous spread has occurred.

Diagnosis

The diagnosis may not be obvious when respiratory distress is minimal and especially when multiple, small abscesses are present. These cases present a syndrome of chronic toxaemia which may be mistaken for splenic or hepatic abscess. Differentiation between tuberculous lesions and non-specific infections may require the use of the tuberculin test. Focal parasitic lesions, such as hydatid cysts, may cause a similar syndrome, but are not usually accompanied by toxaemia or haematological changes.

Treatment

Treatment is not usually successful. If the lesion is not too extensive a combination of broad spectrum antibiotics and parenteral enzymes may effect a cure. The antibiotic should be administered for several days before treatment with the enzyme is commenced.

Pulmonary Neoplasms

Primary neoplasms of the lungs, including carcinomas and adenocarcinomas, are rare in animals (1, 2, 4) and metastatic tumours also are relatively uncommon in large animals. An asymptomatic, squamous-cell type tumour, thought to be a benign papilloma, has been observed in 10 of a series of 1600 adult angora goats (3). The lesions were mostly in the diaphragmatic lobes, were multiple in 50 per cent of the cases and showed no evidence of malignancy although some had necrotic centres. Six cases of 'granular-cell myoblastoma' have been reported in horses, none of whom showed any clinical signs of illness (5). Malignant melanomas in adult grey horses and lymphomatosis in young cattle may be accompanied by pulmonary localization. Clinical findings are those usually associated with a decrease in vital capacity of the lungs, and include dyspnoea which develops gradually, cough and evidence of local consolidation on percussion and auscultation. There is no fever or toxaemia and a neoplasm may be mistaken for a chronic, encapsulated, pulmonary abscess. In the latter there may be no evidence of inflammation, and the total and differential white cell counts may be normal.

Thymoma is not uncommon in cattle and may resemble pulmonary neoplasm but there is usually displacement and compression of the heart resulting in displacement of the apex beat and congestive heart failure. The presence of jugular engorgement, ventral oedema, tachycardia, chronic tympany and hydropericardium may cause a mistaken diagnosis of traumatic pericarditis. Mediastinal tumour or abscess may have a similar effect. Metastasis to the bronchial lymph nodes may cause obstruction of the oesophagus with dysphagia, and in cattle chronic ruminal tympany.

REFERENCES
(1) Monlux, A. W. et al. (1956). *Amer. J. vet. Res.*, *17*, 646.
(2) Cotchin, E. (1956). *Neoplasms of the Domesticated Animals*, Commonwealth Agric. Bureau, Farnham Royal, Bucks.
(3) Pearson, E. G. (1961). *Cornell Vet.*, *51*, 13.
(4) Swoboda, R. (1964). *Path. vet.*, *1*, 409.
(5) Misdorp, W. & Gelder, H. L. N. (1968). *Path. vet.*, *5*, 385.

DISEASES OF THE PLEURA

Hydrothorax and Haemothorax

The accumulation of oedematous transudate or whole blood in the pleural sacs is manifested by respiratory embarrassment caused by collapse of the ventral parts of the lungs.

Aetiology

Hydrothorax accompanies general oedema caused by congestive heart failure and hypo-proteinaemia or may occur independently in lymphomatosis in cattle. Chylous hydrothorax caused by rupture of the thoracic lymph duct is rare. Haemothorax is also rare and occurs when pleural adhesions are ruptured or there is traumatic injury to the chest wall.

Pathogenesis

Accumulation of fluid in the pleural sac causes compression atelectasis of the ventral portions of the lungs and the degree of atelectasis governs the severity of the resulting dyspnoea. Compression of the atria by fluid may cause an increase in venous pressure in the great veins.

Clinical Findings

In both diseases there is an absence of systemic signs although acute haemorrhagic anaemia may be present when extensive bleeding occurs in the pleural cavity. There is dyspnoea, which usually develops gradually, and an absence of breath sounds accompanied by dullness on percussion over the lower parts of the chest. These conditions are always bilateral in the horse but may be unilateral in other species, causing an absence of movement of the ribs on the affected side. In thin animals the intercostal spaces may be observed to bulge. If sufficient fluid is present it may cause compression of the atria, engorgement of the jugular veins, and a jugular pulse of increased amplitude may be present. The cardiac embarrassment is not usually sufficiently severe to cause congestive heart failure although this disease may already be present.

Clinical Pathology

Thoracic puncture will be followed by a flow of clear serous fluid in hydrothorax, or blood in recent cases of haemothorax. The fluid is bacteriologically negative but may contain protein.

Necropsy Findings

In animals which die of acute haemorrhagic anaemia resulting from haemothorax, the pleural cavity is filled with blood which usually has not clotted, the clot having been broken down by the constant respiratory movement. Hydrothorax is not usually fatal but is a common accompaniment of other diseases which are evidenced by their specific necropsy findings.

Diagnosis

Hydrothorax and haemothorax can be differentiated from pleurisy by the absence of pain, toxaemia and fever and by the sterility of an aspirated fluid sample. Other space-occupying lesions of the thorax, including tumours, are not characterized by an accumulation of fluid unless the tumours have implanted on the pleura.

Treatment

Treatment of the primary condition is necessary. If the dyspnoea is severe, aspiration of fluid from the pleural sac causes a temporary improvement but the fluid usually reaccumulates rapidly. Parenteral coagulants and blood transfusion are rational treatments in severe haemothorax.

Pneumothorax

Entry of air into the pleural cavity in sufficient quantity causes collapse of the lung and respiratory embarrassment.

Aetiology

Puncture of the chest wall from the exterior by a sharp foreign body or rupture of the lung are common causes. Rupture of the lung may occur when it is pierced by the sharp end of a broken rib, or it may occur spontaneously. Coughing and exercise are common precipitating causes but prior pulmonary or pleural lesions causing weakness of the parenchymal stroma are probably important predisposing causes. Bullae of emphysema are the common sites at which rupture occurs.

Pathogenesis

Pneumothorax is unilateral except in the horse. Collapse of the lung on the affected side occurs because of the absence of negative pressure in the pleural sac. The degree of collapse varies with the amount of air which enters the cavity, small amounts being absorbed very quickly but large amounts may cause fatal anoxia. Haemothorax may occur simultaneously and pleurisy is a common sequel.

Clinical Findings

There is an acute onset of inspiratory dyspnoea which may terminate fatally within a few minutes in the horse. If the collapse occurs in only one pleural sac, the rib cage on the affected side collapses and shows decreased movement. There is a compensatory increase in movement and bulging of the chest wall on the unaffected side. On auscultation there is complete absence of the normal vesicular murmur but bronchial tones are still audible over the base of the lung. The mediastinum bulges toward the unaffected side and may cause moderate displacement of the heart and the apex beat. The heart sounds on the affected side have a metallic note and the apex beat may be absent. On percussion of the thorax on the affected side the sound is metallic rather than tympanitic. The same sound can be heard with auscultatory percussion.

The entry of air into the sac usually ceases within a short time and the air is absorbed, the lung returning to its normal functional state. The introduction of infection at the time of injury usually causes a serious pleurisy.

Clinical Pathology

Laboratory examinations are of no assistance in diagnosis but roentgenological examination of animals of suitable size shows displacement of the mediastinum and heart, and collapse of the lung.

Necropsy Findings

The lung in the affected sac is collapsed. In cases where spontaneous rupture occurs there is discontinuity of the pleura usually over an emphysematous bulla. Haemothorax may also be evident.

Diagnosis

The clinical findings are usually diagnostic. Diaphragmatic hernia may cause similar clinical signs in small animals but is relatively rare in farm animals. In cattle herniation is usually associated with traumatic reticulitis and is not usually manifested by respiratory distress. Large herniae with entry of liver, stomach and intestines cause respiratory embarrassment, a tympanitic note on percussion and audible peristaltic sounds on auscultation. Roentgenological examination is of value in differentiation if the animal is sufficiently small.

Treatment

Closure of a thoracic wound by surgical means prevents further entrance of air but little can be done when internal laceration or rupture of the lung occurs. The animal should be kept as quiet as possible and permitted no exercise. Prophylactic treatment to avoid the development of pleurisy is advisable.

Diaphragmatic Hernia

Diaphragmatic hernia is rare in farm animals. It occurs in cattle, especially in association with traumatic reticuloperitonitis. Here the hernia is small and causes no respiratory distress, nor are there abnormal sounds in the chest. Occasional cases of acquired hernia not caused by foreign body perforation also occur in cattle and horses (3). In horses colic and dyspnoea are recorded as prominent signs. The presence of intestinal sounds in the thorax can be misleading; they are often present in the normal animal, but their presence, accompanied by dyspnoea and resonance on percussion, should arouse suspicion. Radiological examination is recommended to confirm the diagnosis. Congenital herniae occur in all species. In affected animals abdominal viscera including liver, stomach and intestines, enter the thorax and dyspnoea is evident at birth. In some cases the pericardial sac is incomplete and the diaphragm is rudimentary and in the form of a small fold projecting from the chest wall (1). Affected animals usually survive for a few hours to several weeks. In pigs a number of animals in each litter may be affected (2).

REFERENCES

(1) Horney, F. D. & Cote, J. (1961). *Canad. vet. J.*, 2, 422.
(2) Griffin, R. M. (1965). *Vet. Rec.*, 77, 492.
(3) Sasse, H. H. L. & Kalsbeek, H. C. (1965). *T. Diergeneesk.*, 90, 1327.

Pleurisy

Acute inflammation of the pleura causes pain during respiratory movements, manifested clinically by shallow, rapid respiration. Subacute inflammation is accompanied by empyema causing collapse of the lung and respiratory embarrassment. Chronic pleurisy is usually manifested by the development of fibrous adhesions and minor interference with respiratory movement.

Aetiology

Primary pleurisy occurs rarely and is due usually to traumatic perforation of the thoracic wall. It is more commonly a part of specific diseases including Glasser's disease of swine, contagious bovine pleuropneumonia, pleuropneumonia of sheep and goats, pneumonia caused by *Pasteurella multocida* and *P. haemolytica* in all species, sporadic bovine encephalomyelitis and tuberculosis of cattle. Pleurisy also occurs sporadically as a late sign in many other bacterial pneumonias or in pulmonary abscess when there is spread from the pulmonary parenchyma. In horses this occurs most commonly in infectious equine pneumonia and strangles. Perforation of the diaphragm by a sharp foreign body may cause pleurisy as a sequel to traumatic reticuloperitonitis of cattle. Spread via the lymphatics through the diaphragm may also occur from a primary peritonitis without traumatic perforation.

Pathogenesis

In the early, acute, dry stage of pleurisy contact and movement between the parietal and visceral pleurae causes pain due to stimulation of pain end-organs in the pleura. Respiratory movements are restricted and the respiration is rapid and shallow. The second stage of pleurisy is characterized by the production of serofibrinous inflammatory exudate which collects in the pleural sacs and causes collapse of the ventral parts of the lungs, thus reducing vital capacity and interfering with gaseous exchange. If the accumulation is sufficiently severe there may be pressure on the atria and a damming back of blood in the great veins. Clinical signs may be restricted to one side of the chest in all species with an imperforate mediastinum. In the third stage the fluid is resorbed and adhesions develop, restricting movement of the lungs and chest wall but interference with respiratory exchange is usually minor and disappears gradually as the adhesions stretch with continuous movement.

In all bacterial pleuritides there is an element of toxaemia caused by toxins produced by the bacteria and by tissue breakdown. The toxaemia may be severe when large amounts of pus accumulate.

Clinical Findings

In the early stages the respirations are rapid and shallow and the animal shows evidence of pain and anxiety. Respiratory movements are markedly abdominal and movement of the chest wall is restricted. The animal stands with its elbows abducted and is disinclined to move. On auscultation pleuritic friction sounds are audible. These have a continuous to and fro character, are dry and abrasive, and do not abate with coughing. They may be difficult to identify if there is a coincident pneumonia accompanied by râles and increased vesicular murmur. When the pleurisy involves the pleural surface of the pericardial sac a friction rub may be heard with each cardiac cycle and be confused with the friction rub of pericarditis. However, there is usually in addition a rub synchronous with respiratory movements and the pericardial rub waxes and wanes with expiration and inspiration. Pressure on the chest usually causes pain. The temperature and pulse rate are usually elevated, the degree varying with the virulence of the causative agent. Toxaemia, with anorexia and depression, is also present in most cases.

As exudation causes separation of the inflamed pleural surfaces the pain and friction rub diminish but do not completely disappear. The respiratory rate decreases but is still above normal. On auscultation there may still be friction sounds but they are less evident and usually localized to small areas. Fluid sounds may be audible especially if the animal is shaken or moves. There is dullness on percussion, the dull area having a level topline, and percussion sounds are transmitted clearly through the fluid. Dyspnoea is evident, particularly during inspiration, and a pleuritic ridge develops at the costal arch due to elevation of the ribs and the abdominal-type respiration. If the pleurisy is unilateral movement of the affected side of the chest is restricted as compared to the normal side. Pain is still evident on percussion or deep palpation of the chest and the animal still stands with its elbows abducted, is disinclined to lie down or move but is not as apprehensive as in the early stages. Toxaemia is often more severe during this stage, the temperature is usually high, the pulse rate is increased and the animal eats poorly. Cough is usually present because of the concurrent pneumonia and is painful, short and shallow. Extension of the inflammation to the pericardium may occur. Death may occur at any time and is due to a combination of toxaemia and anoxia caused by pressure atelectasis.

Animals that recover do so slowly. The toxaemia usually disappears first but residual respiratory embarrassment of moderate degree remains for some time because of the presence of adhesions. Rupture of the adhesions during severe exertion may cause fatal haemothorax. Some impairment of respiratory function can be expected to persist and racing animals do not usually regain complete efficiency. Chronic pleurisy, such as that which occurs in tuberculosis in cattle, is usually symptomless, no acute inflammation or fluid exudation occurring.

Clinical Pathology

Thoracic puncture can be used to obtain a sample of the inflammatory fluid for bacteriological examination and determination of the sensitivity of the causative bacteria. Roentgenological examination may reveal the presence of fluid displacement of the mediastinum and heart to the unaffected side and collapse of the lung.

Necropsy Findings

In early acute pleurisy there is marked oedema, thickening and hyperaemia of the pleura, with engorgement of small vessels and the presence of tags and shreds of fibrin. These can be most readily seen between the lobes of the lung. In the exudative stage the pleural cavity contains an excessive quantity of turbid fluid containing flakes and clots of fibrin. The pleura is thickened and the ventral parts of the lung collapsed and dark red in colour. A concurrent pneumonia is usually present and there may be an associated pericarditis. In the later healing stages adhesions connect the parietal and visceral pleurae.

Diagnosis

Identification of pleurisy depends upon the presence of a friction rub or inflammatory exudate in the pleural sac. Pleurisy usually occurs in conjunction with pneumonia and differentiation is difficult and often unnecessary. The râles of pneumonia are less distinct and abrasive, and fluctuate with coughing. Emphysema, especially when bullae are present under the pleura, may be manifested by a friction rub but loud crepitant and sibilant râles are present and the dyspnoea has a characteristic prolongation of expiration. In pleurisy the dyspnoea is largely inspiratory. A tympanitic note on percussion is typical of emphysema, dullness on percussion is typical of pleurisy, and fever and toxaemia usually accompany the latter.

Hydrothorax and haemothorax are not usually accompanied by fever or toxaemia and pain and pleuritic friction sounds are not present. Aspiration of fluid by needle puncture can be attempted if doubt exists. Pulmonary congestion and oedema are manifested by increased vesicular murmur and ventral consolidation without hydrothorax or pleural inflammation.

Treatment

The primary aim of treatment is to control the infection in the pleural sac. This is best achieved by the parenteral or oral administration of antibiotics or sulphonamides, the choice of drug preferably being dictated by bacteriological examination of the pleuritic exudate. When the amount of fluid present is excessive aspiration may cause temporary improvement and the antibacterial agent can be injected directly into the pleural sac. Aspiration is not easy as the drainage needle or cannula tends to become blocked with fibrin, and respiratory movements may result in laceration of the lung. Diuretics are unlikely to aid in the removal of this or any other inflammatory exudate.

Supportive treatment includes the use of mustard plasters or hot blankets to the chest. These may have little effect on healing but they ease discomfort during the acute stages. The administration of ataractic drugs or other analgesics may also be of value in relieving the animal's distress at this time. The injection into the pleural sac of material designed to prevent the formation of adhesions is largely impractical and may interfere with healing. When empyema is present the simultaneous administration of antibiotics plus parenteral enzymes, combined with drainage by an indwelling catheter or repeated needle puncture may hasten recovery.

DISEASES OF THE UPPER RESPIRATORY TRACT

Rhinitis

Acute rhinitis is characterized by sneezing, difficult, stertorous respiration and a serous or mucoid nasal discharge. The discharge becomes more purulent in chronic inflammations.

Aetiology

Rhinitis usually occurs in conjunction with inflammation of other parts of the respiratory tract. It is present as a minor lesion in most bacterial and viral pneumonias but the diseases listed are those in which it occurs as an obvious and important part of the syndrome.

Bacterial causes. Rhinitis is an important lesion in glanders and strangles in horses, necrotic rhinitis of pigs and melioidosis in sheep.

Viral causes. Ulcerative or erosive rhinitis is characteristic of bovine malignant catarrh, mucosal disease and rinderpest of cattle. Catarrhal rhinitis occurs in infectious bovine rhinotracheitis, in equine viral rhinopneumonitis and equine viral arteritis, bluetongue in sheep, and in swine influenza and inclusion body rhinitis of swine. Spread of lesions into the nasal cavities may occur in malignant cases of contagious ecthyma and the poxes.

Fungal causes. Rhinitis affecting the anterior nares is common in epizootic lymphangitis of horses, and rhinosporidiosis of cattle is manifested chiefly by rhinitis.

Metazoan causes. Infestation with the blood fluke *Schistosoma nasalis* in cattle, and larvae of the nasal botfly, *Oestrus ovis*, in sheep are accompanied by rhinitis.

Allergic rhinitis. Although the cause is not well defined the clinical syndrome of 'summer snuffles' in cattle is thought to be allergic in origin. A similar condition has also been observed in sheep.

Rhinitis caused by unknown agents. Atrophic rhinitis of swine and muzzle disease of cattle are important specific diseases in which rhinitis occurs.

Pathogenesis

Rhinitis is of minor importance as a disease process except in severe cases when it causes obstruction of the passage of air through the nasal cavities. Its major importance is as an indication of the presence of some specific diseases. The type of lesion produced is important. The erosive and ulcerative lesions of rinderpest, bovine malignant catarrh and mucosal disease, the ulcerative lesions of glanders, melioidosis and epizootic lymphangitis and the granular rhinitis of the anterior nares in allergic rhinitis all have diagnostic significance.

In atrophic rhinitis of pigs the destruction of the turbinate bones and distortion of the face appear to be a form of devitalization and atrophy of bone caused by a primary, inflammatory rhinitis. Secondary bacterial invasion of facial tissues of swine appears to be the basis of necrotic rhinitis.

Clinical Findings

The cardinal sign in rhinitis is a nasal discharge which is usually serous initially but soon becomes mucoid and, in bacterial infections, purulent. Erythema, erosion or ulceration may be visible on inspection. The inflammation may be unilateral or bilateral. Sneezing is characteristic in the early acute stages and this is followed in the later stages by snorting and the expulsion of large amounts of mucopurulent discharge.

'Summer snuffles' of cattle presents a characteristic syndrome. Cases occur in the spring and autumn when the pasture is in flower and are most common in Channel Island breeds. There is a sudden onset of dyspnoea with a profuse nasal discharge of thick, orange to yellow material which varies from a mucopurulent to caseous consistency. Sneezing, irritation and obstruction are severe. The irritation may cause the animal to shake its head, rub its nose along the ground or poke its muzzle repeatedly into hedges and bushes. Sticks and twigs may be pushed up into the nostrils as a result and cause laceration and bleeding. Stertorous, difficult respiration, accompanied by mouth breathing may be evident when both nostrils are obstructed. In the most severe cases a distinct pseudomembrane is formed which is later snorted out as a complete nasal cast. In the chronic stages multiple nodules about 1 cm. in diameter are present in the anterior nares.

Clinical Pathology

Examination of nasal swabs or scrapings for bacteria, inclusion bodies or fungi may aid in diagnosis. Discharges in allergic rhinitis usually contain many more eosinophils than normal.

Necropsy Findings

Rhinitis is not a fatal condition although animals may die of specific diseases in which rhinitis is a prominent lesion.

Diagnosis

Rhinitis is readily recognizable on clinical grounds. Differentiation of the specific diseases listed under aetiology above is discussed under their respective headings. Rhinitis may be confused with inflammation of the facial sinuses or guttural pouches in the horse in which the nasal discharge is usually purulent and persistent and often unilateral, and there is an absence of signs of nasal irritation.

Treatment

Specific treatment aimed at control of individual causative agents is described under the specific diseases. Medicated inhalations comprising 1 oz. of turpentine, eucalyptus oil or creolin in 2 gallons of boiling water or nasal irrigation with weak solutions of antiseptics may temporarily alleviate discomfort. Animals affected with allergic rhinitis should be taken off the pasture for about a week and treated with antihistamine preparations.

Obstruction of the Nasal Cavities

Nasal obstruction does not occur commonly in farm animals unless caused by acute rhinitis. Large mucus-filled polyps may develop in the posterior nares of cattle and sheep and cause unilateral or bilateral obstruction. Granulomatous lesions caused by a fungus, *Rhinosporidium* spp. and by the blood fluke, *Schistosoma nasalis* may cause chronic obstruction. Foreign bodies may enter the cavities when cattle rub their muzzles in bushes in an attempt to relieve the irritation of acute allergic rhinitis. Neoplasms of the olfactory mucosa are not common but do occur, particularly in sheep in which the incidence in individual flocks may be sufficiently high to suggest an infectious cause (1, 2). The lesions are usually situated just in front of the ethmoid bone, are usually unilateral but may be bilateral and have the appearance of adenocarcinomas of moderate malignancy.

In cattle and pigs there is severe inspiratory dyspnoea when both cavities are blocked. The animals may show great distress and anxiety and breathe in gasps through the mouth. Obstruction is usually not complete and a loud, wheezing sound occurs with each inspiration. A nasal discharge is usually present but varies from a small amount of blood-stained serous discharge when there is a foreign body present, to large quantities of purulent exudate in allergic rhinitis. Shaking of the head and snorting are also common signs. If the obstruction is unilateral the distress is not so marked and the difference in breath streams between the two nostrils can be detected by holding the hands in front of the nose. The signs may be intermittent when the obstruction is caused by a pedunculated polyp in the posterior nares.

Treatment must be directed at the primary cause of the obstruction. Removal of foreign bodies can usually be effected with the aid of long forceps although strong traction is often necessary when the obstructions have been in position for a few days. As an empirical treatment in cattle oral or parenteral administration of iodine preparations is in general use in chronic nasal obstruction.

REFERENCES

(1) Young, S. *et al.* (1961). *Cornell Vet.*, *51*, 96.
(2) Dunan, J. R. *et al.* (1967). *J. Amer. vet. med. Ass.*, *151*, 732.

Epistaxis

Epistaxis or nosebleed is in most instances caused by disease of the mucosae of the upper respiratory tract. Erosion of the mucosa occurs in glanders and in granulomatous and neoplastic lesions in the nasal cavities. Local trauma may be caused by passage of a stomach tube via the nostril, by the entry of foreign bodies in acute allergic rhinitis or by accidental injury to the facial bones. Small amounts of blood may be discharged from the nostrils in purpuric diseases, including purpura haemorrhagica, sweet clover poisoning, bracken fern poisoning and in congestive heart failure. An important occurrence of epistaxis is that which occurs in horses while racing (1, 2). Affected horses stop running immediately and may cause serious accidents by interference with other horses. In severe cases the animal may bleed to death. The cause of the condition is unknown, but it tends to affect young horses which often shake off the tendency as they grow older. It has been suggested that many cases are due to guttural pouch mycosis (3, 4). In some instances a deficiency of platelets leading to thrombocytopenia has been observed with apparent improvement following steroid therapy (5).

REFERENCES

(1) Pfaff, G. (1950). *J. S. Afr. vet. med. Ass.*, *21*, 74.
(2) Scott, M. L. (1953). *Vet. Med.*, *48*, 95.
(3) Boucher, W. B. *et al.* (1964). *J. Amer. vet. med. Ass.*, *145*, 1004.
(4) Cook, W. R. (1968). *Vet. Rec.*, *83*, 336, 422.
(5) Franco, D. A. (1969). *Vet. Med. small Anim. Clin.*, *64*, 1071.

Laryngitis, Tracheitis, Bronchitis

Inflammation of the air passages usually involves all levels and no attempt is made here to differentiate between inflammations of various parts of the tract. They are all characterized by cough, by noisy inspiration and some degree of inspiratory embarrassment.

Aetiology

All infections of the upper respiratory tract cause inflammation, either acutely or as chronic diseases. In most diseases the laryngitis, tracheitis and bronchitis form only a part of the syndrome and the causes listed below are those diseases in which upper respiratory infection is a prominent feature.

Cattle. Infectious bovine rhinotracheitis, and calf diphtheria are the common causes in cattle. A congenital cavitation of the arytenoid is suspected as having contributed to a series of cases of laryngeal abscess in calves (2).

Sheep. Chronic laryngitis caused by infection with *Corynebacterium pyogenes* has been observed in sheep (1).

Horse. Equine viral rhinopneumonitis, equine viral arteritis, infectious equine bronchitis and strangles are all characterized by upper respiratory infection.

Pigs. Upper respiratory infection occurs commonly only in swine influenza in this species.

Pathogenesis

Irritation of the mucosa causes frequent coughing, and swelling causes partial obstruction of the air passages with resulting inspiratory dyspnoea.

Clinical Findings

Cough is the cardinal sign. It is short, dry and harsh in acute affections and is easily induced by pinching the trachea or larynx, or by exposure to cold air or dusty atmospheres. In chronic affections the cough is less frequent and distressing and is usually dry and harsh. If the lesions cause much exudation or ulceration of the mucosa the cough is moist and in the latter case is very painful, the animal making obvious attempts to suppress it.

Inspiratory dyspnoea varies with the degree of obstruction and is usually accompanied by stertor and loud, coarse râles or dry respiratory sounds on each inspiration. These are best heard over the trachea although they are quite audible over the base of the lung, being most distinct on inspiration. The respiratory movements are usually deeper than normal and the inspiratory phase more prolonged and forceful. Additional signs, indicative of the presence of a primary specific disease, may also be present. Laryngoscopic examination is not usually possible without general anaesthesia. Secondary bacterial infection of primary viral diseases, or extension of bacterial infections to the lungs commonly results in pneumonia.

Clinical Pathology

Laboratory examinations may be of value in determining the presence of specific diseases.

Necropsy Findings

Upper respiratory infections are not usually fatal but lesions vary from acute catarrhal inflammation to chronic granulomatous lesions depending upon the duration and severity of the infection. When secondary bacterial invasion occurs a diphtheritic pseudo-membrane may be present and be accompanied by an accumulation of exudate and necrotic material at the tracheal bifurcation and in the dependent bronchi.

Diagnosis

The diagnosis depends on the presence of cough, inspiratory dyspnoea and increased pulmonary sounds during inspiration. Differentiation from pneumonia, especially viral pneumonia, may be difficult if râles are absent and abnormal pulmonary sounds consist solely of bronchial tones. Differentiation is usually necessary in terms of the specific diseases. Obstruction of the upper respiratory tract due to other causes may also be difficult to distinguish unless other signs are present.

Treatment

Treatment of the primary disease is most important. Prevention of exposure to cold air, inclement weather or a dusty atmosphere is essential. Affected animals should not be worked. Treatment with expectorants as discussed under principles of treatment may reduce the distress of the animal and facilitate healing. The administration of antibiotics in the drinking water or topically by a special pharyngeal spray is currently a popular treatment. A combination of dexamethasone and antibiotic therapy is reported to be of value in chronic cases in horses (3).

REFERENCES

(1) Salisbury, R. M. (1956). *N.Z. vet. J.*, *4*, 144.
(2) Lawrence, J. A. (1967). *Vet. Rec.*, *81*, 540.
(3) Gerber, H. (1968). *Schweiz. Arch. Tierheilk.*, *110*, 139.

Obstruction of the Upper Respiratory Tract

Oedema of the larynx may occur as part of an allergic syndrome or because of the inhalation of smoke or fumes and cause upper respiratory tract obstruction. The oedema which occurs in gut oedema of swine is usually not sufficiently severe to do this. Acute cellulitis of the throat (pharyngeal phlegmon) and anthrax in horses and pigs commonly cause acute peripharyngeal cellulitis and oedema. Swelling is readily visible from the exterior and is accompanied by a high fever and profound toxaemia. Obstruction may occur accidentally when cattle or horses vomit and solid food material lodges in the larynx or when sharp pointed foreign bodies lodge in the region of the pharynx or larynx. A specific form of obstruction in sheep is caused by chronic laryngitis associated with a *Corynebacterium pyogenes* infection. Partial obstruction of the larynx during exercise occurs in unilateral paralysis of the vocal cords (roaring) in horses. One of the most important causes of nasal obstruction in farm animals is enzootic nasal granuloma which is discussed under that heading.

Clinically there is marked inspiratory dyspnoea with forceful prolonged elevation of the ribs and sinking of the flanks. Distress is often evident and cyanosis may be marked. Mouth-breathing, respiratory stridor, salivation and extension of the head are prominent signs and manipulation of the head or exercise may cause fatal asphyxia.

Auscultation of the larynx reveals loud, stenotic sounds and fremitus may be detectable on palpa-

tion. Tracheotomy or laryngotomy may be necessary to prevent fatal asphyxia until the obstruction subsides or is relieved.

10

Diseases of the Urinary System

INTRODUCTION

DISEASES of the bladder and urethra are more common and more important in farm animals than diseases of the kidneys but some discussion of renal insufficiency is necessary because of the sporadic cases of pyelonephritis, embolic nephritis, amyloidosis and nephrosis that occur in these species. A knowledge of the physiology of urinary secretion and excretion is also required for a proper understanding of diseases of the bladder and urethra. The principles of renal insufficiency as set out below are derived largely from human medicine and although they probably apply in general terms to farm animals the details of renal function and failure in these animals have not been extensively examined. In the section on manifestations of renal insufficiency only those abnormalities which are known to occur in farm animals are discussed.

Principles of Renal Insufficiency

The two functions of the kidneys are to excrete the end products of tissue metabolism (except for carbon dioxide), and to maintain homeostasis with respect to fluids and solutes by selective excretion of these substances. This latter function is controlled by the capacity of the kidney to vary the volume of fluid excreted and the concentration of solutes. This capacity is dependent upon the functional activity of the tubules while control of excretion of metabolic end products is vested in the glomeruli. Glomerular filtrate is derived from plasma by a process of simple filtration and is identical with it except that it contains little protein or lipids. The absolute volume of filtrate, and therefore its content of metabolic end products, depends upon the hydrostatic pressure and the plasma osmotic pressure in the glomerular capillaries and the proportion of glomeruli which are functional. These factors are not under the control of renal mechanisms and in the absence of disease the rate of filtration through the glomeruli varies little.

It is the function of the tubules actively to reabsorb from the glomerular filtrate those substances which need to be retained for utilization and participation in metabolic processes, while permitting the excretion of waste products. The retention of water by reabsorption in the proximal tubules is the main means whereby control of water homeostasis is achieved. As a result the concentration of solutes in the urine varies widely when the kidneys are functioning normally. The principal mechanism which governs reabsorption of water is the antidiuretic hormone of the posterior pituitary gland, the secretion of which is stimulated by tissue dehydration and an increase in effective osmotic pressure of the tissue fluid. This control is not limitless, functioning only within a restricted range, and can be overcome by the use of diuretics whereby the flow of urine is so increased that maximum tubular reabsorption cannot sufficiently reduce the volume. Thus, an animal in a state of dehydration can be still further dehydrated by the use of diuretics. The tubular epithelium also selectively reabsorbs the solutes in the glomerular filtrate. Glucose is reabsorbed entirely, within the normal range of blood levels; phosphate is reabsorbed in varying amounts depending upon the needs of the body to conserve it; other substances such as inorganic sulphates and creatinine are not reabsorbed at all.

Disease of the kidneys, and in some instances of the ureters, bladder and urethra, reduce the efficiency of these two functions and causes disturbances in protein, solute and water homeostasis and in the excretion of metabolic end products. A relative loss of function is described as renal insufficiency, complete or fatal loss as renal failure.

RENAL INSUFFICIENCY AND RENAL FAILURE

Renal efficiency depends upon the functional integrity of the individual nephrons, and insufficiency can occur because of abnormality in the rate of renal blood flow, the glomerular filtration rate, and the efficiency of tubular reabsorption. Of these the latter two are those which are intrinsic functions of the kidney, the first depending largely upon vaso-motor control and in animals is affected only by emergencies in circulatory dynamics such as shock, dehydration and haemorrhage. Although in these diseases there may be a serious reduction in glomerular filtration the cause is extrarenal and cannot be considered as a true cause of renal insufficiency. However tubular necrosis may follow prolonged renal ischaemia and cause renal insufficiency.

Glomerular filtration and tubular reabsorption may be affected independently of each other in disease states such as haemoglobinuric nephrosis, where glomerular filtration is unaffected but tubular reabsorption is seriously depressed. However, because of the common blood supply of the glomerulus and tubule, damage to any part of the nephron is followed by damage to the remaining parts and it is probably more accurate to think in terms of loss of entire nephrons rather than loss of tubular or glomerular function. At least this is true when the prognosis in a particular case is under discussion. Even when there is loss of entire nephrons rather than selective depression of tubular function, the end result may be the same because of disproportionate compensatory response on the part of the residual nephrons, resulting in an imbalance of glomerular and tubular functions. The progress and the end result of renal disease of any kind thus tend to be very similar. In glomerulonephritis the primary reaction is glomerular but a secondary involvement of the tubules occurs. In nephrosis the primary lesion is in the tubules and in interstitial nephritis tubular degeneration is probably the primary and major lesion but glomerular dysfunction commonly follows.

The development of renal dysfunction is dependent upon the loss of functional renal tissue. If the degree of loss, and therefore the degree of dysfunction, is such that the animal can survive its state can be described as one of renal insufficiency. If the degree of loss is so great that the animal's continued existence is not possible it is said to be in a state of renal failure and the clinical syndrome of uraemia is manifest.

In contrast to the degree of renal dysfunction there is the concept of the form of the insufficiency. The form, including the clinical and clinico-pathological manifestations of the dysfunction, depends upon the anatomical location of the lesion and thus upon the imbalance of residual function between glomeruli and tubules. Renal dysfunction tends to be a dynamic process and the degree and form of the dysfunction are likely to vary from time to time.

Pathologic Physiology of Renal Insufficiency

Damage to the glomerular epithelium permits the passage of plasma proteins into the capsular fluid. The protein is principally albumin, probably because it has a smaller molecule than globulin. Complete cessation of glomerular filtration may occur when there is extensive damage to glomeruli, particularly if there is acute swelling of the kidney, but it is believed that in many instances the anuria of the terminal stages of acute renal disease is caused by back diffusion of all glomerular filtrate through the damaged tubular epithelium. When the kidney damage is of a less severe degree, the compensatory response on the part of residual nephrons is to maintain total glomerular filtration by an increase in filtration per nephron. This may be in excess of the capacity of the tubular epithelium to reabsorb fluid and solutes and achieve normal urine concentration, and therefore urine of a constant specific gravity and daily volume passes into the renal pelvis. This defect may be further exaggerated if there is tubular damage. It is this lack of ability to concentrate urine (isosthenuria), in spite of variations in fluid and electrolyte intake, which is characteristic of developing renal insufficiency.

Loss of glomerular filtration is also reflected by a retention in the blood of urea and other nitrogenous end products of metabolism. Although blood levels of urea are probably not significant in the production of clinical signs they are used as a measure of glomerular filtration rate. Phosphate and sulphate retention also occurs when total glomerular filtration is reduced and may precipitate renal acidosis. Phosphate retention also causes a secondary hypocalcaemia, due in part to an increase in calcium excretion in the urine. Variations in serum potassium levels also occur and appear to depend largely on potassium intake. Hyperpotassaemia is a serious complication in renal insufficiency in man and is one of the principal causes of the myocardial asthenia and fatal heart failure which occurs in uraemia in this species.

Loss of tubular reabsorptive function is evidenced by a continued loss of sodium and a resultant hyponatraemia which eventually occurs in all cases of nephritis. The continued loss of large quantities of fluid in the poorly concentrated urine may cause clinical dehydration but more commonly puts the patient in a position of being particularly susceptible to further fluid loss or to shock or other circulatory emergency.

The Pathogenesis of Renal Failure

The terminal stage of renal insufficiency—renal failure—is the result of the accumulated effects of disturbed renal excretory and homeostatic functions. Continued excretion of large volumes of urine of low concentration causes a degree of dehydration, and if other circulatory emergencies arise acute renal ischaemia results, and is followed by acute renal failure. Hypoproteinaemia may be prolonged and results in rapid loss of body condition and muscle weakness. Acidosis is also a contributing factor. Hyponatraemia and hyperpotassaemia cause skeletal muscle weakness and myocardial asthenia. The hypocalcaemia may be of sufficient degree further to increase circulatory failure and contribute to nervous signs. All of these factors play some part in the production of clinical signs. In some cases one or other of them may be of major importance and the clinical syndrome is therefore subject to a great deal of variation.

Renal failure is manifested by the clinical state of uraemia which can also occur in urinary tract obstruction. It is characterized biochemically by an increase in blood levels of total and urea nitrogen (azotaemia) and by retention of other solutes as described above.

Causes of Renal Insufficiency and Uraemia

The causes of renal insufficiency, and therefore of renal failure and uraemia, can be divided into pre-renal and renal groups. Pre-renal causes include congestive heart failure and acute circulatory failure, either cardiac or peripheral, in which acute renal ischaemia occurs. Haemoglobinuric and myoglobinuric nephrosis are also included in this category. Renal causes include glomerulonephritis, interstitial nephritis, pyelonephritis, embolic nephritis and amyloidosis.

Uraemia may also occur due to post-renal causes, specifically complete obstruction of the urinary tract by vesical or urethral calculus or more rarely by bilateral ureteral obstruction. Internal rupture of any part of the urinary tract will have the same effect.

Principal Manifestations of Urinary Tract Disease

The principal manifestations of disease of the urinary tract include abnormal constituents of the urine, abnormalities of volume, pain and dysuria, rupture of the renal pelvis, bladder and urethra, and defects of nervous control of the bladder.

ABNORMAL CONSTITUENTS OF THE URINE

Proteinuria. Normal urine contains very small amounts of protein derived from desquamating epithelial cells but the amount is insufficient to produce a positive reaction to standard tests for proteinuria. One exception to this rule is the proteinuria observed in normal calves up to 40 hours old if they have received colostrum and in newborn kids and lambs (3). Protein may be present in appreciable amounts in haemoglobinuria, myoglobinuria, and haematuria and when the sample contains necrotic material from the urinary tract. These possibilities should be eliminated as causes before a diagnosis of renal disease is made.

Proteinuria, often designated as albuminuria because of the high proportion of albumin present, occurs in congestive heart failure, glomerulonephritis, renal infarction, nephrosis and amyloidosis. It is also a common finding in cows affected by the 'downer cow' syndrome. The degree of proteinuria varies, the greatest concentration occurring in amyloidosis. Small amounts may be present when mild glomerular damage occurs in fever and toxaemia. In renal disease the concentration may vary during different phases of the disease. Not all of the protein derives from the passage of plasma albumin through damaged glomerular capillaries; appreciable amounts may be contributed by the degeneration of the cells of the tubules in acute cortical necrosis. The significance of proteinuria as an indication of renal disease is much greater when formed elements, including casts, are present in the urine.

If the proteinuria persists there may be sufficient loss to cause hypoproteinaemia but oedema of renal origin as it occurs in man is uncommon in animals. If the protein originates from the lesions of pyelonephritis or cystitis clinical evidence of these diseases can usually be detected.

Casts and cells. Casts appear as organized, tubular structures which vary in appearance according to their composition. They occur only in nephritis and their presence is an indication of inflammatory or degenerative changes in the kidney, the casts having been formed by the agglomeration of desquamated cells and protein. Erythrocytes, leucocytes and epithelial cells may originate in any part of the urinary tract.

Haematuria. Pre-renal causes of haematuria include trauma to the kidney, septicaemias and purpura haemorrhagica accompanied by vascular damage. Renal causes include acute glomerulonephritis, renal infarction, embolism of the renal artery, tubular damage as caused by sulphonamide intoxication, and pyelonephritis. Post-renal haematuria occurs particularly in urolithiasis and cystitis. A special instance is enzootic haematuria of cattle.

In severe cases the blood may be voided in the form of clots but more commonly causes a deep red to brown colouration of the urine. Less severe cases may show only cloudiness which settles to form a red deposit on standing, or the haematuria may be so slight as to be detectable only on microscopic examination of a centrifuged sediment. The origin of the blood may be ascertained by collection of the urine in stages. Blood which originates from the kidneys is usually intimately mixed with the urine and is present in equal concentration in all samples. When the blood originates from a vesical lesion it is usually most concentrated in the final sample and blood from a urethral lesion is most evident in the first part of the flow. It may be necessary to collect a sample by catheterization in females to avoid the chance of contamination of the urine occurring in the vagina.

Urine containing blood gives positive results in biochemical tests for haemoglobin and myoglobin, and as the erythrocytes are often lysed, it is necessary to examine all red coloured urine for the presence of erythrocytes. The presence of a heavy brown deposit is not sufficient basis for a diagnosis of haematuria as this may also occur in haemoglobinuria. Involvement of the bladder or urethra may be detectable on physical examination of the patient. Gross haematuria persisting for long periods may result in severe haemorrhagic anaemia.

Haemoglobinuria. False haemoglobinuria occurs in haematuria when the erythrocytes are broken down and liberate their haemoglobin. Its presence can be determined only by microscopic examination of the urinary sediment for the presence of cellular debris.

True haemoglobinuria is manifested by a deep red coloration of the urine, a positive reaction to chemical tests for haemoglobin and protein, and the absence of cellular debris. There are many causes of intravascular haemolysis, the source of haemoglobinuria. The specific causes are listed under haemolytic anaemia.

Normally, haemoglobin liberated from effete erythrocytes is converted to bile pigments in the cells of the reticulo-endothelial system. When haemolysis occurs in excess of the capacity of this system to remove the haemoglobin, it increases in concentration in the blood until it exceeds a certain renal threshold and then escapes with the urine. There is no evidence as to why the large haemoglobin molecule passes the glomerular filter when smaller molecules are retained. Some haemoglobin is reabsorbed from the glomerular filtrate by the tubular epithelium but probably not in sufficient amounts to appreciably affect the haemoglobin content of the urine. Precipitation of haemoglobin to form casts occurs in the tubules, especially if the urine is acid and some plugging of tubules results,

but the chief cause for the development of uraemia in haemolytic anaemia is the tubular nephrosis which occurs.

Myoglobinuria. The presence of myoglobin (myohaemoglobin) in the urine is evidence of severe muscle dystrophy. The only notable occurrence in animals is in azoturia of horses. In enzootic muscular dystrophy myoglobinuria may occur but there is usually insufficient myoglobin in the muscles of young animals to cause an appreciable degree of abnormality. The myoglobin molecule is much smaller than that of haemoglobin and passes the glomerular filter much more readily so that a detectable dark brown staining of the urine occurs without very high levels of myoglobin being attained in the serum. Thus a detectable discolouration of the serum does not occur as it does in haemoglobinaemia. In inherited congenital porphyria, the other disease in which the urine is discoloured a reddish brown, the plasma is also normal in colour. Differentiation from myoglobinuria is made on the negative reaction to the guaiac test and the characteristic spectrograph. The porphyrins in this disease are the only pigments which fluoresce when illuminated by ultra-violet light.

The presence of the pigment in the urine can be determined accurately by spectrographic examination. The abnormality of the urine is usually accompanied by clinical signs of acute myopathy. Precipitation of myoglobin in the tubules occurs as with haemoglobin and may contribute towards a terminal uraemia.

Pyuria. Pus in the urine indicates inflammatory exudation at some point in the urinary tract, usually the renal pelvis or bladder. It may occur as macroscopically visible clots or shreds, or be detectable only by microscopic examination as leucocytic casts, or as individual cells which are most readily observed in a centrifuged deposit. Pyuria is usually accompanied by the presence of bacteria in the urine.

Crystalluria. The presence of crystals in the urine of herbivorous animals has no special significance unless they occur in very large numbers and are associated with clinical signs of irritation of the urinary tract. Crystals of calcium carbonate and triple phosphate are commonly present in normal urine. Their presence in large numbers may suggest that the concentration of the urine is above normal and the possible future development of urolithiasis.

Glycosuria and ketonuria. Glycosuria together with ketonuria occurs only in diabetes mellitus, a rare disease in large animals. Glycosuria is not common but is associated with enterotoxaemia due to *Clostridium perfringens* type D and occurs after parenteral treatment with dextrose solutions, adrenocorticotrophic hormones or cortisone analogues. It occurs also in nephrosis due to failure of tubular resorption. Ketonuria is a more common finding and occurs in starvation, acetonaemia of cattle and pregnancy toxaemia of ewes.

Indicanuria. The presence of indican (potassium indoxyl sulphonate) in excessive amounts indicates increased absorption of this detoxication product of indole from the large intestine. Indicanuria occurs when the alimentary sojourn is prolonged for any reason.

Creatinuria. Excessive endogenous breakdown of muscle causes an increased concentration of creatine in the urine and some use has been made of this in the detection of muscular dystrophy. However, a degree of creatinuria may be found in normal sheep, cattle and pigs suggesting caution in the use of the creatine to creatinine ratio as a diagnostic aid in these species (4, 5).

VARIATIONS IN DAILY URINE FLOW

An increase or decrease in urine flow is often described in animals but accuracy demands physical measurement of the amount of urine voided over a 24 hour period. This is not often practicable in clinical work and it is often necessary to guess whether the flow is increased or decreased. Care should be taken to differentiate between increased daily flow and increased frequency without increased flow. The latter is much more common.

Polyuria. A transient increase in urine volume may be apparent with excessive water intake. The time taken to excrete an oral water load varies widely between individual animals and between species, being longer in cattle than in the dog (6). Continued polyuria is in most instances the result of decreased tubular reabsorption. This may occur because of absence of the antidiuretic hormone (diabetes insipidus), because of an increase in solutes in the glomerular filtrate beyond the resorptive capacity of the tubular epithelium, or because of damage to the tubules. A transient increase in urine volume may occur due to fear or emotional stress. Diabetes insipidus is rare in farm animals, being reported most commonly in horses in which it is usually caused by a tumour of the pituitary gland. It is characterized by excessive thirst, the passage of a very large volume of urine of low specific gravity (1·002 to 1·006), and a temporary response to the parenteral administration of pitressin. Osmotic diuresis, caused by an increase in solutes in the glomerular filtrate, may result from administration of diuretics comprising substances not reabsorbed by the tubules, or by the excretion of naturally-occurring substances such as urea and glucose in amounts larger than the tubular epithelium can reabsorb. Fluid is lost in both instances because of the osmotic relationship between solutes and water in the urine. Polyuria has been demonstrated to occur in Vitamin A deficiency in sheep but the mechanism is uncertain (11).

Damage to the tubular epithelium and failure of tubular resorption occur in nephrosis and nephritis. This form of polyuria is characterized by inability of the kidney to vary the concentration of the urine with varying intakes of fluid (isosthenuria or hyposthenuria), so that dehydration occurs if fluid intake is reduced. The specific gravity also varies only within narrow limits (1·006 to 1·016) and is usually about 1·010.

Oliguria and anuria. Reduction in the daily output (oliguria) and complete absence of urine (anuria) occur under the same conditions and vary only in degree. Complete anuria occurs most commonly in urethral obstruction, although it may result from acute tubular necrosis such as is caused by mercury poisoning. The anuria of acute glomerulonephritis which is a familiar syndrome in man rarely if ever occurs in animals. Oliguria occurs in the terminal stages of all forms of nephritis. The retention of solutes and disturbances of acid-base balance that follow anuria or severe oliguria contribute to the development of uraemia. In dehydration urine flow decreases due to increased osmotic pressure of the plasma, and congestive heart failure and peripheral circulatory failure may cause such a reduction in renal blood flow that oliguria follows.

PAIN AND DYSURIA

Abdominal pain and dysuria are both expressions of discomfort caused by disease of the urinary tract. Acute abdominal pain due to disease of the urinary tract occurs rarely and is usually associated with sudden distension of the renal pelvis or ureter, or infarction of the kidney. None of these conditions is common in animals, but occasionally in cattle affected with pyelonephritis attacks of acute abdominal pain occur which are thought to be due to either renal infarction or obstruction of the pelvis by necrotic debris. The attacks of pain are acute with downward arching of the back, paddling with the hind feet, rolling and bellowing. Subacute abdominal pain occurs with urethral obstruction and distension of the bladder and is manifested by tail-switching, kicking at the belly, and efforts at urination accompanied by grunting.

Painful or difficult urination occurs in cystitis, vesical calculus and urethritis and is manifested by the frequent passage of small amounts of urine.

Grunting may occur with urination and the animal remains in the typical posture after the act is completed. Differentiation of pain caused by urinary disease from that due to other causes depends largely upon detection of other signs indicative of involvement of the urinary tract.

URAEMIA

The term uraemia is poorly defined but is used here to describe the clinical syndrome which occurs in the terminal stages of renal insufficiency. The physiological basis of the various signs observed is uncertain and in dogs and humans varies from case to case and from time to time in the one patient. This subject has been discussed in general terms under principles of renal failure (p. 181) and details are omitted because they are not available for natural or experimental uraemia in farm animals.

Clinical signs include anuria or oliguria, the latter being more common unless there is complete obstruction of the urinary tract. Chronic renal disease may be manifested by polyuria but this is essentially a compensatory phenomenon and oliguria always appears in the terminal stages when clinical uraemia develops. The animal is depressed, shows muscular weakness and muscle tremor and the respiration is usually deep and laboured. If the disease has been in progress for some time body condition is poor, due probably to continued loss of protein in the urine, to dehydration and to the anorexia which is characteristic of the disease. The respiration is usually increased in rate and depth but is not dyspnoeic; in the terminal stages it may become periodic in character. The heart rate is markedly increased because of the terminal dehydration and myocardial asthenia but the temperature remains normal unless an infectious process is present. An ammoniacal or uriniferous smell on the breath is often described but is usually undetectable.

In the terminal stages the animal becomes recumbent and comatose, the temperature falls to below normal and death occurs quietly, the whole course of the disease having been one of gradual but inexorable intoxication. Necropsy findings apart from those of the primary disease are non-specific and include degeneration of parenchymatous organs, sometimes accompanied by emaciation and moderate gastroenteritis.

Special Examination of the Urinary System

Rectal examination in horses and cattle is essential for examination of the urinary tract and is described in Chapter 1. Roentgenological examination is not usually undertaken but special examination techniques including catheterization, and biochemical and microscopic examination of urine are in routine use. Tests of renal function are available but have not been generally adopted in large animal practice because of the comparative rarity of renal disease. Percutaneous biopsy of the kidney has been successfully carried out in cows and a horse. The left kidney is fixed in position by rectal manipulation and a biopsy needle introduced through the upper flank (9).

CATHETERIZATION

Rams and boars cannot be catheterized because of inaccessibility of the penis and the small diameter of the urethra. A lead wire is used in steers and bulls but is not sufficiently flexible to make the passage easy. Ewes and sows have vulvas which are too small to allow easy access to the urethra. Passage of a catheter in a cow is relatively simple provided a fairly rigid catheter of small diameter (0·5 cm.) is used and a finger can be inserted into the sub-urethral diverticulum to direct the tip of the catheter into the external urethral orifice. Mares are catheterized with ease, the external urethral orifice being large and readily accessible. There is difficulty in bringing the penis of the male horse into view, although the penis is usually relaxed when urethral obstruction occurs. Administration of an ataractic drug makes manipulation of the penis easier and often results in its complete relaxation. A proper male horse catheter, well lubricated, should be used as sufficient rigidity is necessary to pass through the long urethra and around the ischial arch.

URINALYSIS

The reader is referred to a textbook of veterinary clinical pathology for details of the biochemical and microscopic examination of the urine. The occurrence and significance of the more common abnormalities of the urine are described under manifestations of diseases of the urinary system.

RENAL FUNCTION TESTS

The simplest and most important test of urinary function is that aimed at determining whether or not urine is being voided. This is generally accomplished in large animals by restraining them on a clean, dry floor which is examined periodically.

The term renal function tests includes those tests in which various functions of the kidney are measured by biochemical means. They can be considered in groups depending on whether they are based on the examination of blood, urine or both.

Tests conducted on urine. The simplest test is that which measures the capacity of the kidneys to vary the specific gravity of the urine. The normal S.G. is of the order of 1·028 to 1·032. In chronic nephritis this falls to about 1·010 and is not appreciably altered by either deprivation of water for 24 hours or the administration of large quantities of water by stomach tube. Other more complicated tests require the administration of urea or the intravenous injection of a dye such as phenolsulphonphthalein which is excreted in urine. Periodic catheter samples are taken and the time required for excretion of the administered compound determined. Excretion is delayed in renal disease but standards for normality in large animals are not available.

Tests conducted on blood. These tests depend on the accumulation, in cases of renal insufficiency, of metabolites normally excreted by the kidney. The estimation of the level of urea in the blood is most commonly used but tests for non-protein nitrogen or creatinine are also available. All suffer from the disadvantage that blood levels of these substances vary with the rate of protein catabolism and are not dependent entirely on renal function (7). The levels do not rise appreciably above the normal range until 60 to 75 per cent of nephrons are destroyed. The fractional clearance of phenolsulphonphthalein has been suggested as a suitable test for the measurement of renal function in animals and some data are available for cattle (1, 10).

Tests conducted on urine and blood. The capacity of the kidneys to transfer administered urea from the blood stream to the urine is measured against time and is probably the most efficient clearance test available. It suffers from the deficiency that urine samples are often not readily obtainable, especially in male ruminants. This test, together with a test of the ability to increase and decrease the specific gravity of the urine, provides most information on renal efficiency. A good deal of information is available on renal function in the calf (8).

Principles of Treatment of Diseases of the Urinary System

Little can be done other than to treat the primary disease. If an inflammatory or infectious process can be halted the animal may be able to survive on its residual, functional, renal tissue; reversible renal failure is not a common occurrence in animals but the rational treatment of dehydration, haemorrhagic anaemia and shock may prevent renal ischaemia and resulting renal insufficiency.

Supportive treatment, including the parenteral administration of fluid and sodium and possibly calcium salts, may enable an animal to survive an acute renal insufficiency until an infectious process is brought under control. Continuous peritoneal or vascular dialysation as is practised in human medicine has not yet achieved any significant place in veterinary medicine except in small animal work. Once the destruction of nephrons has passed the critical point there is little that can be done other than temporarily to prolong the animal's life. Emergency slaughter is not recommended as the carcass is usually graded as unsuitable for human consumption.

The use of diuretics has no place in renal disease. In chronic uraemia solute diuresis is already in operation and the stimulation of further water flow can only exacerbate the dehydration. In acute uraemia the defect is one of glomerular filtration which is not improved by diuretics, and in the terminal stages of chronic uraemia too many nephrons have been destroyed to enable any functional improvement in nephron efficiency to exert an appreciable effect on the course of the disease.

REFERENCES

(1) Mixner, J. P. & Anderson, R. R. (1958). *J. Dairy Sci.*, *41*, 306.
(2) Kiesel, G. K. (1956). *N. Amer. Vet.*, *37*, 936.
(3) Pierce, A. B. (1961). *Proc. R. Soc. Med.*, *54*, 996.
(4) Blanch, E. & Setchell, B. P. (1960). *Aust. J. biol. Sci.*, *13*, 356.
(5) Aafjes, J. H. & de Groot, T. (1961). *Brit. vet. J.*, *117*, 201.
(6) Dalton, R. G. (1964). *Brit. vet. J.*, *120*, 69.
(7) Campbell, J. R. & Watts, C. (1970). *Vet. Rec.*, *87*, 127.
(8) Dalton, R. G. (1968). *Brit. vet. J.*, *124*, 371, 451, 498; *125*, 367.
(9) Osborne, C. A. *et al.* (1968). *J. Amer. vet. med. Ass.*, *153*, 563.
(10) Osbaldiston, G. W. & Moore, W. E. (1971). *J. Amer. vet. med. Ass.*, *159*, 292.
(11) Webb, K. E. Jr. *et al.* (1968). *J. anim. Sci.*, *27*, 1657.

DISEASES OF THE KIDNEY

Renal Ischaemia

Reduction in the flow of blood through the kidneys is usually the result of a general circulatory failure. There is transitory oliguria followed by anuria and uraemia if the circulatory failure is not corrected.

Aetiology

Acute renal ischaemia occurs during severe circulatory emergencies such as shock, dehydration, acute haemorrhagic anaemia and acute heart failure. Embolism of the renal artery has also been recorded as a cause of acute renal ischaemia in horses. Chronic renal ischaemia is a common accompaniment of congestive heart failure.

Pathogenesis

Acute ischaemia of the kidneys occurs when compensatory vasoconstriction affects the renal blood vessels in response to a sudden reduction in circulating blood volume. There is an immediate reduction in glomerular filtration and an elevation of levels of normally excreted metabolites in the blood stream. For example, an elevation of blood urea nitrogen occurs and gives rise to the name pre-renal uraemia. There is a concomitant reduction in urine flow. If the ischaemia is severe enough and persists for long enough the reduction in glomerular filtration, which has been reversible by a return of normal blood flow, becomes irreversible because of anoxic degenerative lesions in the renal parenchyma. This is most likely to occur in acute circulatory disturbances and is an unlikely event in chronic congestive heart failure.

The parenchymatous lesions vary from tubular necrosis to cortical necrosis in which both tubules and glomeruli are affected. The nephrosis of haemoglobinuria is caused by the vasoconstriction of renal vessels. The uraemia which contributes to a fatal termination in acute haemolytic anaemia and in acute muscular dystrophy with myoglobinuria may be exacerbated by plugging of the tubules with casts of coagulated protein but the nephrosis is the more important factor.

Clinical Findings

Renal ischaemia does not usually appear as a disease entity, largely because it is masked by the clinical signs of a primary disease. However, bilateral cortical necrosis, with anuria and renal colic, has been reported in a mare (1). The oliguria and azotaemia which occur will in most cases go unnoticed if the circulatory defect is corrected in the early stages. However, failure to respond completely to treatment with transfusion or the infusion of other fluids in haemorrhagic or haemolytic anaemia, or in shock or dehydration, may be caused by renal insufficiency. The general clinical picture has been described under uraemia.

Clinical Pathology

Laboratory examinations are of value particularly in determining the degree of residual renal damage after the circulatory defect has been corrected. Estimation of urea nitrogen levels in the blood are most commonly used as an index. Haematological examinations may be undertaken to determine the degree and type of circulatory insufficiency. In the irreversible stage when damage to the parenchyma has occurred there will be proteinuria if the lesion is primarily glomerular. The passage of large volumes of urine of low specific gravity after a period of oliguria is usually a good indication of a return of normal glomerular and tubular function.

Necropsy Findings

Renal ischaemia is manifested chiefly in the cortex which is pale and swollen and there may be a distinct line of necrosis visible macroscopically at the corticomedullary junction. Histologically there is necrosis of tubular epithelium and, in severe cases, of the glomeruli. In haemoglobinuria and myoglobinuria hyaline casts are present in the tubules.

Diagnosis

Evidence of oliguria and azotaemia in the presence of circulatory failure suggests renal ischaemia with the possibility of permanent renal damage. It is important to differentiate the early reversible stage from primary renal disease. In the latter instance there are abnormalities of the urine as described above. When irreversible ischaemic changes have occurred it is impossible to differentiate the disease from glomerulonephritis and nephrosis.

Treatment

Treatment must be directed at correction of the circulatory disturbance at the earliest opportunity. If renal damage has occurred, supportive treatment as suggested for the treatment of renal failure should be instituted.

REFERENCE
(1) Nordstoga, K. (1967). *Path. vet.*, 4, 233.

Glomerulonephritis

Nephritis involving primarily the glomeruli and extending secondarily into the surrounding interstitial tissue and blood vessels is a rare disease in animals, although a high incidence of proliferative glomerulo-nephritis has been recorded in normal sheep and also in cattle and goats, but not pigs or horses (1, 2). The suspected cause in man, in which species the disease occurs commonly, is the development of hypersensitivity to streptococcal protein, and the relative infrequency of systemic streptococcal infections in animals other than the horse and pig may be responsible for the rarity of the disease. The clinical course of the disease in man is marked by an acute onset of uraemia followed by a rapid and complete recovery although some cases persist as a chronic form after partial recovery and terminate fatally at a later date. There is marked oliguria or anuria, and severe uraemia during the acute stage. Proteinuria is present and casts and red cells can be detected in the urine. In the chronic stage the defect of function is largely tubular and urine of low specific gravity and containing no protein is characteristic. There is isosthenuria and a gradual development of uraemia as residual nephrons are destroyed. At necropsy acute cases are characterized by swelling and pallor of the kidney, the pallor being most evident in the cortex. The chronic form is characterized by a shrunken kidney with a granular surface, an adherent capsule and a narrowing of the cortex.

REFERENCES

(1) Lerner, R. A. et al. (1968). Amer. J. Path., 53, 501.
(2) Lerner, R. A. (1968). Fed. Proc., 27, 363.

Nephrosis

Nephrosis includes degenerative and inflammatory lesions of the renal tubules. Uraemia may develop acutely or as the terminal stage after a chronic illness manifested by polyuria, dehydration and loss of weight.

Aetiology

Most cases of nephrosis are caused by exogenous or endogenous toxins. Mercury poisoning is the classical cause but nephrosis also follows poisoning with arsenic, oxalate, highly chlorinated naphthalenes and in overdosing with sulphonamides (1, 2, 3), especially when water intake is restricted. A characteristic nephrosis is produced in pigs (4) and cattle (5, 6) by the feeding of *Amaranthus retroflexus* (Pigweed or Prince of Wales Feather). Minor degrees of nephrosis occur in most toxaemias and in overdosing with parenteral injections of calcium salts in cases of parturient paresis of cattle but are not usually sufficiently severe to appreciably affect the course of the disease. Tubular degeneration is a major lesion in renal ischaemia especially in the presence of haemoglobinuria.

Pathogenesis

In acute nephrosis there is obstruction to the flow of glomerular filtrate through the tubules and an obstructive oliguria and uraemia develop. In chronic cases there may be impairment of tubular resorption of solutes and fluids with an attendant polyuria.

Clinical Findings

Clinical signs are often masked by other signs of the primary disease. In acute nephrosis there is oliguria and proteinuria and the clinical signs of uraemia in the terminal stages. These signs include anorexia, hypothermia, depression, slow heart rate and small weak pulse. In cows there is a continuous mild hypocalcaemia with signs reminiscent of that disease and which respond, in a limited way, to treatment with calcium. Polyuria is characteristic of chronic cases but oliguria usually follows when secondary glomerular damage prevents glomerular filtration.

Clinical Pathology

The presence of protein in a urine of high specific gravity is accompanied by high levels of urea nitrogen in the blood in acute nephrosis. In the chronic stages the urine is of low S.G. and may or may not contain protein but no azotaemia occurs until the terminal stages when uraemia is present.

Necropsy Findings

In acute cases the kidney is swollen and wet on the cut surface and oedema, especially of perirenal tissues, may be apparent. Histologically there is necrosis and desquamation of tubular epithelium, and hyaline casts are present in the dilated tubules.

Diagnosis

Clinical differentiation from glomerulonephritis is difficult except in terms of the specific causes listed above. A combination of polyuria and glycosuria is an uncommon finding in large animals and is usually caused by nephrosis but occasional cases of diabetes mellitus have been recorded in horses (7) and cattle (8).

Treatment

Only those treatments directed at correction of the primary disease and those indicated as supportive treatment during acute uraemia can be recommended.

REFERENCES

(1) Sautter, J. H. & Hoyt, H. H. (1957). J. Amer. vet. med. Ass., 130, 18.
(2) Stowe, C. M. et al. (1957). Amer. J. vet. Res., 18, 511.
(3) Brightenback, G. E. et al. (1958). Amer. J. vet. Res., 19, 794.
(4) Buck, W. B. et al. (1966). J. Amer. vet. med. Ass., 148, 1525.
(5) Jeppesen, Q. E. (1966). J. Amer. vet. med. Ass., 149, 22.
(6) Gay, C. C. (1968–9). Vict. vet. Proc., 27, 71.
(7) Jeffrey, J. R. (1968). J. Amer. vet. med. Ass., 153, 1168.
(8) Kaneko, J. J. & Rhode, E. A. (1964). J. Amer. vet. med. Ass., 144, 367.

Interstitial Nephritis

Interstitial nephritis is a common disease of the dog but less so in other animals. It may be diffuse or focal but is always non-suppurative. Focal interstitial nephritis (white-spotted kidney) is a common incidental finding at necropsy but has no known clinical significance. Diffuse interstitial nephritis is usually associated with infection by *Leptospira* spp. and is important clinically because of the resultant destruction of nephrons which occurs. In the acute stages affected nephrons show chiefly tubular degeneration, and fatal uraemia is uncommon. In the chronic stages much of the renal parenchyma is gradually replaced by scar tissue and although many glomeruli are unaffected the destruction of tubules is eventually almost complete and results in death due to uraemia. Clinically the disease is characterized by a gradual onset of polyuria, urine of low specific gravity, isosthenuria and terminal uraemia.

Embolic Nephritis

Embolic lesions in the kidney cause no clinical signs unless they are very extensive when toxaemia may be followed by terminal uraemia. Transitory periods during which proteinuria and pyuria occur may be observed if urine samples are examined at frequent intervals.

Aetiology

Embolic suppurative nephritis may occur after any septicaemia or bacteraemia when bacteria lodge in renal tissue but is most commonly associated with valvular endocarditis. The common occurrences in systemic infections in large animals are in shigellosis of foals and erysipelas of pigs. Sporadic cases occur in cattle and the lesions usually contain *Corynebacterium pyogenes* originating in suppurative lesions in other organs including the uterus, udder, navel and peritoneal cavity. Sporadic cases also occur in strangles in horses.

Pathogenesis

Localization of single bacterial cells or bacteria in small clumps in renal tissue causes the development of embolic suppurative lesions. Emboli which block vessels larger than capillaries cause infarction in which portions of kidney, the size varying with the calibre of the vessel which is occluded, are rendered acutely ischaemic. These infarcts are not usually so large that the residual renal tissue cannot compensate fully and they usually cause no clinical signs. If the urine is checked repeatedly for the presence of protein and erythrocytes, the sudden appearance of proteinuria, casts, and microscopic haematuria, without other signs of renal disease, suggests the occurrence of a renal infarct. The gradual enlargement of focal embolic lesions leads to the development of toxaemia and gradual loss of renal function. Clinical signs usually develop only when the emboli are multiple and destroy much of the renal parenchyma, although the same result can be produced by one or more large infected infarcts.

Clinical Findings

Usually there is insufficient renal damage to cause signs of renal dysfunction but signs of toxaemia and the primary disease are usually present. Enlargement of the kidney may be palpable on rectal examination. Repeated showers of emboli or gradual spread from several large, suppurative infarcts may cause fatal uraemia. Spread to the renal pelvis may cause a syndrome very similar to that of pyelonephritis. The development of large infarcts may cause bouts of transient abdominal pain.

Clinical Pathology

The urine may contain pus and blood which are visible macroscopically although microscopic examination may be necessary to detect the presence of these abnormalities when the lesions are minor. Culture of urine at the time when proteinuria occurs may reveal the identity of the bacteria infecting the embolus.

Necropsy Findings

In animals which die of intercurrent disease the early lesions are seen as small greyish spots in the cortex. In the later stages these lesions may have developed into large abscesses, which may be confluent and in some cases extend into the pelvis. Much fibrous tissue may surround lesions of long standing and healed lesions consist of areas of scar tissues in the cortex. These areas have depressed surfaces and indicate that destruction of cortical tissue has occurred. When many such lesions are present the shrinking of the cortex may cause an obvious reduction in the size of the kidney.

Diagnosis

Differentiation from pyelonephritis is difficult unless the latter is accompanied by detectable cystitis or urethritis. Enlargement of the kidney occurs in both conditions and the findings on urinalysis are the same when embolic nephritis invades the renal pelvis. Many cases of embolic nephritis go unrecognized clinically because of the absence of overt signs of renal involvement.

The sudden occurrence of bouts of acute abdominal pain in some cases of renal infarction may suggest acute intestinal obstruction but defaecation is usually unaffected and rectal examination of the intestines is negative.

Treatment

If the causative bacteria can be isolated and their sensitivity to standard antibiotics and sulphonamides determined, control of early cases of embolic nephritis can usually be effected. However, unless the primary disease is controlled renal lesions may recur. Antibiotic treatment is usually required over a fairly lengthy period (7 to 10 days) and can be supplemented by the administration of parenteral enzymes during this time. Bacteriological examination of the urine is advisable at intervals after treatment is completed to ensure that the infection has been completely controlled.

Pyelonephritis

Pyelonephritis develops by ascending infection from the lower urinary tract. Clinically it is characterized by pyuria, suppurative nephritis, cystitis and ureteritis.

Aetiology

Pyelonephritis may develop secondarily to any infection of the lower urinary tract but it occurs most commonly as the specific pyelonephritis of cattle and pigs.

Pathogenesis

The development of pyelonephritis depends upon the presence of infection in the urinary tract and the stagnation of urine, permitting the multiplication and progression of the infection up the tract (1) and possibly enhanced by reflux up the ureters from the bladder (2). Urinary stasis may occur as a result of bacterial infection and the blocking of ureters by inflammatory swelling or debris, by pressure from the uterus in pregnant females, and by obstructive urolithiasis. The infection ascends the ureters, not always bilaterally, and invades the renal pelvis. Involvement of the papillae occurs and lesions develop in the renal medulla although the lesions may extend to the cortex. Toxaemia and fever result and if renal involvement is bilateral and sufficiently extensive uraemia develops. Pyelonephritis is always accompanied by pyuria and haematuria because of the inflammatory lesions of the ureters and bladder.

Clinical Findings

The clinical findings in pyelonephritis vary between species. In sows there may be an initial period during which a vaginal discharge is noted but most affected animals die without premonitory illness. The disease in cattle is described in detail in the section on Bovine Pyelonephritis.

Clinical Pathology

Erythrocytes, leucocytes and cell debris are found in the urine on microscopic examination and there may be gross evidence of their presence in severe cases. Culture of the urine is necessary to determine the causative bacteria.

Necropsy Findings

The kidney is usually enlarged and lesions in the parenchyma are in varying stages of development. The characteristic lesions are necrosis and ulceration of the pelvis and papillae and the pelvis is usually dilated and contains clots of pus and turbid urine. Streaks of grey, necrotic material radiate out through the medulla and may extend to the cortex. The affected parenchyma is necrotic but suppuration is unusual and healed lesions appear as contracted scar tissue. Infarction of lobules may also be present, especially in cattle. Histologically the lesions are similar to those of embolic nephritis except that there is extensive necrosis of the apices of the papillae. Necrotic, suppurative lesions are usually present in the bladder and ureters.

Diagnosis

The presence of pus and blood in the urine may suggest cystitis or embolic nephritis, as well as pyelonephritis, and it may be difficult to distinguish between these diseases. Renal enlargement or pain on rectal palpation of the kidney will indicate the presence of renal involvement and if the urine is abnormal at all times pyelonephritis is the more likely cause. Diagnosis at necropsy will depend on the principal location of the lesions; they are most common in the medulla in pyelonephritis and in the cortex in embolic nephritis.

Treatment

The treatment prescribed for cases of suppurative embolic nephritis applies equally well in this disease and is discussed in more detail under bovine pyelonephritis.

REFERENCES

(1) Brumfitt, H. W. & Heptinstall, R. H. (1958). *Brit. J. exp. Path.*, *39*, 610.
(2) Heptinstall, R. H. (1964). *Brit. J. exp. Path.*, *45*, 436.

Hydronephrosis

Cystic enlargement of the kidney due to obstruction of the ureter is a relatively common finding at necropsy but is seldom detected clinically in farm animals, because it is usually unilateral and the unaffected kidney compensates fully for the loss of function. Obstructive urolithiasis is the most common cause although congenital obstructive anomalies of the ureter may have the same effect. Complete obstruction of the urethra causes dilatation and rupture of the bladder. Back pressure in the ureters causes distension of the pelvis and pressure atrophy of the renal parenchyma but this effect is greatest when the obstruction is only partial and develops slowly. Bilateral hydronephrosis results in terminal uraemia; unilateral obstruction may be detectable on palpation per rectum of a grossly distended kidney.

Congenital Defects of the Kidneys

Congenital anomalies of the kidney are rarely recognized clinically. Polycystic kidney is the most common defect. If it is bilateral the affected animal is usually stillborn or dies soon after birth. If it is unilateral no clinical signs appear because of compensatory activity in the other kidney, but in cattle and horses the enormously enlarged kidney may be encountered during rectal examination. A high incidence of renal defects has been recorded in sucking pigs from sows vaccinated during early pregnancy with attenuated hog cholera virus and a bilateral renal hypoplasia has been observed as a probable inherited defect in Large White pigs (1).

REFERENCE

(1) Cordes, D. O. & Dodd, D. C. (1965). *Path. vet.*, 2, 37.

Renal Neoplasms

Primary neoplasms of the kidney are uncommon. Adenomas occur in cattle and horses and nephroblastomas in pigs but they cause little clinical disturbance. Enlargement of the kidney is the characteristic sign and in cattle and horses neoplasms must be considered in the differential diagnosis of renal enlargement. Nephroblastomas in particular may reach a tremendous size and cause visible abdominal enlargement in the pig.

Metastatic neoplasms occur fairly commonly in the kidney, especially in lymphomatosis but again cause little clinical disturbance. They may be palpable as discrete enlargements in the kidneys of cattle but the lesion may be diffuse and cause a general enlargement of the organ.

DISEASES OF THE BLADDER, URETERS AND URETHRA

Cystitis

Inflammation of the bladder is usually caused by bacterial infection and is characterized clinically by frequent, painful urination and the presence of blood, inflammatory cells, and bacteria in the urine.

Aetiology

Cystitis occurs sporadically due to the introduction of infection into the bladder when trauma to the bladder has occurred or when there is stagnation of the urine. It occurs most commonly in association with vesical calculus, late pregnancy, difficult parturition or catheterization. Rarely it is the result of paralysis of the bladder. Cystitis is a common precursor of bovine pyelonephritis. *Corynebacterium renale* is the causative bacterium in these cases; in those due to trauma the bacterial population is usually mixed although *Escherichia coli* is the most common organism. A form of cystitis, accompanied in some cases by ataxia and incoordination of the rear limbs, has been reported as occurring in horses grazing Sudan grass or Sudax (1, 3). An outbreak of cystitis, characterized by incontinence and haematuria, has been reported in Australian horses (2). A fungal toxin was postulated as a cause. Enzootic haematuria is not a true cystitis but rather a chronic hyperplastic inflammation of the vesical mucosa, followed in some cases by the development of benign and malignant tumours.

Pathogenesis

Bacteria frequently gain entrance to the bladder but are removed before they invade the mucosa by the physical emptying of the urine. Injury to the mucosa facilitates invasion but stagnation of urine is the most important predisposing cause. Introduction of bacteria occurs chiefly via the urethra but descending infection from an embolic suppurative nephritis may also occur.

Clinical Findings

The urethritis which usually accompanies a cystitis causes painful sensations and the desire to urinate. Urination occurs frequently and is accompanied by pain and sometimes grunting; the animal remains in the posture adopted for urination for some minutes after the flow has ceased, often manifesting additional expulsive efforts. The volume of urine passed on each occasion is usually small. In very acute cases there may be moderate abdominal pain as evidenced by treading with the hind feet, kicking at the belly and swishing with the tail, and a moderate febrile reaction. Acute retention may develop if the urethra becomes blocked with pus or blood but this is unusual.

Chronic cases show the same syndrome but the abnormalities are less marked. Frequent urination and small volume are the characteristic signs. The small volume is in part due to the inflammatory thickening of the bladder wall which is palpable on rectal examination. In acute cases no palpable abnormality may be detected but pain may be evidenced.

Clinical Pathology

The presence of blood and pus in the urine is typical of acute cases and the urine may have a strong odour. In less severe cases the urine may be only turbid and in chronic cases there may be no abnormality on gross inspection. Microscopic examination for erythrocytes, leucocytes and desquamated epithelial cells, carried out on sedimented or centrifuged deposits, and bacteriological examination, may be necessary to confirm the diagnosis.

Necropsy Findings

Acute cystitis is manifested by hyperaemia, haemorrhage, swelling and oedema of the mucosa. The urine is cloudy and contains mucus. In subacute and chronic cases the wall is grossly thickened and the mucosal surface is rough and coarsely granular. Highly vascular papillary projections may have eroded causing the urine to be bloodstained or contain large clots of blood. In the cystitis associated with Sudan grass, soft masses of calcium carbonate may be found in the bladder and the vaginal wall may be inflamed and coated with the same material.

Diagnosis

The syndrome caused by cystitis resembles that of pyelonephritis and vesical urolithiasis. Pyelonephritis is commonly accompanied by vesical involvement and differentiation depends on whether there are lesions in the kidney. This may be determined by rectal examination but in many cases it is not possible to make a firm decision. Provided the causative bacteria can be identified this is probably not of major importance as the treatment will be the same in either case. However, the prognosis in pyelonephritis is less favourable than in cystitis.

The presence of calculi in the bladder can usually be detected by rectal examination or by roentgenological examination in smaller animals. Urethral obstruction may also cause frequent attempts at urination but the urine flow is greatly restricted, usually only drops are voided, and the distended bladder can be felt on rectal examination.

Treatment

Irrigation of the bladder has been largely discarded as a method of treatment and the usual technique is to depend entirely on parenteral treatment. Antibiotics offer the best chance of controlling the infection and determination of the drug sensitivity of the causative bacteria is virtually essential if recovery is to be anticipated. Sulphonamides, and drugs such as hexamine and mandelic acid which alter the pH of the urine, are at best bacteriostatic and their use is often followed by relapse. Even with antibiotics relapses are common unless the treatment is continued for a minimum of 7 and preferably for 14 days. Persistence of the infection is usually due to failure to destroy small foci of infection in the accessory glands and in the bladder wall.

The prognosis in chronic cases is poor because of the difficulty of completely eradicating the infection and the common secondary involvement of the kidney. Free access to water should be permitted at all times to ensure a free flow of urine.

REFERENCES
(1) Adams, L. G. et al. (1969). J. Amer. vet. med. Ass., 155, 518.
(2) Hooper, P. T. (1968). Aust. vet. J., 44, 11.
(3) Knight, P. R. (1968). Aust. vet. J., 44, 257.

Paralysis of the Bladder

Vesical paralysis is uncommon in large animals, the main cause being lesions in the lumbosacral part of the spinal cord. Lack of tone of the bladder wall may persist for some days after correction of obstructive distension.

In the early stages of paralysis of neurogenic origin the bladder remains full, and dribbling occurs especially during movement although a good flow of urine can be obtained by manual compression of the bladder per rectum or through the abdominal wall. At a later stage the bladder will begin to empty involuntarily although the evacuation is usually incomplete and some urine is retained. The stagnation causes ideal conditions for the multiplication of bacteria, and cystitis is a common sequel. The prognosis in paralysis of the bladder is therefore poor. Regular catheterization is essential and adequate care must be taken to avoid the introduction of infection. The administration of antibiotics as a prophylaxis against the development of cystitis is advisable.

Urolithiasis

Urolithiasis is an important disease of castrated male ruminants, because of the common occurrence of urethral obstruction. Obstruction of the urethra is characterized clinically by complete retention of urine, unsuccessful efforts to urinate, distension of the bladder and the sequelae of urethral perforation and rupture of the bladder.

Aetiology

Urolithiasis occurs in all species but is of greatest economic importance in feeder steers and lambs being fed heavy concentrate rations, and stock running at range in particular problem areas (1, 2). The latter areas may be associated with the presence of pasture plants containing large quantities of oxalate (3, 4), oestrogens (6) or silica (5). At pasture the incidence of obstructive urolithiasis often varies with the seasons; this variation is probably related to variation in one or a number of the aetiological factors described below. Among feedlot cattle in the United States, obstructive urolithiasis is second in importance only to diseases of the respiratory tract.

There are three main groups of causes of urolithiasis; those which favour the development of a nidus about which concretion can occur, those which facilitate precipitation of solutes on to the nidus, and those which favour concretion by cementing the precipitated salts to the developing calculus (7).

Nidus formation. A nidus, usually in the form of a group of desquamated epithelial cells or necrotic tissue, favours the deposition of crystals about itself. The nidus may result from local infection in the urinary tract in occasional cases but when large numbers of animals are affected it is probable that some other factor such as a deficiency of vitamin A or the administration of oestrogens is the cause of excessive epithelial desquamation. A mortality rate of 20 per cent due to obstructive urolithiasis has been recorded in wethers implanted with 30 mg. stilboestrol compared with no mortalities in a control group (4). Diets low in vitamin A have been implicated as a cause of urolithiasis but vitamin A deficiency does not appear to be a major causative factor (8).

Precipitation of solutes. Urine is a highly saturated solution containing a large number of solutes, many of them in higher concentrations than their individual solubilities permit in a simple solution. The reasons why the solutes remain in solution are improperly understood but several factors are known to be important. Probably the most important factor in preventing precipitation is the presence of protective colloids which convert urine into a gel. These colloids are efficient up to a point but their capacity to maintain the solution may be overcome by abnormalities in one or more of a number of other factors. Even in normal animals crystals of a number of solutes may be present in the urine from time to time and urine must be considered to be an unstable solution.

The pH of urine affects the solubility of some solutes, mixed phosphate and carbonate calculi being more readily formed in an alkaline than an acid medium. Addition of ammonium chloride or phosphoric acid to the rations of steers increases the acidity of the urine and reduces the incidence of calculi (9). The mechanism is uncertain but is probably related to the effect of pH on the stability of the urinary colloids. There is evidence that pH of the urine is not an important factor in the formation of siliceous calculi (35). It is of interest that the addition of sodium chloride to the ration prevents their formation (36). Citrate acts as a buffer in urine, maintaining calcium in solution by the formation of soluble citrate complexes which are not dissociated. Depression of the citrate content of the urine thus favours the precipitation of calcium salts.

Concentration of the urine may occur in several ways and also favours precipitation of salts. Continued deprivation of water is often exacerbated by heavy fluid loss by sweating in hot, arid climates. An excessive intake of minerals may occur on highly mineralized artesian water, or on diets containing high concentrations, particularly of phosphates on heavy concentrate diets (10). Diets containing up to 0·33 per cent of phosphorus were not associated with urolithiasis in sheep but concentrations beyond this were, and at levels of 0·8 per cent phosphorus in the diet the incidence of urolithiasis was as high as 73 per cent. Additional calcium in the diet appeared to have a partial protective action against calculus formation (11, 12).

One of the important factors in the development of uroliths in ruminants is the episodic nature of their feeding—short periods of eating followed by long periods of rumination. Urinary function, with respect to concentration and pH, changes markedly depending on whether or not the animal is eating. This is thought to have a considerable influence on the precipitation and concretion of minerals in the urine of sheep (38).

Metabolic defects may also cause increased concentration of the urine. Hypervitaminosis D has been suggested as a cause of excessive urine concentration of calcium especially in hot climates where dehydration may also be a contributing factor. The ingestion of large quantities of oxalic acid, and possibly other organic acids, results in an increased concentration of calcium in the urine, and the oxalates formed in the tubules are relatively insoluble and readily precipitate out of solution. The oxalates are usually ingested in certain herbaceous plants which have an unusually high concentration and these plants may dominate a pasture at certain times of the year. Although pasture of this type appears to be capable of causing a high incidence of urolithiasis without the apparent intervention of other factors (3), the simple feeding of oxalate does not have this effect. A high incidence of siliceous calculi in up to 80 per cent of calves on range in some areas and on certain farms may or may not be related to the ingestion of plants with a high silica content (13, 14). It appears that a high urinary level of silicon is not the only factor involved in the formation of siliceous calculi (8).

Factors favouring concretion. It has been suggested that mucoprotein, particularly its mucopolysaccharide fraction, may act as a cementing agent and favour the formation of calculi. The mucoprotein in the urine of feeder steers and lambs is increased by heavy concentrate-low roughage rations (15), by the feeding of pelleted rations (16), even more so by implantation with diethylstilboestrol (17) and, combined with a high dietary intake of phosphate, may be an important cause of urolithiasis in this class of livestock. These high levels of mucoprotein in urine may be the result of a rapid turnover of supporting tissues in animals which are making rapid gains in weight.

Miscellaneous factors in the development of urolithiasis. Stasis of urine favours precipitation of the solutes, probably by virtue of the infection which commonly follows and provides cellular material for a nidus. Certain feeds, including cottonseed meal and milo sorghum (18), are credited with causing more urolithiasis than other feeds. Alfalfa is in an indeterminate position: by some observers it is thought to cause the formation of calculi, by others to be a valuable aid in preventing their formation. Pelleting appears to increase calculi formation if the ration already has this tendency.

Attempts to produce urolithiasis experimentally by varying any one of the above factors are usually unsuccessful and natural cases most probably occur as a result of the interaction of several factors. In feedlots a combination of high mineral feeding and a high level of mucoprotein in the urine associated with rapid growth are probably the important factors in most instances, but a dietary deficiency of vitamin A or the use of oestrogens as implants may be contributing factors in some. In range animals a high intake of mineralized water, or oxalates or silica in plants, are most commonly associated with a high incidence of urinary calculi, but again other predisposing factors, including deprivation or excessive loss of water, or vitamin A deficiency may contribute to the development of the disease. Restriction of water intake in very cold weather may also be a contributory factor.

Although the occurrence of obstructive urolithiasis is usually sporadic, cases occurring at irregular intervals in a group of animals, outbreaks have been reported in which a large number of animals are affected in a short time (4). In these outbreaks it is probable that some factor operates which favours the development of obstruction as well as the development of calculi.

Composition of calculi. The chemical composition of urethral calculi varies and appears to depend largely on the dietary intake of individual elements. Calcium, ammonium and magnesium carbonate are the common constituents of calculi in cattle and sheep at pasture (3). In particular areas a high incidence of siliceous calculi has been observed in steers (1) and calculi containing calcium carbonate in animals on oxalate-rich pasture (19). Xanthine calculi in sheep (20) are recorded in some areas in New Zealand where pasture is poor (21). Sheep and steers in feedlots usually have calculi composed of calcium, ammonium and magnesium phosphate, the latter being especially prevalent when sorghum products form a major part of the ration. The calculi are usually present as individual stones of varying size. Less commonly there is a sludge-like sediment but no formed calculi. An amorphous sediment is less likely to cause obstruction than a stone but may do so when the animal is shaken up by driving or transport. Although the greatest field problem is that of obstructive urolithiasis caused by mineralized calculi or sediment, obstruction can also be caused by materials containing very little mineral. Soft, moist, yellow calculi containing 2 benzo-coumarins (19, 22) have been observed in sheep grazing pasture dominated by subterranean clover, which has a high content of an oestrogenic substance. A 10 per cent incidence of obstructive urolithiasis has also been recorded in feedlot lambs receiving a supplement of stilboestrol (0·5 mg. per lb. of feed or 2·0 mg. per lamb daily), the obstruction being caused by plugs of mucoprotein (23). The accessory sex glands were enlarged.

Pathogenesis

Urinary calculi are commonly observed at necropsy in normal animals, and in many appear to cause little or no harm. In a few animals pyelonephritis, cystitis, and ureteral obstruction may occur. Obstruction of one ureter causes unilateral hydronephrosis and bilateral obstruction causes death from uraemia. The important effect of urolithiasis is in the production of urethral obstruction, particularly in wethers and steers. This difference between urolithiasis and obstructive urolithiasis is an important one. Simple urolithiasis has relatively little importance but obstructive urolithiasis is a fatal disease unless the obstruction is relieved. Rupture of the urethra or bladder occurs and the animal dies of uraemia or secondary bacterial infection. Rupture of the bladder is more likely to occur with a spherical smooth calculus which causes complete obstruction of the urethra. Rupture of the urethra is more common with irregularly shaped stones which cause partial obstruction and pressure necrosis of the urethral wall.

The common occurrence of urethral obstruction in wethers and steers is due to the relatively small diameter of the urethra in these animals. The obstruction may occur at any site but is most common at the sigmoid flexure in steers and in the vermiform appendage or at the sigmoid flexure in wethers, all sites at which the urethra narrows. The mortality rate in these animals may reach as high as 10 per cent and in special circumstances may be as high as 20 per cent (4). Bulls are not infrequently affected and a high incidence has been observed in rams. Urethral obstruction occurs rarely in horses, most cases being seen in geldings with the calculus lodged in the scrotal region. Urolithiasis is as common in females as in males but obstruction rarely if ever occurs because of the shortness and large diameter of the urethra. Repeated attacks of obstructive urolithiasis are not uncommon in wethers and steers and at necropsy up to 200 calculi may be found in various parts of the tract of one animal.

Clinical Findings

Calculi in the renal pelvis or ureters are not usually diagnosed ante mortem although obstruction of a ureter may be detectable on rectal examination, especially if it is accompanied by hydronephrosis. Occasionally the exit from the renal pelvis is blocked and the acute distension which results may cause acute pain, accompanied by stiffness of the gait and pain on pressure over the loins. Calculi in the bladder commonly cause cystitis and are manifested by signs of this disease. Rectal palpation usually reveals the presence of the calculi and in male horses these may reach a diameter of 15 to 22 cm.

Obstruction of the urethra by a calculus is a common occurrence in steers and wethers and causes a characteristic syndrome of abdominal pain with kicking at the belly, treading with the hind feet and swishing of the tail (24). Repeated twitching of the penis, sufficient to shake the prepuce, is often observed and the animal may make strenuous efforts to urinate, accompanied by straining, grunting and grating of the teeth, but these result in the passage of only a few drops of blood-stained urine. On rectal examination the urethra and bladder are palpably distended and the urethra is painful and pulsates on manipulation. A heavy precipitate of saline crystals is often visible on the preputial hairs or on the inside of the thighs. The passage of a lead wire up the urethra, after relaxing the penis by epidural anaesthesia or by administering an ataractic drug, may make it possible to locate the site of obstruction.

In horses the syndrome is similar but in addition the penis is relaxed during efforts at urination. Passage of a catheter enables the site of obstruction to be determined, the end of the catheter grating on the rough surface of the calculus.

If the obstruction is not relieved perforation of the urethra or rupture of the bladder occurs in about 48 hours. In the first instance the urine leaks into the connective tissue of the ventral abdominal wall and prepuce and causes an obvious fluid swelling which may spread as far as the thorax. The urine is often infected and severe cellulitis may occur with an attendant toxaemia. In occasional animals an area of skin over the swelling sloughs permitting drainage, and the course is rather more protracted in these cases. When the bladder ruptures there is an immediate disappearance of discomfort but anorexia and depression develop as uraemia appears. Distension of the abdomen soon becomes apparent and a fluid thrill is detectable on tactile percussion. The animal may continue in this state for as long as two to three days before it dies in a coma. In occasional cases death occurs soon after rupture of the bladder due to severe internal haemorrhage.

Rupture of the bladder is the most common sequel in horses. There is usually complete emptying of the bladder into the peritoneal cavity but if the rupture occurs at the neck of the bladder the urine accumulates retroperitoneally with the production of a large diffuse, fluid swelling which is palpable per rectum. When rupture occurs the acute signs disappear and are replaced by immobility and pain on palpation of the abdominal wall. The pulse rate rises rapidly and the temperature falls to below normal.

In occasional cases calculi may form in the prepuce of steers. The calculi are top shaped and, by acting as floating valves, cause obstruction of the preputial orifice, distension of the prepuce and infiltration of the abdominal wall with urine (1). These cases may be mistaken for cases of urethral perforation.

Clinical Pathology

Laboratory examinations may be utilized in the diagnosis of the disease in its early stages when the calculi are present in the kidney or bladder. The urine usually contains erythrocytes and epithelial cells and a higher than normal number of crystals, sometimes accompanied by larger aggregations described as sand or sabulous deposit. Bacteria may also be present if secondary invasion of the traumatic cystitis and pyelonephritis has occurred.

Aspiration of fluid from the abdominal cavity after rupture of the bladder or from a subcutaneous aggregation is often practised as an aid to diagnosis but there is some difficulty in identifying the fluid as urine other than by appearance and smell, or by exhaustive biochemical examination.

Necropsy Findings

Calculi may be found in the renal pelvis or bladder of normal animals, or of those dying of other diseases. In the renal pelvis they may cause no abnormality although in occasional cases there is an accompanying pyelonephritis. Unilateral ureteral obstruction is usually accompanied by dilatation of the ureter and hydronephrosis. Bilateral obstruction causes fatal uraemia. Calculi in the bladder are usually accompanied by varying degrees of chronic cystitis. The urethra may be obstructed by one or more stones, or may be impacted for up to 35 cm. with fine sabulous deposit.

When rupture of the urethra has occurred the urethra is eroded at the site of obstruction and extensive cellulitis and accumulation of urine are present in the ventral abdominal wall. When the bladder has ruptured the peritoneal cavity is distended with urine and there is a mild to moderate chemical peritonitis which is more marked in horses than in cattle or sheep. In areas where urolithiasis is a problem it is an advantage to determine the chemical composition of the calculi.

Diagnosis

Non-obstructive urolithiasis may be confused with pyelonephritis or cystitis, and differentiation may be possible only by rectal examination in the case of vesical calculi or by roentgenological examination in small animals. The same comments apply to the diagnosis of obstructive lithiasis in the ureter which on physical examination is indistinguishable from other causes of abdominal pain. Subsequent development of hydronephrosis may enable a diagnosis to be made in cattle.

The syndrome caused by obstruction of the urethra in cattle and sheep is characteristic but if there is doubt a rectal examination should be carried out or the animal kept under observation to see if urine is passed. The syndrome in horses is also typical but the condition is uncommon and the attempted passage of a catheter is necessary for diagnosis.

Treatment

The treatment of obstructive urolithiasis is primarily surgical (25). An urethral calculi retriever has been used with some success in bulls (42). It is not practicable to expect that calculi can be dissolved by medical means although further increase in size of existing stones and the development of new ones may be prevented. The use of agents to relax the urethral muscle and permit the onward passage of an obstructing calculus has not received much attention. In cattle the injection of a protein-free extract of mammalian pancreas (5 to 10 ml. repeated once or twice on successive days) has been reported to produce this effect provided some urine is still dribbling from the urethra (26). Similar doses have been used in sheep with good results (27). Other specific relaxants of plain muscle, e.g. aminopromazine, have given excellent results in feedlot cattle (28, 29). Animals treated medically should be in the early stages of the disease and kept under close observation to ensure that urination continues.

Prevention

A number of agents and management procedures have been recommended in the prevention of urolithiasis in feeder lambs and steers. First, and probably most important, the diet should contain an adequate balance of calcium and phosphorus to avoid precipitation of excess phosphorus in the urine. The ration should have a Ca:P ratio of 1·2:1, but higher calcium inputs (1·5 to 2·0:1) have been recommended (37, 39, 41). The feeding of alfalfa is considered to increase urine flow and lower the incidence of urolithiasis (30) and the inclusion of 4 per cent of sodium chloride in the ration has been shown experimentally to have this effect on both steers (13) and lambs (18, 31). Under practical conditions salt is usually fed at a concentration of 3 to 5 per cent, higher concentrations causing lack of appetite. It is usually necessary to increase the salt gradually to this level over a period of several weeks and incorporate it in pellets to facilitate mixing. It is thought that supplementary feeding with sodium chloride helps to prevent urolithiasis by decreasing the rate of deposition of magnesium and phosphate around the nidus of a calculus (32). The chloride ion appears to be more effective in this regard than the sodium ion. The potassium ion has a mixed press (40, 41) but the consensus is that if anything it increases susceptibility to obstructive urolithiasis. The feeding of ammonium chloride (45 g. per day to steers and 10 g. daily to sheep) has also been found to be satisfactory in the prevention of urolithiasis (33). For range animals the drug can be incorporated in a protein supplement and fed at about two thirds of the above dosage.

The observation that the addition of chlortetracycline to the ration (10 mg. per lb.) significantly reduced deaths from obstructive urolithiasis may be due to alteration in the pH of the urine subsequent to changes in ruminal digestion or the control of urinary tract infection. The latter is not known to be a factor of importance in the aetiology of urolithiasis in animals, except in sporadic cases.

Dangerous pastures can usually be grazed with impunity by females. In areas where the oxalate content of the pasture is high wethers and steers should be permitted only limited access to pastures dominated by herbaceous plants. Adequate water supplies should be available and highly saline waters should be regarded with suspicion. Sheep on lush pasture commonly drink little if any water, apparently because they obtain sufficient in the feed. Although the importance of vitamin A in the production of the disease has been decried in recent years an adequate intake should be ensured, especially during drought periods and when animals are fed grain rations in feedlots. Deferment of castration, by permitting greater urethral dilatation, may reduce the incidence of obstructive urolithiasis (8, 34).

REFERENCES

(1) Connel, R. et al. (1959). Canad. J. comp. Med., 23, 41.
(2) Bennetts, H. W. (1950). J. Dept. Agric. W. Aust., 27, 129.
(3) Sutherland, A. K. (1958). Aust. vet. J., 34, 44.
(4) Udall, R. H. & Jensen, R. (1958). J. Amer. vet. med. Ass., 133, 514.
(5) Forman, S. A. & Sauer, F. (1962). Canad. J. Anim. Sci., 42, 9.
(6) Gardiner, M. R. et al. (1966). Aust. vet. J., 42, 315.
(7) Udall, R. H. & Chow, F. H. C. (1969). Adv. vet. Sci., 13, 29.
(8) Hawkins, W. W. et al. (1965). J. Amer. vet. med. Ass., 147, 1321.
(9) Crookshank, H. R. et al. (1960). J. Anim. Sci., 19, 595.
(10) Robbins, J. D. et al. (1965). J. Anim. Sci., 24, 76.
(11) Bushman, D. H. et al. (1965). J. Nutr., 87, 499.
(12) Bushman, D. H. et al. (1965). J. Anim. Sci., 24, 671.
(13) Whiting, F. et al. (1958). Canad. J. comp. Med., 22, 332.
(14) Mathams, R. H. & Sutherland, A. K. (1951). Aust. vet. J., 27, 68.
(15) Udall, R. H. et al. (1958). Amer. J. vet. Res., 19, 825.
(16) Crookshank, R. H. et al. (1965). J. Anim. Sci., 24, 638.
(17) Cornelius, C. E. (1963). Annals N.Y. Acad. Sci., 104, 638.
(18) Udall, R. H. (1962). Amer. J. vet. Res., 23, 1241.
(19) Bennetts, H. W. (1956). J. Dept. Agric. W. Aust., 5, 421, 425, 429, 433.
(20) Easterfield, T. H. et al. (1930). Vet. J., 86, 251.
(21) Askew, H. O. (1957). Ann. Rep. Cawthron Inst., Nelson, N.Z., pp. 28–30.
(22) Pope, G. S. (1964). Biochem. J., 93, 474.
(23) Marsh, H. (1961). J. Amer. vet. med. Ass., 139, 1019.
(24) Oehme, W. W. (1965). J. Amer. vet. med. Ass., 147, 1331.
(25) Metcalf, F. L. & Hastings, D. H. (1965). J. Amer. vet. med. Ass., 147, 1327, 1329.
(26) Tonken, B. W. (1958). Canad. J. comp. Med., 22, 347.
(27) Prier, J. E. et al. (1952). Vet. Med., 47, 459.
(28) Scheel, E. H. & Paton, I. M. (1960). J. Amer. vet. med. Ass., 137, 665.
(29) Baldwin, R. A. (1960). Vet. Med., 55, 41.
(30) Newsom, I. E. (1938). J. Amer. vet. med. Ass., 92, 495.
(31) Elam, C. J. et al. (1957). Proc. Soc. exp. biol. Med., 95, 769
(32) Udall, R. H. et al. (1965). Cornell Vet., 55, 198 & 538.
(33) Crookshank, H. R. (1970). J. Anim. Sci., 30, 1002.
(34) Belonje, P. C. (1965). J. S. Afr. vet. med. Ass., 36, 381.
(35) Bailey, C. B. et al. (1963). Canad. J. Anim. Sci., 43, 150.
(36) Bailey, C. B. (1967). Science, 155, 696.
(37) Hoar, D. W. et al. (1970). J. Anim. Sci., 31, 118.
(38) Stacy, B. D. (1969). Aust. vet. J., 45, 395.
(39) Vipperman, P. E. et al. (1969). J. Nutr., 97, 449.
(40) Crookshank, H. R. (1966). J. Anim. Sci., 25, 1005.
(41) Hoar, D. W. et al. (1970). J. Anim. Sci., 30, 597.
(42) Oehme, F. W. (1968). Vet. Med. small Anim. Clin., 63, 53.

Urinary Bladder Neoplasms

Tumours of the urinary bladder are uncommon in farm animals. In cattle bladder tumours are commonly associated with bracken poisoning, but they do occur in other circumstances (1).

REFERENCE
(1) Mugera, G. M. et al. (1969). J. comp. Path., 79, 251.

Congenital Defects of the Urinary Tract

Pervious urachus. Failure of the urachus to obliterate at birth occurs most commonly in foals. Urine is discharged through the umbilicus as a continuous dribble and cystitis is a common sequel. The umbilicus fails to heal and omphalophlebitis and polyarthritis may also develop.

Rupture of the bladder. This condition has been described as rupture of the bladder (1, 2, 3) but the general appearance of the lesion suggests that there is a congenital, defective closure of the bladder wall.

It is observed only in newborn colt foals, clinical signs appearing 24 to 36 hours after birth. There is subacute colic which bears some resemblance to that which occurs in retention of the meconium. The foal sucks in a half-hearted manner and makes frequent, moderate straining movements during which the penis may be protruded but no urine is passed, there is upward humping of the back and the legs are bunched under the body. Catheterization is not obstructed but urine does not flow. The temperature and pulse rate are normal in the early stages. The course of the disease is not acute and during the subsequent 48 hours the foal becomes progressively more dull, the temperature falls as uraemia develops, and the abdomen becomes distended. Fluid can be heard in the abdomen if the foal is shaken and paracentesis through the posteroventral abdominal wall, lateral to the umbilicus, reveals free urine in the peritoneal cavity. Surgical repair of the discontinuity has been successfully carried out (4).

REFERENCES

(1) Cosgrove, J. S. M. (1955). *Vet. Rec.*, 67, 961.
(2) du Plessis, J. L. (1958). *J. S. Afr. vet. med. Ass.*, 29, 261.
(3) Leader, G. H. (1952). *Vet. Rec.*, 64, 241.
(4) Darbishire, H. B. (1961). *Vet. Rec.*, 73, 693.

11

Diseases of the Nervous System

INTRODUCTION

THE normal functions of the nervous system are directed at the maintenance, on a short-term basis, of the body's relation with its environment. These functions are performed by the several divisions of the nervous system including the sensorimotor system responsible for the maintenance of normal posture and gait, the autonomic nervous system controlling the activity of plain muscle and endocrine glands, and thereby the internal environment of the body, the largely sensory system of special senses, and the psychic system which controls the animal's mental state. The system is essentially a reactive one geared to the reception of internal and external stimuli and their translation into activity and consciousness, and is dependent upon the integrity of both the afferent and efferent pathways.

The first step in the examination of the nervous system is to determine whether or not the system is functioning normally. This is the most difficult step and for the most part depends upon the elimination from consideration of diseases of other organs. In this way if there is paresis, and neither abnormality of muscles nor a systemic state capable of causing muscle weakness, it can be considered that the defect probably lies with the nervous system. In other words if both the receptor and effector organs appear to be normal the co-ordinating system is probably at fault.

The nervous system itself is not independent of other organs and its functional capacity is regulated to a large extent by the function of other systems, particularly the cardiovascular system. Hypoxia (anoxia), due to cardiovascular disease, quite commonly leads to depressed or increased cerebral function because of the dependence of the brain on an adequate oxygen supply. It is important to distinguish between primary and secondary disease of the nervous system since both the prognosis and the treatment will differ with the cause. In primary disease of the nervous system the lesion is usually an anatomical one with serious, long-range consequences; in secondary disease the lesion, at least in its early stages, is more likely to be functional

and therefore more responsive to treatment, provided the defect in the primary organ can be corrected.

The clinical signs which should arouse suspicion of neurological disturbance include abnormalities in the four main functions of the system.

(i) *Muscle tone*. Skeletal muscle tone should be sufficient to enable the animal to get up, to support its own weight and maintain normal limb and body relationships.

(ii) *Posture and gait*. An animal's ability to maintain a normal posture and to proceed with a normal gait are dependent largely upon the tone of skeletal muscle but also upon the efficiency of its postural reflexes. Abnormalities of posture and gait are among the best indications of nervous system disease because these functions are governed largely by the co-ordination of nervous activity.

(iii) *Sensory perceptivity*. Tests of sensory perception in animals can only be objective, and never subjective as they can be in man, and any test used in animals presupposes integrity of the motor system.

(iv) *Mental state*. Depression or enhancement of the psychic state is not difficult to judge, particularly if the animal's owner is observant and accurate. The difficulty usually lies in deciding whether the abnormality is due to primary or secondary changes in the brain.

Disease of the nervous system should be suspected when there are abnormalities of posture or gait, involuntary muscle movements, aberration of muscle tone including that of viscera and sphincters, abnormality of sensory perceptivity including that of skin and special senses, and mental disturbances.

Although one or more of these abnormalities is suggestive of neurological disease the interpretation of them is subject to the principles given below.

Principles of Nervous Dysfunction

Nervous tissue is limited in the ways in which it can respond to noxious influences because of its essentially co-ordinating function. The transmission of impulses along nerve fibres can be enhanced or depressed in varying degrees, the extreme degree being complete failure of transmission. Because of the structure of the system, in which nerve impulses are passed from neurone to neurone by relays at the nerve cells, there may also be excessive or decreased intrinsic activity of individual cells giving rise to an increase or decrease in nerve impulses discharged by the cells. The end result is the same whether the disturbance be one of conduction or discharge and these are the only two ways in which disease of the nervous system is manifested. Nervous dysfunction can thus be broadly divided into two forms, depressed activity and exaggerated activity. These can be further subdivided into the four common modes of nervous dysfunction given below.

When a disease of the nervous system is under investigation the first step should be to determine the mode of nervous dysfunction as this is the basis for determining the nature of the lesion.

MODES OF NERVOUS DYSFUNCTION

(i) *Excitation or irritation signs*. Increased activity of the reactor organ occurs because of an increase in the number of nerve impulses received either because of excitation of neurones or by facilitation of passage of stimuli. The excitability of nerve cells can be increased by many factors including stimulant drugs, inflammation, and mild degrees of those influences which in a more severe form may cause depression of excitability. Thus early or mild anoxia may result in increased excitability while continued or severe anoxia will cause depression of function or even death of the nerve cell. Hypoglycaemia also may cause increased excitability, as manifested by hypoglycaemic convulsion in insulin therapy, but if sufficiently severe or prolonged causes a fatal hypoglycaemic encephalopathy. Irritation phenomena may result from many causes including inflammation of nervous tissue caused by bacteria or viruses, certain nerve poisons and anoxia. In those diseases which cause an increase in pressure within the cranial cavity, irritation phenomena result from interference with circulation and the development of local anaemic anoxia. The major manifestations of irritation of nervous tissue are convulsions and muscle tremor in the motor system and hyperaesthesia and paraesthesia in the sensory system. For the most part the signs produced fluctuate in intensity and may occur periodically as nervous energy is discharged and reaccumulated in the nerve cells.

The area of increased excitability may be local or sufficiently generalized to affect the entire body. Thus a local lesion in the brain may cause signs of excitatory nervous dysfunction in one limb and a more extensive lesion may cause a complete epileptiform convulsion.

(ii) *Release signs*. Exaggeration of normal nervous system activity occurs when lower nervous centres are released from the inhibitory effects of higher centres. Cerebellar ataxia is a classical example. In the absence of cerebellar control combined limb movements are exaggerated in all modes of action including rate, range, force and direction. In general, release phenomena are present constantly while the causative lesion operates whereas excitatory phenomena fluctuate with the building up and exhaustion of energy in the nerve cells.

(iii) *Paralysis due to tissue destruction*. Degrees of depression of activity can occur with depression of metabolic activity of nerve cells, the terminal stage being complete paralysis when nervous tissue is destroyed. Such depression of activity may result from failure of supply of oxygen and other essential nutrients either directly from their general absence or indirectly because of failure of the local circulation. Infection of the nerve cell itself may cause initial excitation, then depression of function, and finally complete paralysis when the nerve cell dies.

Signs of paralysis are constant and are manifested by muscular paresis or paralysis when the motor system is affected and by hypoaesthesia or anaesthesia when the sensory system is involved. Deprivation of metabolites and impairment of function by actual invasion of nerve cells or by toxic depression of their activity produce temporary, partial depression of function which is completely lost when the neurones are destroyed.

(iv) *Nervous shock*. An acute lesion of the nervous system causes damage to nerve cells in the immediate vicinity of the lesion but there may be, in addition, a temporary cessation of function in parts of the nervous system not directly affected. The loss of function in these areas is temporary and usually persists for only a few hours. Stunning is the obvious example. Recovery from the flaccid unconsciousness of nervous shock may reveal the presence of permanent residual signs caused by the destruction of nervous tissue.

It is because of this limited range of modes of reaction to injury in the nervous system that determination of the type of lesion is so difficult. Irritation signs may be caused by bacterial or virus infection, by pressure, vascular disturbance or general anoxia, by poisons and by hypoglycaemia. It is often impossible to determine whether the disturbance is structural or functional. Degenerative lesions produce mainly signs of paralysis but unless there are signs of local nervous tissue injury, such as facial nerve paralysis, paraplegia or local tremor, the disturbance may only be definable as a general disturbance of a part of the nervous system. Encephalopathy is an all-embracing diagnosis, but it is often impossible to go beyond it unless other clinical data, including epizootiology and systemic signs, are assessed or special tests including roentgenological examination and examination of the cerebrospinal fluid are undertaken.

Some information can be derived from a study of the time relationships in the development of nervous disease. A lesion which develops suddenly tends to produce maximum disturbance of function, sometimes accompanied by nervous shock. Slowly developing lesions permit a form of compensation in that undamaged pathways and centres may assume some of the functions of the damaged areas. Even in rapidly developing lesions partial recovery may occur in time but the emphasis is on maximum depression of function at the beginning of the disease. Thus a slowly developing tumour of the spinal cord will have a different pattern of clinical development to that resulting from an acute traumatic lesion. Another aspect of the rapidity of onset of the lesion is that irritation phenomena are more likely to occur when the onset is rapid and less common when the onset is slow.

Manifestations of Diseases of the Nervous System

The major manifestations of nervous dysfunction include aberrations of mental state, posture, movement, perception and sphincter activity.

MENTAL STATE

Excitation states include mania and frenzy. Mania occurs in the nervous form of acetonaemia in cattle in which licking, depraved appetite, abnormal voice and drunken behaviour are seen, and in liver insufficiency in horses poisoned by certain plants. Frenzy occurs in the early stages of some encephalomyelites including the furious form of rabies and in acute lead poisoning and takes the form of violent uncontrolled movements and the not infrequent tendency to attack. Both mania and frenzy are probably manifestations of general excitation of the cerebral cortex. The areas of the cerebral cortex which govern behaviour, intellect and personality traits in humans are the frontal lobes and the temporal cortex but the importance of these areas, which are poorly developed in animals, to veterinary medicine is unknown.

Depressive mental states include somnolence, lassitude, syncope and coma. They are all manifestations of depression of cerebral cortical function in various degrees and occur as the result of those influences which depress nervous system function generally. They can thus occur in the encephalomyelites, in any disease which causes increase in intracranial pressure, in cerebral anoxia and hypoglycaemia. The onset of unconsciousness is sudden in syncope (fainting) and more gradual in coma. Syncope may be caused by acute cerebral anoxia due to acute heart failure, by spontaneous cerebral haemorrhage, concussion and contusion, and lightning stroke and electrocution. Coma is usually the terminal stage of unconsciousness and occurs subsequent to depression and lethargy in uraemia, heat stroke and most poisonings or infections which affect the brain.

Head-pressing, a syndrome characterized by the animal pushing its head against fixed objects, leaning into a stanchion or between two fence posts, is difficult to explain. It appears to be due to a combination of headache and mania in that it seems to afford the animal some relief and it can be prevented only by the application of considerable force. It occurs in any condition in which intracranial pressure is increased and in many infections of the brain.

INVOLUNTARY MOVEMENTS

Involuntary movements include convulsions and tremor. Tremor is a continuous, repetitive twitching of skeletal muscles which is usually visible and palpable. The muscle units involved may be small and cause only local skin movement in which case the tremor is described as fibrillary, or the muscle units may be extensive, the movement much coarser and sufficient to move the extremities, eyes or parts of the trunk. The tremor may become intensified when the animal undertakes some positive action, this usually being indicative of cerebellar involvement and is the counterpart of intention tremor in humans. Choreiform movements, as they occur in man, are repetitive, relatively slow, purposeless gestures of the limbs or grimaces of the face, and do not appear to have any counterpart in animals.

Convulsions are violent muscular contractions affecting part or all of the body and occurring for relatively short periods as a rule, although in the late stages of encephalitis they may recur with such rapidity as to give the impression of being continuous. They may be clonic, the typical 'paddling' convulsions, in which repeated muscle spasms alternate with periods of relaxation. Epileptiform convulsions have a particular pattern of development which serves to identify them. Tetanic or tonic convulsions are less common and are manifested by prolonged muscular spasm without intervening periods of relaxation. True tetanic convulsions occur only rarely, chiefly in strychnine poisoning and in tetanus, and in most cases they are a brief introduction to a clonic convulsion. Convulsions always originate in the cerebral cortex but the primary cause may be a dysfunction in a system other than the nervous system. Convulsions are therefore often subdivided into central and peripheral types although there is no purely neurological method of differentiating the groups on clinical grounds.

Central convulsions occur particularly in diseases in which there is inflammation of the brain or a sudden increase in intracranial pressure. Space-occupying lesions, including haemorrhage, abscess and tumour, and concussion or contusion are among the common causes. Acute cerebral oedema occurs in polioencephalomalacia and water intoxication; compression of the brain, by failure of the cranial cavity to expand is the cause of convulsions in vitamin A deficiency in calves. Encephalitis is most commonly caused by a virus although cerebral vascular lesions caused by bacterial infections may also cause convulsions.

Peripheral convulsions are commonly the result of anoxia, for example in cyanide and nitrite poisoning, in acute heart failure and pneumonia. Hypoglycaemic convulsions may occur in baby pig disease and pregnancy toxaemia. Convulsions characterize lactation tetany and hypomagnesaemic tetany of calves.

Convulsions may occur in various intoxications including those caused by lead, organic arsenicals, organic mercurials and organic phosphates, the toxins of Clostridium perfringens type D. and Cl. tetani, chlorinated hydrocarbon insecticides, strychnine and nicotine and a variety of poisonous plants. The pathogenesis of the convulsions in many of these intoxications has not been satisfactorily explained.

POSTURE AND GAIT

Abnormal postures may be adopted intermittently by animals in pain but in disease of the nervous system the abnormality is usually continuous. Deviation or rotation of the head and drooping of the lips, eyelids, cheeks and ears, and opisthotonus and orthotonus are examples al-though the latter two are often intermittent in that they occur as part of a convulsive seizure. Head-pressing and assumption of a dog-sitting posture are further examples.

Disturbances of posture, other than those more accurately defined as disturbances of balance caused by lesions of the cerebellum and vestibular tract, are rarely diagnosed in farm animals and are not discussed here. The importance of vision and thalamic and cortical control in the maintenance of posture by statotonic and statokinetic reflexes have not been extensively studied in animals other than the dog and cat.

The vestibular influence on balance can be affected at the vestibular canals, along the vestibular nerve or at the vestibular nucleus in the medulla. Unilateral excitation or loss of function can be caused by lesions at any of these points. Rotation of the head occurs and the animal falls to one side. When the lesion affects the vestibules, as it may do in otitis media, the affected side is turned down, the animal falls to that side and there is usually facial paralysis on the same side. When the vestibular nucleus is affected, which may occur in listeriosis, there is deviation without rotation of the head and the animal falls to the opposite or normal side. Nystagmus and forced circling are common when there is irritation of the vestibular nucleus or the medial longitudinal fasciculus.

When cerebellar function is lacking a typical syndrome of ataxia results. In general terms there are defects in the rate, range, force and direction of movement. In true cerebellar ataxia the affected animal stands with the legs wide apart, sways and falls in any direction. The head oscillates and cannot be maintained in the normal spatial relationship with the rest of the body. The limbs do not move in unison, the movements are grossly exaggerated and there is a lack of proper placement of the feet so that falling is common. Attempts to proceed to a particular point are usually unsuccessful and the animal cannot accurately reach its feed or drinking bowl. Nystagmus may also be present. Cerebellar ataxia may occur in encephalomyelitis together with other signs of brain involvement but it is the only sign in congenital cerebellar hypoplasia and in poisoning with Claviceps paspali. Occasional cases of cerebellar dysfunction develop in animals after birth (6) and may be due to a congenitally derived demyelination or to nematode invasion. Ataxia must be differentiated from incoordination which is manifested by inability to walk in a straight line, by staggering and by falling and which may be caused by a variety of lesions in various parts of the nervous system.

PARALYSIS

PARALYSIS

The motor system comprises the pyramidal tracts, originating in the motor cortex, the extrapyramidal system originating in the corpus striatum, red nucleus, the vestibular nucleus and the roof of the midbrain, and the peripheral nerves originating in the ventral horn cells. In hoofed animals (ungulates) the pyramidal tracts are of minor importance, reaching only to the fourth cervical segment. The main motor nuclei in these animals are subcortical and comprise the extrapyramidal system and most combined movements are controlled by nerve stimuli originating in the corpus striatum. The pyramidal and extrapyramidal tracts comprise the upper motor neurones which reach to the ventral horn cells of the spinal cord, which cells together with their peripheral axons form the lower motor neurones. Paralysis is a physiological end result in all cases of motor nerve injury, which if severe enough is expressed clinically. The type of paralysis is often indicative of the site of the lesion. A lesion of the upper motor neurone causes a spastic paralysis with loss of voluntary movement, increased tone of limb muscles and increased tendon jerks or clonus. These are all release phenomena resulting from liberation of spinal reflex arcs from higher control. A lesion of the lower motor neurone causes a flaccid paralysis, with loss of voluntary movement, decreased tone of the limb muscles, absence of the tendon jerks and wasting of the affected muscle (*neurogenic atrophy*). Injuries to peripheral nerves are not dealt with in this book, being considered more relevant to a textbook of surgery. The common injuries have been reproduced experimentally and extensively reviewed (5). Most paralyses seen in farm animals are flaccid and are caused by lesions in the spinal cord.

There are several other features of paralysis which may aid in localizing diagnosis. Unilateral lesions of the upper motor neurone cause paralysis of the limb muscle on the opposite side of the body and the facial muscles of the same side when they are above the medullary decussation of the fibre tracts. Below this level the limb paralysis and the lesions are on the same side.

The spasticity of an upper motor neurone lesion may occur with the affected limb in flexion or in extension. The limb is flexed when both corticospinal and vestibulospinal tracts are damaged and is extended when only the corticospinal tract is damaged.

DISTURBANCES IN SENSATION

Lesions of the sensory system are rarely diagnosed in animals, except for those affecting sight and the vestibular apparatus, because of the impossibility of measuring subjective responses. Lesions of the peripheral sensory neurones cause hypersensitivity or decreased sensitivity of the area supplied by the nerve. Lesions of the spinal cord may affect only motor or only sensory fibre tracts or both, or may be unilateral.

Although it is often difficult to decide whether failure to respond to a normally painful stimulus is due to failure to perceive or inability to respond, certain tests may give valuable information. The test commonly used is pricking with a pin or needle and observing the reaction. In exceptional circumstances light stroking may elicit an exaggerated response. The reaction in sheep affected with scrapie is a striking example of hypersensitivity.

In every test of sensitivity it must be remembered that there is a great deal of variation between animals and in an individual animal from time to time, and much discretion must be exercised when assessing the response. In any animal there are also cutaneous areas which are more sensitive than others. The face and the cranial cervical region are highly sensitive, the caudal cervical and shoulder regions less so, with sensitivity increasing over the posterior thorax and lumbar region to a high degree on the perineum. The proximal parts of the limbs are much less sensitive than the distal parts and sensitivity is highest over the digits, particularly on the medial aspect.

Absence of a response to the application of a painful stimulus to the limbs (absence of the withdrawal reflex) indicates interruption of the reflex arc; absence of the reflex with persistence of central perception, as indicated by groaning or body movement, indicates interruption of motor pathways. Increased sensitivity is described as hyperaesthesia, decreased as hypoaesthesia, and complete absence as anaesthesia. Special cutaneous reflexes include the anal reflex, in which spasmodic contraction of the anus occurs when the anus is touched, and the corneal reflex, in which there is closure of the eyelids on touching the cornea. Examination of the eye reflexes and hearing are discussed under examination of the cranial nerves (see below).

MANIFESTATIONS OF DISEASE OF THE AUTONOMIC NERVOUS SYSTEM

Lesions affecting the cranial parasympathetic outflow do so by involvement of the oculomotor, facial, vagus and glossopharyngeal nerves or their nuclei and the effects produced are discussed under examination of the individual nerves. In general the lesions cause abnormality of pupillary constriction, salivation and involuntary muscular activity in the upper part of the alimentary and respiratory tracts. Lesions affecting the craniocervical branch of the sympathetic system also cause abnormalities of salivation and pupillary constriction. Lesions of the spinal sympathetic system interfere with normal motility of all viscera including heart and alimentary tract. For the most part affections of the autonomic nervous system are of minor importance in farm animals. Central lesions of the hypothalamus can cause abnormalities of heat exchange, manifested as neurogenic hyperthermia or hypothermia and obesity, but they are also of minor importance.

Some manifestations of autonomic disease are important. Autonomic imbalance is usually described as the physiological basis for spasmodic colic of horses; paralysis of the recurrent laryngeal nerve is the cause of roaring in horses; grass sickness of horses is characterized by degenerative lesions in the sympathetic ganglia; involvement of the vagus nerve in traumatic reticulitis of cattle causes impairment of motility of the stomachs and the development of vagus indigestion.

Defects of sphincter control and motility of the bladder and sphincter may also be of importance in the diagnosis of defects of lumbosacral parasympathetic outflow and the spinal sympathetic system. The parasympathetic nerve supply to the bladder stimulates the detrusor muscle and relaxes the sphincter; the sympathetic nerve supply has the reverse function. A spinal cord lesion may cause loss of the parasympathetic control and result in urinary retention. Incontinence, if it occurs, does so from overflow. When the sympathetic control is removed incontinence occurs but the bladder is always empty. Similar disturbances of defaecation occur. Both micturition and defaecation are controlled by medullary and spinal centres but some measure of control is regained even when the extrinsic nerve supply to the bladder and rectum is completely removed. Incontinence of faeces and urine is almost impossible to determine, except in house-trained cats and dogs.

Special Examination of the Nervous System

Many of the techniques used in the special examination of the nervous system in humans and in dogs or cats are not applicable to farm animals because of their size and because they are unaccustomed to being handled. Young lambs and pigs may be satisfactory subjects because of their size but the result of many tests, particularly those involving tonic and kinetic postural reflexes, cannot be interpreted and are not dealt with here.

HISTORY

Special attention should be given to the recording of an accurate history. The duration of signs, the mode of onset—particularly whether acute with later subsidence, or chronic with gradual onset—the progression of involvement and the description of signs which occur only intermittently should be ascertained. When the disease is a herd problem the morbidity and mortality rates and the method of spread may indicate an intoxication when all affected animals show signs within a very short period. Changes in behaviour and mental state can often be assessed only on the history. Traumatic injury is often a cause of nervous disease and may not be detectable other than from the history.

When obtaining a history of convulsive episodes an estimate should be made of their duration and frequence. The pattern is also of importance, and may be diagnostic, for example in salt poisoning in swine. Abnormal behaviour prior to a convulsion, suggestive of the apprehensive aura in human epilepsy, is a common precedent to grand mal epilepsy. The occurrence of pallor or cyanosis during the convulsion is of particular importance in the differentiation of cardiac syncope and a convulsion originating in the nervous system.

EXAMINATION

Many of the general techniques of examination of the central nervous system have already been dealt with in Chapter 1 and in the section on Manifestations of Nervous System Disease in this chapter. They include assessment of the mental state, gait, posture, balance and sensory perception and the presence of involuntary and compulsive movements. Special aspects of examination of the nervous system include examination of muscle tone, muscle wasting, reflex arcs, cranial and spinal nerves and the bony encasement of the central nervous system (CNS). Examination of the cerebrospinal fluid and roentgenological examination are also included.

Examination of muscle tone. The tone of skeletal muscle may be examined by passively moving the limbs and the neck. Increased muscle tone, tetany or spasticity may be so great that the limb cannot be flexed or the resistance may be in varying degree greater than normal. The spasticity may occur with the limb fixed in extension or less commonly in flexion. Both are expressions of upper-motor-neurone lesions which leave the spinal reflex arcs intact. Flaccidity, or decreased tone, indicates the presence of a lower-motor-neurone lesion with interruption of the spinal reflex arc.

Muscle wasting. Localized atrophy of muscles may be myogenic or neurogenic and the difference can be determined only by the response to a galvanic current, a technique not well suited to large animal practice. If the atrophic muscle corresponds to the distribution of a peripheral nerve it is usually assumed that the atrophy is neurogenic.

Examination of reflex arcs. Much of the examination already described depends upon the integrity of reflex arcs. Additional tests include the pupillary light reflex (see below), postural reflexes which are not described here because of their limited use in farm animals, and the tendon reflexes. Of the tendon reflexes, the patella reflex is the only one which can be consistently applied and then only to the smaller species and when they are recumbent. A light tap on the patella tendon elicits reflex extension of the limb. Absence of the response is caused by interruption of the reflex arc by damage to the peripheral nerve or to the relevant spinal cord segment. An enhanced response, characterized by an exaggeration of the limb extension, or by clonus, a rapid series of muscle twitches, is caused by an upper-motor-neurone lesion in which the relevant spinal cord segment is not directly involved but is released from the inhibitory effects of higher centres.

Examination of cranial and spinal peripheral nerves. Special examination of most peripheral nerves is possible using tests of sensory perceptivity and examination of muscle tone and function. Special attention should be given to the cranial nerves.

Olfactory nerve. Tests of smell are unsatisfactory in animals because of their response to food by sight and sound.

Optic nerve. The only tests of visual acuity applicable in animals are testing the eye preservation reflex, consisting of provoking closure of the eyelids and withdrawal of the head by stabbing the finger at the eye, and by making the animal run a contrived obstacle course. Both tests are often difficult to interpret and must be carried out in such a way that other senses are not used to determine the presence of the obstacles or threatened injury. Ophthalmoscopic examination is an integral part of an examination of the optic nerve. It is not discussed here because of limitations of space.

Oculomotor nerve. This nerve supplies the pupilloconstrictor muscle of the iris and all of the extrinsic muscles of the eyeball except the superior oblique, the lateral rectus and the retractor muscles. Loss of function of the nerve results in defective pupillary constriction when the light is increased and abnormal position or defective movement of the eyeballs. The pupillary light reflex is best tested by shining a flashlight into the eye, preferably in a darkened stall. Testing of ocular movements can be carried out by moving the hand about in front of the face. In paralysis of the oculomotor nerve there may also be deviation from the normal ocular axes and rotation of the eyeball.

Trochlear nerve. This nerve supplies only the superior oblique muscle of the eye so that external movements and position of the eyeball are abnormal when the nerve is injured.

Trigeminal nerve. The sensory part of the trigeminal nerve supplies sensory fibres to the face and can be examined by testing the corneal reflex and the sensitivity of the face. The motor part of the nerve supplies the muscles of mastication and observation of the act of chewing may reveal abnormal jaw movements and asymmetry of muscle contractions. There may also be atrophy of the muscles. All of these abnormalities are best observed when the lesion is unilateral.

Abducent nerve. Because the abducent nerve supplies motor fibres to the retractor and lateral rectus muscles of the eyeball, injury to the nerve may result in protrusion and medial deviation of the globe.

Facial nerve. The seventh cranial nerve supplies motor fibres to the muscles of the face and ears. The symmetry and posture of the ears, eyelids and lips are the best criteria for assessing the function of the nerve. Ability to move the muscles in question can be determined by creating a noise or stabbing a finger at the eye. Absence of the eye preservation reflex may be due to facial nerve paralysis or blindness.

Acoustic nerve. The auditory part of the acoustic nerve is not easily tested but failure to respond to sudden sharp sounds, created out of sight and without creating air currents, suggests deafness. Abnormalities of balance and carriage of the head (rotation around the long axis and not deviation laterally) usually accompany lesions of the vestibular part of the acoustic nerve and nystagmus is usually present.

Glossopharyngeal nerve. Because of its motor function for the muscles of the pharynx and larynx, defects in this nerve are usually accompanied by paralysis of these organs with signs of dysphagia or inability to swallow, regurgitation through the nostrils, abnormality of the voice and interference with respiration.

Vagus nerve. The motor nerve supply to the pharynx and larynx also contains fibres from the vagus nerve and abnormalities of swallowing, voice and respiration may also occur when the vagus nerve is injured. Because of the additional role of this nerve in supplying parasympathetic fibres to the upper alimentary tract, loss of its function will lead to paralysis of the pharynx, oesophagus and stomach.

Spinal accessory nerve. Loss of function of this nerve will lead to paralysis of the trapezius, brachiocephalic and sternocephalic muscles.

Hypoglossal nerve. As the motor supply to the tongue the function of this nerve can be best examined by observing the motor activity of the tongue. There may be protrusion, deviation or fibrillation of the organ, all resulting in difficulty in prehending food and drinking water.

The testing of individual cord segments and their peripheral nerves depends upon a knowledge of the anatomical distribution of each nerve. The tests usually used are the skin reflexes tested with a pin, and tendon reflexes where they are applicable.

Palpation of the bony encasement of the central nervous system. Palpable or visible abnormalities of the cranium or spinal column are not commonly encountered in diseases of the nervous system but this examination should not be neglected. There may be displacement, abnormal configuration or pain on deep palpation. Abnormal rigidity or flexibility of the vertebral column may also be evident.

Examination of the cerebrospinal fluid (CSF). CSF can be collected from the cysterna magna or the lumbosacral space. The anatomical site for introduction of the needle requires careful consideration and the technique is not easy. A special spinal needle containing a stilette should be used as ordinary hypodermic needles readily block with fat. A primary puncture of the skin with a hypodermic needle makes the introduction of the spinal needle much easier. The needle must be introduced in a vertical position relative to the plane of the animal's back because of the danger of entering one of the lateral blood-vessels in the vertebral canal. General anaesthesia is advisable for puncture of the cysterna magna and local anaesthesia for lumbosacral puncture.

The CSF pressure can be determined by the use of a special manometer attached to the spinal needle (1). When the fluid system is properly connected occlusion of both jugular veins causes a marked rise in a water manometer. CSF pressure is increased in a number of diseases including polio-encephalomalacia, bacterial meningitis and thromboembolic meningo-encephalitis. As a rule pressures are higher during the early stages of the disease (7). Normal pressures are of the order of 120 mm. of Ringer's solution. CSF can be collected and examined for the presence of protein, cells and bacteria. The number of cells present in normal animals is usually less than 5 per cmm. but they may be present in large numbers in cases of meningitis. Samples which show visible turbidity usually contain large numbers of cells and much protein.

Brain biopsy. A technique for obtaining small samples of brain from cattle has been described (2) and may have value in clinical work when animals have to be salvaged for meat.

Roentgenological examination. Examination of the central nervous system by the use of X-rays is not readily applicable to farm animals except sheep, pigs and young animals. Its principal use is in the detection of fractures but it has also found some application in the early detection of chondrodystrophic dwarf calves. The injection of contrast media into the vertebral canal may have some application when localization of a lesion is being attempted.

Electroencephalography (EEG). Because of the sensitivity of the recording instruments used, artifacts occur commonly in electroencephalographs made on animals not conditioned to electroencephalography (3) and the technique is unlikely to be of much value in clinical cases. The method has been used successfully in dogs (4) and recommendations have been made on the standardization of EEG techniques for animals (8).

Principles of Treatment in Diseases of the Nervous System

Treatment of disease of the nervous system presents some particular problems because of the failure of nervous tissue in the brain and spinal cord to regenerate and because of the impermeability of the blood–brain barrier to many drugs.

When peripheral nerves are severed regeneration occurs if the damage is not extensive but no specific treatment, other than surgical intervention, can be provided to facilitate repair. When neurones are destroyed in the brain and spinal cord no regeneration occurs and the provision of nervous system stimulants can have no effect on the loss of function that occurs. The emphasis in treatment of diseases of the nervous system must be on prevention of further damage. On occasion this can be done by providing specific or ancillary treatments.

Control of infection. Viral infections are not highly susceptible to any drug, but the larger, psittacoid viruses may be controlled by the broad spectrum antibiotics including the tetracyclines and chloramphenicol. Bacterial infections of the central nervous system are usually manifestations of a general systemic infection either as a bacteraemia or a septicaemia. Treatment of such infections is limited by the existence of the blood–brain barrier which prevents penetration of some substances into nervous tissue. Its practical importance in modifying treatment does not appear to be very great because diffusion of any antibiotic into nervous parenchyma is limited and chronic suppurative processes are unlikely to respond. The cerebrospinal fluid is probably of little importance as a means of bringing antibacterial agents to brain tissue. The levels of sulphonamides and antibiotics in CSF are low unless meningitis is present, when their concentration increases but not to the degree attained in blood. Thus in cases of meningitis it may be advisable to supplement parenteral treatment with intrathecal injection but the latter is unlikely to be of value in infection of the nervous tissue.

Decompression. Increased intracranial pressure probably occurs in most cases of inflammation of the brain but it is only likely to be severe enough to cause physical damage in acute cerebral oedema and hypovitaminosis A. In these circumstances some treatment should be given to withdraw fluid from the brain tissue and reduce the pressure. Hypertonic solutions of glucose, saline or sucrose have been injected intravenously and with good but transitory results. Sucrose produces a longer-term depression than the other substances. The usual dose rate of sucrose in man is 100 ml. of a 50 per cent solution given intravenously but it is not without toxicity. Care should be exercised if the patient is dehydrated or has renal involvement. Repeated injection or overdosage may cause tubular nephrosis. Diuretics, including acetazoleamide, have been used for the same purpose and appear to have some beneficial effect.

Central nervous system stimulants. These substances are used to excess in many instances. They exert only a transitory improvement in nervous function and are indicated only in nervous shock and after anaesthesia or other short-term reversible anoxias such as cyanide or nitrate poisoning. It is unlikely that terminal respiratory failure caused by anoxia over a long period, and in which anoxia is likely to continue, will respond permanently to their use.

Central nervous system depressants. The same general considerations as apply in the use of CNS stimulants also apply to the use of depressants except that here there is greater point in their use in that sedation does prevent extreme exhaustion caused by muscle activity and prevents the animal doing itself physical injury. Nevertheless, unless the exciting cause is removed there will be little permanent effect.

REFERENCES

(1) Anonymous (1965). *Mod. vet. Pract.*, *46: 13*, 44.
(2) Johnston, L. A. Y. & Callow, L. L. (1963). *Aust. vet. J.*, *39*, 22.
(3) Klemm, W. R. (1965). *Amer. J. vet. Res.*, *26*, 1237.
(4) Delahunter, A. & Cummings, J. F. (1965). *J. Amer. vet. med. Ass.*, *146*, 954.
(5) Vaughan, L. C. (1964). *Vet. Rec.*, *76*, 1293.
(6) Dungworth, D. L. & Fowler, M. E. (1966). *Cornell Vet.*, *61*, 17.
(7) Howard, J. R. (1969). *J. Amer. vet. med. Ass.*, *154*, 1174.
(8) Klemm, W. R. (1968). *Amer. J. vet. Res.*, *29*, 1895.

DISEASES OF THE BRAIN

In the following discussion of diseases of the brain the terms 'irritation', 'release', 'paralysis' and 'nervous shock' are used to describe groups of signs. These terms are used in accordance with their definitions under the Principles of Nervous Dysfunction (p. 201).

Diffuse Diseases of the Brain

Cerebral Anoxia

Cerebral anoxia occurs when the supply of oxygen to the brain is reduced for any reason. An acute or chronic syndrome develops depending on the acuteness of the deprivation. Initially there are irritation signs followed terminally by signs of loss of function.

Aetiology

All forms of anoxia, including anaemic, anoxic, histotoxic and stagnant forms cause some degree of cerebral anoxia but signs referable to cerebral dysfunction occur only when the anoxia is severe. In animals the most common occurrences of cerebral anoxia are in acute hydrocyanic acid and nitrite poisoning, acute heart failure due to severe copper deficiency in adult cattle and the terminal stages of pneumonia and congestive heart failure. The syndrome known as barkers and wanderers in thoroughbred foals is thought to be a special example of cerebral anoxia caused by acute blood loss. In all of these circumstances the signs of cerebral anoxia will be part of a syndrome which includes the signs of the primary disease. Local anoxia of the brain also occurs in any condition in which intracranial pressure is increased; thus acute cerebral oedema leads to swelling of the brain and embarrassment of the vascular supply. Again the effects of anoxia are secondary only.

Pathogenesis

The central nervous system is extremely sensitive to anoxia, and degeneration occurs if the deprivation is extreme and prolonged for more than a few minutes. Complete anoxia for 15 seconds is usually fatal. The effects of the anoxia vary with the speed of onset and with the severity (1). When the onset is sudden there is usually a transitory period during which excitation phenomena occur and this is followed by a period of loss of function. If recovery occurs a second period of excitation usually develops as function returns. In more chronic cases the excitation phase is not observed, the signs being mainly those of loss of function. These signs include dullness and lethargy when deprivation is moderate, and unconsciousness when it is severe. All forms of nervous activity are depressed but the higher centres are more susceptible than medullary centres and the pattern of development of signs may suggest this.

Clinical Findings

Acute and chronic syndromes occur depending on the severity of the anoxia. Acute cerebral anoxia is manifested by a sudden onset of signs referable to paralysis of all brain functions, including flaccid paralysis and unconsciousness. Muscle tremor, beginning about the head and spreading to the trunk and limbs, followed by recumbency, clonic convulsions and death or recovery after further clonic convulsions is the most common pattern although affected animals may fall to the ground without premonitory signs. In chronic anoxia there is lethargy, dullness, ataxia, weakness and in some cases muscle tremor or convulsions. In both acute and chronic anoxia the signs of the primary disease will also be evident.

Clinical Pathology and Necropsy Findings

There is no distinctive clinical pathology or characteristic necropsy lesions other than those of the primary disease.

Diagnosis

Clinically there is little to differentiate cerebral anoxia from hypoglycaemia in which similar signs occur. Irritation and paralytic signs follow one another in many poisonings including lead and arsenic and in most diffuse diseases of the brain including encephalitis and encephalomalacia. The differential diagnosis of cerebral anoxia depends upon the detection of the cause of the anoxia.

Treatment

The provision of oxygen is essential and can usually only be provided by removing the causative agent. A respiratory stimulant may be advantageous in acute cases and artificial respiration may keep the animal alive for a few minutes.

REFERENCE

(1) Terlecki, S. *et al.* (1967). *Acta neuropath.*, 7, 185.

Hydrocephalus

Hydrocephalus may be congenital or acquired and is manifested in both cases by a syndrome referable to a general increase in intracranial pressure. Irritation signs of mania, head-pressing, muscle tremor and convulsions occur when the onset is rapid, and signs of paralysis including dullness, blindness and muscular weakness are present when the increased pressure develops slowly.

Aetiology

Hydrocephalus may be congenital or acquired but in both instances it is due to defective drainage of cerebrospinal fluid. In the congenital disease there is an embryological defect in the drainage canals and foraminae between the individual ventricles or between the ventricles and the subarachnoid space. It may occur as a congenital defect alone, with lateral narrowing of the mesencephalon (2), or with chondrodysplasia. Many congenital cases occur as a result of conditioning by an inherited factor. Vitamin A deficiency is also thought to contribute as a cause and other cases occur, sometimes at a high level of incidence (2), without known cause. When the disease is acquired it is always because of obstruction of drainage by some local space-occupying lesion or inflammation. In acquired hydrocephalus the obstruction may occur acutely or even transiently; cholesterol granulomas (cholesteatoma) in the choroid plexuses of the lateral ventricles of the horse may produce transient, acute hydrocephalus on a number of occasions before the tumour reaches sufficient size to cause permanent obstruction.

Compression of the brain occurs in hypovitaminosis A in calves due to failure of growth and sculpturing of the cranial vault to accommodate the growing brain.

Pathogenesis

Increased intracranial pressure in the foetus and before the syndemoses of the skull have fused causes hydrocephalus with enlargement of the cranium. After fusion of the suture lines the skull acts as a rigid container and an increase in the volume of its contents increases intracranial pressure. Although the increase in volume of the contents may be caused by the development of a local lesion such as an abscess, tumour, haematoma, or cestode cyst, which interferes with drainage of the CSF, the more common lesion is a congenital defect of CSF drainage. The general effects in all cases are the same, the only difference being that local lesions may produce localizing signs as well as signs of increased intracranial pressure. These latter signs are caused by compression atrophy of nervous tissue and ischaemic anoxia due to compression of blood vessels and impairment of blood supply to the brain. In congenital hydrocephalus the signs observed are usually those of paralysis of function while acquired hydrocephalus, being more acute, is usually manifested first by irritation phenomena followed by signs of paralysis. Oedema of the optic papilla is one of the characteristic signs of increased intracranial pressure and can usually be detected ophthalmoscopically. Bradycardia occurs inconstantly and cannot be considered to be diagnostic.

Clinical Findings

In hydrocephalus there is, in most cases, a gradual onset of general paralysis. Initially there is depression, disinclination to move, an expressionless stare and a lack of precision in acquired movements. A stage of somnolence follows and is most marked in horses. The animal stands with half closed eyes, lowered head and a vacant expression and often leans against or supports itself upon some solid object. Chewing is slow, intermittent and incomplete and animals are often observed standing with food hanging from their mouths. The reaction to cutaneous stimulation is reduced, and abnormal postures are frequently adopted. Frequent stumbling, faulty placement of the feet and inco-ordi-

nation are evidenced when the animal moves, and circling may occur in some cases. Bradycardia and cardiac arrhythmia have been observed.

Although the emphasis is on depression and paralysis, signs of brain irritation may occur particularly in the early stages. These signs often occur in isolated episodes during which a wild expression, charging, head-pressing, circling, tremor and convulsions appear. These episodes may be separated by quite long intervals, sometimes of several weeks duration. In vitamin A deficiency in calves blindness and papilloedema are the early signs and an acute convulsive stage occurs terminally.

Congenitally affected animals are usually alive at birth but are unable to stand and most die within 48 hours. The cranium is domed, the eyes protrude and nystagmus is often evident.

Clinical Pathology

Examination of the constitution and pressure of the CSF will be of value. The fluid is usually normal biochemically and cytologically but the pressure is increased. A marked increase in serum enzyme levels has been observed in calves with congenital hydrocephalus, due probably to an accompanying muscular dystrophy (1).

Necropsy Findings

The cranium may be swollen and soft in congenital hydrocephalus. The ventricles are distended with CSF under pressure and the overlying cerebral tissue is thinned if the pressure has been present for some time.

Diagnosis

Congenital hydrocephalus may be mistaken for vitamin A deficiency in newborn pigs, toxoplasmosis and hydranencephaly if there is no distortion of the cranium.

Acquired hydrocephalus needs to be differentiated from other diffuse diseases of the brain, including encephalitis and encephalomalacia, and from hepatic dystrophies which resemble it very closely. In these latter diseases there may be other signs of diagnostic value, including fever in encephalitis, and jaundice in hepatic dystrophy. In most cases it is necessary to depend largely on the history and recognition of individual disease entities.

REFERENCES

(1) Rhodes, M. B. *et al.* (1962). *Proc. Soc. exp. Biol., N.Y., 111,* 735.
(2) Barlow, R. M. & Donald, L. G. (1963). *J. comp. Path., 73,* 410.

Diffuse Cerebral Oedema

Diffuse cerebral oedema always occurs acutely and causes a general increase in intracranial pressure. It is a transient phenomenon and may be fatal but complete recovery or recovery with residual nervous signs also occurs. It is manifested clinically by blindness, opisthotonus, muscle tremor, paralysis and clonic convulsions.

Aetiology

The most important occurrence of diffuse cerebral oedema is in polioencephalomalacia of ruminants and in salt poisoning of swine. In these diseases the oedema is primary and due probably to alterations in the concentration of cations in brain tissue and the sudden passage of water into the brain to establish ionic equilibrium.

Diffuse cerebral oedema also occurs after most traumatic injuries to the brain, in most encephalitides and in many poisonings but in these circumstances it is only of minor degree although it probably contributes to development of the clinical signs.

Pathogenesis

An increase in intracranial pressure occurs suddenly and, as in hydrocephalus, there is a resulting ischaemic anoxia of the brain due to compression of blood vessels and impairment of blood supply. This may not be the only factor which interferes with cerebral activity in polioencephalomalacia and salt poisoning. The clinical syndrome produced by the rapid rise in intracranial pressure is manifested by irritation phenomena followed by signs of paralysis. If the compression of the brain is severe enough and of sufficient duration ischaemic necrosis of the superficial layers of the cortical grey matter may occur, resulting in permanent nervous defects in those animals which recover. Opisthotonus and nystagmus are commonly observed and are probably due to the partial herniation of the cerebellum into the foramen magnum.

Clinical Findings

Although the rise of intracranial pressure in diffuse cerebral oedema is usually more acute than in hydrocephalus the development of clinical signs takes place over a period of 12 to 24 hours and cerebral shock does not occur. There is central blindness, and periodic attacks of abnormality occur in which opisthotonus, nystagmus, muscle tremor and convulsions are prominent. In the intervening periods the animal is dull, depressed, and blind and papilloedema can be observed on ophthalmoscopic examination. The irritation signs of tremor, convulsions and opisthotonus are usually not extreme but this varies with the rapidity of onset of the oedema. As the disease progresses, muscle weakness appears, the animal becomes ataxic, goes down and is unable to rise and the early signs persist. Clonic convulsions occur terminally and animals that survive may have residual defects of mentality and vision.

Clinical Pathology

Clinico-pathological observations have not been recorded in the specific diseases.

Necropsy Findings

Macroscopically the gyrae are flattened and the cerebellum is partially herniated into the foramen magnum with consequent distortion of its posterior aspect. The brain has a soft, swollen appearance and tends to sag over the edges of the cranium when the top has been removed.

Diagnosis

Diffuse cerebral oedema causes a syndrome not unlike that of encephalitis although there are rather fewer irritation phenomena. Differentiation from encephalomalacia and vitamin A deficiency may be difficult if the history does not give a clue to the cause of the disease. Metabolic diseases, particularly pregnancy toxaemia, hypomagnesaemic tetany of calves and lactation tetany resemble it closely, as do some cases of acute ruminal impaction. In the history of each of these diseases there are distinguishing features which aid in making a tentative diagnosis. Some of the poisonings, particularly lead, organic mercurials and arsenicals and enterotoxaemia caused by *Clostridium perfringens* Type D produce similar nervous signs and gut oedema of swine may be mistaken for diffuse cerebral oedema.

Treatment

Decompression of the brain is necessary in acute cerebral oedema. This is best effected by the intravenous injection of hypertonic solutions, either saline, glucose or sucrose, the latter being preferred because it maintains the hypertonicity over a long period. Diuretics usually produce tissue dehydration too slowly to be of much value in acute cases but they may be useful as an adjunct to hypertonic solutions, or in early or chronic cases. Temporary relief may also be achieved by drainage of the CSF but the technique is not without danger especially if the patient is convulsive.

Encephalitis

Encephalitis is, by definition, inflammation of the brain but in general usage it is taken to include those diseases in which inflammatory lesions occur in the brain, whether there is inflammation of the nervous tissue or primarily of the vessel walls. Clinically encephalitis is characterized by initial irritation signs followed by signs caused by loss of nervous function.

Aetiology

Most animal encephalitides are caused by viruses. *Listeria monocytogenes* is the most widespread bacterial cause and occurs in all species. Infectious bovine meningo-encephalitis is caused by bacterial infection. In swine, salmonellosis is often, and erysipelas is sometimes, accompanied by severe encephalitis. Toxoplasmosis is not a common cause but occurs occasionally in all species. A number of virus infections cause encephalitis. *All Species:* Rabies, pseudorabies and Japanese B. encephalitis. *Cattle:* Bovine malignant catarrh and sporadic bovine encephalomyelitis. *Swine:* Viral encephalomyelitis, hog cholera and African swine fever. *Horses:* Infectious encephalomyelitis and Borna disease. *Sheep:* Scrapie, louping ill and visna.

Pathogenesis

With the exception of the viruses of bovine malignant catarrh and sporadic bovine encephalomyelitis, which exert their effects principally on the vasculature, those viruses which cause encephalitis do so by invasion of cellular elements, usually the neurones, and cause initial stimulation and then death of the cells. Those bacteria which cause diffuse encephalitis also exert their effects primarily on vascular endothelium.

Entrance of the viruses into the nervous tissue occurs in several ways. Normally the blood–brain barrier is an effective filtering agent but when there is damage to the endothelium infection readily occurs. The synergistic relationship between the rickettsiae of tick-borne fever and the virus of louping ill probably has this basis. Entry may also occur by progression of the agent up a peripheral nerve trunk as occurs with the viruses of rabies and pseudorabies and with *L. monocytogenes*. Entry via the olfactory nerves is also possible.

The clinical signs of encephalitis are usually referable to a general stimulatory or lethal effect on neurones in the brain. This may be in part due to the general effect of inflammatory oedema and partly due to the direct effects of the agent on nerve cells. In any particular case one or other of these factors may predominate but the tissue damage and therefore the signs are generalized. This is not the case in listeriosis in which damage is usually localized in the medulla with restriction of signs to the head and neck. Localizing signs may appear in the early stages of generalized encephalitis and remain as residual defects during the stage of convalescence. Visna is the only demyelinating encephalitis which occurs in farm animals.

Clinical Findings

Because the encephalitides are caused by infectious agents they are usually accompanied by fever and its attendant signs of anorexia, depression and increased heart rate. This is not the case in the very chronic diseases such as scrapie. In those diseases caused by agents which are not truly neurotropic there are characteristic signs which are not described here.

There may be an initial period of excitement or mania. The animal is easily startled and responds excessively to normal stimuli. It may exhibit viciousness and uncontrolled activity including blind charging, bellowing and pawing. Mental depression, including head-pressing, may occur between episodes. Irritation signs include convulsions, usually clonic and accompanied by nystagmus, champing of the jaws and excessive frothy salivation, and muscle tremor especially of the face and limbs. Unusual irritation phenomena are the paraesthesia and hyperaesthesia of pseudorabies and scrapie. Signs caused by loss of nervous function follow and may be the only signs in some instances. The loss of function varies in degree from paresis with knuckling at the lower limb joints, to spasticity of the limbs with resultant ataxia, to complete paralysis. More restricted pareses do occur and may be manifested by deviation of the head, walking in circles, abnormalities of posture, ataxia and inco-ordination but these are more commonly residual signs after recovery from the acute stages. Residual lesions affecting the cranial nerves do not commonly occur, except in listeriosis.

Clinical Pathology

Clinical pathology may be of considerable assistance in the diagnosis of encephalitis but the techniques used are for the most part specific to the individual diseases.

Necropsy Findings

There are no gross lesions in most encephalitides apart from those which occur in organs other than the brain and which are typical of the specific disease. Histological lesions vary with the type and mode of action of the causative agent. Material for laboratory diagnosis should include the fixed brain and portions of fresh brain material for culture and for transmission experiments.

Diagnosis

The diagnosis of encephalitis cannot depend entirely on the recognition of the typical syndrome because similar syndromes may be caused by many other brain diseases. Acute cerebral oedema and focal space-occupying lesions of the cranial cavity, a number of poisonings including salt, lead, arsenic, mercury, rotenone and chlorinated hydrocarbons all cause similar syndromes as do hypovitaminosis A, hypoglycaemia, encephalomalacia and meningitis. Fever is common in encephalitis but does not occur for example in rabies and scrapie, but it may occur in the non-inflammatory diseases if convulsions are severe. To a great extent, the clinical diagnosis rests upon the recognition of the specific encephalitides and the elimination of the other possible causes on the basis of the history and clinical pathology, especially in poisonings, and on clinical findings characteristic of the particular disease. In many cases a definite diagnosis can only be made on necropsy. For differentiation of the specific encephalitides reference should be made to the diseases listed under aetiology above.

Treatment

Specific treatments are dealt with under each disease. Generally the aim should be to provide supportive treatment by intravenous or stomach tube feeding during the acute phase. Sedation during the excitement stage may prevent the animal from injuring itself, and nervous system stimulants during the period of depression may maintain life through the critical phase. Although there is an increase in intracranial pressure no attempt is usually made to relieve this because of the deleterious effects of the procedure on other affected tissues.

Encephalomalacia

The degenerative diseases of the brain are grouped together under the name encephalomalacia. By definition encephalomalacia means softening. Here it is used to include all degenerative changes, particularly demyelination and necrosis of the grey matter. Leuco-encephalomalacia and polio-encephalomalacia refer to softening of the white and grey matter respectively. The syndrome produced is essentially one of loss of function.

Aetiology

Some indication of the diversity of causes of encephalomalacia can be obtained from the examples which follow but many sporadic cases occur in which the cause cannot be defined. Swayback and enzootic ataxia of lambs are caused by copper deficiency. Leuco-encephalomalacia of horses occurs when mouldy corn is fed and nigropallidal encephalomalacia occurs in horses fed on Yellow Star Thistle (*Centaurea solstitialis*). Focal symmetrical encephalomalacia of lambs is thought to be a residual lesion after intoxication with the toxin of *Clostridium perfringens* type D and malacial lesions associated with damage to blood vessels in pigs is thought to be due to sub-clinical attacks of enterotoxaemia similar to oedema disease (1). Encephalomalacia also occurs in poisonings caused by organic arsenicals and mercurials and by salt and in some instances by lead. Polioencephalomalacia is a disease of unknown aetiology which occurs in cattle, sheep and pigs. Leuco-encephalomalacia also occurs in mulberry heart disease of pigs. Degenerative brain lesions are described in bracken and horsetail poisoning in horses in which the major defect is a conditioned thiamine deficiency. In none of these diseases is there any evidence of an infectious agent, nor are the common causes in humans including the vascular lesions of infarction, haemorrhage and ischaemic necrosis, in evidence. In most instances the diseases are due to nutritional deficiencies or are associated with probable plant or bacterial toxins.

Pathogenesis

The pathogenesis of leuco-encephalomalacia is completely obscure although there is some indication that it may occur as a result of endothelial injury. Polioencephalomalacia appears to be, in some cases at least, a consequence of acute oedematous swelling of the brain and cortical ischaemia. The defect in swayback appears to be one of defective myelination probably caused by interference with phospholipid formation.

Whether the lesion is in the grey matter (polioencephalomalacia) or in the white matter (leuco-encephalomalacia) the syndrome is largely one of loss of function, although as might be expected irritation signs are more likely to occur when the grey matter is damaged.

Clinical Findings

Paralysis of varying degree is accompanied by dullness or somnolence, blindness, ataxia, head-pressing, circling and terminal coma. In the early stages, particularly in polio-encephalomalacia there are irritation signs including muscle tremor, opisthotonus, nystagmus and convulsions. The course may be one of gradual progression of signs or more commonly a level of abnormality is reached and maintained for a long period, often necessitating sacrifice of the animal.

Clinical Pathology

There are no clinico-pathological tests specific for encephalomalacia but various tests may aid in the diagnosis of some of the specific diseases mentioned above under aetiology.

Necropsy Findings

Gross lesions including areas of softening, cavitation and laminar necrosis of the cortex may be visible. The important lesions are described under each of the specific diseases.

Diagnosis

The syndromes produced by encephalomalacia resemble very closely those caused by most lesions which elevate intracranial pressure. The onset is quite sudden and there is depression of consciousness and loss of motor function. One major difference is that the lesions tend to be non-progressive and affected animals may continue to survive in an impaired state for long periods.

Treatment

Encephalomalacia is irreversible and the best that can be hoped for is that the patient can be maintained by supportive treatment through the initial stages so that it can be fattened for slaughter.

REFERENCE

(1) Harding, J. D. J. (1966). *Path. vet.*, 3, 83.

Traumatic Injury to the Brain

The effects of trauma to the brain vary with the site and extent of the injury but initially nervous shock is likely to occur followed by death, recovery, or the persistence of residual nervous signs.

Aetiology

Direct trauma to the head is an uncommon cause of brain injury in farm animals because of the force required to damage the cranium. Occasional cases may be seen in horses following accidental collisions or on falling backwards after rearing and in all animals following bizarre accidents. Cerebral nematodiasis causes brain damage occasionally in all species. *Setaria* spp. (1) and *Elaphostrongylus tenuis* (2, 3) are two of the causative filarid worms.

Many larval nematodes accidentally migrate through the brain, especially those which have a somatic migration route and when they are in an atypical host. A distinction should be made between the occasional presence in the central nervous system (CNS) of nematode larvae which have followed an aberrant course, and a large-scale invasion of nervous tissue by a worm whose larvae undergoes a somatic type of migration. The latter is described as 'visceral larva migrans', and the CNS is only one of the organs invaded. *Hypoderma bovis* and *Oestrus ovis* larvae occasionally migrate to brain and spinal cord. Animals trapped in bogs, cellars, sumps and water holes are sometimes dragged out by the head with dire consequences to the medulla and cervical cord. Spontaneous cerebral haemorrhage is rare in animals but has been observed in cows at parturition, in which multiple small haemorrhages occur in the medulla and mid-brain.

Pathogenesis

The initial reaction in severe trauma or haemorrhage is nervous shock. Slowly developing subdural haematoma, a common development in man, is accompanied by the gradual onset of signs of a space-occupying lesion of the cranial cavity but this seems to be a rare occurrence in animals (4).

If structural injury to nervous tissue does not occur there are no residual effects, but in most cases damage has been done and the residual signs vary with the site and extent of the lesion. There may be haemorrhage or a depressed fracture, both of which cause local pressure effects; there may be bruising (contusion) or damage to nerve cells without macroscopic change (concussion). In nematodiasis traumatic destruction of nervous tissue may occur in many parts of the brain and in general the severity of the signs depends upon the size and mobility of the parasites and the route of entry (5). One exception to this generalization is the experimental 'visceral larva migrans' produced by *Toxocara canis* in pigs in which the nervous signs occur at a time when lesions in most other organs are healing. The signs are apparently provoked by a reaction of the host to static larvae rather than trauma due to migration (6). Nematodes not resident in nervous tissues may cause nervous signs due possibly to allergy or the formation of toxins (5).

Clinical Findings

The syndrome usually follows the pattern of greatest severity initially with recovery occurring quickly but incompletely to a point where a residual defect is evident, this defect persisting unchanged for a long period and often permanently. This failure to improve or worsen after the initial phase is a characteristic of traumatic injury.

With severe injury there is cerebral shock in which the animal falls unconscious with or without a transient clonic convulsion. Consciousness may never be regained but in animals that recover it returns in from a few minutes up to several hours. During the period of unconsciousness clinical examination reveals dilatation of the pupils, absence of the eye preservation and pupillary light reflexes, and a slow, irregular respiration, the irregularity being phasic in many cases. There may be evidence of bleeding from the nose and ears and palpation of the cranium may reveal a site of injury. Residual signs vary a great deal, blindness is present if the optic cortex is damaged; hemiplegia may be associated with lesions in the midbrain; traumatic epilepsy may occur with lesions in the motor cortex.

Necropsy Findings

In most cases a gross haemorrhagic lesion will be evident but in concussion and nematodiasis the lesions may be detectable only on histological examination.

Diagnosis

Unless a history of trauma is available diagnosis may be difficult. Infestation with nematode larvae causes a great variety of signs depending on the number of invading larvae and the amount and location of the damage.

Treatment

Surgical treatment may be possible in injuries where depressed fractures of cranial bones can be detected. Central nervous system stimulants or artificial respiration may be necessary if cerebral shock is severe or prolonged and respiratory failure seems imminent. Parenteral coagulants are advisable if extensive haemorrhage is suspected.

REFERENCES
(1) Innes, J. R. M. (1951). *Brit. vet. J.*, *107*, 187.
(2) Kennedy, P. C. *et al.* (1952). *Cornell Vet.*, *42*, 118.
(3) Whitlock, J. (1959). *Cornell Vet.*, *49*, 3.
(4) Leonard, E. (1947). *Cornell Vet.*, *37*, 381.
(5) Sprent, J. F. A. (1955). *Parasitology*, *45*, 31 & 41.
(6) Done, J. T. *et al.* (1960). *Res. vet. Sci.*, *1*, 133.

Focal Diseases of the Brain
Brain Abscess

Brain abscesses produce a great variety of clinical signs depending on their situation and size. Basically the syndrome produced is one of a space-occupying lesion of the cranial cavity.

Aetiology

Intracranial abscesses may occur as extensions from local suppurative processes in cranial sinuses, nasal cavities, hypophysis or the middle ear. In all these instances the lesion is usually single and accompanied by meningitis. Haematogenous metastases, deriving from suppurative lesions in other organs, which periodically produce a bacteraemia, may be multiple (1). *Actinobacillus mallei* may occur in brain abscesses in horses affected with glanders and *Streptococcus equi* as a complication of strangles. *Act. bovis* and *Mycobacterium tuberculosis* have been observed in metastatic focal cerebral lesions in cattle and *Sphaerophorus necrophorus* in similar lesions in calves. *Staphylococcus aureus* is present in brain lesions of tick pyaemia of lambs. Granulomas may occur in the brain in systemic fungal infections. Listeriosis is the one specific disease characterized by the development of micro-abscesses in the brain.

Pathogenesis

Single abscesses cause local pressure effects on nervous tissue and may produce some signs of irritation including head-pressing and mania but the predominant effect is one of loss of function due to destruction of nerve cells. Multiple abscesses have much the same effect but whereas in single abscesses the signs usually make it possible to define the location of the lesion, multiple lesions present a confusing multiplicity of signs and variation in their severity from day to day suggesting that damage has occurred at a number of widely distributed points and at different times.

Clinical Findings

General signs include mental depression, clumsiness, head-pressing and blindness often preceded or interrupted by transient attacks of motor irritation including excitement, uncontrolled activity, and convulsions. Localizing signs depend on the location of lesions and may include cerebellar ataxia, deviation of the head with circling and falling, hemiplegia or paralysis of individual or groups of cranial nerves often in a unilateral pattern. In the later stages there is usually papilloedema.

Clinical Pathology

Roentgenological examination will not detect brain abscesses unless they are calcified or cause erosion of bone. Leucocytes, protein and bacteria may be present in the CSF and it may be possible to determine the drug sensitivity of the causative organisms.

Necropsy Findings

The abscess or abscesses may be visible on gross examination and if superficial are usually accompanied by local meningitis. Large abscesses may penetrate to the ventricles and result in a diffuse ependymitis. Micro-abscesses may be visible only on histological examination. A general necropsy examination may reveal the primary lesion.

Diagnosis

Brain abscess is manifested by signs of irritation and loss of function which can occur in many other diseases of the brain especially when local lesions develop slowly. This occurs more frequently with tumours and parasitic cysts but it may occur in encephalitis. There may be evidence of the existence of a suppurative lesion in another organ, and a high cell count and detectable infection in the cerebrospinal fluid to support the diagnosis of abscess. Fever may or may not be present. The only specific disease in which abscess occurs is listeriosis in which the lesions are largely confined to the medulla and the characteristic signs include circling and unilateral facial paralysis. Occasional cases may be caused by fungal infections including cryptococcosis. Toxoplasmosis is an uncommon cause of granulomatous lesions in the brain of most species.

Many cases have a superficial resemblance to otitis media but there is, in the latter, rotation of the head rather than deviation, a commonly associated facial paralysis and an absence of signs of cerebral depression (2).

Treatment

Parenteral treatment with antibacterial drugs offers the best chance of curing the animal but the results are generally unsatisfactory because of the inaccessibility of the lesion.

REFERENCES

(1) Griner, L. A. *et al.* (1956). *J. Amer. vet. med. Ass., 129*, 417.
(2) Blood, D. C. (1960). *Canad. vet. J., 1*, 437 & 476.

Neoplasms of the Brain

Neoplasms in the brain or meninges produce a syndrome indicative of a general increase in intracranial pressure and local destruction of nervous tissue.

Aetiology

The reader is referred to references 1 and 5 for a summary of available reports on the neoplasms of the brain in animals. Some other observations include an ependymoma in a cow with signs resembling listeriosis but which persisted over a period of 6 months (2), a cerebral glioma in the lateral ventricle which also caused persistent circling in a cow for 6 weeks (3), a squamous cell carcinoma of the leptomeninges and brain in a cow (6), a schwannoma of the intracranial part of a vagus nerve in a heifer (7), a medullablastoma in a newborn calf with opisthotonus and tonic convulsions (8) and 2 cases involving the acoustic nerve in young cattle (4). The acoustic and vagal nerve lesions were associated with circling, deviation of the head and inco-ordination. The much quoted cholesteatoma of horses is a chronic granulomatous lesion containing massive deposits of cholesterol but due to its gradual growth it produces a syndrome similar to that of a brain tumour.

Pathogenesis

The development of the disease parallels that of any space-occupying lesion with the concurrent appearance of signs of increased intracranial pressure and local tissue destruction.

Clinical Findings

The clinical picture is very similar to that produced by a slowly developing abscess and localizing signs depend on the location, size and speed of development of the tumour.

Clinical Pathology

There are no positive findings in clinico-pathological examination which aid in diagnosis.

Necropsy Findings

The brain should be carefully sectioned after fixation if the tumour is deep-seated.

Diagnosis

Differentiation is required from the other diseases in which space-occupying lesions of the cranial cavity occur. The rate of development is usually much slower in tumour than with the other lesions.

Treatment

Surgical removal of a tumour is unlikely to be attempted in a farm animal.

REFERENCES

(1) Innes, J. R. M. & Saunders, L. Z. (1957). *Advances in Veterinary Science*, Vol. 3, New York: Academic Press.
(2) Rees Evans, E. T. & Palmer, A. C. (1960). *J. comp. Path., 70*, 305.
(3) Luginbuhl, H. (1956). *Vet. Rec., 68*, 1032.

(4) Sullivan, D. J. & Anderson, W. A. (1958). *Amer. J. vet. Res.,* *19*, 848.

(5) Luginbuhl, H. (1963). *Ann. N.Y. Acad. Sci., 108*, 702.

(6) Peterson, J. E. (1963). *J. comp. Path., 73*, 163.

(7) Palmer, A. C. & Spratling, F. R. (1964). *Brit. vet. J., 120*, 105.

(8) McGavin, M. D. (1961). *Aust. vet. J., 37*, 390.

Coenurosis

(Gid, Sturdy)

Coenurosis is the disease caused by invasion of the brain and spinal cord by the intermediate stage of a tapeworm believed to be *Taenia multiceps*. The syndrome produced is one of localized, space-occupying lesions of the central nervous system. In most countries the disease is much less common than it used to be and relatively few losses occur.

Aetiology

The disease is caused by *Coenurus cerebralis* which is commonly considered to be the intermediate stage of the tapeworm *Taenia multiceps* which inhabits the intestine of dogs and wild Canidae. However, it has also been suggested that *Coenurus cerebralis* is the intermediate stage of *Taenia serialis* which normally occurs in the subcutaneous tissues of rabbits. The embryos, which hatch from eggs ingested in food contaminated by the faeces of infested dogs, hatch in the intestine and pass into the blood stream. Only those embryos which lodge in the brain or spinal cord survive and continue to grow to the coenurid stage. *Coenurus cerebralis* (*Multiceps multiceps*) can mature in the brain and spinal cords of sheep, goats, cattle, horses and wild ruminants and occasionally man but clinical coenurosis is primarily a disease of sheep and occasionally cattle (3). Infection in newborn calves, acquired prenatally, has been observed occasionally (2).

Pathogenesis

During their early stages of migration through nervous tissue the migrating embryos may cause signs of irritation including mania and convulsions but most signs are caused by the mature coenurus which may take 6 to 8 months to develop to its full size of about 5 cm. The cyst-like coenurus develops gradually and causes pressure on nervous tissue resulting in its irritation and eventual destruction. It may cause sufficient pressure to rarefy and soften cranial bones.

Clinical Findings

Some affected sheep show an acute onset of irritation phenomena including a wild expression, salivation, frenzied running and convulsions. De-

viation of the eyes and head may also occur. Some animals may die in this stage but the greater proportion go on to the second stage of loss of function phenomena, the only stage in most affected animals. Dullness, clumsiness, head-pressing, ataxia, incomplete mastication and periodic epileptiform convulsions are the usual signs. Papilloedema may be present. Localizing signs comprise chiefly deviation of the head and circling and sometimes unilateral blindness. In young animals local softening of the cranium may occur over a superficial cyst and rupture of the cyst to the exterior may follow with final recovery. When the spinal cord is involved there is a gradual development of paresis and eventually inability to rise. Death usually occurs after a long course of several months.

Clinical Pathology

Clinico-pathological examinations are not generally used in diagnosis in animals but a haemagglutination test has been used with some success in sheep and goats (4).

Necropsy Findings

Thin-walled cysts may be present anywhere in the brain but are most commonly found on the external surface of the cerebral hemispheres. In the spinal cord the lesions are most common in the lumbar region but can be present in the cervical area. Local pressure atrophy of nervous tissue is apparent and softening of the overlying bone may occur.

Diagnosis

The condition needs to be differentiated from other local space-occupying lesions of the cranial cavity and spinal cord including abscess, tumour and haemorrhage. In the early stages the disease may be confused with encephalitis because of the signs of brain irritation. Clinically there is little difference between them and it is often necessary to depend upon local knowledge of the incidence of these diseases when making a diagnosis.

Treatment and Control

Surgical drainage of the cyst may make it possible to fatten the animal for slaughter (1). The life cycle can be broken most satisfactorily by control of mature tapeworm infestation in dogs. Periodic treatment with a taenicide of all farm dogs is essential for control of this and other more pathogenic tapeworms. Carcases of livestock infested with the intermediate stages should not be available to dogs.

REFERENCES

(1) de Villiers, S. W. (1950). *J. S. Afr. vet. med. Ass.*, *21*, 155.
(2) McManus, D. (1963). *Vet. Rec.*, *75*, 697.
(3) Dent, C. H. R. (1965). *Aust. vet. J.*, *42*, 28.
(4) Biswal, G. *et al.* (1962). *Indian vet. J.*, *39*, 153.

Diseases of the Meninges

Meningitis

Inflammation of the meninges occurs most commonly as a complication of a pre-existing disease. It is usually caused by a bacterial infection and clinically is manifested by fever, cutaneous hyperaesthesia and rigidity of muscles. Although it may affect the spinal cord or brain specifically it commonly affects both and is dealt with here as a single entity.

Aetiology

A mild degree of meningitis occurs in most viral encephalitides and may dominate the initial symptomatology. In bovine malignant catarrh and sporadic bovine encephalomyelitis the meningitis is morphologically dominant. Bacterial meningitis is more common and important than that caused by viruses and is usually haematogenous. Some of the more common bacterial diseases in which meningitis may occur are strangles (*Streptococcus equi*) in horses, listeriosis (*Listeria monocytogenes*), streptococcal and coliform septicaemias in newborn animals, Glasser's disease (*Haemophilus suis*) in pigs, pasteurellosis (*Pasteurella multocida*) in calves and (*Past. haemolytica*) in lambs, leptospirosis (*L. pomona*) in cattle and tuberculosis. Minor serous meningitis and vasculitis occur in erysipelas (*Erysipelothrix insidiosa*) and salmonellosis (*Salmonella* spp.) in pigs.

Sporadic cases occur as a result of penetrating wounds of the skull, otitis media and frontal sinusitis usually after dehorning. The latter is particularly likely to occur by the excessive application of a hot iron used as a cautery.

Pathogenesis

Inflammation of the meninges causes local swelling, interference with blood supply to the brain and spinal cord, but as a rule penetration of the inflammation along blood vessels and into nervous tissue is of minor importance and causes only superficial encephalitis. Failure to treat meningitis caused by pyogenic bacteria often permits the development of a fatal choroiditis, with exudation into CSF, and ependymitis. There is also inflammation around the nerve trunks as they pass across the subarachnoid space. The signs produced by meningitis are thus a combination of those resulting from irritation of both central and peripheral nervous systems. In spinal meningitis there is muscular spasm with rigidity of the limbs and neck, arching of the back and hyperaesthesia with pain on light touching of the skin. When the cerebral meninges are affected, irritation signs, including muscle tremor and convulsions are the common manifestations. Since meningitis is usually bacterial in origin, fever and toxaemia can be expected if the lesion is sufficiently extensive.

Defects of drainage of CSF occur in both acute and chronic inflammation of the meninges and produce signs of increased intracranial pressure. The signs are general although the accumulation of fluid may be localized to particular sites such as the lateral ventricles.

Clinical Findings

Acute meningitis usually develops suddenly and is accompanied by fever and toxaemia in addition to nervous signs. Vomiting is common in the early stages in pigs. There is trismus, opisthotonus and rigidity of the neck and back. Motor irritation signs include tonic spasms of the muscles of the neck causing retraction of the head, muscle tremor and paddling movements. Cutaneous hyperaesthesia is present in varying degrees, even light touching of the skin causing severe pain in some cases. There may be disturbance of consciousness manifested by excitement or mania in the early stages, followed by drowsiness and eventual coma. In uncomplicated meningitis the respiration is usually slow and deep, and often phasic in the form of Cheyne-Stokes's or Biot's breathing.

Although meningitis in farm animals is usually diffuse affecting particularly the brain stem and upper cervical cord, it may be quite localized and produce localizing signs including involvement of the cranial or spinal nerves. Localized muscle tremor, hyperaesthesia and rigidity may result. Muscles in the affected area are firm and board-like on palpation. Anaesthesia and paralysis usually develop caudal to the meningitic area. Spread of the inflammation along the cord is usual.

Reference should be made to the specific diseases cited under aetiology for a more complete description of their clinical manifestations.

Clinical Pathology

Cerebrospinal fluid collected aseptically under anaesthesia contains protein, has a high cell-count and usually contains bacteria. Culture and determination of drug sensitivity of the bacteria is advisable because of the low concentrations of anti-bacterial drugs achieved in CSF.

Necropsy Findings

Hyperaemia, the presence of haemorrhages, thickening and opacity of the meninges, especially over the base of the brain, are the usual macroscopic findings. The CSF is often turbid and may contain fibrin. A local, superficial encephalitis is a common accompaniment. Additional morbid changes are described under the specific diseases and are often of importance in differential diagnosis.

Diagnosis

Hyperaesthesia, muscle rigidity and fever are the major diagnostic signs in meningitis but it may be confused with encephalitis and myelitis. Examination of the CSF is the only means of confirming the diagnosis before death. Spinal cord compression is usually more insidious in onset, is seldom accompanied by fever, hyperaesthesia is less marked or absent and there is flaccidity rather than spasticity.

Treatment

The infection is usually bacterial, and parenteral treatment with antibiotics or sulphonamides is necessary. Large doses over a long period (7 to 10 days) are usually required as relapses occur commonly. The passage of drugs into the CSF does not occur readily and high concentrations cannot be anticipated. Intrathecal administration is sometimes undertaken to ensure a better response in severe or intractable cases. Analgesics may be advisable if pain is severe. Oral salicylates are effective especially in chronic cases. Animals recumbent for long periods require careful nursing to avoid pressure sores.

Functional Diseases of the Brain

There are a number of diseases in which manifestations of involvement of the nervous system occur but in which no histological lesion can be found. Because most of these are dealt with as specific diseases they are not described in detail here.

Psychoses or neuroses are extremely rare in farm animals although the vices of crib-biting and weaving in horses could be included in this category. Hysteria in sows at farrowing is a common occurrence. Affected animals attack the piglets as soon as they approach to suckle and cause serious, often fatal injury. Cannibalism is not a feature, the sow making no attempt to eat the piglets. Administra-tion of an ataractic drug to the sow usually causes sufficient sedation to permit suckling by the piglets and there is no further trouble although in occasional cases hysteria persists and the piglets are lost.

Idiopathic epilepsy appears to be very rare in farm animals. It is recorded as an inherited condition in Brown Swiss cattle. Residual lesions after encephalitis may cause symptomatic epileptiform seizures but there are usually other localizing signs. A true grand mal epileptiform seizure is manifested by an initial period of alertness, the counterpart of the aura in human seizures, followed by falling in a state of tetany which gives way after a few seconds to a clonic convulsion with paddling, opisthotonus and champing of the jaws. The clonic convulsions may last for some minutes and are followed by a period of relaxation. The animal is unconscious throughout the seizure but appears normal shortly afterwards. Some fits may be preceded by a local motor phenomenon such as tetany or tremor of one limb or of the face. The convulsion may spread from this initial area to the rest of the body. This form is referred to as Jacksonian epilepsy and the local sign may indicate the whereabouts of the local lesion or point of excitation. The attacks are always recurrent and the animal is normal in the intervening periods.

Liver dystrophies including those caused by plant poisons are often accompanied by nervous signs. Severe mental depression occurs in poisoning by *Crotalaria* spp. and other plants. Hydrophobia may occur in photosensitivity of hepatic origin in sheep: affected animals develop clonic convulsions when driven through water or immersed in dipping tanks.

Poisons. Many poisons cause neurological disturbances without the production of detectable lesions in the brain. Most of these are organic and include rotenone, chlorinated hydrocarbons, organophosphates, nicotine sulphate, carbon tetrachloride and strychnine. Many plants produce purely nervous signs. *Indigophera enneaphylla* is the cause of a functional nervous derangement of horses known as Birdsville Horse Disease; *Phalaris tuberosa*, perennial rye grass, marshmallow, stagger weed and many other plants too numerous to mention here cause ataxia when animals graze on them. Rape causes a syndrome of blindness, wandering, head-pressing and occasional excitement in cattle.

Bacterial toxins, including those of *Clostridium botulinum*, *Cl. tetani* and *Cl. perfringens* type D, produce marked neurological signs without detectable lesions and in gut oedema of swine there are severe nervous signs without an apparent structural cause other than a mild oedema. Infestations with ticks, including *Ixodes holocyclus* and *Dermacentor andersoni* may cause mortality in young farm animals. Posterior paralysis and respiratory embarrassment occur and affected animals die of respiratory paralysis, thirst and starvation. Lightning stroke and electrocution cause death by severe cerebral shock without the appearance of lesions in most cases.

Inherited diseases. In many of the inherited defects of the CNS there are no demonstrable lesions to account for the clinical signs observed and the defects appear to be mainly functional. These diseases are dealt with in more detail under the specific disease and are only listed here:

Inherited Idiopathic Epilepsy of cattle
Inherited Spastic Paresis of cattle
Inherited Periodic Spasticity of cattle
Inherited Myotonia Congenita of goats
Inherited Exophthalmus and Strabismus of cattle

DISEASES OF THE SPINAL CORD

Traumatic Injury

Sudden severe trauma to the spinal cord causes a syndrome of immediate, complete, flaccid paralysis caudal to the injury because of spinal shock. This is soon followed by flaccid paralysis in the area supplied by the injured segment and spastic paralysis caudal to it.

Aetiology

Dislocation of vertebrae or fracture of the arch or body are the usual causes. As in the brain, concussion or contusion may occur without structural damage to the bones of the vertebral column. Horses with osteodystrophia fibrosa in a mild form may suffer spontaneous fractures of lumbar vertebrae while galloping or jumping and lactating sows may suffer the same injury when they climb up on low fences at feeding time. Horses and cattle falling through barn floors are among the more common subjects for vertebral fracture. A special occurrence is in old bulls in insemination centres. With increasing age these bulls are prone to calcification of the ventral vertebral ligaments and the development of a 'spondylitis.' With a vigorous ejaculation the calcified ligament may fracture, the discontinuity extending up through a vertebral body. Less severe degrees of spondylitis have been recorded in a high proportion of much younger (2 to 3 years) bulls but the lesions appear to cause no clinical signs (5). Cerebrospinal nematodiasis is thought to be the cause of myelomalacia in a number of exotic diseases characterized by posterior paralysis in horses, goats and sheep (1, 2). *Stephanurus dentatus* larvae cause similar lesions in swine, as do the larvae of *Hypoderma bovis* in cattle. Experimental visceral larva migrans in pigs caused by infestation with larvae of *Toxocara canis* may also result in ataxia and posterior paralysis (3). The lesion is essentially traumatic and the diseases are included here rather than under myelomalacia.

Trauma due to excessive mobility of upper cervical vertebrae may contribute to the spinal cord lesion in wobbles in horses.

Pathogenesis

The lesion may consist of disruption of nervous tissue or its compression by displaced bone or haematoma. Minor degrees of damage may result in local oedema or hyperaemia, or in the absence of macroscopic lesions, transitory injury to nerve cells classified as concussion. The initial response is that of spinal shock which affects a variable number of segments on both sides of the injured segment, and is manifested by complete flaccid paralysis. The lesion must affect at least the ventral third of the cord before spinal shock occurs. When the shock wears off the effects of the residual lesion remain. These may be temporary in themselves and completely normal function may return as the oedema or the haemorrhage is resorbed. In man, if structural damage persists, there is usually hyperaesthesia in the area of the lesion, flaccid paralysis in the same general area and spastic paralysis caudally. Whether the same pattern holds for animals, especially ruminants, is open to doubt. In sheep extensive experimental damage to the cord may be followed by recovery to the point of being able to walk (4).

Traumatic lesions usually affect the whole cross section of the cord and produce a syndrome typical of complete transection. Partial transection signs are more common in slowly developing lesions.

Clinical Findings

Spinal shock develops immediately after severe injury and is manifested by flaccid paralysis to a variable degree up and down the cord. There is a concurrent fall in local blood pressure due to vasodilatation and there may be local sweating. Stretch reflexes and cutaneous sensitivity disappear but reappear within a half to several hours.

Residual signs may remain when the shock passes off. Paralysis occurs and varies in severity and extent with the severity of the lesion. The extremities are affected in most cases and the animal is unable to rise and may be in sternal or lateral recumbency. The muscles of respiration may also be affected resulting in interference with respiration. The body area supplied by the affected segments will show flaccid paralysis, disappearance of reflexes and muscle wasting—a lower motor neurone lesion. When the lesion is situated in the cervical cord there will be spastic paralysis in all four extremities, the reflexes will be exaggerated and there will be no muscle wasting.

Anaesthesia occurs at and caudal to the lesion and hyperaesthesia may be observed in a girdle-like zone at the anterior edge of the lesion due to irritation of sensory fibres by local inflammation and oedema. Because of interference with the sacral autonomic nerve outflow there may be paralysis of the bladder and rectum although this is not usually apparent in large animals. The vertebral column should be examined carefully for signs of injury. Excessive mobility, pain on pressure, and mal-alignment of spinous processes may indicate bone displacements or fractures. Rectal examination may also reveal damage or displacement particu-larly in fractures of vertebral bodies and in old bulls with spondylitis. There is usually no systemic disturbance but pain may be sufficiently severe to cause an increase in heart rate and prevent eating.

Recovery may occur in 1 to 3 weeks if nervous tissue is not destroyed but when extensive damage has been done to a significantly large section of the cord there is no recovery and disposal is advisable. In rare cases animals which suffer a severe injury continue to be ambulatory for up to 12 hours before paralysis appears. In such instances it may be that a fracture occurs but displacement follows at a later stage during more active movement.

Clinical Pathology

Roentgenological examination may reveal the site and extent of the injury.

Necropsy Findings

The abnormality is always visible on macrosco-pic examination.

Diagnosis

Differentiation from other spinal cord diseases is not usually difficult because of the speed of onset and the history of trauma although spinal myelitis and meningitis may also develop rapidly. Other causes of recumbency may be confused with trauma especially if the animal is not observed in the imme-diate pre-clinical period. In most diseases charac-terized by recumbency, such as azoturia, acute rumen impaction and acute coliform mastitis there are other signs to indicate the existence of a lesion other than spinal cord trauma.

Treatment

Treatment is expectant only, surgical treatment rarely being attempted. Careful nursing on deep bedding with turning at 3-hourly intervals, massage of bony prominences and periodic slinging may help to carry an animal with concussion or other minor lesion through a long period of recumbency. In cattle especially, recumbency beyond a period of about 48 hours is likely to result in widespread necrosis of the posterior muscles of the thigh and recovery in such cases is improbable.

REFERENCES

(1) Innes, J. R. M. & Saunders, L. Z. (1957). *Advances in Veterinary Science.* Vol. 3, New York: Academic Press.
(2) Nielsen, S. W. & Aftosmis, J. (1964). *J. Amer. vet. med. Ass.,* *144,* 155.
(3) Done, J. T. *et al.* (1960). *Res. vet. Sci.,* *1,* 133.
(4) Tietz, W. J. (1964). *Amer. J. vet. Res.,* *25,* 1500.
(5) Bane, A. & Hansen, H. J. (1962) *Cornell Vet.,* *52,* 362.

Spinal Cord Compression

The gradual development of a space-occupying lesion in the vertebral canal produces a syndrome of progressive paralysis.

Aetiology

Tumours, protruding abscesses of the vertebrae and exostoses are the common causes. Migrating parasite larvae and the cysts of *Coenurus cerebralis* may also produce a gradually developing lesion. The only commonly occurring tumour in animals is lymphomatosis which infiltrates the nerve trunks and invades the vertebral canal, usually in the lumbosacral region and less commonly in the brachial and cervical areas. A rare case of angioma in the spinal cord of a horse, causing ataxia, is also reported (1). Abscesses may develop by haemato-genous spread from other lesions in actinomycosis of cattle, caseous lymphadenitis of sheep and in infections with *Corynebacterium pyogenes*. It most commonly occurs in young farm animals, the infec-tion usually gaining entrance through an infected navel. There may or may not be accompanying signs of liver abscess, arthritis or endocarditis. In most cases the development of a spinal cord abscess takes several weeks or even months and the original navel lesion may have disappeared by this time (2). Local spread from vertebral osteomyelitis is prob-ably the most common cause of spinal cord abscess and is usually accompanied by local pachymenin-gitis but spinal cord abscesses not involving verte-bral bodies have also been described in lambs (3). These vertebral lesions occur commonly in brucel-losis of swine. Exostoses may develop over prolapsed intervertebral discs although these do not seem to be common lesions in animals other than dogs. An exostosis over an incomplete fracture of a vertebral body has been observed to cause partial cord injury in individual cases and in groups of lambs grazing around old lead mines. Hypovitaminosis A, particularly in young growing swine, causes compression of the spinal cord and of the nerve roots as they pass through vertebral foraminae.

Pathogenesis

The development of any of the lesions listed above results in the gradual appearance of motor paralysis or anaesthesia depending on whether the lesion is ventrally or dorsally situated. In most cases there is involvement of all tracts but care is necessary in examination if the more bizarre lesions are to be accurately diagnosed. There may be hemiplegia if the lesion is laterally situated. Paraplegia is caused by a bilateral lesion in the thoracic or lumbar cord and monoplegia by a unilateral lesion in the same area. Bilateral lesions in the cervical region cause quadriplegia.

Clinical Findings

Pain and hyperaesthesia may be evident before motor paralysis appears. The pain may be constant or occur only with movement. Motor paralysis develops gradually; difficulty in rising is the first sign, then unsteadiness during walking due to weakness which may be more marked in one of a pair of limbs. The toes are dragged along the ground while walking and the animal knuckles over on the fetlocks when standing. Finally the animal can rise only with assistance and then becomes permanently recumbent. These stages may be passed through in a period of 4 to 5 days. The paralysis will be flaccid or spastic depending on the site of the lesion and reflexes will be absent or exaggerated in the respective states.

Considerable variation in signs occurs depending on the site of the lesion. There may be local hyperaesthesia around the site of the lesion and straining to defaecate may be pronounced. Retention of the urine and faeces may occur. There is usually no detectable abnormality of the vertebrae on physical examination.

Clinical Pathology

Roentgenological examination of the vertebral column should be carried out if the animal is of a suitable size.

Necropsy Findings

The abnormality is usually visible.

Diagnosis

Differentiation between abscess, tumour and exostosis in the vertebral canal is usually not practicable without roentgenological examination. In lymphomatosis of cattle there may be signs caused by lesions in other organs. A history of previous trauma may suggest exostosis. The history usually serves to differentiate the lesion from acute trauma. Spinal myelitis, myelomalacia and meningitis may resemble cord compression but are much less common. They are usually associated with encephalitis, encephalomalacia and cerebral meningitis respectively. Meningitis is characterized by much more severe hyperaesthesia and muscle rigidity. Rabies in the dumb form may be characterized by a similar syndrome but ascends the cord and is fatal within a 6-day period. Iliac thrombosis in the horse appears during exercise and is manifested by vascular changes in the affected limbs.

Treatment

Treatment is usually not possible and in most cases it is advisable to sacrifice the animal for meat.

REFERENCES
(1) Palmer, A. C. & Hickman, J. (1960). Vet. Rec., 72, 611.
(2) Downey, N. E. (1957). N.Z. vet. J., 5, 47.
(3) Dodd, D. C. & Cordes, D. O. (1964). N.Z. vet. J., 12, 1.

Myelitis

Inflammation of the spinal cord is usually associated with viral encephalitis and, as in that disease, the initial signs of irritation are followed by signs of loss of function. Hyperaesthesia or paraesthesia may result if the dorsal nerve nuclei are involved. This is particularly noticeable in pseudorabies and to a lesser extent in rabies. Paralysis is the more usual result. There are no specific myelitides in animals. Myelitis resembles myelomalacia and space-occupying lesions of the vertebral canal.

Myelomalacia

Myelomalacia occurs rarely as an entity separate from encephalomalacia. One recorded occurrence is focal spinal poliomalacia of sheep and in enzootic ataxia the lesions of demyelination are often restricted to the spinal cord. In both instances there is a gradual development of paralysis without signs of irritation and with no indication of brain involvement. Degeneration of spinal cord tracts has also been recorded in poisoning by Phalaris *tuberosa* in cattle and sheep. Poisoning of cattle by plants of *Zamia* spp. produces a syndrome suggestive of injury to the spinal cord but no lesions have been reported. Pantothenic acid or pyridoxine deficiencies also cause degeneration of spinal cord tracts in swine.

Sporadic cases of demyelination of spinal tracts have been observed in pigs. One outbreak is recorded in the litters of sows on lush clover pasture (1). The piglets were unable to stand, struggled violently on their sides with rigid extension of the limbs and although able to drink usually died of starvation. A moderately high prevalence of a focal myelitis–encephalitis is recorded in horses in the U.S.A. (2). Impairment of function of one limb begins gradually or suddenly and then appears in one or more other legs so that ataxia develops. This may be so severe that horses are unable to stand without assistance. Inability to walk backwards and sinking of the back on light pressure are other signs. At necropsy, gross lesions of circumscribed haemorrhage and necrosis are visible.

The disease requires to be differentiated from myelitis and spinal cord compression caused by space-occupying lesions of the vertebral canal.

REFERENCES

(1) McClymont, G. L. (1954). *Aust. vet. J.*, *30*, 345.
(2) Rooney, J. R. *et al.* (1970). *Cornell vet.*, *60*, 494.

Spinal Meningitis

Spinal meningitis is usually an accompaniment of cerebral meningitis and when it does occur locally in association with spinal cord abscess it produces local hyperaesthesia and rigidity characteristic of meningitis. The commonest occurrence is in lambs after infection of docking wounds. The treatment is as for cerebral meningitis.

CONGENITAL DEFECTS OF THE CENTRAL NERVOUS SYSTEM

The pathogenesis of congenital defects, including those of the central nervous system, has been dealt with in general terms in the section on diseases of the newborn. Inheritance, nutrition and virus infections in early pregnancy all play a part in the genesis of these defects but in many instances sporadic cases occur in which no specific aetiological agent can be invoked. Among those which may be encountered are meningocele, in which the meninges protrude through the unclosed fontanelles, spina bifida in which there is complete posterior paralysis, sometimes accompanied by marked flexion and contracture of the hind limbs,

together with atrophy of the muscles of the thigh (2), and micrencephaly (3) characterized by stillbirth or weak calves which soon die. In the latter there is no visible abnormality of the cranium but the cerebral hemispheres, cerebellum and brain stem are reduced in size and the corpus callosum and fornix are absent. It is suggested that the defect may be conditioned by inheritance. Micrencephaly has also been recorded in sheep (7). Other less common defects include dysplasia of the olfactory lobes and lateral ventricles in calves (4) and multiple neurofibromatosis causing subcutaneous swellings and transmitted from cow to calf (6). Some disease processes begin at or before birth but do not cause clinical signs until some days or weeks later. Two such congenital diseases are cerebellar atrophy in cattle and foals (5).

The following list is arranged on an aetiological classification and is not complete. A check list of familial and inherited diseases of the CNS of pigs (8), and one of all species have been compiled (1) and includes several exotic conditions not listed here.

(1) *Congenital Defects Conditioned by Inheritance*
Inherited congenital hydrocephalus
Inherited congenital chondrodystrophy
Inherited cerebellar hypoplasia of calves
Inherited cerebellar atrophy of lambs
Inherited congenital spasms of cattle
Inherited congenital posterior paralysis of cattle
Inherited congenital posterior paralysis of swine
Inherited congenital meningocele of swine
Inherited neuraxial oedema

(2) *Congenital Defects Caused by Nutritional Deficiency*
Swayback and enzootic ataxia of lambs
Brain compression caused by vitamin A deficiency

(3) *Congenital Defects Caused by Virus Infections in Early Pregnancy*
After vaccination with attenuated hog cholera virus
After vaccination with attenuated bluetongue virus
Possibly cerebellar hypoplasia in calves after infection with mucosal disease virus, and in piglets after infection with hog cholera virus

(4) *Congenital Defects caused by Infection of the Brain*
Toxoplasmosis

(5) *Congenital Defects Caused by Toxic Agents*
Poisoning of sheep by *Veratrum californicum*

(6) *Congenital Defects due to Unknown Causes*
Myoclonia congenita of pigs
Arthrogryposis and hydranencephaly of
calves
'Barkers' and 'wanderers' in foals
Spina bifida
Micrencephaly

REFERENCES

(1) Saunders, L. Z. (1952). *Cornell Vet.*, *42*, 592.
(2) McFarland, L. Z. (1959). *J. Amer. vet. med. Ass.*, *134*, 32.
(3) Fielden, E. D. (1959). *N.Z. vet. J.*, 7, 80.
(4) Morsier, C. de (1962). *Acta neuropath.* (*Berl.*), *1*, 433.
(5) Dungworth, D. L. & Fowler, M. E. (1966). *Cornell Vet.*, *61*, 17.
(6) Simon, J. & Brewer, R. L. (1963). *J. Amer. vet. med. Ass.*, *142*, 1102.
(7) Hartley, W. J. & Kater, J. C. (1965). *Aust. vet. J.*, *41*, 107.
(8) Done, J. T. (1968). *Lab. Animals*, *2*, 207.

12

Diseases of the Musculoskeletal System

DISEASES of the organs of support, including muscles, bones and joints, have much in common in that the major clinical manifestations of diseases which affect them are lameness, failure of support and insufficiency of movement. Insufficiency of movement affects all voluntary muscles, including those responsible for respiratory movement and mastication, but lameness and failure of support are manifestations of involvement of the limbs.

Various classifications of the diseases of the musculoskeletal system, based on clinical, pathological and aetiological differences are in use but the simplest is that which divides the diseases into degenerative and inflammatory types. The degenerative diseases of muscles, bones and joints are distinguished as myopathy, osteodystrophy and arthropathy, respectively, and the inflammatory diseases as myositis, osteomyelitis and arthritis.

DISEASES OF MUSCLES

Myopathy

The term myopathy describes the non-inflammatory degeneration of skeletal muscle which is characterized clinically by muscle weakness and at necropsy by hyaline degeneration of the muscle fibres which gives to affected muscles the appearance of fish flesh. Myoglobinuria is a common accompaniment.

Aetiology

Myopathies in man are largely of unknown aetiology and for the most part occur as inherited defects of muscle, or degenerative lesions caused by interruption of their nerve supply (1). In animals the myopathies have achieved a position of economic importance because of the high incidence of enzootic muscular dystrophy in lambs and calves.

The factors which appear to be of most importance in the aetiology of myopathy in farm animals (2) are: a primary or secondary deficiency of vitamin E, the absence of a protective level of selenium in the diet, unaccustomed muscular exertion, and the presence of certain legumes or highly unsaturated fatty acids in the diet. Because of their close association with primary or secondary deficiency of vitamin E, these factors have been discussed in the section on vitamin E deficiency and are generally referred to as white muscle disease (WMD).

Muscular dystrophy, as distinct from WMD (8), includes a number of disease entities whose aetiology is obscure. They include a congenital myopathy of lambs which affects the dorsal cervical muscles, cod liver oil poisoning and paralytic myoglobinuria (azoturia) of horses. 'Tying-up' or polymyositis is a poorly defined but not uncommon condition in saddle horses. In susceptible horses it occurs with dramatic suddenness during exercise. For this reason it is often bracketed with azoturia but the relationship between the two has not been defined (11). Polymyositis of horses (5) has occurred in enzootic proportions in Scandinavia with acute myonecrosis developing in the hind quarters and to a lesser extent in the masseter muscles. A similar condition has been described in sucking foals in New Zealand (4). Herztod of swine has much in common with enzootic muscular dystrophy of ruminants but its aetiology is even more obscure. More is known of an hereditary metabolic myopathy, which is characterized by the development of fatal hyperpyrexia in pigs submitted to halothane anaesthesia. Apart from these deaths the disease may cause undesirable changes in pork meat (12). Pale, soft musculature is an increasingly important problem in swine but the relationship of the above hereditary condition to the overall problem is not clear. A common and often fatal myopathy occurs in the hind limbs of cattle which are recumbent for periods of more than about 48 hours, although here the cause is probably ischaemia resulting from compression of the blood vessels to the hind limbs. The occurrence of severe myopathy in man after heavy dosing with cortisone analogues (3) arouses some interest although animals are not likely to receive such heavy doses. Many poisonous plants have been suggested as causes of myopathy in animals and two, *Cassia occidentalis* and *Karwinskia humboldtiana*, have been shown to contain myotoxins (9).

Although neurogenic myopathy occurs sporadically in animals, as it does in man, there is also a record of its occurrence in an epizootic congenital disease as arthrogryposis and hydranencephaly of calves. Also of interest is the observation of skeletal myopathy in sheep, sometimes but not always associated with scrapie.

Pathogenesis

Secondary myopathy may occur as a result of interruption of the nerve or blood supply to the part. In primary myopathy the lesion is present only in the muscle fibres and the histological and biochemical changes which occur in the muscle are remarkably similar irrespective of the cause. Variations in the histological lesions occur but indicate variation in the severity and rapidity of onset of the change rather than different causes.

The characteristic change in most cases of primary myopathy varies from hyaline degeneration to coagulative necrosis, affecting particularly the heavy thigh muscles and the muscles of the diaphragm. Myocardial lesions are also commonly associated with the degeneration of skeletal muscle. The visible effects of the lesions are asthenia of the muscles of the limbs and of the diaphragm and an accompanying myocardial weakness. Because of the necrosis of muscle, myoglobin is excreted in the urine. In myopathy in adult animals other than the horse and pig, and occasionally in cattle, the muscles, because of their low content of myoglobin, do not liberate sufficient to colour the urine. In all species the renal threshold of myoglobin is so low that discolouration of the serum does not occur.

In azoturia of adult horses myoglobinuria may precipitate nephrosis and cause fatal uraemia. Two other biochemical manifestations of myopathy are the increased excretion of creatine in the urine and an elevation of the level of muscle enzymes in serum. Serum glutamic oxalacetate transaminase and creatinine phosphokinase are both elevated in myopathy.

Clinical Findings

The clinical findings in enzootic muscular dystrophy in calves and lambs have been described in detail under vitamin E deficiency, and those of azoturia under that heading. In general terms there is a sudden onset of weakness and pseudo-paralysis of the affected muscles, causing paresis and recumbency and, in many cases, accompanying respiratory and circulatory insufficiency. The skeletal muscles in acute cases are swollen, hard and rubbery. Cardiac irregularity and tachycardia may be evident. In 'tying-up' in horses there is a very sudden onset of muscle soreness during exercise. The degree of soreness varies from mild, in which the horse moves with a short, shuffling gait, to acute, in which there is a great disinclination to move at all. Recovery is usual, much improvement occurring within a few hours. Recurrences in the same horse are common (6).

A special occurrence of myopathy has been recorded in sucking thoroughbred foals up to five months of age (4). The disease occurs in the spring and early summer in foals running at pasture with their dams and is unassociated with excessive exercise. In peracute cases there is a sudden onset of dejection, stiffness, disinclination to move, prostration and death three to seven days later. Lethargy and stiffness of gait are characteristic of less acute cases. There is also a pronounced swelling and firmness of the subcutaneous tissue at the base of the mane and over the gluteal muscles. There may be excessive salivation, desquamation of lingual epithelium and board-like firmness of the masseter muscles. The foals are unable to suck because of inability to bend their necks. Spontaneous recovery occurs in mild cases but most of the severely affected foals die.

Clinical Pathology

Creatinuria and an increase in serum glutamic oxalacetate transaminase (SGO-T) are characteristic findings. In the absence of hepatic injury SGO-T levels of over 1000 SF (Sigma-Frankel) units are strongly indicative of myopathy. Horses which are resting usually have SGO-T levels of about 150 SF units. Those in training have levels of about 250 units and these rise to 300 to 600 units immediately after exercise (10). In some normal horses levels slightly in excess of 1000 units may occur after strenuous exercise (6). In abnormal horses subject to 'tying-up' levels of 4000 and much higher are not uncommon after exercise. Many other serum enzymes are at present being investigated as indicators of muscular and hepatic damage. They have been shown to give significant diagnostic assistance in the detection of cows with myonecrosis due to recumbency at calving time (7). Myoglobinuria does not always occur. It is a common finding in azoturia of horses but not in enzootic muscular dystrophy in calves. The myoglobinuria may be clinically detectable as a red or chocolate brown discolouration of the urine. This discolouration can be differentiated from that caused by haemoglobin only by spectrographic examination, although discolouration of the plasma suggests the presence of haemoglobinuria. Both myoglobin and haemoglobin give positive tests for protein and positive guaiac tests. Porphyria causes a similar discolouration although this may not be evident until the urine has been exposed to light for some minutes. The colouration is lighter, pink to red rather than brown, and the urine is negative to the guaiac test and fluoresces with ultra-violet light.

Necropsy Findings

Affected areas of skeletal muscle have a white, waxy, swollen appearance like fish flesh. Commonly only linear strips of large muscle masses are affected and the distribution of lesions is characteristically bilaterally symmetrical. Histologically the lesion varies from a hyaline degeneration to a severe myonecrosis, and subsequently by the disappearance of large groups of muscle fibres and replacement by connective and adipose tissue. Calcification of the affected tissue may be present to a mild degree in these cases.

Diagnosis

Myopathy occurs acutely in most cases and may be manifested by palpable abnormality of skeletal muscles. A history of exercise after a period of inactivity, and of dietary abnormality may also be provided. It may only be on this basis that a differentiation from peripheral nerve paralysis can be made. Biochemical examination of the blood and urine may provide data of diagnostic value. Myositis may present a similar syndrome but is usually present as a secondary lesion in a clinically distinguishable primary disease or is accompanied by obvious trauma or toxaemia.

Treatment

Specific treatments for vitamin E deficiency and azoturia are described under those headings. Supportive treatment comprises adequate care of a recumbent animal and includes slinging, ample bedding, frequent turning and provision of a palatable, nutritious diet.

REFERENCES

(1) Innes, J. R. M. (1951). Brit. vet. J., 107, 131.
(2) Blaxter, K. L. (1957). Vet. Rec., 69, 1150.
(3) Williams, R. S. (1959). Lancet, 276, 698, 701 & 718.
(4) Hartley, W. J. & Dodd, D. C. (1957). N.Z. vet. J., 5, 61.
(5) Alstrom, I. (1948). Skand. vet. Tidskr., 38, 593.
(6) Cornelius, C. E. et al. (1963). J. Amer. vet. med. Ass., 142, 639.
(7) Boyd, J. W. et al. (1964). Vet. Rec., 76, 567.
(8) Hartley, W. J. (1963). Aust. vet. J., 39, 338.
(9) Dollahite, J. W. & Henson, J. B. (1965). Amer. J. vet. Res., 26, 749.
(10) Cardinet, G. H. et al. (1963). Amer. J. vet. Res., 24, 980.
(11) Steel, J. D. (1969). Aust. vet. J., 45, 162.
(12) Berman, M. C. et al. (1971). S. Afr. Med. J., 45, 580 & 590.

Myositis

Myositis may arise from direct or indirect trauma to muscle and occurs as part of a syndrome in a number of specific diseases including blackleg, foot and mouth disease, blue tongue, sarcosporidiosis and trichinosis, although clinical signs of myositis are not usually evident in the latter. An asymptomatic eosinophilic myositis is not uncommon in beef cattle and may cause economic loss through carcass condemnation (2). The cause has not been determined.

Acute myositis of limb muscles is accompanied by severe lameness, swelling, heat and pain on palpation. There may be accompanying toxaemia and fever. In chronic myositis there is much wasting of the affected muscles and this is difficult to differentiate clinically from atrophy due to other causes. Biopsy of the muscle may be necessary to confirm the diagnosis. In horses traumatic myositis of the posterior thigh muscles may be followed by the formation of fibrous adhesions between the muscles (fibrotic myopathy) and by subsequent calcification of the adhesions (ossifying myopathy). Occasionally similar lesions may be seen in the foreleg. The lesions cause a characteristic abnormality of the gait in that the stride is short in extension and the foot is suddenly withdrawn as it is about to reach the ground. The affected area is abnormal on palpation (1). An inherited disease of pigs, generalized myositis ossificans, is also characterized by deposition of bone in soft tissues (3).

REFERENCES

(1) Adams, O. R. (1961). J. Amer. vet. med. Ass., 139, 1089.
(2) Reiten, A. C. et al. (1966). Amer. J. vet. Res., 27, 903.
(3) Seibold, H. R. & Davis, C. L. (1967). Path. vet., 4, 79.

DISEASES OF BONES

Osteodystrophy

Osteodystrophy includes those diseases of bones in which there is failure of normal bone development, or abnormal growth of bone which is already mature. The major clinical manifestations include distortion and enlargement of the bones, susceptibility to fractures and interference with gait and posture.

Aetiology

Deficiencies of calcium, phosphorus and vitamin D, or imbalance of calcium and phosphorus in the diets of animals are common causes of rickets, osteomalacia and osteodystrophia fibrosa. A condition with a much more complicated aetiology is 'cappi' or 'double scalp' of young sheep in the U.K. The disease is essentially a generalized osteoporosis which may be accompanied by rachitic lesions (6). In recent years there has been an obvious increase in cases of moderate osteodystrophy and arthropathy in pigs on diets which appear to contain adequate amounts of vitamin D, and calcium and phosphorus in their correct proportions. Cases are most common in pigs which are growing very rapidly and which are being fed ground grain in self-feeders. It has been suggested that a dietary deficiency of protein of high biological value may be a causative factor (5). 'Leg-weakness' of pigs appears to be a closely related condition and occurs in the same circumstances of heavy feeding. It is thought to be caused by excessive weight-bearing on joints which are predisposed to injury by unspecified nutritional deficiencies (7). A significant weakening of bones also occurs when there is a dietary deficiency of copper. A deformity of limb bones occurs in bowie of sheep but there is no apparent osteodystrophy. Chronic lead poisoning has been related to the occurrence of osteomalacia and paralysis in lambs. Fluorosis is commonly accompanied by exostoses of the limb bones.

Achondroplasia and chondrodystrophy are inherited defects which occur in achondroplastic dwarfism in cattle and in some types of prolonged gestation. A fibrous dysplasia of bone, probably an inherited defect, has also been recorded in swine (1), and a congenital absence of bones may also be inherited. Osteogenesis imperfecta as it occurs in man is not common in animals, but a very similar condition manifested by marked bone fragility and characteristic radiological changes has been recorded in newborn lambs (8, 10). Chondrodystrophic changes have also been recorded in a congenital defect of cattle known colloquially as 'acorn calves'. Vertebral exostoses are not uncommon in old bulls and usually affect the last two or three thoracic and first two or three lumbar vertebrae. The exostoses occur mainly on the ventral aspects of the vertebral bodies, fusing to cause immobility of the region. Fracture of the ossification may occur and cause injury or compression of the spinal cord or peripheral nerves (2, 3). The disease is commonly referred to as spondylitis or vertebral osteochondrosis and also occurs less commonly in adult cows and in pigs. The pathogenesis suggested for the disease is that the annulus fibrosus degenerates and the resulting malfunctioning of the disc allows excessive mobility of the vertebral bodies leading to the stimulation of new bone formation (11). A similar lesion occurs commonly in horses and may affect racing performance, particularly in hurdle races and cross-country events (9). The initial lesion may be a degeneration of the intervertebral disc (4).

Pathogenesis

There are some species differences in the abnormalities which occur with dietary deficiencies of calcium, phosphorus and vitamin D. Rickets and osteomalacia develop in ruminants and osteodystrophia fibrosa in horses, and pigs may develop either. In rickets there is a failure of provisional calcification of the osteoid and cartilaginous matrix of developing bone. The epiphyseal plate increases in width due to hypertrophy of the cartilage, resulting in enlargement of the joints. The poorly calcified diaphyseal bones bend easily, and weight-bearing causes deformity of the long bones. In osteomalacia the demineralized bone lacks strength and fractures easily and the deposition of uncalcified osteoid around the diaphysis may cause some thickening. In osteodystrophia fibrosa a fibrous dysplasia occurs around the affected bones.

Congenital defects of bone include complete (achondroplasia) and partial (chondrodystrophy) failure of normal development of cartilage. Growth of the cartilage is restricted and disorganized, and mineralization is reduced. The affected bones fail to grow, leading to gross deformity, particularly of the bones of the head.

Clinical Findings

In general terms there is weakening of the bones due to defective mineralization and osteoporosis so that fractures occur more readily and normal weight or tension stresses cause distortion of the normal axial relationships of the bones. Fractures are more likely to occur in mature animals and distortions in growing animals. Thickening of the bones may be detectable clinically if the deposition of osteoid or fibrous tissue is excessive, or if exostoses develop. Compression of the spinal cord or spinal nerves may lead to paraesthesia, paresis or paralysis which may be localized in its distribution. Details of the clinical findings in the osteodystrophies caused by nutritional deficiency are provided in Chapter 28.

The fibrous dysplasia of pigs which is thought to be inherited is manifested by swelling of the anterior aspect of the face at about four months of age. The distortion is accompanied by dyspnoea and snoring and there is stiffness of the limbs with enlargement of the joints. Swelling of the face extends from the snout to the eyes and is spongy or firm in patches.

Clinical Pathology and Necropsy Findings

Clinico-pathological and necropsy findings vary with the cause and are dealt with in detail under the specific diseases. The inherited fibrous dysplasia of swine is manifested by gross thickening of the nasal bones and to a less extent the mandibles, maxillae and the lacrimal, palatine, frontal and temporal bones. The swollen bones have a smooth surface and are soft enough to be cut with a knife. Cavitation of the bones is present and there is compression of the turbinate bones and partial occlusion of the nasal cavities. Enlargement of the epiphyses of the long bones is accompanied by local thickening of the periosteum.

Diagnosis

The osteodystrophies produce characteristic clinical findings and are unlikely to be confused with other conditions. Differentiation of the causes may be more difficult and depends largely upon the dietary history and clinico-pathological findings which should suggest one of the causes listed under aetiology above. The presence of bony deformities at birth suggests a chondrodystrophy, some of which appear to be inherited and some due to environmental influences.

Treatment

The treatment of osteodystrophy must be determined by the causative agent and no general supportive measures can be recommended.

REFERENCES

(1) Kowalczyk, T. et al. (1958). J. Amer. vet. med. Ass., 133, 601.
(2) McEntee, K. (1958). J. Amer. vet. med. Ass., 132, 328.
(3) Rourke, G. J. et al. (1959). Canad. J. comp. Med., 23, 122.
(4) Hansen, H. J. (1959). Lab. Invest., 8, 1242.
(5) Platt, B. S. & Stewart, R. J. C. (1962). Brit. J. Nutr., 16, 483.
(6) Nisbet, D. I. et al. (1962). J. comp. Path., 72, 270.
(7) Walker, T. et al. (1966). Vet. Rec., 79, 472.
(8) Holmes, J. R. et al. (1964). Vet. Rec., 76, 980.
(9) Smythe, R. H. (1962). Med. vet. Pract., 43, No. 9, 50.
(10) Kater, J. C. et al. (1963). N.Z. vet. J., 11, 41.
(11) Thomson, R. G. (1969). Path. vet., 6, Suppl. 46.

Hypertrophic Pulmonary Osteo-arthropathy

(*Marie's Disease, Achropachia Ossea*)

Although hypertrophic pulmonary osteo-arthropathy is more common in dogs than in the other domestic animals it has been observed in horses (1, 3, 4), cattle (2) and sheep (5). The disease is characterized by proliferation of the periosteum leading to the formation of periosteal bone, and bilateral symmetrical enlargement of bones, usually the long bones of limbs. The enlargement is quite obvious, and in the early stages is usually painful and often accompanied by local oedema. On roentgenological examination there is a shaggy periostitis and evidence of periosteal exostosis. The pathogenesis is obscure but the lesion appears to be neurogenic in origin, unilateral vagotomy causing regression of the bony changes (6). Stiffness of gait and reluctance to move are usually present, and there may be clinical evidence of the pulmonary lesion with which the disease is almost always associated. Such lesions are usually chronic, neoplastic or suppurative processes such as tuberculosis (7). The disease is considered to be incurable, unless the thoracic lesion can be removed, and affected animals are usually euthanized. At necropsy the periostitis, exostosis and pulmonary disease are evident. There is no involvement of the joints.

REFERENCES

(1) Alexander, J. E. et al. (1965). J. Amer. vet. med. Ass., 146, 703.
(2) Hofmeyr, C. F. B. (1964). Berl. Münch. tierärztl. Wschr. 77, 319.
(3) Goodbarry, R. F. & Hage, T. J. (1960). J. Amer. vet. med. Ass., 137, 602.
(4) Holmes, J. R. (1961). Vet. Rec., 73, 333.
(5) Carre, H. et al. (1936). C. R. Soc. Biol., Paris, 123, 557.
(6) Holling, H. E. et al. (1961). Lancet, 7215, 1269.
(7) Kersjes, A. W. et al. (1968). Neth. J. vet. Sci., 1, 55.

Osteomyelitis

Inflammation of the bone marrow is uncommon in farm animals except when infection is introduced by traumatic injury. Specific diseases which may be accompanied by osteomyelitis include actinomycosis of cattle, and brucellosis, atrophic rhinitis, and necrotic rhinitis of pigs. Non-specific, haematogenous infection with other bacteria occurs sporadically and is often associated with omphalitis, abscesses from tail-biting in pigs or infection of castration or docking wounds in lambs. Osteomyelitis is usually accompanied by severe, persistent pain. Erosion of the bone occurs and pus discharges into surrounding tissues causing a cellulitis or phlegmon, and to the exterior through sinuses which persist for long periods. The affected bone is often greatly swollen and fractures easily because of weakening of its structure. When the bones of the jaw are involved, the teeth are often shed and this, together with pain and the distortion of the jaw, interferes with prehension and mastication. Involvement of vertebral bodies may lead to the secondary involvement of the meninges and the development of paralysis. Lameness and local swelling are the major manifestations of involvement of the limb bones.

Medical treatment is rarely completely successful because of the poor vascularity of the affected solid bone and the inaccessibility of the infection. A long course of antibiotics administered parenterally may control the infection but local surgical treatment is usually advisable.

DISEASES OF THE JOINTS

Arthropathy

(Osteo-arthritis)

Non-inflammatory lesions of the joint cavities occur in a number of diseases. They may occur in a proportion of cases of rickets, osteomalacia, bowie and osteodystrophia fibrosa. Degenerative arthropathy also occurs unassociated with obvious defects of the bones, particularly in beef bulls and aged dairy cows (5) and is described under calcium deficiency diseases. Traumatic injury of the joints and surrounding tissues is common in horses but is not dealt with here on the grounds that it is a surgical disease. It has been extensively reviewed (4). Chronic zinc poisoning in pigs is characterized by degenerative lesions of the articular surface of the head of the humerus. Lesions of the articular surfaces of the cervical vertebrae occur in a proportion of horses affected by enzootic inco-ordination. Similar involvement of intervertebral joints in the caudal thoracic and cranial lumbar regions have been recorded in the osteomalacic condition—the so-called spondylitis—which occurs in old bulls. Degenerative lesions of the articular surfaces in the limb joints have also been observed in bulls affected by inherited spasticity (1) and in cattle affected with Manchester Wasting Disease. In sporadic cases injury to the joint surfaces, menisci and ligaments, especially the cruciate ligaments of the stifle joints, may be followed by continuous damage to the articular cartilages. Falls and sprains may be the precipitating causes, especially in aged cattle (2). In cattle the hip or stifle joints are most commonly affected and when there is a dietary cause, both joints in both legs are usually involved. The causes of osteo-arthritis in horses are of great importance to the racing industry. Poor conformation, nutritional deficiencies (particularly calcium, phosphorus, vitamin A and copper) and the type of running surface or terrain are thought to be important but there is little supporting evidence (3).

When the limb joints are affected there is lameness and, in severe cases, crepitus and distension of the joint capsule with synovial fluid. The disease has much in common with chronic arthritis and differentiation between the two may be difficult without a history suggestive of dietary deficiency, or the presence in the herd of other signs which suggest dietary deficiency or injury. Clinical pathology may be of assistance, especially estimations of the calcium and phosphorus or phosphatase levels of the blood which may reveal the existence of a mineral imbalance or deficiency. Examination of aspirated joint fluid may be of value but is often inconclusive as the causative bacteria and inflammatory cells may be present in very small numbers in chronic arthritis.

Involvement of intervertebral articulations may cause pain and restriction of movement but the clinical syndrome is more commonly one of compression of the spinal cord or peripheral nerves by periarticular ossification or prolapsed intervertebral discs.

At necropsy the changes are not generalized but are localized to certain joints and to parts of them. The joint cartilage is thin or patchily absent and polished bone is evident. The articular surfaces are irregular and sometimes folded. Exposed bone may be extensively eroded and osteophytes (small bony excrescences) may be present on the non-articular parts of the bone around the articular surface. There is often an excess of turbid, brown-coloured joint fluid, menisci, cartilages and ligaments may be entirely absent and there may be areas of calcification in the joint capsule and particles of cartilage free in the synovium. When the stifle is affected fractures of the head of the tibia occur commonly, usually a chip of the lateral condyle having become separated. In such cases fracture of the lateral condyle of the distal end of the femur may follow. With either of these fractures lameness is extreme and the animal may often refuse to rise. When the hip-joint is affected the head of the femur becomes much smaller and more flattened than normal, the acetabulum is shallower and the round ligament usually ruptured.

The treatment of arthropathy depends largely upon correction of the cause but in most cases the damage is irreparable and the animal should be sent for slaughter. Relief of pain may be accomplished by the use of the ancillary treatments prescribed for arthritis.

REFERENCES

(1) McEntee, K. (1958). *J. Amer. vet. med. Ass.*, *132*, 328.
(2) Vaughan, L. C. (1960). *Vet. Rec.*, *72*, 534.
(3) Sokoloff, L. (1960). *Advances in Veterinary Science*, Vol. 6. New York: Academic Pub. Inc.

(4) Ravdin, I. S. *et al.* (1962). *J. Amer. vet. med. Ass.*, *141*, 1231.
(5) Pelt, R. W. van (1966). *J. Amer. vet. med. Ass.*, *148*, 535.

Arthritis

Inflammation of the synovial membrane and articular surfaces occurs commonly in animals as a result of bacterial infection. It is characterized by lameness and local pain, heat and swelling in the joint.

Aetiology

Sporadic cases of arthritis are caused by trauma with perforations of the joint capsule or by extension of an infection from surrounding soft tissues such as occurs in footrot of cattle and pigs (5) and interdigital abscess of sheep, or by haematogenous spread from suppurative lesions in the udder or uterus, from diaphragmatic abscess or endocarditis in the cow, from an infected navel, or infected, bitten tails or castration wounds of pigs. The invading bacteria vary but commonly include *Escherichia coli*, *Corynebacterium pyogenes*, *Sphaerophorus necrophorus*, *Streptococcus* and *Staphylococcus* spp. Specific infections in farm animals in which localization occurs in the joints from a bacteraemia or septicaemia include particularly the infections of newborn animals which arise from navel or intrauterine infection. *E. coli* and *Streptococcus* spp. cause arthritis in all species; *Actinobacillus equuli*, *Cor. equi* and *Salmonella abortivoequina* are important causes in newborn foals. *Erysipelothrix insidiosa* may cause arthritis in newborn and recently docked lambs but occurs more commonly at other times in pigs and rarely in calves. *Salm. dublin* and *Salm. typhimurium* may occasionally cause arthritis in calves. Sporadic outbreaks and individual cases of arthritis in the newborn may also arise from infection of the navel by *Cor. pyogenes*, *Sph. necrophorus* and *Staphylococcus.* spp. *Cor. pseudotuberculosis*, *Haemophilus agni* and *Pasteurella haemolytica* have also been observed as causes of arthritis in lambs. Arthritis also occurs commonly in tick pyaemia of lambs but is associated with extensive suppurative lesions elsewhere.

Specific diseases of older animals in which infectious arthritis occurs as a prominent sign include Glasser's disease of pigs and serositis-arthritis of sheep and goats. Occasional cases may also occur in young calves vaccinated against contagious bovine pleuropneumonia with cultures of *Mycoplasma mycoides*, and arthritis, caused by *Mycoplasma* spp., has been observed in most animal species (2). Because of the absence of bacteria from some arthritic joints of pigs, a viral infection has also been suggested as a cause in this species, but most of such cases are probably caused by residual lesions after the subsidence of an infection with *Ery. insidiosa* (1, 3, 6). An infectious polyarthritis of lambs and calves is described in a later section. Infection with *Brucella suis* may also cause involvement of bones and joints, particularly the vertebrae, in adult pigs.

Pathogenesis

The predilection of blood-borne infections for localization in the joints in young animals is probably related to the prior occurrence of moderate trauma to the articular surfaces caused by early weight bearing. There may be a similar explanation for the common occurrence of arthritis in animals soon after transport. Pain, heat and swelling of the joint usually occur. The arthritis may be suppurative or serofibrinous depending on the causative organism. In chronic cases, erosion of joint cartilages, periarticular proliferation of bone and villi of granulation tissue may develop.

Clinical Findings

Inflammation of the synovial membrane causes pain and lameness in the affected limb, sometimes to the point that the animal will not put it to the ground. Pain and heat are usually detectable on palpation and passive movement of the joint is resented. The joint may be swollen but the degree will depend on the type of infection. Pyogenic bacteria cause the greatest degree of swelling and may result in rupture of the joint capsule. Some enlargement of the epiphysis is usual and this may be the only enlargement in non-pyogenic infections, particularly that caused by *Ery. insidiosa*.

In many of the neonatal infections there will also be an accompanying omphalophlebitis and evidence of lesions in other organs, particularly the liver, endocardium and meninges. Arthritis in older animals may also be accompanied by signs of inflammation of the serous membranes and endocardium when the infection is the result of haematogenous localization.

The joints most commonly involved are the hock, stifle and knee but infection of the fetlock, interphalangeal and intervertebral joints is not uncommon. In chronic cases there may be physical impairment of joint movement because of fibrous thickening of the joint capsule, periarticular ossification, and rarely ankylosis of the joints. Crepitus may be detectable in joints where much erosion has occurred. In newborn and young animals, involvement of several joints is common. The joints may become inflamed simultaneously or serially. Lameness is often so severe that affected foals lie down in lateral recumbency most of the time and may have to be assisted to rise. The gait may be so impaired as to suggest ataxia of central origin.

The prognosis in cases of acute suppurative arthritis is never good. Neglected animals may die or have to be destroyed because of open joints or pressure sores. The subsequent development of chronic arthritis and ankylosis may greatly impede locomotion and interfere with the usefulness of the animal.

Clinical Pathology

Aspiration of exudate from the joint may be attempted if the swelling is marked and free fluid is present. Careful disinfection of the skin and the use of sterile equipment is essential to avoid the introduction of further infection. If the navel is infected, examination of swabs taken from the exudate may provide the necessary information about the bacteria present and their sensitivity to antibacterial drugs. Serological tests may be of value in determining the presence of specific infections with *Myco. mycoides*, *Salmonella* spp., *Brucella* spp. and *Ery. insidiosa*. Roentgenological examination may aid in diagnosing the presence of joint lesions and may in some cases suggest the presence of either inflammatory or degenerative changes. Although its application may be limited to experimental studies, the measurement of joint movements by electronic means—electrogoniometry—offers an opportunity for advancement in the study of diseases of joints (10).

Necropsy Findings

The nature of the lesions varies with the causative organism. The synovial membrane is thickened and roughened and there is inflammation and erosion of the articular cartilage. There is usually an increase in the amount of synovial fluid present, varying from a thin, clear, serous, brownish fluid through a thicker, serofibrinous fluid to pus. There may be some inflammation of the periarticular tissues in acute cases and proliferation of the synovial membrane in chronic cases. In the latter, plaques of inspissated necrotic material and fibrin may be floating free in the synovial fluid. There may be a primary omphalophlebitis in newborn animals and metastatic abscesses may be present in other organs.

Diagnosis

Lameness and stiffness of gait caused by myositis, myopathy and lesions affecting the peripheral nerves or spinal cord may be confused with arthritis unless the joints are examined carefully. Joint involvement may not be obvious in the early stages and lameness associated with septicaemia or omphalophlebitis in the newborn should be considered as an infectious arthritis unless there is good evidence to the contrary.

Traumatic sprains of tendons or ligaments, and fractures of the epiphyses may cause lameness and local pain and when they involve periarticular tissues, may be difficult to differentiate from arthritis. These lesions are largely of surgical interest and their differentiation is not discussed here. The greatest confusion in the diagnosis of arthritis is in differentiating it from arthropathy which resembles chronic arthritis in most clinical respects. In both there is lameness, an absence of heat or pain in the joint and osseous enlargement at the epiphysis. If roentgenological examination is impossible, one usually has to depend upon the history. In young animals, chronic arthritis is more probable especially if there is a history of omphalophlebitis or septicaemia. In pigs, infection with *Ery. insidiosa* is the most probable cause. In adult cattle and horses and particularly in overfat beef bulls the lesion is more commonly a degenerative arthropathy. Arthritis is never present at birth and apparent fixation of the joints should arouse suspicion of a congenital anomaly.

Treatment

Control of an infection in a joint is difficult to achieve because of the poor blood supply to the part and the low levels of antibacterial drugs which develop in synovial fluid after their parenteral administration. It is customary to administer broad spectrum antibiotics, or a combination of penicillin and streptomycin, intramuscularly if the causative bacteria is not identified. The probability that the bacteria in suppurative lesions are streptococci and staphylococci permits economy in many cases in that long-acting penicillin alone may be used. Intra-articular injection is not usually practised unless synovial exudate is aspirated for diagnosis or in treatment. In both cases careful asepsis and an accurate technique are required (7, 8, 9).

The tendency for arthritis to progress to a chronic stage has encouraged the use of two ancillary forms of treatment. The parenteral or intra-articular administration of cortisone or hydrocortisone or the oral or parenteral administration of phenylbutazone (1 g. intravenously for 1 or 2 days in horses and 2 to 4 g. orally each day for 5 days in cattle (4)) are widely used in an attempt to reduce pain and facilitate healing by permitting normal movement of the affected joint. The treatment has the disadvantage that an acute exacerbation of the inflammation may occur if the infection is not under control when the cortisone is administered. If the arthritis is suppurative, enzymes may be administered parenterally in an attempt to facilitate the removal of the pus. Results are not usually good and there is again a tendency for the inflammation to become acute if the infection is not controlled. Enzymes have more value when administered locally in an open joint. With both cortisone and enzymes it is wisest to begin a course of treatment with antibiotics and if the temperature and local signs subside by the third or fourth day to then commence enzyme or cortisone therapy.

The local application of heat, by hot fomentations or other physical means, is laborious, but if practised frequently and vigorously will reduce the pain and local swelling quickly. The local application of liniments may also be advantageous in chronic cases. Analgesics are often advisable if the animal is recumbent much of the time. Sodium salicylate (1 to 2 oz. twice daily in large animals) can be left for administration by the owner. Persistent recumbency is one of the problems in the treatment of arthritis, particularly in foals. The animal spends little time feeding or sucking and loses much condition. Compression necrosis over bony prominences are a common complication and require vigorous preventive measures.

REFERENCES

(1) Sikes, D. (1960). *Canad. J. comp. Med.*, *24*, 347.
(2) Sokoloff, L. (1964). *Proc. 101st. Ann. Mtg Amer. vet. med. Ass., Chicago, Illinois*, p. 251.
(3) Duthie, I. F. & Lancaster, M. C. (1964). *Vet. Rec.*, *76*, 263.
(4) Ebert, E. F. (1962). *Vet. Med.*, *57*, 33.
(5) Penny, R. H. C. (1963). *Vec. Rec.*, *75*, 1225.
(6) Crimmins, L. T. & Siks, D. (1965). *Canad. J. comp. Med.*, *29*, 312.
(7) Kruiningen, H. J. van (1963). *J. Amer. vet. med. Ass.*, *143*, 1079.
(8) Pelt, R. W. van (1970). *J. Amer. vet. med. Ass.*, *156*, 84, 457.
(9) Pelt, R. W. van & Riley, W. F. (1969). *J. Amer. vet. med. Ass.*, *155*, 1467.
(10) Taylor, B. M. *et al.* (1966). *Amer. J. vet. Res.*, *27*, 85.

Congenital Defects of Muscles, Bones and Joints

A number of inherited congenital defects of the musculo-skeletal system are described in Chapter 33. They include achondroplastic dwarfism, prolonged gestation with cyclopian deformity, umbilical and scrotal herniae, cryptorchidism, reduced phalanges, deformity of the tail and taillessness, multiple joint ankylosis, multiple joint contracture, 'leg weakness', congenital thickleg and congenital splay-leg (myofibrillar hypoplasia) of piglets, displaced molar teeth, osteopetrosis, mandibular prog-

nathism and muscular hypertrophy. A number of non-inherited congenital defects including enzootic muscular dystrophy, acorn calves, a cyclopian-type deformity in lambs due to poisoning with *Veratrum californicum*, and arthrogryposis with hydranencephaly in calves have been described in other chapters. A less common defect is a non-inherited absence or development of rudimentary limbs. This has occurred naturally in calves in outbreak form (1) and has also been produced experimentally by radiation injury of sows, cows and ewes during early pregnancy (3). A high incidence of deformed, newborn calves has occurred for many years on Kodiak Island, Alaska (2). Defects include cleft palate, anopia, cyclopia, scoliosis, kyphosis, torticollis, anal atresia and abnormally straight hind limbs. The cause is unknown but the cows had access to lupins and similarly affected calves have been produced experimentally by feeding their dams lupins and lead during pregnancy (4). The birth of calves with crooked, deformed limbs (crooked calf disease) has also been attributed to a manganese deficiency. A similar condition in foals, referred to as 'contracted foals' or congenital axial and appendicular contractures of the foal, has been reported from the USA (5). Again the aetiology is unknown but the condition is not thought to be inherited. The deformities include torticollis, scoliosis, thinning of the ventral abdominal wall, sometimes accompanied by eventration, asymmetry of the skull, and flexion-contracture of the distal limb joints. Deformed foals with ankylosed limb joints are reported in mares grazing hybrid Sudan grass pastures but no cause–effect relationship has been established (7). A congenital progressive myopathy affecting merino sheep has been recorded in Australia (8). The muscles of the pelvic and pectoral girdles are worst affected and cause great difficulty in locomotion. There is inability to flex joints and, in some cases, prostration. Recovery does not occur and affected animals usually starve to death. A general review of congenital defects of the skeleton of animals conditioned by inherited factors (6) and a smaller review (9) are available.

Sporadic cases of joint deformity at birth are not unusual in animals. Many sporadic cases occur in foals and calves, most commonly manifested by excessive flexion of the metacarpophalangeal joints causing affected animals to knuckle at the fetlock. Many mild cases recover spontaneously but surgical treatment may be required in badly affected animals. The cause in these sporadic cases is unknown and necropsy examination fails to reveal lesions other than excessive flexion of the joints caused by shortening of the flexor tendons. Fixation of the joints in the newborn may be associated with absence of ventral horn cells in the spinal cord and with spina bifida.

REFERENCES

(1) Harbutt, P. R. *et al.* (1965). *Aust. vet. J.*, *41*, 173.
(2) King, J. A. (1965). *J. Amer. vet. med. Ass.*, *147*, 239.
(3) McFee, A. F. *et al.* (1965). *J. Anim. Sci.*, *24*, 1130.
(4) Shupe, J. L. *et al.* (1967). *J. Amer. vet. med. Ass.*, *151*, 191, 198.
(5) Rooney, J. R. (1966). *Cornell Vet.*, *56*, 172.
(6) Greeneberg, H. (1963). *The Pathology of Development. A Study of Inherited Skeletal Disorders in Animals*, Oxford: Blackwell Scientific Publications.
(7) Pritchard, J. T. & Voss, J. L. (1967). *J. Amer. vet. med. Ass.*, *150*, 871.
(8) McGavin, M. D. & Baynes, I. D. (1969). *Path. vet.*, *6*, 513.
(9) Hutt, F. B. (1968). *Cornell vet.*, *58*, Suppl. 104.

13

Diseases of the Skin

INTRODUCTORY

DISEASES of the skin may be primary or secondary in origin. In primary skin disease the lesions are restricted initially to the skin although they may spread from the skin to involve other organs. On the other hand cutaneous lesions may be secondary to disease originating in other organs. Differentiation between primary and secondary skin diseases can be accomplished by making a complete clinical examination of the patient. If there is no evidence that organs other than the skin are affected it can be assumed that the disease is primary. When involvement of other organs is suspected, it is necessary to determine whether the involvement constitutes the primary state or whether it has developed secondarily to the skin disease. The chronology of the signs, elicited by careful history taking, is the most efficient guide in making a correct decision, although a detailed knowledge of the individual diseases likely to be encountered is of the utmost importance. When a careful clinical examination has been made and an accurate history taken it is then necessary to make a careful examination of the skin itself. Using the proper technique of examination and making accurate observations and then the application of one's knowledge of pathology of the skin make it possible to determine the basic defect, whether it be inflammatory or due to malfunction, and thus to define the type of lesion present.

The purpose of this chapter is to describe the basic skin lesions so that the differential diagnosis up to the point of defining the type of lesion can be accomplished. Final determination of the exact cause requires further examination and is included in the discussion of the specific disease. The present section will describe in sequence the various steps in clinical examination of the skin, beginning with the exact definition of the lesions, then the interpretation of the findings and finally the physiological effects of the disease and the consequential principles of treatment.

Special Examination

A general clinical examination should be carried out first. This is followed by the special examination of the skin and must include inspection, and in many cases, palpation. Additional information can be provided by the taking of swabs for bacteriological examinations, by taking scrapings for examination for dermatophytes and metazoan parasites and by biopsy for histological examination. The biopsy material should include abnormal, marginal, and normal skin. Special staining techniques are of considerable assistance in the histological examination of skin. The use of Wood's lamp in the examination of the skin for dermatophytes is discussed under ringworm.

The description of lesions should include their size, the depth to which they penetrate, their distribution over the body surface, and the area covered. Abnormalities of sebaceous and sweat secretion, or changes in the hair or wool coat, and alterations in colour of the skin should be noted. The presence or absence of pain or pruritus should be observed. The manifestations of skin disease are set out below and the common lesions are defined.

Lesions. Lesions may be discrete or diffuse. *Discrete lesions* are defined as follows: *papules* (pimples), *nodules* and *nodes* are solid elevations and are listed here in order of increasing size; *vesicles* are small swellings containing serum or lymph, and *blebs*, *bullae* or *blisters* are similar lesions of greater size. *Pustules* are similar swellings containing pus. Circumscribed swellings caused by local oedema and erythema, as in urticaria, are classified as *wheals*. *Scabs* comprise dried exudates or other inflammatory products. *Diffuse lesions* include *scales*, which are dry exfoliations of skin in the form of flakes, *excoriations*, which are superficial discontinuities in the skin surface caused by trauma; and *fissures*, which are cracks which penetrate more deeply, usually into the subcutaneous tissues.

Abnormal Colouration. Abnormal colourations including jaundice, pallor and erythema may be visible. These signs are best seen in the oral or vaginal mucosae or in the conjunctiva. In animals with light-coloured skins they may be visible at first glance. The red to purple discolouration of the skin of white pigs affected by various septicaemias may be extreme and no diagnostic significance can be attached to its degree because the same colour can be observed in cases of salmonellosis, pasteurellosis, erysipelas and hog cholera. Early erythema is a common finding where more definite skin lesions are to develop, as in early photosensitization. The blue colouration of early gangrene is characterized by coldness and loss of elasticity. This is particularly evident on the udder and teat skin of cows in the early stages of acute mastitis caused by *Staphylococcus aureus*.

Pruritus. Pruritus or itching is the sensation which gives rise to the desire to scratch. It must be differentiated from hyperaesthesia, which is increased sensitivity to normal stimuli. Paraesthesia or perverted sensation is subjective in nature and can hardly be defined in animals. All sensations which give rise to rubbing or scratching are therefore included with pruritus. The abnormality is more properly defined as scratching. There are two kinds of itching, peripheral and central, and care must be taken to distinguish between them. Damage to cells in the deeper layer of the skin (the dermis or corium) causes stimulation of pain end-organs and is the anatomical basis of itching of peripheral or cutaneous origin. Itching does not occur in the centre of deep ulcerations nor in very superficial lesions, such as those of ringworm, where only the hair fibres and keratinized epithelium are involved. Although itching can be elicited over the entire skin surface, it is most severe at the mucocutaneous junctions because of the concentration of pain end-organs at these sites.

Itching of central origin derives in the main from the scratch centre below the acoustic nucleus in the medulla. It may have a structural basis as in scrapie and pseudorabies, or it may be functional in origin as in the nervous form of acetonaemia. The only lesions observed are those of a traumatic dermatitis with removal of the superficial layers to a variable depth, breakage or removal of the hairs, and a distribution of lesions in places where the animal can bite or rub easily.

One other cause for scratching is mnemodermia or 'skin memory'. This is a special form of hyperaesthesia in which hypersensitivity to innocuous stimuli persists after the initial lesions have subsided. There are numerous examples of this in humans as a result of plant and insect stings. The persistent scratching which gives rise to dry eczema along the backs of dogs may have a similar basis.

Abnormalities of sweat secretion. The activity of the sweat glands is controlled by the sympathetic nervous system and is for the most part a reflection of body temperature. Excitement and pain may cause sweating before the body temperature rises; here the sweating is due to cerebral cortical activity. A form of hyperhydrosis, apparently inherited, has been recorded in Shorthorn calves (4). Local areas of abnormal sweating may arise from peripheral nerve lesions or obstruction of sweat gland ducts. A generalized anhidrosis is recorded in horses and occasionally in cattle.

Abnormalities of sebaceous gland secretion. Excessive sebum secretion causes oiliness of the skin. It occurs in several diseases of animals including greasy heel of horses and exudative epidermitis of pigs but the cause of the abnormality is unknown.

Abnormalities of wool and hair fibres. Deficiency of hair or wool in comparison to the normal pilosity of the skin area is referred to as alopecia. There are two kinds of alopecia. One is caused by follicle dysfunction and the other by injury to the fibre, as in ringworm and trauma. The capacity of the follicular epithelium to produce a fibre may be congenitally defective or may be temporarily reduced because of nutritional deficiency or severe systemic disease. Bands of weak fibre through a hair coat or fleece may result in 'breaks' and loss of the major part of the coat. Special note should be taken of whether the fibre is completely absent or has been broken off along the shaft.

Bands of depigmentation in an otherwise black wool fleece are the result of a transitory deficiency of copper in the diet. Cattle on diets containing excess molybdenum and deficient copper show a peculiar speckling of the coat caused by an absence of pigment in a proportion of hair fibres. The speckling is often most marked around the eyes giving the animal the appearance of wearing spectacles. Vitiligo, premature greying of the hair, is not uncommon in cattle and horses (1). The usual manifestation is the appearance of patches of grey or white hair—'snowflakes'—in an otherwise pigmented coat. The defect is aesthetic only. The cause is unknown but the condition may be inherited. Depigmentation can also be brought about by the application of 'super-cooled' instruments which selectively destroy melanocytes (2). Pressure and X-irradiation may have a similar effect.

The character of the fibre may also vary with variations in the internal environment. In copper deficiency the crimp of fine wool fibres is lost and the wool becomes straight and 'steely'.

Special Pathology

The reaction of the skin to noxious stimuli varies with the severity and depth of the injury (3). In the corium or dermis the reaction is the same as that in other tissues because of the presence of blood and lymphatic vessels, nerve fibres, and connective tissue. The epidermis, because of its purely cellular composition, reacts differently. If the reaction is acute, the development of lesions begins with swelling and oedema of the cells of the prickle cell layer—the so-called 'spongiosis'. If the oedema is severe enough, cells rupture and fluid collects to form foci which gradually emerge through the stratum corneum and appear on the surface as vesicles. Should the foci rupture before reaching the surface the result is weeping of the affected area. In less acute inflammations, the intracellular oedema in the prickle cell layer interferes with the normal functioning of the granular layer and gives rise to abnormal formation of cornified epithelium. As a result the epidermis becomes thickened. All layers are affected, particularly the stratum corneum, because of improper keratinization and failure of exfoliation. This lesion is described histologically as parakeratosis. It may be accompanied by acanthosis which consists of pronounced thickening of the prickle cell layer and prolongation of the interpapillary processes. The disease state is usually described as pachydermia. Acanthosis in conjunction with the deposition of melanin is known as acanthosis nigricans, a disease in dogs and man commonly associated with thyroid dysfunction.

It should be possible to distinguish clinically between acute inflammatory changes and those caused by chronic inflammation or malfunction of skin tissue due to other causes by observing the type of reaction in the skin. Both acute and chronic inflammation may be caused by bacterial, viral, metazoan and protozoan agents, and also by chemical and physical agents including light sensitization and allergy. Chronic inflammation may also arise from any of these causes and the inflammation interferes with normal skin metabolism. Similar lesions can be produced by nutritional deficiency; thus parakeratosis may arise from chronic inflammation or from a dietary deficiency of zinc. Further identification of the type of lesion necessitates classification and the various categories are set out in the subsequent parts of this chapter.

Skin diseases of allergic origin are not well understood, but two manifestations require mention here. When an allergen is applied to skin sensitized to it, it causes a local increase in tissue histamine levels and an accumulation of eosinophils. If the quantity of histamine liberated is in excess of the detoxifying capacity of the eosinophil aggregation, histamine escapes into the vascular system, and the blood histamine levels rise. This elevation of total blood histamine levels and the accompanying eosinophilia are quite transitory. The levels return to normal in one to eight hours after removal of the allergen, the time varying with the severity and duration of the allergic reaction. Examination of histamine levels or eosinophil counts in the blood may be of diagnostic value although negative results do not preclude the possibility of an allergic aetiology. The local skin reaction to the allergen is due to the vasodilatory effects of histamine. If the reaction is severe enough, other organs may show the effects of histamine toxicity. An ingested allergen may produce reactions in other organs in addition to those in the skin.

Physiological Effects of Diseases of the Skin

The major functions of the skin are to maintain a normal body temperature and a normal fluid and electrolyte balance within the animal. In general these functions are not greatly impeded by most diseases of the skin although failure of the sweating mechanism does seriously interfere with body temperature regulation, and severe burns or other skin trauma may cause fatal fluid and electrolyte loss.

The major effects of skin diseases in animals are aesthetic and economic. The unsightly appearance of the animal distresses the owner. Discomfort and scratching interfere with normal rest and feeding and when the lips are affected there may be interference with prehension. There is loss of the economic coat and the protective function of the skin is reduced.

Another cause of loss may be the serious depletion of protein stores when extensive loss of epithelium occurs. The epithelial cells and appendages have a high content of sulphur-containing amino-acids and if these are not available in the diet they will be withdrawn from protein molecules in other tissues and serious tissue wasting may result. The intervention of secondary infection may, of course, lead to grave consequences.

Principles of Treatment of Diseases of the Skin

Removal of hair coat and debris to enable topical applications to come into contact with the causative agent is desirable. Accurate diagnosis of the cause must precede the selection of any topical or systemic treatment. In bacterial diseases sensitivity tests on cultures of the organism are advisable. Specific skin disease due to bacteria, fungi and metazoan parasites are reasonably amenable to treatment. Removal of the causative agent in allergic diseases and photosensitization may be impossible and symptomatic treatment may be the only practicable solution. In many cases, too, the primary disease may be confounded by the presence of a secondary agent, which can lead to confusion in diagnosis. Treatment may be unsuccessful if both agents are not treated. In addition to specific treatments the following measures should be considered. Prevent secondary infection by the use of bacteriostatic ointments or dressings. Prevent further damage from scratching by the application of local anaesthetic ointments or the administration of centrally-acting sedatives. When large areas of skin are involved prevent the absorption of toxic products by continuous irrigation or the application of absorptive dressings. Losses of fluid and electrolytes can be made good by the parenteral administration of isotonic fluids containing the necessary electrolytes. Ensure an adequate dietary intake of protein, particularly sulphur-containing amino-acids to facilitate the repair of skin tissues.

Many preparations are used empirically in the treatment of skin diseases. Preparations containing arsenic, antimony, gold, and manganese given orally or, more commonly, parenterally, are in common use in human medicine. Arsenic, sulphur and antimony are deposited preferentially in the skin and hair in high concentrations and in addition arsenic has activity against spirochaetes and protozoa.

REFERENCES

(1) Meijer, W. C. P. (1965). *Vet. Rec.*, 77, 1046.
(2) Farrell, R. K. *et al.* (1966). *J. Amer. vet. med. Ass.*, *149*, 745.
(3) Head, K. W. (1970). *Vet. Rec.*, *87*, 460.
(4) Larson, P. W. & Prior, R. W. (1971). *Vet. Med. small Anim. Clin.*, *66*, 667.

DISEASES OF THE EPIDERMIS AND DERMIS
Pityriasis

Pityriasis or dandruff is a condition characterized by the presence of bran-like scales on the skin surface.

Aetiology

Pityriasis may be of dietary, parasitic, fungal or chemical origin. Dietary pityriasis occurs in the later stages of avitaminosis A, in deficiency of most factors of the vitamin B complex, particularly nicotinic acid and riboflavine, and when there is a deficiency of essential unsaturated fatty-acids such as linolenic acid. Parasitic pityriasis often accompanies infestations with external parasites including fleas, lice and mange mites. Pityriasis is often pronounced in fungal infections of the skin, particularly the early stages of ringworm. In cases of iodism one of the most obvious signs is the shedding of large bran-like scales from the skin.

Pathogenesis

The scales of pityriasis are keratinized epithelial cells. These are sometimes softened and made greasy by the exudation of serum or sebum. Overproduction of keratinized epithelial cells, as in vitamin A deficiency, or excessive desquamation, caused for example by scratching in parasitic infestations, lead to the accumulation of scales on the skin surface. When hyperkeratinization occurs it begins around the orifices of the hair follicles and spreads to the surrounding stratum corneum.

Clinical Findings

Primary pityriasis comprises the accumulation of scales without itching or other skin lesions. The scales are superficial in origin. They accumulate most readily where the coat is long and their presence is usually associated with a dry lustreless coat. Secondary pityriasis is usually accompanied by the lesions of the primary disease.

Clinical Pathology

The definition of primary pityriasis depends upon the examination of skin scrapings to eliminate other primary agents, particularly parasites and fungi.

Diagnosis

Pityriasis is one of the commonest accompaniments of skin disease. Further differentiation of primary causes will not be discussed here although it is necessary to distinguish pityriasis from hyperkeratosis and parakeratosis.

Treatment

Correction of the primary cause is the first necessity. Non-specific treatment should commence with a thorough washing. This is followed by alternating applications of a bland, emollient ointment and an alcoholic lotion. Salicylic acid is frequently incorporated into a lotion or ointment with a lanolin base.

Parakeratosis

Parakeratosis is a condition of the skin in which keratinization of the epithelial cells is incomplete.

Aetiology

Non-specific, chronic inflammation of the cellular epidermis causes faulty keratinization of the horny cells. A specific dietary deficiency of zinc produces the same results in pigs and possibly in cattle.

Pathogenesis

The initial lesion comprises oedema of the prickle cell layer, dilatation of the intercellular lymphatics, and leucocyte infiltration. Imperfect keratinization of epithelial cells at the granular layer of the epidermis follows. When keratinization is thus interfered with the horn cells produced are sticky and soft and retain their nuclei. They tend to stick together to form large masses. These either stay fixed to the underlying tissues or fall off as large scales.

Clinical Findings

The lesions may be extensive and diffuse but are often confined to the flexor aspects of joints. Initially there is reddening followed by thickening of the skin and the development of a grey colouration. The scales are often held in place by hairs. The lesions usually crack and fissure, and removal of the scales leaves a raw, red surface. Psoriasis, mallenders and sallenders are clinical terms describing various forms of parakeratosis.

Clinical Pathology

For a definite diagnosis of parakeratosis a biopsy or a skin section at necropsy is necessary.

Diagnosis

Histologically, the imperfect keratinization is evident and differentiates the condition from hyperkeratosis. In contrast to hyperkeratosis the crusts are soft and have a raw skin surface beneath them.

Treatment

In nutritional parakeratosis the deficiency must be corrected. The abnormal tissue is first removed by the use of a keratolytic ointment (e.g. salicylic acid ointment) or by vigorous washing with soapy water. This is followed by the application of an astringent preparation (e.g. white lotion paste). The astringent preparation must be applied frequently and for some time after the lesions have disappeared.

Hyperkeratosis

Hyperkeratosis is a condition in which excessively keratinized epithelial cells accumulate on the surface of the skin.

Aetiology

Chronic arsenic poisoning and poisoning with highly chlorinated naphthalene compounds are specific causes of hyperkeratosis. Local areas of hyperkeratosis occur at pressure points, such as the elbows, in animals lying on hard surfaces. Congenital ichthyosis (fish-scale disease) is a cutaneous hyperkeratosis of newborn animals, especially calves.

Pathogenesis

The continued adhesion of epithelial scales, which is characteristic of hyperkeratosis, is caused by excessive keratinization of epithelial cells and intercellular bridges and by hypertrophy of the stratum corneum. The excessive keratinization encountered in cases of poisoning with highly chlorinated naphthalenes is due to a deficiency of vitamin A and interference with normal cell division in the granular layer of the epidermis. Local compression also leads to the accumulation of keratinized epithelial cells.

Clinical Findings

The skin becomes thicker than normal and is usually corrugated and hairless. Dryness and scaliness of the external surface are characteristic. Fissures develop in a grid-like fashion giving a scaly appearance. Secondary infection of the fissures may occur if the area is continually wet. However, the lesion is usually dry and the plugs of hyperkeratotic material can be removed leaving the underlying skin intact.

Clinical Pathology

Histological examination of a biopsy section shows the characteristically thickened stratum corneum.

Diagnosis

The differentiation of hyperkeratosis from parakeratosis has already been described.

Treatment

Treatment of the primary condition is essential. The use of keratolytic agents (e.g. salicylic acid ointment) may effect some improvement.

Pachydermia

Pachydermia is a thickening of the skin affecting all layers. Frequently the subcutaneous tissue is also involved. Scleroderma is also included in this classification.

Aetiology

Non-specific chronic or recurrent inflammation of the skin is the cause of most cases of pachydermia. The lesion is usually local in origin although the affected area may be of considerable size as in lymphangitis and greasy heel in the horse and in baldy calves.

Pathogenesis

The cells in all layers are usually normal but the individual layers are increased in thickness. There is hypertrophy of the prickle-cell layer of the epidermis and enlargement of the interpapillary processes.

Clinical Findings

The hair-coat is thin or absent and the affected skin is thicker and tougher than usual. The skin appears tight and, because of its thickness and the diminution of subcutaneous tissue, cannot be picked into folds or moved over underlying tissue as readily as in normal areas. There are no discontinuities in the skin surface.

Diagnosis

In pachydermia the thickening of the skin is usually confined to localized areas. There are no superficial skin lesions and no accumulation of cell debris. These findings serve to differentiate the condition from the other chronic skin thickenings, parakeratosis and hyperkeratosis.

Treatment

In chronic cases little improvement can be anticipated. The administration of cortisone preparations locally or parenterally in the early stages of the disease may cause recovery. When small areas are involved surgical removal may be attempted.

Impetigo

Impetigo is a superficial eruption of thin-walled, usually small, vesicles surrounded by a zone of erythema. The vesicles develop into pustules and rupture to form scabs.

Aetiology

In humans impetigo is specifically a streptococcal infection but lesions are often invaded secondarily by staphylococci. In animals the main organism found is usually a staphylococcus. Impetigo as a primary disease occurs most commonly on cows' udders, especially on the lower areas where the hair is scanty. It is described in greater detail under the heading of miscellaneous abnormalities of the udder. In piglets it is the main lesion in 'infectious dermatitis' caused by bite wounds when the milk teeth are not cut.

Pathogenesis

The causative organism appears to gain entry through minor abrasions. Rupture of lesions causes contamination of the surrounding skin and the appearance of more lesions. Spread from animal to animal occurs readily. Udder impetigo in cows is particularly infectious.

Clinical Findings

Vesicles appear chiefly on the relatively hairless parts of the body. They remain as small (3 to 6 mm.) discrete lesions and do not become confluent. In the early stages a zone of erythema is evident around the vesicle. There is no irritation. Rupture of the vesicles occurs readily although they may persist and become pustules which form yellow scabs. Involvement of hair follicles is common and leads to the development of acne and much deeper, more extensive lesions. Individual lesions heal rapidly in about a week but successive crops of vesicles may occur and prolong the duration of the disease.

Clinical Pathology

Culture of vesicular fluid should be carried out to determine the causative bacterium and its sensitivity.

Diagnosis

Impetigo must be differentiated from pox lesions particularly in cattle. Cowpox lesions occur mainly on the teats and pass through the characteristic stages of pox. Pseudo-cowpox is unlikely to develop as a true pox lesion and its distribution on the udder is its major diagnostic feature. The early, vesicular stages of eczema may be confused with impetigo but in eczema irritation is intense and the lesions show a marked tendency to coalesce. The vesicles are also much smaller in size.

Treatment

Local treatment is usually all that is required. Individual lesions heal so rapidly that the main aim of treatment is to prevent the occurrence of new lesions and spread of the disease to other animals. Twice daily bathing with an efficient germicidal skin wash is usually adequate.

Urticaria

Urticaria is an allergic condition characterized by the appearance of wheals on the skin surface.

Aetiology

Primary urticaria occurs as a result of insect bites, from contact with stinging plants, in association with the ingestion of unusual food or on the administration of some drugs, e.g. penicillin. A sudden change of feed immediately preceding the attack is a common history, especially if the new diet has a high protein content. Warble larvae are an occasional cause. Secondary urticaria occurs in association with other diseases, particularly those in which other manifestations of allergy are common. Upper respiratory tract infections in horses, particularly the viral infections and strangles, and erysipelas in pigs, are typical examples.

Pathogenesis

The lesions of urticaria are characteristic of an allergic reaction. A primary dilatation of capillaries causes erythema of the skin. Exudation from the damaged capillary walls results in local oedema of the dermis, with swelling and pallor due to compression of the capillaries. The lesion usually remains red at the edges. Only the dermis, and sometimes the epidermis, is involved.

Clinical Findings

Urticarial lesions appear very rapidly and often in large numbers, particularly on the body. They vary from 0·5 to 5 cm. in diameter, are elevated with a flat top and are tense to the touch. There is usually no itching, except with plant or insect stings, nor discontinuity of the epithelial surface. Colour changes in the wheals can be observed only in unpigmented skin. No exudation or weeping occurs. Other allergic phenomena, including diarrhoea and slight fever, may accompany the eruption. Subsidence of the lesions within a few hours is common but the disease may persist for 3 to 4 days. Such persistence is usually due to the appearance of fresh lesions.

Clinical Pathology

Tissue histamine levels are increased and there is a local accumulation of eosinophils. Blood histamine levels and eosinophil counts may show transient elevation.

Diagnosis

Urticaria can be differentiated from angioneurotic oedema because in urticaria the lesions can be palpated in the skin itself. Angioneurotic oedema involves the subcutaneous tissue rather than the skin and the lesions are much larger and more diffuse.

Treatment

Spontaneous recovery is common. Antihistamines provide the best and most rational treatment. Parenteral injections of adrenaline may also be used. One treatment is usually sufficient. Lesions may recur if the diet is not changed or exposure to the causal insects or plants not prevented. A mild purgative is recommended, and the local application of cooling astringent lotions such as calamine or white lotion or a dilute solution of sodium bicarbonate is favoured. In large animal practice parenteral injections of calcium salts are used with apparently good results.

Eczema

Eczema is an inflammatory reaction of the epidermal cells to substances to which the cells are sensitized. These substances may be present in the external or internal environment.

Aetiology

Eczema occurs when the skin cells are brought into contact with allergens (1). These allergens are described as exogenous when they are applied to the skin surface or as endogenous when they are carried in the blood stream. Endogenous allergens usually enter the circulation by absorption from the gut. Identification of the allergens is impossible in most cases in animals. Suspected exogenous allergens include external parasites, some soaps and some antiseptic washes. Endogenous allergens may be ingested, usually as proteins, or they may be formed in the gut, as in auto-intoxication due to overeating or constipation or by digestion of internal parasites.

Predisposition to eczema is marked in some animals and in some cases appears to be inherited. In others it appears to be environmental and is commonly associated with repeated wetting or dampness as in continued sweating. Constant scratching, due to the presence of external parasites, appears to predispose and so does soiling and the accumulation of dirt.

Pathogenesis

The primary lesion is erythema, followed by inter- and intra-cellular oedema, the characteristic 'spongiosis' lesion of eczema. The accumulation of oedematous fluid causes the formation of small vesicles which are characteristic of the early stages of eczema. Rupture of the vesicles and exfoliation of epidermal cells result in weeping and the subsequent development of scabs. In some cases a general outpouring of fluid without the appearance of vesicles occurs. This acute stage may disappear quickly or a chronic inflammation may persist with either parakeratosis or, in the very chronic form, pachydermia.

Clinical Findings

True eczema is rare in large animals. In the acute form the earliest observable change is a patch of erythema, followed by the appearance of small vesicles which rupture and cause weeping of the surface. Scab formation follows. The lesions may occur in isolated patches or be diffuse over large areas and in some cases are symmetrical. Itching and irritation are usually intense and scratching and rubbing exacerbate the condition. Chronic eczema may follow an acute attack or, because of a persistent low-grade irritation, be chronic from the beginning. Because of the scratching and rubbing there is alopecia, some scaling and hypertrophy of all skin layers with resultant pachydermia, but there is no discontinuity of the skin.

Clinical Pathology

Because of the expense involved, skin tests to determine the sensitizing agent are not used. The clinical pathology of the condition consists of the elimination of other causes of superficial dermatitis, particularly ectoparasites.

Diagnosis

A definite diagnosis of eczema is difficult to make because differentiation between it and dermatitis poses a problem, especially in an individual case. In eczema the lesions are superficial, follow a fairly regular pattern of development and recur when the skin is exposed to the same or other sensitizing substances which are not recognized irritants and are innocuous to normal animals.

Treatment

The basis of treatment is to prevent exposure to the sensitizing substance. Because detection of the allergen is often impossible, changes in environment, including a change in diet, changes of bedding and in the surroundings, the removal of internal and external parasites, the avoidance of wetting and unnecessary irritation, and the protection of the skin are often instituted. A light, high-protein, laxative diet is generally recommended. In the early acute stages sedation is an advantage because it avoids further damage by scratching. Antihistamine preparations are used extensively in the treatment of eczema and give good results in acute cases. Non-specific protein injections, including autogenous whole blood or boiled skim milk, and cortisone preparations are also used to stimulate healing.

Local treatment varies with the stage of development of the disease. In the early, weeping stage astringent antiseptic lotions are required. In the later, scabby stage, protective ointments or pastes, particularly those containing local anaesthetic agents, should be applied at frequent intervals.

REFERENCE

(1) Walton, G. S. (1968). *Vet. Rec.*, **82**, 204.

Dermatitis

The term dermatitis includes those conditions characterized by inflammation of the dermis and epidermis.

Aetiology

The important types of dermatitis in animals include the following:

Bacterial dermatitis. Mycotic dermatitis of cattle, horses and sheep due to *Dermatophilus congolense* and *Derm. dermatonomus.*

Strawberry footrot due to *Derm. pedis.*

Infectious dermatitis of pigs due to *Streptococcus* spp. and *Staphylococcus aureus.*

Ulcerative granuloma of pigs due to *Borrelia suilla.*

Viral dermatitis. The poxes, cowpox and pseudocowpox, swine pox, horse pox, sheep pox.

Contagious ecthyma of sheep and mammillitis of cattle.

Knopvelsiekte or lumpy skin disease of cattle.

Ulcerative dermatosis of sheep.

There are also several viral diseases in which secondary skin lesions occur particularly around the natural orifices and the coronet. Some of the more common are foot and mouth disease, rinderpest, vesicular exanthema, vesicular stomatitis, bovine malignant catarrh, mucosal disease and bluetongue.

Fungal dermatitis. Ringworm in all species is rarely a dermatitis, since it affects only the stratum corneum.

Sporotrichosis of horses.

Metazoan dermatitis. Mange and mite dermatitis, elaeophoriasis, cutaneous habronemiasis and stephano-filariasis are the common metazoan dermatidites. Cutaneous myiasis includes infestations with the maggots of blowflies and screwworm flies.

Dermatitis due to physical agents. Sunburn, excessive heat or cold are common causes of dermatitis. Trauma, excessive wetting, as in fleece rot of sheep, photosensitization and beta-radiation are also causes of dermatitis in animals. Skin necrosis has become a disease of major importance in newborn and young pigs. Worst affected parts are those which contact the floor and preliminary investigations suggest that the disease is commonly caused by this contact, resulting in trauma or contact dermatitis.

Chemical dermatitis. Irritant chemicals applied to the skin and chemical poisons taken orally or absorbed percutaneously, such as arsenic, cause dermatitis.

Allergic dermatitis. Sensitivity of the epidermis to substances which are innocuous to normal individuals typically results in the development of eczema. More extensive lesions may cause dermatitis, e.g. allergic dermatitis of horses.

Dermatitis due to nutritional deficiency. Deficiency of some of the B vitamin complex produces dermatitis in pigs.

Dermatitis of undetermined cause. The aetiology of exudative epidermis of pigs and of hyperplastic dermatitis of horses (2) is unknown. Dermatitis is commonly recorded in cattle on diets of potatoes.

Pathogenesis

Dermatitis is basically an inflammation of the deeper layers of the skin involving the blood vessels and lymphatics. The purely cellular layers of the epidermis are involved only secondarily. The noxious agent causes cellular damage, often to the point of necrosis, and depending on the type of agent responsible, the resulting dermatitis varies in its manifestations. It may be acute or chronic, suppurative, weeping, seborrhoeic, ulcerative or gangrenous. In all cases there is increased thickness and increased temperature of the part. Pain or itching is present and erythema is evident in unpigmented skin. Histologically there is vasodilatation and infiltration with leucocytes and cellular necrosis. These changes are much less marked in chronic dermatitis.

Clinical Findings

Affected skin areas first show erythema and increased warmth. The subsequent stages vary according to the type and severity of the causative agent. There may be development of discrete vesicular lesions or diffuse weeping. Oedema of the skin and subcutaneous tissues may occur in severe cases. The next stage may be the healing stage of scab formation or, if the injury is more severe, there may be necrosis or even gangrene of the affected skin area. Spread of infection to subcutaneous tissues may result in a diffuse cellulitis or phlegmonous lesion.

A systemic reaction is likely to occur when the affected skin area is extensive. Shock, with peripheral circulatory failure, may be present in the early stages. Toxaemia due to absorption of tissue breakdown products, or septicaemia, due to invasion via unprotected tissues, may occur in the later stages.

Clinical Pathology

Examination of skin scrapings or swabs for parasitic, bacterial or other agents is essential. Culture and sensitivity tests for bacteria are advisable to enable the best treatment to be selected. Skin biopsy may be of value in determining the causal agent. In allergic or parasitic states there is usually an accumulation of eosinophils in the inflamed area. In mycotic dermatitis organisms are usually detectable in the deep skin layers although they may not be cultivable from superficial specimens.

Diagnosis

The clinical features of dermatitis are apparent. Differentiation from eczema may be difficult unless there is a history of exposure to a probable allergen. The characteristic features of the aetiological types of dermatitis are described under each specific disease.

Treatment

The primary aim of treatment must be to remove the noxious stimulus. Removal of the physical or chemical agent from the environment or supplementation of the diet to repair a nutritional deficiency are an essential basis for treatment. The choice of a suitable treatment for infectious skin disease will depend upon the accurate identification of the aetiological agent. For example, in bacterial infections the sensitivity of the organism will influence the choice of antibacterial drugs.

Supportive treatment includes both local and systemic therapy. Local applications may need to be astringent either as powders or lotions in the weeping stage or as greasy salves in the scabby stage. The inclusion of antihistamine preparations is recommended in allergic states and it is desirable to prescribe anaesthetic agents when pain or itching is severe.

If shock is present, parenteral fluids should be administered. When tissue destruction is extensive or the dermatitis is allergic in origin, antihistamines are of value. If the lesions are extensive or secondary bacterial invasion is likely to occur, parenterally-administered antibiotics or antifungal agents may be preferred to topical applications. To facilitate skin repair, a high protein diet or the administration of protein hydrolysates or amino-acid combinations may find a place in the treatment of valuable animals.

The use of vaccines as prophylaxis in viral and bacterial dermatitides must not be neglected. Autogenous vaccines may be most satisfactory in bacterial infections.

REFERENCES

(1) Penny, R. H. C. et al. (1971). Aust. vet. J., 47, 529.
(2) Binninger, C. E. & Piper, R. C. (1968). J. Amer. vet. med. Ass., 153, 69.

Photosensitization

Photosensitization is the disease caused by the sensitization of the superficial layers of lightly pigmented skin to light of certain wave-lengths. Dermatitis develops when the sensitized skin is exposed to strong light.

Aetiology

If photosensitizing substances (photodynamic agents) are present in sufficient concentration in the skin dermatitis occurs when the skin is exposed to light (1). Photodynamic agents are substances which are activated by light and may be ingested preformed (and cause primary photosensitization), be products of abnormal metabolism (and cause photosensitization due to aberrant synthesis of pigment) or be normal metabolic products which accumulate in tissues, because of faulty excretion through the liver (and cause hepatogenous photosensitization). Faulty excretion through the liver is usually due to hepatitis, caused in most instances by poisonous plants, but in rare cases is due to biliary obstruction by cholangiohepatitis or biliary calculus.

(1) *Primary photosensitization*. Photosensitization due to the ingestion of exogenous photodynamic agents usually occurs when the plant is in the lush green stage and is growing rapidly. Livestock are affected within 4 to 5 days of going onto pasture and new cases cease to appear soon after the animals are removed. In most cases the plant responsible must be eaten in large amounts and will therefore usually be found to be a dominant inhabitant of the pasture. All species of animals are affected by photodynamic agents although susceptibility may vary between species and between animals of the same species. Photosensitizing substances which occur naturally in plants include hypericin in St John's Wort (*Hypericum perforatum*) and possibly other members of *Hypericum* spp., and fagopyrin in the seeds and dried mature plants of buckwheat (*Polygonum fagopyrum*). An unidentified photosensitizing agent also occurs in *Cymopterus watsoni* (wild carrot) and is capable of causing photosensitization of sheep (5). Miscellaneous compounds which act similarly are phenothiazine whose metabolic end-product phenothiazine sulphoxide is photodynamic, rose bengal, acridine dyes, perloline from perennial rye-grass (*Lolium perenne*), and a photodynamic agent in the aphids which commonly infest *Medicago denticulata* (burr trefoil).

(2) *Photosensitization due to aberrant pigment synthesis*. The only known example in domestic animals is inherited congenital porphyria in which there is an excessive production in the body of porphyrins which are photodynamic.

(3) *Hepatogenous photosensitization*. The photosensitizing substance is in all instances phylloerythrin—a normal end-product of chlorophyll metabolism excreted in the bile. When biliary secretion is obstructed by hepatitis or biliary duct obstruction phylloerythrin accumulates in the body and may reach levels in the skin which make it sensitive to light. Although hepatogenous photosensitization is more common in animals grazing green pasture it can occur in animals fed entirely on hay or other stored feeds. There appears to be sufficient chlorophyll, or breakdown products of it, in such feed to produce critical tissue levels of phylloerythrin in affected animals (1). The following list includes those substances or plants which are common causes of hepatogenous photosensitization. The individual plants are discussed in more detail in the section on poisonous plants. *Pithomyces chartarum*, a fungus on perennial rye-grass which causes facial eczema; *Lantana camara*; *Lippia rehmanni*; *Tribulus terrestris* (Caltrops); *Agave*

lecheguilla (Lecheguilla); *Microcystis flosaquae* (water-bloom, alga); *Panicum* spp. (panic and millet grasses); *Nolina texana* (Sacahuiste); *Tetradymia* spp. (coal oil bush, etc.); *Holocalyx glaziovii* (Alecrim); *Lupinus angustifolius* (Lupin); and *Myoporum laetum* (Ngaio). A number of other suspected poisonings which may cause hepatogenous photosensitization are the fungus *Periconia* spp. on mouldy or frosted Bermuda grass (2) and phenanthridium used as a treatment against several trypanosomiases. In some cases animals affected with hepatitis caused by carbon tetrachloride. *Crotalaria retusa* and *Senecio jacobeus* may also show mild evidence of photosensitization. Inherited photosensitization of Southdowns is caused by a congenital defect in the excretion of biliary pigment.

(4) *Photosensitization of uncertain aetiology.* Photosensitive dermatitis has also been observed in animals fed on *Brassica rapa* (rape), kale, *Medicago denticulata* (burr trefoil, burr medic), *Medicago sativa* (lucerne, alfalfa), *Medicago minima*, *Trifolium hybridium* (Alsike clover, Swedish clover), *Erodium cicutarium* and *Erodium moschatum* (lambs' tongue, plantain). Whether the photosensitization is primary or due to hepatitis has not been definitely ascertained. Extensive outbreaks of photosensitive dermatitis have occurred in cattle fed on water-damaged alfalfa hay, but whether the observed hepatic injury was due to fungal infestation of the hay was not determined (3). Many clinical cases of severe photosensitive dermatitis occur in adult cattle grazing green pasture without the cause being identified. In most cases the photosensitization is hepatogenous. A similar situation exists less commonly in sheep (4) and in the condition in horses known as bluenose (6).

Pathogenesis

Sensitization of skin tissues to light of particular wavelengths can only result in dermatitis if the skin is exposed to sunlight and if the light rays can penetrate the superficial layers of skin. Thus lesions occur only on the unpigmented skin areas and on these only when they are not covered with a heavy coat of hair or wool. Lesions are thus more severe on the dorsal parts of the body and on those underparts exposed to sunlight when the animal lies down. The penetration of light rays to sensitized tissues causes the liberation of histamine, local cell death and tissue oedema. Irritation is intense because of the oedema of the lower skin level and loss of skin is common in the terminal stages. Nervous signs may occur and are caused either by the photodynamic agent as in buckwheat poisoning or by liver dysfunction.

Clinical Findings

The clinical findings in liver insufficiency are described elsewhere and may accompany photosensitive dermatitis when it is secondary to liver damage. The skin lesions show a characteristic distribution. They are restricted to the unpigmented areas of the skin and to those parts which are exposed to solar rays. They are most pronounced on the dorsum of the body, diminishing in degree down the sides and are absent from the ventral surface. The demarcation between lesions and normal skin is often very clear cut, particularly in animals with broken-coloured coats. Predilection sites for lesions are the ears, eyelids, muzzle, face, the lateral aspects of the teats and, to a lesser extent, the vulva and perineum. The first sign is erythema followed by oedema. Irritation is intense and the animal rubs the affected parts, often lacerating the face by rubbing it in bushes. When the teats are affected the cow will often kick at her belly and will walk into ponds to immerse the teats in water, sometimes rocking backwards and forwards to cool the affected parts. In nursing ewes there may be resentment to the lambs sucking and heavy mortalities due to starvation can occur. The oedema is often severe and may cause drooping of the ears, dyspnoea due to nasal obstruction and dysphagia due to swelling of the lips. Exudation commonly occurs and results in matting of the hair and, in severe cases, closure of the eyelids and nostrils. In extreme cases, necrosis and gangrene, sometimes with sloughing of affected parts, is the terminal stage.

The skin lesions may be severe enough to cause shock in the early stages. There is an increase in the pulse rate with ataxia and weakness. Subsequently a considerable elevation of temperature (41 to 42 °C or 106 to 107 °F) may occur. Dyspnoea is often marked, and nervous signs including ataxia, posterior paralysis, blindness and depression or excitement are often observed. A peculiar sensitivity to water is sometimes seen in sheep with facial eczema.

Clinical Pathology

There are no suitable field tests to determine whether or not photosensitivity is present. In experimental work the application of filter-containing screens to the skin is used to determine which light wavelengths activate the sensitized cells. An important step in diagnosis is the differentiation of primary from hepatogenous photosensitization. The use of serum enzyme tests, as described under the heading of diseases of the liver, is recommended as the most valuable procedure.

Necropsy Findings

Liver lesions may be present if the photodynamic agent is phylloerythrin. In congenital bovine porphyria there is a characteristic pink-brown pigmentation of the teeth and bones. In other forms of the disease the lesions are confined to the skin and are manifested by dermatitis of varying degree.

Diagnosis

The determination of photosensitivity depends almost entirely on the distribution of the lesions. It can be readily confused with other dermatitides if this restriction to unpigmented and hairless parts is not kept in mind. Mycotic dermatitis is often mistaken for photosensitization because of its tendency to commence along the backline and over the rump. Bighead of rams caused by *Clostridium novyi* infection may also be confused with this disease but the local swelling is an acute inflammatory oedema and many clostridia are present in the lesion.

To differentiate between the aetiological types of photosensitization one must first determine whether the photodynamic agent is exogenous or endogenous, and, if it is exogenous, whether or not its accumulation is due to liver damage.

Treatment

In cases of photosensitization general treatment includes immediate removal from direct sunlight, prevention of ingestion of further toxic material and the administration of laxatives to eliminate toxic materials already eaten. In areas where the disease is enzootic the use of dark-skinned breeds may make it possible to utilize pastures which would otherwise be too dangerous.

Local treatment will be governed by the stage of the lesions. Antihistamines should be administered immediately and adequate doses maintained. To avoid septicaemia the prophylactic administration of antibiotics may be worth while in some instances.

REFERENCES

(1) Clare, N. T. (1955). *Advances in Veterinary Science* Vol. 2. New York: Academic Pub. Inc.

(2) Kidder, R. W. *et al.* (1961). *Bull. Florida agric. exp. Stn*, 630, 21.

(3) Monlux, A. W. *et al.* (1963). *J. Amer. vet. med. Ass.*, *142*, 989.

(4) Ford, E. J. H. (1964). *J. comp. Path.*; 74, 37.

(5) Binns, W. *et al.* (1964). *Vet. Med.*, 59, 375.

(6) Greatorex, J. C. (1969). *Equ. vet. J.*, *1*, 157.

DISEASES OF THE HAIR, WOOL, FOLLICLES AND SKIN GLANDS
Alopecia

Alopecia or baldness is deficiency of the hair or wool coat.

Aetiology

Alopecia may be due to lack of hair production or to damage to hairs already produced. The follicle fails to produce a fibre in the inherited diseases described in a later chapter as congenital hypotrichosis, symmetrical alopecia, baldy calves and adenohypophyseal hypoplasia. The same mechanism operates in hypothyroidism due to iodine deficiency (goitre) and in a possibly inherited generalized alopecia of newborn Holstein-Friesian calves (1). In the latter disease the thyroid glands are much smaller than normal and the affected calves usually die soon after birth. Nervous alopecia is the result of peripheral nerve injury. Infection of a follicle has a similar effect. Deep skin lesions and subsequent scarring may destroy the follicle, a condition known as cicatricial alopecia.

Loss of pre-formed fibre is characteristic of the dermatomycoses and fleece rot of sheep. Metabolic alopecia occurs during or subsequent to a period of malnutrition or a period of impaired nutrition associated with severe illness. The feeding of excessive amounts of whale, palm or soya oil in milk replacers to calves is also thought to encourage the development of alopecia (2). Fibres grown during this time contain a zone of weakness and are easily broken. In traumatic alopecia fibres are broken and lost because of scratching or rubbing. Toxic alopecia occurs in cases of thallium poisoning and in poisoning by the 'Jumbey' plant (*Leucaenia glauca*). Loss of hair from the tail switch is relatively common in well-fed beef bulls in the U.S.A. but the cause has not been determined. In some cases ergotism is suspected.

Pathogenesis

Normal shedding of hair fibres is a constant process. It occurs most rapidly when there are changes in environmental temperature. The long winter coat is shed in response to warmer spring temperatures and increased hours of sunlight. The hair coat rapidly grows again as environmental temperatures fall in the autumn. Whether these variations in growth rate are due to the effects of temperature variations, of longer sunlight hours or of specific light wavelengths is unknown. Nor is it certain in what manner the response is mediated.

Possibilities that suggest themselves are variations in capillary blood supply to the skin, or variations in the nutritive quality of the blood to the hairs. The fact that *alopecia areata* of humans occurs without diminution in capillary blood supply and is often associated with psychic disturbances suggests that there is at least some element of nervous control. In most cases of congenital alopecia there is reduction of all cellular elements of the epidermis. In some congenital conditions there is an absence of hair follicles.

Clinical Findings

When alopecia is due to breakage of the fibre, the stumps of old fibres or developing new ones may be seen. When fibres fail to grow the skin is shiny and in most cases is thinner than normal. In cases of congenital follicular aplasia, the ordinary covering hairs are absent but the coarser tactile hairs about the eyes, lips and extremities are often present. Absence of the hair coat makes the animal more susceptible to sudden changes of environmental temperature. There may be manifestations of a primary disease and evidence of scratching or rubbing.

Clinical Pathology

Unless the cause of the alopecia is apparent after the examination of skin scrapings or swabs, a skin biopsy should be taken to determine the status of the follicular epithelium.

Diagnosis

Alopecia is readily recognizable, the main diagnostic problem being to determine the primary cause of the hair or fibre loss.

Treatment

The primary condition should be treated but in most animal cases little is done to stimulate hair growth. The most logical treatment is to improve the blood supply to the skin by the use of an ultraviolet lamp or mild rubefacients (e.g. 1 in 20 parts biniodide of mercury or cantharides).

REFERENCES

(1) Shand, A. & Young, G. B. (1964). *Vet. Rec.*, 76, 907.
(2) Grunder, H. D. & Musche, R. (1962). *Dtsch. tierärztl. Wschr.*, 69, 437.

Seborrhoea

Seborrhoea is an excessive secretion of sebum on to the skin surface.

Aetiology

Primary or true seborrhoea as it occurs in humans is rarely recorded in animals. Secondary seborrhoea associated with dermatitis and skin irritation, e.g. in some types of eczema, appears to be more common. The common forms of seborrhoea encountered in animals are seborrhoea oleosa (exudative epidermitis) of baby pigs, greasy heel of horses and flexural seborrhoea of cattle. These conditions probably originate as a dermatitis or eczema, the increased sebaceous exudate being secondary rather than primary.

Pathogenesis

Increased blood supply to the skin and increased hair growth appear to stimulate the production of sebum. The reason why skin irritation should provoke seborrhoea in some individuals and not in others is unknown.

Clinical Findings

In primary seborrhoea there are no lesions, the only manifestation being excessive greasiness of the skin. The sebum may be spread over the body surface like a film of oil or be dried into crusts which can be removed easily. Hypertrophy of the sebaceous glands may be visible. Secondary infection can lead to the development of acne.

Flexural seborrhoea of cattle occurs most commonly in dairy cows which have calved recently. Lesions are present in the groin between the udder and the medial surface of the thigh, or in the median fissure between the two halves of the udder. There is a profuse outpouring of sebum. Extensive skin necrosis may develop and it is the pronounced odour of decay which may first attract the owner's attention. Irritation may cause the cow to attempt to lick the part. Shedding of the oily, malodorous skin leaves a raw surface beneath and causes lameness.

Greasy heel occurs most commonly in the hind legs of horses which are allowed to stand for long periods in wet unsanitary stables, although cases do occur under good management conditions. Cattle, especially those animals kept on muddy pasture or in dirty barns, may develop lesions similar to those in horses. The first signs seen are lameness and soreness due to excoriations called 'scratches' which appear on the back of the pastern and extend down to the coronary band. There is thickening and pronounced greasiness of the skin of the part which is painful to the touch and causes lameness. If the disease is neglected, it usually spreads around to the front and up the back of the leg. When the thickening of the skin and subcutaneous tissue is very marked it can interfere with normal movements of the limbs.

Clinical Pathology

The primary cause of the seborrhoea may be parasitic or bacterial and suitable diagnostic procedures should be employed.

Diagnosis

The principal difficulty is to determine whether the seborrhoea is primary or secondary. The safest procedure is to treat all cases as being secondary and to search carefully for the primary cause. Flexural seborrhoea of cattle may be mistaken for injury and greasy heel of horses for chorioptic mange.

Treatment

The skin must be kept clean and dry. Affected areas should be defatted with hot soap and water washes, then properly dried, and an astringent lotion, e.g. white lotion, applied daily. In acute cases of greasy heel the application of an ointment made up of 5 parts salicylic acid, 3 parts boric acid, 2 parts phenol, 2 parts mineral oil and 2 parts petroleum jelly at 5-day intervals is recommended.

Acne

When correctly used the term acne refers specifically to an infection of hair follicles by the acne bacillus—a diphtheroid organism. In the present context 'acne' is used to include all infections of hair follicles caused by suppurative organisms, including staphylococci (more properly termed sycosis). Boils or furuncles are acneiform lesions which progress to penetrate the deeper skin layers and subcutaneous tissue.

Aetiology

Non-specific acne is a sporadic disease and is more common in horses than in other animals. Lesions are usually present on areas where pressure is exerted by harness or saddles. Staphylococci are usually present in the lesions.

Specific acnes include Canadian horse pox caused by infection with *Corynebacterium pseudotuberculosis* and demodectic mange. Both these infections are easily spread among a group of animals.

Pathogenesis

When sebaceous gland ducts are blocked by inspissated secretion and epithelial debris they are predisposed to infection. Pressure is likely to cause such obstruction. Seborrhoea with hypertrophy of the glands and dilatation of the ducts also predisposes to acne.

Clinical Findings

Lesions begin as nodules around the base of the hair and then develop into pustules. The lesions are painful and rupture under pressure. This leads to contamination of the surrounding skin and the lesions spread as further follicles become infected. The hair in the affected follicle is usually shed.

Clinical Pathology

Swabs should be taken for bacteriological and parasitological examination.

Diagnosis

Acne is an infection of the hair follicles and should not be confused with impetigo in which the lesions arise on the surface of the skin.

Treatment

Clean the skin by washing and follow this with a disinfectant rinse. Affected areas should be treated with antibacterial ointments or lotions. If the lesions are extensive the parenteral administration of antibiotics is recommended. In stubborn cases an autogenous vaccine may be helpful. Infected animals should be isolated and grooming tools and blankets disinfected.

DISEASES OF THE SUBCUTIS

Oedema

The accumulation of oedema fluid in the subcutaneous tissue is called anasarca when the accumulation is extensive.

Aetiology

Subcutaneous oedema or anasarca often occurs as a manifestation of general oedema and has the same aetiology. It is brought about either by increased venous pressure or by reduced osmotic pressure of the blood. In congestive heart failure of old horses, traumatic pericarditis in cattle, and severe udder engorgement in cows, particularly heifers about to calve, subcutaneous oedema may be a sign of increased venous pressure. On the other hand it may be a sign of reduced osmotic pressure which occurs when there is hypoproteinaemia due to liver damage, as in acute fascioliasis, and when there is hypoproteinaemia in heavy parasitic infestations or dietary deficiency. Anasarca associated with vitamin A deficiency has been observed in beef cattle, but anasarca due to renal injury is rare in animals.

Inflammatory oedema due to clostridial infection is common in large animals. Angioneurotic oedema of allergic origin presents rather different features and is dealt with elsewhere.

Pathogenesis

The accumulation of fluids symptomatic of oedema may be due either to increased venous pressure, to decreased osmotic pressure of the blood or to damage to capillary walls. Reduced osmotic pressure is often associated with hypoproteinaemia. When capillary walls are damaged, as in malignant oedema and angioneurotic oedema, there is leakage of fluid or plasma into local tissue spaces.

Clinical Findings

There is visible swelling, either local or diffuse. The skin is puffy and pits on pressure; there is no pain unless inflammation is also present. In large animals the oedema is usually confined to the ventral aspects of the trunk and is seldom seen on the limbs.

Clinical Pathology

The differentiation between obstructive and inflammatory oedema can be made on the basis of the location of the oedematous area, and the presence or absence of fever, anorexia or local pain, and by bacteriological examination of the fluid.

Diagnosis

Subcutaneous oedema may be confused with infiltration of the belly wall with urine as a result of urethral obstruction and with subcutaneous haemorrhage.

Treatment

Unless the primary condition is repaired, removal of the fluid by drainage methods such as intubation or multiple incision or by the use of a diuretic will be of little value.

Angioneurotic Oedema

The sudden appearance of transient subcutaneous oedema due to allergic cause is known as angioneurotic oedema.

Aetiology

Endogenous and exogenous allergens provoke either local or diffuse lesions. Angioneurotic oedema occurs most frequently in cattle and horses on pasture, especially during the period when the pasture is in flower. This suggests that the allergen is a plant protein. Fish meals may also provoke an attack. Recurrence in individual animals is common.

Pathogenesis

Local vascular dilatation with damage to capillary walls is apparently caused by the liberation of histamine. Leakage of plasma through damaged vessels produces oedema after an initial erythema.

Clinical Findings

There are usually no general signs except in rare cases where bloat, diarrhoea and dyspnoea are manifest. In angioneurotic oedema local lesions most commonly affect the head although the perineum and udder are also involved in some cases. There is diffuse oedema of the muzzle, eyelids and sometimes the conjunctiva and cheeks. Occasionally the conjunctiva is the only part affected, and in this case the eyelids are puffy, the nictitating membrane is swollen and protrudes, and lacrimation is profuse. There is no pain on touching affected parts but there is some irritation, evidenced by shaking the head and rubbing against objects. There may be salivation and nasal discharge.

When the perineum is involved, the vulva is swollen, often asymmetrically, and the perianal skin, and sometimes the skin of the udder, is swollen and oedematous. When the udder alone is affected, the teats and base of the udder are oedematous. There is some irritation and the cow may paddle with the hind legs. Sometimes there is oedema of the lower limbs, usually from the knees or hocks down to the coronets.

Clinical Pathology

The blood eosinophil count is often within the normal range, but may be elevated from a normal level of 4 to 5 per cent up to 12 to 15 per cent.

Diagnosis

The sudden onset and equally sudden disappearance of oedema at the predilection sites typifies this condition. Subcutaneous oedema due to vascular pressure occurs mostly in dependent parts and is not irritating. In horses, and rarely in cattle, angioneurotic oedema may be simulated by purpura haemorrhagica but in the latter disease haemorrhages are usually visible in the mucosae.

Treatment

Local applications are seldom necessary. Spontaneous recovery is the rule, but treatment is often administered. Antihistamine drugs are favoured, and usually one injection of 0·5 to 1·0 g. intramuscularly is adequate for an adult cow or horse. For more rapid response intravenous injection is advisable. Adrenaline or epinephrine (3 to 5 ml. of a 1:1000 solution intramuscularly) is also satisfactory. A purgative may be administered to hasten the elimination of exogenous allergens.

Affected animals should be removed from the source of allergens. Cattle running at pasture should be confined and fed on dry feed for at least a week to prevent a recurrence.

Emphysema

The term emphysema denotes the presence of free gas in the subcutaneous tissue.

Aetiology

Emphysema occurs when air or gas accumulates in the subcutaneous tissue. This may be the result of air entering through accidental or surgical wounds of the skin; of lung puncture by rib fracture or penetrating injury especially traumatic reticulitis; of rumen gases seeping through trocarization sites; or the result of extension of interstitial emphysema. Infections with gas gangrene organisms are often accompanied by emphysema but these cases always show severe systemic signs.

Pathogenesis

When a lung is punctured air escapes under the visceral pleura and passes to the hilus of the lung, hence to beneath the parietal pleura, between the muscles and into the subcutis. The extension of an interstitial pulmonary emphysema occurs in the same way.

Clinical Findings

Visible swellings occur over the body. They are soft, fluctuating and obviously crepitant to the touch. There is no pain and no external skin lesion except in gas gangrene, when discolouration, coldness and oozing of serum may be evident.

Clinical Pathology

If a severe systemic reaction is evident a bacteriological examination of fluid from the swelling should be carried out to determine the organism present.

Diagnosis

The crepitus and the extreme mobility of the swelling distinguish emphysema from other superficial swellings.

Treatment

Sterile emphysema requires no treatment, unless it is extensive and incapacitating when multiple skin incisions may be necessary. The primary cause of the condition should be ascertained and treated. Gas gangrene requires immediate and drastic treatment with antibiotics.

Lymphangitis

The term lymphangitis denotes inflammation and enlargement of the lymph vessels and is usually associated with lymphadenitis.

Aetiology

Lymphangitis is due in most cases to local skin infection with subsequent spread to the lymphatic system. In horses, glanders, epizootic lymphangitis, sporadic lymphangitis and ulcerative lymphangitis are the forms most often encountered. In cattle, skin farcy caused by *Nocardia farcinica* and skin tuberculosis are the commonest causes. In both horses and cattle non-specific infections of the skin and subcutaneous tissues may lead to local lymphangitis.

Pathogenesis

Spread of infection along the lymphatic vessels causes chronic inflammation of the vessel walls. Abscesses often develop and discharge to the skin surface through sinuses.

Clinical Findings

An indolent ulcer usually exists at the original site of infection. The lymph vessels leaving this ulcer are enlarged, thickened and tortuous and often have secondary ulcers or sinuses along their course. Local oedema may result from lymphatic obstruction. In chronic cases considerable fibrous tissue may be laid down in the subcutis and chronic thickening of the skin may follow. The medial surface of the hind leg is the most frequent site, particularly in horses.

Clinical Pathology

In lymphangitis laboratory examination is largely a matter of the bacteriological examination of discharges for the presence of the specific bacteria or fungi which commonly cause the disease.

Treatment

The focus of infection must be removed by surgical excision or specific medical treatment. Early treatment is essential to prevent the widespread involvement of lymphatic vessels and nodes.

Haemorrhage

Subcutaneous haemorrhage occurs as the result of extravasations of whole blood into the subcutaneous tissues.

Aetiology

Accumulation of blood in the subcutaneous tissues beyond the limit of that normally caused by trauma may be due to defects in the coagulation mechanism or to increased permeability of the vessel wall. Included among the causes of such haemorrhage in animals are dicoumarol poisoning due to the ingestion of mouldy sweet clover hay, purpura haemorrhagica, bracken fern poisoning and poisoning by trichloroethylene-extracted soya bean meal.

Pathogenesis

Defects in the clotting system are seldom encountered except in dicoumarol poisoning. The damage to capillary walls which occurs in allergic states such as purpura haemorrhagica is probably due to liberation of histamine.

Clinical Findings

Subcutaneous swellings resulting from haemorrhage are diffuse and soft with no visible effect on the skin surface. There may be no evidence of trauma and the diagnosis can only be confirmed by opening the swelling.

Clinical Pathology

In cases where haemorrhage is excessive the determination of the primary cause may be helped by ascertaining platelet counts, the levels of histamine in the blood, and prothrombin, clotting and bleeding times.

Diagnosis

Subcutaneous haemorrhages are usually associated with haemorrhages into other tissues, both manifestations being due to defects in clotting or capillary wall continuity as listed above.

Treatment

Removal of the cause is of first importance. The haemorrhages should not be opened until clotting is completed. If blood loss is severe, blood transfusions may be required. Parenteral injection of coagulants is advisable if the haemorrhages are recent.

Gangrene

Gangrene is the result of death of tissues with subsequent sloughing of the affected part and when it occurs in the skin it usually involves the dermis, epidermis and the subcutaneous tissue.

Aetiology

Severe or continued trauma (as in pressure sores and saddle or harness galls), damage by strong chemical agents, or severe heat or cold may cause local or diffuse gangrene of the skin. Bacterial infections, especially erysipelas in pigs and staphylococcal mastitis and cutaneous gangrene of the udder in cattle, may cause local areas of skin gangrene. Local vascular obstruction by thrombi or arteriolar spasm, e.g. ergotism, causes skin gangrene but as a rule deeper structures are also involved. In flexural seborrhoea in cows and in severe dermatitis due to photosensitization there is often a terminal stage of gangrene and sloughing of skin.

Pathogenesis

The basic cause of gangrene is interference with local blood supply. This is often brought about by external pressure or by severe swelling of the skin, as in photosensitization. Arteriolar spasm or damage to vessels by bacterial toxins has the same effect.

Clinical Findings

If the arterial supply and drainage systems are involved the initial lesion will be moist. The area is swollen, raised, discoloured and cold. Separation occurs at the margin and sloughing may occur before drying of the affected skin is apparent. The underlying surface is raw and weeping. If, on the other hand, the veins and lymphatics remain patent, the lesion is dry from the beginning and the area is cold, discoloured and sunken. Sloughing may take a considerable time and the underlying surface usually consists of granulation tissue. Secondary bacterial invasion may occur in either type of gangrene.

Treatment

Local treatment comprises the application of astringent and antibacterial ointments to facilitate separation of the gangrenous tissue and to prevent bacterial infection. The primary condition must also be treated.

CUTANEOUS NEOPLASMS

Neoplasms arising from the epidermis, dermis and subcutaneous tissue are not rare in animals (1). A brief description of the more common types is given here.

PAPILLOMA

Papillomatosis of horses and cattle has been described elsewhere.

SARCOID

This tumour is transplantable and occurs in horses on the lower limbs and around the base of the ears. It is a fibroid tumour consisting mainly of connective tissue. The lesions occur singly or in groups and have the appearance of rather large warts. They show moderate malignancy in that they frequently recur after excision but do not metastasize. Similar tumours can be produced by the intradermal inoculation of bovine papillomatosis virus.

SQUAMOUS CELL CARCINOMA

This neoplasm is common on the eyelids and the eyeball in horses and cattle and is colloquially referred to as 'cancer eye'. The initial lesion may be on the third eyelid, the cornea or the eyelid. The tumours grow rapidly and show considerable invasiveness, often metastasizing to the local lymph nodes. Considerable discussion has revolved about the aetiological factors. Hereford cattle seem to be more commonly affected than other breeds but the relative importance of heredity, lack of pigment in the eye structures, sunlight and viruses is still uncertain (4, 5). There does appear to be a strong correlation between absence of pigmentation of the eyelids and a high incidence of the disease, and because of the apparent high heritability of this pigmentation in Hereford cattle it is suggested that a breeding programme aimed at increasing the degree of pigmentation of eyelids could quickly reduce the incidence of the disease in this breed (9). On the other hand selection on the basis of the occurrence of lesions results in only limited reduction in incidence (13). In early cases excision is often successful and treatment by the use of radioactive implants has also aroused favourable comment (2, 3). A favourable response to a single injection of a saline phenol extract of fresh tumour tissue has been reported recently (12).

Squamous cell carcinomas also occur on the skin and penis of the horse. The common 'cancer of the horn core' in cattle is a squamous cell carcinoma arising from the mucosa of the frontal sinus and invading the horn core (7, 8). The horn becomes loosened and falls off leaving the tumour exposed. Cancer of the ear in sheep is in most cases a squamous cell carcinoma. The lesion commences around the free edge of the ear and then invades the entire ear which becomes a large cauliflower shaped mass. Less commonly the perineum and muzzle are involved. A high incidence of epitheliomas has been recorded in some families of Merino sheep in Australia. The lesions occurred on the woolled skin and were accompanied by many cutaneous cysts. It was suggested that predisposition to the neoplasm was inherited (18, 19, 20). In both of the above cases metastasis into local lymph nodes is common. Squamous cell carcinomata also occur on the vulva of cattle and a greater incidence has been observed on unpigmented than on pigmented vulvas (14). The so-called 'brand cancer', which occurs as a granulomatous mass at the site of a skin fire brand, is of chronic inflammatory rather than neoplastic origin.

MELANOMA

Superficially situated melanomata are most often seen in aged, grey horses and also occur rarely in dark-skinned cattle. Those of horses are usually malignant and metastasize widely. In horses the common site is at the root of the tail. The skin is usually intact but ulceration may occur if the tumour is growing rapidly. Melanomata in cattle are usually benign and are only removed if they spoil the animal's appearance. Malignant melanomata have been observed rarely in sheep (10) and goats (11). In pigs the incidence is low, but a very high rate of occurrence has been observed in young pigs of the Duroc-Jersey breed (15) and the tumours have been present at birth (16).

CUTANEOUS ANGIOMATOSIS

This condition is recorded only in dairy cattle in the U.K. (17) and France (21). It is manifested clinically by recurrent profuse haemorrhage from small single cutaneous lesions usually situated along the dorsum of the back. The lesions are relatively inconspicuous and consist of what appears to be protruding granulation tissue about 1·0 to 1·5 cm. diameter. In most instances the life of the cow does not appear to be endangered. Surgical excision is an effective treatment.

LYMPHOMATOSIS

In this disease of cattle the skin lesions commonly occur as nodules under the skin. They are situated in the subcutaneous tissue and are most common in the paralumbar fossae and the perineum. In all cases they are a secondary manifestation of the disease and are associated with lesions in other organs. Biopsy of a node may reveal a considerable increase in immature lymphocytes. A diffuse thickening of the skin itself is a rare form of this neoplasm.

MAST CELL TUMOURS

Cutaneous mastocytoma is recorded rarely in cattle (6). It appears as a rapidly-growing intradermal nodule, which may become widely disseminated if excised.

REFERENCES

(1) Cotchin, E. (1956). *Neoplasms of the Domesticated Mammals.* Review Series No. 4, Cwlth Bur. Anim. Hlth, Farnham Royal, Bucks.
(2) Vigue, R. F. (1955). *J. Amer. vet. med. Ass., 126,* 23.
(3) Wheat, J. *et al.* (1954). *J. Amer. vet. med. Ass., 125,* 357.
(4) Anderson, D. E. (1970). *Mod. vet. Pract., 51,* No. 5, 43.
(5) Russell, W. D. *et al.* (1956). *Cancer, 9,* 1.
(6) McGavin, M. D. & Leis, T. J. (1968). *Aust. vet. J., 44,* 20.
(7) Pachauri, S. P. & Pathak, R. C. (1969). *Amer. J. vet. Res., 30,* 475.
(8) Patra, B. N. (1959). *Vet. Rec., 71,* 844.
(9) French, G. T. (1959). *Aust. vet. J., 35,* 474.
(10) Baxter, J. T. (1960). *Brit. vet. J., 116,* 67.
(11) Omar, A. R. & Colins, G. W. (1961). *J. comp. Path., 71,* 183.
(12) Manilla, G. T. *et al.* (1972). *Fed. Proc., 31,* No. 2, 768.
(13) Vogt, D. W. & Anderson, D. E. (1964). *J. Hered., 55,* 133.
(14) Burdin, M. L. (1964). *Res. vet. Sci., 5,* 497.
(15) Hjerpe, C. A. & Theilen, G. H. (1964). *J. Amer. vet. med. Ass., 144,* 1129.
(16) Case, M. T. (1964). *J. Amer. vet. med. Ass., 144,* 254.
(17) Cotchin, E. & Swarbrick, O. (1963). *Vet. Rec., 75,* 437.
(18) Lloyd, L. C. (1961). *Brit. J. Cancer, 15,* 780.
(19) Lloyd, L. C. (1961). *J. Path. Bact., 88,* 219.
(20) Carne, H. R. *et al.* (1963). *J. Path. Bact., 86,* 305.
(21) Lombard, C. & Levesque, L. (1964). *C. R. Acad. Sci. (Paris), 258,* 3137.

PART TWO

SPECIAL MEDICINE

14

Mastitis

THE TERM mastitis refers to inflammation of the mammary gland regardless of the cause. It is characterized by physical, chemical and usually bacteriological changes in the milk and by pathological changes in the glandular tissue. The most important changes in the milk include discolouration, the presence of clots and the presence of large numbers of leucocytes. Although there is swelling, heat, pain and induration in the mammary gland in many cases, a large proportion of mastitic glands are not readily detectable by manual palpation nor by visual examination of the milk using a strip cup. Because of the very large numbers of such subclinical cases the diagnosis of mastitis has come to depend largely on indirect tests which depend, in turn, on the leucocyte content of the milk. In the present state of knowledge it seems practicable and reasonable to define mastitis as a disease characterized by the presence of a significantly increased leucocyte content in milk from affected glands. More exact definition of the type of mastitis depends on the identification of the causative agent whether it be physical or infectious.

Incidence

Although mastitis occurs sporadically in all species, it assumes major economic importance only in dairy cattle. In terms of economic loss it is undoubtedly the most important disease with which the dairying industry has to contend. This loss is occasioned much less by fatalities, although fatal cases do occur, than from the reduction in milk production from affected quarters. Moreover, it is the one major infectious disease of cattle against which no real progress had been made for many years. In the past decade, as described at the end of this chapter, effective control programmes have at last been developed. The clinical syndrome may vary from a peracute inflammation with toxaemia to a fibrosis which develops so gradually that it may escape observation until most of the secretory tissue has been destroyed. There is the additional danger that the bacterial contamination of milk from affected cows may render it unsuitable for human consumption, or interfere with manufacturing process or, in rare cases, provide a mechanism of spread of disease to humans. Tuberculosis, streptococcal sore throat and brucellosis may be spread in this way.

In most countries surveys of the incidence of mastitis, irrespective of cause, show comparable figures of about 40 per cent morbidity amongst cows and a quarter incidence of about 25 per cent. The incidence is similar in goats and buffaloes kept in dairies (1).

Most estimates show that on the average an affected quarter suffers a 30 per cent reduction in productivity and an affected cow is estimated to lose 15 per cent of its production. Experimental infection of quarters during the dry period causes 35 per cent reduction in yield in these quarters during the next lactation. Quarters found to be infected in late lactation had a 48 per cent reduction in yield but if the infection was caused in the dry period the depression of yield after calving was only 11 per cent (2). These losses are supplemented by a loss of about 1 per cent of total solids by changes in composition (fat, casein and lactose are reduced and glycogen, whey proteins, pH and chlorides are increased) which interfere with manufacturing processes, loss due to increased culling rates and costs of treatment.

A good deal more has been written on the biological effects of mastitis on total milk production and the chemical composition of milk from mastitic quarters (3, 4). This information is of very great importance when attempting to plan a control programme but its compilation and analysis awaits a chapter on quantitative pathology in a textbook of preventive veterinary medicine. If, as has been suggested, it is necessary to control mastitis to maintain or increase the solids not fat content of milk to comply with minimum legal standards for milk as a food, the control programmes may be in operation before the book is written (5).

AETIOLOGY

Many infective agents have been implicated as

causes of mastitis and these are dealt with separately as specific entities:

Cattle: *Streptococcus agalactiae, Str. uberis, Str. zooepidemicus, Str. dysgalactiae, Str. faecalis* and *Str. pneumoniae, Staphylococcus aureus, Escherichia coli, Klebsiella* spp., *Corynebacterium pyogenes, Cor. bovis, Mycobacterium tuberculosis, Mycobacterium* spp., *Bacillus cereus, Pasteurella multocida, Pseudomonas pyocyaneus, Sphaerophorus necrophorus, Serratia marcescens, Mycoplasma* spp., and *Nocardia* spp., a fungus *Trichosporon* spp., and yeasts *Candida* spp., *Cryptococcus neoformans, Saccharomyces* and *Torulopsis* spp. The disease in milking buffaloes in India is caused by the same bacteria as in cattle (1). Some viruses may cause mastitis in cattle (6) but present knowledge suggests that this is of very little practical significance.

Sheep: *Pasteurella haemolytica, Staph. aureus, Actinobacillus lignieresi, E. coli, Str. uberis* and *Str. agalactiae.* Suppurative lesions due to *Cor. pseudotuberculosis* occur commonly but are not true mastitis although function of the gland may be lost.

Goats: *Str. agalactiae, Str. dysgalactiae, Str pyogenes* and *Staph. aureus.*

Pigs: *Aerobacter aerogenes, E. coli, Str. agalactiae, Str. dysgalactiae, Str. uberis* and *Staph. aureus.* Mammary actinomycosis is not a true mastitis and is dealt with under the heading of actinomycosis.

Surveys of the incidence of the various infections in cattle show a great deal of similarity in different countries. The predominant position of *Str. agalactiae* as a cause of bovine mastitis has been usurped in recent years by *Staph. aureus,* especially in areas where the treatment of mastitis with penicillin has been practised intensively and where machine milking has replaced hand milking. In such areas a relative incidence of *Str. agalactiae,* other streptococci and *Staph. aureus* of 1:1:2 is a common finding.

The importance of bacteria as the primary cause of mastitis in cattle is still debated, largely because of the absence of bacteria from a proportion of clinical cases and their presence in many clinically normal glands. There is, too, the common field observation that the incidence of mastitis varies widely with different environmental conditions. Undoubtedly factors other than exposure to bacteria are of importance but these factors are unable to produce mastitis without the presence of bacteria and so must be considered as predisposing or precipitating causes only. The absence of bacteria from

some clinical cases is probably due to control of the infection by natural protective mechanisms.

There are two main sources of infection in mastitis, the infected udder and the environment. In dairy cattle and milking goats, the important infections are those which persist readily in the udder, especially *Str. agalactiae* and *Staph. aureus.* Bacteria which are normal inhabitants of the environment, such as *E. coli* and *Ps. pyocyaneus* cause mastitis much less frequently but when they do, the disease is much more resistant to hygienic control measures. The contamination of milkers' hands, wash cloths and milking machine cups by milk from infected quarters may quickly lead to the spread of infection to the teats of other animals.

In sheep, the only other species in which outbreaks occur, spread appears to be due to contamination of sheep bedding grounds by discharges from affected glands. Surveys of the incidence of the disease in this species do not appear to have been carried out in areas other than those in which ewes' milk is used extensively for human consumption. In such countries *Str. agalactiae* is the common cause. In most other areas either *Staph. aureus* or *Past. haemolytica* is the common pathogen. One Norwegian survey (7) records a total incidence of mastitis in 6000 sheep at 2 per cent per year, 86 per cent of these being caused by *Staph. aureus,* 10 per cent by *E. coli,* 3 per cent by *Str. agalactiae* and 1 per cent by *Past. haemolytica.* In a New Zealand survey the incidence of mastitis was 1·65 per cent. In recently lambed ewes *Staph. aureus* was the common bacterial cause, in post-weaning ewes streptococci were most common (8).

The predisposing causes of mastitis include injury to and sores on the teats and udder and variations in susceptibility which depend upon inheritance, management, and possibly feeding practices. The management of these causes is described in the section on control of mastitis.

PATHOGENESIS

Except in the case of tuberculosis, where the method of spread may be haematogenous, infection of the mammary gland always occurs via the teat canal and on first impression the development of inflammation after infection seems a natural sequence. However, the development of mastitis is more complex than this and can be most satisfactorily explained in terms of the three stages—invasion—infection—inflammation (9). Invasion is the stage at which organisms pass from the exterior of the teat to the milk inside the teat canal. Infection is the stage in which the organisms multiply rapidly and invade the mammary tissue. After invasion a bacterial population may be established in the teat canal and, using this as a base, a series of multiplications and extensions into mammary tissue may occur, with infection of mammary tissue occurring frequently or occasionally depending on its susceptibility (10). This in turn causes inflammation, the stage at which clinical mastitis appears or a greatly increased leucocyte count is apparent in the milk. Investigations of the factors governing the cell count in milk have been extensively reviewed (11). One might expect that the introduction of organisms into the udder would naturally result in the development of mastitis but this is not necessarily the case. There are considerable variations in the ease with which mastitis can be set up in individual animals and with different bacteria. These variations are due to different responses at each of the three stages of development of the disease. It is possible that repeated infection, or resurgence of existing infection, may result in the development of a state of tissue hypersensitivity which renders the gland more susceptible to attacks of acute inflammation.

In the context of the above general description of the development of mastitis the following factors suggest themselves as being involved in the development of the disease in individual cows and in the herd.

Invasion Phase

(i) The presence and population density of the causative bacteria in the milking shed environment. The quarter infection rate and the degree of contamination of the teat skin are commonly used as indices of this factor.

(ii) The frequency with which the cow's teats, particularly the apices, are contaminated with these bacteria. This depends largely on the efficiency of milking hygiene.

(iii) The degree of damage to the teat sphincters facilitating entry of bacteria into the teat canal. Milking machine design, adjustment, maintenance and proper use, and teat care are the important contributors to this factor and to the possible reflux of milk back into the udder from the liner of the milking cup during milking.

(iv) Tone of the teat sphincter, particularly in the period directly after milking when the sphincter is most relaxed. Slackness of the sphincter facilitates invasion by permitting both suction and growth of bacteria into the teat.

(v) The presence of antibacterial substances in the teat duct.

Infection Phase

(vi) The type of bacteria which determines its capacity to multiply in the milk.

(vii) The susceptibility of the bacteria to the commonly used antibiotics. This may depend on natural or acquired resistance resulting from the improper use of antibiotics.

(viii) The presence of protective substances in the milk. Immune substances may be natural or be present as a result of previous infection or vaccination.

(ix) A pre-existing high leucocyte count due to intercurrent mastitis or physical trauma.

(x) The stage of lactation, infection occurring more readily in the dry period because of the absence of physical flushing. There has been general acceptance that this is so but a careful analysis suggests that susceptibility is high at drying off, but is much less in the quarter which has been dried off for some time (12).

Inflammation Phase

(xi) The pathogenicity and tissue-invasive powers of the causative bacteria.

(xii) The susceptibility of the mammary tissue to the bacteria. This may vary from resistance, due to the presence of fixed tissue antibody, to hypersensitivity as a result of previous infection.

Of the three phases, prevention of the invasion phase offers the greatest potential for reducing the incidence of mastitis by good management, notably in the use of good hygienic procedures.

Because of the difficulties encountered in the control of the disease any factor capable of reducing the severity of the response to infection is worthy of examination. Immunity to infection, because of the promise it holds as a control measure, has attracted much attention but in spite of the resistance to mammary infection which is known to occur naturally in a small proportion of cows little is known of its mechanism. There is a division of opinion on whether immunity is produced locally or by the secretion of immune globulins from the blood (13). Whichever is the case, and either one may be important in different situations, the artificial production of immunity is at present of very limited practical value.

CLINICAL FINDINGS

Dependent upon the resistance of the mammary tissue and the virulence of the invading bacteria, there may be all degrees of variation in signs from the gradual onset of fibrosis, through acute inflammation without systemic signs, to severe toxaemia with systemic signs.

Details of the clinical findings are provided under each bacteriological type of mastitis. These may be taken as a guide but because many species of bacteria can cause chronic, acute and peracute forms of the disease, clinical differentiation of bacteriological types of mastitis is generally impossible. The clinical findings in mastitis include abnormalities of secretion, abnormalities of the size, consistency and temperature of the mammary glands and frequently a systemic reaction. The clinical forms of mastitis are usually classified according to their severity; severe inflammation of the quarter with a marked systemic reaction is classified as peracute; severe inflammation without a marked systemic reaction as acute; mild inflammation with persistent abnormality of the milk as subacute; and recurrent attacks of inflammation with little change in the milk as chronic.

Proper examination of the milk requires the use of a strip cup, preferably one which has a shiny, black plate permitting the detection of discolouration as well as clots, flakes and pus. Milk is drawn on to the plate in pools and comparisons made between the milk of different quarters. Discolouration may be in the form of blood staining or wateriness, the latter usually indicating chronic mastitis when the quarter is lactating. Little significance is attached to barely discernible wateriness in the first few streams but if this persists for 10 streams or more, it can be considered to be an abnormality. Clots or flakes are usually accompanied by discolouration and they are always significant, usually indicating a severe degree of inflammation, even when small and present only in the first few streams. Blood clots are of little significance, nor are the small plugs of wax which are often present in the milk during the first few days after calving, especially in heifers. Flakes at the end of milking are often indicative of mammary tuberculosis in cattle. During the dry period in normal cows, the secretion changes from normal milk to a clear watery fluid, then to a secretion the colour and consistency of honey and finally to colostrum in the last few days before parturition. Some variation may occur between individual quarters in the one cow and if this is marked, it should arouse suspicion of infection.

The strip cup has been a valuable adjunct to the detection of mastitis and still has its place in the cursory examination of suspicious quarters. However, it has been almost completely superseded by the more accurate indirect tests listed below. Because the herdsman frequently has little time to examine milk for evidence of mastitis it is customary to milk the first few streams onto the floor, in some parlours onto black plates in the floor. The practice does not appear to be harmful, especially where the floor is kept washed down. To avoid the difficulties arising from foremilk stripping in-line filters have been introduced which detect the presence of clots in the milk (14).

Abnormalities of size and consistency of the quarters may be seen and felt. Palpation is of greatest value when the udder has been recently milked, whereas visual examination of both the full and empty udder may be useful. The udder should be viewed from behind and the two back quarters examined for symmetry. By lifting up the back quarters, the front quarters can be viewed. A decision on which quarter of a pair is abnormal may depend on palpation, which should be carried out on adjacent quarters simultaneously. Although in most forms of mastitis the observed abnormalities are mainly in the region of the milk cistern, the whole of the quarter must be palpated, particularly if tuberculosis is suspected. Moreover, the teats and supramammary lymph nodes should be palpated and the teats examined for sores especially about the sphincter.

Palpation and inspection of the udder are directed at the detection of fibrosis, inflammatory swelling and the atrophy of mammary tissue. Fibrosis occurs in various forms. There may be a diffuse increase in connective tissue, giving the quarter a firmer feel than its opposite number and usually a more nodular surface on light palpation. It should be remembered, however, that some cows and some families of cattle normally have firm quarters and little attention is paid to this unless there is marked induration or one of a pair differs from the other. Error may occur when the anterior part of a front quarter or the posterior part of a hind quarter are palpated. The loose attachment of these parts in many cows may give the impression of diffuse fibrosis. Local areas of fibrosis may also occur in a quarter, and vary in size from pea-like lesions to masses as large as a fist. Acute inflammatory swelling is always diffuse and is accompanied by heat and pain and marked abnormality of the secretion. In severe cases there may be areas of gangrene, or abscesses may develop in the glandular tissue. The terminal stage of chronic mastitis is atrophy of the gland. On casual examination an atrophied quarter may be classed as normal because of its small size, while the normal quarter is judged to be hypertrophic. Careful palpation may reveal that, in the atrophic quarter, little functioning mammary tissue remains.

A systemic reaction comprising toxaemia, fever, general depression and anorexia may or may not be present, depending upon the type and severity of the infection. The details of the different types of mastitis in cattle are given in the subsequent sections.

CLINICAL PATHOLOGY

In the diagnosis and control of mastitis, laboratory procedures are of value in the examination of milk samples for cells, bacteria and chemical changes, and for testing for sensitivity of bacteria to specific drugs. Because of the expense of laboratory examination of large numbers of milk samples, much attention has been given to the development of field tests based on physical and chemical changes in the milk. Because these tests are indirect and detect only the presence of inflammatory changes, they are of value only as screening tests and must be supplemented by bacteriological examination for determination of the causative organism and, if necessary, its sensitivity to antibiotics and chemotherapeutic agents.

Milk sampling for cultural examination must be carried out with due attention to cleanliness since samples contaminated during collection are worthless. The technique of cleaning the teat is of considerable importance. If the teats are dirty, ensure that they are properly dried after washing or water will run down the teat and infect the milk sample. Cleanse the end of the teat with a swab dipped in 70 per cent alcohol, extruding the external sphincter by pressure to ensure that dirt and wax are removed from the orifice. Brisk rubbing is advisable, especially of teats with inverted ends. The first streams are collected as the bacterial population is usually higher in these than in later samples. If tuberculosis is suspected, the last few streams should be collected. In sows where the amount of secretion may be small, a few drops of milk may be collected on to a sterile swab.

Individual quarter samples are preferable to composite samples unless cost is a major factor; with the former, the status of each quarter is determined, while with the latter, all four quarters have to be treated if the sample is positive. Composite samples are often collected directly on to culture medium without the need of an intermediate collection technique. If individual quarter samples are collected, screw-cap vials with rubber wads are most satisfactory. During collection the vial is canted to avoid as far as possible the entrance of dust, skin scales and hair. If there is delay between the collection of samples and laboratory examinations, the specimens should be kept cool. The laboratory techniques used vary widely and depend to a large extent on the facilities available. Incubation on blood agar is most satisfactory, selective media for *Str. agalactiae* having the disadvantage that other pathogens may go undetected. Smears of incubated milk are generally unsatisfactory as not all bacteria grow equally well in milk.

Cell counts are usually performed on the same sample as that used for cultural examination and serious errors are avoided if the samples are always taken at the same stage of milking. There is a great deal of variation in the cell counts at various times during milking and the most significant sample is the one taken just before the evening milking (15, 16). In chronic mastitis the highest counts are in the strippings. When foremilk counts are highest the lesion is probably in the teat. Leucocytes break down readily in stored milk and for preference, smears should be made, fixed and stained within an hour or two of collection of the sample. Cell counts, now a practical reality because of the development of electronic cell-counting machines (17), are of considerable value in determining the presence of inflammation. Counts of less than 250,000 per ml. are considered to be below the limit indicative of inflammation although most normal quarters show less than 100,000 per ml. Cows in early and late lactation may show high counts but all four quarters are equally affected, an unusual state in mastitis. The degree of elevation also varies with the type of mastitis, *Str. agalactiae* infections being associated with higher counts than other types of infection.

Leucocyte counts on bulk milk collected at the farm or the milk depot are satisfactory as a screening test for the presence of mastitis in the herd of origin. In several countries a count of more than 300,000 leucocytes per ml. is accepted as indicating the presence of significant mastitis in the herd (12) but this is considered to be too low a level for standard use (11).

Differential counts have not received much attention because of the difficulty of identifying the cell types. The total count reflects the amount of gland involved in the inflammatory process, whereas the neutrophil count reflects the stage of the inflammation. A high total count (e.g. 10 million per ml.) and a high proportion of neutrophils (e.g. 90 per cent) indicate acute inflammation affecting much of the quarter. A low total count (e.g. 500,000 per ml.) and a low proportion of neutrophils (e.g. less than 40 per cent) indicate a small, chronic lesion (18).

Indirect tests for the detection of mastitis, and designed principally for use in the field, are now restricted almost entirely to those which determine the quantity of DNA, and therefore approximately the number of leucocytes, in the sample. The California (Rapid) Mastitis Test is most commonly used and has proved to be highly efficient, especially in the hands of a skilled operator. It reflects accurately the total leucocyte and the polymorph count of the milk (19, 20, 21). After mixing milk and the prepared reagent in a white container, the result is read as a negative, trace, 1, 2 or 3 reaction depending on the amount of gel formation in the sample. Cows in the first week after calving or in the last stages of lactation always give a strong positive reaction.

The relationship between the CMT reaction and the leucocyte count of milk and the reduced productivity of affected cows is set out in the table below (22). The test has also been shown to be a reliable indicator of the cell count of ewe's milk (23).

CMT Reaction	Leucocyte count per ml.	Loss of milk yield for lactation, per cent
Trace	500,000	6·0
1	1,000,000	10·0
2	2,000,000	16·0
3	4,000,000	24·5

Other tests which depend on the same principle as the CMT but use different reagents are the Whiteside test (24), the Michigan Mastitis Test (25), one developed in the U.K. (21) and the Negretti Field Mastitis Test (26). A comparison of the efficiency of the various tests as indicators of the cell count has been made (27, 28).

Because of the tediousness of cell counting, modifications of indirect field tests have been devised for use in the laboratory. These include the Brabant test, which measures the viscosity produced in a CMT-like reaction by the rate of flow through a capillary tube, a modification of the Feulgen reaction for DNA (11), and the Wisconsin Mastitis Test which also measures viscosity objectively (29). A method of making approximate counts with a Coulter Counter is also available (30). The Wisconsin test is highly accurate and repeatable. For every increase of 1 mm. in the WMT viscosity test there is a daily milk yield loss of 0·065 kg. (31).

The California Mastitis Test has the advantage that it can be used on the bulk milk from the cow, from individual cans and from a herd bulk tank as well as on individual quarters (17, 32). Of course the results become less accurate as greater dilution occurs and bulk samples from the herd will tolerate on the average about 18 per cent positive cows before showing a 1 reaction. A grade 1 reaction on herd milk suggests that mastitis is present, a grade 2 or 3 that a serious situation exists. CMT scores of N, T, 1, 2 and 3 have been found to equate to mean cow cell counts of 100,000, 300,000, 900,000, 2,700,000 and 8,100,000 respectively. When a positive test is obtained on a herd or individual sample a bacteriological examination of those quarters showing a positive CMT is indicated.

A laboratory report on milk samples should include identification of the organisms and some estimate of their numbers. Additional valuable information includes an estimate of the pathogenicity and drug sensitivity of the bacteria. Some information on the presence of inflammation is required either in the form of a cell count or the result of one of the indirect tests mentioned above. In about 10 per cent of clinical cases a negative bacterial result will be obtained because the infection is at the time under control by natural defence mechanisms. Resampling in such cases is recommended.

NECROPSY FINDINGS

Necropsy findings are not of major interest in the diagnosis of mastitis and are omitted here, and included in the description of specific infections.

DIAGNOSIS

The diagnosis of mastitis presents little difficulty if a careful clinical examination is carried out. Examination of the udder is often omitted unless called for, particularly when animals are recumbent. The diagnosis of mastitis depends largely upon the detection of clinical abnormality of the milk. Other mammary abnormalities, including oedema, passive congestion, rupture of the suspensory ligament and haematomata, are not accompanied by abnormality of the milk unless there is haemorrhage into the udder. The presence of 'free' electricity in the milking plant should not be overlooked in herds where the sudden lowering of production arouses an unfounded suspicion of mastitis. The presence of more than 3 volts on the power earth and on the milk line is not unusual and it may require more than one examination to detect it. Levels as low as this would not be a cause for concern to an electricity supply authority but can cause lowered milk production (33). Clinical differentiation of the various bacteriological types of mastitis is not easy but may have to be attempted, especially in peracute cases, as specific treatment has to be given before results of laboratory examinations are available.

TREATMENT

Special bacterial types of mastitis require specific treatments and these are discussed under the aetiological entities, but there are some general principles that apply to all forms (34).

Degree of Response

The treatment of mastitis can be highly effective in removing infection from the quarter and returning the milk to normal composition. However, the yield of milk, although it can be improved by the removal of congestion in the gland and inflammatory debris from the duct system, is unlikely to be returned to normal, at least until the next lactation. The degree of response obtained depends particularly on the type of causative agent, the speed with which treatment is commenced and to other factors as set out below.

Parenteral treatment is advisable in all cases of mastitis in which there is a marked systemic reaction, to control or prevent the development of a septicaemia or bacteraemia and to assist in the treatment of the infection in the gland. The systemic reaction can usually be brought under control by standard doses of antibiotics or sulphonamides but complete sterilization of the affected quarters is seldom achieved because of the relatively poor diffusion of the antibiotic from the blood stream into the milk. The rate of diffusion is greater in damaged than in normal quarters and can be further increased in the case of penicillin by the use of the penicillin ester, penethamate. Parenteral injections of 2 million units of penethamate are sufficient to achieve bacteriostatic levels in milk.

Udder Infusions

Because of convenience and efficiency, udder infusions are the preferred method of treatment. Disposable tubes containing suitable drugs in a water-soluble ointment base are best suited for dispensing and the treatment of individual cows but aqueous infusions are adequate, are much cheaper and are indicated when large numbers of quarters are to be treated. The degree of diffusion into glandular tissue is the same when either water or ointment is used as a vehicle for infusion.

Strict hygiene is necessary during treatment to avoid the introduction of bacteria, yeasts and fungi into the treated quarters. Care must be taken to ensure that bulk containers of mastitis infusions are not contaminated by frequent withdrawals and that individual, sterilized teat cannulae are used for each quarter. Because of the bad record of spread of pathogens by bulk treatments they are best avoided if possible.

Diffusion of infused drugs is often impeded by the blockage of lactiferous ducts and alveoli with inflammatory debris. Complete emptying of the quarter before infusion by the parenteral injection of oxytocin is advisable in cases of acute mastitis. This can be further aided by hourly stripping of the quarter, the intramammary infusion being left until right after the last stripping has been carried out.

After an intramammary infusion avoid emptying the gland, and thus losing the antibiotic or other drug, for as long as possible by treating immediately after milking, preferably in the evening.

Treatment of Dry Cows

Chronic cases, particularly those caused by *Staph. aureus*, are often cleared up most satisfactorily by treatment when the cow is not lactating. Treatment at this time is also a good prophylaxis. Because of interference with diffusion of an infused drug by the viscid secretion of much of the dry period, infusion at the time of the last milking or at the beginning or end of the dry period is recommended. The material is introduced and allowed to remain permanently.

Intraparenchymal Injections

Intraparenchymal injection of drugs into mammary tissue by passing a needle through the skin into the mass of the gland is not widely used. It is sometimes recommended when the gland is so swollen that no diffusion is likely to occur from the milk cistern but in this case, diffusion from a parenchymal injection may also be greatly impeded.

Choice of Drug

Use the drug most likely to control the particular infection in adequate dosage. When the type of infection is not determined, use a broad spectrum drug or a combination of narrow spectrum drugs. Although there are contrary views, it is generally held to be necessary to maintain an effective concentration of the drug in the udder for about 6 days to obtain good results. This can be done by multiple infusions of a water-soluble preparation or of one or two infusions of the drug in a slow release base e.g. mineral oil and aluminium monostearate (37). This is in conflict with the present policy of ensuring rapid excretion of the drug from the mammary gland to avoid rejection of milk. A recent examination of treatment of infected quarters during lactation showed that the use of a slow-release base was significantly better than a quick-release preparation (35). Sodium cloxacillin was used and showed almost complete cure of *Str. agalactiae* and *Str. dysgalactiae* infections, 80 per cent against *Str. uberis*, and in a slow-release base 60 per cent effective against *Staph. aureus*.

Adjuvants in Udder Infusions

The use of hyaluronidase to promote the diffusion of an infused agent has not been generally adopted but the use of enzymes to break down necrotic tissue and liquefy pus has given good results. Mixtures of streptokinase (20,000 units) and streptodornase (5,000 units), given as infusions on two occasions at 48-hour intervals, or stabilized trypsin (50 mg. daily for 3 days), together with antibiotics, appear to be safe and beneficial, particularly if the quarters are thoroughly stripped out beforehand. The parenteral administration of enzyme preparations may also be of value. Treatment with enzymes is probably best restricted to the treatment of acute cases in which there is no systemic reaction, and to chronic cases which discharge pus or clots continuously. Immunoglobulins extracted from blood have been combined with antibiotics and used in the treatment of mastitis with reported excellent results (36).

Corticosteroids in Mastitis

Cortisone and allied compounds have been used to facilitate the reduction of inflammation in acute mastitis. A reduction in convalescent time of 25 per cent and increase in cures of 20 per cent have been claimed. Delta-1-cortisone (prednisone) and its acetate, hydrocortisone and its acetate (50 to 100 mg.), and fluorohydrocortisone (10 to 25 mg.) have been used combined with adequate doses of antibiotics as infusions in cattle with apparently good results. Experimental work with mastitis caused by *Aerobacter aerogenes* has failed to show any advantage in cows treated systemically or by intramammary infusion with corticosteroids (37).

Drug-resistant Bacteria

The widespread use of antibiotics for the treatment of mastitis has coincided with the detection of large numbers of strains of bacteria which are resistant to the antibiotic in use. This has been much more noticeable with staphylococci and penicillin than with other combinations. Inefficient, indiscriminate use of penicillin is to be avoided and the determination of drug sensitivity of the causative bacteria is becoming increasingly necessary.

Antibiotic Residues in Milk

Of great consequence is the effect of antibiotics in milk on the manufacture of dairy products and the development of sensitivity syndromes in human beings. In some countries the maximum intra-mammary dose of antibiotics is limited by legislation and the presence of detectable quantities of antibiotics in milk constitutes adulteration. Attention has also been directed to the excretion of antibiotics in milk from untreated quarters, after treatment of infected quarters and after their administration by parenteral injection or by insertion into the uterus. The degree to which this excretion occurs varies widely between animals and in the same animal at different points in the lactation period, and differs from one antibiotic to another. It is not possible to lay down rigid rules to avoid antibiotics appearing in milk but at least 96 hours should be allowed to elapse before milk from an infected quarter is put into the bulk supply. Milk from any cow treated systemically should be retained for 72 hours but it is not a common practice to do so. The problem is an involved one and several detailed reviews of the subject are available (38, 39).

In order to avoid the rejection of milk containing antibiotics a good deal of attention has been given to the dispensing of active agents in bases which permit rapid excretion of the antibiotic from the udder. This policy is directly opposed to the basis of antibiotic therapy which encourages retention of the drug for as long as possible.

Acid-resistant penicillins e.g. phenoxymethyl-penicillin, are probably best not used as mammary infusions because of their ability to pass through the human stomach, thus presenting a more serious potential threat to humans drinking contaminated milk.

Drying off Chronically Affected Quarters

If a quarter does not respond to treatment and is classified as incurable, the affected animal should be isolated from the milking herd or the affected quarter may be permanently dried off by producing a chemical mastitis. Methods of doing this, arranged in decreasing order of severity, are infusions of 30 to 60 ml. of 3 per cent silver nitrate solution, 20 ml. of 5 per cent copper sulphate solution, 100 to 300 ml. of 1 in 500, or 300 to 500 ml. of a 1 : 2000 acriflavine solution. If a severe local reaction occurs, the quarter should be milked out and stripped frequently until the reaction subsides. If no reaction occurs, the quarter is stripped out 10 to 14 days later. Two infusions may be necessary.

Supportive Therapy

Supportive treatment, including the parenteral injection of large quantities of isotonic fluids, particularly those containing glucose, and of antihistamine drugs, is indicated in cases where extensive tissue damage and severe toxaemia are present. The application of cold, usually in the form of crushed ice in a canvas bag suspended around the udder, may reduce absorption of toxins in such cases.

CONTROL

A discussion of the methods used in the control of all types of bovine mastitis is included at the end of this chapter.

REFERENCES

(1) Kalra, D. S. & Dhanda, M. R. (1964). *Vet. Rec.*, 76, 219.
(2) Smith, A. *et al.* (1968). *J. Dairy Res.*, 35, 287.
(3) Janzen, J. J. (1970). *J. Dairy Sci.*, 53, 1151.
(4) King, J. O. L. (1969). *Brit. vet. J.*, 125, 57, 63.
(5) Rathore, A. K. (1970). *Brit. vet. J.*, 126, xvi.
(6) Afshar, A. & Bannister, G. L. (1970). *Vet. Bull.*, 40, 681.
(7) Saeter, E. A. & Eieland, E. (1961). *Nord. Vet.-Med.*, 13, 32.
(8) Quinlivan, T. D. (1968). *N.Z. vet. J.*, 16, 149, 153.
(9) Murphy, J. M. (1945). *Proc. 49th ann. gen. Mtg U.S. live Stock sanit. Ass.*, Memphis, U.S.A., 30–43.
(10) Forbes, D. (1969). *Vet. Bull.*, 39, 529.
(11) Cullen, G. A. (1966). *Vet. Bull.*, 36, 337.
(12) Reiter, B. *et al.* (1970). *Res. vet. Sci.*, 11, 18.
(13) McDowell, G. H. & Lascelles, A. K. (1971). *Res. vet. Sci.*, 12, 258.
(14) Hoyle, J. B. & Dodd, F. H. (1970). *J. Dairy Res.*, 37, 133.
(15) Schalm, O. W. & Lasmanis, J. (1968). *J. Amer. vet. med. Ass.*, 153, 1688.
(16) Cullen, G. A. (1967). *Vet. Rec.*, 80, 649.
(17) Cullen, G. A. (1968). *Vet. Rec.*, 83, 125.
(18) Macadam, I. (1958). *J. comp. Path.*, 68, 106.
(19) Daniel, R. C. W. *et al.* (1966). *Canad. vet. J.*, 7, 80, 99.
(20) Miller, D. D. & Kearns, J. V. (1967). *J. Dairy Sci.*, 50, 683.
(21) Nageswararao, G. & Derbyshire, J. B. (1969). *J. Dairy Res.*, 36, 359.
(22) Schneider, R. & Jasper, D. E. (1964). *Amer. J. vet. Res.*, 25, 1635.
(23) Ziv, G. *et al.* (1968). *Refuah vet.*, 25, 179, 133.
(24) Nageswararao, G. & Derbyshire, J. B. (1970). *J. Dairy Res.*, 37, 77.
(25) Paape, M. J. *et al.* (1962). *Quart. Bull. Mich. St. Univ. agric. Exp. Stn*, 45, 255.
(26) Blackburn, P. S. (1965). *Brit. vet. J.*, 121, 154.
(27) Schneider, R. *et al.* (1966). *Amer. J. vet. Res.*, 27, 1169.
(28) Astermark, S. *et al.* (1969). *Acta vet. scand.*, 10, 146.
(29) Kroger, D. & Jasper, D. E. (1967). *J. Dairy Sci.*, 50, 1226.
(30) Phipps, L. W. & Newbould, F. H. S. (1966). *J. Dairy Res.*, 33, 51.
(31) Daniel, R. C. W. & Fielden, E. D. (1971). *N.Z. vet. J.*, 19, 155, 157.
(32) Pearson, J. K. L. *et al.* (1971). *Vet. Rec.*, 88, 488.
(33) Salisbury, R. M. & Williams, F. M. (1967). *N.Z. vet. J.*, 15, 206.
(34) Uvarov, O. (1971). *Vet. Rec.*, 88, 674.
(35) Wilson, C. D. (1972). *Brit. vet. J.*, 128, 71.
(36) Bates, H. J. W. (1970). *J. S. Afr. vet. med. Ass.*, 41, Suppl. 44.
(37) Schalm, O. W. *et al.* (1965). *Amer. J. vet. Res.*, 26, 851, 858.
(38) Eberhart, R. J. *et al.* (1963). *J. Amer. vet. med. Ass.*, 143, 390, 395.
(39) Siddique, I. H. *et al.* (1965). *J. Amer. vet. med. Ass.*, 146, 594.

Mastitis Caused by *Streptococcus agalactiae*

Infection of the mammary gland with *Streptococcus agalactiae* produces a specific mastitis in cattle, sheep and goats.

Incidence

The disease occurs in cattle wherever dairying is practised and usually at about the same level of incidence. In any large cattle population where the disease is not controlled in any way, most herds will be found to be infected and the average morbidity rate among the cows will be about 25 per cent. Where good hygienic measures and efficient treatments are in general use, the morbidity rate in the cattle population will be considerably below this. In fact, since the advent of antibiotic treatment, *Str. agalactiae* has been supplanted by *Staphylococcus aureus* as the major cause of bovine mastitis.

This disease is of major importance as a brake on the economic production of milk. In individual cows, the loss of production caused by *Str. agalactiae* mastitis is about 25 per cent during the infected lactation, and in affected herds the loss may be of the order of 10 to 15 per cent of the potential production. Reduction of the productive life probably represents approximately an average loss of one lactation per cow in an affected herd. Deaths rarely if ever occur due to *Str. agalactiae* infection and complete loss of productivity of a quarter is uncommon, the losses being incurred in the less dramatic but no less important fashion of decreased production per cow.

Aetiology

The disease can be reproduced by the introduction of *Str. agalactiae* into the mammary glands of cattle, goats and sheep. Goats are uniformly susceptible but only about 50 per cent of cows can be infected experimentally. Although the disease is most common under natural conditions in cattle, it occurs to a lesser extent in goats and has been recorded in pigs, and in sheep used as milking animals (1). The mortality in the latter species may be severe, approaching 10 per cent in some herds. In cattle there is no particular breed susceptibility but infection does become established more readily in older cows (2) and in the early part of each lactation.

Transmission

The main source of the infection is the udder of infected cows although, when hygiene is poor, contamination of the environment may provide a ready source of infection. The teats and skin of cattle, milkers' hands, floors, utensils and clothes are often heavily contaminated. Sores on teats are the commonest sites outside the udder for persistence of the organism. The infection may persist for up to 3 weeks on hair and skin and on inanimate materials such as dung and bricks. The importance of environmental contamination as a source of infection is given due recognition in the general disinfection technique of eradication. Transmission of infection from animal to animal occurs most commonly by the medium of milking machine liners, hands, udder cloths and possibly bedding.

Only the teat canal is important as a portal of entry, although there is doubt as to how the invasion occurs through the sphincter. Suction into the teat during milking or immediately afterwards does occur, but growth of the bacteria into the canal between milkings also appears to be an important method of entry (1). It is difficult to explain why heifers which have never been milked may be found to be infected with *Str. agalactiae* although sucking between calves after ingestion of infected milk or contact with infected inanimate materials are the probable sources of infection.

Pathogenesis

When the primary barrier of the teat sphincter is passed, either naturally or experimentally, many of the introduced bacteria are washed out by the physical act of milking. In many animals the bacteria proliferate and in some, invasion of the udder tissue follows. There is considerable variation between cows in the developments which occur at each of these three stages. The reasons for this variation are not clear but resistance appears to depend largely on the continuity of the lining of the teat cistern (2). After the introduction of infection into the teat, the invasion, if it occurs, takes from 1 to 4 days and the appearance of inflammation 3 to 5 days. Again there is much variation between cows in the response to tissue invasion, and a balance may be set up between the virulence of the organism and the undefined defence mechanisms of the host so that very little clinically detectable inflammation may develop, despite the persistence of a permanent bacterial flora.

The development of mastitis caused by *Str. agalactiae* is essentially a process of invasion and inflammation of lobules of mammary tissue in a series of crises, particularly during the first month after infection, each crisis developing in the same general pattern (3). Initially there is a rapid multiplication of the organism in the lactiferous ducts, followed by passage of the bacteria through the duct walls into lymphatic vessels and to the supramammary lymph nodes, and an outpouring of neutrophils into the milk ducts. At this stage of tissue invasion, a short-lived systemic reaction occurs and the milk yield falls sharply due to inhibition and stasis of secretion caused by damage to acinar and ductal epithelium. Fibrosis of the interalveolar tissue and involution of acini result even though the tissue invasion is quickly cleared. Subsequently, similar crises develop and more lobules are affected in the same way resulting in a step-wise loss of secretory function with increasing fibrosis of the quarter and eventual atrophy.

The clinico-pathological findings vary with the stage of development of the disease. Bacterial counts in the milk are high in the early stages but fall when the cell count rises at the same time as swelling of the quarter becomes apparent. In some cases bacteria are not detectable culturally at this acute stage. The febrile reaction is often sufficiently mild and short lived enough to escape notice. When the inflammatory changes in the epithelial lining of the acini and ducts begin to subside, the shedding of the lining results in the clinical appearance of clots in the milk. Thus the major damage has already been done when clots are first observed. At the stage of acute swelling, it is the combination of inflamed interalveolar tissue and retained secretion in distended alveoli which cause the swelling. Removal of the retained secretion at this stage may considerably reduce the swelling and permit better diffusion of drugs infused into the quarter. Inflammatory reactions also occur in the teat wall of affected quarters.

The variation in resistance between cows and the increased susceptibility with advancing age are unexplained. Hormonal changes and hypersensitivity of mammary tissue to streptococcal protein have both been advanced as possible causes of the latter. Local immunity of mammary tissue after an attack probably does not occur but there is some evidence to suggest that a low degree of general immunity may develop. At least in goats, vaccination causes a rise in serum antibodies which may provide a degree of immunity. The rapid disappearance of the infection in a small proportion of cows in contrast to the recurrent crises which are the normal pattern of development suggests that immunity does develop in some animals (4). The antibodies are hyaluronidase inhibitors and are markedly specific for specific strains of the organism. A non-specific rise in other antibodies may occur simultaneously and this is thought to account for the field observations that coincident streptococcal and staphylococcal infections are unusual and that the elimination of one infection may lead to an increased incidence of the other.

Difficulty is likely to be encountered in the application of the known facts about immunity to the artificial production of immunity in the field because of the multiplicity of strains involved and the known variability between animals in their reaction to mammary infection.

Clinical Findings

In the experimentally produced disease, there is initially a sudden attack of acute mastitis, accompanied by a transient fever, followed at intervals by similar attacks, usually of less severity. In natural cases, fever, lasting for a day or two, is occasionally observed with the initial attack, but the inflammation of the gland persists and the subsequent crises are usually of a relatively mild nature. These degrees of severity may be classified as peracute when the animal is febrile and off its feed, acute when the inflammation of the gland is severe but there is no marked systemic reaction, and chronic when the inflammation is mild. In the latter instance, the gland is not greatly swollen, pain and heat are absent, and the presence of clots in watery foremilk may be the only apparent abnormality. The induration is most readily palpable at the cistern and in the lower part of the udder and varies in degree with the stage of development of the disease.

The milk yield of affected glands is markedly reduced during each crisis but with proper treatment administered early, the yield may return to almost normal. Even without treatment the appearance of the milk soon becomes normal but the yield is significantly reduced and subsequent crises are likely to reduce it further.

Clinical Pathology

Most of the information on the clinical pathology of mastitis in general applies in this form of the disease. The number of bacteria present in the milk sample is of importance, infected glands usually yielding more than 200 colonies per ml. of milk, with smaller counts suggesting the invasion phase before the infection becomes established, or of contamination of the sample from the skin of the teat (5). It is characteristic of mastitis caused by *Str. agalactiae* that bacteria may virtually disappear from the milk during the acute phase when they invade mammary tissue, the count subsequently rising and then falling as involution and fibrosis develop. Conversely the cell counts of milk from infected quarters are highest at the acute inflammatory stage.

Large scale mastitis programmes are faced with the problem of deciding which of the available methods to use in order to determine the type of streptococci present. Agglutination tests are most accurate but are too laborious. Selective media, such as the sodium hippurate-arginine-aesculin (HAA) medium, are simple to use but the results may require confirmation. The CAMP test, which utilizes the lytic phenomenon shown by Lancefield's group B streptococci in the presence of staphylococcal beta-toxin, is sufficiently accurate for the routine presumptive identification of *Str. agalactiae* in large scale eradication schemes.

Necropsy Findings

The gross and microscopic pathology of mastitis caused by *Str. agalactiae* are not of importance in the diagnosis of the disease and are not reported here, although detailed information is available (5).

Diagnosis

The diagnosis of mastitis has already been described and the identification of this particular form of the disease depends entirely on the isolation of *Str. agalactiae* from the milk. Differentiation from other types of acute and chronic mastitis is not possible clinically.

Treatment

Procaine-penicillin G is universally used as a mammary infusion at a dose rate of 100,000 units. There seems to be no advantage in using higher dose rates especially as they have the disadvantage of increasing penicillin residues in the milk (6). A moderate increase in efficiency is obtained by using procaine penicillin rather than crystalline penicillin and a significant increase can be obtained by the use of a slow-release base, particularly mineral oil and aluminium monostearate. Using 100,000 units of penicillin in a long-acting base the cure rate (95·5 per cent) was significantly better than with quick-acting preparations (83 per cent). There is a place for both preparations (7, 8), the short-acting being best in a contaminated environment when reinfection is likely, and the long-acting when a control programme is in operation.

The duration and frequency of treatment are subject to variation. On the understanding that it is necessary to maintain adequate milk levels for 72 hours, three infusions at intervals of 24 hours are recommended but dosing with two infusions 72 hours apart, or one infusion of 100,000 units in a base containing mineral oil and aluminium monostearate (9) give similar results. As a general rule clinical cases should be treated with three infusions and subclinical cases, particularly those detected by routine examination in a control programme, with one infusion. If a combined infection with streptococci and staphylococci is encountered, four infusions of 100,000 units each, at 48-hour intervals, may be administered. Infusions of procaine penicillin give more prolonged levels in the milk than the crystalline salts but the proportion of cures effected is approximately the same for each.

Recovery, both clinically and bacteriologically, should be achieved in at least 90 per cent of quarters if treatment has been efficient. In dry cows, one infusion is sufficient, milk levels of penicillin remaining high for 72 hours. Failure of penicillin to cure *Str. agalactiae* infections is encountered occasionally. On rare occasions a penicillin resistant strain of streptococci is encountered, mixed infection with bacteria which produce penicillinase, e.g. *E. coli*, *B. subtilis*, may inactivate the penicillin, and treatments administered after the morning milking in highly productive cows may not maintain an adequate milk level of penicillin for long enough if the morning and evening milkings are close together. Failure to respond to treatment may be countered as follows. Quarters treated previously with one infusion of penicillin G should be re-treated with a two or three infusion course of penicillin. In the absence of a laboratory diagnosis of drug sensitivity, quarters which do not respond to a three infusion course of treatment with penicillin G should be treated with one of the tetracyclines or with spiramycin.

Penicillin can be administered parenterally and is effective against this form of mastitis but it is expensive as compared to intramammary infusions. An initial dose of six million units of procaine-penicillin G injected intramuscularly, followed by 12 injections of three million units at 12-hour intervals, is an efficient treatment regimen (10) but lighter doses of three daily injections of 5,000 units per lb. body weight are also claimed to be satisfactory (12). Benzathine penicillin administered parenterally has been only moderately effective when given at an initial dose level of 6 million units followed by two injections of 3 million units each at 24-hour intervals (11).

Other drugs used in the treatment of *Str. agalactiae* infections include the tetracyclines, which are as effective as penicillin and have the added advantage of a wider antibacterial spectrum, an obvious advantage when the type of infection is unknown. Neomycin (12) and Hibitane are reported to be inferior to penicillin in the treatment of *Str. agalactiae* mastitis while tylosin (13) and erythromycin (14) appear to have equal efficiency.

Treatment of mastitis in other animal species can utilize the same drugs. Ewes and does can be treated locally with infusion tubes prepared for bovine use but sows are best treated parenterally.

Control

Eradication on a herd basis of mastitis caused by *Str. agalactiae* is an accepted procedure and has been undertaken on a large scale in some countries. The control measures as outlined elsewhere in this chapter are applicable to this disease and should be adopted in detail. If suitable hygienic barriers against infection can be introduced and if the infection can be eliminated from individual quarters by treatment, the disease is eradicable fairly simply and economically (6, 9).

In general it can be anticipated that about 80 per cent of herds can be rid of infection within a year of commencing the programme. In herds where the initial incidence of infection is very high, the reinfection rate may be too rapid to permit elimination of the infection by this means, and in these circumstances the *General Disinfection Technique* (15) has given good results. The essential steps in this method are (a) treatment of all quarters of all cows in the herd with infusions of 100,000 units of penicillin after five successive evening milkings, (b) the application of penicillin cream to the hands of milkers and the teats of all cows for 14 days commencing on the first day of treatment, (c) spraying of the cows with a solution of sodium hypochlorite, and cleaning and disinfection with a phenolic disinfectant of the stable on the fifth day of treatment, and (d) the provision of sterilized udder cloths and clothing for the milkers at the last treatment.

Some other problem herds are those in which the recommendations are not strictly followed. One of the disquieting reasons for failure of the control programme is the development of 'L forms' of *Strep. agalactiae* which are not susceptible to benzathine cloxacillin (16). The extent to which this occurs and the seriousness of the breakdowns it causes in control programmes merits investigation.

As with any eradication programme a high degree of vigilance is required to maintain a 'clean' status. This is particularly so with mastitis due to *Str. agalactiae*. Breakdowns are usually due to the introduction of infected animals, even heifers which have not yet calved (17), or the employment of milkers who carry infection with them.

There are many reports of breakdowns in herds in which the disease has been eradicated. The cause is always the introduction of an infected animal and the relaxation of hygienic precautions. With increasing awareness of the need for continuous prophylaxis such breakdowns should diminish greatly.

Vaccination against *Str. agalactiae* is in the experimental stage. Some resistance to infection results after repeated vaccination with an homologous bacterin but the method is unlikely to be used in practice. Experimentally, an autogenous vaccine injected into the area of the supramammary lymph node on four occasions at weekly intervals caused a significant fall in the quarter infection rate (18).

REFERENCES

(1) Murphy, J. M. & Stuart, O. M. (1955). *Cornell Vet.*, *45*, 262.
(2) Murphy, J. M. (1959). *Cornell Vet.*, *49*, 411.
(3) Pattison, I. H. (1958). *Vet. Rec.*, *70*, 114.
(4) Howell, D. G. *et al.* (1954). *J. comp. Path.*, *64*, 335.
(5) Neave, F. K. *et al.* (1952). *J. Dairy Res.*, *19*, 14.
(6) Roberts, S. J. *et al.* (1963). *J. Amer. vet. med. Ass.*, *143*, 1193.
(7) Sanderson, C. J. (1966). *Vet. Rec.*, *79*, 328.
(8) Frost, A. J. (1966). *Aust. vet. J.*, *42*, 401.
(9) Frost, A. J. & Sanderson, C. J. (1965). *Aust. vet. J.*, *41*, 97.
(10) Murphy, J. M. & Stuart, O. M. (1954). *Cornell Vet.*, *44*, 139.
(11) Quadri, C. A. D. *et al.* (1959). *J. Amer. vet. med. Ass.*, *135*, 224.
(12) Simon, J. *et al.* (1954). *J. Amer. vet. med. Ass.*, *124*, 89.
(13) Barnes, L. E. & Hennessey, J. A. (1961). *J. Amer. vet. med. Ass.*, *139*, 548.
(14) Schultz, E. J. (1968). *J. Amer. vet. med. Ass.*, *152*, 376.
(15) Stableforth, A. W. (1950). *Vet. Rec.*, *62*, 219.
(16) Wilson, C. D. *et al.* (1971). *Brit. vet. J.*, *127*, 253.
(17) Hale, H. H. *et al.* (1961). *Cornell Vet.*, *51*, 200.
(18) Johnson, S. D. & Norcross, N. L. (1971). *Cornell Vet.*, *61*, 258.

Mastitis Caused by Miscellaneous Streptococci

Mastitis caused by these streptococci has assumed increased importance in recent years, particularly in dairy herds where infection with *Str. agalactiae* has been greatly reduced or eliminated.

Incidence

As in most forms of the disease, there is no geographical restriction of mastitis caused by these organisms. All recent work and experience points to the increasing importance of the types of mastitis under discussion. The disease resembles mastitis caused by *Str. agalactiae*, and losses resulting from it are due to loss of production rather than to fatalities. *Str. zooepidemicus*, *Str. pneumoniae* and streptococci of Lancefield's group O are rare causes of mastitis in cattle although mastitis caused by the latter two can occur as outbreaks affecting up to 50 per cent of a herd. Existing knowledge about *Str. uberis* has been extensively reviewed recently (1).

Aetiology

Str. dysgalactiae and *Str. zooepidemicus* belong to Lancefield's group C, and *Str. uberis* are unclassified. None of these bacteria are common residents of the bovine udder and, in the case of *Str. zooepidemicus* and *Str. pneumoniae*, infections in other species may act as reservoirs. The naturally occurring disease is common only in dairy cows, although sporadic cases occur in sows, and goats can be infected experimentally with *Str. dysgalactiae*. *Str. pyogenes*, apparently of human origin, has been identified as the cause in a few outbreaks of mastitis.

Transmission

Details of the epizootiology of these infections are lacking but there appears to be a definite causal relationship between infection and teat injuries caused by milking technique and improper housing (2). *Str. uberis* has been shown to be a common inhabitant of the skin, lips and tonsils of cows in infected herds. Contrary to expectations teat skin appears to be refractory to colonization. However, infection of the milk appears to be secondary to infection of the skin and both occur more commonly in the cooler part of the year (3). *Str. pneumoniae* infection may originate from respiratory tract infections in human attendants.

Pathogenesis

Infections with *Str. dysgalactiae*, artificially induced in goats, are indistinguishable from mastitis caused by *Str. agalactiae* and the pathogenesis is probably similar in all streptococcal mastitides.

Clinical Findings

In bovine mastitis caused by *Str. dysgalactiae*, *Str. uberis* and streptococci of Lancefield's group O the syndrome is usually acute, with severe swelling of the quarter and abnormality of the milk, and occasional cases show a moderate systemic reaction. Mastitis caused by *Str. zooepidemicus* is usually subacute or chronic, and that caused by *Str. pneumoniae* is peracute with a high fever in most cases but can cause chronic disease (7).

Diagnosis

There are no significant differences between the clinico-pathological and necropsy findings in mastitis caused by these streptococci and those in mastitis caused by *Str. agalactiae*. Diagnosis depends on cultural examination of the milk.

Treatment

Mastitis caused by *Str. dysgalactiae* and *Str. uberis* responds well to penicillin, erythromycin or tetracyclines but reinfection may occur quickly if the contributory causes are not corrected. Infections with *Str. zooepidemicus* do not respond well to treatment with penicillin. Mastitis caused by *Str. pneumoniae* responds well to local treatment with penicillin in large doses (300,000 units per infusion) but complete loss of function results in quarters allowed to go without treatment for any length of time. All cases of mastitis caused by this organism should receive parenteral treatment with penicillin (4).

Control

The general control measures are recommended, with particular attention to milking technique, housing and avoidance of injury to teats. Infected quarters should be treated vigorously. However, once the infection has become established in a herd, sporadic cases are likely to occur in spite of good hygenic precautions. Vaccination by the intraperitoneal injection of killed cultures of *Str. dysgalactiae* gives good protection in goats against subsequent experimental exposure (5), but the vaccine has not been subjected to field trials. Vaccination of cows with a killed *Str. dysgalactiae* vaccine in the area of the supramammary lymph node appears to provide some protection (6).

REFERENCES

(1) Cullen, G. A. (1969). *Vet. Bull., 39*, 155.
(2) Hughes, D. L. (1954). *Vet. Rec., 66*, 235.
(3) Cullen, G. A. & Little, T. W. A. (1969). *Vet. Rec., 85*, 115.
(4) Smith, H. W. & Stables, J. W. (1958). *Vet. Rec., 70*, 986.
(5) Smith, I. M. *et al.* (1954). *J. comp. Path., 64*, 206.
(6) Stark, D. M. & Norcross, N. L. (1970). *Cornell Vet., 60*, 604.
(7) Romer, O. (1962). *Pneumococcus Infections of Animals*. Copenhagen: Mortensen.

Mastitis Caused by *Staphylococcus aureus*

Mastitis caused by *Staph. aureus* occurs in cattle, sheep and pigs, and in the former appears to be increasing in importance.

Incidence

Staphylococcal mastitis in cattle assumes equal importance with mastitis caused by *Str. agalactiae* or other miscellaneous streptococci in most surveys of the disease. As in other forms of mastitis, loss of production is the major cause of economic loss, but in some herds there may be fairly heavy death losses. Response to treatment is comparatively poor and satisfactory methods for the eradication of staphylococcal mastitis from infected herds have yet to be devised. The presence of *Staph. aureus* in market milk may be considered to present a degree of risk to the consumer.

In sheep the disease can be a serious problem because the morbidity rate may be as high as 20 per cent; the mortality rate varies between 25 and 50 per cent and affected quarters in surviving ewes are usually destroyed. The disease can be a very important one in those countries in which ewes' milk is a staple article of diet (1). Sporadic cases occur in sows.

Aetiology

Haemolytic, coagulase-positive *Staph. aureus* is the usual cause although it may be difficult to demonstrate the presence of the organism in peracute cases especially when necrotic tissue is invaded by *E. coli* and *Clostridium* spp. The beta-toxin, or a combination of alpha- and beta-toxins, are produced by most pathogenic strains isolated from cattle. Staphylococcal antibodies are found in the blood of infected cows but they appear to afford little protection against mastitis due to these bacteria. This may be due to the low titre of the antibodies in the milk. Antibody titres in the serum rise with age and after an attack of mastitis. Experimental mastitis caused by *Staph. aureus* causes a significant reduction in milk yield and rate of milking (2).

Non-haemolytic coagulase-negative staphylococci have in general been disregarded as mammary pathogens, but because of the intense investigation of staphylococcal mastitis they have come under closer scrutiny. It does appear that although these bacteria are capable of causing microscopic lesions, and in some cases increased leucocyte counts in the milk, they are not nearly as pathogenic as haemolytic staphylococci (4). The tissue reaction is usually so mild that the California Mastitis Test is negative. If the infection is capable of causing loss of productivity, current standards for the diagnosis of mastitis will need to be reassessed. They appear to have the advantage that they resist colonization of the teat duct and teat skin by coagulate positive staphylococci (4).

Transmission

All the evidence suggests that in cattle this form of mastitis is infectious, the main source of the infection being the quarter infected with the organism, and the method of spread being by infected hands and teat cups. Although staphylococci can multiply on the surface of the skin and provide a source of infection for the udder, the cutaneous lesions are usually infected originally from the udder (6). There is some controversy over the age susceptibility to this type of mastitis in cattle but there does not seem to be an increase in susceptibility with advancing age as there is in *Str. agalactiae* mastitis, the disease tending to reach a peak in the younger age groups (7). In sows the infection appears to gain entrance most commonly through cutaneous wounds.

Pathogenesis

Although the disease can be reproduced experimentally by the injection of *Staph. aureus* organisms into the udder of cattle and sheep, there is considerable variation in the type of mastitis produced. This does not seem to be due to differences in virulence of the strains used, although strain variations do occur (8), but it may be related to the size of the inoculum used or more probably the lactational status of the udder at the time of infection. Infection during early lactation often results in the appearance of the peracute form, with gangrene of the udder due to the acute necrotizing action of the alpha toxin (9). During the later stages of lactation or during the dry period, new infections are not usually accompanied by a systemic reaction but result in the chronic or acute forms.

The pathogenesis of acute and chronic staphylococcal mastitis in the cow is the same, the variation occurring only in degree of involvement of mammary tissue. In the chronic form there are less foci of inflammation and the reaction is milder. In both forms each focus commences with an acute stage characterized by proliferation of the bacteria in the collecting ducts and, to a lesser extent, in the alveoli. In acute mastitis the small ducts are quickly blocked by fibrin clots leading to more severe involvement of the obstructed area. In chronic mastitis the inflammation is restricted to the epithelium of the ducts. The inflammation subsides within a few days and is replaced by connective tissue proliferations around the ducts, leading to their blockage and atrophy of the drained area (9).

In the experimentally produced disease in goats the pathogenesis is very similar except that there is a marked tendency for the staphylococci to invade and persist in foci in the interacinar tissue (10). In some cases abscesses develop and botryomycosis of the udder, in which granulomata develop containing Gram positive cocci in an amorphous eosinophilic mass, is also seen. In the gangrenous form the death of tissue is precipitated by thrombosis of veins causing local oedema and congestion of the udder. Staphylococci are the only bacteria which commonly cause this reaction in the udder of the cow and the resulting toxaemia is due to bacterial toxins and tissue destruction. Staphylo-

coccal gangrenous mastitis in ewes is identical to that in cattle.

Clinical Findings

In cows the peracute form is more dramatic, but the most important losses are caused by the chronic form. Although 50 per cent of cattle in a herd may be affected by the latter, only a few may show sufficient signs to be recognized by the average dairyman. Many cases are characterized by a slowly developing induration and atrophy with the occasional appearance of clots in the milk or wateriness of the first streams. The cell count of the milk is increased but, unless strip cup or indirect tests and palpation of the udder are carried out regularly, the disease may go unnoticed until much of the functional capacity of the gland is lost. The infection can persist and the disease progress slowly over a period of many months.

Acute staphylococcal mastitis occurs most commonly in early lactation. There is severe swelling of the gland and the milk is purulent or contains many thick clots. Extensive fibrosis and severe loss of function always result.

The peracute form occurs usually in the first few days after calving and is highly fatal. There is a severe systemic reaction with elevation of the temperature to 41 to 42 °C (106 to 107 °F), rapid heart rate (100 to 120 per minute), complete anorexia, profound depression, absence of ruminal movements, and muscular weakness, often to the point of recumbency. The onset of the systemic and local reactions is sudden. The cow may be normal at one milking and recumbent and comatose at the next. The affected quarter is grossly swollen, hard and sore to touch, and causes severe lameness on the affected side. Gangrene is a constant development and may be evident very early. A bluish discolouration may develop and this may eventually spread to involve the floor of the udder and the whole or part of the teat, but may be restricted to patches on the sides and floor of the udder. Within 24 hours the gangrenous areas become black and ooze serum and may be accompanied by subcutaneous emphysema and the formation of blisters. The secretion is reduced to a small amount of blood-stained serous fluid without odour, clots or flakes. Unaffected quarters in the same cow are often swollen, and there may be extensive subcutaneous oedema in front of the udder caused by thrombosis of the mammary veins. Toxaemia is profound and death usually occurs if early, appropriate treatment is not provided. Even with early treatment the quarter is invariably lost and the gangrenous areas slough. Separation begins after 6 or 7 days, but without interference the gangrenous part may remain attached for weeks. After separation, pus drains from the site for many more weeks before healing finally occurs.

Staphylococcal mastitis in ewes is clinically identical with the peracute form in cattle and the oedema and gangrene often spread along the belly as far as the front legs. The disease in sows is always chronic and is characterized by the presence of large, fibrous nodules in the gland and the discharge through sinuses of thin pus, containing granules.

Clinical Pathology

The laboratory diagnosis of staphylococcal mastitis has been made much easier by the observation that pathogenic staphylococci grown on sheep or cow blood-agar plates produce alpha-, beta- or alpha-beta-haemolysis. Such bacteria are always coagulase positive and produce alpha and beta toxins of high potency. Bacterial counts of more than 200 per ml. are commonly used as a criterion for a positive diagnosis of infection and leucocyte counts of more than 500,000 per ml. of milk are usually considered to indicate the presence of inflammation. The California Mastitis Test, although not specific to any causative agent, is of great value in attracting attention to a chronically infected quarter which may show no clinical abnormality.

Necropsy Findings

Necropsy examinations are not often carried out on mastitis cases except where an animal dies of acute toxaemia. Histologically there are marked differences between streptococcal and staphylococcal mastitis. In the latter the bacteria persist in the interacinar tissue and set up foci of chronic inflammation which may be visible macroscopically and are referred to as botryomycosis of the udder. In mastitis caused by *Str. agalactiae*, the invasion of mammary tissue is transitory. In peracute staphylococcal mastitis, the affected quarter is grossly swollen, may contain blood-stained milk in the upper part of the udder but only serosanguineous fluid in the ventral part. There is extreme vascular engorgement and swelling, and haemorrhage of the mammary lymph nodes. Bacteria are not isolated from the blood stream or tissues other than the mammary tissue or regional lymph nodes. Histologically there is severe coagulation necrosis and thrombosis of veins.

Diagnosis

Because of the occurrence of the peracute form in the first few days after parturition, the intense depression and inability to rise, the owner may conclude that the cow or ewe has parturient paresis. The heart rate is much faster than in parturient paresis and a cursory examination of the udder will indicate the true source of the trouble. Other bacterial types of mastitis, particularly *E. coli* and *Cor. pyogenes*, may cause severe systemic reactions but gangrene of the quarter does not occur. The chronic and acute forms are indistinguishable clinically from many other bacterial types of mastitis and bacteriological examination is necessary for identification.

In sheep there is a strong similarity between this form of mastitis and that caused by *Pasturella haemolytica*. They are both peracute, gangrenous infections. In sows the disease is chronic and has to be differentiated from the granulomatous lesions of the ventral abdominal wall caused by *Actinomyces* spp.

Treatment

Although most staphylococci isolated from quarters affected with mastitis are sensitive to penicillin and tetracyclines *in vitro*, the results of treatment with these drugs in infected quarters are often disappointing. The poor results are probably due to the inaccessibility of the bacteria in the interacinar tissue or obstructed ducts and alveoli. Resistant strains of staphylococci appear to be increasing but their incidence varies widely. In the U.K. 70 per cent were resistant (11) and in Australia 100 per cent of strains in some herds were resistant (12).

Because of the increasing incidence of staphylococcal mastitis, and the high proportion of bacteria which are resistant to penicillin and streptomycin, a great deal of work has been directed to finding a satisfactory programme of treatment for chronic and acute cases. Novobiocin (250 mg. per infusion for 3 infusions) or sodium cloxacillin (0·2 to 0·6 g. in a slow-release base per infusion for three infusions at 48-hour intervals) appear to be most effective and in early cases can be expected to achieve cure rates of 60 to 80 per cent (13).

The following treatment programmes, all of 3 infusions at 24-hour intervals, appear to be about 60 to 80 per cent effective in lactating cows:

Tetracyclines (400 mg.), penicillin-streptomycin combination (100,000 units—250 mg.), penicillin-nitrofurazone combination (100,000 units —150 mg.), penicillin-tylosin combination (100,000 units—240 mg.), furaltodone (500 mg.), erythromycin (300 to 600 mg.), spiramycin (250 mg.).

Because of the increasing availability of laboratory

services the final choice of the antibiotic to be used can often be decided on a drug sensitivity test. One of the major problems in mastitis control is the variation in response to treatment or control between herds. Preliminary examination of the problem with respect to *Staph. aureus* shows that this infection is less likely to respond when it occurs in an older cow, when the cow has several infected quarters, in cows treated in early lactation and so on (13).

It has become a common practice to leave chronic cases until they are dried off before attempting to eliminate the infection. Milk need not be discarded and results are always better in non-lactating quarters. All of the above preparations can be used provided they are used with slow release bases and can be expected to achieve about 80 per cent of cures. The material is infused either early or late in the dry period and left in situ. The treatment of chronic cases by parenteral injection is unlikely to achieve popularity but has been used in valuable animals that do not respond to intramammary infusion.

Early parenteral treatment of peracute cases with adequate doses of sulphonamides or penicillin will save the lives of most animals. When penicillin is used the initial intramuscular injection should be supported by an intravenous injection of crystalline penicillin, and subsequent intramuscular injections should aim at maintaining a blood level of the drug over a four- to six-day period. Intramammary infusions or intraparenchymal injections appear to be of little value in such cases because of failure of the drugs to diffuse into the gland. Transient improvement may follow the injection of large doses of antihistamine drugs and their administration may help to combat the effects of toxaemia. The administration of large quantities of electrolyte solutions is also recommended. Frequent massage and stripping exert a beneficial effect by aiding drainage of the quarter; the administration of Pitressin exerts little effect. Total amputation of the quarter or ligation of the mammary vessels (14) is often indicated but the animal may be a poor surgical risk because of toxaemia. Amputation of the teat is frequently practised to encourage drainage but multiple incision of the gland has little beneficial effect.

Control

Because of the relatively poor results obtained in the treatment of staphylococcal mastitis, any attempt at control must depend heavily on effective methods of preventing the transmission of infection from cow to cow. Hygiene in the milking shed attains great importance, especially as the organism is capable of such persistence in the environment, and a great deal of attention is being devoted to possible production of a suitable method of vaccination. Eradication is not possible and only control programmes aimed at restraining the infection rate should be instituted.

Until recent years satisfactory control of staphylococcal mastitis was impossible. Nowadays the quarter infection rate can be rapidly and cheaply reduced from the average level of 30 per cent to 10 per cent or less. The measures set down under Control of Bovine Mastitis (p. 284) must be intensively applied (15) and the disinfection of hands or use of rubber gloves provides additional advantages. The programme helps to eliminate infected quarters and reduces the new infection rate by 50 to 65 per cent compared to controls.

The inconclusive nature of the results of experimental work on vaccines against staphylococcal mastitis (16) is not reflected by the claims of manufacturers of commercial vaccines nor by the very large quantities of their products used in dairy cows. A number of major principles have been defined which must be considered when the preparation of a vaccine is under consideration. (*a*) Antibodies and antitoxins present in the serum of vaccinated cows do not appear in the milk, other than in the colostrum or during drying off, unless the mammary epithelium is damaged. Thus any parenteral vaccine is unlikely to be completely effective, although it could reduce the severity of an attack—a common finding in field practice. This difficulty has aroused interest in the possibility of intramammary vaccines (17) but the frequence of local reactions and the short duration of immunity make the method impracticable at the present time. Because of the relative importance of the inguinal and supramammary lymph nodes in the production of staphylococcal antibodies, it has been suggested that subcutaneous vaccination in the area draining them may be advantageous (18). In ewes the use of intramammary vaccine during the dry period gives good protection against infection in the subsequent lactation (19). On the other hand the infusion of immune serum into the udder with staphylococci does not prevent nor lessen the severity of the experimentally produced mastitis (20). (*b*) Some cross-immunity between strains of staphylococci does occur but this is not sufficiently extensive to permit the use of a single strain in a commercial vaccine. As a result autogenous vaccines are preferred but their use is limited by obvious practical difficulties. (*c*) The antibody required to prevent damage to mammary tissue by staphylococci varies between strains, so that most vaccines now contain killed cells and detoxicated toxin (bacterin-toxoids) and these preparations appear to be more effective, especially if they contain a safe adjuvant. (d) Superiority has been claimed for vaccines prepared from disrupted bacteria over whole-cell, killed bacterins but there appears to be little difference between the methods (21). (e) Large repeated doses of even the most efficient vaccines are necessary initially to achieve effective levels of antibodies and revaccination every 3 to 6 months is necessary to maintain them. (f) No vaccination programme can hope to succeed unless other control measures of sanitation and proper milking management are instituted.

The disease in ewes is probably spread from infected bedding grounds, the infection gaining entry through teat injuries caused by sucking lambs. It is possible that vaccination could be an effective method of control. A bacterin-toxoid has proved moderately effective in reducing the incidence of the disease. Two injections of the vaccine were necessary (22). The frequent changing of pasture areas and culling of affected ewes should also help to control the spread of infection.

REFERENCES

(1) Butozan, V. & Mihajlovic, S. (1963). *Bull. Off. int. Epizoot.*, *60*, 1041.
(2) Prasad, L. B. M. & Newbould, F. H. S. (1968). *Canad. vet. J.*, *9*, 170.
(3) Stabenfeldt, G. H. & Spencer, G. R. (1966). *Path. vet.*, *3*, 27.
(4) Edwards, S. J. & Jones, G. W. (1966). *J. Dairy Res.*, *33*, 261, 271.
(5) Davidson, I. (1961). *Res. vet. Sci.*, *2*, 22.
(6) Stableforth, A. W. (1953). *Vet. Rec.*, *65*, 709.
(7) Edwards, S. J. (1958). *Vet. Rec.*, *70*, 139.
(8) Schalm, O. W. (1944). *Vet. Med.*, *39*, 279.
(9) Stabenfeldt, G. H. & Spencer, G. R. (1965). *Path. vet.*, *2*, 585.
(10) Derbyshire, J. B. (1958). *J. comp. Path.*, *68*, 449.
(11) Sanderson, C. J. (1965). *Aust. vet. J.*, *42*, 47.
(12) Frost, A. J. (1962). *Aust. vet. J.*, *38*, 110.
(13) Wilson, C. D. *et al.* (1972). *Brit. vet. J.*, *128*, 71.
(14) Brewer, R. L. (1963). *J. Amer. vet. med. Ass.*, *143*, 44.
(15) Newbould, F. H. S. (1968). *J. Amer. vet. med. Ass.*, *153*, 1683.
(16) Oehme, F. W. & Coles, E. H. (1967). *J. Dairy Sci.*, *50*, 1792.
(17) Derbyshire, J. B. & Smith, G. S. (1969). *Res. vet. Sci.*, *10*, 559.
(18) Willoughby, R. A. (1966). *Amer. J. vet. Res.*, *27*, 522.
(19) Outteridge, P. L. *et al.* (1968). *Res. vet. Sci.*, *9*, 416.
(20) Skeen, J. D. & Overcast, W. W. (1969). *J. Dairy Sci.*, *52*, 47.
(21) Slanetz, L. W. *et al.* (1965). *Amer. J. vet. Res.*, *26*, 688.
(22) Contini, A. (1968). *Vet. ital.*, *19*, 62.

Mastitis Caused by *Corynebacterium pyogenes*

Sporadic cases of mastitis caused by *Cor. pyogenes* occur but its major importance is in relation to endemic 'summer mastitis' of cattle.

Incidence

In many countries bovine mastitis caused by *Cor. pyogenes* occurs only sporadically and is most common in dry cows or pregnant heifers, although lactating cows may also be affected. In the United Kingdom there is a much higher incidence of suppurative 'summer mastitis' during the summer months when dry cows are left at pasture and not kept under close observation. The incidence is much higher in wet summers and on heavily wooded and low lying farms when the fly population is high (1). The disease is a serious one in that the mortality rate without adequate treatment is probably about 50 per cent and the affected quarters of surviving cows are always totally destroyed.

Aetiology

Cor. pyogenes is a common cause of suppurative lesions in cattle and other species and can often be isolated from normal animals. It is probable that devitalization of tissues is necessary for infection to occur. *Cor. pyogenes* can cause sporadic cases of suppurative mastitis but the specific cause of 'summer mastitis' is not necessarily this bacterium alone. Streptococci and staphylococci, and other unspecified cocci, are commonly present and may play some part in the development of the disease (2). *Cor. bovis* is a common inhabitant of the bovine udder and is usually considered to be non-pathogenic but has been suggested as a cause of mastitis in some herds (3). *Cor. ulcerans* is an uncommon cause of a subacute mastitis (8).

Transmission

The method of spread is uncertain in sporadic cases but flies appear to play an important role in outbreaks of 'summer mastitis' (1). *Cor. pyogenes* has been identified in the viscera of flies collected from the teats of cows in areas where the disease is endemic (4).

Pathogenesis

It is suggested that massive invasion of the mammary tissue occurs and that the greater part of the gland is affected at the first attack causing a severe systemic reaction and loss of function of the entire quarter. The disease has been produced experimentally in goats with udder lesions being typical of acute suppurative mastitis (5). Non-lactating goats developed a severe mastitis, lactating animals only a moderate one. It has also been produced experimentally, a diffuse suppurative mastitis, in sheep (6).

Clinical Findings

Corynebacterial mastitis is always peracute with a severe systemic reaction, including fever (40 to 41 °C or 105 to 106 °F), rapid heart rate, complete anorexia, severe depression and weakness. Abortion may occur during this stage. The quarter is very hard, swollen and sore and the secretion is watery and later purulent, with a typical, putrid odour. If the cow survives the severe toxaemia, the quarter becomes extremely indurated and abscesses develop, later rupturing through the floor of the udder, commonly at the base of the teat. True gangrene, such as occurs in staphylococcal mastitis, rarely if ever occurs in uncomplicated infections with *Cor. pyogenes* but quarters may be so severely affected that sloughing occurs. The function of the quarter is permanently lost and cows which have calved recently may go completely dry. Severe thelitis with obstruction of the teat is a common sequel. Partial or complete obstruction of the teat and damage to the teat cistern can also occur independently of an acute attack of mastitis (7).

Clinical Pathology

Isolation of the organism and determination of its sensitivity to antibacterial drugs is the only special examination required.

Necropsy Findings

Details of the pathology of the disease are not available.

Diagnosis

The seasonal incidence of the disease in some areas, the acute inflammation of the quarter, the suppurative nature and putrid odour of the milk, the development of abscesses and the severe systemic reaction make this form of mastitis one of the easiest to diagnose clinically in cattle.

Treatment

Although the organism is usually susceptible to penicillin in vitro, response to treatment with this drug is poor. In peracute cases parenteral treatment with sodium sulphadimidine or one of the tetracyclines is preferable and should be accompanied by repeated stripping of the quarter. Broad spectrum antibiotics are usually given by intramammary infusion but the quarter is almost always rendered functionless. Treatment with *Cor. pyogenes* antiserum in the acute stages and toxoid in the later, chronic, suppurative stage has been used but with little effect.

The use of parenteral or local enzyme preparations is of some value especially in the later stages. Crystalline trypsin (1 g.) incorporated in an infusion containing 500,000 units of penicillin and 0·5 g. streptomycin in 50 ml. physiological saline has been found to be an efficient treatment in dry cows when administered daily for 5 to 7 days (9). In lactating cows multiple treatments (3 to 14) with intramammary infusions containing oxytetracycline, penicillin or chloramphenicol and either a combination of 25 units fibrolysin and 15,000 units desoxyribonuclease or a streptokinase-streptodornase-plasminogen preparation or crystalline trypsin gives much better results than antibiotics alone (10). Even with this intensive therapy at least 50 per cent of quarters are rendered useless and many of those which respond are greatly reduced in productivity.

Control

The question of control of this form of mastitis centres largely around 'summer mastitis'. Many prophylactic measures, including infusion of the quarter when the cow is dried off, sealing the teat ends with collodion and vaccination with toxoid, have been tried but with inconclusive results. Two infusions of procaine penicillin (30,000 units) in mineral oil 3 weeks apart during the dry period are commonly practised in Great Britain and appear to be effective (1). Careful, daily examination of dry cows during the summer may enable affected quarters to be identified and treated at an early stage and thus limit the spread of infection. The spraying of the udder and coat of dry cows at pasture with various contact insecticides has afforded a good degree of protection (11).

REFERENCES

(1) Derbyshire, J. B. (1962). *Vet. Bull.*, *32*, 1.
(2) Stuart, P. *et al.* (1951). *Vet. Rec.*, *63*, 451.
(3) Duckitt, S. M. & Woodbine, M. (1963). *Vet. Bull.*, *33*, 67.
(4) Bahr, L. (1953). *Proc. 15th int. vet. Congr.*, *2*, 849.
(5) Jain, N. C. & Sharma, G. L. (1964). *Indian vet. J.*, *41*, 379, 516; *42*, 231.
(6) El Etreby, M. F. & Abdel-Hamid, Y. M. (1970). *Path. vet.*, *7*, 246.
(7) Renk, W. (1961). *Zbl. vet. Med.*, *8*, 1141.
(8) Higgs, T. M. *et al.* (1967). *Vet. Rec.*, *81*, 34.
(9) Forscher, E. (1956). *Dtsch. tierärztl. Wschr.*, *63*, 377.
(10) Heidrich, H. J. & Fiebiger, E. (1965). *Berl. Munch. tierärztl. Wschr.*, *78*, 324, 341, 389, 401.
(11) Aehnelt, E. (1956). *Dtsch. tierärztl. Wschr.*, *62*, 493.

Mastitis Caused by Coliform Bacteria

Coliform bacteria are a relatively uncommon cause of mastitis in cattle but are frequently incriminated in mastitis in sows.

Incidence

While coliform mastitis is rare in cattle as a clinical syndrome, bacteriological surveys of cattle often show a surprisingly high incidence of infection unassociated with clinical signs (1). The disease is more common in cattle that are housed during the winter than in animals which remain at pasture. Of the three clinical forms the peracute is most common and the major loss caused is by the death of animals (up to 20 per cent) or the complete loss of function of affected quarters.

In pigs the disease appears to be more common when sows are fed heavily and farrow with excessive udder engorgement, and when farrowing pens are used without adequate disinfection between farrowings (4). Losses may be heavy in pigs, not only because of deaths of sows but also because of the heavy mortality in sucking pigs.

Aetiology

E. coli (non-haemolytic, haemolytic and mucoid types), Aero. aerogenes and intermediate types are the common causative agents in cattle (10) and sows. Paracolon bacteria have also been isolated (2). The strains isolated from the milk in cases of bovine mastitis possess a distinct capsule which is not apparent in non-pathogenic strains (3). A high proportion of cases occur in cows soon after calving—within 2 to 3 days—and many of those which occur at other times are related to severe teat injuries (10). Repeated experimental exposure of quarters to infection with Aero. aerogenes fails to produce any detectable antibodies.

Transmission

Coliform mastitis has usually been considered as an accidental infection of the udder by a common environmental contaminant. Failure to wash the udder before milking, the use of contaminated teat siphons and mastitis tubes, and constant soiling of the udder in dirty bedding or muddy yards, are considered to be some of the important causative factors. When only occasional animals become infected, this chance invasion of quarters is probably the important method of spread but other factors may have to be considered when, as sometimes happens, a high incidence (up to 25 per cent) of coliform infections associated with chronic and acute attacks of clinical mastitis is found in individual herds. The higher relative susceptibility of older cows appears to be related to the increased patency of the streak canal which occurs with age. Because of the difficulty encountered in producing the disease experimentally in quarters with high leucocyte counts, it has been suggested that efficient mastitis control, by encouraging the production of milk containing few leucocytes, may provide favourable conditions for the development of coliform mastitis (11).

Pathogenesis

E. coli is a potent toxin producer and the extracted endotoxin has been shown experimentally to produce a marked increase in serum albumin and leucocytes in the milk (12), acute swelling, fever of 41–42 °C (106–107 °F), serous fluid with flakes or clots in lieu of milk, rapid pulse rate, depression, shivering and recumbency (13). All clinical signs disappeared at 48 to 96 hours. Some pre-existing infections in the quarters, resistant to chemotherapeutic agents, were cured by the infusion. A marked change in vascular permeability was the most apparent lesion. It is probable that the variability in the severity of clinical cases is due to variations in degree of tissue invasion and toxin production of different strains of the organism or to variations in the susceptibility of udder tissue. Septicaemia occurs also in cattle and pigs but the absorption of endotoxins is probably the more important factor and may be the cause of the transient attacks of severe diarrhoea which occur in some cases.

Clinical Findings

Peracute, acute and chronic forms occur. The peracute form is most common in cattle and is the only form in sows. The onset is sudden and the systemic reaction severe; the temperature is high (40 to 41 °C or 105 to 106 °F) and the pulse rate fast (100 to 120 per minute), there is complete anorexia, ruminal stasis, severe depression and weakness causing either muscle trembling or recumbency. In advanced cases the cow is comatose. At this stage, which may occur very quickly, the temperature is often subnormal and there may be a superficial resemblance to parturient paresis. The secretion is thin, yellow and serous in consistency and contains small, meal-like flakes. There may be some enlargement of the quarter but this is often deceptively small. Without proper treatment affected cows may die, and even with treatment the quarter often loses its function. Unless treatment is vigorous and begun early, the cow may go dry for the lactation. Additional quarters may become affected within a day or two of the first attack and a transient attack of severe diarrhoea is not uncommon. In the acute form there is mild inflammation and clots appear in the milk but there is no systemic reaction and the chronic form is still less severe and recurs intermittently.

In sows the disease resembles the peracute form in cows except that there is considerable swelling, hardness, discolouration and pain in the affected gland. The pain may be so severe that the sow lies on her belly to prevent the piglets from sucking, and marked lameness may be observed (5). Very little milk can be expressed and it is usually discoloured and stringy. The systemic reaction is severe and the sow may be unable to get up. With *E. coli* infections there may be an accompanying metritis, with the bacteria present in the vaginal discharge. Outbreaks of enteritis in the piglets may also occur but death losses in piglets are more frequently due to starvation. Severe mammary induration may occur in sows and interfere with their future usefulness as breeding animals (5).

Clinical Pathology

Isolation of the organism and determination of its sensitivity is most necessary in coliform mastitis because of the common occurrence of resistance to particular antibiotics by bacteria in this group.

Necropsy Findings

In all species there is oedema and hyperaemia of the mammary tissue. Haemorrhages are present and are accompanied by thrombus formation in the blood and lymphatic vessels and there is necrosis of the parenchyma (9).

Diagnosis

In cows the severe systemic reaction, the characteristic appearance of the milk and the moderate swelling of the gland may suggest a diagnosis in some cases but a definite diagnosis can only be made on cultural examination. In many cases in cattle, especially soon after calving, there is no fever, the cow is recumbent and dull, and in many instances the disease can be mistaken for parturient paresis. The rapid heart rate should arouse suspicion of a toxaemia rather than a hypocalcaemia. Peracute mastitis in sows is usually due to coliform bacteria.

Treatment

Bovine mastitis caused by infections with *E. coli* and *Aero. aerogenes* can be satisfactorily treated by infusion with streptomycin (500 mg. once or twice daily for 3 days), oxytetracycline (400 mg. once daily for 3 days), but neomycin has not been found to be highly effective (6, 7, 8). Cases showing systemic involvement require parenteral treatment either with streptomycin (10 g. daily intramuscularly in 2 divided doses) or one of the tetracyclines (2 mg. per lb. body weight daily for 3 days). Because of their efficiency in the treatment of other coliform infections, nitrofurazone and chloramphenicol are also recommended in the treatment of this form of mastitis. Prophylactic infusions in the other quarters are worth while because of their common secondary involvement. Paracolon infections often do not respond to these standard treatments. Supportive treatment should include the parenteral administration of large volumes of isotonic fluids and standard doses of antihistamines. Treatment of the disease in sows is along the same general lines as that used in cattle.

Control

Because of the paucity of information on the epizootiology of the infection and because of the failure of standard hygienic precautions to prevent spread in a herd, a control programme is difficult to outline. Scrupulous cleanliness at milking, the provision of adequate bedding and avoidance of soiling of the udder in muddy barnyards suggest themselves as logical control measures. In affected swine herds, proper disinfection of farrowing pens is recommended and some advantage may be gained by reducing the diet of sows during the last two weeks of pregnancy to avoid over-distension of the udder.

Vaccination of sows before farrowing with an autogenous bacterin or a polyvalent *E. coli* antiserum (4) may reduce losses in herds where the disease is enzootic. Similar preparations have been used in cattle but are not generally recommended.

REFERENCES

(1) Murphy, J. M. & Hanson, J. J. (1943). *Cornell Vet.*, *33*, 61.
(2) Johnson, S. D. *et al.* (1951). *Cornell Vet.*, *41*, 283.
(3) Plastridge, W. N. (1958). *J. Dairy Sci.*, *41*, 1141.
(4) Sumner, G. R. (1957). *Vet. Rec.*, *69*, 131.
(5) Smith, H. C. (1965). *J. Amer. vet. med. Ass.*, *147*, 626.
(6) Tucker, E. W. & Johnson, S. D. (1953). *J. Amer. vet. med. Ass.*, *123*, 332.
(7) Schalm, O. W. & Woods, G. M. (1952). *J. Amer. vet. med. Ass.*, *120*, 385.
(8) Barnes, L. E. (1955). *Amer. J. vet. Res.*, *16*, 386.
(9) Renk, W. (1962). *Zbl. Vet.-Med.*, *9*, 264.
(10) Radostits, O. M. (1961). *Canad. vet. J.*, *2*, 401.
(11) Schalm, O. W. & Lasmanis, J. (1964). *Amer. J. vet. Res.*, *25*, 75, 83 & 90.
(12) Carroll, E. J. *et al.* (1964). *Amer. J. vet. Res.*, *25*, 720.
(13) Schalm, O. W. & Ziv-Silberman, G. (1968). *Vet. Rec.*, *82*, 100.

Mastitis Caused by *Klebsiella* Spp.

Klebsiella mastitis occurs rarely in cattle but it may appear in peracute, acute or chronic forms.

Incidence

Klebsiella mastitis has been recorded in isolated herds in the United Kingdom and in North

America. Losses are due to occasional deaths and to severe loss of production. In some instances a fatal pneumonia and septicaemia occur in calves fed infected milk or in contact with infected cows. The disease may occur sporadically or affect a large proportion of a herd (1, 5).

Aetiology

Klebsiella pneumoniae is the common causative agent.

Transmission

The method of spread has not been studied in detail but when spread occurs, it probably does so by means of contaminated milking equipment.

Clinical Findings

Peracute, acute and chronic forms occur. In the peracute form there is a severe systemic reaction including high fever (40 to 41 °C or 105 to 106 °F), severe weakness, depression and anorexia accompanied by a sudden, severe swelling of the quarter. The secretion is reduced to small amounts of serous fluid containing a few flakes of pus. A concurrent infection of the respiratory tract may occur and is manifested by dyspnoea, cough, nasal discharge and lacrimation. Swelling and pain in the joints, particularly the hind legs, may also occur (2). In the acute form there is severe swelling of the udder, yellow-brown secretion with clots and, in spite of treatment, the cow often goes dry (3). The chronic form is characterized by the gradual development of mild fibrosis and the presence of clots in the foremilk (4).

An acute form has been described in sows, accompanied by septicaemia and a high mortality (6).

Clinical Pathology

Culture of the organism from the milk should be supplemented by bacteriological examination of nasal swabs in calves or adult cattle showing respiratory signs.

Necropsy Findings

There are no characteristic necropsy findings in cattle affected with mastitis but pneumonia from which the bacteria may be isolated may be observed in the associated calves. There may be anaemic infarcts in the udder and other organs.

Diagnosis

Bacteriological examination is essential for diagnosis.

Treatment

In the chronic form, intramammary infusion with either oxytetracycline (400 mg. daily for 2 days), neomycin (once daily for 3 days), chlortetracycline and chlortetracycline-dapsone gives good results. In peracute cases the intravenous injection of chlortetracycline or tetracycline (2 mg. per lb. body weight) is recommended. Parenteral treatment with streptomycin or sodium sulphadimidine, combined with intramammary infusion with streptomycin, neomycin, chlortetracycline or tetracycline, is also effective.

Control

No specific programme can be recommended. In addition to the hygienic measures usually used in the control of mastitis, some attention should be devoted to elimination of the respiratory tract infection in affected animals.

REFERENCES

(1) Hinze, P. M. (1956). *Vet. Med.*, *51*, 257.
(2) Barnes, L. E. (1954). *J. Amer. vet. med. Ass.*, *125*, 50.
(3) White, F. (1957). *Vet. Rec.*, *69*, 566.
(4) Buntain, D. and Field, H. I. (1953). *Vet. Rec.*, *65*, 91.
(5) Easterbrooks, H. L. & Plastridge, W. N. (1956). *J. Amer. vet. med. Ass.*, *128*, 502.
(6) Lake, S. G. & Jones, J. E. T. (1970). *Vet. Rec.*, *87*, 484.

Mastitis Caused by *Pasteurella* Spp.

Mastitis caused by *Pasteurella* spp. is common in ewes, occurring in a peracute gangrenous form, but it is comparatively rare in cattle.

Incidence

In sheep the disease occurs in the western U.S.A., Australia and in Europe in ewes kept under systems of husbandry varying from open mountain pasture to enclosed barns. It is most common in ewes suckling big lambs 2 to 3 months old. In cattle the disease is encountered rarely but may be a problem in individual herds, particularly where calves are reared by nurse cows (1).

Aetiology

Past. haemolytica, the causative organism in ewes, can be isolated from affected quarters and the disease can be reproduced by the intramammary infusion of cultures of the organism (2). *Staph. aureus*, *Cor. pyogenes* and streptococci are often present as secondary invaders (3). In cattle *Past. multocida* is the causative organism.

Transmission

Infection is thought to occur through injuries to teats perhaps caused by over-vigorous suckling by big lambs or calves. The occurrence of this form of mastitis is not related to hygiene, many outbreaks occurring in sheep at range, but because of the sheep's habit of sleeping at night on bedding grounds, it is possible that transmission occurs by contact with infected soil or bedding. The disease in both sheep and cattle is sporadic in occurrence.

Clinical Findings

In ewes an acute systemic disturbance, with a high fever (40 to 42°C or 105 to 107°F), anorexia and dyspnoea, accompanies acute swelling of the gland and severe lameness on the affected side. This lameness is an important early sign and is useful in picking affected animals from a group. The udder is at first hot, swollen and painful and the milk watery, but within 24 hours the quarter becomes blue and cold, the milk shows clots and a profound toxaemia is evident. The temperature subsides in 2 to 4 days, the secretion dries up entirely and the animal either dies of toxaemia on the third to seventh day or survives with sloughing of a gangrenous portion of the udder, followed by the development of abscesses and the continual draining of pus. Usually only one side is affected. During outbreaks of this type of mastitis, cases of pneumonia due to the same organism may occur in lambs.

In cattle the mastitis is severe with fever, marked swelling, abnormal secretion, complete cessation of milk flow in affected and unaffected quarters and subsequent fibrosis and atrophy. Calves allowed to suck affected cows may die of pasteurellosis (5).

Clinical Pathology

Culture of the organism in the milk is necessary to confirm the diagnosis.

Necropsy Findings

The disease is not fatal in cows but in ewes there is marked oedema of the ventral abdominal wall and severe engorgement and oedema of the mammary tissue.

Diagnosis

In sheep the peracute nature of the disease makes it similar to mastitis caused by *Staph. aureus* although gangrene of the udder is more typical in the latter disease. A similar disease in ewes has been ascribed to *Actinobacillus lignieresi* but the causative organism closely resembles the *Pasteurella* spp., described here (7). Suppurative mastitis caused by *Cor. pseudotuberculosis* is chronic in type and no systemic signs occur. Mastitis caused by *Str. agalactiae* in ewes resembles the same disease in

cattle. Bovine mastitis caused by *Past. multocida* must be differentiated from the many other forms of acute mastitis in this species and this can be done only by bacteriological examination of the milk.

Treatment

Sulphadimidine administered intravenously and orally is effective in ewes if given in the early stages of the disease (2). Streptomycin and the broad spectrum antibiotics should be equally effective. In cattle, streptomycin administered by intramammary infusion is effective but a tetracycline is preferred. Recurrence in quarters which appear to have recovered is not infrequent (6) and poor response to treatment has been observed (8).

Control

Removal of sources of infection in sheep flocks necessitates culling some ewes with affected udders but even rigid culling usually fails to completely eradicate the disease. Polyvalent hyperimmune serum and a formolized vaccine have been shown to be of value in prophylaxis (4) and an autogenous vaccine may be effective in a flock where the disease is occurring.

REFERENCES

(1) Barnum, D. A. (1954). *Canad. J. comp. Med.*, *18*, 113.
(2) Tunnicliff, E. A. (1949). *Vet. Med.*, *44*, 498.
(3) Simmons, G. C. & Ryley, J. W. (1954). *Qd J. agric. Sci.*, *11*, 29.
(4) Mura, D. & Manca, A. (1955). *Vet. ital.*, *6*, 1003.
(5) Packer, R. A. & Merchant, I. A. (1946). *N. Amer. Vet.*, *27*, 496.
(6) Pascoe, R. R. (1960). *Aust. vet. J.*, *36*, 408.
(7) Laws, L. & Elder, J. K. (1969). *Aust. vet. J.*, *45*, 401.
(8) Pepper, T. A. *et al.* (1968). *Vet. Rec.*, *83*, 211.

Mastitis Caused by *Nocardia asteroides*

Nocardial mastitis is an uncommon occurrence in cattle and is manifested as an acute or subacute mastitis accompanied by extensive granulomatous lesions in the udder.

Incidence

Nocardial mastitis is a sporadic disease affecting only one or two cows in a herd, unless there is accidental introduction of the causative bacteria into udders when infusions are being administered when it may appear as a herd problem (1, 2).

Until a recent report of the disease as a herd problem, nocardial mastitis in cattle had been recorded only as a sporadic infection. The disease is a serious one in that there is extensive destruction of tissue, loss of production and occasionally death of a cow. Also, there is a possibility that human infection may occur as the organism may not be destroyed by usual pasteurization procedures.

Aetiology

Nocardia asteroides can be cultured from the milk of affected quarters and the disease can be produced experimentally by this organism. One case of chronic mastitis caused by *N. braziliensis* (3) and two caused by *N. farcinicus* (4) have also been recorded.

Transmission

The organism is a common soil contaminant and probably gains entrance to the udder when udder washing is ineffective or udder infusion is not carried out aseptically. The disease is most common in freshly calved adult cows particularly if infusion of the udder with contaminated materials is carried out in the dry period (6). *N. asteroides* is capable of surviving in mixtures used for intramammary infusion for up to 7 weeks.

Pathogenesis

The inflammation of the teat sinus and lower parts of the gland suggest invasion via the teat canal. Infection of mammary tissue results in the formation of discrete granulomatous lesions and the development of extensive fibrosis, the spread of inflammation occurring from lobule to lobule. Infected animals are not sensitive to tuberculin.

When infection occurs early in lactation (the first 15 days) the reaction is a systemic one with fever and anorexia. At other times the lesions take the form of circumscribed abscesses and fibrosis (8). There may also be infected foci in supramammary and mesenteric lymph nodes (9).

Clinical Findings

Affected animals may show a systemic reaction with high fever, depression and anorexia but an acute or subacute inflammation is more usual. Fibrosis of the gland and the appearance of clots in greyish, viscid secretion, which also contains small, white particles, is the usual clinical picture. The fibrosis may be diffuse but is usually in the form of discrete masses 2 to 5 cm. in diameter. Badly affected glands may rupture or develop sinus tracts to the exterior.

Clinical Pathology

The organism can be detected on culture of the milk. Small (1 mm. diameter) specks are visible in the milk and, on microscopical examination, these prove to be felted masses of mycelia. Intradermal injection of antigens prepared from the organism has shown some promise as a diagnostic test (7).

Necropsy Findings

Grossly diffuse fibrosis and granulomatous lesions containing pus are present in mammary tissue. The lining of milk ducts and the teat sinus are thick and roughened. On histological examination the granulomatous nature of the lesions is evident (1). Metastatic pulmonary lesions have been found in occasional long-standing cases (5).

Diagnosis

The appearance of the milk is distinctive but cultural examination is necessary for positive identification.

Treatment

The disease does not respond to treatment with the common antibiotics but novobiocin (500 mg.) combined with 25 to 40 ml. of 0·2 per cent nitrofurazone solution shows promise (1). Isoniazid (10), chloramphenicol and neomycin are also effective (8).

Control

Because of the probable invasion via the teat canal from a soil-borne infection, proper hygiene at milking and strict cleanliness during intramammary infusion are necessary on farms where the disease is enzootic. The organism appears to be sensitive to sodium hypochlorite (200 p.p.m. of free chlorine). Treatment in late cases is unlikely to be of value because of the nature of the lesions, and in affected herds particular attention should be given to the early diagnosis of the disease.

REFERENCES

(1) Pier, A. C. *et al.* (1958). *Amer. J. vet. Res.*, *19*, 319.
(2) Eales, J. D. *et al.* (1964). *Aust. vet. J.*, *40*, 321.
(3) Ditchfield, J. *et al.* (1959). *Canad. J. comp. Med.*, *23*, 93.
(4) Awad, F. I. (1960). *Vet. Rec.*, *72*, 341.
(5) Pier, A. C. *et al.* (1961). *Amer. J. vet. Res.*, *22*, 502.
(6) Pier, A. C. *et al.* (1961). *Amer. J. vet. Res.*, *22*, 698.
(7) Pier, A. C. & Enright, J. B. (1962). *Amer. J. vet. Res.*, *23*, 284.
(8) Schulz, W. & Wester, G. (1968). *Mh. Vet.-Med.*, *23*, 601.
(9) Nicolet, J. *et al.* (1968). *Schweiz. Arch. Tierheilk.*, *110*, 289.
(10) Wendt, K. *et al.* (1969). *Mh. Vet.-Med.*, *24*, 254, 293.

Bovine Mastitis Caused by *Mycoplasma* Spp.

Bovine mastitis caused by *Mycoplasma* spp. is characterized by sudden onset, involvement of all four quarters usually, a precipitous drop in milk production, severe swelling of the udder and gross abnormality of the milk without obvious signs of systemic illness.

Incidence

The disease has been recorded in the U.K. (1), the U.S.A. (5), and Israel (4) and has been observed in Australia. Details of the incidence of the disease are lacking because of its relatively recent identification. It is tempting to suggest that recognition of the disease has been delayed until bacteriological techniques for the isolation of the causative bacteria have been developed, but the clinical picture is so different from that of any other mastitis that it seems probable that it is a new disease.

The disease is a disastrous one because of the high incidence in affected herds and the almost complete cessation of production for the lactation and failure in many cows to ever return to milking. As many as 75 per cent of affected cows may have to be culled.

Aetiology

Several strains of a *Mycoplasma* spp. (tentatively identified as *Myco. genitalium* or *Myco. agalactiae* var. *bovis*) have been isolated from clinical cases and have been used to produce the disease experimentally. Antibodies to the bacteria have not been detectable in sera or whey from animals infected with some strains, but complement fixing antibodies are present in the sera of animals recovered from infection with other strains.

Cows of all ages and at any stage of lactation are affected, cows which have recently calved showing the most severe signs.

Transmission

Little is known of the epidemiology of the disease. It occurs most commonly in herds where milking hygiene is poor and when cows are brought in from other farms or from public saleyards. Mycoplasma mastitis usually breaks out subsequently after a delay of weeks or even months. The delay in development of an outbreak may be related to the long term persistence of the organism (up to 13 months) in some quarters, and some cows become shedders of the organism without ever evidencing severe clinical mastitis. The use of bulk mastitis treatments using a common syringe and cannula may be included in the immediate past history. There is one record (5) of a very close relationship between a high incidence of the disease and faulty milking machines.

The disease is readily transmitted by inoculation of the bacteria into a quarter or by external application of infected secretion to the teat skin. Although the disease occurs first in the inoculated quarter there is usually rapid spread to all other quarters. It seems likely that the infection is spread between cows in the same manner as are other mastitis organisms, by contamination of the teats during milking, but other means, particularly inhalation, have been suggested.

Pathogenesis

This is a purulent interstitial mastitis and although infection probably occurs via the teat canal, the rapid spread of the disease to other quarters of the udder and occasionally to joints suggests that systemic invasion may occur. The presence of the infection in heifers milked for the first time also suggests that systemic invasion may be followed by localization in the udder (3).

Experimental production of the disease (6, 7) has produced little tissue necrosis but mycoplasma are detectable in many tissues including blood, vagina and foetus, suggesting again that systemic invasion occurs.

Clinical Findings

In lactating cows there is a sudden onset of swelling of the udder, a sharp drop in milk production and grossly abnormal secretion in one or more quarters. In most cases all four quarters are affected and a high-producing cow may fall in yield to almost nil between one milking and the next. Dry cows show little swelling of the udder. Although there is no overt evidence of systemic illness and febrile reactions are not observed in most field cases in lactating cows, those which have recently calved show most obvious swelling of the udder and may be off their feed and have a mild fever. However, cows infected experimentally show fever up to 41 °C (105·5 °F) on the third or fourth day after inoculation, at the same time as the udder changes appear. The temperature returns to normal in 24 to 96 hours. In some cases the supramammary lymph nodes are greatly enlarged. A few cows, with or without mastitis, develop arthritis in the knees and fetlocks. The affected joints are swollen, with the swelling extending up and down the leg. Lameness may be so severe that the foot is not put to the ground. Mycoplasma may be present in the joint.

The secretion from affected quarters is deceptive in the early stages in that it appears fairly normal at collection, but on standing a deposit which may be in the form of fine, sandy material, flakes or floccules settles out leaving a turbid whey-like supernatant. Subsequently the secretion becomes scanty and resembles colostrum or soft cheese curd in thin serum. It may be tinged pink with blood or show a grey or brown discolouration. Within a few days the secretion is frankly purulent or curdy but there is an absence of large, firm clots. This abnormal secretion persists for weeks or even months.

Affected quarters are grossly swollen but the swelling is smooth, hard and almost painless and quite unlike the uneven fibrosis which occurs in most other types of mastitis, except that caused by *Myco. lacticola*. Response to treatment is very poor and the swollen udders become grossly atrophied. In infection with one strain of the mycoplasma, many cows do not subsequently come back into production although some may produce moderately well at the next lactation. With other strains there is clinical recovery in one to four weeks without apparent residual damage to the quarter.

Clinical Pathology

The causative organism can be cultured without great difficulty and concurrent infection with other bacteria is common. A marked leucopenia, with counts as low as 1800 to 2500 per cmm., is present when clinical signs appear and persists for up to 2 weeks. Leucocyte counts in the milk are very high, usually over 20 million per cmm. In the acute stages the organisms can usually be demonstrated by the examination of a milk film stained with giemsa or Wright-Leishman stain. The fluorescent antibody technique may also be of value (3).

Necropsy Findings

The disease is a purulent interstitial mastitis with granuloma formation as a common feature. There is cortical hyperplasia in the local lymph nodes and organisms are plentiful in the mammary tissue, subcutaneous oedema fluid and in the lymph nodes.

Diagnosis

A presumptive diagnosis can be made on clinical grounds because of the unusual clinical findings but laboratory confirmation by culture of the organism is desirable. The fact that the organism does not grow on standard media and other pathogenic bacteria are commonly present may lead to errors in the laboratory unless attention is drawn to the characteristic field findings.

Mycoplasma mastitis resembles that caused by *Myco. lacticola*. They both occur commonly after intramammary infusion with oily materials and both show marked, smooth, painless hypertrophy of the udder. The secretions differ, however, and cultural examination serves to differentiate them accurately.

Treatment

None of the commonly used antibiotics are effective and oil–water emulsions used as infusions appear to increase the severity of the disease. Parenteral treatment with oxytetracycline (5 g. daily for 3 days intravenously) has been shown to cause only temporary improvement. Because of the general sensitivity of *Mycoplasma* spp. to tylosin and erythromycin (2), these two antibiotics should be tried but unless treatment is administered very early the damage will already have been done.

Control

Prevention of introduction of the disease into a herd appears to depend upon avoidance of introductions, or of isolating introduced cows until they can be checked for mastitis. The disease spreads rapidly in a herd and affected animals should be culled immediately or placed in strict isolation until sale. Intramammary infusions must be carried out with great attention to hygiene and preferably with individual tubes rather than multidose syringes. The need for a suitable vaccine has been stressed.

REFERENCES

(1) Stuart, P. *et al.* (1963). *Vet. Rec.*, *75*, 59.
(2) Soeci, A. *et al.* (1970). *Arch. vet. ital.*, *21*, 235.
(3) Karbe, E. & Mosher, A. H. (1968). *Zbl. Vet.-Med.*, *15B*, 372, 817.
(4) Bar-Moshe, R. (1964). *Refuah. vet.*, *21*, 99.
(5) Jasper, D. E. *et al.* (1966). *J. Amer. vet. med. Ass.*, *148*, 1017.
(6) Kehoe, J. M. *et al.* (1967). *J. infect. Dis.*, *117*, 171.
(7) Jain, N. C. *et al.* (1969). *Cornell vet.*, *59*, 10.

MISCELLANEOUS MASTIDITES

Mastitis Caused by *Sphaerophorus necrophorus*

A high incidence of mastitis in one dairy herd has been attributed to infection with *Bacteroides funduliformis* (*Sph. necrophorus*). Affected quarters showed viscid, clotty, stringy secretion but little fibrosis. No systemic reaction was apparent but treatment with a variety of antibiotics was unsuccessful (12).

Mastitis Caused by *Pseudomonas aeruginosa*

Mastitis in cattle caused by *Pseudomonas aeruginosa* is rare and occurs usually as sporadic cases after intramammary infusion with contaminated material, *Pseudomonas* spp. being common in the environment of cattle (1). Occasionally it may be encountered as a herd problem with a number of animals affected and in this instance the infection may originate in contaminated water used for washing udders (13). Clinically there is acute swelling and the appearance of clotted, discoloured milk; function of the gland is usually completely lost at the first attack but recurrent crises may occur. Rarely, strains of this organism are highly virulent and cause fatal mastitis with generalized lesions (2). Experimentally the disease in goats is acute with extensive necrosis and fatal septicaemia in some (23). Treatment with antibiotics is generally unsuccessful. Daily infusions of streptomycin (1 g.) or neomycin (0·5 g.), or both combined with polymixin B, for 4 days are most commonly employed. Carbenicillin (Pyopen) should be effective but has given poor results, probably because of inaccessibility of the bacteria (24). Gentamicin has some activity (25). The oral administration of an organic iodine compound and vaccination with a killed autogenous vaccine are credited with bringing the disease under control in one herd (21).

Mastitis Caused by *Mycobacterium* Spp.

Tuberculous mastitis has been dealt with under tuberculosis. Other mycobacteria, especially *Myco. lacticola*, have been isolated from cases of mastitis in cattle which occur after the intramammary infusion of therapeutic agents in oils (3, 4). The disease can be reproduced by the intramammary injection of the organism in oil but not in watery suspension. Subsequent oily infusions exacerbate the condition. Clinically there is tremendous hypertrophy of the quarter with the appearance of clots in discoloured milk but there is no systemic reaction. Affected animals do not show sensitivity to avian or mammalian tuberculin. No effective treatment is recorded.

Myco. fortuitum has been encountered as a cause of a severe outbreak of bovine mastitis (20). Infected quarters were seriously damaged, did not respond to treatment and affected cows died or were salvaged. The disease was reproduced experimentally and affected animals showed positive reactions to mammalian and avian tuberculosis and some sensitivity to johnin.

Mastitis Caused by *Bacillus cereus*

This saprophytic organism is usually considered to have little pathogenicity but a few cases of mastitis from which it has been isolated have been recorded in cattle, usually subsequent to injury of the teat (5, 22). There is a severe systemic reaction accompanied by gangrene and haemorrhage of the udder. Chlortetracycline is of some value in treatment.

Mastitis Caused by *Serratia marcescens*

A mild chronic mastitis in which clinical signs of swelling of the quarter with the presence of clots in the milk appeared periodically, has been observed to occur naturally and was produced experimentally (14). Neomycin (2 g. initially followed by three daily doses of 1 g. by intramammary infusion) was successful as a treatment.

Mastitis Caused by Fungi and Yeasts

Trichosporon spp. can cause mastitis in cattle and is manifested clinically by swelling of the gland and clots in the milk. The infection rate is low and the fungi disappear spontaneously. Experimental transmission of the disease has been effected (6).

Cryptococcus neoformans, the yeast which causes human cryptococcosis, has caused acute mastitis in cattle (7). Contaminated infusion material and spread from other infected quarters are the probable source of infection. Infection in humans drinking the milk is unlikely to occur because the yeast does not withstand pasteurization but there may be some hazard to farm families. While there is no systemic reaction, the mastitis may be acute with marked swelling of the affected quarter and the supramammary lymph node, a severe fall in milk yield and the appearance of viscid, mucoid, grey-white secretion. Clinical mastitis persists for some weeks and, in many cases, subsides spontaneously, but in others the udder is so severely damaged that the cow has to be slaughtered. Systemic involvement occurs rarely. At necropsy, there is dissolution of the acinar epithelium and in chronic cases a diffuse or granulomatous reaction in the mammary tissue and lymph node. Similar lesions have been found in the lungs (10).

Many other yeasts, including *Candida* spp., *Saccharomyces* spp., *Pichia* spp. and *Torulopsis* spp. (16), have also caused mastitis in cattle, the infection probably being introduced with contaminated intramammary infusions (8, 17) or teat cup liners (9). Establishment of the infection is encouraged by damage to the mammary epithelium and stimulated by antibiotic therapy; for example *Candida* spp. utilize penicillin and tetracyclines as sources of nitrogen (19). A fever (41 °C or 106 °F) is accompanied by a severe inflammation of the quarter, enlargement of the supramammary lymph nodes, and a marked fall in milk yield. The secretion consists of large yellow clots in a watery, supernatant fluid. Usually the disease is benign and spontaneous recovery in about a week is the rule.

None of these infections respond well to anti-biotic therapy but treatment with iodides, either sodium iodide intravenously, organic iodides by mouth, or iodine in oil as an intramammary infu-sion, might be of value. A number of drugs, in-cluding Actidione, cycloheximide, nystatin, poly-mixin B, neomycin and isoniazid, have been tested for efficiency against mastitis in cattle produced experimentally by the infusion of *Cryptococcus neoformans* but did not alter the clinical course of the disease (11). Merthiolate (20 ml. of a 0·1 per cent solution) as an infusion daily for 2 to 3 days is reported to have a beneficial effect if administered early in the course of the disease (18).

Traumatic Mastitis

Injuries to the teats or udder which penetrate to the teat cistern or milk ducts, or involve the ex-ternal sphincter are commonly followed by mastitis. Any of the organisms which cause mastitis may invade the udder after such injury and in such cases mixed infections are usual. All injuries to the teat or udder, including surgical interference, should be treated prophylactically with wide spectrum anti-biotics.

REFERENCES

(1) Tucker, E. W. (1950). *Cornell Vet.*, *40*, 95.
(2) Winter, H. & O'Connor, R. F. (1957). *Aust. vet. J.*, *33*, 83.
(3) Stuart, P. & Harvey, P. (1951). *Vet. Rec.*, *63*, 881.
(4) Richardson, A. (1970). *Vet. Rec.*, *86*, 497.
(5) Brown, R. W. & Scherer, R. K. (1957). *Cornell Vet.*, *47*, 226.
(6) Murphy, J. M. & Drake, C. H. (1947). *Amer. J. vet. Res.*, *8*, 43.
(7) Pounden, W. D. *et al.* (1952). *Amer. J. vet. Res.*, *13*, 121.
(8) Weigt, U. (1970). *Dtsch. tierärztl. Wschr.*, *77*, 538.
(9) Simon, J. & Hall, R. (1955). *J. Milk Technol.*, *18*, 298.
(10) Innes, J. R. M. *et al.* (1952). *Amer. J. vet. Res.*, *13*, 469.
(11) Redaelli, G. & Rosaschino, F. (1957). *Arch. vet. ital.*, *8*, 311.
(12) Simon, J. & McCoy, E. (1958). *J. Amer. vet. med. Ass.*, *133*, 165.
(13) Curtis, P. E. (1969). *Vet. Rec.*, *84*, 476.
(14) Barnum, D. A. *et al.* (1958). *Canad. J. comp. Med.*, *22*, 392.
(15) Loftsgard, G. & Lindquist, K. (1960). *Acta vet. scand.*, *1*, 201.
(16) Bolck, G. *et al.* (1967). *Mh. Vet.-Med.*, *22*, 289.
(17) Loken, K. I. *et al.* (1959). *J. Amer. vet. med. Ass.*, *134*, 401.
(18) Immer, J. (1965). *Schweiz. Arch. Tierheilk.*, *107*, 206.
(19) Mehnert, B. *et al.* (1964). *Zbl. Vet.-Med.*, *11A*, 97.
(20) Peterson, K. J. (1965). *J. Amer. vet. med. Ass.*, *147*, 1600.
(21) Kruiningen, H. J. van. (1963). *Cornell Vet.*, *53*, 240.
(22) Gloor, H. (1968). *Schweiz. Arch. Tierheilk.*, *110*, 63.
(23) Lepper, A. W. D. & Matthews, P. R. J. (1966). *Res. vet. Sci.*, *7*, 151.
(24) Ziv, G. *et al.* (1969). *Refuah. vet.*, *26*, 152.
(25) Ziv, G. & Risenberg-Tirer, R. (1970). *Zbl. Vet.-Med.*, *17B*, 963.

THE CONTROL
OF BOVINE MASTITIS

Although mastitis due to *Str. agalactiae* has been eradicated from individual herds, bovine mastitis is not, in terms of practicality, an eradicable disease at the herd or area level. For this reason it does not lend itself to legislative control but rather to volun-tary involvement by dairymen in programmes aimed at reducing its incidence and maintaining the infection rate at a low level. Because the justi-fication for control of the disease is purely eco-nomic, any control programme must be based on its applicability on each individual farm. Generally area control is not a feasible objective and a national programme can only be in the form of providing incentives and assistance to individual dairymen who wish to participate.

To be effective a mastitis control programme must

(1) Provide an economic advantage.
(2) Be within the scope of the dairyman's tech-nical skill and understanding.
(3) Be capable of introduction into the manage-ment system employed.

Most of the control programmes of the past have not satisfied these criteria, and on most dairy farms in developed areas, even today, mastitis control de-pends on the treatment of clinical cases and the use of relatively ineffective hygiene techniques in the milking parlour. As a result, subclinical cases go undetected and the continuous spread to further quarters goes on relatively unchecked. In most dairy populations the percentage of quarters infected is in the range of 25 to 50 per cent and the resulting financial losses are very heavy. What is required is a control programme which satisfies the above cri-teria and is capable of being applied at various levels of intensity to accommodate various levels of profit-ability, with the object of limiting the quarter in-fection rate to a predetermined level. The two criteria necessary to the biological objective of limit-ing the quarter infection rate are (*a*) reduction of the new infection rate and (*b*) reduction in the duration of the infected status of infected quarters.

All of these criteria are satisfied in the N.I.R.D. mastitis control programme which has the capacity of quickly reducing the quarter infection rate (from 30 to 10 per cent) and the number of clinical cases by half (30, 42).

The N.I.R.D. Programme. The basic control pro-gramme in use today is the one developed at the National Institute for Research in Dairying at Reading, England (1, 2, 3, 42). It has the virtues of simplicity, cheapness (estimated cost of £1·50 or $3·50 per cow per year) and widespread applicability because it does not depend on laboratory diagnosis. It is set out in detail below but it is also suggested that the programme is susceptible to desirable modification for individual farms by the inclusion of veterinary surveillance and laboratory diagnosis.

There is no doubt from the many reports available and from our personal experience of the N.I.R.D. programme that its application for a very large population of dairy cattle could be very rapid indeed and could reduce the wastage due to mastitis by 65 per cent within the space of a year and at very low cost. But from our experience two problems can arise and, in the provision of an individually tailored service to a farmer, some attempt should be made to overcome them, provided this can be done in a financially rewarding manner. The most important problem is that the N.I.R.D. programme is unsupervised and the average farmer, having witnessed the dramatic reduction in clinical cases which usually occurs, is likely to relax the intensity of the several techniques and allow a recrudescence of the disease. A monitoring system is desirable, if not essential. Bulk Milk Cell counts do provide such a system but they are seriously inaccurate and a very bad mastitis situation could develop in a herd before a warning was given (44). Periodic sampling of a portion of the herd is a suitable alternative.

The second problem with the N.I.R.D. programme is that it is designed for the control of the common mastitis pathogens and at the average level of incidence. Absence of a diagnostic examination could result in the application of a control programme to a herd with a 'free electricity' problem rather than mastitis, or to infection with *Nocardia* spp. or with a quarter infection of less than 10 per cent, in none of which is measurable improvement likely to occur. The frequency of such occurrences will be so small that they will be nationally insignificant but they could be very significant to individual farmers. Whether the problem herds are revealed by the failure of the programme or by a preliminary diagnostic examination may be immaterial but in terms of providing the best available veterinary service to a client the latter course is recommended.

The basic programme is:
(*a*) Reduction of duration of infection.
   (i) Treat all quarters of all cows at drying off.
   (ii) Treat clinical cases as they occur. Detect clinical cases by in-line filter.
   (iii) Cull chronic clinical cases.

(*b*) Reduction of new infection rate.
   (iv) Dip all teats after each milking.
   (v) Adequately service and maintain milking machine.
   (vi) Backflush cups after each milking and rinse off udder before milking, both with running water.

There are many additional options and these are set down in the following paragraphs.

Detection of Infected Quarters

This is the most important option. A programme to include milk-sampling of cows is expensive and, if generally applied, puts a great strain on laboratory resources. A decision on whether to attempt this detection of infected quarters can probably be made on the following lines. If a herd owner has a problem and calls for assistance, a herd survey, or at least an examination of a significant sample of the herd, should be carried out. However, where it is intended to encourage the general use of a control programme it is satisfactory to omit the procedure until those farms on which the programme does not work well become noticeable. This will be at about the end of the first year, when it will be apparent that the clinical mastitis rate is not significantly reduced. The detection of infected quarters can then proceed.

The recommended procedure which gives satisfactory results at a reasonable cost under field conditions is:

   (i) Submission of quarter samples from all cows to the California Mastitis Test (CMT).
   (ii) Bacteriological examination of CMT positive quarters.
   (iii) Identification of coagulase-positive staphylococci and CAMP-test positive streptococci.
   (iv) Determination of the sensitivity of the pathogens.

Treatment of Infected Quarters

If an *ad hoc* quarter sampling is done it is usual to leave those quarters infected with *Staphylococcus aureus* until the next dry period before treating them. Quarters infected with other organisms are treated, as set down for those bacteria, either immediately or at drying off, depending on the anticipated cure rate and the cost versus benefit comparison. In the case of *Str. agalactiae* treatment may be administered under the general disinfection technique described under the control of that type of mastitis.

Dry-period treatment is carried out at the end of

the last milking before the cow is turned out. In seasonal dairying areas farmers would prefer to dry their cows off over a two or three week period, bring them all in when the last one is dry and treat them all. This method permits a large number of infections to develop in the period right after drying off, the most dangerous period. It also provides an opportunity for a flare-up of chemical mastitis when the treatment is infused into a quarter which has no secretion in it. Some medicaments are more irritant than others and this is not always a problem.

Because of the preponderance of *Staphylococcus aureus* infection the recommended antibiotics are benzathine cloxacillin and novobiocin but more important is the need for the antibiotic to be in a long-acting base. A longer-acting base than those generally available would be an advantage, so that the protected period could be longer than it is.

One of the undecided questions about dry-period treatment is whether or not all quarters should be treated. The general recommendation is that all quarters be treated and this is fine when the infection rate is 40 to 50 per cent of quarters. But the resulting complete sterilization of quarters and a fall in leucocyte count possibly leading to infection just before or at calving with a potent pathogen such as *Escherichia coli* is what the herd owner fears most. There is no proof that this is a significant occurrence but it is admitted that it could be (1, 21). Also the treatments are not inexpensive and if the infected quarters are 10 per cent or less the reduction of the treatment cost by 75 per cent would be a useful saving. The alternative method is to sample the cows before drying off and treat only the infected quarters.

The range of suitable products for use as dry-cow therapy is not wide. Benzathine cloxacillin (0·5 to 1 g.) in a long-acting base gives excellent results (36, 37, 38). A mixture of sodium novobiocin (250 mg.) and penicillin (200,000 units) is equally effective. Procaine penicillin G alone has a mixed reputation. In a long-acting base it does prevent new infections with *Cor. pyogenes* during the dry period (39) but is of mediocre efficiency in eliminating staphylococci and streptococci (41). Spiramycin (500 mg.) is less effective (38).

Monitoring Quarter Infection Rate

Once a programme is under way it becomes a matter of importance to monitor the results. This is for two purposes. One is to check that the programme is working against the causative agents in the particular herd; the other is to check that the programme is being properly applied. There are three ways of applying such surveillance. The cheapest and least satisfactory is to keep check on the number of clinical cases treated, often by monitoring consumption of treatment tubes. An effective monitoring method is to have cell counts or California Mastitis Tests carried out on bulk milk samples at regular, say weekly, intervals. This probably should be done at the milk depot anyway as a check point in quality milk control. The technique is not inexpensive and although it is generally favoured (4) as a monitoring system it lacks accuracy (2) as a monitor for individual herds. For a control programme which is under veterinary supervision the method is not good enough. The only available alternative is to periodically sample a portion of the herd. The obvious group to use is cows about to be dried off. The results can be used in the dry period treatment technique described above.

Detection of Infected Quarters

When cows are tied in and milked *in situ* the use of a strip cup before milking is mandatory. In a milking parlour, especially when there is plenty of running water, squirting of the foremilk onto a black plate in the floor is adequate. To avoid reflux of milk during squirting (see below) stainless steel in-milk-line filters are now available. The clots can be readily seen (45).

Teat Dipping

Excellent results in preventing new infections are obtained by the use of suitable teat dips. This effectiveness includes herds infected with *Staph. aureus* and the technique is the basis of modern control programmes. All teats of all cows are dipped or sprayed after each milking. At present the only satisfactory method of application is complete immersion of the teat and the base of the udder in the solution. But dipping is just too time-consuming in fast herringbone sheds and diluted dipping solutions are sprayed on. Coverage of the teat is incomplete and much of the costly solution is wasted. There is a great need for an efficient automatic method.

The teat dipping solution must be as cheap as possible, be effective at killing bacteria on the teat skin and remain effective until the next milking, even if cows are walking through long, wet grass, but be non-irritant to the skin of teats and hands. Iodophors solutions containing 1 per cent available iodine (46), hypochlorite solutions containing 4 per cent free chlorine and with negligible free alkali, and chlorhexidine (Hibitane) 0·5 or 1 per cent in polyvinylpyrrolidone solution (40) or as 0·3 per cent aqueous solution (33) have been shown to be effective in these circumstances (8). Iodophor dips are expensive but efficient. If chapping or teat sores develop the inclusion of 33 per cent glycerol in the dip provides a very satisfactory emollient action. A commercial bleach (Chlorox) in the U.S.A. meets the requirements of a 4 per cent available chlorine dip (of 0·08 per cent sodium hydroxide, 0·3 per cent sodium carbonate, 0·17 per cent sodium chlorate and 4·5 per cent sodium chloride) but other commercially available products generally contain too much alkali and cause severe skin irritation. Although the efficiency of a solution containing 1 per cent available chlorine is less, it is as efficient as 0·5 per cent iodophor and can be inexpensively prepared by diluting commercial dairy hypochlorite solution 1 in 9. The alkalinity is at a suitably low level but teat chapping occurs in some herds. The addition of lanoline may help prevent this (35).

Udder Washing and Teat Stripping

It has been adequately shown that the new infection rate is reduced significantly if the teats are stripped (a few squirts milked out) before pre-milking washing rather than after (26), and if the stripping is done in such a way that there is no chance of refluxing milk from the teat cup into the udder (27). In areas where water supplies are limited chemical sanitization is necessary. Individual paper towels are used, or cloth towels boiled after each use on one cow. The same procedure may also be adopted in addition to udder washing when a 'partial hygiene' programme is attempted. In these circumstances it is usual to wear disinfected rubber gloves during milking.

The chemical to be used is important but more harm is usually done by the inappropriate use of an effective agent than by the use of poor preparations. Detailed information on udder disinfection is available (7) but some recommendations are generally applicable. The cost of some highly efficient disinfectants for application to the udder is prohibitive in some circumstances. Hibitane, a diguanide compound, in a solution containing a detergent (alkylaryl polyether alcohol) is highly efficient when used in the proportion of 4 to 8 g. per litre of water, i.e. 1:5000. Quarternary ammonium compounds as 0·2 per cent solutions, compounds containing iodine and phosphorus (iodophors) used in solutions containing at least 100 ppm of available iodine, and sodium hypochlorite solutions containing 800 to 1200 ppm of free chlorine are efficient against *Str. agalactiae*. Since all of these compounds are likely to lose much of their efficiency when contaminated with organic matter, udders should be cleaned carefully before disinfection and the wash-water changed frequently.

Teat Cup Disinfection/Back-flushing

Three methods are available. The conventional method is to rinse the cups and dip them in disinfectant wash water between cows, ensuring that the disinfectant gets well up into the cups by dipping a pair of each cluster in turn. Short term immersion in hot water (76·5 to 82°C or 170 to 180°F for 10 seconds) is effective (3, 34), but has physical disadvantages in a fast-moving line. Chemical sanitization has the same disadvantages as those for udder washing and the same alternative procedure is now extensively used—the back flushing of the milking tube and cups with cold water for 15 seconds after each cow (5, 6). In herringbone sheds automatic equipment is available and very little time is wasted.

Milking Machine Design and Management

The milking machine is an essential part of the dairying industry but it is assumed that its use, proper or improper, has been the principal factor in the increase of sub-clinical (largely staphylococcal) mastitis in recent years. In spite of this assumption reports persist which show that quarters which are not milked become infected more readily than those which are, provided all quarters are repeatedly exposed to infection (28). The following features of machine milking are generally accepted as those which need to be examined in a control programme (8). An annual examination by a qualified technician is the minimum.

With respect to failure of the control programme described here it will be found that most failures are due to machine faults. The desirable standards for machines are (32, 42): reserve vacuum pump capacity 1 c.f.m. free air per unit; vacuum level 15 in. mercury; pulsation rate 40 to 60 per minute; ratio vacuum/rest 50:67; clawpiece airbleed 1/4 c.f.m. free air per unit; vacuum level inches of mercury high-line 14 to 15, low-line 12·5 to 13·5; milking vacuum at teat cup under full load 11 to 12; minimum vacuum residual for massage 6; milk to rest ratio 35:65 to 65:35 (32).

Vacuum pressure in milking machines. Although excessive vacuum level is generally considered to be the most obvious cause of injury by milking machines, there is much conflicting evidence about it and no general agreement that vacuum pressure *per se* is associated with the incidence of infection. However, there are many clinical reports which indicate that an unsuspected high vacuum has resulted in outbreaks of severe clinical mastitis and that a reduction in vacuum level was followed by an improvement in the disease situation. These conflicting views probably depend upon differences in the rate of infection in the respective herds initially.

Vacuum pressure in a machine should not exceed that recommended by the manufacturer. With most machines a pressure of 37·5 cm. of mercury is sufficient and pressures in excess of this are likely to cause injury, as are large fluctuations of pressure caused by inadequate vacuum reserve. In any eradication or control programme the milking technique should be observed and the pressure checked as obstructions may be present in the air line permitting the pressure between the obstruction and the pump to be greatly in excess of normal. The gauge on the machine should also be checked. The small air vent at the end of the claw which permits onward movement of the milk may be blocked, causing milk to accumulate in the liner and exert excessive pressure on the teat. When this occurs the teat ends show redness and prominence of the external meatus, and in severe cases, sores or chapped, rosette formations at the tip. This may progress to eversion of the teat lining with fissuring of the teat sphincter and warty or hair-like growths around it. Such teats are extremely sore at milking and predispose to permanent obstruction or mastitis caused by mixed bacterial infections. Small, firm teats are most susceptible to this form of trauma.

Vacuum stability and reserve. Excessive variation in vacuum level may be an important factor contributing to the development of mastitis but conflicting views are expressed (19, 20, 24). The consensus is that severe aberrations are of great importance. Fluctuation of more than 5 cm. of pressure in bucket systems and more than 7·5 cm. in pipeline systems is considered to be undesirable. Vacuum stability can be checked by inserting a vacuum gauge in one cup of a cluster on a cow while the rest of the units are in use. Excessive fluctuations in vacuum pressure which last for 5 seconds should indicate the need for a close check on the equipment by a serviceman.

Reverse flow of milk in high-line milkers, when the milk line is too small in calibre to take peak milk flows, can result in the transfer of contaminated milk from one set of cups to another during the milking process. In the same way reflux back into the udder may also be encouraged. Such errors can occur suddenly when a dairyman changes to Friesians from Jerseys or increases the size of his shed without increasing milking machine capacity (26).

Teat cup design and management. Abnormalities in size and shape of teat cup liners are also likely to cause damage. Small diameter (0·75 in.) tension liners are preferable to wide (1 to 1·25 in.) moulded slack liners as they cause less injury. In the same way, liners which are allowed to lose their resilience and shape are also dangerous. Proper care of liners includes rinsing after milking, weekly boiling in caustic soda or lye solution (1 oz. per gallon) for 15 minutes, followed by rinsing in boiling water, and discarding liners when they lose shape or become rough or cracked. When one liner is discarded, the others in the set should also be changed because a new liner will milk more efficiently and may work on a dry teat for some time while the inefficient liners are still milking. Although there are conflicting reports on the relationship between overmilking and mastitis it is generally assumed that if a milking machine is adjusted so that it is likely to cause damage, then the effect will be aggravated by any delay in removing the cups after milk flow has ceased. Overmilking, particularly for long periods, causes severe damage to the lining of the teat cistern and streak canal (10) and could contribute to the development of mastitis.

Milking technique. Excessive machine stripping and removal of the teat cups too violently or before the vacuum is released are two common causes of teat injury. Such errors can only be detected if the milking shed is visited at milking time.

Removal of the cups at the appropriate time is important since, if the cups are left on too long, the teat is sucked into the cup and the lining of the teat canal may be injured. This can be adequately controlled by having a sight-glass between each cup and the claw, and removing the cups individually from each quarter as milk ceases to flow. Cups are apt to be left on too long when too many cows are being milked by one person. One of the best measures of milking machine efficiency is the average milking time per cow. Four minutes is considered to be optimum and 6 minutes can be considered as evidence of defective procedure or inefficient equipment or both. Provided adequate hygiene precautions are taken, careful hand-milking is probably the technique least likely to cause damage to the udder and predisposition to mastitis.

The number of sets of teat cups that one man can handle is critical. Labour costs demand that it be high. Mastitis control requires it to be sufficiently low that significant overmilking does not occur (26). What determines how many sets can be handled by one man is the time required for the necessary chores for each cow, bringing in, preparation and so on. Under existing conditions one man can look after 2 sets in a long static milk line, up to 4 sets in a doubled-up walk through, and 6 sets in a herringbone. To increase this number automation of the chores, e.g. automatic cluster removers, are necessary.

Another potentially important factor in the milking process is the development of a higher negative pressure in the udder than at the apex of the teat. This can occur during overmilking, with vacuum fluctuation and because of failure of let-down. In this event there is a possibility of a reflux of contaminated milk back into the udder (22). One of the important recent advances in milking machine technology is the automatic teat cup remover which operates on the rate of milk flow and completely avoids overmilking.

Pulsation rate. The pulsation rate is of doubtful importance in so far as mastitis is concerned. Too rapid pulsation (the optimum is about 40 per minute but varies with different machines) results in incomplete filling of the teat and a tendency for the teats to be crammed into the cup with resulting injury to the soft tissues (12, 13).

In recent years more and more attention has been given to the construction, installation and handling of the milking machine in such a way as to avoid mastitis. Some of the major points are discussed above but more detailed information is available (9, 14, 15, 16).

Drying Off

Cows are commonly dried off at the end of a lactation by abrupt cessation of milking or by milking them at gradually increasing intervals. Many new infections occur during this period due to flareups of infections not apparent during lactation or to the fall in bactericidal and bacteriostatic qualities of the milk which are at their lowest ebb during the dry period. The method of drying off has no effect on subsequent milk yields but in herds where mastitis is common the incidence of infection during the dry period is higher when milking is terminated abruptly, particularly if the cow is milking well when she is dried off. Withdrawal of milk during the dry period does not appear to increase the chance of infection. These factors are of considerable importance as many of the infections, particularly those caused by *Str. agalactiae*, which commence during the dry period, persist and cause clinical mastitis when the next lactation begins. Dipping of the teats for 20 seconds in 5 per cent tincture of iodine, after preliminary washing with sodium hypochlorite, on several occasions at drying off effectively reduces the subsequent rate of new infections with *Staph. aureus* (17).

Nutrition and Inheritance

It is commonly believed that the incidence of mastitis increases when cattle go on to lush pasture or are fed diets high in protein. There is no proof of either contention but reduction of diet is commonly practised when clinical mastitis occurs. The commonly reported increased incidence of mastitis when cows are turned out to pasture has led to the suggestion that a high intake of oestrogenic compounds may precipitate mastitis but investigations into the role of these substances have been inconclusive (18, 23). Genetic variations in resistance to mastitis have been proven with regard to *Str. agalactiae* mastitis of cows and may well hold for other forms of the disease but it is unlikely that selection for resistance to mastitis will ever be a practical measure.

Vaccination

Vaccination has so far proved to be of limited value in the control of mastitis. Its efficiency will depend largely upon the antigenicity of the causative organisms. While the vaccination story is by no means complete and further research is indicated, it seems safe to say that vaccination against *Str. agalactiae* mastitis is unlikely to be effective since most recovered animals have little if any immunity. The use of an autogenous bacterin against *Staph. aureus* may be of some value in herds where the infecting organism is highly antigenic. In these herds it is unlikely to be sufficiently effective to completely prevent infection but it may reduce the incidence and severity of clinical mastitis. Recent developments in vaccines against staphylococcal mastitis are discussed under that heading and the possible use of vaccination in the control of mastitis in sows caused by coliform organisms, and in ewes caused by staphylococci and pasteurella, is discussed under those headings. The development of local immunity in the udder is currently being investigated (47). Its application refers largely to staphylococcal mastitis and it is discussed in that section of this chapter.

In considering the general problem of mastitis control, it should be remembered that, by definition, mastitis is an inflammation of the mammary gland and may be caused by a wide variety of bacteria. It cannot therefore be considered to be a specific infectious disease. Many of the causative bacteria cannot be eradicted from the environment and, although strong measures may succeed in bringing widespread infection in a herd under control, little permanent benefit will result unless a continuous mastitis control programme can be incorporated into the management practices of the herd.

Milking Order

Known infected cows should be milked last and in general young cows should be milked before older ones. Newly introduced animals should be milked separately until their status is determined. The California Mastitis Test offers a quick and efficient method of screening cows before admitting them to the milking herd.

Miscellaneous Procedures

The ability of certain bacteria to colonize the teat skin, and thus be in advantageous position to invade the mammary gland, is well recognized. Although the factors determining the ability to colonize in this way, and great variations do occur (25), are not determined, any practical procedure which keeps it under control is likely to reduce the prevalence of mastitis. Teat sores are common sites for such colonization but few dairymen appreciate their importance in mastitis control. Vigorous treatment with a suitable antiseptic cream after each milking is recommended. The preferred antiseptics are chlorhexidine and iodophors. Iodophor teat dip containing glycerine often clears up sore and chapped teats. Disinfection of the hands is necessary only where hand stripping or hand milking is practised. In these circumstances the hands should be dipped in a disinfectant wash water between cows and rubbed with a disinfectant cream at the end of the milking period. The latter procedure is most important because of the persistence of the causative organism on the skin.

Hand stripping should be avoided when possible and only machine stripping by bearing down on the milking cups permitted. Sucking by calves may spread infection from quarter to quarter or cow to cow and may also be a factor in the spread of the disease to other calves if they are allowed to suck each other. Infected milk must be disposed of hygienically. The addition of 5 per cent phenol or an equivalent disinfectant is a satisfactory method of destroying the infectivity of small quantities of milk.

Quarters which do not respond to treatment should be permanently dried up as described above or the affected cows culled. Valuable breeding cows may be retained if they are isolated and milked with strict hygienic precautions.

Amputation of the tail has been used in an attempt to reduce the prevalence of mastitis but without apparent effect (31).

REFERENCES

(1) Dodd, F. H. & Neave, F. K. (1970). *Natn. Inst. Res. Dairying, Biennial Review*, NIRD Paper No. 3559.
(2) Dodd, F. H. & Jackson, E. R. (1971). *Control of Mastitis*. Reading, Berks.: British Cattle Veterinary Association, NIRD.
(3) Barnum, D. (1962). *Canad. vet. J.*, *3*, 161.
(4) Pearson, J. K. L. *et al.* (1971). *Vet. Rec.*, *88*, 488.
(5) Wilkinson, F. C. (1965). *Aust. vet. J.*, *41*, 93.
(6) Brookbanks, E. O. (1965). *N.Z. vet. J.*, *13*, 163.
(7) Newbould, F. H. S. (1965). *Canad. vet. J.*, *6*, 29.
(8) Newbould, F. H. S. & Barnum, D. A. (1960). *J. Milk Fd Technol.*, *23*, 374.
(9) Fell, L. R. (1964). *Dairy Sci. Abstr.*, *26*, 551.
(10) Peterson, K. J. (1964). *Amer. J. vet. Res.*, *25*, 1003.
(11) Meigs, E. B. *et al.* (1949). *U.S.A. Dept. Agric. tech. Bull.*, *992*, 1–51.
(12) Whittlestone, W. G. & Olney, G. R. (1962). *Aust. J. Dairy Tech.*, *17*, 205.
(13) Bratlie, O. *et al.* (1962). *Nord. vet. Congr.*, *1*, 654.
(14) Noorlander, D. O. (1960). *Mod. vet. Pract.*, *41*, (16) 33, (20) 42, (18) 30, (41) 64; (1961). *Mod. vet. Pract.*, *42*, (3) 33, (5) 41.
(15) Wilson, C. D. (1963). *Vet. Rec.*, *75*, 1311.
(16) McDonald, J. S. (1971). *J. Amer. vet. med. Ass.*, *158*, 184.
(17) Oliver, J. *et al.* (1956). *J. Dairy Res.*, *23*, 194, 197, 204, 212.
(18) Frank, N. A. *et al.* (1967). *J. Amer. vet. med. Ass.*, *150*, 503.
(19) Eberhardt, R. J. *et al.* (1968). *J. Dairy Sci.*, *51*, 1026.
(20) Kirkbride, C. A. & Erhart, A. B. (1969). *J. Amer. vet. med. Ass.*, *155*, 1499.
(21) Schalm, O. W. & Lasmanis, J. (1968). *J. Amer. vet. med. Ass.*, *153*, 1688.
(22) Forbes, D. (1969). *Vet. Bull.*, *39*, 529.
(23) Bourland, C. T. *et al.* (1967). *J. Dairy Sci.*, *50*, 978.
(24) Nyhan, J. F. & Cowhig, M. J. (1967). *Vet. Rec.*, *81*, 122.
(25) Cullen, G. A. & Hebert, C. N. (1967). *Brit. vet. J.*, *123*, 14.
(26) Brookbanks, E. O. (1971). *Aust. vet. J.*, *47*, 226.
(27) Phillips, D. S. M. *et al.* (1969). *N.Z. vet. J.*, *17*, 90.
(28) Neave, F. K. *et al.* (1968). *J. Dairy Res.*, *35*, 127.
(29) O'Shea, J. & Walshe, M. J. (1970). *Irish J. agric. Res.*, *9*, 279.
(30) Ziv, G. (1971). *Refuah. vet.*, *28*, 1.
(31) Elliott, R. E. W. (1969). *N.Z. vet. J.*, *17*, 89.
(32) Schroder, R. J. *et al.* (1968). *J. Amer. vet. med. Ass.*, *153*, 1676.
(33) Schultze, W. D. & Smith, J. W. (1970). *J. Dairy Sci.*, *53*, 38.
(34) McDonald, J. S. (1970). *Amer. J. vet. Res.*, *31*, 233.
(35) Anon. (1970). *Vet. Rec.*, *86*, Info. Supp. No. 41, p. 78.
(36) Rosenzuaig, A. & Mayer, E. (1970). *Refuah. vet.*, *27*, 129.
(37) Smith, A. *et al.* (1967). *Vet. Rec.*, *81*, 504.
(38) Loosmore, R. M. *et al.* (1968). *Vet. Rec.*, *83*, 358.
(39) Edwards, S. J. & Smith, G. S. (1967). *Vet. Rec.*, *80*, 486.
(40) Gerring, E. L. *et al.* (1968). *Vet. Rec.*, *83*, 112.
(41) Daniel, R. C. W. & Seffert, I. J. (1969). *Aus. vet. J.*, *45*, 530.
(42) Kingwill, R. G. *et al.* (1970). *Vet. Rec.*, *87*, 94.
(43) Roberts, S. J. *et al.* (1969). *J. Amer. vet. med. Ass.*, *155*, 157.
(44) Westgarth, D. R. *et al.* (1970). *Int. Dairy Congr.*, 18, Sydney, *1E*, 615.
(45) Hoyle, J. B. & Dodd, F. H. (1970). *J. Dairy Res.*, *37*, 133.
(46) Wesen, D. P. & Schultz, L. H. (1970). *J. Dairy Sci.*, *53*, 1391.
(47) Norcross, N. L. & Stark, D. M. (1970). *J. Dairy Sci.*, *53*, 387.

Miscellaneous Abnormalities of the Udder

Blood in the Milk. Blood in the milk is usually an indication of a rupture of a blood vessel in the gland by direct trauma, or of capillary bleeding in a congested udder soon after calving. Although in the latter circumstance the bleeding usually ceases in 2 to 3 days it may persist beyond this period and render the milk unfit for human consumption. The discolouration varies from a pale pink to a dark chocolate brown and may still be present 7 to 8 days after parturition. In these circumstances, treatment is often requested although the cow is clinically normal in all other respects. Calcium borogluconate injected intravenously is a standard treatment but better results are likely to be obtained by the injection of parenteral coagulants. Difficulty may be experienced in milking the clots out of the teats but if they are broken up by compressing them inside the teat, they will usually pass easily. The presence of blood-stained milk in all four quarters at times other than immediately postpartum should arouse suspicion of leptospirosis, and possibly other diseases in which intravascular haemolysis or capillary damage occurs.

Oedema and Congestion of the Udder. Congestion of the udder at parturition is physiological but it may be sufficiently severe to cause oedema of the belly, udder and teats in cows and mares. In most cases the oedema disappears within a day or two of calving, but if it is extensive and persistent, it may interfere with sucking and milking (9). No treatment is recommended unless the condition is severe. Milking may be started some days before parturition. After parturition, frequent milking, massage and the use of diuretics are recommended. Acetazolamide (1 to 2 g. twice daily orally or parenterally for 1 to 6 days) gives excellent results in a high proportion of cases (6), the oedema often disappearing within 24 hours. Chlorothiazide (2 g. twice daily by mouth or 0·5 g. twice daily by intravenous or intramuscular injection, each for 3 to 4 days) is also effective (7). The use of diuretics before calving may be dangerous if considerable fluid is lost. Although interference with venous drainage resulting from pressure of the foetus in the pelvic cavity is thought to be the primary cause, hypoproteinaemia has been proposed as a predisposing cause. The administration of plasma protein, although unlikely to be used as a practical measure, is reported to be an effective treatment (2). It is a common recommendation that the amount of grain fed in the last few weeks of pregnancy be limited and there is evidence that heavy grain feeding predisposes to the condition, at least in heifers (9).

Simple congestion causing a hard, localized plaque along the floor of a quarter is most common after parturition in heifers and is relatively innocuous but may interfere with milking. If repeated for a number of lactations it may cause permanent thickening of the skin (scleroderma) of the lateral aspect of the udder (8). Hot fomentations, massage and the application of liniments are of value in reducing the hardness and swelling.

Rupture of the Suspensory Ligaments of the Udder. Rupture of the suspensory ligaments occurs most commonly in adult cows and develops gradually over a number of years. When it occurs acutely, just before or after parturition, the udder drops markedly, is swollen and hard, and serum oozes through the skin. Severe oedema occurs at the base of the udder. It may be confused with gangrenous mastitis on cursory examination. Partial relief may be obtained with a suspensory apparatus but complete recovery does not occur.

Agalactia. Partial or complete absence of milk flow may affect one or more mammary glands and is of major importance in sows although it occurs occasionally in cattle. The importance of the disease in sows derives from the fact that piglets are very susceptible to hypoglycaemia. The condition may be due to failure of 'let-down' or absence of milk secretion (1, 11).

The causes of failure of 'let-down' include painful conditions of the teat, sharp teeth in the piglets, inverted nipples which interfere with sucking, primary failure of milk ejection especially in gilts and excessive engorgement and oedema of the udder. In many sows the major disturbance seems to be hysteria which is readily cured by the use of ataractic drugs. Treatment of the primary condition and the parenteral administration of oxytocin, repeated if necessary, is usually adequate.

Absence of milk secretion is commonly due to severe toxaemia. Affected sows show fever (39·5 to 41 °C or 103 to 106 °F), lack of appetite, constipation, swelling and congestion of the udder, a moderate, often creamy vaginal discharge, disinclination to rise and a stiff gait. The course of the disease is usually 3 or 4 days, recovered sows coming back onto their feed but rarely back to full milk production so that the piglets are stunted and many may die. Some sows are sick for several weeks and have a protracted convalescence; a few die. *E. coli* is often present in pure cultures in milk and vaginal discharges, but whether mastitis and metritis are present is uncertain. In many instances a series of sows in a piggery will be affected one after the other and a specific infectious disease is suspected. In one instance a mycoplasma was isolated and the syndrome was reproduced by injection of the organism into pathogen-free sows (13). The most commonly used treatment in such cases is a combination of broad spectrum antibiotic and oxytocin. When animals have been affected for several days the response in milk flow is often quite transitory and many of the sucking pigs die. A combination of antibiotic and corticosteroid has also been recommended (5) but results obtained are not greatly improved.

Ergotism may be a specific cause of agalactia in sows and has been recorded in animals fed on bull-rush millet infested with ergot (12).

Apparent hormonal defects do occur, particularly in cattle. In heifers and gilts there may be complete absence of mammary development and, in such cases, no treatment is likely to be of value. In animals which have lactated normally after previous parturitions, the parenteral administration of chorionic gonadoptrophin has been recommended but often produces no apparent improvement.

Cutaneous Gangrene. This condition occurs sporadically and usually in heifers with distended udders which show marked congestion and oedema. There is little or no systemic effect but the lesions may interfere with milking. The clinical description of this disease suggests that it is probably identical with ulcerative bovine mammillitis and is also described there.

'Black Pox'. This is a clinical entity only, although a pure culture of *Staphylococcus aureus* is frequently isolated from the lesions. The lesions occur only on the teats and take the form of deep, crater-shaped ulcers with raised edges and a black spot in the centre. The lesions are confined almost entirely to the tip of the teat, usually invade the sphincter and are responsible for a great deal of mastitis. Treatment is usually by topical application of ointments. Whitfield's, 10 per cent salicylic, 5 per cent sulphathiazole and 5 per cent salicylic, 5 per cent copper sulphate are all recommended. An iodophors ointment, or iodophor teat dip with 35 per cent added glycerol, are also effective but treat-ment needs to be thorough and repeated and milking machine errors need to be corrected (4).

Udder Impetigo. This disease is of importance because of the discomfort it causes, its common association with staphylococcal mastitis, its not uncommon spread to milkers' hands (10) and the frequency with which it is mistaken for cowpox. The lesions are usually small pustules (2 to 4 mm. diameter) but in occasional animals they extend to the subcutaneous tissue and appear as furuncles or boils. The commonest site is the hairless skin at the base of the teats but the lesions may spread from here on to the teats and over the udder generally. Spread in the herd appears to occur during milking and a large proportion of a herd may become affected over a relatively long period. The institution of suitable sanitation procedures, such as dipping teats after milking, washing of udders before milking and treatment of individual lesions with a suitable antiseptic ointment as described under the control of mastitis usually stops further spread. An ancillary measure is to vaccinate all cows in the herd with an autogenous bacterin produced from the *Staph. aureus* which is always present. Good immunity is produced for about 6 months but the disease recurs unless satisfactory sanitation measures are introduced.

Neoplasms of the Udder. Neoplasms of the bovine udder are particularly rare (3). Mammary carcinoma occurs occasionally in mares and is characterized by great malignancy. Neoplasms of the skin of the udder may spread to involve mammary tissue.

REFERENCES

(1) Hebeler, H. F. (1954). *Vet. Rec.*, *66*, 871.
(2) Larson, B. L. & Hays, R. L. (1958). *J. Dairy Sci.*, *41*, 995.
(3) Povey, R. C. & Osborne, A. D. (1969). *Path. vet.*, *6*, 502.
(4) Jackson, E. R. (1970). *Vet. Rec.*, *87*, 2.
(5) Noble, W. A. *et al.* (1960). *Vet. Rec.*, *72*, 60, 225, 266.
(6) Gouge, H. E. *et al.* (1959). *Vet. Med.*, *54*, 342.
(7) Snider, G. W. *et al.* (1962). *Canad. vet. J.*, *3*, 150.
(8) Cadwallader, W. P. & McEntee, K. (1966). *Cornell Vet.*, *56*, 353.
(9) Emery, R. S. *et al.* (1969). *J. Dairy Sci.*, *52*, 345.
(10) Zinn, R. D. (1961). *J. Amer. vet. med. Ass.*, *138*, 382.
(11) Loveday, R. K. (1964). *J. S. Afr. vet. med. Ass.*, *35*, 229.
(12) Shone, D. K. *et al.* (1959). *Vet. Rec.*, *71*, 129.
(13) Moore, R. W. *et al.* (1966). *Vet. Med.*, *61*, 883.

15

Diseases Caused by Bacteria—I

DISEASES CAUSED BY
STREPTOCOCCUS Spp.

MASTITIS caused by *Streptococcus agalactia*, *Str. dysgalactiae*, *Str. uberis* and *Str. zooepidemicus* is dealt with in the section on mastitis. Strangles in horses, neonatal streptococcal infections and streptococcal cervical abscesses of pigs are dealt with in this section.

Other miscellaneous diseases in which streptococci appear to have aetiological significance include septicaemic infections of swine, sheep and calves, pneumonia in calves, meningo-encephalitis and otitis media in feeder pigs, lymphangitis in foals, and infectious dermatitis of piglets.

Acute streptococcal septicaemia of adult sows and their litters occurs sporadically (1, 9). The onset is sudden and death occurs in from 12 to 48 hours. Clinically there is weakness, prostration, fever, dyspnoea, dysentery and haematuria. At necropsy, petechial and ecchymotic haemorrhages are present throughout all organs. Animals which survive for several days show extensive oedema and consolidation of the lungs. The infection spreads rapidly and the mortality rate may be very high unless the drug sensitivity of the organism, usually *Str. zooepidemicus*, is determined and appropriate treatment instituted.

Septicaemia with sudden deaths in calves has also been recorded in which *Str. pneumoniae* was the apparent cause (2). *Str. zooepidemicus* has also caused heavy losses in sheep, up to 90 per cent mortality occurring in groups of lambs (3). Pneumonia in calves may be caused commonly by *Str. pneumoniae* in some areas (4) and unidentified streptococci are common invaders in viral pneumonia of calves. Infections in calves with *Str. pneumoniae* may have public health significance; the isolation of identical strains of the organism from the lungs of calves dying of the disease and from the throats of their human attendants suggests that interspecies transmission may occur (10). Calves may be immunized either by the use of antiserum (11) or through vaccination of their dams

with a polyvalent aluminium hydroxide adsorbed vaccine (12). Good therapeutic results have been obtained with chloramphenicol (13). Meningo-encephalitis is a common complication of streptococcal septicaemia of the newborn but it has also occurred in feeder pigs of five to six months of age (5). An ulcerative lymphangitis, caused in many instances by *Str. zooepidemicus*, has been observed in foals from six months to two years of age (6) and may be confused with ulcerative lymphangitis. Infectious dermatitis (contagious pyoderma) of pigs is characterized by the formation of pustules about the face and neck and, to a less extent the trunk (7). Streptococci and staphylococci are present in the lesions and spread appears to occur through abrasions, especially in young pigs which fight and have not had their needle teeth removed. The disease may be confused with exudative epidermitis.

Streptococcal infections of the genital tract occur commonly, especially in mares, in which the disease is thought to be spread by coitus, and is accompanied by a high incidence of abortion, sterility and neonatal infection in foals. Foals from infected mares may be affected each year. Although streptococcal metritis occurs in sows, there appears to be no relationship between uterine infection and neonatal septicaemia. Abortions in sows may be due in some instances to infection with beta-haemolytic streptococci (8).

REFERENCES

(1) Bryant, J. B. (1945). *J. Amer. vet. med. Ass.*, *106*, 18.
(2) Donald, I. G. & Mann, S. O. (1950). *Vet. Rec.*, *62*, 257.
(3) Rafyi, A. & Mir Chamsy, H. (1953). *Bull. Acad. vét. Fr.*, *26*, 145.
(4) Hammer, D. (1956). *Zbl. Bakt.* 1, *161*, 269, cited in (1956), *Vet. Bull.*, *26*, 1.
(5) Jansen, J. A. C. & van Dorssen, C. A. (1951). *T. Diergeneesk.*, *76*, 815.
(6) Stepkowski, S. & Woloszyn, S. (1958). *Ann. Univ. M. Curie, Sklodowska*, Sect. DD. *11*, 229.
(7) Hjarre, A. (1948). *Skand. Vet.-Tidskr.*, *38*, 662.
(8) Saunders, C. N. (1958). *Vet. Rec.*, *70*, 965.
(9) Baker, W. L. (1960). *Vet. Med.*, *55*, 32.
(10) Romer, O. (1960). *Nord. Vet.-Med.*, *12*, 73.

(11) Romer, O. (1959). *Nord. Vet.-Med.*, *11*, 653.
(12) Fey, H. & Richle, R. (1961). *Schweiz. Arch. Tierheilk.*, *103*, 349.
(13) Wachnik, Z. (1963). *Med. Wet.*, *19*, 156.

Strangles

(*Distemper*)

Strangles is an acute disease of horses caused by infection with *Streptococcus equi*. It is characterized by inflammation of the upper respiratory tract and abscessation in the adjacent lymph nodes.

Incidence

The distribution of strangles is world wide although, with the decline in horse numbers and improvement in therapy, it has become of minor importance in most countries. The major epidemics which used to occur in mounted units of the armed forces, in remount depots and draught horse stables are now reduced for the most part to minor outbreaks in polo and racing stables and to individual horses taken to fairs and riding schools.

When an outbreak does occur in a large group of horses, it is usually restricted to the younger age groups and the morbidity rate may be as low as 10 per cent. Under adverse climatic conditions, and when shelter is inadequate, or when the group is made up of predominantly young horses, up to 100 per cent may be affected. Such a high incidence is often encountered soon after large numbers of susceptible horses, which may have come from many localities, are stabled together.

The mortality rate with adequate early treatment is very low but may reach 1 to 2 per cent due to occasional extension of infection to other organs. Purpura haemorrhagica may also be an important sequel.

Aetiology

Str. equi is present in the nasal discharge and abscesses and young, pure cultures of the organism are capable of producing the disease (1). Horses are the only species affected, the disease occurring in animals of any age but particularly in the one to five year age group. Outbreaks can occur at any time of the year but are most likely to happen in cold, wet weather. The movement of horses has more influence on the occurrence of outbreaks than the climate. Although strong immunity occurs immediately after an attack, a horse may suffer repeated attacks at intervals of about six months if the infection is a virulent one and persists in the group.

Transmission

The source of infection in strangles is the nasal discharge from infected animals which contaminates pasture and feed and water troughs. Such animals can spread infection for at least 4 weeks after a clinical attack. The organism is relatively resistant to environmental influences and mediate contagion can occur in infected premises for about a month after affected animals have been removed. Infection occurs by ingestion or by inhalation of droplets.

Pathogenesis

Infection of the pharyngeal and nasal mucosae causes an acute pharyngitis and rhinitis. Drainage to local lymph nodes results in abscessation and the infection may spread to other organs causing the development of suppurative processes in the kidney, brain, liver, spleen, tendon sheaths and joints.

Clinical Findings

After an incubation period of 4 to 8 days, the disease develops suddenly with complete anorexia, fever (39·5 to 40·5 °C or 103 to 105 °F), a serous nasal discharge, which rapidly becomes copious and purulent, and a severe pharyngitis and laryngitis. Rarely there is a mild conjunctivitis. The pharyngitis may be so severe that the animal is unable to swallow, and attempts to swallow food or water are often followed by regurgitation through the nostrils. A soft, moist cough which causes apparent pain and is easily stimulated by compression of the pharynx is constant. The head may be extended to ease the pain in the throat.

A febrile reaction commonly subsides in 2 to 3 days but soon returns as the characteristic abscesses develop in the lymph nodes of the throat region. The affected nodes become hot, swollen and painful. The purulent nasal discharge increases and there may be obstruction to swallowing and respiration. Obvious swelling of the nodes may take 3 to 4 days to develop and, in many cases, if treatment is not effective, the glands begin to exude serum at about 10 days and rupture to discharge thick, cream-yellow pus soon afterwards.

If the infection is particularly severe, many other lymph nodes, including the pharyngeal, submaxillary and parotid nodes may abscess at the same time. Local abscesses may also occur at any point on the body surface, particularly on the face and limbs, and the infection may spread to local lymphatic vessels causing obstructive oedema. This occurs most frequently in the lower limbs where extreme oedema may cause the part to swell to three or four times the normal size. It is probable that abscess formation in other organs also occurs at this time. Purpura haemorrhagica and empyema of the guttural pouches are occasional sequels after an attack of strangles.

Atypical forms of the disease occur as a result of metastasis and abscess formation in other organs; metastatic spread to the lungs may cause the development of acute pneumonia; cerebral involvement usually takes the form of purulent meningitis with signs of excitation, hyperaesthesia, rigidity of the neck and terminal paralysis; infected thrombi in veins occur rarely and cause local signs of vascular obstruction; abscesses may develop in the liver, spleen or visceral lymph nodes and may cause death if rupture occurs weeks or months after apparent recovery from the acute form of the disease. A specific syndrome has been described in which pericarditis and arthritis occur and from which *Str. faecalis* has been isolated. Clinically there are severe lameness, dyspnoea and an increased cardiac impulse.

The disease in burros is manifested by different signs and lesions from those in horses (4). Strangles in burros is a slowly developing, debilitating disease. At post mortem examination the characteristic lesions consist of caseation and calcification of abdominal lymph nodes.

Clinical Pathology

Nasal swabs and discharges from abscesses can be examined for the presence of *Str. equi* and sensitivity tests carried out on the cultures. There is a leucocytosis with a neutrophilia reaching a peak as the lymph nodes abscess. There may or may not be an anaemia due to the haemolytic effect of the streptococci or to toxic depression of haemopoiesis.

Necropsy Findings

In the rare fatalities that occur, necropsy examination usually reveals extensive suppuration in internal organs, especially the liver, spleen, lungs, pleura, large vessels and the peritoneum. When the latter is involved, it is usually due to extension from abscesses in the mesenteric lymph nodes.

Diagnosis

An upper respiratory tract infection with purulent nasal discharge and enlargement of the lymph nodes of the throat region are diagnostic of strangles. In the early stages of the disease it may be confused with equine viral rhinopneumonitis, equine viral arteritis and equine bronchitis but in these diseases there is usually no marked enlargement of the lymph nodes. Occasionally non-specific syndromes with purulent nasal discharges but no enlargement of the lymph nodes are found to be associated with infection by *Str. zooepidemicus*.

Treatment

Infected horses should be isolated and treatment commenced as soon as possible. Specific treatment comprises the parenteral administration of suitable antibiotics. The sulphonamides are quite effective but have been largely replaced by penicillin. The first injection should combine crystalline and procaine penicillin (1000 and 3000 units per lb. body weight respectively is not excessive) and be followed by procaine penicillin alone for two further injections at 24-hour intervals. Chlortetracycline is also effective. Provided treatment is commenced early, penicillin is quite adequate but at a later stage intravenous injections of one of the tetracyclines (5 mg. per lb. body weight per day) will be more effective (5) but must be continued over a longer time, say 4 to 5 days. The systemic involvement at least can be controlled but if abscessation in lymph nodes is advanced, the nodes may continue to enlarge and eventually rupture.

General treatment consists in providing good warm shelter, blanketing if necessary, a soft, palatable diet, keeping the nostrils and muzzle clean and, if time is available, giving steam inhalations. Surgical treatment of abscessed nodes is usually not necessary unless pressure causes dyspnoea.

Control

Infected animals should be isolated immediately. If the animal has been housed the stall should be thoroughly cleaned and disinfected and the bedding burned. Pails, brooms, grooming brushes and blankets should also be disinfected. Vaccination should be considered if a number of horses are exposed but infected horses should not be vaccinated.

A commercial vaccine, prepared by carefully killing young cultures of *Strep. equi* (2, 3), is administered in gradually increasing doses on two or three occasions at 10- to 14-day intervals. Vaccination should not be commenced until the foals are 12 weeks of age. Reactions at the site of vaccination are not unknown and careful skin preparation and after-injection massage are strongly recommended. Annual boosters of one injection are also recommended. The most that can be expected from such a vaccination programme is a reduction in the number of cases and in the severity of the illness in the cases that do occur. On the other hand the immunity produced may be sufficient to slow down or stop an outbreak.

REFERENCES

(1) Bryans, J. T. *et al.* (1964). *Cornell Vet.*, *54*, 198.
(2) Bazeley, P. L. (1942). *Aust. vet. J.*, *18*, 141 & 189, & (1943) *19*, 62.
(3) Engelbrecht, H. (1969). *J. Amer. vet. med. Ass.*, *155*, 425, 427.
(4) Wisecup, W. G. *et al.* (1967). *J. Amer. vet. med. Ass.*, *150*, 303.
(5) Sheetz, H. O. (1951). *Vet. Med.*, *46*, 38.

Neonatal Streptococcal Infection

Streptococcal infection of the newborn is characterized by involvement of the navel and the subsequent development of a bacteraemia resulting in localization of the infection in other organs, particularly the joints.

Incidence

Streptococci are the commonest cause of postnatal infections of foals, representing 50 per cent of such cases in some surveys (1). Up to 20 per cent of abortions in mares are found in similar surveys to be due to streptococci. Affected foals may die or be worthless because of permanent injury to joints.

In pigs, lambs (5) and calves the disease is sporadic but a high incidence may occur on individual farms.

Aetiology

Str. genitalium (*Str. pyogenes equi*) is usually recovered from the joints of infected foals and may also be present in the uterus of the mare and in aborted foetuses. The streptococcus isolated from clinically affected piglets and their normal litter mates (7), and which is capable of producing the disease experimentally (2), is in group D but it has not been accurately identified and it is proposed that it be called *Streptococcus suis*. In one survey *Str. equisimilis* was found to be the predominant streptococcus causing disease in pigs (8). Group C streptococci and *Str. faecalis* have been isolated from cases of polyarthritis and endocarditis in lambs (6) and *Str. pyogenes* from swollen joints in calves (7).

Transmission

The source of the infection is usually the environment which may be contaminated by uterine discharges from infected dams or by discharges from lesions in other animals. The portal of infection in most instances appears to be the umbilicus, and continued patency of the urachus is thought to be a contributing factor in that it delays healing of the navel. Contamination of the umbilicus may result from infected soil or bedding, although in the special occurrence of the disease in calves in the southern U.S.A., the screwworm fly (*Cochlyomyia americana*) is known to act in a passive carrier (7).

Pathogenesis

The infection spreads from the navel to cause an acute, fatal septicaemia, or a bacteraemia with suppurative localization in various organs, particularly the joints. Arthritis is the most common manifestation but other complications may be encountered. These include ophthalmitis in foals, meningitis and endocarditis in piglets, meningitis in calves and endocarditis in lambs.

Clinical Findings

Horses: Foals do not usually show signs until 2 to 3 weeks of age. The initial sign is usually a painful swelling of the navel and surrounding abdominal wall, often in the form of a flat plaque which may be 15 or 20 cm. in diameter. A discharge of pus may or may not be present and a patent urachus is a frequent accompaniment. A systemic reaction occurs but this is often mild with the temperature remaining at about 39·5°C (103°F). Lameness becomes apparent and is accompanied by obvious swelling and tenderness in one or more of the joints. The hock, stifle and knee joints are most commonly affected but in severe cases the distal joints are involved and there is occasionally extension to tendon sheaths. Lameness may be so severe that the foal lies down most of the time, sucks rarely and becomes extremely emaciated. There may be hypopyon in one or both eyes.

If treatment is begun in the early stages, recovery occurs but when joint involvement is severe, particularly if the abscesses have ruptured, the animal may have to be destroyed because of the resulting ankylosis. Death from septicaemia may occur in the early stages of the disease.

Pigs: Arthritis and meningitis may occur alone or together and are most common in the 2 to 6 weeks age group. The arthritis is identical with that described in foals above. With meningitis there is a systemic reaction comprising fever, anorexia and depression. The gait is stiff, the piglets standing on their toes and there is swaying of the hindquarters. The ears are often retracted against the head. Blindness and gross muscular tremor develop followed by inability to maintain balance, lateral recumbency, violent paddling and death. In many cases there is little clinical evidence of omphalophlebitis. With endocarditis the young pigs are usually found dead without premonitory signs having been observed.

Sheep: The incubation period is short, usually 2 to 3 days, and outbreaks occur soon after birth or docking. There is intense lameness with swelling of one or more joints appearing in a day or two. Pus accumulates and the joint capsule often ruptures. Recovery usually occurs with little residual enlargement of the joints, although there may be occasional deaths due to toxaemia.

Calves show polyarthritis, meningitis, ophthalmitis and omphalophlebitis. The ophthalmitis may appear very soon after birth. The arthritis is often chronic and causes little systemic illness. Calves with meningitis show hyperaesthesia, rigidity and fever.

Clinical Pathology

Pus from any source may be cultured to determine the organism present and its sensitivity to the drugs available. Bacteriological examination of the uterine discharges of the dam may be of value in determining the source of infection. The success rate with blood cultures is not very high but an attempt is worthwhile. The identification of the causative bacteria is important but the sensitivity of the organism may mean the difference between success and failure in treatment.

Examination of synovial fluid may be of value in estimating the extent of joint damage.

Necropsy Findings

In affected foals, calves and lambs, suppuration at the navel and severe suppurative arthritis affecting one or more joints are usual, and multiple abscesses may also be present in the liver, kidneys, spleen and lungs. Valvular endocarditis may be present in the lambs. Acute cases may die without suppurative lesions having had time to develop. Pigs show the same range of necropsy findings but in addition there will be large vegetative lesions on the heart valves in those dying of endocarditis (3, 4). Necropsy findings in the meningitic form in pigs include turbidity of the cerebrospinal fluid, congestion and inflammation of the meninges and an accumulation of whitish, purulent material in the subarachnoid space. In most cases the choroid plexuses are severely affected and the ventricles, aqueduct and central canal of the medulla and the cord may be blocked by exudate, in some cases sufficient to cause internal hydrocephalus. The nervous tissue of the spinal cord, cerebellum and brain stem may show liquefaction necrosis (2).

Diagnosis

Omphalophlebitis and suppurative arthritis in foals may be due to infection with *Escherichia coli*, *Actinobacillus equuli* or *Salmonella abortivoequina*, but these infections tend to take the form of a fatal septicaemia within a few days of birth whereas streptococcal infections are delayed in their onset and usually produce a polyarthritis. In pigs there may be sporadic cases of arthritis due to staphylococci but the streptococcal infection is the common one. Glasser's disease occurs usually in older pigs and is accompanied by pleurisy, pericarditis and peritonitis. Erysipelas in very young pigs is usually manifested by septicaemia. Nervous diseases of piglets may resemble arthritis on cursory examination but there is an absence of joint enlargement and lameness. However, the meningitic form of the streptococcal infection can easily be confused with viral encephalitides. Meningitis in young calves may also be caused by *Pasteurella multocida*. Polyarthritis in calves, lambs and piglets may also be caused by infection with *Corynebacterium pyogenes* and *Sphaerophorus necrophorus*.

The response of streptococcal infections to treatment with penicillin may be of value in the differentiation of the arthritides, and the microscopic and histological findings at necropsy enable exact differentiation to be made. In lambs suppurative arthritis occurs soon after birth and after docking. The other common arthritis in the new-born lamb is that caused by *Erysipelothrix insidiosa* but this usually occurs later and is manifested by lameness without pronounced joint enlargement. Calves may also develop erysipelatous arthritis.

Treatment

Penicillin is successful as treatment in all forms of the disease provided irreparable structural damage has not occurred. In new-born animals the dosage rate should be high (10,000 units per lb. body weight) and should be repeated at least once daily for 3 days. If suppuration is already present, a longer course of antibiotics will be necessary, preferably 7 to 10 days, and may be accompanied by the parenteral administration of enzymes on the last 4 days. Local or parenteral treatment with cortisone or similar drugs may also be provided if the infection is adequately controlled with antibiotics. General aspects of treatment are dealt with in the section on diseases of the newborn.

Control

The principles of control of diseases of the newborn are dealt with elsewhere. Because the most frequent source of infection in foals is the genital tract of the dam, some attempt should be made to treat the mare and limit the contamination of the environment. Mixed bacterins have been widely used to establish immunity in mares and foals against this infection but no proof has been presented that they are effective. On heavily infected premises the administration of long-acting penicillin at birth may be advisable. A major factor in the control of navel and joint-ill in lambs is the use of clean fields or pens for lambing, as umbilical infection originating from the environment seems to be more important than infection from the dam in this species. Docking should also be done in clean surroundings and, if necessary, temporary yards should be erected. Instruments should be chemically sterilized between lambs. Regardless of species and where practicable, all parturition stalls and pens should be kept clean and disinfected and the navels of all new-born animals disinfected at birth. Where screwworms are prevalent, the unhealed navels should be treated with a reliable repellent.

REFERENCES

(1) Gunning, O. V. (1947). *Vet. J.*, *103*, 47.
(2) Field, H. I. *et al.* (1954). *Vet. Rec.*, *66*, 453.
(3) Hont, S. & Banks, A. W. (1944). *Aust. vet. J.*, *20*, 206.
(4) Cotchin, E. & Hayward, A. (1953). *J. comp. Path.*, *63*, 68.
(5) Dennis, S. M. (1968). *Vet. Rec.*, *82*, 403.
(6) Jamieson, S. & Stuart, J. (1950). *J. Path. Bact.*, *62*, 235.
(7) Elliott, S. D. (1966). *J. Hyg.*, *Camb.*, *64*, 205, 213.

Streptococcal Cervical Abscess of Pigs

Cervical or 'jowl' abscess of pigs is observed mainly at slaughter. Clinically there is obvious enlargement of the lymph nodes of the throat region, particularly the mandibular nodes. It is of considerable importance because of the losses due to rejection of infected carcases at meat inspection.

Beta-haemolytic streptococci of Lancefield's Group E are the most common organisms found in the lesions (1) although *Past. multocida*, *E. coli* and *Cor. pyogenes* may also be present. The disease has been produced by feeding or the intranasal or intrapharyngeal instillation of the streptococci (2) and they are thought to be the cause, infection occurring through the pharyngeal mucosa from contaminated food and water. In herds where cervical abscess is a problem, streptococci can commonly be isolated from the vaginas of pregnant sows. Chlortetracycline fed at the rate of 50 g. per ton of feed is claimed to be an effective preventive (3) and vaccination of pregnant sows with an autogenous or commercial bacterin containing streptococci and staphylococci is

thought to be of value in protecting the litters of the vaccinated sows (4). Vaccination of young pigs appears to have no protective effect (5). A recent report indicating that pigs under 6 weeks of age are resistant to infection points to early weaning as a useful control measure, possibly combined with a short period of chlortetracycline feeding (6).

REFERENCES

(1) Collier, J. R. & Noel, J. (1971). *Amer. J. vet. Res.*, *32*, 1501, 1507.
(2) Armstrong, C. H. *et al.* (1970). *Amer. J. vet. Res.*, *31*, 1595.
(3) Gouge, H. E. *et al.* (1957). *J. Amer. vet. med. Ass.*, *131*, 324.
(4) Conner, G. H. *et al.* (1965). *J. Amer. vet. med. Ass.*, *147*, 479.
(5) Shuman, R. D. & Wood, R. L. (1968). *Cornell vet.*, *58*, 21.
(6) Schmitz, J. A. & Olson, L. D. (1972). *Amer. J. vet. Res.*, *33*, 1995.

DISEASES CAUSED BY *STAPHYLOCOCCUS* Spp.

Mastitis caused by *Staphylococcus aureus* is dealt with in the section on mastitis and udder impetigo of cattle in the section on miscellaneous abnormalities of the udder. Staphylococcal infection of the newborn, especially lambs, is relatively common and may be manifested by a high incidence of lesions in the myocardium. Infection may occur via marking wounds but in most cases the portal of entry appears to be the navel (1).

REFERENCE

(1) Dennis, S. J. (1966). *Vet. Rec.*, *79*, 38.

Tick Pyaemia of Lambs

(*Enzootic Staphylococcosis of Lambs*)

Tick pyaemia is a staphylococcal infection of lambs spread by the bites of ticks and is manifested by septicaemia, or by bacteraemia with subsequent localization occurring in many organs. The disease has been recorded only in the United Kingdom (1). It occurs in the early summer and causes serious losses in areas where tick infestations are heavy. Lambs are affected soon after birth and die quickly of septicaemia or show signs of arthritis or meningitis in the period between the second and fourth weeks of life. In cases where localization has occurred, suppurative lesions may be found in the skin, muscles, tendon sheaths, joints, viscera and meninges.

Tick pyaemia may occur in association with a number of other diseases including enterotoxaemia, louping-ill, lamb dysentery and tick-borne fever, and a concurrent infection with the last is thought to predispose to its development (2).

Tick pyaemia resembles other suppurative infections of the newborn, including infections caused by *Streptococcus* spp., but the lesions are much more extensive and infection enters through bites of the ticks rather than navel or docking wounds. The ticks are not thought to provide portals of entry for, nor to act as carriers of, the infection but to act as a precipitating cause possibly by causing intercurrent disease. *Staph. aureus* can be isolated from the lesions, and in affected flocks there is a high incidence of lambs carrying the same infection on their nasal mucosa (5). Cutaneous infection shows no such relationship. Although spread of the infection from the ewes to the lambs is not proven, the lambs acquire the infection during the first few days of life and the incidence of infection is highest in flocks kept in confined quarters. Control of the tick population is the obvious method of controlling the disease and dipping the lambs every 3 weeks in an organophosphatic insecticide is capable of greatly reducing the incidence of the clinical disease and increasing the weight gains of clinically normal lambs (6). Failing this, vaccination of the ewes with an autogenous bacterin during late pregnancy may be practised but is of doubtful value (3). Treatment with penicillin should be effective, provided lesions are not too advanced (4). Effective prophylaxis is obtained by the injection of 1 million units of benzathine penicillin but administration has to be timed at just before the period of greatest risk (7).

REFERENCES

(1) Watson, W. A. (1964). *Vet. Rec.*, *76*, 743, 793.
(2) Foster, W. M. N. & Cameron, A. E. (1968). *J. comp. Path.*, *78*, 243.
(3) Foggie, A. (1948). *J. comp. Path.*, *58*, 24.
(4) Foggie, A. (1953). *Vet. Rec.*, *65*, 169.
(5) Watson, W. A. (1965). *Vet. Rec.*, *77*, 477.
(6) Watson, W. A. (1966). *Vet. Rec.*, *79*, 101.
(7) Watt, J. A. (1968). *Vet. Rec.*, *83*, 507.

Exudative Epidermitis

(*Greasy Pig Disease*)

Exudative epidermitis of sucking pigs is a poorly defined disease thought to be caused by an unidentified bacteria. Clinically it is distinguished by the appearance of an acute, generalized, seborrhoeic dermatitis.

Incidence

The disease appears under various names. It is referred to as a non-specific 'eczema' in the United Kingdom, as exudative epidermitis and seborrhoea oleosa in the United States. It has also been recorded in Australia and Europe. The incidence is not high but many of the affected pigs die.

Aetiology

The disease can be reproduced by the inoculation of a Gram-positive organism designated as *Staphylococcus hyos* or *Staph. hyicus* (1, 2, 3, 8). It resembles closely a non-pathogenic staphylococcus but can be differentiated serologically (9). Field evidence suggests that environmental stress of various kinds, including agalactia in the sow and intercurrent infection, predisposes to the disease.

In many cases lesions develop first about the head, apparently in association with bite wounds which occur when the needle teeth have not been cut. Within litters the incidence is high, often all piglets being affected. Most cases occur in animals under 6 weeks of age but occasionally groups of pigs up to 3 months of age suffer from the disease.

Pathogenesis

The principal lesion is an inflammatory–exudative reaction in the corium and the upper layers of the epidermis (4).

Clinical Findings

Initially there is depression and a dull, lustreless hair coat, covered with thin dry scales. The skin becomes thickened, damp and oily, the appetite diminishes and the pig loses condition rapidly. There is no irritation or pruritis. In severe cases, the entire skin is covered with moist, greasy exudate and there is marked cutaneous erythema. The exudate may dry to form scabs which lift, leaving a raw skin surface. Progressive weakness is followed by death in a few days. In more chronic cases, the skin lesions are not so widespread and the course is longer; small vesicles and ulcers may be observed as the initial lesions and the skin subsequently become thickened and wrinkled. The scabs are also thicker and crack along flexion lines, forming deep fissures. Most affected pigs die in from 1 to 3 weeks.

Clinical Pathology

Bacteriological examination of skin swabs may reveal the presence of streptococci but their aetiological significance is doubtful.

Necropsy Findings

At necropsy there are macroscopic lesions in the skin and kidneys. A white precipitate is found in the papillary ducts and the renal pelvis, and the kidneys are pale and wet. There are degenerative changes in the renal tubular epithelium, retention of urine within the kidneys and blockage of the ureters. Lesions in the central nervous system have also been described (5).

Diagnosis

Parakeratosis may be confused with this disease, but there is no seborrhoea and the crusts are thick and crumbly. Older pigs are affected, not sucklings, and there is response to supplementation of the diet with zinc. Swine pox affects pigs of this age and the presence of lice and the appearance of vesicular or discrete scabby lesions, usually beginning about the head, should serve to identify it. Other miscellaneous skin conditions, including infestation with harvest mites, are not accompanied by seborrhoea and can be diagnosed on examination of skin scrapings. A congenital dermatosis of pigs characterized by the development of lesions on the lower extremities and interference with hoof growth is also recorded (6). The lesions spread over the body and are often accompanied by a giant-cell tumour of the lungs. Affected pigs usually die at about 6 weeks of age.

Treatment

Treatment should include the administration of a wide-spectrum antibiotic, tylosin being specially recommended (3), and the alleviation of the environmental stress whatever its nature. If topical applications are to be used cloxacillin ointment in conjunction with parenteral treatment with penicillin is reported as a successful combination (7). In all treatments early applications are essential. Advanced cases respond very poorly.

Control

No positive control measures can be recommended. Supplementary feeding of piglets when milk is short, and the cutting of the needle teeth at birth are advised. Immunity develops within a herd and the use of an autogenous vaccine on pregnant sows could be a logical procedure in severely affected herds.

REFERENCES

(1) Mebus, C. A. et al. (1968). Path. vet., 5, 146.
(2) L'Ecuyer, C. (1967). Canad. J. comp. Med., 31, 243.
(3) Van Os, J. L. (1967). T. Diergeneesk., 92, 662.
(4) Bollevahn, W. et al. (1970). Dtsch. tierärztl. Wschr., 77, 601.
(5) Blood, D. C. & Jubb, K. V. (1957). Aust. vet. J., 33, 126.
(6) Hjarre, A. (1953). Dtsch. tierärztl. Wschr., 60, 105.
(7) L'Ecuyer, C. & Alexander, D. C. (1969). Canad. J. vet. Med., 10, 227.
(8) Schulz, W. (1969). Arch. exp. vet. Med., 23, 415.
(9) Hunter, D. et al. (1970). Brit. vet. J., 126, 225.

DISEASES CAUSED BY CORYNEBACTERIUM Spp.

Cor. pyogenes is an ubiquitous organism and occurs in many animal diseases either as a primary cause or as a secondary invader. Its role in the production of mastitis in cattle is described in the section on mastitis, and as a secondary invader in calf and sheep pneumonia in the descriptions of the viral pneumonias of calves and sheep. Infection of the uterus of mares and cows is commonly associated with sterility and abortion or in the birth of infected young. The disease must be differentiated from those caused by Salm. abortivoequina and Str. genitalium, and equine viral rhinopneumonitis and equine viral arteritis. The bacteriology, occurrence, method of transmission and susceptibility of the organism to various drugs have been reviewed (1). Most corynebacteria have been recorded as causes of perinatal deaths of lambs (12). The bizarre occurrence in cattle of abscessation of the pituitary gland both by itself and in association with other lesions has been recorded (13).

Cor. pseudotuberculosis has been determined to cause a nonsuppurative arthritis and bursitis in lambs in an area where caseous lymphadenitis does not occur (2). The joints are only slightly enlarged and many animals show only mild clinical signs. Recovery occurs if the lambs are fed and confined. This bacterium may also be present in outbreaks of foot abscess in sheep (8).

Cor. pseudotuberculosis has been isolated from deer and from engorged female ticks (Dermacentor albipictus) feeding on the deer. Transmissibility between sheep and deer, possibly by means of the bites of ticks, is suggested (3). The occurrence of ulcerative lymphangitis in an isolated group of horses has also suggested that wild animals may act as vectors of the organism (4). Suppurative orchitis in rams caused by Cor. pseudotuberculosis has been recorded in South Africa (7), New Zealand (5) and the U.S.A. (6) and may be confused with epididymitis caused by Brucella ovis. The corynebacterial infection is considered to be a specific transmissible disease of sheep.

In horses in California (9, 10, 11) Cor. pseudotuberculosis infections have also been associated with a high incidence of chronic abscesses, chiefly in the pectoral region but in some animals extending as far back as the mammary gland. The abscesses appear to develop in a deep site and may reach a diameter of 10 to 20 cm., with a surrounding area of oedema, before they rupture 1 to 4 weeks later. Occasional generalized cases occur, the internal lesions being located chiefly in the abdominal cavity and being palpable rectally particularly in and around the kidney. The disease occurs in an area where caseous lymphadenitis is common in sheep but the portal of entry of infection is unknown. Because of the seasonal occurrence of the disease its transmission by insect vectors has been suggested but not confirmed.

REFERENCES

(1) Purdom, M. R. et al. (1958). Vet. Rev. Annot., 4, 55.
(2) Marsh, H. (1947). Amer. J. vet. Res., 8, 294.
(3) Humphreys, F. A. & Gibbons, R. J. (1942). Canad. J. comp. Med., 6, 35.
(4) Mitchell, C. A. & Walker, R. V. L. (1944). Canad. J. comp. Med., 8, 3.
(5) Dodd, D. C. & Hartley, W. J. (1955). N.Z. vet. J., 3, 105.
(6) McGowan, B. & Shultz, G. (1956). Cornell Vet., 46, 277.
(7) Belonje, C. W. A. (1951). J. S. Afr. vet. med. Ass., 22, 165.
(8) Gardner, D. E. (1961). N.Z. vet. J., 9, 59.
(9) Hughes, J. P. & Biberstein, E. L. (1959). J. Amer. vet. med. Ass., 135, 559.
(10) Hughes, J. P. et al. (1962). Cornell Vet., 52, 51.
(11) Knight, H. D. (1969). J. Amer. vet. med. Ass., 155, 446.
(12) Dennis, S. M. & Bamford, V. W. (1966). Vet. Rec., 79, 105.
(13) Taylor, P. A. & Meads, E. B. (1963). Canad. Vet. J., 4, 208.

Contagious Bovine Pyelonephritis

Contagious bovine pyelonephritis is a specific infection of the urinary tract of cattle caused by *Cor. renale* and characterized by chronic purulent inflammation in the bladder, ureters and kidneys.

Incidence

The disease is widespread in Europe and North America although it seldom constitutes an important problem in any herd or area. As a rule, clinical cases appear sporadically, even in herds found to harbour a significant number of carriers. Unless appropriate treatment is instituted early, the disease is highly fatal and economic loss is due mainly to deaths of the affected animals.

Aetiology

Cor. renale, the specific aetiological agent, has little apparent resistance to physical or chemical agents. It is readily isolated from the urine of affected or carrier animals. It has been shown that *Cor. pseudotuberculosis, Cor. pyogenes, Act. equuli, E. coli* and *Staph. aureus* are capable of producing renal lesions in mice following intravenous injection (1) and some of these organisms are sometimes found in the urinary tract of cattle and pigs affected with pyelonephritis, either alone or associated with *Cor. renale*. Because of the ease with which pyelonephritis can be produced by causing stagnation of

urine, it is likely that the primary cause of the disease is temporary or permanent obstruction of part of the urinary tract. *Cor. renale*, because of its particular ability to grow in urine, is the most common pathogen present in these circumstances.

Although pyelonephritis is considered to be essentially a bovine disease, sheep are occasionally affected (5). Cattle are seldom affected before maturity and cows appear to be much more susceptible than bulls. An increase in clinical cases is usually found in the colder seasons of the year and heavily fed, high-producing dairy herds appear to show an increased susceptibility.

Transmission

Although the intravenous injection of *Cor. renale* has been shown to produce renal lesions in mice (2), the vulva is thought to be the portal of entry in the cow. Typical lesions can be established in some animals by the introduction of the organism into the bladder (1). Clinically affected or clinically normal 'carrier' cows are probably the principal source of infection, the disease being transmitted by direct contact, brushing the vulva of clean cows with contaminated brushes, service by infected or contaminated bulls or by the careless use of catheters. The incidence of cows excreting *Cor. renale* in their urine is higher in herds where the disease occurs than in herds where the disease is unknown (3).

Pathogenesis

Pyelonephritis usually appears to develop as an ascending infection involving successively the bladder, ureters and kidneys. The destruction of renal tissue and obstruction of urinary outflow ultimately result in uraemia and the death of the animal.

Clinical Findings

Early signs vary considerably from case to case. The first sign observed may be the passage of blood-stained urine in an otherwise normal cow. In other cases, the first sign may be an attack of acute colic, passing off in a few hours. Such attacks are caused by obstruction of a ureter or renal calyx by pus or tissue debris and may be confused with acute intestinal obstruction. More often the onset is gradual with a fluctuating temperature (about 39·5 °C or 103 °F), capricious appetite, loss of condition and fall in milk yield over a period of weeks. Other than this, there is little systemic reaction and the diagnostic signs are associated with the urinary tract. The most obvious sign is the presence of blood, pus, mucus and tissue debris in the urine, particularly in the last portion voided. Urination is frequent and may be painful. Periods during which the urine is abnormal may be followed by apparent recovery with later remissions. In the early stages, rectal examination may be negative but later there is usually detectable thickening and contraction of the bladder wall and enlargement of one or both ureters. The terminal portion of the latter may be palpated through the floor of the vagina over the neck of the bladder. One or both of the kidneys may show enlargement, absence of lobulation and pain on palpation. The course is usually several weeks or even months and the terminal signs are those of uraemia.

Clinical Pathology

The presence of *Cor. renale* in suspected urine can be confirmed by culture or direct microscopic examination. Blood constituents remain normal until the later stages when the waste products ordinarily eliminated by the kidneys will be increased. The urine will contain blood cells and protein. A diagnostic serological test has been reported (1).

Necropsy Findings

Characteristic necropsy findings are limited to the kidneys, ureters and bladder. The kidneys are usually enlarged and the lobulation less evident than normal. Light coloured necrotic areas may be observed on the surface and the pelvis and grossly enlarged ureters will contain blood, pus and mucus. Abscesses and necrotic areas may be observed in the cut lobules. The bladder and urethra are thick-walled and their mucous membranes are haemorrhagic, oedematous and eroded.

Diagnosis

The gross changes in urine, together with palpable abnormalities in the urinary tract and the presence of bacteria including *Cor. renale* in the urine, are sufficient basis for a diagnosis of contagious bovine pyelonephritis. Cases characterized by acute colic can be differentiated from acute intestinal obstruction by the absence of a palpable obstruction and the disappearance of abdominal pain within a few hours. Chronic cases may be confused with traumatic reticulitis but may be differentiated by the urine changes present in pyelonephritis. Sporadic cases of non-specific cystitis can only be differentiated by culture of the urine. Other causes of haematuria must be considered but, for the most part, they are not associated with pyuria. Enzootic haematuria resembles contagious bovine pyelonephritis clinically but it occurs only

in certain areas, the lesions are confined to the bladder, and the urine is sterile. Death in this disease usually results from haemorrhagic anaemia.

Treatment

Prior to the introduction of penicillin, treatment of pyelonephritis was seldom undertaken successfully. Acidification of the urine by the administration of monobasic sodium phosphate (4 oz. daily for several days) was frequently followed by clinical improvement but seldom by permanent recovery.

Although several antibiotics appear to inhibit *Cor. renale*, penicillin remains the antibiotic of choice for treatment of pyelonephritis. Large doses (5,000,000 units of procaine penicillin G) are recommended every second day for five injections. In early cases where little structural damage has occurred, permanent recovery can be expected following such a course of treatment. In general, a good prognosis is suggested by an improvement in condition, appetite and milk yield and clearing of the urine. However, in well-established cases, relapse is not uncommon and, where tissue destruction has been extensive, relief through antibiotic therapy is only temporary. The parenteral injection of enzyme preparations may improve the usual recovery rate of 50 per cent when penicillin alone is used (4).

Control

No specific control measures are usually practised but isolation of affected animals and destruction of infected litter and bedding should reduce the population of the organism in the local environment and minimize the opportunity for transmission.

REFERENCES

(1) Hitamune, T. *et al.* (1972). *Res. vet. Sci., 13*, 82.
(2) Lovell, R. & Cotchin, E. (1952). *J. comp. Path., 62*, 245.
(3) Morse, E. V. (1950). *Cornell Vet., 40*, 178.
(4) Arthur, G. H. (1949). *Vet. Rec., 61*, 257.
(5) Allen, R. C. *et al.* (1959). *J. Amer. vet. med. Ass., 134*, 235.

Cystitis and Pyelonephritis of Pigs

This disease is well recognized in swine practice but little accurate information is available about it. In many cases adult sows become ill quite suddenly, show profound depression and circulatory collapse and die within 12 hours. In the early stages of the disease, the frequent passage of blood-stained, turbid urine accompanied by vaginal discharge, occurs in sows 3 to 4 weeks after service (1). Infection may be introduced at mating or be residual from the previous farrowing. The relationship to mating has been well-established and it has been suggested that sows which bleed or show pain after service should be treated prophylactically with a broad-spectrum antibiotic (4). Haematuria for a few days has also been observed in boars in the early stages of the disease. The appetite is normal or slightly reduced and there is no febrile reaction but excessive thirst may occur. At necropsy, cystitis is the main lesion with ureteritis and pyelonephritis occurring in some pigs. *Cor. suis* can be isolated from the urine of the live pig and the lesions of the urinary tract at necropsy, in some cases in conjunction with other bacteria (2). Because of the occurrence of the disease after service, the presence of *Cor. suis* in the urine, semen and sheath of normal boars but only in association with pathological conditions in sows (3), and the apparent ascending nature of the disease, venereal transmission seems likely. Early treatment with penicillin should be effective but, if lesions are well advanced, relapse commonly occurs.

REFERENCES

(1) Soltys, M. A. & Spratling, F. R. (1957). *Vet. Rec.*, 69, 500.
(2) Weidlich, N. (1954). *Zbl. Vet.-Med.*, 1, 455.
(3) Soltys, M. A. (1961). *J. Path. Bact.*, 81, 441.
(4) Biering-Sorensen, U. (1967). *Medlemsbl. danske Dyrlægeforen.*, 24, 1103.

Caseous Lymphadenitis of Sheep

Caseous lymphadenitis is a chronic disease of sheep characterized by the formation of abscesses in lymph nodes and exerting little effect on the general health of the sheep unless the disease becomes generalized.

Incidence

The disease appears to be of importance whereever sheep are raised in large numbers. In most cases the disease has little effect on the health of affected sheep but in rare instances generalization may occur and cause death. The important losses are caused by restriction on the use of affected carcases. The morbidity in flocks of adult sheep may be as high as 70 per cent.

Aetiology

Corynebacterium pseudotuberculosis is the specific cause of the disease. It is also the cause of ulcerative lymphangitis of cattle and horses, contagious and suppurative arthritis of lambs, suppurative orchitis of rams and contagious acne of horses, but these have been dealt with as separate diseases because they do not occur in association with caseous lymphadenitis.

Caseous lymphadenitis in sheep reaches a peak of incidence in adults because of repeated exposure to infection at each shearing. The disease has also been observed in goats (1).

Transmission

The source of infection is the discharges from ruptured lymph nodes. Contamination of the soil on bedding grounds or in shelters may result in persistence of the organism in the environment for very long periods. Infection gains entrance to the body through shearing wounds and less commonly through the navel and docking wounds. At shearing time, affected nodes may be ruptured and contamination of the shears leads to contamination of subsequent skin wounds unless the shears are properly cleaned and disinfected.

Pathogenesis

Spread of infection from infected skin wounds leads to involvement of local lymph nodes and the development of abscesses. Less commonly, bloodborne infection may result in abscess formation in many organs including lung, liver, kidney, brain and spinal cord (2).

Clinical Findings

There is palpable enlargement of one or more of the superficial lymph nodes. Those most commonly affected are the submaxillary, prescapular, prefemoral, supramammary and popliteal nodes. The abscesses commonly rupture and thick, green pus is discharged. In rare cases in which systemic involvement occurs, chronic pneumonia, pyelonephritis, ataxia and paraplegia may be present. In ewes, local spread from the supramammary lymph node to the mammary tissue is common. The resulting fall in milk yields leads to poor growth and even death of lambs and this may be a serious economic feature in badly affected flocks.

Clinical Pathology

Examination of pus for the presence of *Cor. pseudotuberculosis* is the only laboratory aid available. Allergic tests have been used but are unreliable (3). Agglutination (8) and anti-haemolysininhibition (7) tests on serum have been reported to be reliable and practical.

Necropsy Findings

Caseous abscesses filled with greenish yellow pus occur chiefly in lymph nodes and to a lesser extent in internal organs. In the early stages the pus is soft and pasty but in the later stages it is firm and dry and has a characteristic laminated appearance. Diffuse bronchopneumonia, with more fluid pus of a similar colour, may also be present.

Diagnosis

Palpable enlargements of peripheral lymph nodes as a flock problem in sheep are usually due to this disease. The caseous, greenish pus is diagnostic. Caseous lymphadenitis runs a much more chronic course than that of meliodosis although the lesions in the two diseases have a superficial similarity. Suppurative lymphadenitis in lambs has been found to be caused by infection with *Past. multocida* (4) and a disease characterized by the presence of yellow-green pus in abscesses situated in close proximity to the lymph nodes of sheep is caused by a Gram-positive micrococcus. The latter disease occurs in France and Kenya and is referred to as Morel's disease (9).

Treatment

Treatment is not usually attempted although the organism is susceptible to penicillin. The local formation of abscesses is unlikely to respond to other than surgical treatment and the usual non-progressive nature of this disease makes treatment unnecessary in most cases.

Control

Attempts to develop a vaccine have been largely unsuccessful (5). Control must depend upon elimination of the source of infection by culling all sheep with enlarged lymph nodes, preferably at shearing time when palpation is easier. Lambing and docking should be carried out in clean surroundings or in fresh fields (6). All docking implements and shears used for the Mules operation should be dipped in strong disinfectant before each use. Similar attention should be given to shears at shearing time and pus spilt on the shearing floor should be cleaned up and all shearing cuts disinfected. The younger age groups should be shorn first as the chance of infection is less among the lambs.

REFERENCES

(1) Dhanda, M. R. & Singh, M. M. (1955). *Indian vet. J.*, *32*, 43.
(2) Carne, H. R. *et al.* (1956). *Nature, Lond.*, *178*, 701.
(3) Carne, H. R. (1932). *Aust. vet. J.*, *8*, 42.
(4) Madeyski, S. *et al.* (1957). *Méd. vét. Varsovie*, *13*, 75.
(5) Quevedo, J. M. *et al.* (1957). *Rev. invest. Ganad.*, *1*, 47.
(6) Belonje, C. W. A. (1951). *J. S. Afr. vet. med. Ass.*, *22*, 165.
(7) Zaki, M. M. (1968). *Res. vet. Sci.*, *9*, 489.
(8) Benham, C. L. *et al.* (1962). *Vet. Bull.*, *32*, 645.
(9) Shirlaw, J. F. & Ashford, W. A. (1962). *Vet. Rec.*, *74*, 1025.

Ulcerative Lymphangitis of Horses and Cattle

Ulcerative lymphangitis is a mildly contagious disease of horses and cattle characterized by lymphangitis of the lower limbs.

Incidence

The disease was of considerable importance and widely distributed during the horse era. The mortality rate was negligible but among affected horses there was interference with their ability to perform. Ulcerative lymphangitis has also been recorded in cattle (1, 2).

Aetiology

Corynebacterium pseudotuberculosis causes the classical disease but similar lesions may be due to infection with other pyogenic organisms including streptococci, staphylococci, *Cor. equi* (2, 6), and *Pseudomonas aeruginosa* (3).

Transmission

Infection occurs through abrasions on the lower limbs and is more likely to occur when horses are crowded together in dirty, unhygienic quarters. As a rule only sporadic cases occur in a stable.

Pathogenesis

Infection of skin wounds is followed by invasion of lymphatic vessels and the development of abscesses along their course. Lymph node involvement is unusual.

Clinical Findings

In horses the initial wound infection is followed by swelling and pain of the pastern, often sufficient to cause severe lameness. Nodules develop in the subcutaneous tissue particularly around the fetlock. These may enlarge to 5 to 7 cm. in diameter and rupture to discharge a creamy green pus. The resulting ulcer has ragged edges and a necrotic base. Lymphatics draining the area become enlarged and hard and secondary ulcers may develop along them. Lesions heal in 1 to 2 weeks but fresh crops may occur and cause persistence of the disease for up to 12 months. In rare cases there is a slight systemic reaction and a bacteraemia may result in localization in other organs (5). The lesions in cattle are similar to those in horses except that there may be lymph node enlargement and the ulcers discharge a gelatinous, clear exudate (1).

Clinical Pathology

The isolation of *Cor. pseudotuberculosis* from discharging lesions is necessary to confirm the diagnosis.

Diagnosis

Differentiation of ulcerative lymphangitis from the other diseases causing similar lesions is important because of the serious nature of such diseases as glanders and epizootic lymphangitis in horses. Restriction of the lesion to the lower limbs and absence of lymph node involvement are important features although these are shared by sporotrichosis.

Treatment

Local treatment of ulcers is usually sufficient although parenteral injections of penicillin may be necessary in severe cases (4). In the early stages an autogenous bacterin may have value as treatment.

Control

Good hygiene in stables and careful disinfection of injuries to the lower limbs usually afford adequate protection against the disease.

REFERENCES

(1) Purchase, H. S. (1944). *J. comp. Path.*, *54*, 238.
(2) Neave, R. M. S. (1951). *Vet. Rec.*, *63*, 185.
(3) Azizuddin, I. M. & Chandrasekharan, N. K. P. (1954). *Madras vet. Coll. Ann.*, *12*, 17.
(4) Delestre, R. (1953). *Rev. vet. milit.* (*B. Aires*), *8*, 171.
(5) Gallo, G. G. (1954). *Rev. vet. milit.* (*B. Aires*), *2*, 258.
(6) Bain, A. M. (1963). *Aust. vet. J.*, *39*, 116.

Contagious Acne of Horses

(*Canadian Horse Pox, Contagious Pustular Dermatitis*)

Contagious acne of horses is characterized by the development of pustules particularly where the skin comes in contact with harness.

Incidence

Contagious acne is of limited occurrence and causes temporary inconvenience when affected horses are unable to work.

Aetiology

Corynebacterium pseudotuberculosis is the specific cause of this disease.

Transmission

Spread from animal to animal is by means of infected grooming utensils or harness. An existing seborrhoea or folliculitis due to blockage of seba- ceous gland ducts by pressure from harness probably predisposes to infection. Inefficient grooming may also be a contributing cause.

Pathogenesis

Infection of the hair follicle leads to local suppuration and the formation of pustules which rupture and contaminate surrounding skin areas. Occasional lesions penetrate deeply and develop into indolent ulcers.

Clinical Findings

The skin lesions usually develop in groups in areas which come into contact with harness. The lesions take the form of papules which develop into pustules varying in diameter from 1 to 2·5 cm. There is no pruritus but the lesions may be painful to touch. Rupture of the pustules leads to crust formation over an accumulation of greenish-tinged pus. Healing of lesions occurs in about one week but the disease may persist for four or more weeks if successive crops of lesions develop.

Clinical Pathology

Swabs of the lesions can be taken to determine the presence of *Cor. pseudotuberculosis*.

Diagnosis

Contagious acne bears some similarity to other skin diseases, particularly some forms of ringworm, bursatti and non-specific pyogenic infections including those caused by staphylococci. Bursatti, or swamp cancer, is caused by the larvae of the nematode worm, *Habronema megastoma*. Nodules which develop into ulcers occur below the eyes, and on the legs and belly. Isolation of *Cor. pseudotuberculosis* from lesions is necessary to confirm the diagnosis of contagious acne.

Treatment

Affected animals should be rested until all lesions are healed. Frequent washing with a mild skin disinfectant solution followed by the application of antibacterial ointments to the lesions should facilitate healing and prevent the development of further lesions. Parenteral administration of antibiotics may be advisable in severe cases.

Control

Infected horses should be rigidly isolated and all grooming equipment, harness and blankets disinfected. Grooming tools must be disinfected before each use. Vaccination is not likely to be effective because of the poor antigenicity of the organism.

Corynebacterial Pneumonia of Foals

This is a well-recognized infectious disease of young foals with localization in many organs but particularly in the lungs with clinical manifestations of pneumonia.

Incidence

The disease appears to occur in most countries comprising about 5 per cent of infectious disease in foals in the U.K. (1) and probably a similar proportion in other countries. It is generally restricted to particular farms where it may cause considerable death loss in thoroughbred studs. A mortality of about 80 per cent is usual, although the number of deaths decreases markedly in foals more than 3 months of age. The disease is most common in foals 1 to 2 months of age but can occur in older foals up to 6 months old (4). Foals which survive the acute stages of the disease seldom develop normally.

Aetiology

Corynebacterium equi affects horses principally but may also be found in lymph node abscesses in the pig and in ulcerative lymphangitis in cattle. Predisposing causes in the horse are unknown but the disease can be produced experimentally in foals by oral or intranasal inoculation of the organism (3). The possibility of infection from the dam has been suggested. Although the organism is not highly resistant and is unlikely to persist in the environment it has been found to survive in moist soil for periods of longer than 12 months. *Cor. pseudotuberculosis* and *Cor. pyogenes* can also cause the disease.

Transmission

The mode of transmission of the disease is unknown. A genital mode has been proposed with infection occurring either prenatally or by invasion via the navel soon after birth (2). Other experience points to migrating parasitic larvae as carriers of infection through the body (4). The proponents of this theory are most enthusiastic that control of strongylosis writes finis to endemic pneumonia in affected studs.

Pathogenesis

After an initial bacteraemia, suppurative foci may develop in many organs, particularly the lungs and to a lesser extent in the joints and subcutaneous tissues (4). When the pulmonary involvement reaches a sufficiently advanced stage, the standard clinical picture becomes apparent.

Clinical Findings

The clinical picture in foals varies with the age at which foals become affected. Those affected at a month of age have a more acute form of the disease than those affected subsequently. Thus young foals may suddenly become acutely ill with the appearance of signs of pneumonia, fever, anorexia and in some cases acute arthritis affecting one or more joints. Subcutaneous abscesses may develop. In older foals a subacute pneumonia develops slowly with cough, an increase in the depth of respiration with obvious dyspnoea developing in the late stages and characteristic loud, moist râles, or 'rattles', on auscultation. The foal continues to suck and the temperature is normal but the foal becomes emaciated. Severe diarrhoea may follow or accompany the respiratory signs (5). Nasal discharge and lymph node enlargement in the throat regions are absent. In most cases there is continued emaciation even with treatment and severely affected animals die in 1 to 2 weeks.

Clinical Pathology

Cervical swabs for cultural purposes should be taken from the cervix of repeat-breeding mares and those that abort or produce infected foals. Nasal swabs from infected foals in the later stages of the disease may reveal the presence of respiratory tract infection with *Cor. equi*. The use of a filtrate from a culture of the organism has been used as an allergic skin test, a positive result being an oedematous plaque at the injection site 18 hours later (2).

Necropsy Findings

With pulmonary involvement there is suppurative bronchopneumonia with multiple abscesses along the ventral borders of the lungs and in the bronchial lymph nodes. Occasionally abscesses are also present in the mesenteric lymph nodes, the intestinal wall, and subcutaneous tissue, and there is sometimes suppurative arthritis.

Diagnosis

The age group affected, the suppurative bronchopneumonia, the long subacute course and the association with infected mares all help in field diagnosis of the disease. Other respiratory tract infections including equine viral rhinopneumonitis, equine viral arteritis and strangles have a short course and affect upper respiratory tract rather than lungs. The other foal septicaemias and bacteraemias including infections with *Act. equuli*, *E. coli*, *Str. pyogenes equi*, *Salm. abortivoequina* and *Salm. typhimurium* may show joint lesions but there is rarely serious involvement of the lungs.

Treatment

Because of the chronic suppurative nature of the disease, treatment with antibiotics alone is rarely successful. Combined use of antibiotics and parenteral enzymes is suggested as a possible method of treatment. Chloromycetin or tetracyclines are preferred in treatment but a penicillin-streptomycin combination or a sulphonamide should be effective in early cases.

Control

If the infection can be shown to be present in the mares, control of the disease should aim at removal of the infection from the group, either by treatment or culling affected animals. In badly affected studs, hygiene at foaling, particularly muzzling the foal and allowing it to suckle only when the mare has been washed down, is recommended. When an outbreak is in progress on a farm prophylactic injections of long-acting penicillin for the first week of each foal's life appear to prevent further cases. A programme to reduce infestation with helminth parasites is recommended as a control measure (4).

REFERENCES

(1) Gunning, O. V. (1947). *Vet. J.*, *103*, 47.
(2) Wilson, M. M. (1955). *Aust. vet. J.*, *31*, 175.
(3) Harakawa, T. & Morita, S. (1949). *Jap. J. vet. Sci.*, *11*, 63.
(4) Bain, A. M. (1966). *Aust. vet. J.*, *39*, 116.
(5) Rooney, James R. (1966). *Mod. vet. Pract.*, *47*, 43.
(6) Sippel, W. L. *et al.* (1968). *J. Amer. vet. med. Ass.*, *153*, 1610.

DISEASES CAUSED BY *LISTERIA* Spp.

Listeriosis

Listeriosis is an infectious disease caused by *Listeria monocytogenes* and characterized by either meningo-encephalitis, abortion or septicaemia.

Incidence

The disease has been of most importance in New Zealand, North America, Europe, the United Kingdom and Australia. It is much less common in tropical and subtropical than in temperate climates. Losses due to this disease, both from abortion and fatal meningo-encephalitis, have been reported more frequently in recent years. The disease is of greatest economic importance in sheep and cattle but its host range includes 37 mammals in addition to man, 17 fowls, a fly, fish and crustaceans. In man the disease is serious, often fatal, and the fact that the organism occurs commonly in the milk of infected animals and may withstand pasteurization adds a further reason for the prompt recognition and control of this disease. Extreme care should be exercised by veterinarians when infected material, particularly from abortions, is handled. Animals of any age, including the newborn, may be affected and in a herd the infection rate may reach 10 per cent. The mortality rate without treatment in listerial septicaemia and listerial meningo-encephalitis approaches 100 per cent.

Aetiology

List. monocytogenes is the causative organism and can be isolated in pure culture from affected animals. Several strains of the organism have been identified, the commonest in natural cases in farm animals being 4B. *List. monocytogenes* is of high infectivity but low pathogenicity and the disease is not readily produced unless the animal's resistance is reduced. A number of predisposing agents have been suggested as causing such reductions in resistance. Although gross nutritional deficiency is the commonest precursor of outbreaks, heavy silage feeding is also well recognized as a predisposing influence. Silage may exert this effect by increasing the susceptibility of the host or by providing a suitable medium for the growth and maintenance of the bacteria. *L. monocytogenes* does not multiply in good ensilage (pH 4·0 to 4·5) but it may not be killed. In spoiled silage with incomplete fermentation and a pH above 5·5 the bacteria survives and may multiply (2, 3). Outbreaks which occur in sheep after introduction to silage usually commence about 3 weeks later (4).

Sheep, cattle, buffalo, goats, horses, pigs, cats, rabbits and some wild animals and man are susceptible to infection. There is one report of the isolation of *List. monocytogenes* from the brain of a moose and it is suggested that the disease may be prevalent in this species and cause many losses (5). The presence of listeria in mice and deer in association with its presence in sheep and ensilage (6) and its frequent occurrence in birds (7) suggest possible feral reservoirs of infection.

Transmission

Experimentally meningo-encephalitis can be produced by intranasal instillation, inoculation of the conjunctival sac, or intra-neural, intracerebral or intracarotid injections of the organism. Intravenous and subcutaneous injections have caused septicaemia (8), oral dosing has produced visceral infection (9) and intravenous injection in pregnant heifers has caused abortion (10). Experimental inoculation into rams has resulted in localization in testis and epididymis and suggest the possibility of venereal transmission (11). The portal of infection in natural cases is uncertain but the prevalence of the particular forms of the disease under different environmental conditions suggests that infection may gain entrance by several portals. It seems probable that meningo-encephalitis results from inhalation or conjunctival contamination, and the visceral infection with abortion from ingestion of infected material. Venereal transmission may also lead to abortion.

Infective material derives from infected animals in the faeces, urine, aborted foetuses and uterine discharge and in the milk. Although immediate spread among animals in a group has been demonstrated, field observations suggest that mediate contagion by means of inanimate objects also occurs and this has been substantiated under experimental conditions (1). The organism persists for as long as 3 months in sheep faeces and has been shown to survive for up to $11\frac{1}{2}$ months in damp soil, up to $16\frac{1}{2}$ months in cattle faeces, up to 207 days on dry straw and for more than 2 years in dry soil and faeces. The bacterium is also resistant to temperatures of $-20\,°C$ for 2 years and is still viable after repeated freezing and thawing. It appears from the epizootiological pattern of the disease that carrier animals play a part in its transmission and normal animals from infected herds appear to bring the disease into herds to which they are introduced (7).

Pathogenesis

There are a number of manifestations of the disease and these have an irregular distribution among the animal species. Visceral listeriosis with or without meningitis occurs most commonly in monogastric animals and in young ruminants; the meningo-encephalitic form of the disease is more common in adult ruminants (7). Infection of the uterus causing abortion and intra-uterine infection occurs in all mammals. Visceral listeriosis affects organs other than the brain and the principal clinical manifestations are those of abortion or septicaemia. In listerial meningo-encephalitis the lesions are confined to the brain and the clinical picture is referable only to these lesions.

When the disease is produced experimentally by injection, both visceral and meningo-encephalitis forms may occur in the one animal and organisms can be isolated from brain, spinal cord and viscera. Pregnant ewes abort in 7 to 11 days, the foetuses are often decomposed and *List. monocytogenes* is present in the foetal tissues and placenta.

In naturally occurring cases usually only the one clinical form, either the meningo-encephalitic or the visceral, occurs in a particular group of animals. In the nervous form the organism is present in the brain only in most cases but a localized myelitis, manifested clinically by posterior paralysis of one limb, has been recorded in lambs (12). In the visceral form the viscera and sometimes the spinal cord, but never the brain, are infected. These observations lend weight to the hypothesis that different portals of entry may result in involvement of different organs. The pathway by which *List. monocytogenes* enters the brain is still under debate. It has been shown experimentally that the bacteria can ascend the trigeminal nerve to produce meningo-encephalitis, in which the lesions are confined to the brain stem in the region of the trigeminal nerve nucleus, and lesions occur along the nerve trunk and its branches (11). It is presumed that the organism reaches peripheral branches of the nerve by way of wounds in the oral mucosa. However, a study of natural cases suggests that infection occurs by way of the blood vessels, the bacteria lodging in and about the reticular formation of the brain stem with lesions developing in the mid-brain, pons and medulla (13) with subsequent extension to the meninges, ependyma and occasionally the eye. It is possible that both portals of entry are important.

Ingestion of the organism, with penetration of the mucosa of the intestine, is thought to lead either to an inapparent infection with prolonged faecal excretion of the organism (14), or to a bacteraemia with localization in various organs, or to development to a fatal septicaemia. The pregnant uterus appears to be particularly susceptible to infection. Infection early in pregnancy causes abortion but infection late in pregnancy results in stillbirths or the delivery of young which rapidly develop a fatal septicaemia. Maternal metritis is constant and if the foetus is retained a fatal listerial septicaemia may follow (1, 8).

The peculiar localization of the infection to the brain stem in cases of meningo-encephalitis is often unilateral and accounts for the localizing signs of facial paralysis and circling. The additional signs of dullness, head-pressing and delirium are referable to the more general effects of inflammation of the brain. Spread of the infection along the optic nerve may result in endophthalmitis in sheep and cattle.

Clinical Findings

One can expect to find the meningo-encephalitic form and the visceral form (chiefly as abortion or neonatal septicaemia) in different outbreaks of the disease, and rarely the two forms together in the one outbreak.

Listerial meningo-encephalitis. This form has been observed in all species and presents a standard syndrome except that in pigs there are more involuntary muscle movements of the jaws and salivation than in the other species. In adult cattle the course of the disease is usually 1 to 2 weeks but in sheep and calves the disease is more acute, death occurring in 3 to 4 days. Basically the clinical picture combines the signs of the 'dummy' syndrome, with pressing against fixed objects, and unilateral facial paralysis. Affected animals are dull, often to the point of somnolence, and isolate themselves from the rest of the group. Prehension and mastication are slow and the animal may stand for long periods drooling saliva and with food hanging from its mouth. The position of the head and neck varies. In most cases there is deviation of the head to one side with the poll–nose relationship undisturbed (i.e. there is no rotation of the head as in a middle ear infection). However, the head may be retro- or ventro-flexed depending on the localization of the lesions in the brain stem and in some cases may be in a normal position. The deviation of the head cannot be corrected actively by the animal and if it is corrected passively the head returns to its previous position as soon as it is released. Progression is usually in a circle in the direction of the deviation and the circle is of small diameter. Unilateral facial paralysis is also a common localizing sign, the ear, eyelids and lips on the affected side showing a flaccid paralysis. Panophthalmitis, with pus evident in the anterior chamber of one or both eyes, is not uncommon in cattle which have been affected for a number of days. The affected animal becomes recumbent and is unable to rise although often still able to move its legs. Death is due to respiratory failure. Fever (usually 40°C or 104°F, but occasionally as high as 42°C or 107°F) is usual in the early stages of the disease but the temperature is usually normal when frank clinical signs are present.

Listerial abortion. In cattle many sporadic abortions due to *List. monocytogenes* are recorded and outbreaks of abortion due to this organism are recorded in cattle, sheep and in goats. In cattle there may be stillbirths or abortions at about the seventh month of pregnancy or later, retention of the afterbirth occurs commonly, there is no evidence of clinical meningo-encephalitis but there is commonly clinical illness and a fever of up to 40·5°C (105°F) and *List. monocytogenes* is present in the foetal stomach. The disease has been observed soon after the commencement of silage feeding. In sheep and goats abortions occur from the twelfth week of pregnancy onwards and the afterbirth is retained; meningo-encephalitis does not occur although there may be some deaths of ewes due to septicaemia if the foetus is retained. In both species the incidence of abortion in a group is low but may reach as high as 15 per cent and on some farms recurs each year, sometimes more than once in the one animal (10).

Septicaemic listeriosis. Acute septicaemia due to *List. monocytogenes* is not common in adult ruminants but does occur in monogastric animals including foals, young pigs (16) and new-born lambs and calves. There are no signs suggestive of nervous system involvement, the syndrome being a general one comprising depression, weakness, emaciation, pyrexia and diarrhoea in some cases, with hepatic necrosis and gastroenteritis at necropsy. The same syndrome is also seen in ewes and goats after abortion if the foetus is retained. A rather better defined but less common syndrome has been described in calves 3 to 7 days old. Corneal opacity is accompanied by dyspnoea, nystagmus and mild opisthotonus. Death follows in about 12 hours. At necropsy there is ophthalmitis and sero-fibrinous meningitis.

Clinical Pathology

Attempts may be made to isolate the organism from the faeces, urine and milk of infected animals and from aborted foetuses. All organs of the foetus, including the stomach, should be examined as well as the placenta and uterine discharges, if they are available, because the organisms tend to be very patchy in their distribution. The organism can be cultivated from vaginal secretions for up to 2 weeks after abortion and a proportion of aborting cows also have *List. monocytogenes* in the milk and faeces (15). Reculture of tissues is recommended if listeriosis is suspected.

Haematological examination is not of much value as the monocytosis of laboratory animals does not occur in the domestic animals. A nondiagnostic neutrophilia does occur in sheep. Examination of the cerebrospinal fluid for inflammatory cells and the presence of bacteria may be worth while. Serological tests (agglutination and complement fixation tests) are used but are unreliable because of a high proportion of false negatives (15). The interpretation of serological tests for antibodies against *List. monocytogenes* is made difficult by the presence of positive reactions of up to 1:200 in clinically normal animals. Titres higher than this are usually associated with listerial infection but are commonly encountered in normal cattle in herds where clinical cases have been seen. In sheep the antibody titre may persist for several years but after abortion in cattle it may return to normal in as short a time as one month (10).

Necropsy Findings

The cerebrospinal fluid may be cloudy, there may be some congestion of meningeal vessels and in some bovine cases there is panophthalmitis but in general the macroscopic findings are not marked. Histological examination of brain tissue is necessary to demonstrate the micro-abscesses which are characteristic of the disease. Heavy inoculation of media with material which has been macerated and refrigerated for long periods is advisable when attempting to isolate the organisms which are often present in small numbers (1). Visceral lesions occur as multiple foci of necrosis in the liver, spleen, endocardium and myocardium especially in the septicaemic form and in aborted foetuses.

Diagnosis

Listerial meningo-encephalitis may be confused with the nervous form of acetonaemia in cattle and with early cases of pregnancy toxaemia in sheep. In these diseases dullness, isolation, apparent blindness and circling are also characteristic but there is no facial nerve paralysis and no endophthalmitis. However, acetonaemia occurs in cattle soon after parturition and in ewes pregnancy toxaemia is observed only during late pregnancy and usually in association with multiple pregnancy and a declining nutritional status. Also circling in these diseases is accompanied by muscle twitching, particularly of the face, champing of the jaw and blinking of the eyelids and these signs appear only intermittently. As soon as the convulsive episode has passed a normal posture is adopted and the animal can walk in a straight line. Pregnancy toxaemia may be accompanied by a rise in body temperature if muscular activity is much increased. Both of these metabolic diseases are accompanied by marked ketonuria. Brain abscess, while rare, may be clinically indistinguishable from listeriosis. Cerebrospinal fluid and blood leucocyte examinations may yield little or no basis for differentiation. The course is usually much longer, the animal often surviving for some weeks. Rabies should be considered in the differential diagnosis but there are no localizing signs as there are in listeriosis.

Listerial abortion must be differentiated from the other causes of abortion in cattle and sheep and in goats from *Br. melitensis* infection. Acute septicaemias of new-born animals are due to many causes but association with abortion and stillbirths may suggest the possible presence of listeriosis. The necropsy lesions are distinctive and positive cultural findings confirm the diagnosis.

Treatment

List. monocytogenes is resistant to many drugs but is sensitive to chlortetracycline. The intravenous injection of chlortetracycline (5 mg. per lb. body weight per day for 5 days) is reasonably effective in meningo-encephalitis of cattle but less so in sheep. The recovery rate depends largely on the speed with which treatment is commenced. If severe clinical signs are already evident death usually follows in spite of treatment. Usually the course of events in an outbreak is that the first case dies but subsequent cases are picked out sufficiently early for treatment to arrest further development of the disease. Chloramphenicol and a combination of streptomycin and penicillin (0·25 g. and 0·3 million units) have also been used successfully in the septicaemic form in lambs.

Control

Most attempts to produce a satisfactory killed vaccine have been unsuccessful although field trials with a killed bacterin are reported to reduce the incidence in sheep flocks. Virulent living culture or attenuated bacteria are also under investigation as immunizing agents (17). A common recommendation is to reduce the amount of ensilage fed and in animals in the feedlot the constant feeding of low levels of tetracyclines is recommended for the duration of the fattening period. There may be some merit in the recommendation that a change of diet to include heavy feeding of ensilage should be made slowly, particularly if the ensilage is spoiled or if listeriosis has occured on the premises previously.

REVIEW LITERATURE

Gray, M. L. & Killinger, A. H. (1966). *Bact. Rev.*, *30*, 309.

REFERENCES

(1) Gray, M. L. *et al.* (1956). *Amer. J. vet. Res.*, *17*, 510.
(2) Irvin, A. D. (1968). *Vet. Rec.*, *82*, 115.
(3) Blenden, D. C. *et al.* (1968). *Amer. J. vet. Res.*, *29*, 223.
(4) Blenden, D. C. *et al.* (1967). *Proc. 3rd int. Symposium Listeriosis, Bilthoven*, pp. 214–44.
(5) Archibald, R. McG. (1960). *Canad. vet. J.*, *1*, 225.
(6) Killinger, A. H. & Mansfield, M. E. (1970). *J. Amer. vet. med. Ass.*, *157*, 1318.

(7) Gray, M. L. (1958). *Listeriosen Symposion, Beiheft 1 zum Zentralblatt fur Veterinarmedizin.* Berlin: Paul Parey.

(8) Urbaneck, D. & Rittenbach, P. (1963). *Arch. exp. Vet.-Med., 17,* 35, 117.

(9) Paulsen, M. & Moule, G. R. (1953). *Aust. vet. J., 29,* 133.

(10) Osebold, J. W. *et al.* (1960). *J. Amer. vet. med. Ass., 137,* 221, 227.

(11) Smith, R. E. *et al.* (1968). *Cornell vet., 58,* 389.

(12) Gates, G. A. *et al.* (1967). *J. Amer. vet. med. Ass., 150,* 200.

(13) Cordy, D. R. & Osebold, J. W. (1959). *J. infect. Dis., 104,* 164.

(14) Lehnert, C. (1964). *Arch. exp. Vet.-Med., 18,* 981.

(15) Dijkstra, R. G. (1967). *Proc. 3rd int. Symp. Listeriosis, Bilthoven,* pp. 215–24, 275–82.

(16) Meyer, E. P. & Gardner, J. M. (1970). *Aust. vet. J., 10,* 514.

(17) Asahi, O. (1963). *Proc. 2nd Symp. Listeric Infections, Montana,* 1962, 49–56.

DISEASES CAUSED BY *ERYSIPELOTHRIX INSIDIOSA*

Erysipelas of pigs is the major disease of animals caused by this bacterium but there are several other minor conditions which require mention.

Erysipelas in Cattle

Arthritis caused by *Erysipelothrix insidiosa* has been observed in calves (1). There is a non-suppurative arthritis with ulceration of articular cartilages. Polyarthritis is manifested by lameness, recumbency, fluctuating joint capsules and severe loss of condition. Clinical erysipelas in adult cattle has not been recorded but the organism has been isolated from the tonsils of healthy cattle and from endocardial lesions at post-mortem examination (2).

Erysipelas in Sheep

Erysipelas in sheep is manifested as arthritis or laminitis.

ARTHRITIS IN LAMBS

A non-suppurative arthritis of lambs caused by *Ery. insidiosa* occurs commonly after docking, less commonly after birth as an umbilical infection and has occurred accidentally by the use of contaminated serum (3). Phenol in the concentration ordinarily used in serum will not kill the organism. It persists for long periods in soil and if lambing or docking are carried out in an infected environment the organism gains entry through wounds or the umbilicus and causes polyarthritis. Up to 50 per cent of a flock may become affected and although the mortality rate is low, about 5 per cent of the affected lambs lose much weight and may have permanently swollen joints.

Signs appear about 14 days after birth or dock-ing. Lameness develops suddenly with minor swelling of affected joints, usually the carpal, hock and stifle joints. Recovery is slow and there is a high incidence of swollen joints and chronic lameness. At necropsy the synovium is turbid and present in excessive amounts but there is no suppuration as in arthritis of lambs due to streptococcal infection. There is thickening of the joint capsule and erosion of articular cartilages. Penicillin is effective in treatment if given early. Hygiene in lambing and docking areas and the use of clean instruments will reduce the incidence of the disease considerably. Vaccination should be considered on farms where the disease is a problem.

LAMINITIS AFTER DIPPING

The use of plunge baths as dips for sheep may be followed by a high incidence of laminitis if the insecticide solution used does not contain a suitable disinfectant (4). Dips that become grossly contaminated with organic matter are most likely to cause the disease. Infection occurs through skin abrasions and causes a cellulitis with extension to the laminae of the feet but without involving the joints. Up to 90 per cent of a flock may be affected although the incidence is usually about 25 per cent. Similar outbreaks of laminitis caused by *Ery. insidiosa* have occurred unassociated with dipping and usually in circumstances where sheep have to walk through muddy areas likely to be contaminated with the organism (5).

Severe lameness begins 2 to 4 days after exposure, usually in one leg, sometimes in all four. The affected legs are hot and slightly swollen from the coronet to halfway up the metatarsus or metacarpus and the hair over the affected area usually falls out. Much bodily condition is lost but deaths are rare, except in recently weaned lambs where a septicaemia may develop. The lambs show fever, malaise and anorexia.

At necropsy there is subcutaneous oedema of the area, sometimes accompanied by haemorrhage. The inflammation usually extends into the laminae of the feet. Most cases recover spontaneously in 10 to 14 days but penicillin should facilitate recovery. Inclusion of a bacteriostatic agent such as copper sulphate (0·04 per cent) in the dipping fluid is usually sufficient to prevent spread of the disease (6). There is no underrunning of the hoof as in foot rot, no abscessation as in foot abscess and no proliferative dermatitis as in strawberry foot rot.

REFERENCES

(1) Moulton, J. E. *et al.* (1953). *J. Amer. vet. med. Ass., 123,* 335.

(2) Roemmele, O. (1952). *Liebensm. Tierärzt., 3,* 43.

(3) Rowlands, W. T. & Edwards, C. M. (1950). *Vet. Rec.*, *62*, 213.
(4) Whitten, L. K. *et al.* (1948). *Aust. vet. J.*, *24*, 157.
(5) Whitten, L. K. (1952). *Aust. vet. J.*, *28*, 6.
(6) Thompson, G. E. *et al.* (1968). *J. S. Afr. med. Ass.*, *38*, 420.

Erysipelas in Swine

Erysipelas is an infectious disease of pigs and appears in an acute, septicaemic form often accompanied by diamond shaped skin lesions and a chronic form manifested by a non-suppurative arthritis and a vegetative endocarditis.

Incidence

Erysipelas in pigs occurs generally throughout the world and in most countries reaches a level of incidence sufficient to cause serious economic loss due to deaths of pigs and devaluation of pig carcases due to arthritis. The importance of the disease is increased by the difficulties encountered in controlling and eradicating it. Because of man's susceptibility swine erysipelas has some public health significance. Veterinarians particularly are exposed to infection when vaccinating with virulent culture.

Spread of the infection to most other species can also occur. Morbidity and mortality rates in swine vary considerably from place to place largely due to variations in virulence of the particular strain of the organism involved. On individual farms or in areas the disease may occur as a chronic arthritis in fattening pigs, or as extensive outbreaks of the acute septicaemia, or both forms may occur together.

Aetiology

Ery. insidiosa (*E. rhusiopathiae*) is the causative bacterium and the disease can be produced in either chronic or acute, septicaemic forms by the injection of cultures of the organism. There is considerable variation in the ease with which the disease can be reproduced and in its severity (1, 2, 3, 4). Many factors such as age, health and intercurrent disease, exposure to erysipelas, and heredity govern the ease of both natural and artificial transmission. Virulence of the strain is probably the most important factor. Smooth strains can be used successfully to produce the disease experimentally but rough strains appear to be non-pathogenic (3). This variation in virulence between strains of the organism has been utilized in the production of living, avirulent vaccines.

Pigs of all ages are susceptible although adult pigs are most likely to be affected if the local strain is of relatively low virulence. Recently farrowed sows seem to be particularly susceptible. When the strain is virulent pigs of all ages, even sucklings a few weeks old, develop the disease. Piglets from an immune sow may get sufficient antibodies in the colostrum to give them immunity for some weeks (7).

Transmission

Soil contamination occurs through the faeces of affected or carrier pigs. Other sources of infection include infected animals of other species, and birds. The clinically normal carrier group represents the most important source of infection, the tonsils being the predilection site for the organism in such cases. Since the organism can pass through the stomach without loss of viability, carrier animals may reinfect the soil continuously (8).

The persistence in soil is variable and may be governed by many factors including temperature, pH and the presence of other bacteria (8) and this may account in part for the variable incidence of the disease. The organism is highly resistant to most environmental influences and is not readily destroyed by chemical disinfection.

Experimentally the disease can be produced by oral dosing, by intradermal, intravenous and intra-articular injection and by application to scarified skin, conjunctiva and nasal mucosa. Under natural conditions skin abrasions and the alimentary tract mucosa are considered to be the probable portals of entry and transmission is by ingestion of contaminated food. Flies are known to transmit the disease (19). Occasional outbreaks occur after the use of virulent and incompletely avirulent cultures as vaccines.

Pathogenesis

Invasion of the blood stream occurs in all infected animals in the first instance. The subsequent development of either an acute septicaemia, or a bacteraemia with localization in organs and joints, is dependent on undetermined factors. Virulence of the particular strain may be important and this may depend upon the number of recent pig passages experienced (9). Concurrent viral infection, especially hog cholera, may increase susceptibility of the host (1).

Localization in the chronic form is commonly in the skin, joints and on the heart valves with probable subsequent bacteraemic episodes. In joints the initial lesion is an increase in synovial fluid and hyperaemia of the synovial membrane followed in several weeks by the proliferation of synovial villi, thickening of the joint capsule and enlargement of the local lymph nodes (20).

The observation that repeated injections of the organism are necessary to produce the chronic form experimentally may be of great importance (2). It has been suggested that sensitivity to the bacteria may play some part in the development of arthrodial and endocardial lesions (18, 28). This has been advanced as an explanation of the frequent failure to isolate *Ery. insidiosa* from typically affected joints (22). Controversy still rages on the question of whether the common polyarthritis of pigs is due primarily to invasion by *Ery. insidiosa* or because of sensitivity to these bacteria or other agents. It seems safest at the moment to consider that the lesion is due to the primary effects of *Ery. insidiosa* and that there is no relationship between this disease and rheumatoid arthritis of humans (21, 29).

Clinical Findings

Acute Form. After an incubation period of 1 to 7 days there is a sudden onset of high fever (up to 42 °C or 108 °F) which is followed some time later by severe prostration, complete anorexia, thirst and occasional vomiting (10). Initially, affected pigs may be quite active and continue to eat even though the temperature is high. A marked conjunctivitis with profuse ocular discharge may be present. Skin lesions are almost pathognomonic but may not always be apparent. These may take the form of the classical diamond-shaped, red, urticarial plaques of about 2·5 to 5 cm. square or a more diffuse oedematous eruption with the same appearance. In the early stages the lesions are often palpable before they are visible. The lesions are most common on the belly, inside the thighs, on the throat, neck and the ears and appear usually about 24 hours after the initial signs of illness. After a course of 2 to 4 days the pig recovers or dies with diarrhoea, dyspnoea and cyanosis evident terminally. The mortality rate may reach 75 per cent but wide variation occurs.

The so-called 'skin' form is usually the acute form with more prominent skin localization but less severe signs of septicaemia and with a low mortality. The skin lesions disappear in about 10 days without residual effects. In the more serious cases the plaques spread and coalesce, often over the back, to form a continuous, deep purple area extending over a greater part of the skin surface. The affected skin becomes black and hard, the edges curl up and separate from an underlying, raw surface. The dry skin may hang on for a considerable time and rattle while the pig walks.

Chronic Form. Signs are vague and indistinct except for the joint lesions characteristic of this form of the disease. There may be alopecia, sloughing of the tail and tips of the ears, and a dermatitis

in the form of hyperkeratosis of the skin of the back, shoulders and legs, and growth may be retarded. Joint lesions are commonest in the elbow, hip, hock, stifle and knee joints and cause lameness and stiffness. The joints are obviously enlarged and are usually hot and painful at first but in 2 to 3 weeks are quite firm and without heat. This is especially the case when the arthritis has been present for some time, allowing healing and ankylosis to develop. Paraplegia may occur when intervertebral joints are involved or when there is gross distortion of limb joints.

Endocarditis also occurs as a chronic form of the disease with or without arthritis. Suggestive clinical signs are often absent, the animals dying suddenly without previous illness. In others there is progressive emaciation and inability to perform exercise. With forced exercise dyspnoea and cyanosis occur. The cardiac impulse is usually markedly increased, the heart rate is faster and a loud murmur is audible on auscultation.

Clinical Pathology

In the acute form examination of blood smears may reveal the presence of the bacteria, particularly in the leucocytes, but blood culture is likely to be more successful as a method of diagnosis. Repeated examinations in the chronic form of the disease may by chance give a positive result during a bacteraemic phase. Final identification of the organism necessitates mouse or pigeon inoculation tests, and protection tests in these animals using anti-erysipelas serum.

In the early stages of the acute form there is first a leucocytosis followed by a leucopenia and a monocytosis (3, 25). The leucopenia is of moderate degree (40 per cent reduction in total leucocyte count at most) compared with that occurring in hog cholera. The monocytosis is quite marked, varying from a 5- to 10-fold increase (2·5 to 4·5 per cent normal levels rise to 25 per cent). Agglutinins appear in the blood 2 to 4 days after the first signs of illness and titres of 1:25 are usually considered to be positive. The efficiency of agglutination tests for *Ery. insidiosa* is not clear. They appear to be satisfactory for herd diagnosis but not sufficiently accurate for identification of individual affected pigs, particularly clinically normal carrier animals. A more accurate complement fixation test is available.

Necropsy Findings

Acute Form. Skin lesions may be absent although the 'diamond skin' lesions are pathognomonic when they occur. The more diffuse, purplish oedema of the belly is common to other septicaemic diseases of pigs. Large ecchymotic haemorrhages throughout the body are reported by some observers but others find only minor degrees of petechiation. They are best observed under the kidney capsule, pleura and peritoneum. Venous infarction of the stomach is accompanied by swollen, haemorrhagic mesenteric lymph nodes and there is congestion of the lungs and liver. Infarcts may be present in the spleen and kidney. The organism can be isolated from blood and tissues.

Chronic Form. A non-suppurative proliferative arthritis involving limb and intervertebral joints is characteristic. A synovitis, with a serous or sero-fibrinous, amber-coloured, intra-articular effusion occurs first (2, 10) and degenerative changes in the subendochondral bone, cartilages and ligaments follow. When the synovial changes predominate, the joint capsule and villi are thickened. They are enlarged, dark red pedunculations or patches of vascular granulation tissue which spread as a pannus on to the articular surface. When bony changes predominate the articular cartilages are detached from the underlying bone causing abnormal mobility of the joint. Ulceration of the articular cartilages may also be present. Local lymph node enlargement is usual. The joint lesions in time often repair by fibrosis, adhesions and ankylosis sufficiently to permit use of the limb. Such joints are often sterile on bacteriological examination. Joints in which changes are still progressing may also be sterile.

Endocardial lesions, when present, are large, crumbly vegetations on the valves, often sufficiently large to apparently block the valvular orifice. Infarcts occur in the kidney.

Isolation of *Ery. insidiosa* from the joints should be attempted. Many affected joints may be sterile and secondary bacterial invaders may cause an atypical necrosis and an excess of turbid joint fluid. Culture of apparently normal joints in affected pigs is positive in approximately half the joints examined. Endocardial vegetations and kidney infarcts yield pure cultures of the organism as a rule.

Diagnosis

Erysipelas in pigs is not ordinarily difficult to diagnose because of the characteristic clinical and necropsy findings. The acute disease may be confused with the other septicaemias affecting pigs, but pigs with erysipelas usually show the characteristic skin lesions and are less depressed than pigs with hog cholera or salmonellosis. In salmonellosis there is usually gross skin discolouration, some evidence of enteritis, and respiratory difficulty. In both hog cholera and salmonellosis signs of cerebral involvement including muscle tremor and convulsions are also common.

The chronic disease occurs in pigs of all ages but less commonly in adults. Streptococcal septicaemia and arthritis is almost entirely confined to sucking pigs in the first few weeks of life. Streptococcal endocarditis has a similar age distribution to erysipelas endocarditis and bacteriological examination is necessary to differentiate them. Glasser's disease in pigs is accompanied by a severe painful dyspnoea and at necropsy there is serositis and meningitis. Rickets and chronic zinc poisoning produce lameness in pigs but they occur under special circumstances, are not associated with fever, and rickets is accompanied by abnormalities of posture and gait which are not seen in erysipelas. Foot rot of pigs is easily differentiated by the swelling of the hoof and the development of discharging sinuses at the coronet.

In recent years there has been a marked increase in chronic osteoarthritis and various forms of 'leg weakness' in growing swine, probably related to the increased growth rate resulting from modern feeding and management practices. In many instances differentiation from erysipelas can be accomplished only by bacteriological methods.

Treatment

Penicillin and anti-erysipelas serum comprise the standard treatment, often administered together by dissolving the penicillin in the serum. Penicillin alone is usually adequate when the strain has only mild virulence. Some diagnostic indication can be gained from the response of acute cases to 20 to 30 ml. of serum given intravenously because of the considerable improvement which occurs within 24 hours. The serum can also be administered by the subcutaneous or the intramuscular routes. This method of administration is facilitated by the use of dried serum which requires a much smaller injection volume. Chronic cases do not respond well to either treatment because of the structural damage which occurs to the joints and the inaccessibility of the organism in the endocardial lesions. Cortisone (75 mg. daily) administered subcutaneously produces marked clinical improvement of the arthritis without complete recovery but adrenocorticotrophic hormones appear to be of no therapeutic value (11).

Control

Eradication is virtually impossible because of the ubiquitous nature of the organism and its resistance to adverse environmental conditions. Complete removal of all pigs and leaving the yards unstocked is seldom satisfactory and eradication by slaughter of reactors to the agglutination test is not recommended because of the uncertain status of the test.

General hygienic precautions should be adopted. Clinically affected animals should be disposed of quickly and all introductions isolated and examined for signs of arthritis and endocarditis. This procedure will not prevent the introduction of clinically normal carrier animals. All animals dying of the disease should be properly incinerated to avoid contamination of the environment. Although thorough cleaning of the premises and the use of very strong disinfectant solutions are advisable, these measures are unlikely to be completely effective. Whenever practicable contaminated feed-lots or paddocks should be cultivated.

Immunization. Because of the difficulty of eradication biologic prophylactic methods are in common use. Immunizing agents available include hyperimmune serum and vaccines.

Anti-erysipelas serum. The parenteral administration of 5 to 20 ml. of serum, the amount depending on age, will protect in-contact pigs for 1 to 2 weeks during an outbreak. Sucking pigs in herds where the disease is enzootic should receive 10 ml. during the first week of life and at monthly intervals until they are actively vaccinated which can be done as early as 6 weeks provided the sows have not been vaccinated. Repeated administration of the serum may cause anaphylaxis because of its equine origin.

Vaccination. The observation that infected pigs are refractory to subsequent infection has led to the development of active vaccination procedures using living *Ery. insidiosa* cultures as the vaccine. This measure is not permitted in many countries because of the risk of variation in virulence of the strains used and the possibility of spreading infection.

Vaccination against erysipelas is in a state of flux. Immunity is produced by injection of living or dead organisms but the best balance between a strong immunity and low pathogenicity is still being sought. One of the major difficulties is to assess the value of each vaccine under standard conditions because of variation in the severity of the challenge. As far as possible a standard 'preparation' of experimental pigs should be followed to ensure that their susceptibility is not a variable in challenge experiments (5). A definite criterion of response must also be followed. The usual method

of testing resistance is by swabbing virulent cultures on skin scarifications, by intradermal injection or by conjunctival instillation. A local or systemic reaction with only primary lesions at the inoculation site, or these accompanied by secondary skin lesions elsewhere, represent different degrees of severity of infection (6).

Serum-simultaneous vaccination is the method most commonly used. The strain of the organism used is often of lower virulence than field strains. Immunity for about 6 months is usually achieved. Vaccination of baby pigs 2 to 5 days after farrowing affords no appreciable protection but vaccination at 2 months is followed by durable immunity for 3 to 5 months (12). A 'booster' injection, culture alone or with serum, was formerly recommended 10 to 12 weeks after the initial vaccination but gives no appreciable increase in immunity.

Avirulent living vaccines produce some immunity and are gaining acceptance (13). Simultaneous serum is not required. One such vaccine which has been field tested recently is claimed to produce effective immunity for 6 months and to virtually eliminate arthritis in young pigs if they are vaccinated at 8 to 12 weeks of age (17). Difficulty is often encountered in maintaining the low virulence of the vaccine. An avirulent vaccine given orally has been shown to be an effective vaccination procedure and seems to have practical application in large pig-raising units. The vaccine can be administered in troughs, its efficiency is not reduced by concurrent feeding of antibiotics and overdosing has no adverse effect (26, 27).

Killed bacterins consisting of formalin-killed cultures of *Ery. insidiosa*, absorbed on to aluminium hydroxide have been widely tested with generally favourable results. Immunity persists for 12 weeks, and much longer after use of an emulsified bacterin (15). In field tests the emulsified products have markedly reduced the incidence of arthritis and deaths due to erysipelas especially if a 'booster' injection is given 3 to 6 weeks after the first injection (16). However, protection against arthritis is less apparent when the vaccinates are challenged experimentally (18). A local reaction may occur at the site of the injection with these products. The axilla or flank are the sites most commonly used.

All of the above methods are in use at the moment (14) and opinions on their relative efficiencies vary. An accurate assessment is difficult unless standard methods of challenge are used. Field experiments usually use two criteria, proportion of deaths due to the acute form and the incidence of arthritis after vaccination. The choice of the most satisfactory immunizing agent is not easy to make. Virulent living vaccines give the longest and most durable immunity but may cause the disease and their use is not without risk to the vaccinator. Avirulent, or modified virulent, living vaccines satisfy the needs of duration of immunity and should be safe provided that their virulence is properly stabilized. Killed bacterins produce a less durable immunity but are completely safe. 'Breaks' in vaccination do occur after use of all the products.

General recommendations for vaccination include the use of serum in all pigs during outbreaks, and active immunization procedures in herds where the disease has become established. The optimum age for active immunization is 5 to 8 weeks, although if the disease is common in sucking pigs in a herd, the sows should be vaccinated 4 to 6 weeks before farrowing, or the piglets may be given serum until they reach vaccination age. Vaccination of baby pigs from a vaccinated sow is unlikely to be effective if carried out before the pigs are 12 weeks of age because of the passive immunity derived from the sow (23). Vaccination of all breeding stock should be carried out every 6 months preferably with an adsorbed killed bacterin or living avirulent vaccine. Every effort should be made to maintain a closed herd (24).

Vaccination against hog cholera does increase susceptibility to erysipelas so that simultaneous vaccination is not possible if virulent culture is being used. Simultaneous vaccination with hog cholera virus and avirulent or killed erysipelas vaccines is safe and is commonly used.

REFERENCES

(1) Doyle, T. M. (1947). *Vet. J.*, *103*, 11.
(2) Hughes, D. L. (1955). *Brit. vet. J.*, *111*, 183.
(3) Sikes, D. *et al.* (1955). *Amer. J. vet. Res.*, *16*, 349.
(4) Sikes, D. *et al.* (1956). *J. Amer. vet. med. Ass.*, *128*, 277.
(5) Thomson, A. & Gledhill, A. W. (1953). *Vet. Rec.*, *65*, 40.
(6) Shuman, R. D. & Schoening, H. W. (1953). *J. Amer. vet. med. Ass.*, *123*, 301.
(7) Wellman, G. & Heuner, F. (1957). *Zbl. Vet.-Med.*, *4*, 557.
(8) Rowsell, H. C. (1958). *J. Amer. vet. med. Ass.*, *13*, 357.
(9) Rowsell, H. C. (1955). *Proc. 92nd ann. Mtg Amer. vet. med. Ass.*, 143.
(10) Connell, R. *et al.* (1952). *Canad. J. comp. Med.*, *16*, 104.
(11) Sikes, D. *et al.* (1955). *Amer. J. vet. Res.*, *16*, 367.
(12) Shuman, R. D. (1953). *J. Amer. vet. med. Ass.*, *123*, 304 & 307.
(13) Ose, E. E. (1972). *J. Amer. vet. med. Ass.*, *160*, 603.
(14) Ray, J. D. (1958). *J. Amer. vet. med. Ass.*, *132*, 365.
(15) Jungk, N. K. & Murdock, F. M. (1957). *Amer. J. vet. Res.*, *18*, 121 & 126.
(16) Gouge, H. E. (1957). *J. Amer. vet. med. Ass.*, *131*, 523.
(17) Lawson, K. F. *et al.* (1958). *Canad. J. comp. Med.*, *22*, 164.
(18) Neher, G. M. *et al.* (1958). *Amer. J. vet. Res.*, *19*, 5.
(19) Wellman, G. (1955). *Zbl. Bakt. l.*, *162*, 261 & 265.
(20) Corhs, P. & Schulz, L. C. (1960). *Mh. Vet.-Med.*, *15*, 608.
(21) Sokoloff, L. (1960). *Advances in Veterinary Science*, pp. 194–250. New York: Academic Press.
(22) Sikes, D. (1960). *Canad. J. comp. Med.*, *24*, 347.
(23) Shuman, R. D. (1961). *J. Amer. vet. med. Ass.*, *139*, 776.
(24) Doyle, T. M. (1960). *Vet. Rev. Annot.*, *6*, 95.
(25) Dougherty, R. W. *et al.* (1965). *Cornell Vet.*, *55*, 87.
(26) Sampson, G. R. *et al.* (1965). *J. Amer. vet. med. Ass.*, *147*, 484.
(27) Lawson, K. F. *et al.* (1966). *Canad. vet. J.*, *7*, 13.
(28) Freeman, M. J. *et al.* (1964). *Amer. J. vet. Res.*, *25*, 135, 145 & 151.
(29) Ajmal, M. (1970). *Vet. Bull.*, *40*, 1.

DISEASE CAUSED BY BACILLUS ANTHRACIS

Anthrax

Anthrax is a peracute disease characterized by septicaemia and sudden death with the exudation of tarry blood from the body orifices of the cadaver. Failure of the blood to clot, absence of rigor mortis and the presence of splenomegaly are the most important necropsy findings.

Incidence

The disease is world wide in distribution although the incidence varies with the soil, climate and the efforts put forward to suppress it. It is often restricted to particular areas, the so-called 'anthrax belts', where it is enzootic. In most countries vaccination of susceptible animals in affected areas has reduced the incidence of the disease to negligible proportions on a national basis but heavy losses may still occur in individual herds. The morbidity rate may be high among all farm animals although susceptibility is highest among ruminants followed by horses and swine in that order. The disease is almost invariably fatal except in swine and even in this species the death rate is high. Anthrax in man takes the form of a localized cutaneous infection although a fatal septicaemic form does occur. Serious outbreaks of anthrax and persistence of the infection in the soil is most commonly encountered in tropical and subtropical countries. For example the annual financial loss due to anthrax in animals in Indonesia is estimated to be $6\frac{1}{2}$ million dollars (23). In temperate cool climates sporadic outbreaks due to accidental ingestion of contaminated bone meal or tannery effluent are more common although permanently infected areas do exist. In this circumstance outbreaks are few and the number of animals affected is small (2).

Aetiology

Bacillus anthracis is the specific cause of the disease. When material containing anthrax bacilli is exposed to the air, spores are formed which protract the infectivity of the environment for very long periods. The spores are resistant to most external influences including the salting of hides, normal environmental temperatures and standard disinfectants. Anthrax bacilli have remained viable in soil stored for 60 years in a rubber stoppered bottle (27), and field observations indicate a similar duration of viability in exposed soil, particularly in the presence of organic matter, in an undrained alkaline soil and in a warm climate. Outbreaks originating from soil-borne infection always occur in warm weather when the environmental temperature is over 15°C (60°F) (17). The occurrence of outbreaks at isolated points when environmental conditions are warm and humid has made it possible to predict 'anthrax years' (8) and has led to the suggestion that vegetative proliferation may occur in the soil. Putrefaction in the carcase destroys the bacteria and provided the carcase is unopened and no discharges appear, contamination of the soil will not occur.

Predisposing causes include close grazing of tough scratchy feed in dry times, which results in abrasions of the oral mucosa, and confined grazing on heavily contaminated areas around water holes. The disease occurs in all vertebrates but is most common in cattle and sheep and occurs less frequently in goats and horses. Man occupies an intermediate position between this group and the relatively resistant swine, dogs and cats. Algerian sheep are said to be resistant and, within all species, certain individuals seem to possess sufficient immunity to resist natural exposure. Whether or not this immunity has a genetic basis has not been determined. The most interesting example of natural resistance is the dwarf pig in which it is impossible to establish the disease (28). Spores remain in tissues ungerminated and there is complete clearance from all organs by 48 hours. This ability to prevent spore germination appears to be inherited in this species.

An atypical form of anthrax has been observed in pigs in Papua, New Guinea (20). Severe outbreaks with heavy mortalities occur in pigs but, except for guinea pigs, the disease is not transmissible to other species in spite of the apparent classical identity of the bacteria.

In most developed countries anthrax is no longer a significant cause of livestock wastage because of appropriate control measures. However it still holds an important political position and, largely because of its potential as a zoonosis, the cry 'anthrax' is almost as evocative as 'mad dog'.

Transmission

Infection gains entrance to the body by ingestion, inhalation or through the skin. While the exact mode of infection is often in doubt, it is generally considered that animals are infected by the ingestion of contaminated food or water. It is true that experimental transmission by the ingestion of virulent anthrax spores has not always been successful. Injury to the mucous membrane of the digestive tract will facilitate infection but there is little doubt that infection can take place without such injury. The increased incidence of the disease on sparse pasture is probably due both to the ingestion of contaminated soil and to injury to the oral mucosa facilitating invasion by the organism. Spores can be picked up directly from the soil or from fodder grown on infected soil, from contaminated bone meal or protein concentrates or from infected excreta, blood or other material. Outbreaks in swine can usually be traced to the ingestion of infected bone meal or carcases. Water can be contaminated by the effluent from tanneries, infected carcases and by flooding anthrax-infected soil.

Inhalation infection is thought to be of minor importance in animals although the possibility of infection through contaminated dust must always be considered (24). 'Woolsorter's disease' in man is due to the inhalation of anthrax spores by workers in the wool and hair industries, but even in these industries cutaneous anthrax is much more common.

Biting flies and other insects have often been found to harbour anthrax organisms and their ability to transmit the infection has been demonstrated experimentally (1). The transmission is mechanical only and a local inflammatory reaction is evident at the site of the bite. The tendency in infected districts for the heaviest incidence to occur in the late summer and autumn is probably due to the increase in the fly population at that time. An outbreak of anthrax has been recorded following the injection of infected blood for the purpose of immunization against anaplasmosis (6). There have been a number of reports of the occurrence of anthrax after vaccination due probably to inadequately attenuated spores. Wound infection occurs occasionally.

Spread of the organism within an area may be accomplished by streams, insects, dogs and other carnivores, and wild birds and by faecal contamination from infected animals. Introduction of infection into a new area is usually through contaminated animal products such as bone meal, fertilizers, hides, hair and wool or by contaminated concentrates or forage.

Pathogenesis

Upon ingestion of the spores infection may occur through the intact mucous membrane, through defects in the epithelium around erupting teeth or through scratches from tough, fibrous food materials. After entry the bacteria are moved to the local lymph nodes by motile phagocytes. After proliferation in this site the bacilli pass via the lymphatic vessels into the blood stream and septicaemia, with massive invasion of all body tissues, follows (21). *B. anthracis* produces a lethal toxin which causes oedema and tissue damage, death resulting from shock and acute renal failure (18), and terminal anoxia mediated by the central nervous system (11). The pathology of anthrax and the mode of action of the toxin have always been matters of great scientific interest, largely because of the great speed with which the infection kills animals. For further information on these subjects two recent reviews should be consulted (15, 21).

In pigs localization occurs in the lymph nodes of the throat after invasion through the upper part of the digestive tract. Local lesions often lead to a fatal septicaemia.

Clinical Findings

The incubation period after field infection is not easy to determine but is probably 1 to 2 weeks.

Cattle and Sheep. Only two forms of the disease occur in these species, the peracute and the acute. The peracute form of the disease is most common at the beginning of an outbreak. The animals are usually found dead without premonitory signs, the course being probably only 1 to 2 hours, but fever, muscle tremor, dyspnoea and congestion of the mucosae may be observed. The animal soon collapses, and dies after terminal convulsions. After death, discharges of blood from the nostrils, mouth, anus and vulva are common. The acute form runs a course of about 48 hours. Severe depression and listlessness are usually observed first although they are sometimes preceded by a short period of excitement. The body temperature is high, up to 42 °C (107 °F), the respiration rapid and deep, the mucosae congested and haemorrhagic and the heart rate much increased. No food is taken and ruminal stasis is evident. Pregnant cows may abort. In milking cows the yield is very much reduced and the milk may be blood-stained or deep yellow in colour. Alimentary tract involvement is usual and is characterized by diarrhoea and dysentery. Local oedema of the tongue and oedematous lesions in the region of the throat, sternum, perineum and flanks may occur.

Pigs. In pigs anthrax may be acute or subacute. There is fever, with dullness and anorexia and a characteristic inflammatory oedema of the throat and face. The swellings are hot but not painful and may cause obstruction to swallowing and respiration. Blood-stained froth may be present at the mouth when pharyngeal involvement occurs. Petechial haemorrhages are present in the skin and when localization occurs in the intestinal wall there is dysentery, often without oedema of the throat. An outbreak of a pulmonary form of the disease has been observed in baby pigs which inhaled infected dust. Lobar pneumonia and exudative pleurisy were characteristic (24). Death usually occurs after a course of 12 to 36 hours although individual cases may linger for several days.

Horse. Anthrax in the horse is always acute but varies in its manifestations with the mode of infection (3). When infection is by ingestion there is septicaemia with enteritis and colic. When infection is by insect transmission, hot, painful, oedematous, subcutaneous swellings appear about the throat, lower neck, floor of the thorax and abdomen, prepuce and mammary gland. There is high fever and severe depression and there may be dyspnoea due to swelling of the throat or colic due to intestinal irritation. The course is usually 48 to 96 hours.

Clinical Pathology

In the living animal the organism may be detected in a stained smear of peripheral blood. The blood should be carefully collected in a syringe to avoid contamination of the environment. When local oedema is evident smears may be made from the oedema fluid. For a more certain diagnosis, especially in the early stages when bacilli may not be present in the blood stream in great numbers, blood culture or the injection of syringe-collected blood into guinea pigs is satisfactory. Fluorescent antibody techniques are available for use on blood smears and tissue sections. In cases where antibiotic therapy has been used the identification from blood smears or culture may be difficult and animal passage may be necessary (4).

Necropsy Findings

At necropsy there is a striking absence of rigor mortis and the carcase undergoes rapid gaseous decomposition and quickly assumes the characteristic 'sawhorse' attitude. All natural orifices usually exude dark, tarry blood which does not clot and putrefaction and bloating are rapid. If there is good reason to suspect the existence of anthrax the carcase should not be opened. However, if a necropsy is carried out, the failure of the blood to clot, the presence of ecchymotic haemorrhages throughout the body tissues, the presence of blood-stained serous fluid in the body cavities, severe enteritis and gross enlargement of the spleen with softening and liquefaction of its structure are almost certain indications of the presence of anthrax. Subcutaneous swellings containing gelatinous material and enlargement of the local lymph nodes are features of the disease as it occurs in horses and pigs.

To confirm the diagnosis on an unopened carcase smears of peripheral blood or local oedema fluid should be collected by needle puncture. If possible, blood or oedema fluid should also be collected for guinea pig or mouse inoculation. If decomposition of a carcase is advanced an ear or a portion of spleen should be sent to the laboratory for the preparation of an Ascoli precipitin test and for culture. If experimental animal inoculation is not possible, microscopic examination of smears should be supported by blood culture (12). Care must be taken when suspected material is sent through the post to ensure that no hazard is created for persons handling the package.

Diagnosis

Although sudden death is uncommon amongst animals there are many causes and differentiation is often difficult. Lightning stroke is usually evidenced by singeing of the hair and by a history of electrical storms. Peracute blackleg may resemble anthrax but it is largely restricted to young animals and the crepitating swellings which are characteristic of blackleg do not occur in anthrax. Other clostridial infections may simulate anthrax, especially in pigs.

Acute leptospirosis usually occurs only sporadically and is characterized by haemoglobinuria. Bacillary haemoglobinuria is featured by haemoglobinuria and the presence of characteristic infarcts in the liver. Blood culture and smear will serve to differentiate the conditions. Peracute lead poisoning and hypomagnesaemic tetany are usually accompanied by obvious nervous signs and a completely different necropsy picture. Snake-bite is characterized by the presence of local swelling around obvious fang marks.

Animals dying of acute bloat show gaseous distension and exudation of blood from orifices as in anthrax. The probability of either disease occurring can usually be assessed and laboratory examination must be used if there is any doubt.

Treatment

Antibiotics and anti-anthrax serum are most commonly used in treatment. Severely ill animals are unlikely to recover but in the early stages, particularly when fever is detected before other signs are evident, recovery can be anticipated. Penicillin (5 million units twice daily) has had considerable vogue (5, 6) but streptomycin (8 to 10 g. daily in 2 doses intramuscularly for cattle) is much more effective (7). Oxytetracycline (2 mg. per lb. body weight daily) parenterally has also proved superior to penicillin in the treatment of clinical cases after vaccination in cattle (8, 9) and sheep (10). In spite of the observations made on clinically affected animals, a strong case has been made for the use of procaine penicillin and streptomycin in large doses at 12-hour intervals plus antiserum for at least 5 days (21). The need to prolong treatment to at least 5 days to avoid a recrudescence of the disease is stressed (26). While anti-anthrax serum intravenously in doses of 100 to 250 ml. daily is effective and may be given in conjunction with an antibiotic, it is too expensive for routine use.

Control

Hygiene is the biggest single factor in the prevention of spread of the disease. Careful disposal of infected material is most important. Infected carcases should not be opened but immediately burned or buried, together with bedding and soil contaminated by discharges. Burial should be at least 6 feet deep with an ample supply of quicklime added. All suspected cases and in-contact animals must be segregated until cases cease and for 2 weeks thereafter and the affected farm placed in quarantine to prevent the movement of livestock. The administration of hyperimmune serum to in-contact animals may prevent further losses during the quarantine period. The disinfection of premises, hides, bone meal, fertilizer, wool and hair requires special care. When disinfection can be carried out immediately, before spore formation can occur, ordinary disinfectants or heat ($60\,°C$ or $140\,°F$ for a few minutes) are sufficient to kill vegetative forms. This is satisfactory when necropsy room or abattoir floors are contaminated. When spore formation occurs (i.e. within a few hours of exposure to the air), disinfection is almost impossible by ordinary means. Strong disinfectants such as 5 per cent lysol require to be in contact with spores for at least 2 days. Strong solutions of formalin or sodium hydroxide (5 to 10 per cent) are probably most effective. Infected clothing should be sterilized by soaking in 10 per cent formaldehyde. Shoes may present difficulty and sterilization is most efficiently achieved by placing them in a plastic bag and introducing ethylene oxide. Contaminated materials should be damp and left in contact with the gas for 18 hours (21). Hides, wool and mohair are sterilized commercially by gamma-irradiation usually from a radioactive cobalt source. Special care must be taken to avoid human contact with infected material and if such contact does occur the contaminated skin must be thoroughly disinfected. The source of the infection must be traced and steps taken to prevent further spread of the disease. Control of the disease in a feral animal population presents major problems. Attempts to control anthrax in wild bison have been recorded (25).

Immunization of animals as a control measure is extensively used and many types of vaccine are available. Those vaccines which consist of living attenuated strains of the organism with low virulence but capable of forming spores, have been most successful. The sporulation character has the advantage of keeping the living vaccine viable over long periods. These vaccines have the disadvantage that the various animal species show varying susceptibility to the vaccine and anthrax may result in some cases from vaccination. This has been largely overcome by preparing vaccines of differing degrees of virulence for use in different species and in varying circumstances. Another method of overcoming the virulence is the use of saponin or saturated saline solution in the vehicle to delay absorption (14). This is the basis of the Carbozo vaccine. The avirulent spore vaccine described by Stern has overcome the risk of causing anthrax by vaccination and produces a strong immunity which lasts for at least 26 months in sheep (13). It appears probable that this vaccine will supersede others in current use. A febrile reaction does occur after vaccination and the milk yield of dairy cows will be depressed and pregnant sows will probably abort (19).

An additional vaccination method utilizes a cell-free filtrate of a culture of a non-encapsulated, spore-forming strain of *B. anthracis*, either injected as an aqueous solution intradermally, or injected subcutaneously as an antigen adsorbed on to colloidal aluminium hydroxide. The vaccine is incapable of causing anthrax but the duration of the immunity produced in cattle (3 to 6 months) leaves something to be desired (16). Two injections of the vaccine produce a longer period of immunity but the procedure is rather costly.

In enzootic areas annual revaccination of all stock is necessary. When the disease occurs for the first time in a previously clean area, all in-contact animals should either be treated with hyperimmune serum or be vaccinated. Vaccination before this is not usually recommended because of the possibility of introducing infection on to the farm. This is unlikely to happen with the newer, avirulent vaccines. The measures used to control outbreaks and the choice of a vaccine depend largely on local legislation and experience. If a large feed supply becomes suspect of being contaminated by anthrax spores, a reasonable procedure is to vaccinate the livestock and resume feeding the material 2 to 3 weeks later (19). There is some risk of contamination of the environment if this is done.

REFERENCES

(1) Sen, S. K. & Minett, F. C. (1944). *Indian J. vet. Sci.*, *14*, 149.
(2) Campbell, A. D. (1969). *Vet. Rec.*, *85*, 89.
(3) McNellis, R. (1943). *Bull. U.S. Army med. Dept.*, *71*, 84–86.
(4) Clarenburg, A. *et al.* (1956). *T. Diergeneesk.*, *81*, 216.
(5) Riggs, C. W. & Tew, A. C. (1947). *J. Amer. vet. med. Ass.*, *111*, 44.
(6) Wessels, C. C. & de Kock, J. A. (1947). *J. S. Afr. vet. med. Ass.*, *18*, 163.
(7) Miller, E. S. *et al.* (1946). *J. Immun.*, *53*, 371.
(8) Flynn, D. M. (1968/69). *Vict. vet. Proc.*, *27*, 32.
(9) Bailey, W. W. (1954). *J. Amer. vet. med. Ass.*, *124*, 296.
(10) Johnson, W. P. & Percival, R. C. (1955). *J. Amer. vet. med. Ass.*, *127*, 142.
(11) Remmele, N. S. *et al.* (1968). *J. infect. Dis.*, *118*, 104.
(12) Thompson, P. D. (1955). *J. comp. Path.*, *65*, 1.
(13) Israil, M. & Quader, M. A. (1955). *Pakist. J. sci. Res.*, *7*, 38.
(14) Bone, J. R. (1957). *N. Amer. Vet.*, *38*, 10, 12a (Oct.).
(15) Nungester, W. J. (1967). *Fed. Proc.*, *26*, 1483.
(16) Jackson, F. C. *et al.* (1957). *Amer. J. vet. Res.*, *18*, 771.
(17) van Ness, G. B. (1961). *S.W. Vet.*, *14*, No. 4, 290.
(18) Harris-Smith, P. W. *et al.* (1958). *J. gen. Microbiol.*, *19*, 91.
(19) Spears, H. N. & Davidson, J. C. (1959). *Vet. Rec.*, *71*, 637.
(20) Egerton, J. R. (1966). *Papua N. Guinea agric. J.*, *17*, 136, 141.
(21) Lincoln, R. E. *et al.* (1964). *Advances in Veterinary Science*, Vol. 9, New York: Academic Press.
(22) Greenough, P. R. (1965). *Vet. Rec.*, *77*, 784.
(23) Mansjoer, M. (1961). *Commun. vet.*, *5*, 61.
(24) Ratalics, L. & Toth, L. (1964). *Magy. allatorv. Lap.*, *19*, 203.
(25) Cousineau, J. G. & McClenaghan, R. J. (1965). *Canad. vet. J.*, *6*, 22.
(26) Greenough, P. R. (1965). *Vet. Rec.*, *77*, 784.
(27) Wilson, J. B. & Russell, K. E. (1964). *J. Bact.*, *87*, 237.
(28) Walker, J. S. *et al.* (1967). *J. Bact.*, *93*, 2031.

16

Diseases Caused by Bacteria—II

DISEASES CAUSED BY
CLOSTRIDIUM Spp.

THE clostridia are of major importance in farm animals as primary causes of disease. They rarely act as secondary invaders except where gangrene is already present. They are all potent producers of exotoxins upon which their pathogenicity depends. The toxins of the different organisms vary in their effects and in the manner in which they gain entry to the circulation; they may be ingested preformed in the feed as in botulism; be absorbed from the gut after abnormal proliferation of the causative organism in the alimentary tract as in enterotoxaemia or be elaborated in a more proper infection of the tissues such as blackleg. Other clostridial infections develop as local infections with elaboration of toxins in minor lesions such as in tetanus, black disease, braxy and bacillary haemoglobinuria.

Pathogenic clostridia are commonly present in soils rich in humus. They are also found in the intestinal contents of normal animals and cause disease only in special circumstances. The ubiquitous character of these organisms makes eradication of the clostridial diseases virtually impossible and necessitates control by prophylactic measures. Fortunately diseases of this group are unique among bacterial diseases in that they can be effectively prevented in almost all instances by vaccination with killed culture vaccines. Because of the common occurrence of a number of clostridial infections in an area, it has become a common practice in recent years to use multiple vaccines capable of immunizing against as many as five separate diseases. The vaccines, if carefully prepared, appear to be highly effective and, in situations where the extra expense can be justified, worthy of recommendation.

Tetanus

Tetanus is a highly fatal, infectious disease of all species of domestic animals caused by the toxin of *Clostridium tetani*. It is characterized clinically by hyperaesthesia, tetany and convulsions.

Incidence

Tetanus occurs in all parts of the world and is most common in closely settled areas under intensive cultivation. It occurs in all farm animals mainly as individual, sporadic cases, although outbreaks are occasionally observed in young pigs and lambs. The mortality rate is usually about 80 per cent.

Aetiology

Cl. tetani forms spores which are capable of persisting in soil for a number of years. The spores are resistant to many standard disinfection procedures including steam heat at 100 °C (212 °F) for 30 to 60 minutes but can be destroyed by heating to 115 °C (239 °F) for 20 minutes.

The neurotoxin of *Cl. tetani* is exceedingly potent but there is a great deal of variation in susceptibility between the animal species, the horse being the most susceptible and cattle the least. The variation in incidence of the disease in the different species is partly due to this variation in susceptibility but also because exposure is more likely to occur in some species than in others.

Transmission

Cl. tetani organisms are commonly present in the faeces of animals, especially horses, and in the soil contaminated by these faeces. The portal of entry is usually through deep puncture wounds but the spores may lie dormant in the tissues for some time and produce clinical illness only when tissue conditions favour their proliferation. For this reason the portal of entry is often difficult to determine. Puncture wounds of the hooves are common sites of entry in horses. Introduction to the genital tract at the time of parturition is the usual portal of entry in cattle. A high incidence of tetanus may occur in young pigs following castration, and in lambs following castration, shearing and docking. Docking by the use of elastic band ligatures appears to be especially hazardous (1).

Pathogenesis

The tetanus bacilli remain localized to their site of introduction and do not invade surrounding tissues. They start to proliferate and produce neurotoxin only if certain environmental conditions are attained, particularly a lowering of the local tissue oxygen tension. This may occur immediately after introduction if the accompanying trauma has been sufficiently severe, or may be delayed for several months until subsequent trauma to the site causes tissue damage. The original injury may have completely healed by this time.

The toxin reaches the central nervous system by passing up peripheral nerve trunks and not by passage from the blood stream through the blood–brain barrier. The exact means by which the toxin exerts its effects on nervous tissue is not known. No structural lesions are produced but there is central potentiation of normal sensory stimuli so that a state of constant muscular spasticity is produced and normally innocuous stimuli cause exaggerated responses (2). Death occurs by asphyxiation due to fixation of the muscles of respiration.

Clinical Findings

The incubation period varies between one and three weeks with occasional cases occurring as long as several months after the infection is introduced. In sheep and lambs cases appear 3 to 10 days after shearing or docking. The clinical picture is similar in all animal species. A general increase in muscle stiffness is observed first and is accompanied by muscle tremor. There is trismus with restriction of jaw movements, prolapse of the third eyelid, stiffness of the hind legs causing an unsteady, straddling gait and the tail is held out stiffly especially when backing or turning. The prolapse of the third eyelid is one of the earliest signs and can be exaggerated by sharp lifting of the muzzle or tapping the face below the eye. Additional signs include an anxious and alert expression contributed to by an erect carriage of the ears, retraction of the eyelids and dilatation of the nostrils, and exaggerated responses to normal stimuli. The animal may continue to eat and drink in the early stages but mastication is soon prevented by tetany of the masseter muscles and saliva may drool from the mouth. If food or water are taken attempts at swallowing are followed by regurgitation from the nose. Constipation is usual and the urine is retained, due in part to inability to assume the normal position for urination. The temperature and pulse rate are within the normal range in the early stages but may rise later when muscular tone and activity are further increased. In cattle, particularly young animals, bloat is an early sign, but is not usually severe and is accompanied by strong, frequent rumen contractions.

As the disease progresses muscular tetany increases and the animal adopts a 'saw-horse' posture. Uneven muscular contractions may cause the development of a curve in the spine and deviation of the tail to one side. There is great difficulty in walking and the animal is inclined to fall, especially when startled. Falling occurs with the limbs still in a state of tetany and the animal can cause itself severe injury. Once down it is almost impossible to get a large animal to its feet again. Tetanic convulsions begin in which the tetany is still further exaggerated. Opisthotonus is marked, the hind limbs are stuck out stiffly behind and the forelegs forward. Sweating may be profuse and the temperature rises, often to 42°C (107°F). The convulsions are at first only stimulated by sound or touch but soon occur spontaneously.

The course of the disease varies both between and within species. The duration of a fatal illness in horses and cattle is usually 5 to 10 days but sheep usually die about the third or fourth day. Although tetanus is almost always fatal a long incubation period is usually associated with a mild syndrome, a long course and a favourable prognosis. In fatal cases there is often a transient period of improvement for several hours before a final, severe tetanic spasm during which respiration is arrested. Mild cases which recover usually do so slowly, the stiffness disappearing gradually over a period of weeks or even months.

Clinical Pathology

A satisfactory ante-mortem test is the injection of serum from infected animals into mice as a check on the amount of toxin in the blood stream.

Necropsy Findings

There are no gross or histological findings by which a diagnosis can be confirmed although a search should be made for the site of infection, and culture of the organism attempted.

Diagnosis

Fully developed tetanus is so distinctive clinically that it is seldom confused with other diseases. The muscular spasms, the prolapse of the third eyelid and a recent history of accidental injury or surgery are characteristic findings. However, in its early stages, tetanus may be confused with other diseases. Strychnine poisoning is uncommon in farm animals, usually affects a number at one time or results from overdosing, and the tetany between convulsive episodes is not so marked. Hypo-calcaemic tetany (eclampsia) of mares also resembles tetanus but is confined to lactating mares and responds to treatment with calcium salts. Acute laminitis resembles tetanus also, but there is no tetany nor prolapse of the third eyelid. Cerebrospinal meningitis causes rigidity, particularly of the neck, and hyperaesthesia to touch but the general effect is one of depression and immobility rather than excitement and hypersensitivity to sound and movement. Lactation tetany of cattle and whole milk tetany of calves are accompanied by tetany and convulsions but these are more severe than those seen in tetanus, and prolapse of the third eyelid and bloat are absent. Enzootic muscular dystrophy may be mistaken for tetanus because of the marked stiffness but there is an absence of tetany. Enterotoxaemia of lambs is accompanied by other more marked nervous signs.

Treatment

The response to treatment in horses and sheep is poor but cattle frequently recover.

The main principles in the treatment of tetanus are to eliminate the causative bacteria, neutralize residual toxin, relax the muscle tetany to avoid asphyxia, and maintain the relaxation until the toxin is eliminated or destroyed. There are no structural changes in the nervous system and the management of cases of tetanus depends largely on keeping the animal alive through the critical stages.

Elimination of the organism is usually attempted by the parenteral administration of penicillin in large doses. If the infection site is found it should be treated locally but preferably only after anti-toxin has been administered, because debridement, irrigation with hydrogen peroxide and the local application of penicillin may facilitate the absorption of the toxin.

Tetanus antitoxin is usually administered but is of little value once signs have appeared. For optimum results horses should receive 300,000 units 12-hourly for 3 injections (19). Local injection of some of the anti-toxin around the wound is advised.

Relaxation of the muscle tetany can be attempted with various drugs. Chloral hydrate and magnesium sulphate injections have been in use for many years but suffer from the deficiency of short term action and depression of the respiratory centre. Muscle-relaxing agents including tubo-curarine and succinylcholine have found some use in the treatment of equine (5) and human (6, 7) tetanus but require to be given by continuous

intravenous drip or at frequent intervals. Ataractic drugs have given excellent results in equine and bovine tetanus. Chlorpromazine has been most widely used (8, 9, 10, 11, 20) and injections at 8- or 12-hour intervals are given until tetany disappears 8 to 12 days later. The daily doses administered are of the order of 0·4 mg. per lb. body weight by intravenous injection or 1·0 mg. per lb. body weight intramuscularly.

Additional supportive treatment includes slinging of horses during the recovery period when hyperaesthesia is diminishing, and intravenous or stomach-tube feeding during the critical stages when the animal cannot eat or drink. Because of the disturbance caused each time the stomach tube is passed, the use of an in-dwelling tube should be considered. Positive respiratory control by tracheal intubation is an important feature of treatment in humans but is unlikely to be attempted in animals. Affected animals should be kept as quiet as possible and provided with dark, well-bedded quarters with plenty of room to avoid injury if convulsions occur. Administration of enemas and catheterization may relieve the animal's discomfort.

Control

Many cases of tetanus could be avoided by proper skin and instrument disinfection at castrating, docking and shearing time. These operations should be carried out in clean surroundings and in the case of lambs docked in the field, temporary pens are to be preferred to permanent yards for catching and penning. For short-term prophylaxis passive immunity can be achieved by the injection of antitoxin. Doses of 1500 to 3000 I.U. of antitoxin are injected subcutaneously in horses, the dose varying with the extent and duration of the injury. On farms where the incidence of tetanus in lambs is high antitoxin is usually given at docking and a dose rate of 200 I.U. has been shown to be effective (21). The immunity is transient, persisting for only 10 to 14 days. The antitoxin can be combined with the toxoid to provide long term immunity and the toxoid can be administered simultaneously with pulpy kidney vaccine without reduction of the antibody response to either vaccine (16).

In enzootic areas all susceptible animals should be actively immunized with 'toxoid', an alum-precipitated, formalin-treated toxin. One injection gives immunity in 10 to 14 days lasting for a year and revaccination in 12 months gives solid immunity for life. A more vigorous programme of two vaccinations 6 to 8 weeks apart followed by annual booster vaccinations has also been recommended

(12) and may be necessary for valuable horses or in bad areas (18). A transient phase of reduction of antibody titre occurs after this booster injection in horses and the animal may be more susceptible at this time (15). In spite of the known efficiency of vaccination, animals which suffer injury subsequently are usually given an injection of antitoxin to ensure complete protection. Antitoxin does not interfere with the production of antibodies by toxoid so that both can be administered at the one time, the antitoxin providing short-term passive immunity until an active immune status is attained (16). In some areas the incidence of tetanus in young foals is high and repeated doses of antitoxin at weekly intervals is not always completely effective. Provided foals get an adequate supply of colostrum they can be passively immunized during the first few weeks of life by active vaccination of the mare during the last weeks of pregnancy. The foal should be vaccinated with toxoid at five to six weeks of age (13). The toxoid is usually injected subcutaneously but intramuscular injection produces less local inflammation and an increased immune response (14). Reactions to absorbed toxoid in horses, which take the form of severe local swelling, can be avoided by using a product containing minimal amounts of aluminium hydroxide (16). All horses which suffer wounds likely to be contaminated with the spores of *Cl. tetani* should receive a combined injection of toxoid and antitoxin. An injection of a long-acting penicillin preparation is commonly given at the same time. Prevention of tetanus in newborn lambs is also best effected by vaccination of the ewe in late pregnancy. Because the duration and degree of immunity are dependent on the titre of antibodies in the ewe's serum, optimum protection is obtained by vaccinating the ewes in the last two or three weeks of pregnancy. The greatest response is obtained in ewes which have received a prior vaccination, for example as a lamb or in a preceding pregnancy (17), and annual revaccination of late-pregnant ewes is highly recommended (21).

REFERENCES

(1) Mahoney, M. (1949). *J. Amer. vet. med. Ass.*, *115*, 352.
(2) Wright, G. P. (1955). *Mechanisms of Microbial Pathogenicity*, pp. 78–102, London: Cambridge University Press.
(3) Fedotov, A. I. (1948). *Veterinariya* (*Moscow*), *25*, 34 cited in (1949) *J. Amer. vet. med. Ass.*, *114*, 37.
(4) Couvy, M. L. (1947). *Bull. Acad. nat. Med.*, *131*, 143.
(5) Booth, N. H. & Pierson, R. E. (1956). *J. Amer. vet. med. Ass.*, *128*, 257.
(6) Woolmer, R. & Cates, J. E. (1952). *Lancet*, *263*, 808.
(7) Lassen, H. C. A. *et al.* (1954). *Lancet*, *267*, 1040.
(8) Troughton, S. E. *et al.* (1955). *Vet. Rec.*, *67*, 903.
(9) Tait, A. R. & Ryan, F. B. (1957). *Aust. vet. J.*, *33*, 237.
(10) Owen, L. N. *et al.* (1959). *Vet. Rec.*, *71*, 61.
(11) Lundwall, R. L. (1958). *J. Amer. vet. med. Ass.*, *132*, 254.
(12) Löhrer, J. & Radvila, P. (1970). *Schweiz. Arch. Tierheilk.*, *112*, 307.
(13) Lemétayer, E. *et al.* (1953). *Proc. 15th int. vet. Cong.*, *1*, Pt. 1, 57–61.
(14) Montgomerie, R. F. (1940). *Vet. Rec.*, *52*, 539.
(15) Lemétayer, E. *et al.* (1955). *Bull. Acad. vét. Fr.*, *28*, 425.
(16) Chodnik, K. S. *et al.* (1959). *Vet. Rec.*, *71*, 904.
(17) Wallace, G. V. (1964). *N.Z. vet. J.*, *12*, 61.
(18) Fessler, J. F. (1966). *J. Amer. vet. med. Ass.*, *148*, 399.
(19) Radvila, P. & Lohrer, J. (1965). *Schweiz. Arch. Tierheilk.*, *107*, 123 & 319.
(20) Morrow, D. A. (1963). *Cornell Vet.*, *53*, 445.
(21) Cooper, B. S. (1966). *N.Z. vet. J.*, *14*, 186.

Botulism

Botulism is a rapidly fatal, motor paralysis caused by the ingestion of the toxin of *Cl. botulinum*, which organism proliferates in decomposing animal matter and sometimes in plant material.

Incidence

Botulism has no geographical limitations, sporadic outbreaks occurring in most countries. In farm animals it assumes major economic importance, however, only in areas where sheep and cattle suffer from a phosphorus or protein deficiency on range. Most such outbreaks have been reported from South Africa, Australia and the Gulf Coast area of the U.S.A. The disease usually occurs in a number of animals at one time and is almost invariably fatal.

Aetiology

Botulism is most common in birds, particularly the domestic chicken and wild waterfowl. Cattle, sheep and horses are susceptible but pigs (17), dogs and cats appear to be resistant.

The causative organism is the spore-forming anaerobe *Cl. botulinum* which proliferates only in decaying animal or plant material. Under favourable conditions of warmth and moisture it multiplies rapidly elaborating a relatively stable and highly lethal toxin which, when ingested, causes the disease. There are a number of antigenically distinct types of *Cl. botulinum*, classified as A, B, C, D and E. Cattle are usually affected by types C and D. The geographical distribution of these types varies considerably—an important feature when prophylactic vaccination is under consideration (13).

Botulism in range animals has a seasonal distribution. Outbreaks are most likely to occur during drought periods when feed is sparse, phosphorus intake is low and carrion is plentiful. The spores of *Cl. botulinum* are extremely resistant and survive for long periods in most environmental circumstances. The toxin is also capable of surviving for long periods, particularly in bones or if protected from leaching (9). The disease has also occurred in horses fed on spoiled vegetables and potatoes contaminated by *Cl. botulinum* (12).

Transmission

The causative organism is a common inhabitant of the alimentary tract of Herbivora and may be introduced into new areas in this way. It occurs commonly in soils in affected areas, and soil and water contamination occurs from faeces and decomposing carcases. The source of infection for animals is almost always carrion, which includes domestic and wild animals and birds. Where cattle subsist on a phosphorus deficient diet, and manifest osteophagia and the ingestion of carrion, the disease is likely to occur in outbreak form. In sheep pica is more usually associated with a dietary deficiency of protein or nett energy. Occasional outbreaks occur due to drinking of water contaminated by carcases of dead animals. Dead rodents in haystacks (14) or ensilage pits (15) may provide a source of toxin. Chicken manure has also caused mortality when the organism was present in the intestinal tract of the birds. Although decomposing animal carcases are by far the commonest source of toxin, proliferation of the organism can occur in decaying vegetable material. Decaying grass at the base of old tussocks and in trampled stubble are reputed to be suitable sites for growth of *Cl. botulinum* (1). Silage and hay may spoil to a stage suitable for the growth of *Cl. botulinum*. Toxin has also been demonstrated in oat grain which caused toxic effects when fed to horses (5).

Pathogenesis

The toxins of *Cl. botulinum* are neurotoxins and produce functional paralysis without the development of histological lesions. When toxin is injected parenterally much smaller doses are required to cause death than when it is ingested. This is probably due to digestion of the toxin by proteolytic enzymes in the alimentary tract. The site at which neuromuscular transmission is impeded is probably at the synapses of efferent parasympathetic and somatic motor nerves where there is interference with the secretion of acetylcholine, the chemical mediator of nerve impulse transmission (3). A true flaccid paralysis develops and the animal dies of respiratory paralysis.

Clinical Findings

Cattle and Horses. Signs usually appear three to seven days after the animals gain access to the toxic material, the incubation period being shorter as the amount of toxin available is increased. Peracute cases die without prior signs of illness although a few fail to take water or food for a day beforehand. The disease is not accompanied by fever and the characteristic clinical picture is one of progressive muscular paralysis affecting particularly the limb muscles and the muscles of the jaw and throat. Muscle weakness and paralysis commence in the hindquarters and progress to the forequarters, the head and the neck. In most cases the disease is subacute. Restlessness, inco-ordination, stumbling, knuckling, and ataxia are followed by inability to rise or to lift the head. Skin sensation is retained. Affected animals lie in sternal recumbency with the head on the ground or turned into the flank, not unlike the posture of a cow with parturient paresis. The tongue becomes paralysed and hangs from the mouth, the animal is unable to chew or swallow and drools saliva. Defaecation and urination are usually unaffected although cattle may be constipated. Paralysis of the chest muscles results in a terminal abdominal-type respiration. Sensation and consciousness are retained until the end which usually occurs quietly, and with the animal in lateral recumbency, 1 to 4 days after the commencement of illness. Occasional field cases and some experimental cases in cattle show mild signs and recover after an illness of 3 to 4 weeks (11). The survivors can eat concentrate and ensilage but have difficulty prehending hay. The defect may persist for three weeks (15).

Sheep. Sheep do not show the typical flaccid paralysis of other species until the final stages of the disease (4). There is stiffness while walking, inco-ordination and some excitability in the early stages. The head may be held on one side or bobbed up and down while walking. Lateral switching of the tail, salivation, and serous, nasal discharge are also common. In the terminal stages there is abdominal respiration, limb paralysis and rapid death.

Pigs. Authentic reports in this species are rare (6, 16, 17). Clinical signs include staggering followed by recumbency, vomiting, and pupillary dilation. The muscular paralysis is flaccid and affected animals do not eat or drink.

Clinical Pathology

Little if any ante-mortem data can be assembled to aid in diagnosis, although mild to marked indicanuria, albuminuria and glycosuria have been observed in cattle (2) and albuminuria and glycosuria in pigs (6). Marked hypoglycaemia has also been recorded in experimental cases in horses (8). In cattle these biochemical changes occur intermittently and only in some animals and they do not provide satisfactory clinico-pathological tests. In peracute cases toxin can be detected in the blood by mouse inoculation tests (11).

Necropsy Findings

There are no specific changes detectable at necropsy although the presence of suspicious, foreign material in the forestomachs or stomach may be suggestive. There may be non-specific sub-endocardial and sub-epicardial haemorrhages and congestion of the intestinal mucosa and serosa. Perivascular haemorrhages have been recorded in the brain, especially in the corpus striatum, cerebellum and cerebrum and there may be destruction of Purkinje cells in the cerebellum. The presence of *Cl. botulinum* in the alimentary tract is of little significance and examination of gut contents for the presence of toxin is often misleading because the toxin may have already been absorbed.

Diagnosis

Although sporadic cases of botulism are often suspected it is seldom possible to establish the diagnosis by demonstrating the presence of toxin in the suspected food. Filtrates of the stomach and intestinal contents should be tested for toxicity to experimental animals but a negative answer may not be proof that the disease has not occurred. The main contributory evidence is provided by the feeding of suspect material to susceptible animals. When the disease occurs in ruminants at pasture the occurrence of pica is of diagnostic significance. Clinically and at necropsy the disease resembles parturient paresis in cattle, and hypocalcaemia in sheep but the conditions under which the diseases occur are quite different. Many other diseases of the nervous system may present a clinical picture similar to that of botulism. Paralytic rabies in cattle and equine encephalomyelitis and ragwort poisoning in horses may present similar clinical pictures. In sheep louping ill, some cases of scrapie and miscellaneous plant poisonings may also be confused with botulism.

Treatment

Specific or polyvalent antitoxic serum may be used in very early cases but their efficacy is questionable. Purgatives to remove the toxin from the alimentary tract, and central nervous system stimulants are sometimes administered (7). These treatments are usually confined to horses which may also be supported in slings and fed by stomach tube. In general, treatment should only be undertaken in subacute cases in which signs develop slowly and which have some chance of recovery. The remainder of the animals in the group should be vaccinated immediately.

Control

In range animals correction of dietary deficiencies by supplementation with phosphorus or protein should be implemented if conditions permit. Hygienic disposal of carcases is advisable to prevent further pasture contamination but may not be practicable under range conditions. Vaccination with type-specific or combined (bivalent C and D) toxoid is practised in enzootic areas. A single dose, precipitated toxoid is available which gives good immunity after two weeks and the immunity is solid for about 24 months (18). Since the disease in horses is usually due to accidental contamination of feed or water, and the incidence is low, vaccination is seldom practised in this species. Some local reactions are encountered after vaccination in horses but they are seldom serious (10).

REFERENCES

(1) Bennetts, A. W. and Hall, H. T. B. (1938). *Aust. vet. J.*, *14*, 105.
(2) Noyan, A. (1958). *Amer. J. vet. Res.*, *19*, 840.
(3) Wright, G. P. (1955). *Mechanisms of Microbial Pathogenicity*, pp. 78–102, London: Cambridge University Press.
(4) Seddon, H. R. (1953). *Diseases of Domestic Animals in Australia*, Vol. 1, Cwlth. Aust., Dept. of Hlth., Service Publ. No. 9.
(5) Mitchell, C. A. *et al.* (1939). *Canad. J. comp. Med.*, *3*, 245.
(6) Simintzis, G. & Durin, L. (1950). *Bull. Soc. Sci. vét. Lyon*, *52*, 71.
(7) Steyn, D. G. (1950). *J. S. Afr. vet. med. Ass.*, *21*, 81.
(8) Jacquet, J. (1954). *Bull. off. int. Épiz.*, *42*, 473.
(9) Fourie, J. M. (1946). *J. S. Afr. vet. med. Ass.*, *17*, 85.
(10) White, P. G. & Appleton, G. S. (1960). *J. Amer. vet. med. Ass.*, *137*, 652.
(11) Simmons, G. C. & Tammemagi, L. (1964). *Aust. vet. J.*, *40*, 123.
(12) Tamarin, R. & Neeman, L. (1962). *Refuah vet.*, *19*, 45 & 49.
(13) Scholtens, R. G. & Coohon, D. B. (1964). *Proc. 101st Ann. Mtg Amer. vet. med. Ass.*, Chicago, 224–230.
(14) Muller, J. (1963). *Bull. Off. int. Épiz.*, *59*, 1379.
(15) Fjolstad, M. & Klund, T. (1969). *Nord. Vet.-Med.*, *21*, 609.
(16) Beiers, P. R. & Simmons, G. C. (1967). *Aust. vet. J.*, *43*, 270.
(17) Smith, L. D. S. *et al.* (1971). *Amer. J. vet. Res.*, *32*, 1327.
(18) Tammemagi, L. & Grant, K. McD. (1967). *Aust. vet. J.*, *43*, 368.

Blackleg

Blackleg is an acute, infectious disease caused by *Cl. chauvoei* and characterized by inflammation of muscles, severe toxaemia and a high mortality.

True blackleg is common only in cattle but infection initiated by trauma occurs occasionally in other animals.

Incidence

Blackleg is a cause of severe financial loss to cattle raisers in many parts of the world. For the most part major outbreaks are prevented by vaccination although outbreaks still occur, occasionally in vaccinated herds but more frequently in herds where vaccination has been neglected. When the disease occurs it is usual for a number of animals to be affected within the space of a few days. The disease is enzootic in particular areas, especially when they are subject to flooding; such an area may vary in size from a group of farms to an individual field. The mortality rate in blackleg approaches 100 per cent.

Aetiology

True blackleg is caused by *Cl. (feseri) chauvoei*, a Gram positive spore-forming, rod-shaped bacterium. The spores are highly resistant to environmental changes and disinfectants and persist in soil for many years. 'False blackleg' may be caused by *Cl. septicum*, *Cl. novyi* and *Cl. perfringens* but this disease is more accurately classified as malignant oedema. Mixed infections with *Cl. chauvoei* and *Cl. septicum* are not uncommon (1) but the significance of *Cl. septicum* as a cause of the disease is open to doubt (8). True blackleg is usually thought of as a disease of cattle and occasionally sheep but outbreaks of the disease have been recorded in deer (9). In cattle the disease is largely confined to young stock between the ages of 6 months and 2 years. In the field the disease appears to occur most frequently in rapidly growing cattle on a high plane of nutrition. Elevation of the nutritional status of sheep by increased protein feeding increases their susceptibility to blackleg (12). In sheep there is no restriction to age group.

In pigs blackleg does not occur commonly, although a gas gangrene type of lesion may be caused by *Cl. chauvoei* (2, 7) or *Cl. septicum* (13) infection. Typical blackleg of cattle has a seasonal incidence with most cases occurring in the warm months of the year. The highest incidence may vary from spring to autumn, depending probably on when calves reach the susceptible age group.

Transmission

Blackleg is a soil-borne infection but the portal by which the organism enters the body is still in dispute. However, it is presumed that the portal of entry is through the alimentary mucosa after ingestion of contaminated feed. The bacteria may be found in the spleen, liver (15) and alimentary tract of normal animals, and contamination of the soil and pasture may occur from infected faeces or decomposition of carcases of animals dying of the disease. True blackleg develops when spores which are not lodged in normal tissues are caused to proliferate by mechanisms which have not been identified.

In sheep the disease is almost always a wound infection. Infection of skin wounds at shearing and docking and of the navel at birth may cause the development of local lesions. Infection of the vulva and vagina of the ewe at lambing may cause serious outbreaks and the disease has occurred in groups of young ewes and rams up to a year old, usually as a result of infection of skin wounds caused by fighting. Occasional outbreaks have occurred in sheep after vaccination against enterotoxaemia (4). Presumably the formalinized vaccine causes sufficient tissue damage to permit latent spores of the organism to proliferate. A special occurrence has been recorded in foetal lambs (3). Ewes exposed to infection at shearing developed typical lesions but ewes treated with penicillin were unaffected except that the pregnant ewes in the latter group showed distended abdomens, weakness and recumbency due to oedema and gas formation in the foetus from which *Cl. chauvoei* was isolated.

Pathogenesis

In true blackleg the stimulus which results in growth of the latent bacterial spores is unknown. Toxin formed by the organism produces a severe necrotizing myositis locally, and a systemic toxaemia which is usually fatal.

Clinical Findings

Cattle. If the animal is observed before death there is marked lameness, usually with pronounced swelling of the upper part of the affected leg. On closer examination the animal will be found to be very depressed, have complete anorexia and ruminal stasis and a high temperature (41°C or 106°F) and pulse rate (100 to 120 per minute). In the early stages the swelling is hot and painful to the touch but soon becomes cold and painless, and oedema and emphysema can be felt. The skin is discoloured and soon becomes dry and cracked. Although the lesions are usually confined to the upper part of one limb occasional cases are seen where the lesions are present in other locations such as the base of the tongue, the heart muscle, the diaphragm and psoas muscles, the brisket and udder. Lesions are sometimes present in more than one of these locations in the one animal. The condition develops rapidly and the animal dies quietly 12 to 36 hours after the appearance of signs. Many animals die without signs having been observed.

Sheep. When blackleg lesions occur in the limb musculature in sheep, there is a stiff gait and the sheep is disinclined to move due to severe lameness in one or, more commonly, in several limbs. The lameness may be severe enough to prevent walking in some animals but be only moderate in others. Subcutaneous oedema is not common and gaseous crepitation cannot be felt before death. Discolouration of the skin may be evident but skin necrosis and gangrene do not occur.

In those cases where infection occurs through wounds of the skin, vulva or vagina there is an extensive local lesion. Lesions of the head may be accompanied by severe local swelling due to oedema and there may be bleeding from the nose. In all instances there is high fever, anorexia, depression and death occurs very quickly (14).

Clinical Pathology

The disease is usually so acute that necropsy material is readily available but failing this it may be possible to obtain material suitable for cultural examination by needle puncture or swabs from wounds.

Necropsy Findings

Cattle found dead of blackleg are often in a characteristic position, lying on the side with the affected hind limb stuck out stiffly. Bloating and putrefaction occur quickly and blood stained froth exudes from the nostrils and anus. Clotting of the blood occurs rapidly. Incision of the affected muscle mass reveals the presence of dark, discoloured, swollen tissue with a rancid odour, a metallic sheen on the cut surface and an excess of thin, sanguineous fluid containing bubbles of gas. All body cavities contain excess fluid which contains variable amounts of fibrin and is usually blood stained. The solid organs show some degree of degeneration, and post-mortem decomposition with the production of gas in the liver occurs rapidly.

Sheep show a similar picture at necropsy but the muscle lesions are more localized and deeper and the subcutaneous oedema is not so marked except around the head. Gas is present in the affected muscles but not in such large amounts as in cattle. When the disease has resulted from infection of skin wounds the lesions are more obvious superficially, with subcutaneous oedema and swelling, and involvement of the underlying musculature. When invasion of the genital tract occurs, typical lesions are found in the perineal tissues and in the walls of the vagina and occasionally the uterus. In the special case of pregnant ewes which develop infection of the foetus, typical lesions involve the entire foetus and cause marked abdominal distension in the ewe.

In all cases of suspected blackleg smears of affected tissue should be made and material collected for bacteriological examination. Pasteur pipettes from muscle tissue and heart blood, and sections of muscle removed aseptically are suitable specimens for laboratory examination.

Diagnosis

In typical cases of blackleg in cattle a definite diagnosis can be made on the clinical signs and the necropsy findings. However, in many cases the diagnosis may be in doubt because of failure to find extensive, typical lesions. Such cases may be confused with other acute clostridial infections, with lightning stroke and with anthrax although in the latter the characteristic splenic lesion is usually present. Bacillary haemoglobinuria produces a rather similar necropsy picture with rapidly developing post-mortem changes in muscle but the liver infarcts and haemoglobinuria should identify the disease. Lactation tetany and acute lead poisoning may also cause sudden deaths in a number of cattle but the typical lesions of blackleg are not present.

In establishing a diagnosis when a number of animals are found dead in a group not kept under close observation one must depend on one's knowledge of local disease incidence, season of the year, age group affected and pasture conditions, and on a close inspection of the environment in which the animals have been maintained. Necropsy findings are most valuable if the cadavers are still fresh but, on many occasions, post-mortem decomposition is so advanced that little information can be obtained.

Treatment

Treatment of affected animals with penicillin is logical if the animal is not moribund but results are generally only fair because of the extensive nature of the lesions. Large doses (5000 units per lb. body weight) should be administered, commencing with crystalline penicillin intravenously and followed by longer-acting preparations some of which should be given into the affected tissue if it is accessible. The tetracyclines given intravenously or intraperitoneally may have some slight advantage over penicillin (10). Blackleg antiserum is unlikely to be of much value in treatment unless very large doses are given.

Control

On farms where the disease is enzootic annual vaccination of all cattle between 6 months and 2 years of age should be carried out just prior to the anticipated danger period, usually spring and summer. Vaccination of calves at three weeks of age has been recommended when the incidence of the disease is very high. Subsequent revaccination may be advisable (11). Of the available preparations the formalin-killed, alum-precipitated bacterin is most satisfactory. Immunity does not develop for 14 days and deaths may continue for some days if vaccination is carried out during an outbreak. When the disease is present in a group other measures are necessary to protect the remainder of the group until immunity has developed. Movement of the cattle from the affected pasture is advisable. Constant surveillance and the early treatment of cases is about all that can be done. Antiserum is expensive and may interfere with the later development of a strong immunity.

In sheep the use of alum-precipitated bacterin is also highly recommended but a good immunity does not develop in sheep vaccinated when less than a year old (5). In areas where the disease is enzootic the following vaccination programme is recommended. To prevent infection of the ewes at lambing they are vaccinated three weeks before lambing on one occasion only. This vaccination will give permanent protection. In subsequent years the young ewes are vaccinated. This vaccination will also protect lambs against umbilical infection at birth (16) and infection of the tail wound at docking, provided the tail is docked before the lamb is 3 weeks old. Vaccination can also be carried out 2 to 3 weeks before shearing or crutching if infection is anticipated. Because of the common occurrence of the disease in young sheep, vaccination before they go on to pasture and are exposed to infection of skin wounds from fighting is recommended in danger areas. The duration of the immunity in these animals, vaccinated at about 7 months of age, is relatively short and ewes in particular must be revaccinated before they lamb for the first time. If an outbreak commences in a flock of ewes at lambing time prophylactic injections of penicillin and antiserum to ewes requiring assistance has been recommended (6, 14).

The constitution of the vaccine is important. A bacterin prepared from a local strain of *Cl.* *chauvoei* is preferred. It is advisable to use a combined bacterin containing *Cl. chauvoei* and *Cl.* *septicum* if both organisms occur in the area. Attenuated organisms are also used in the preparation of vaccines for use in cattle and the same attenuated strain of bovine origin or a recently isolated, virulent, ovine strain may be used to prepare vaccines for use in sheep.

It is important that carcases of animals dying of blackleg be destroyed by burning or deep burial to limit soil contamination.

REFERENCES

(1) Ryff, J. F. & Lee, A. M. (1947). *J. Amer. vet. med. Ass.*, *111*, 283.
(2) Sterne, M. & Edwards, J. B. (1955). *Vet. Rec.*, *67*, 314.
(3) Butler, H. C. & Marsh, H. (1956). *J. Amer. vet. med. Ass.*, *128*, 401.
(4) Seddon, H. R. *et al.* (1931). *Aust. vet. J.*, 7, 2.
(5) Buddle, M. B. (1954). *N.Z. J. sci. Tech.*, Sec. A., *35*, 395.
(6) Buddle, M. B. (1952). *N.Z. vet. J.*, *1*, 13.
(7) Gualandi, G. L. (1955). *Arch. vet. ital.*, *6*, 57.
(8) Smith, L. D. S. (1957). *Advances in Veterinary Science*, Vol. 3, pp. 465–524, New York: Academic Press.
(9) Armstrong, H. L. & MacNamee, J. K. (1950). *J. Amer. vet. med. Ass.*, *117*, 212.
(10) Afzal, H. *et al.* (1966). *Bull. Off. int. Épizoot.*, *66*, 825.
(11) Wayt, L. K. (1953). *N. Amer. Vet.*, *34*, 506.
(12) Minett, F. C. (1948). *J. comp. Path.*, *58*, 245.
(13) Clay, H. A. (1960). *Vet. Rec.*, *72*, 265.
(14) Watt, J. A. A. (1960). *Vet. Rec.*, *72*, 998.
(15) Kerry, J. B. (1964). *Vet. Rec.*, *76*, 396.
(16) Oxer, D. T. *et al.* (1967). *Aust. vet. J.*, *43*, 25.

Malignant Oedema

(Gas Gangrene)

Malignant oedema is an acute wound infection caused by organisms of the genus *Clostridium*. There is acute inflammation at the site of infection and a profound systemic toxaemia.

Incidence

The clostridia which cause malignant oedema are common inhabitants of the animal environment and intestinal tract and although some of the causative species have a restricted distribution, the disease is general in most parts of the world. The disease occurs sporadically, affecting individual animals except in special circumstances when outbreaks may occur. The disease 'swelled head', a form of malignant oedema, occurs in young rams six months to two years old when they are run in bands and fight among themselves. After shearing, docking or lambing a high incidence may occur in sheep especially if they are dipped soon afterwards. Castration wounds in pigs and cattle may also become infected. Unless treatment is instituted in the early stages the death rate is extremely high.

Aetiology

Clostridium septicum, Cl. chauvoei, Cl. perfringens, Cl. sordellii and *Cl. novyi* have all been isolated from lesions typical of malignant oedema of animals. *Cl. sordellii* has been associated chiefly with malignant oedema of cattle but it has been found to be a cause of malignant oedema and swelled head in sheep (5). Swelled head of rams, in which the lesions of malignant oedema are restricted to the head, is almost always caused by *Cl. novyi* infection.

All ages and species of animals are affected. In most cases a wound is the portal of entry and a dirty environment which permits contamination of wounds with soil is the common predisposing cause. Hog cholera infection has also been suggested as a predisposing cause in swine (4). The occurrence of malignant oedema due to *Cl. chauvoei* has been discussed in the section on blackleg.

Transmission

The infection is usually soil-borne and the resistance of spores of the causative clostridia to environmental influence leads to persistence of the infection for long periods in a local area. Deep puncture wounds accompanied by severe trauma offer the most favourable conditions for growth of anaerobes and malignant oedema occurs most frequently under such conditions. Infection may occur through surgical or accidental wounds, following vaccination or venepuncture, or through the umbilical cord in the newborn. Outbreaks have been observed in both cattle and sheep following parturition, sometimes, though not always, associated with lacerations of the vulva. An unusual method of infection occurs when crows which have eaten infected carrion carry the infection to live, weak sheep and to lambs when they attack their eyes. The practice of dipping sheep immediately they are shorn may cause a high incidence of malignant oedema if the dip is heavily contaminated.

Pathogenesis

Potent toxins are produced in the local lesion and cause death when absorbed into the blood stream.

Clinical Findings

Clinical signs appear within 12 to 48 hours of infection. There is always a local lesion at the site of infection consisting of a soft, doughy swelling with marked local erythema. At a later stage the swelling becomes tense and the skin dark and taut. Emphysema may or may not be present depending on the type of infection and may be so marked as to cause extensive frothy exudation from the wound. With *Cl. novyi* infections there is no emphysema. A high fever (41 to 42 °C or 106 to 107 °F) is always present and affected animals are depressed, weak, show muscle tremor and usually stiffness or lameness. The illness is of short duration and affected animals die within 24 to 48 hours of the first appearance of signs. New cases continue to appear for 3 to 4 days after shearing or other precipitating cause.

When infection occurs at parturition swelling of the vulva accompanied by the discharge of a reddish brown fluid occurs within 2 to 3 days. The swelling extends to involve the pelvic tissues and perineal region. The local lesions are accompanied by a profound toxaemia and death occurs within 1 to 2 days.

In 'swelled head' of rams the oedema is restricted initially to the head. It occurs first under the eyes, spreads to the subcutaneous tissues of the head and down the neck. In pigs the lesions are usually restricted to the axilla, limbs and throat and are oedematous with very little evidence of emphysema. Local skin lesions consisting of raised, dull red plaques distended with clear serous fluid containing *Cl. septicum*, and causing no systemic illness have also been observed in pigs at abattoirs (1).

Clinical Pathology

Ante-mortem examination of affected animals is not usually undertaken in the laboratory although aspirated fluid from oedematous swellings or swabs from wounds may give an early diagnosis of the type of infection involved.

Necropsy Findings

Tissue changes occur rapidly after death, particularly in warm weather, and this must be kept in mind when evaluating post-mortem findings. There is usually gangrene of the skin with oedema of the subcutaneous and intermuscular connective tissue around the site of infection. There may be some involvement of underlying muscle but this is not marked. The oedema fluid varies from thin serum to a gelatinous deposit. It is usually blood stained and contains bubbles of gas except in *Cl. novyi* infections when the deposit is gelatinous, clear and contains no gas. A foul, putrid odour is often present in infections with *Cl. perfringens* and *Cl. sordellii*.

Subserous haemorrhages and accumulations of serosanguineous fluid in body cavities are usual. In 'swelled head' of rams the oedema of the head and neck may extend into the pleural cavity and also involve the lungs. Material from local lesions should be examined bacteriologically to determine the specific bacteria present.

Diagnosis

The association of profound toxaemia with local inflammation and emphysema is characteristic. The disease is differentiated from blackleg by the absence of typical muscle involvement and the presence of wounds. A history of prior vaccination against blackleg and the age of the animal may be of assistance in diagnosis. Anthrax in pigs is often accompanied by subcutaneous gelatinous oedema of the throat region. The problem in malignant oedema is to determine the identity of the organism or organisms and this can only be done by laboratory procedures. In this connection it must be remembered that clostridia are present in the alimentary tract of normal animals and under favourable conditions post-mortem invasion of the tissues may occur rapidly.

Treatment

Affected animals should be treated as emergency cases because of the acuteness of the disease. Specific treatment requires the administration of penicillin or a broad spectrum antibiotic. Antitoxin is effective in controlling the toxaemia (2) but is usually too expensive for practical use and must be given very early in the course of the disease. Local treatment of the wound with hydrogen peroxide has been widely practised and the application of cold packs to the area may limit the absorption of toxins.

Control

Hygiene at lambing, shearing, castration and docking is essential to the control of the infection in sheep. The flavine and acridine disinfectants are most effective for prophylactic application to wounds (3). Vaccination with the specific or combined, formalinized bacterin is satisfactory in preventing the occurrence of the disease in enzootic areas. If the probability of infection appears great the administration of adequate doses of penicillin will prevent its occurrence.

REFERENCES

(1) McDonald, I. W. & Collins, F. V. (1947). Aust. vet. J., 23, 50.
(2) Evans, D. G. (1945). Brit. J. exp. Path., 26, 104.
(3) McIntosh, J. & Selbie, F. R. (1946). Brit. J. exp. Path., 27, 46.
(4) Steward, J. S. (1944). Vet. Rec., 56, 321.
(5) Smith, L. D. S. et al. (1962). Cornell Vet., 52, 63.

Braxy

(Bradsot)

Braxy is an acute infectious disease of sheep characterized by inflammation of the abomasal wall, toxaemia and a high mortality rate.

Incidence

The disease occurs in the U.K., various parts of Europe and has been reported in the southern part of Australia (1) but appears to be rare in North America. It is not of major importance because of its low incidence although at one time it was sufficiently common to be an important cause of loss in some countries. In affected sheep the mortality rate is usually about 50 per cent and in enzootic areas an annual loss of 8 per cent has been reported (2).

Aetiology

Clostridium septicum, the common cause of malignant oedema in animals, is generally regarded as the causative bacterium. The disease occurs only in mid-winter when heavy frosts and snow occur and usually only in weaner and yearling sheep. Adult animals in an enzootic area appear to have acquired immunity.

Transmission

Cl. septicum is a soil-borne organism and in many areas can be considered as a normal inhabitant of the ovine intestinal tract.

Pathogenesis

Presumably a primary abomasitis, caused by the ingestion of frozen grass or other feed, permits invasion by Cl. septicum resulting in a fatal toxaemia.

Clinical Findings

There is a sudden onset of illness with segregation from the group, complete anorexia, depression and high fever (42°C or 107°F or more). The abdomen may be distended with gas and there may be signs of abdominal pain. The sheep becomes recumbent, comatose and dies within a few hours of first becoming ill.

Clinical Pathology

Ante-mortem laboratory examinations are of little value in establishing a diagnosis.

Necropsy Findings

There are localized areas of oedema, congestion, necrosis and ulceration of the abomasal wall. Congestion of the mucosa of the small intestine may also be present and there may be a few sub-epicardial petechiae. *Cl. septicum* can be isolated by smear from the cut surface of the abomasal wall or by culture from the heart blood and other organs of fresh carcases. Bacteriological examination of tissues must be carried out within an hour of death if the diagnosis is to be confirmed.

Diagnosis

Clinically the diagnosis of braxy is most difficult. At necropsy the lesions of abomasitis are characteristic especially if the disease occurs under conditions of severe cold. Overeating on grain may cause local patches of rumenitis and reticulitis but there are no lesions in the abomasum. Braxy may resemble infectious necrotic hepatitis but there are no liver lesions in braxy. The final diagnosis depends on isolation of *Cl. septicum* from typical alimentary tract lesions.

Treatment

No treatment has been found to be of value.

Control

Management of the flock is important. The sheep should be yarded at night, and fed hay before being let out on to the frosted pasture each morning. Vaccination with a formalin-killed whole culture of *Cl. septicum* (3), preferably two injections 2 weeks apart, is also an effective preventive.

REFERENCES

(1) Dumaresq, J. A. (1939). *Aust. vet. J.*, *15*, 252.
(2) Gaiger, S. H. (1922). *J. comp. Path.*, *35*, 191 & 235.
(3) Gordon, W. S. (1934). *Vet. Rec.*, *14*, 1.

Infectious Necrotic Hepatitis

(Black Disease)

Infectious necrotic hepatitis is an acute toxaemia of sheep, cattle and sometimes of pigs caused by the toxin of *Clostridium novyi* elaborated in damaged liver tissue. Under field conditions it is usually associated with fascioliasis.

Incidence

The disease is world wide in distribution but is of particular importance in Australia and New Zealand, and to a lesser extent in the U.K., the U.S.A. and in Europe. In sheep the morbidity rate is usually about 5 per cent in affected flocks but may be as high as 10 to 30 per cent and in rare cases up to 50 per cent. The disease is always fatal in both sheep and cattle. Details of the incidence in cattle (2, 4) and pigs (10, 11) are scanty but the disease is becoming more common in some areas.

Aetiology

The disease occurs in sheep and cattle and rarely in pigs. *Cl. novyi*, especially Type B, is the cause of the disease but the intervention of a necrotic process in the liver, which causes the organism to proliferate and produce lethal amounts of toxin, is commonly stated to be the precipitating cause. Although field outbreaks of the disease are usually precipitated by invasion of the liver by immature liver fluke (1) it is possible that other causes of local hepatic injury, e.g. invasion by cysts of *Cysticercus tenuicollis* (8) or hepatitis may precipitate the disease and an increasing number of cases are being observed in which no specific precipitating lesion can be detected (10, 12). This is especially so in cattle and pigs when they are heavily fed on grain, and infection with *Cl. novyi* should be considered in the differential diagnosis of sudden death in these circumstances. Well-nourished adult sheep in the 2 to 4 year age group are particularly susceptible, lambs and yearlings rarely being affected. A seasonal occurrence is marked because of fluctuation in the liver fluke and host snail population. Outbreaks are most common in the summer or autumn months and cease soon after frosts occur because of destruction of encysted metacercariae. Exposure to fluke infestation, as occurs when sheep graze on marshy ground during drought, is commonly associated with outbreaks of black disease, although they can occur in winter (5). Fatal infection with *Cl. novyi* can also occur through the navel in lambs and the uterus in ewes (13).

Transmission

Faecal contamination of the pasture by carrier animals is the most important source of infection although the cadavers of sheep dead of the disease may cause heavy contamination. Many normal animals in flocks in which the disease occurs carry *Cl. novyi* in their livers, not all strains being pathogenic (14). The spread of the infection from farm to farm occurs via these sheep and probably also by infected wild animals and birds (6) and by the carriage of contaminated soil during flooding. Spores of the causative clostridia are ingested and are presumably carried to the liver in the portal blood stream. Sheep removed from a black disease farm may die of the disease up to 6 weeks later because of the time lag required for migration of the flukes. Heavy irrigation of pastures, by creating favourable conditions for the development of flukes, lends itself to a high incidence of the disease and the occurrence of the disease in cattle is limited largely to irrigated farms (4).

Pathogenesis

Under local anaerobic conditions, such as occur in the liver when migrating fluke cause severe tissue destruction, the organisms already present in the liver proliferate, liberating toxins which cause local liver necrosis and more diffuse damage to the vascular system. The nervous signs observed may be due to this general vascular disturbance or to a specific neurotoxin.

Clinical Findings

Deaths of sheep usually occur at night and the sheep are found dead without having exhibited previous signs of illness. When observation is possible clinically affected sheep are seen to segregate from the rest of the flock, lag behind and go down if driven. There is some hyperaesthesia, respiration is rapid and shallow, the sheep remains in sternal recumbency and often dies within a few minutes while still in this position. The course from first illness to death is never more than a few hours and death usually occurs quietly, without evidence of struggling.

Clinical findings are the same in cattle as in sheep but the course is longer, the illness lasting for 1 to 2 days (4). Outstanding clinical findings in cattle include a sudden severe depression, reluctance to move, coldness of the skin, absence of rumen sounds, a low or normal temperature, and weakness and muffling of the heart sounds. There is abdominal pain, especially on deep palpation over the liver, and the faeces are semi-fluid. Periorbital oedema may also develop.

Cl. novyi is becoming more frequently recognized as a cause of sudden death in pigs.

Clinical Pathology

Ante-mortem laboratory examinations are not usually possible because of the peracute nature of the disease.

Necropsy Findings

Blood stained froth may exude from the nostrils. The carcase undergoes rapid putrefaction. There is pronounced engorgement of the subcutaneous vessels and a variable degree of subcutaneous oedema. The dark appearance of the inside of the skin, particularly noticeable on drying, has given rise to the name black disease. Gelatinous exudate may be present in moderate quantities in the fascial planes of the abdominal musculature. There is a general engorgement of the liver which has a dark, grey-brown appearance and exhibits characteristic areas of necrosis. These are yellow areas, 1 to 2 cm. in diameter, and surrounded by a zone of bright red hyperaemia. They occur mostly under the capsule of the diaphragmatic surface of the organ but may be more deeply seated and can easily be missed unless the liver is sliced carefully. In cattle they are linear in shape and may be difficult to find (4). There is usually evidence of recent invasion with liver fluke with channels of damaged liver tissue evident on the cut surface of the liver. These may be mistaken for subcapsular haemorrhages when viewed from the surface. Mature flukes are not ordinarily observed. Blood stained serous fluid is always present in abnormally large amounts in the pericardial, pleural and peritoneal cavities. Subendocardial and subepicardial haemorrhages are frequent. Unusual lesions such as a large area of inflammation in the wall of the abomasum (9) and congestion of the subcutaneous tissue and muscle in the shoulder and withers (10) have been observed in some cattle dying of the disease.

Material for laboratory examination should include a piece of necrotic liver removed aseptically and packed in a sterile jar, smears made from the periphery of the lesion and a piece of liver packed in formalin for histological examination. The critical observation in the diagnosis of black disease is the finding of *Cl. novyi* in the typical liver lesion and the demonstration of preformed toxin in peritoneal fluid and the liver lesion (3). However the use of fluorescent antibody techniques is almost as accurate and much less time-consuming (10).

Diagnosis

In sheep acute fascioliasis can cause heavy mortalities due to massive liver destruction at the same time and under the same conditions as does black disease. The course in fascioliasis is longer, affected sheep showing depression and anorexia for 2 to 3 days before death. At necropsy excess serous fluid is present only in the peritoneal cavity, the necrotic areas characteristic of black disease are absent and the liver is enlarged, friable and mottled, and penetrated by many small blood-filled channels of liver destruction and these may perforate through the liver capsule producing small, subcapsular haemorrhages. Young flukes may be visible through the capsule. Other acute clostridial infections such as blackleg and malignant oedema, and also anthrax cause similar heavy mortalities in sheep with a brief period of illness and specific lesions may be sufficient to make a diagnosis possible at necropsy. However, laboratory examination is necessary for a definite diagnosis.

Treatment

No effective treatment is available. In cattle the longer course of the disease suggests the possibility of controlling the clostridial infection by the parenteral use of penicillin or wide spectrum antibiotics.

Control

Control of the disease can be effected by control of the liver fluke. The host snail must be destroyed in streams and marshes by the use of a molluscicide and the flukes eliminated from the sheep by treatment with carbon tetrachloride or other drug. Pasture contamination from cadavers should be minimized by burning the carcases.

Vaccination with an alum-precipitated toxoid is highly effective and can be carried out during the course of an outbreak. The mortality begins to subside within 2 weeks. On an affected farm the initial vaccination is followed by a second vaccination 1 month later and subsequently by annual vaccinations. To provide maximum immunity at the time when the disease is most likely to occur, vaccination as a prophylactic measure should be carried out in early summer. A single vaccination of toxoid has also been reported to give lifelong immunity (7).

REFERENCES

(1) Turner, A. W. (1931). *Counc. sci. industr. Res., Aust., Pamphlet No. 19.*
(2) Herbert, T. G. G. & Hughes, L. E. (1956). *Vet. Rec., 68,* 223.
(3) Williams, B. M. (1962). *Vet. Rec., 74,* 1536.
(4) Gee, R. W. (1958). *Aust. vet. J., 34,* 352.
(5) Osborne, H. G. (1958). *Aust. vet. J., 34,* 301.
(6) Jamieson, S. (1949). *J. Path. Bact., 61,* 389.
(7) Tunnicliff, E. A. (1943). *J. Amer. vet. med. Ass., 103,* 368.
(8) Hreczko, I. (1959). *Aust. vet. J., 35,* 462.
(9) Ditchfield, J. & Julian, R. J. (1960). *Canad. vet. J., 1,* 542.
(10) Batty, I. *et al.* (1964). *Vet. Rec., 76,* 115.
(11) Bourne, F. J. & Kerry (1965). *Vet. Rec., 77,* 1463.
(12) Williams, B. M. (1964). *Vet. Rec., 76,* 591.
(13) Wallace, G. V. (1966). *N.Z. vet. J., 14,* 24.
(14) Roberts, R. S. *et al.* (1970). *Vet. Rec., 86,* 628.

Bacillary Haemoglobinuria

This acute, highly fatal intoxication of cattle and sheep is characterized clinically by a high fever, haemoglobinuria and jaundice, and by the presence of necrotic infarcts in the liver.

Incidence

Bacillary haemoglobinuria has been reported principally from the western part of the U.S.A. (1) although the disease has also been observed in the southern states, Mexico, Venezuela (2), Chile (3), Turkey (4), Australia (12), New Zealand (10) and Great Britain (5). The disease is not a common one but on infected farms death losses, which are usually less than 5 per cent, may reach as high as 25 per cent. Recovery without treatment is rare. The highest incidence of bacillary haemoglobinuria is on irrigated or poorly drained pasture, especially if the soil is alkaline in reaction (13). Some outbreaks have occurred in feedlots where hay cut from infected fields was fed. The disease is rare on dry, open range country. Heavy mortalities may occur when cattle from an uninfected area are brought on to an infected farm, cases beginning to occur 7 to 10 days later.

Aetiology

Cl. haemolyticum (*Cl. novyi* Type D), a soil-borne anaerobe, is present in the lesions. Cultures of the organism produce severe muscle necrosis and haemoglobinuria when injected intramuscularly into cattle and experimental animals, but the typical disease, including liver infarcts and subperitoneal haemorrhage has not been produced experimentally. In infected areas the organism is often found in the livers of healthy cattle. In field outbreaks cattle are the usual species involved although occasional cases occur in sheep and rare cases in pigs. It is a disease of the summer and autumn months and the high incidence on irrigated pasture suggests an environmental precipitating cause. Telangiectasis and fascioliasis have been suggested as precipitating causes but evidence on this point is incomplete (7, 8). The disease has been produced experimentally by infecting calves orally and precipitating a clostridial toxaemia by carrying out liver biopsis (15). As is the case in many clostridial diseases animals in good condition are more susceptible. The longevity of the spores in soil is unknown but the isolation of the organism from bones at least a year after the death of an animal from bacillary haemoglobinuria has been reported (9).

Cl. haemolyticum is serologically identifiable by an agglutination reaction between specific antiserum and young cultures of the organism. However, antigenically similar but less virulent organisms may produce a positive agglutination test and a positive reaction is not proof of the presence of the disease (6). Immunity appears to develop as a result of subclinical infection or continued exposure under field conditions.

Transmission

The disease is spread from infected to non-infected areas by flooding, natural drainage, by contaminated hay from infected areas or by carrier animals. The carriage of bones or meat by dogs or other carnivora could also effect spread of the infection. Contamination of pasture may occur from faeces or from decomposing cadavers. Although attempts to produce the disease by feeding the organism have been unsuccessful it is probable that under natural conditions invasion occurs from the alimentary tract after ingestion of contaminated material.

Pathogenesis

As in black disease of sheep the bacteria are carried to the liver and lodge there until damage to the parenchyma of the liver and the resulting hypoxia create conditions suitable for their proliferation. The development of an organized thrombus in a sub-terminal branch of the portal vein produces the large anaemic infarct which is characteristic of the disease. Most of the bacteria are to be found in this infarct and it is presumed that under the anaerobic conditions prevailing there, toxin is elaborated in large amounts and causes the severe toxaemia which is the basis of the signs produced. Two toxins, a haemolysin and a necrotizing agent, are formed by the bacterium, the haemolytic agent being responsible for the acute haemolytic anaemia which develops (7). In the later stages bacteraemia also develops and, combined with the anoxia resulting from the severe haemolysis, results in endothelial damage, and extravasations of blood into the tissues, and plasma into serous cavities (11).

Clinical Findings

The experimental disease occurs as early as 15 hours following the intramuscular injection of cultures. When animals are brought into contact with the infection in the field losses seldom start until 7 to 10 days later. The illness is of short duration and cattle at pasture may be found dead without signs having been observed. More often there is a sudden onset, with complete cessation of rumination, feeding, lactation and defaecation. Abdominal pain is evidenced by disinclination to move and an arched-back posture. Grunting may be evident on walking. Respiration is shallow and laboured and the pulse is weak and rapid. Fever (39·5 to 41°C or 103 to 106°F) is evident in the early stages but the temperature subsides to subnormal before death. Oedema of the brisket is a common finding. The faeces are dark brown; there may be diarrhoea with much mucus and some blood. The urine is dark red. Jaundice is present but is never very obvious. The duration of the illness varies from 12 hours in dairy cows in advanced pregnancy, to 4 days in dry stock. Pregnant cows often abort. Severe dyspnoea is evident just before death.

Clinical Pathology

The red colour of the urine is due to the presence of haemoglobin; there are no free red cells. In the later stages the blood is thin, the erythrocyte count being depressed to one to four million per cmm. and the haemoglobin to 3 to 8 g. per cent. Leucocyte counts vary considerably from 6700 to 34,800 per cmm. but are mostly above normal in the range of 10,000 to 16,000 per cmm. Differential counts vary similarly with a tendency to neutrophilia in severe cases. Serum calcium and phosphorus levels are normal but blood glucose levels may be elevated (100 to 120 mg. per cent) in some cases.

Blood cultures during the acute stages of the disease may be positive. Serum agglutinins against *Cl. haemolyticum* may be detectable at low levels (1:25 or 1:50) during the clinical illness and if the animal recovers rise to appreciable levels (1:50 to 1:800) a week later. Titres greater than 1:400 are usual at this time. As pointed out previously a positive agglutination test is not conclusive evidence of the presence of the disease.

Necropsy Findings

Rigor mortis develops quickly. The perineum is soiled with blood stained urine and faeces. Subcutaneous, gelatinous oedema which tends to become crepitant in a few hours, and extensive petechial or diffuse haemorrhages in subcutaneous tissue are characteristic. There is a variable degree of jaundice. Excessive amounts of fluid, varying from clear to blood stained and turbid, are present in the pleural, pericardial and peritoneal cavities. Generalized subserous haemorrhages are also present. Similar haemorrhages appear under the endocardium. Haemorrhagic abomasitis and enteritis are accompanied by the presence of blood stained ingesta or free blood. The characteristic lesion of bacillary haemoglobinuria is an anaemic infarct in the liver. One or more may be present in any part of the organ and vary from 5 to 20 cm. in diameter. The infarct is pale, surrounded by a zone of hyperaemia and has the general appearance of local necrosis. Red urine is present in the kidneys and bladder and petechiation is evident throughout the kidney.

Cl. haemolyticum can be isolated from heart blood, the liver infarct and many other organs from a fresh carcase although post-mortem invaders quickly obscure its presence.

Diagnosis

The diagnosis of bacillary haemoglobinuria is largely a question of differentiation from other diseases in which haemoglobinuria, myoglobinuria and haematuria are cardinal signs. Acute leptospirosis is likely to occur under the same environmental conditions and present a similar clinical picture. Necropsy findings will differentiate the two and clinical pathology may help but in acute outbreaks it may be impossible to make a positive clinical diagnosis in time to save individual animals. Post-parturient haemoglobinuria, haemolytic anaemia caused by cruciferous plants including rape, kale and chou moellier are not accompanied by a severe febrile reaction. Babesiasis and anaplasmosis are geographically limited and the causative protozoa are detectable in blood smears. The course of all of the above diseases may be as short as that of bacillary haemoglobinuria.

Enzootic haematuria, pyelonephritis and cystitis are recognizable by the presence of red cells in the urine. In sheep chronic copper poisoning presents a clinical picture similar to that of bacillary haemoglobinuria but there are no infarcts in the liver. Other causes of sudden death in cattle and sheep including anthrax, blackleg and infectious necrotic hepatitis may confuse the diagnosis especially if terminal haematuria occurs.

Treatment

Specific treatment includes the immediate use of penicillin or tetracyclines in full doses and antitoxic serum (500 to 1000 ml.). Prompt treatment is essential and provided the serum is administered in the early stages of the disease, haemoglobinuria may disappear within 12 hours. Supportive treatment, including blood transfusion, parenteral fluid and electrolyte solutions, is of considerable importance. Care is required during treatment and examination as undue excitement or exercise may cause sudden death. Bulls should not be used for service until at least 3 weeks after recovery because of the danger of liver rupture. Convalescence is often prolonged and animals should be protected from nutritional and climatic stress until they are fully recovered. Haemopoiesis should be facilitated by the provision of mineral supplements containing iron, copper and cobalt.

Control

As a general rule a formalin-killed whole culture adsorbed on aluminium hydroxide gives good protection for a year in cattle. Vaccination is carried out 4 to 6 weeks before the expected occurrence of the disease. Annual revaccination of all animals over 6 months of age is necessary in enzootic areas. In some locations of extreme risk a second vaccination during the grazing season is recommended. To obviate the local reaction which occurs at the site of injection the inoculum may be administered at several sites and distributed under the skin by massage. The injection must be subcutaneous, as intradermal and intramuscular injections are likely to produce severe reactions. A formalin killed bacterin, emulsified in mineral oil, gives promise of more prolonged immunity but has not been completely evaluated (14). In the absence of a type-specific vaccine the use of black disease vaccine appears to be a satisfactory alternative. The carcases of animals dying of the disease should be disposed of by burning or deep burial.

REFERENCES

(1) Records, E. & Vawter, L. R. (1945). *Univ. Nev. agric. exp. Stn, Bull.*, *173*, 9–48.
(2) Dumith, Arteaga, G. (1955). *Bol. Inst. Invest. vet.*, (*Caracas*), *7*, 3.
(3) Anderson, E. H. (1950). *Nord. Vet.-Med.*, *2*, 688.
(4) Gurturk, S. (1952). *Z. Immun.-Forsch.*, *109*, 462.
(5) Soltys, M. A. & Jennings, A. R. (1950). *Vet. Rec.*, *62*, 5.
(6) Smith, L. D. S. & Jasmin, A. M. (1956). *J. Amer. vet. med. Ass.*, *129*, 68.
(7) Roberts, R. S. *et al.* (1970). *J. comp. Path.*, *80*, 9.
(8) Smith, L. D. S. (1957). 'Clostridial Diseases of Animals' in *Advances in Veterinary Science*, Vol. 3, pp. 465–524, New York: Academic Press.
(9) Jasmin, A. M. (1947). *Amer. J. vet. Res.*, *8*, 341.
(10) Quinlivan, T. D. & Wedderburn, J. F. (1959). *N.Z. vet. J.*, *7*, 113 & 115.
(11) Williams, B. M. (1964). *Vet. Rec.*, *76*, 591.
(12) Wellington, N. A. M. & Perceval, A. (1966). *Aust. vet. J.*, *42*, 128.
(13) van Ness, G. B. & Erickson, K. (1964). *J. Amer. vet. med. Ass.*, *144*, 492.
(14) Claus, K. D. (1964). *Amer. J. vet. Res.*, *25*, 699.
(15) Olander, H. J. *et al.* (1966). *Path. vet.*, *3*, 421.

Enterotoxaemia Caused by *Clostridium perfringens* Type A

The role of *Cl. perfringens* Type A in the pathogenesis of diseases of animals is uncertain because the organism forms part of the bacterial flora of the alimentary tract in many normal animals. However, there are isolated reports of mortalities caused by the organism. There are reports of a highly fatal haemolytic disease in sheep and cattle in Australia (1) and in lambs in California (2). An acute haemorrhagic enteritis in calves (3) and adult cattle (4) has been recorded in the United Kingdom.

In the haemolytic disease there is an acute onset of severe depression, collapse, mucosal pallor, jaundice, haemoglobinuria and dyspnoea. Temperatures range from normal to 41°C (106°F). The disease is highly fatal, most affected animals dying within 12 hours of the onset of illness although occasional animals survive for several days. At necropsy the cardinal features are pallor, jaundice and haemoglobinuria. The kidneys are swollen, dark brown in colour and may contain infarcts, the liver is pale and swollen and there may be hydropericardium and pulmonary oedema. Clostridia dominate the bacterial population of the small intestine as indicated by smears made from the contents and alpha-toxin is present in large quantities. The toxin is a lecithinase and is actively haemolytic, and its presence in large quantities in the intestine is indicative of the existence of the disease. The syndrome is very similar to that caused by chronic copper poisoning and leptospirosis in calves.

In the haemorrhagic enteritis of calves and adult cattle the syndrome observed is indistinguishable from that caused by *Cl. perfringens* Types B and C. The disease in adult cattle occurs most commonly in the period shortly after calving. The experimental disease in lambs, produced by the intravenous injection of toxin, is characterized by transitory diarrhoea and hyperaemia of the intestinal mucosa (5). Type A antiserum has been effective in prevention of the disease in calves (1) and a formalinized vaccine has shown some immunizing capacity in sheep (6).

REFERENCES

(1) Rose, A. L. & Edgar, G. (1936). *Aust. vet. J.*, *12*, 212.
(2) McGowan, B. *et al.* (1958). *J. Amer. vet. med. Ass.*, *133*, 219.
(3) MacRae, D. R. *et al.* (1943). *Vet. Rec.*, *55*, 203.
(4) Shirley, G. N. (1958). *Vet. Rec.*, *70*, 478.
(5) Niilo, L. (1971). *Infect. Immun.*, *3*, 100.
(6) Niilo, L. *et al.* (1971). *Canad. J. Microbiol.*, *17*, 391.

Enterotoxaemia Caused by *Clostridium perfringens* Types B, C and E

Infection with *Cl. perfringens* Types B and C results in severe enteritis with diarrhoea and dysentery in young lambs, calves, pigs and foals. A number of diseases caused by these clostridia occur in different parts of the world and are given specific names but are dealt with here as a group. They include lamb dysentery (*Cl. perfringens* Type B), struck (*Cl. perfringens* Type C), and haemorrhagic enterotoxaemia (*Cl. perfringens* Type C). Necrotic haemorrhagic enteritis due to *Cl. perfringens* Type E has been recorded in calves (17).

Incidence

Enterotoxaemia caused by *Cl. perfringens* Type B is encountered only sporadically except for lamb dysentery which occurs fairly extensively in Britain, Europe and South Africa. In affected groups of lambs, the morbidity may reach as high as 20 to 30 per cent. A characteristic of the disease is the tendency of the morbidity rate on infected farms to increase year by year and to affect older lambs up to 2 to 3 weeks of age. The mortality rate approaches 100 per cent. Lamb dysentery is most prevalent in cold weather and on farms where ewes are kept closely confined in small yards or fields for lambing. Gross contamination of the surroundings with the causative bacteria is likely to occur in these circumstances. Haemorrhagic enterotoxaemia caused by *Cl. perfringens* Type C has been reported most commonly from certain areas in the U.S.A. and Britain. Struck is limited in its occurrence to certain localities in Britain. In all species, these diseases are likely to occur in outbreaks affecting a number of animals and death losses are high. Outbreaks in pigs usually affect most susceptible litters on the farm and the majority of pigs in each litter are affected.

Aetiology

The causative clostridia occur commonly in soil and the alimentary tract of normal animals, and, as in enterotoxaemia caused by *Cl. perfringens* Type D, the disease appears to be precipitated by factors still incompletely understood. The bacteria are capable of forming spores which survive for long periods in soil. In general rapidly growing, well-nourished animals are most susceptible.

The diseases as they occur in the different animal species are as follows:

Lamb dysentery caused by *Cl. perfringens* Type B occurs in young lambs up to 3 weeks of age. An enterotoxaemia of young lambs may also be caused by *Cl. perfringens* Type C (7).

Struck (11) caused by *Cl. perfringens* Type C affects adult sheep, particularly when feed is abundant.

Goat enterotoxaemia has been caused by *Cl. perfringens* Type C (12).

Calf enterotoxaemia caused by *Cl. perfringens* Types B and C (1, 2, 3, 4, 8) occurs in young calves up to 10 days of age.

Pig enterotoxaemia caused by *Cl. perfringens* Type C is recorded in sucking pigs during the first week of life (5, 16) and has been produced experimentally by feeding whole cultures of *Cl. perfringens* Type C (14).

Foal enterotoxaemia caused by *Cl. perfringens* (type unknown) and Type B has occurred in foals within the first few days of life (6, 9).

Transmission

The organisms occur in the faeces of infected animals and contamination of the soil and pasture is followed by ingestion of the bacteria. The toxins produced are *alpha*, *beta* and *epsilon* in Type B, and *alpha* and *beta* in Type C. In pigs the organisms are recoverable from the skin of sows and the faeces of affected piglets and infection probably occurs during suckling (5). The predominance of these diseases in very young animals may be due to the immaturity of their alimentary tracts, the beta-toxin being readily inactivated by trypsin. It is probable that many animals become infected but do not show clinical illness as antitoxin has been detected in clinically normal animals (8).

Pathogenesis

The characteristic effect of the beta-toxin, the important toxin produced by *Cl. perfringens* Types B and C, is the production of haemorrhagic enteritis and ulceration of the intestinal mucosa. Beta toxin is inactivated by proteolytic enzymes and these are decreased or absent in affected swine (18).

Clinical Findings

The syndrome of lamb dysentery usually occurs in lambs less than 2 weeks old and is manifested by sudden death without premonitory signs in peracute cases. In the more common acute form, there is severe abdominal pain, recumbency, failure to suck and the passing of brown, fluid faeces sometimes containing blood. Death usually occurs after a period of coma and within 24 hours of the onset of illness. On farms where the disease has become established cases may occur in older lambs up to 3 weeks of age and occasional cases may survive for several days.

As a rule the syndrome known as struck in adult sheep is manifested only by sudden death, clinical signs not being observed beforehand. Occasionally death is preceded by abdominal pain and convulsions.

In calves, the disease usually occurs as outbreaks of severe dysentery with some deaths in calves 7 to 10 days old although calves up to 10 weeks of age may be affected. The signs include diarrhoea, dysentery and acute abdominal pain accompanied by violent bellowing and aimless running. There may be additional nervous signs including tetany and opisthotonus. In very acute cases, death occurs in a few hours, sometimes without diarrhoea being evident. In less severe cases, the illness lasts for about 4 days and recovery is slow, usually requiring 10 to 14 days.

Affected pigs are normal at birth but become dull and depressed and exhibit diarrhoea, dysentery and gross reddening of the anus. Most affected pigs die within 24 hours. Frequently the majority of litters born during an outbreak will be affected although affected litters may include some normal pigs. The disease tends to recur on the same premises in succeeding years (13). Occasionally weaned pigs are affected. Foals usually show severe depression, abdominal pain, diarrhoea and dysentery, and die within a few hours. In both piglets and foals, the disease occurs in the first few days of life.

The disease is an intoxication and there is usually no fever in any of the species. A chronic form with debilitating diarrhoea and failure to grow is suspected in calves (10).

Clinical Pathology

The disease in all species is so acute and highly fatal that the diagnosis is usually made on necropsy material. Ante-mortem laboratory examinations are not widely used in diagnosis but the predominance of clostridia in a faecal smear may suggest a diagnosis of haemorrhagic enterotoxaemia. Specific antitoxins are detectable in the sera of recovered animals. A severe hypoglycaemia has been observed in baby pigs dying of the disease (14) but this is not specific to this infection.

Necropsy Findings

A haemorrhagic enteritis, with ulceration of the mucosa in some cases, is the major lesion in all species. The intestinal mucosa is congested and dark red, and the ulcers are large (2·5 cm. in diameter) and penetrate almost to the serosa. The lesions are usually most severe in the ileum. Blood stained contents are present in the intestine and there is an excess of serous fluid in the peritoneal cavity. Subendocardial and subepicardial haemorrhages are often present. In sheep affected with struck in addition to the above lesions there is often peritonitis and the skeletal muscles have the appearance of malignant oedema if necropsy is delayed for several hours. In pigs in the 7 to 10 days age group, in which the disease is less acute than in newborn pigs, the haemorrhagic enteritis is not so evident, the major lesion being a yellow, fibrinous deposit on the intestinal mucosa accompanied by large quantities of watery, lightly blood stained ingesta in the lumen.

A portion of small intestine with its contents is suitable for laboratory diagnosis. Smears of intestinal contents can be stained and examined for large numbers of clostridia, and filtrates of the contents tested for toxin content. Cultural examination of the ingesta may also be attempted.

Diagnosis

The early age at which this disease occurs, the rapid course and typical necropsy findings suggest the diagnosis, which can be readily confirmed by laboratory examination. Other acute diseases of newborn animals which may be confused with lamb dysentery and haemorrhagic enterotoxaemia include particularly enteritis and septicaemia caused by *Escherichia coli* and *Salmonella* spp., *Actinobacillus equuli* and porcine transmissible gastroenteritis. In most instances, it is necessary to confirm the diagnosis of these diseases by laboratory examination of faecal material or intestinal contents collected at necropsy. Struck is strictly regional in distribution and in affected areas can usually be diagnosed on the basis of necropsy lesions.

Treatment

Hyperimmune antiserum is the only treatment likely to be of value. Doses of 25 ml. of Type C antiserum have been used successfully in calves (8) but in other species death usually occurs too quickly for treatment to be effective. Oral administration of broad spectrum antibiotics may prevent further proliferation of organisms and production of toxins. Chelating agents as described in the section on enterotoxaemia may offer some promise in treatment.

Control

Vaccination, preferably with type-specific toxoid or bacterin, is the only preventive measure available. Because of the need for rapid action, it is usually necessary to proceed with vaccination before typing of the organism can be carried out. Cross-protection occurs between *Cl. perfringens* Types B and C because of the importance of beta-toxin in both strains, and the efficiency of lamb dysentery antiserum in protection against Type C infections has been recorded. Type C toxoid and antiserum are also available.

When an outbreak occurs, active vaccination may be impracticable because of the acute nature of the disease and the immaturity of the exposed animals. Antiserum will protect susceptible animals and should be administered immediately after birth. When the disease is enzootic in a herd, vaccination of the dams should be carried out. To initiate the programme two injections of vaccine are necessary one month apart, the second injection being given 2 weeks before parturition. For the prevention of lamb dysentery the two vaccinations of ewes may be spaced from 2 to 5 weeks apart and the second injection can be given as early as 2 months before lambing, thus avoiding handling of heavily pregnant ewes (15). In subsequent years, cows and ewes require only one booster injection immediately prior to parturition. With the use of clostridial toxoids and antisera, attention should be given to the unitage of the antigen or antitoxin present in the preparation used. These vary widely and the manufacturer's instructions should be followed closely. Anaphylaxis may occur because of the equine origin of the antisera and treated animals should be kept under close observation for 24 hours and treated quickly if signs of dyspnoea and muscle shivering occur.

REFERENCES

(1) Hepple, J. R. (1952). *Vet. Rec., 64*, 633.
(2) McRae, D. R. *et al.* (1943). *Vet Rec., 55*, 203.
(3) Griner, L. A. (1958). *Amer. J. vet. Sci., Sec. 1, 39*, 27.
(4) Smith, L. D. (1957). *Advances in Veterinary Science*, Vol. 3, pp. 465–524, New York: Academic Press.
(5) Field, H. I. & Gibson, E. A. (1955). *Vet. Rec., 67*, 31.
(6) Leader, G. H. (1952). *Vet. Rec., 64*, 241.
(7) Griner, L. A. & Johnson, H. W. (1954). *J. Amer. vet. med. Ass., 125*, 125.
(8) Griner, L. A. & Baldwin, E. M. (1954). *Proc. 91st ann. Mtg Amer. vet. med. Ass.*, 45–51.
(9) Mason, J. H. & Robinson, E. M. (1938). *Onderstepoort, J. vet. Sci., 11*, 333.
(10) Baldwin, E. (1959). *Vet. Med., 54*, 123.
(11) McEwen, A. D. & Roberts, R. S. (1931). *J. comp. Path., 44*, 26.
(12) Barron, N. S. (1942). *Vet. Rec., 54*, 82.
(13) Moon, H. W. & Bergeland, M. E. (1965). *Canad. vet. J., 6*, 159.
(14) Field, H. I. & Goodwin, R. F. W. (1959). *J. Hyg. (Camb.), 57*, 81.
(15) Jansen, B. C. (1961). *Onderstepoort, J. vet. Res., 28*, 495.
(16) Högh, P. (1969). *Acta vet. scand., 10*, 57, 84.
(17) Hart, B. & Hooper, P. T. (1967). *Aust. vet. J., 43*, 360.
(18) Bergeland, M. E. (1972). *J. Amer. vet. med. Ass., 160*, 568.

Enterotoxaemia Caused by *Clostridium perfringens* Type D

(Pulpy Kidney)

This is an acute toxaemia of ruminants caused by the proliferation of *Cl. perfringens* Type D in the intestines and the liberation of toxins. Clinically the disease is characterized by diarrhoea, convulsions, paralysis and sudden death.

Incidence

Enterotoxaemia caused by *Cl. perfringens* Type D is world wide in its distribution principally as a disease of lambs. It causes heavy losses particularly in flocks managed for lamb and mutton production. In North America it ranks as one of the main causes of loss among feedlot lambs. Morbidity rates vary a great deal but seldom exceed 10 per cent. The mortality rate approximates 100 per cent. A proportion of lambs and calves appear to be exposed to subclinical but antigenic levels of *Cl. perfringens* toxin so that they become immune without having shown signs of illness or without having been vaccinated (34). It is a common belief among cattlemen and veterinarians that many unexplained sudden deaths in feedlot cattle are due to this type of enterotoxaemia. This view is based largely on the reduction in mortality after vaccination and the recovery of some animals after treatment with *Cl. perfringens* Type D antitoxin (29). It has also been observed that *Cl. perfringens* can be isolated from the gut contents of 50 per cent of fattening cattle (39).

Aetiology

Cl. perfringens Type D normally inhabits the alimentary tract of sheep (1) and probably other ruminants but only in small numbers. The extent to which it occurs in the alimentary tract varies widely between flocks, although this accounts only in part for the variable incidence. The organism does not persist for very long in the soil. Under certain conditions, the organisms proliferate rapidly in the intestines and produce lethal quantities of toxin (1). The husbandry conditions in which the disease occurs include grazing on lush, rapidly growing pasture or young cereal crops, and heavy grain feeding in feedlots. Lambs on well-fed heavy-milking ewes are particularly susceptible. The high incidence under these conditions has given rise to the name of 'overeating' disease. An increased incidence of the disease has been reported after dosing with phenothiazine and experimental evidence suggests that such dosing may precipitate outbreaks in lambs (25). The disease can be produced experimentally in susceptible sheep and cattle by the injection into the duodenum of whole culture of *Cl. perfringens* Type D and dextrin (26, 35).

While enterotoxaemia is most common in lambs it also occurs in adult sheep, in goats (3), in calves (4, 5) and rarely in adult cattle (6, 28). In most, if not all circumstances, the affected animals are on highly nutritious diets and are in very good condition. The highest incidence of the disease is in sucking lambs between 3 and 10 weeks of age and single lambs are more susceptible than twins. Feeder lambs are most commonly affected soon after they are introduced into feedlots. Immunity is readily produced by suitable vaccination and a degree of natural immunity may be attained by non-lethal exposure to the toxin (31). A blood level of 0·15 Wellcome unit of epsilon antitoxin per ml. of serum is sufficient to protect sheep against further doses of toxin (26).

Transmission

Enterotoxaemia is not a contagious disease in that the presence of the causative bacteria in the intestine does not in itself produce the disease. Under natural conditions the ingestion of feed contaminated by infected faeces introduces the organism into the alimentary tract but the disease does not occur unless other factors intercede.

Pathogenesis

In the normal course of events, ingested *Cl. perfringens* Type D are destroyed in large numbers in the rumen and abomasum although some survive to reach the duodenum where multiplication occurs and toxin is produced. Intoxication does not occur because the movement of ingesta keeps the bacterial population and toxin content down to a low level. In certain circumstances, this does not hold and multiplication of the organisms and the production of toxin proceeds to the point where intoxication occurs. One of the circumstances has been shown to be the passage of large quantities of starch granules into the duodenum when sheep overeat on grain diets or are changed suddenly from a ration consisting largely of roughage to one consisting mainly of grain (2). Other factors such as heavy milk feeding may have the same effect. A slowing of alimentary tract movement has also been thought to permit excess toxin accumulation (7) and it may be that any factor which causes intestinal stasis will predispose to the disease. The importance of diet in the production of ruminal stasis has been discussed in diseases of the forestomachs of ruminants. In a number of instances outbreaks have followed the administration of phenothiazine. A high incidence has been observed in association with heavy tapeworm infestation (20).

The epsilon-toxin of *Cl. perfringens* Type D increases the permeability of the intestinal mucosa to this and other toxins, thereby facilitating its own absorption (8). The first effect of the toxin is to cause a profuse, mucoid diarrhoea, and secondarily, to produce a stimulation and then depression of the central nervous system. In sheep acute cases are characterized by the development in the brain of degeneration of vascular endothelium, perivascular and intercellular oedema and micro-scopic foci of necrosis in the basal ganglia, thalamus, internal capsule, substantia nigra, subcortical white matter and cerebellum (30). The situation of the lesions is similar to those which can be seen macroscopically in the brains of sheep affected by focal symmetrical encephalomalacia, a disease thought to be a sequel to enterotoxaemia. A terminal effect of the toxin is an unexplained, extreme hyperglycaemia in sheep (2).

Clinical Findings

In lambs, the course of the illness is very short, often less than 2 hours and never more than 12 hours, and many are found dead without previously manifesting signs. In closely observed flocks the first signs may be dullness, depression, yawning, facial movements and loss of interest in feed. Acute cases may show little more than severe clonic convulsions with frothing at the mouth and sudden death. Cases which survive for a few hours show a green, pasty diarrhoea, staggering, recumbency, opisthotonus and severe clonic convulsions. The temperature is usually normal but may be elevated if convulsions are severe. Death occurs during a convulsion or after a short period of coma.

Adult sheep usually survive for longer periods, up to 24 hours. They lag behind the flock, show staggering and knuckling, champing of the jaws, salivation and rapid, shallow, irregular respiration. There may be bloat in the terminal stages. Irritation signs, including convulsions, muscle tremor, grinding of the teeth and salivation, may occur but are less common than in lambs.

In calves and adult cattle the syndrome is similar to that seen in adult sheep, with nervous signs predominating. Peracute cases are found dead without having shown premonitory signs of illness and with no evidence of struggling. The more common, acute cases show a sudden onset of bellowing, mania and convulsions, the convulsions persisting until death occurs 1 to 2 hours later. Subacute cases, many of which recover, do not drink, are quiet and docile and appear to be blind, although the eye preservation reflex persists. They may continue in this state for 2 to 3 days and then recover quickly and completely. In an outbreak of the disease in calves all three forms of the disease may be seen. Diarrhoea is a prominent sign in affected goats especially in those which survive for more than a few days (19). In acute cases, there are convulsions after an initial attack of fever (40·5°C or 105°F) with severe abdominal pain and dysentery, and death occurs in 4 to 36 hours. In subacute cases, the goats may be ill for several weeks and show anorexia, intermittent severe diarrhoea and, in some cases, dysentery and the presence of epithelial shreds in the faeces. Chronic cases manifested by emaciation, anaemia and chronic diarrhoea are also recorded in goats.

Clinical Pathology

A high blood-sugar level of 150 to 200 mg. per cent and marked glycosuria are characteristic of the terminal stages of enterotoxaemia in sheep (9). However, similar observations can be made in sheep dying of a number of diseases, especially when there is hepatic injury (24).

Necropsy Findings

The carcase is usually in good condition. In peracute cases there may be no gross lesions. More frequently there is an excess of clear, straw-coloured pericardial fluid and many petechiae are present in the epicardium and endocardium. Patchy congestion of the abomasal and intestinal mucosae is characteristic and the intestine usually contains a moderate amount of thin, custardy ingesta. If the examination is delayed for a few hours, there is rapid decomposition, purple discolouration of the woolless skin, and the wool is easily plucked. A characteristic change is the presence of soft, pulpy kidneys a few hours after death. The liver is dark and congested and the pericardial fluid may be gelatinous and blood stained. The rumen and abomasum of feedlot lambs may be overloaded with concentrates.

Smears of ingesta should be taken from several levels in the small intestine and stained to determine the presence of Gram-positive rods. In affected animals the short, fat, Gram-positive rods dominate the slide to the almost complete exclusion of other bacteria. Attempts should be made to isolate the clostridia by cultural means and bowel filtrates should be tested for toxicity by injection into mice. If the filtrate is toxic, the type of toxin can be determined by protection of the mice with specific antisera but this does not determine the type of clostridia. The presence of beta-toxin indicates the presence of types B or C and epsilon-toxin the presence of B or D. Final identification depends upon agglutination tests with specific antisera (15). Intestinal contents to be examined for the presence of toxin should be milked out into a glass container, not left in a loop of intestine. At average temperatures one can expect to be able to isolate the toxin from the intestine of a sheep dead for up to 12 hours. The addition of one drop of chloroform to each 10 ml. of ingesta will stabilize the toxin for periods of up to a month (24). Hyperglycaemia and glycosuria may also be detected in necropsy material.

Diagnosis

In lambs, the circumstances, clinical syndrome and necropsy findings are diagnostic. Other causes of sudden death in lambs include acute pasteurellosis, hypocalcaemia with hypomagnesaemia, and septicaemia caused by *Haem. agni*. Focal symmetrical encephalomalacia, which may be a chronic form of enterotoxaemia, is accompanied by blindness, inco-ordination and paralysis. In live animals, enterotoxaemia may be confused with polioencephalomalacia in which the syndrome is similar but less acute and the course longer. There is no hyperglycaemia or glycosuria. Acute rumen impaction due to overeating may occur in the same circumstances but there are no convulsions or glycosuria although the animals may be recumbent. The course in acute ruminal impaction is much longer (1 to 3 days) than in enterotoxaemia (about 1 hour). In adult sheep and calves, the syndrome is readily confused with rabies, acute lead poisoning, hypomagnesaemic tetany, pregnancy toxaemia or louping ill. Clinically there may be little difference between these diseases although generally they are less acute and are not restricted to lambs. The history should be examined carefully. In rabies, there is usually a history of exposure; in acute lead poisoning access to toxic material should be evident; pregnancy toxaemia occurs only in late pregnancy in ewes on a falling plane of nutrition, and louping ill has a seasonal occurrence related to the activities of the vector ticks. Biochemical tests are of value in determining the presence of ketonuria in pregnancy toxaemia and the hypomagnesaemia of hypomagnesaemic tetany. Chemical tests of faeces, urine and blood aid in the diagnosis of lead poisoning.

The 'sudden death syndrome' in feedlot cattle includes a number of clinical entities and, while enterotoxaemia may be suspected, a definite diagnosis is often difficult to make. Response to vaccination is slow but is often used as a diagnostic aid despite its doubtful accuracy.

Treatment

Hyperimmune serum is an efficient short term prophylactic but is unlikely to be of much value in sick animals because of the acute nature of the disease, although serum (50 ml. twice daily) combined with orally administered sulphadimidine is reported to be effective in goats (19). Chelating agents are highly effective in neutralizing the toxins of *Cl. perfringens* in experimental animals. The mode of action is the temporary removal of metallic ions necessary for toxin activity. The toxins are capable of causing irreversible effects and the chelating compounds must be given soon after the administration of the toxin (14).

Control

There are two major control measures available, reduction of the food intake and vaccination. Vaccination is highly effective but not completely so and it is often necessary to reduce the food intake if best results are to be obtained (10). This will cause a setback in the growth of the lambs and for this reason farmers tend to rely more on vaccination as a control measure. The best advice is to both adjust the food intake and vaccinate, but to avoid interference with growth as much as possible.

Sheep running at pasture should be allowed access to a haystack or rough pasture; it may be necessary to shut them out of very good pasture fields at night and provide them with hay. Lambs or calves should be brought on to full concentrate feed gradually over a period of about 2 weeks and the amount of hay fed increased if deaths occur. A method of reducing the grain intake of lambs self-fed in feedlots is to mix elemental sulphur (7·5 g. per day per lamb) in the feed (11). In similar circumstances chlortetracycline fed continuously at a level of 10 mg. per lb. of feed prevents death but feeding at higher levels (25 mg. per lb. of feed) for short periods (12 days) does not (16). Another helpful practice in feedlots is to sort lambs into groups according to size so that there is equal competition for available food, and large, forward lambs are not so likely to gorge themselves. When an outbreak is developing in sucking lambs it is also a common practice to dock them, providing a temporary setback which usually stops further cases for several weeks.

Vaccination. Alum-precipitated, formalin-killed, whole culture (anaculture) is in general use but a similar vaccine activated by trypsin (activated alum-precipitated toxoid) is thought to give better results (12, 18). All vaccines in current use are alum-precipitated but the advantage gained by alum precipitation has been questioned (17). Many multiple vaccines are in use and the latest variation in the battle of vaccination against clostridia is the use of combined vaccines suspended in oil–water emulsions (37) and injected intraperitoneally. The vehicle ensures a continuing high level of antibodies, the route avoids local lesions in muscle. Single injections of individual toxins in Freund adjuvant give protection for as long as two years (38).

Alum-precipitated anaculture. For protection of lambs, the ewes are vaccinated twice, at 6 and 2 weeks before the anticipated lambing date. In subsequent years, vaccinated ewes need be revaccinated only once. The lambs become passively immune via the colostrum and are protected for the first few weeks of life (22) but must be vaccinated to obtain a durable immunity. This can be done at docking, although it can be done at any time if losses occur (21). Vaccination of very young lambs is not very effective in passively immune lambs because of a poor immune response. Immunity does not develop for 10 days after vaccination and, if losses are heavy, the prophylactic use of serum may be preferred. The vaccine may cause transient lameness and the development of a small, subcutaneous blemish. After the danger period in the young lamb stage, it may be necessary to revaccinate before the lambs go into feedlots. Only one injection is usually given at this time.

Activated alum-precipitated toxoid is used in the same manner but smaller doses are required (2 ml. as against 5 ml.) and the response to vaccination in young lambs immunized passively via the ewe is better (13). The standard anaculture produces no immunity in very young lambs but the activated toxoid administered when the lambs are 3 days old produces good immunity although a second injection at 1 month of age is recommended. The simultaneous administration of hyperimmune serum with this vaccine does not interfere with the stimulation of antibody production. Revaccination at 6-monthly intervals provides permanent protection (12). Sheep vaccinated for three consecutive years can be considered to be permanently immune and to require no further vaccination (32).

The recommended vaccination programme for fat lamb flocks which are exposed to maximum risk is as follows (23). If an outbreak occurs administer antiserum and toxoid (preferably the activated alum-precipitated product) immediately and repeat the toxoid in a month's time. Revaccinate breeding ewes with toxoid at 6-month intervals thereafter attempting to time one of the two annual injections to fall during the penultimate month of pregnancy. The lambs will derive passive immunity from the colostrum but should be vaccinated with toxoid when 4 to 10 weeks of age and again a month later. If a vaccination programme is initiated at a time other than when an outbreak is in progress the initial injection of antitoxin can be omitted. Most vaccination programmes fall far short of this ideal and recommendations need to be adapted to suit local conditions of economy and degree of risk; for example in New Zealand vaccination of the ewes before lambing is often sufficient to protect fat lambs through to sale time (33). In areas where the disease occurs only sporadically it is customary to administer serum to all sheep as soon as an outbreak commences. Although the immunity lasts for only 2 weeks further immediate losses are prevented, and in most instances the disease does not recur. Toxoid is cheaper, but to administer it alone at such times may result in further serious losses before active immunity develops.

Any vaccination of sheep is not without danger of precipitating blackleg or other clostridial disease and if these are a severe problem in an area it may be wise to vaccinate a portion of the flock as a pilot test and proceed with vaccination of the remainder only when no complications arise. A multiple vaccine (including toxoids of enterotoxaemia, tetanus, blackleg and braxy) is recommended for use in sheep in those circumstances where all of these diseases are likely to occur (27). Effective responses are obtained and the only difficulty is the additional cost (36).

Vaccination with toxoid has been effective in calves (4) but is not highly effective in goats (3, 19) and should be repeated in this species at 6-monthly intervals. The use of serum must be carried out with caution in goats, particularly Saanens, which are very prone to anaphylactic reactions.

REFERENCES

(1) Bullen, J. J. (1952). *J. Path. Bact.*, *64*, 201.
(2) Bullen, J. J. & Batty, I. (1957). *Vet. Rec.*, *69*, 1268.
(3) Oxer, D. T. (1956). *Aust. vet. J.*, *32*, 62.
(4) Blood, D. C. & Helwig, D. M. (1957). *Aust. vet. J.*, *33*, 144.
(5) Griner, L. A. *et al.* (1956). *J. Amer. vet. med. Ass.*, *129*, 375.
(6) Keast, J. C. & McBarron, E. J. (1954). *Aust. vet. J.*, *30*, 305.
(7) Bennetts, H. W. (1932). *Counc. sci. indust. Res., Aust., Bull. No. 57*, p. 72.
(8) Bullen, J. J. & Batty, I. (1957). *J. Path. Bact.*, *73*, 511.
(9) Gordon, W. S. *et al.* (1940). *J. Path. Bact.*, *50*, 251.
(10) Whitlock, J. H. & Fabricant, J. (1947). *Cornell Vet.*, *37*, 211.
(11) Christensen, J. F. *et al.* (1947). *J. Amer. vet. med. Ass.*, *111*, 144.
(12) Thomson, A. & Batty, I. (1953). *Vet. Rec.*, *65*, 659.
(13) Batty, I. *et al.* (1954). *Vet. Rec.*, *66*, 249.
(14) Moskowitz, M. (1958). *Nature, Lond.*, *181*, 550.
(15) Frank, F. W. (1956). *Amer. J. vet. Res.*, *17*, 492.
(16) Johnson, W. P. *et al.* (1956). *J. Anim. Sci.*, *15*, 781.
(17) Smith, L. D. S. (1957). *Advances in Veterinary Science*, Vol. 3, pp. 465–524, New York: Academic Press.
(18) Smith, L. D. S. & Matsuoka, T. (1954). *Amer. J. vet. Res.*, *15*, 361.
(19) Shanks, P. L. (1949). *Vet. Rec.*, *61*, 262.
(20) Thomas, P. L. *et al.* (1956). *N.Z. vet. J.*, *4*, 161.
(21) Hepple, J. R. *et al.* (1959). *Vet. Rec.*, *71*, 201.
(22) Smith, L. D. S. & Matsuoka, T. (1959). *Amer. J. vet. Res.*, *20*, 91.

(23) Montgomerie, R. F. (1960). *Vet. Rec.*, *72*, 995.
(24) Jansen, B. C. (1960). *J. S. Afr. vet. med. Ass.*, *31*, 15.
(25) Jansen, B. C. (1960). *J. S. Afr. vet. med. Ass.*, *31*, 209.
(26) Jansen, B. C. (1960). *J. S. Afr. vet. med. Ass.*, *31*, 205.
(27) Hepple, J. R. *et al.* (1960). *Vet. Rec.*, *72*, 766 (corresp.).
(28) Mumford, D. H. (1961). *Aust. vet. J.*, *37*, 122.
(29) Montgomerie, R. F. (1961). *Canad. vet. J.*, *2*, 439.
(30) Griner, L. A. (1961). *Amer. J. vet. Res.*, *22*, 429 & 443.
(31) Griner, L. A. (1961). *Amer. J. vet. Res.*, *22*, 447.
(32) Jansen, B. C. (1967). *Onderstepoort J. vet. Res.*, *34*, 333.
(33) Wallace, G. V. (1963). *N.Z. vet. J.*, *11*, 39.
(34) Griner, L. A. (1963). *Bull. Off. int. Épizoot.*, *59*, 1443.
(35) Niilo, L. *et al.* (1963). *Canad. vet. J.*, *4*, 31 & 288.
(36) Oxer, D. T. *et al.* (1971). *Aust. vet. J.*, *47*, 134.
(37) Thomson, R. O. *et al.* (1969). *Vet. Rec.*, *85*, 81 & 84.
(38) Jansen, B. C. (1967). *Bull. Off. int. Épizoot.*, *67*, 1539.
(39) Vance, H. N. (1967). *Canad. J. comp. Med.*, *31*, 260.

17

Diseases Caused by Bacteria—III

DISEASES CAUSED BY
ESCHERICHIA COLI

COLIBACILLOSIS of newborn animals occurs in all species and is a major cause of losses in this age group. Gut oedema, enteric colibacillosis of feeder pigs and mastitis caused by *Escherichia coli* are also important diseases and metritis (puerperal fever) of sows immediately after farrowing is commonly caused by this organism.

Colibacillosis of Newborn Animals

By far the commonest disease entity of newborn farm animals is colibacillosis caused by *E. coli*. In calves the disease occurs in three forms—enteric colibacillosis manifested by diarrhoea; septicaemic colibacillosis manifested by bacteraemia and sudden death; and enteric-toxaemic colibacillosis also characterized by sudden death but without significant bacteraemia. In other species the disease is often septicaemic but enteric forms also occur.

Incidence

The disease occurs wherever farm animals are maintained, but it increases in incidence and severity as husbandry methods are intensified. When newborn animals are kept in groups in close confinement, the disease is likely to assume serious proportions. It is difficult to give details on morbidity and mortality but the disease is common in calves, baby pigs and lambs (1), and accounts for up to 25 per cent of septicaemias in foals. In infected pig breeding establishments every litter may be affected with a mortality rate reaching 50 per cent or more of all pigs born. Between 25 and 30 per cent of deaths in dairy calves are due to colibacillosis, most of them occurring during the first week of life. The incidence in beef calves is less than in dairy calves, due mainly to differences in husbandry practices. However, there has been a pronounced increase in prevalence in beef herds in recent years in most countries.

The development of the disease is rapid and the mortality rate is high in all species, particularly in the septicaemic and enteric-toxaemic forms. Apart from actual deaths, there is considerable expense involved in treatment and control of the disease and in loss of condition in recovered animals.

Aetiology

It is evident that specific serotypes of *E. coli* are associated with colibacillosis, some with the septicaemic form of the disease, and another different series with the development of diarrhoea and dilation of an isolated loop of calf gut (1). The disease has been reproduced experimentally by the administration of relevant specific serotypes. Conversely the challenge of experimental animals by specific serotypes has been resisted by the administration of antibodies to those specific serotypes. In the presence of these serotypes the factors suspected to lead to the development of outbreaks of the disease include enhancement of virulence due to rapid passage, increased susceptibility of animals due to lack of specific antibodies from colostrum and other protective substances, and the presence of a large number of animals less than 2 weeks of age.

The organism is very common in the environment and most adults develop an immunity to it. As a result, colostrum is usually rich in antibodies to the K antigen of *E. coli* and passive immunity is passed to the offspring in the colostrum. Thus, any factor which reduces the supply of colostrum to the newborn animal during the first 24 hours of life, or reduces the antibody content of colostrum, is a predisposing cause of the disease. Ability of immune globulins in colostrum to pass the intestinal epithelium is at a maximum at 12 hours after birth in calves and decreases rapidly thereafter. In some calves the permeability of the intestinal epithelium to antibodies disappears in as short a time as 6 to 8 hours. Multiple small intakes of colostrum give significantly greater serum antibody levels than a single, large intake (2) and calves with continuous access to their mothers are in the most favourable position (3). Young sows lacking contact with endemically infected environments, recently established herds or herds into which new strains of *E. coli* have been introduced often have low levels of antibodies (4). Factors which reduce the intake of colostrum include prepartum milking of the dam, agalactia for any reason, and intercurrent disease of the newborn. Anaemia due to iron deficiency, particularly in piglets (5), vitamin A deficiency, gross contamination of the environment and poor hygiene are other predisposing causes.

There is an apparent effect of age, with a much higher susceptibility at birth than later. This has been demonstrated but the mechanism is unknown (39, 40). When *E. coli*, with other bacteria, is introduced into the sterile gut of the neonate there is an initial colonization which disappears from the upper part of the intestine because of the development of acidity. In some animals this does not happen and colibacillosis develops.

The role of viruses as contributory factors in the aetiology of colibacillosis is a moot question. A virus capable of causing diarrhoea in young calves has been reported as occurring in widely separated areas of the U.S.A. (26). When administered to bacteria-free calves it causes a relatively mild enteric disorder but, with *E. coli*, it may cause fatalities. Certain strains of bovine viral diarrhoea virus act in a similar manner (42). The significance of these or other viruses in outbreaks of colibacillosis as observed in the field has not been determined.

The importance of feeding methods in the aetiology of enteritis of the newborn is discussed in the section on enteritis. Diarrhoea of dietetic origin may contribute to the development of colibacillosis but is often a very important disease in its own right, and may in many circumstances heavily outweigh infection as a cause of sickness and death.

Transmission

Colibacillosis can be readily produced in calves and piglets by the feeding of a pathogenic strain in the first milk consumed after birth. In most species the source of infection is the faeces of infected animals, although the organism may be cultured from the vagina or uterus of sows whose litters become affected. It can also be found extensively in the environment (4). Most piglets do not show illness until at least 24 hours after birth and it is probable that the organism derives from the bedding rather than from the uterus. In foals the infection is regarded as being intra-uterine in most cases. Ingestion is the most likely portal of entry in other species although infection via the navel and naso-pharyngeal mucosa can occur. It has been suggested that certain serotypes of *E. coli* may enter by the latter route and lead to the development of meningitis (6). Spread from group to group is by the introduction of animals carrying pathogenic strains of *E. coli*. Within a group, overcrowding and poor husbandry permit spread by contamination of udders, feeding pails and troughs.

Pathogenesis

Although details of the pathogenesis of colibacillosis in animals are incomplete, the two major factors which are important in the understanding of the disease in calves, and probably in colibacillosis in other animals, are the immune status of the calf and the properties of the strain of *E. coli*, particularly its capacity to invade tissues and its capacity to produce toxin (7). The three common forms of the disease are:

Septicaemic colibacillosis results from the presence in the gut of serotypes of *E. coli* which are capable of invading tissues of calves which are deficient in gamma-globulins, usually because they are deprived of colostrum. For unknown reasons other calves are hypogammaglobulinaemic in spite of having taken colostrum and are also susceptible to this form of the disease.

Enteric-toxaemic colibacillosis results from the massive proliferation of potent toxin-producing strains of *E. coli* in the intestine. These strains may form part of the intestinal flora in normal calves and their pathogenicity appears to depend on their numbers. The factors which affect their proliferation have not been determined but their endotoxins are capable of producing hypotension, vascular collapse and hypothermia—the cardinal signs of the disease in calves (8).

Enteric colibacillosis develops when specific serotypes which cause diarrhoea, with or without enteritis, proliferate in the anterior part of the intestine, in calves which have received colostrum.

In calves, the taking of colostrum in the first 24 hours of life, and the presence of normal plasma levels of gamma-globulin, provide good protection against at least the septicaemic and enteric–toxaemic forms of colibacillosis until the development of the calf's own antibodies at about 3 weeks of age. While these circulating antibodies are probably vital in protecting against invasion by bacteria or toxin, their importance in restraining the multiplication of *E. coli* in the gut is doubtful (9). However, it is probable that the continued secretion of immuno-globulins in colostrum for the first week of life does provide this resource. Work with pigs (1) shows that IgA becomes the dominant immuno-globulin in sow colostrum after the first few days of lactation, and this is the immunoglobulin which is not absorbed but is retained in, and reaches a high level in, the gut and must play an important role in restraining the multiplication of *E. coli* at least in germ-free pigs the establishment of colibacillosis is significantly reduced by the continuous presence of adequate levels of antibodies in the intestinal lumen (10, 11). On the other hand, IgG is at a peak in colostrum in the first few days, is readily absorbed and is vital in combating the pyrogenic and lethal effects of the bacterial toxin.

The immunoglobulins in the plasma of calves which have received colostrum are IgG, IgM (probably the more important of the two for the prevention of septicaemia) and IgA (or a globulin resembling IgA in man). Calves which have taken colostrum usually have levels of 7·5 to 8 mg. per ml.; calves which have been deprived have levels of less than 1 mg. per ml. (12).

On the basis of the clinical entities observed three types of toxin have been postulated; one which causes the acute hypotension so characteristic of the enteric-toxaemic form of the disease; one which causes damage to vascular endothelium leading to transudation from vessels, especially into serous cavities as occurs in septicaemic colibacillosis; and a third which causes the enteric form of the disease. Work with pigs shows that gastric hypotonicity and hypomotility are primary responses in the enteric form of the disease and that the resulting gastric distension precedes the appearance of diarrhoea. In young animals the disease is reproduced easily, and the absorbed resulting abnormalities of gut function are known to be due to the organisms' enterotoxin (13). The presence of enterotoxins in individual serotypes of *E. coli* is usually measured by the strain's performance in the ligated gut test (14).

The important abnormality of function which ensues is the outpouring of fluid and sodium and bicarbonate ions leading to fatal dehydration. This is not necessarily accompanied by inflammation which accounts for the usually low protein content of the fluid.

In pigs the pathogenesis of colibacillosis includes three forms of the disease (15)—neonatal colibacillary diarrhoea, weaning colibacillary diarrhoea and gut oedema (oedema disease). The disease of newborn pigs under discussion here is comparable with the enteric–toxaemic form of the disease in calves and the more acute cases of the enteric form. Whether the effects produced by the enterotoxin in these circumstances are direct or indirect, via the medium of anaphylactic shock, is debatable (16). A great deal of work has been done on the effects of various toxins from a variety of strains or serotypes of *E. coli* on gnotobiotic pigs. Histopathological changes in intestinal epithelium vary from villus atrophy to severe inflammation (17, 18). Fever, bradycardia, shock and hypomotility and dilatation of the gut are generally observed (19, 20, 21).

When the disease is confined to the gut, the condition responds reasonably well to treatment, and death, when it occurs, is due to dehydration and electrolyte imbalance. Animals which recover from the septicaemia may develop lesions due to localization in other organs. Arthritis is a common sequel in foals, calves and lambs. Meningitis and pneumonia may also occur. Enteritis or septicaemia may occur in all species but, in lambs and foals, septicaemic colibacillosis is more common. Experimentally the enteric–toxaemic syndrome has been produced in ponies (22) but the arterial hypotension and shock which occur appear naturally only in very young foals.

Clinical Findings

Calves

Three distinct forms of the disease have been identified in calves but these are not necessarily mutually exclusive and one may follow the other in an individual animal.

Enteric-toxaemic colibacillosis. Affected newborn animals collapse and die in as short a time as 2 to 6 hours. Outstanding clinical signs include coma, subnormal temperature, a cold clammy skin, pale mucosae, wetness around the mouth, collapse of superficial veins, slowness and irregularity of the heart, mild convulsive movements and periodic apnoea. No scouring is evident.

Septicaemic colibacillosis. The septicaemic form is most common in animals during the first four days of life. The illness is acute, the course varying from 24 to 96 hours. There are no diagnostic clinical signs. Affected animals are depressed and weak, anorexia is complete, there is a marked increase in heart rate and, although the temperature may be high initially, it falls rapidly to sub-normal levels when diarrhoea and sometimes dysentery appear.

Post-septicaemic localization may cause arthritis with lameness, pain and swelling in the joints. Meningitis is also common in calves and is often accompanied by panophthalmitis (23, 24). Clinical signs include recumbency, opisthotonus, clonic, paddling convulsions, nystagmus and pus in the anterior chamber of the eye. Pneumonia is a less common sequel.

Enteric colibacillosis. The enteric form of the disease is most common in calves but may occur in the other species. It occurs chiefly during the first three weeks of life and particularly during the first week. The faeces are watery or pasty and usually chalk-white to yellow in colour and occasionally are streaked with blood. Defaecation is frequent, the tail and buttocks are soiled and the faeces have an offensive, rancid smell. There is usually a systemic reaction with a temperature up to 40·5 °C (105 °F) and an increase in pulse rate. The animal ceases to drink, is dull and listless and rapidly becomes dehydrated. There may be abdominal pain on palpation, sometimes tenesmus is evident and the back may be arched. Without treatment, death usually occurs in 3 to 5 days. All cases of colibacillosis should be carefully examined for evidence of omphalophlebitis.

Lambs

Although some cases manifest enteric signs and chronic cases may occur, colibacillosis in lambs is almost always septicaemic and peracute (1). Two age groups appear to be susceptible; lambs of one to two days of age and lambs 3 to 8 weeks old. Peracute cases are found dead without premonitory signs. Acute cases show collapse and occasionally signs of acute meningitis manifested by a stiff gait in the early stages, followed by recumbency with hyperaesthesia and tetanic convulsions (25). Chronic cases are usually manifested by arthritis.

Piglets

The piglets are born healthy but illness commences abruptly at 12 hours of age. Some die without showing signs. Others collapse very quickly and are moribund when first seen. The remainder are dull, listless and show diarrhoea, even though they continue to suck. The diarrhoea is profuse and stains the hindquarters yellow. The pigs are shrunken and dehydrated. A weak stumbling gait and, in the later stages, recumbency with weak paddling movements is evident. The temperature is then usually subnormal. Most are dead within 24 hours of the first signs of illness. In newborn pigs the disease is largely enteric and bacteraemia is not usually a feature.

Enteric colibacillosis of pigs 8 to 16 weeks old is described elsewhere.

Clinical Pathology

Faecal swabs and blood should be taken for culture, the latter if septicaemia is suspected, and the organism tested for drug sensitivity. If possible, the serotype should be determined. It is becoming increasingly important to determine the immunoglobulin status of calves, both to assess the need for prophylaxis and the quality of the neonatal care provided (2). A zinc sulphate turbidity test for serum globulins is of value in this connection (43).

Necropsy Findings

In cases of enteric-toxaemic and septicaemic colibacillosis, there may be no gross lesions and diagnosis may depend upon isolation of the bacteria from the abdominal viscera and in the latter from the heart blood. In less severe cases, there may be subserous and submucosal petechial haemorrhages, and a degree of enteritis and gastritis is usually present. Occasionally fibrinous exudates may be present in the joints and serous cavities, and there may be omphalophlebitis, pneumonia or meningitis. In the latter instance, the meningeal vessels are engorged and the cerebrospinal fluid is turbid.

In enteric colibacillosis in piglets the hypotonicity of the gut is evident and although the tissues may be dehydrated the alimentary tract can be distended with fluid and clotted milk. In animals that survive for longer periods there may be gastroenteritis, with oedema of the mesenteric lymph nodes (1). Attempts should be made to culture the organism from the gut, the mesenteric lymph nodes, spleen, heart blood and cerebrospinal fluid.

Diagnosis

Septicaemic colibacillosis presents some difficulty in field diagnosis especially in foals where a similar syndrome may occur in infections with *Actinobacillus equuli*, *Salmonella abortivoequina* and *Salm. typhimurium*. In newborn calves, septicaemia is due largely to this organism although it may be due to infection with *Salmonella* spp. The common neonatal infections are listed in the section on diseases of the newborn.

In enteric colibacillosis, the major difficulty is to determine whether or not the condition is due to infection. The criteria which should be satisfied include the isolation of large numbers of pathogenic *E. coli* in the anterior part of the gut of a euthanized or freshly dead animal, the presence of normal gut acidity and the presence of clinical signs and necropsy lesions which fit the disease. Diarrhoea of dietetic origin is common when animals are overfed on milk. Calves and particularly foals may develop diarrhoea when the dam's milk flow is profuse, but initially there is no systemic reaction and the animal continues to feed. Diarrhoea is sometimes observed in calves on cows feeding on very lush pasture. Whether this is due to a surplus of milk or to some substance from the pasture which passes through the milk has not been determined.

A major development in calf diseases in recent

years, and in most countries, has been a rapidly increasing prevalence of diarrhoea in young (1 to 3 weeks old) beef calves, running at pasture with their dams. The scour is yellow to begin with but soon becomes white, is voluminous and smelly. It pastes up the hindquarters of the calf and lies in pools on the ground where the calf has lain. Most recover spontaneously but suffer a setback in growth. The morbidity rate is often 100 per cent, but the mortality, although occasionally reaching 10 per cent, is usually about 2 to 5 per cent. The disease is commonly referred to as colibacillosis but the diagnosis is unsure. As might be anticipated a virus has been suggested and sought, but no significant identifications have been made.

Other infections which cause diarrhoea in calves are *Salmonella* spp., *Providencia stuartii* (11), *Clostridium perfringens* Type C, the pneumonenteritis virus and *Eimeria* spp. In foals *Salm. typhimurium* and *Cl. perfringens* Type B are likely causes. Transmissible gastroenteritis, vomiting and wasting disease, *Cl. perfringens* Type C and anaemia caused by a dietary deficiency of iron have to be considered as causes of diarrhoea in young pigs. In vomiting and wasting disease, constipation is more likely but diarrhoea may occur in some outbreaks.

Treatment

Antibiotics, including streptomycin, tetracyclines, neomycin and chloramphenicol, are highly effective against *E. coli* although the sensitivity of strains of the organism to the different antibiotics varies widely. This may be because of inherent variations between strains, or to variations induced by previous exposure to low levels of antibiotics, either as feed additives or as prophylactics against scours. In herds where antibiotics and sulphonamides are used prophylactically, it is not uncommon to find that strains of *E. coli* with multiple resistance to streptomycin, tetracyclines, chloramphenicol and sulphadimidine dominate the faecal flora and make treatment extremely difficult (27). For this reason it is advisable to have sensitivity tests carried out on all material sent to the laboratory for culture. The most satisfactory drugs in use at present are chloramphenicol, neomycin, Hibitane and nitrofurazone. The tetracyclines, neomycin and streptomycin are still in widespread use but resistance of the *E. coli* to these drugs is commonly encountered. The sulphonamide drugs still have their place in the treatment of neonatal diarrhoea but fear of kidney damage has seriously restricted their use, especially if dehydration is severe. One of the important factors determining whether or not calves survive colibacillosis is the antibody status of the animal. Most of the literature on therapy omits this information and is therefore difficult to assess (28).

In septicaemic colibacillosis, irrespective of the drug used, the aim should be to achieve an adequate blood level and if possible a high level in the intestinal contents. The rate of excretion of most drugs is high in newborn animals, necessitating a high level of dosage in relation to body weight. For parenteral administration, streptomycin should be administered at the rate of 20 mg. per lb. body weight daily (preferably in two or more divided doses), the tetracyclines, neomycin and chloramphenicol at 5 to 10 mg. per lb. body weight daily and treatment should be continued for three days. It is standard practice to administer oral preparations of these drugs in conjunction with the parenteral treatment. Nitrofurazone or furazolidone, administered orally, are also effective against *E. coli* and doses of 25 mg. per lb. body weight of furazolidone to pigs and 2 g. of nitrofurazone to calves daily in two divided doses by mouth give good results (29). In enteric colibacillosis, it is usual to administer only the oral preparations of these drugs. When treatments are administered orally they should be given at least twice daily and continued for 4 days.

While the primary aim of treatment is to control the infection, appropriate supportive treatment will often make the difference between success and failure. A transfusion of whole blood is most valuable as a fluid replacement and as a source of additional antibodies; 500 to 1000 ml. given intravenously, intraperitoneally or even subcutaneously brings many moribund calves back into the survivor group. Additional fluid should be given to repair the loss of sodium, potassium and calcium, and to combat the acidosis which develops. Recommended dose rates are 1 to 2 litres for moderately affected calves, and for severely dehydrated calves 5 litres administered by continuous infusion over a 3 to 6 hour period followed by smaller doses for a further 2 to 3 days. Intravenous infusion gives best results and although physiological saline is beneficial, a properly balanced electrolyte solution is superior (30, 41).

In an attempt to reduce fluid loss a number of oral preparations containing an antiparasympathetic drug as well as astringents and antibacterial agents are available for the treatment of colibacillosis. Their use seems rational but the apparent clinical effect is meagre. In those animals with the enteric-toxaemic syndrome which show collapse and circulatory failure, some attention should be given to repairing the hypotension. Parenteral fluids and blood transfusions will help but a vaso-pressor agent, such as epinephrine, or a corti-costeroid are more likely to achieve a successful response. There is some controversy over the use of corticosteroids, some feeling that a fulminating septicaemia will develop if the infection is not properly controlled by the antibiotic being used on the case. Antihistamines do not have this dis-advantage and are used extensively in calves with enteric-toxaemic colibacillosis. Alimentary tract astringents and demulcents are also used, usually in conjunction with antibiotics.

Feeding management is important and calves with diarrhoea should receive no milk, or at most one third of the usual amount made up to the usual volume with warm water, until they recover. The restricted fluid intake should be compensated by parenteral fluid therapy or by oral dosing with electrolyte solutions.

Control

The most important control measure in neonatal colibacillosis is to ensure that colostrum is taken in good quantity, early. In calves the critical period appears to be eight hours (31). It is not sufficient to know that a calf is up and could suck. In a com-pletely controlled operation the calf must be seen to suck vigorously before it is 8 hours old, or it must be hand-fed with dam's colostrum, or deep-frozen colostrum from the home farm. The injection of gamma-globulin preparations or hyperimmune sera is also satisfactory or a transfusion of dam's blood may be of value. A general recommendation about colostrum is: dry off the cow at least 4 weeks before calving, avoid pre-partum milking, and feed at least 2 kg. of colostrum soon after birth (32). No absorption blocks are known to occur and the only possible risks are related to low antibody content of colostrum.

Control depends also on proper housing and hy-giene although heavy mortalities may occur under the best possible conditions of husbandry. Over-crowding should be avoided and animals should be run together in as small groups as possible. The ideal is an individual pen for each calf or each litter, whether the animals are housed or at pasture. When they have to be run as groups, only those animals of approximately equal age should be to-gether. Each pen or paddock should be disinfected or rested after each batch of animals leaves it so that infection is not passed from one group to the next. Animals that are run in the open should be in small yards or paddocks of sufficient number to allow some to remain empty for a month after a batch of animals moves out. Individual portable pens or tethering of calves is a practicable and worthwhile method of rearing. The pens or tether-ing pins are moved weekly. A suitable sloping site should be selected to permit good drainage and to allow the animals to be moved uphill gradu-ally. If range cows must calve during cold and wet weather every effort should be made to have the calving area well drained and not overcrowded and to ensure that the newborn calf gets colostrum promptly. With piglets and foals, farrowing pens and foaling boxes should be disinfected between occupants.

Feeding and drinking troughs should be placed so as to minimize the chance of faecal contamina-tion. Feeding pails must be properly cleaned and disinfected after each use and feeding should be done from outside the pens to avoid carrying infec-tion on boots and feed cans.

Special care is needed on farms which specialize in raising veal calves. On these farms newborn calves are often brought in without having had sufficient colostrum. They are also often exposed to inclement weather and to exotic strains of *E. coli* in sale barns or conveyances. Such calves should be kept in isolation for a week and preferably receive some prophylactic medication on arrival. Purchase of very young calves should be avoided.

Prophylactic medication with sulphonamides or antibiotics for the first week or 10 days of life in calves and the first 4 weeks in pigs has the ad-vantage that infection is prevented and growth rate increased but has the disadvantage that resist-ant strains of *E. coli* may develop at the dose rates commonly recommended. In very many circum-stances this is the only practicable procedure but when antibiotics are used they should be given orally, twice daily and at full therapeutic levels. Neomycin, 100 mg. daily by mouth for 5 days, has been shown to be optimum, non-toxic prophylac-tic drug for pigs (33). No drug resistant strains emerge on this regimen. In pigs the administration of broad spectrum antibiotics to the suckling sows is recommended, the results being very much bet-ter if the drug is given parenterally than if given orally and if given 8 to 12 hours before farrowing.

Although the importance of vitamins, particu-larly vitamin A, in the protection of mucosae against infection is well known, the use of vitamin supplements, other than those normally required, has largely gone out of fashion as the result of well controlled trials which have shown their inability to prevent the development of scours in calves.

Biological measures may also be used in a con-trol programme. The standard recommendation is to vaccinate the cows or sows at 2 to 4 weeks before calving or farrowing to stimulate the production of antibodies which will then be present in the colostrum. Vaccination of the neonate itself is usually too late because of the early occurrence of colibacillosis after birth and the failure to develop antibodies. In pigs vaccination before 5 weeks of age causes only a small antibody response (34). Commerical vaccines containing *E. coli* are available, but have not received general approval in spite of the excellent results recorded in some countries, especially with adjuvant vaccines (35). Autogenous vaccines, usually killed bacterins derived from *E. coli* isolated from faecal cultures or lymph nodes of necropsy specimens, have been extensively used and commented on favourably in herds of pigs and cattle where colibacillosis occurs at a high level of incidence. However, in two well-controlled trials in pigs (36) and cattle (37) autogenous vaccines failed to reduce significantly the incidence of scours. Such vaccines are not likely to exert much effect on the occurrence of scours, but they may be of value in preventing the heavy mortalities and sudden deaths caused by the enteric-toxaemic and septicaemic forms of the disease. These occur so quickly that there is little time to institute satisfactory treatment, especially in beef calves running free with their dams. There are several difficulties in the preparation of an autogenous bacterin. The primary one is to select the serotype or serotypes, and there may be a number in a herd, which are causing the mortality. This selection is made much more satisfactorily if a necropsy specimen is available and cultures can be taken from the mesenteric lymph nodes of an untreated calf which has died of the disease. If a series of serotypes follow one another in a herd little protection from a monovalent vaccine can be anticipated (38). Another difficulty is the poor antibody response in the colostrum and serum of cattle to killed vaccines containing some serotypes of *E. coli*. Even after two vaccinations 2 weeks apart antibody titres are often insignificantly elevated. The possibility of stimulating greater antibody response by the use of adjuvant vaccines has been recommended but is subject to the limitations imposed by the need for specific serotypes in the vaccine (29). In pigs the antibody response to vaccination is more evident than in cattle, and the response is better with a formalin-killed bacterin than one in which the cells are destroyed by heat. The antibodies are detectable in the sows' colostrum and the serum of the sucking pigs for up to 4 weeks after weaning (44). In cattle the antibody content of colostrum falls very rapidly after birth and type-specific antibodies may have fallen to negligible levels by as soon as the fourth milking (41). If adequate colostrum is not available, specific antisera, blood transfusion or oral dosing with blood or serum as described in the section on neonatal infections is advised. The preparation of an IgM-rich fraction from pooled bovine sera has been described. The material has excellent prophylactic properties against septicaemia when given parenterally to calves (9).

REFERENCES

(1) Sojka, W. J. (1971). *Vet. Bull.*, *41*, 509.
(2) McBeath, D. G. *et al.* (1971). *Vet. Rec.*, *88*, 266.
(3) Selman, I. E. *et al.* (1971). *Vet. Rec.*, *88*, 460.
(4) Arbuckle, J. B. R. (1968). *Brit. vet. J.*, *124*, 152, 229.
(5) Osborne, J. C. & Davis, J. W. (1968). *J. Amer. vet. med. Ass.*, *152*, 1630.
(6) Glantz, P. J. & Rothenbacher, H. (1965). *Amer. J. vet. Res.*, *26*, 258.
(7) Gay, C. C. (1965). *Bact. Rev.*, *29*, 75.
(8) Tikoff, G. *et al.* (1966). *Amer. J. Physiol.*, *210*, 847.
(9) Logan, E. F. (1971). *Vet. Rec.*, *88*, 222; *89*, 623, 628, 663.
(10) Kohler, E. M. (1967). *Canad. J. comp. med.*, *31*, 277, 283.
(11) Waldhalm, D. G. *et al.* (1969). *Amer. J. vet. Res.*, *30*, 1573.
(12) Penhale, W. J. *et. al.* (1970). *Brit. vet. J.*, *126*, 30.
(13) Kohler, E. M. (1971). *Amer. J. vet. Res.*, *32*, 731.
(14) Gyles, C. L. & Barnum, D. A. (1967). *J. Path. Bact.*, *94*, 189.
(15) Nielsen, N. O. *et al.* (1968). *J. Amer. vet. med. Ass.*, *153*, 1590.
(16) Shreeve, B. J. & Thomlinson, J. R. (1970). *Brit. vet. J.*, *126*, 444; *127*, 57.
(17) Moon, H. W. *et al.* (1970). *Amer. J. vet. Res.*, *31*, 103.
(18) Kenworthy, R. (1970). *J. comp. Path.*, *80*, 53.
(19) Truszczynski, M. & Pilaszek, J. (1970). *Res. vet. Sci.*, *11*, 117.
(20) Smith, H. Williams & Gyles, C. L. (1970). *J. med. Microbiol.*, *3*, 387.
(21) Wachtel, W. & Lyhs, L. (1969). *Arch. exp. Vet. Med.*, *23*, 633.
(22) Burrows, G. E. (1971). *Amer. J. vet. Res.*, *32*, 243.
(23) Moon, H. W. *et al.* (1966). *Amer. J. vet. Res.*, *27*, 1007.
(24) Mosher, A. H. *et al.* (1968). *Amer. J. vet. Res.*, *29*, 1483.
(25) Bates, H. J. W. (1966). *J. S. Afr. vet. med. Ass.*, *37*, 1.
(26) White, R. G. *et al.* (1970). *Vet. Med.*, *65*, 487.
(27) Williams Smith, H. (1967). *Vet. Rec.*, *80*, 464.
(28) Fisher, E. W. & Fuente, G. H. (1971). *Vet. Rec.*, *89*, 579.
(29) Callear, J. F. F. & Smith, I. M. (1966). *Brit. vet. J.*, *122*, 169.
(30) Radostits, O. M. (1965). *J. Amer. vet. med. Ass.*, *147*, 1367.
(31) Selman, I. E. *et al.* (1970). *J. comp. Path.*, *80*, 419.
(32) Kruse, V. (1970). *Anim. Prod.*, *12*, 661.
(33) Kenworthy, R. & Crabb, W. E. (1965). *Vet. Rec.*, *77*, 1504.
(34) Miniats, O. P. & Ingram, D. G. (1967). *Canad. vet. J.*, *8*, 260.
(35) Schoengers, F. *et al.* (1967). *Annl. Méd. vét.*, *111*, 3.
(36) Jones, J. E. T. *et al.* (1962). *Vet. Rec.*, *74*, 202.
(37) Sellers, K. C. *et al.* (1962). *Vet. Rec.*, *74*, 203.
(38) Lemcke, R. M. & Hurst, A. (1961). *J. comp. Path.*, *71*, 268.
(39) Drees, D. T. *et al.* (1970). *Amer. J. vet. Res.*, *31*, 1147, 1159.
(40) Moon, H. W. & Whipp, S. C. (1970). *J. infect. Dis.*, *122*, 220.
(41) Tennant, B. *et al.* (1972). *J. Amer. vet. med. Ass.*, *161*, 993.
(42) Lambert, G. & Fernelius, A. L. (1968). *Canad. J. comp. Med.*, *32*, 440.

(43) Boyd, J. W. (1972). *Vet. Rec.*, *90*, 645.
(44) Gay, C. C. *et al.* (1964). *Canad. vet. J.*, *5*, 248, 297, 314.

Gut Oedema of Swine
(*Enterotoxaemia, Oedema Disease, Bowel Oedema*)

Gut oedema is a disease of young, feeder pigs characterized by subcutaneous and subserous oedema, paralysis and a high mortality rate. Because of the common occurrence of gastroenteritis in pigs of the same age and under the same conditions as those in which gut oedema occurs, and because the same serotypes of *Escherichia coli* appear to be common to both diseases, it has been suggested that they be grouped together under the heading of 'colitoxocosis' (14). The two diseases are dealt with separately here, the latter under the heading of enteric colibacillosis of feeder pigs, because of their different clinical manifestations. That they are closely related is undoubted: they may both occur on the one farm at the one time and an outbreak of one disease may merge into an outbreak of the other in the same pen of pigs.

Incidence

The disease was first reported from Ireland and has come to assume considerable economic importance in the United Kingdom and North America and in most other countries because of its high incidence and mortality rate which may vary between 20 per cent and 100 per cent (average 64 per cent). The disease is sporadic in occurrence, affecting individual pens of pigs without necessarily involving other pens on the same farm. The morbidity rate in affected herds averages 15 per cent (10 to 35 per cent). In an affected group, it is usual to find a number of pigs in the various stages of the disease.

Aetiology

The specific and predisposing causes have not been completely determined. The bulk of evidence available suggests that gut oedema is caused by a toxin formed in the intestinal tract of affected pigs and that the toxin is antigenic and produced by bacterial activity. Extracts of haemolytic strains of *E. coli* isolated from cases of gut oedema are capable of causing the disease and pigs receiving hyperimmune serum against the disease-producing strains are unaffected by the toxin (1). Only some serotypes of haemolytic *E. coli* are capable of producing the disease (2, 3, 10, 17, 18) and these strains differ from the enteropathogenic strains that cause enteritis.

Different serotypes may occur in different outbreaks on the same farm. Serotypes which are not capable of causing gut oedema because they do not produce the toxin may have greater invasive powers and cause enteritis (11).

Gut oedema occurs only in pigs and, although it is most common in young pigs in the 8 to 12 weeks age group soon after weaning, it can occur in very young pigs (9) and older pigs up to market weight and even in adult sows. No details are available on the development of immunity but it seems probable that antibacterial antibodies do not protect against the disease whereas antitoxins may do so (4). In recovered animals there is no increase in specific O antibodies but there is an increase in K antibodies and the disease does not recur in the same pig.

The predisposing causes appear to be nutritional. It is the fastest-growing, thriftiest pigs in the group which are most likely to be affected and the disease is most likely to occur on heavy concentrate rations fed dry in self-feeders.

Transmission

Until more is known of the cause of the disease, any suggestions on transmission must be speculative. The epidemiology of the disease in an affected herd is not characteristic of a highly contagious disease (21). However, it is probable that the significant serotypes of *E. coli* are spread by the movement of pigs and infection, which may not necessarily result in the production of the disease, occurs by ingestion.

Pathogenesis

As knowledge of the disease increases, its resemblance to enterotoxaemia caused by *Cl. perfringens* Type D in lambs becomes more apparent. Specific serotypes of *E. coli* which are capable of causing the disease are introduced into a piggery and become part of the normal intestinal flora. They may not cause trouble until a particular set of environmental conditions arises, in this case heavy feeding with concentrate after weaning, when the bacteria proliferate excessively (13) and produce large quantities of toxin. Variation of the protein content of the ration appears to have no effect on susceptibility, but it is not possible to infect pigs given a restricted diet or fed on barley fibre (23). It is possible that changes in other environmental factors such as recent transport, change from a starting to growing ration or recent vaccination, especially against hog cholera (8), may have the same effect. The mechanism by which the toxin causes the lesions has not been established although there is a hypoproteinaemia in affected litters (5). Although neurotoxins have been isolated from the relevant serotypes of *E. coli* (19) the parenteral administration of extracts of these bacteria produces hypotension and no oedema. To overcome this discrepancy it has been suggested that gut oedema, and the enteric form of colibacillosis in pigs, may be caused by anaphylactic reactions to the polysaccharides of *E. coli* (22). The way in which affected pigs respond to antihistamines and diuretics and the residual vasculitis and eosinophilia support the thesis that allergy is the basic mechanism in the aetiology (24). The proposed pattern of pathogenesis is that most pigs become sensitized to these polysaccharides and those which develop gut oedema do so when they suffer an anaphylactic reaction subsequently when very rapid proliferation of *E. coli* occurs in the gut because of changes in or very high quality of the diet (12). It seems likely, in view of the oedema of other tissues, that the nervous signs are due to cerebral oedema.

Clinical Findings

The disease strikes suddenly in a group, often affecting a number of pigs within a few hours, and shows no tendency to spread from group to group. Outbreaks are shortlived, averaging 8 days and not exceeding 15 days, and commence and end abruptly. However, the disease may recur in the same herd at subsequent farrowing seasons. The thriftiest pigs are most likely to be affected and once the diagnosis is made, all pigs in the pen should be examined in an attempt to detect other animals in the early stages of the disease. The incidence in a litter will vary up to 50 per cent or more.

The earliest and most obvious sign is inco-ordination of the hind limbs, although this may be preceded by an attack of diarrhoea. The pig has difficulty in standing and sways and sags in the hindquarters. There is difficulty in getting up and in getting the legs past each other when walking because of a stiff, stringhalt-like action affecting either the fore or hind legs. In some cases there are obvious signs of nervous irritation manifested by muscle tremor, aimless wandering and clonic convulsions. Complete flaccid paralysis follows.

On close examination, oedema of the eyelids and conjunctiva may be visible. This may also involve the front of the face and ears but cannot usually be seen until necropsy. The voice is often hoarse and may become almost inaudible. Blindness may be apparent. The faeces are usually firm and rectal temperatures are almost always below normal. The course of the disease may be very short with some pigs being found dead without signs having been observed. In most cases, illness is observed for 6 to 36 hours, with a few cases being more prolonged. Recovery does sometimes occur but some degree of inco-ordination may persist (6).

Clinical Pathology

As an aid to diagnosis, while affected animals are still alive, faecal samples should be cultured to determine the presence of haemolytic *E. coli*. Knowledge of the drug sensitivity of the organism may be important in prescribing control measures.

Necropsy Findings

Oedema of the eyelids, forehead, belly, elbow and hock joints, throat and ears is accompanied by oedema of the stomach wall and colonic mesentery in classical cases. Excess pleural, peritoneal and pericardial fluid are also characteristic and the skeletal muscles are paler than normal. The oedema may often be slight and quite localized so that examination of suspected areas should be carried out carefully, using multiple incisions especially along the greater curvature of the stomach near the cardia. Haemolytic *E. coli* can be cultured in almost pure culture from the intestine, particularly the colon and the rectum (13), and in some cases from the mesenteric lymph nodes. Histopathologically, the important lesions in subacute and chronic cases are necrotic arteritis and encephalomalacia affecting principally the brain stem (24).

Diagnosis

Although there are a number of diseases of pigs in the susceptible age group in which nervous signs predominate, gut oedema is usually easy to diagnose because of the rapidity with which the disease strikes, the number of pigs affected at one time, the short duration of the outbreak and oedema of tissues. Affected pigs are usually in prime condition. Rather than attempt to differentiate them here, the reader is referred to the section on diseases of the brain for a list of nervous diseases of pigs. Mulberry heart disease of pigs is often confused with gut oedema. There is in fact some doubt that the diseases are separate entities but, because of the primarily haemorrhagic nature of the lesions of mulberry heart disease, it is described elsewhere. The two diseases may occur coincidentally in the one animal. In poisoning by *Amaranthus* spp. and *Chenopodium album*, the signs may be roughly similar but the oedema is limited to the perirenal tissues.

Treatment

Many treatments have been tried, recommended and discarded and many veterinarians find that treatment has little effect on the outcome of the disease. If cases can be treated early, antihistamines given intravenously may be effective (15), with or without the addition of an antibiotic and a diuretic. Streptomycin is usually used but the tetracyclines or chloramphenicol should give equal or better results. Acetazolamide at the rate of 2 to 5 mg. per lb. body weight intramuscularly or in the drinking water is recommended for treatment or prevention (20) but cost usually limits its administration to individual pigs. When cases are showing advanced nervous signs, little response can be expected. Elimination of the toxin-producing bacteria may be attempted by an antibiotic or oral purgative. Treatment with *E. coli* antiserum has been followed by death due to anaphylaxis (6). Thiamine hydrochloride in 100 mg. doses has also been suggested as a satisfactory treatment (7). The unaffected pigs in the group should be placed on the control programme set out below.

Control

Feed consumption should be reduced immediately, either by reducing the amount fed or, if the pigs are on self-feeders, by mixing more roughage, such as shorts or bran, with the ration in the ratio of 1:1 or 1:2. Emptying of the alimentary tract by placing mineral oil on the drinking water or feeding Epsom salts in a thin gruel may be of value. An antibacterial drug should be provided in the feed or the drinking water. Neomycin, the tetracyclines, streptomycin and nitrofurazone are all used for this purpose. The organism may be susceptible to sulphadimidine and sulphathiazole (3). A sensitivity test on the causative organism is worth while because the sensitivities may vary considerably, many strains being resistant to the tetracyclines (6) and other drugs.

No vaccine is available and experimental work suggesting that a toxoid might stimulate sufficient antitoxin production to protect animals against the disease (1, 19), has not as yet been supported (16).

REFERENCES

(1) Timoney, J. F. (1957). *Vet. Rec., 69*, 1160.
(2) Erskine, R. G. *et al.* (1957). *Vet. Rec., 69*, 301.
(3) Gregory, D. W. (1958). *Vet. Med., 53*, 77.
(4) Gitter, M. & Lloyd, M. K. (1957). *Brit. vet. J., 113*, 168 & 212.
(5) Luke, T. & Gordon, W. M. (1950). *Nature, Lond., 165*, 286.
(6) Lemcke, R. M. *et al.* (1957). *Vet. Rec., 69*, 601.
(7) Ward, V. C. (1958). *Vet. Rec., 70*, 240.
(8) Woods, G. T. & Beamer, P. D. (1951). *J. Amer. vet. med. Ass., 119*, 436.
(9) Austvoll, J. (1957). *Vet. Rec., 69*, 104.
(10) Pickrell, J. A. *et al.* (1969). *Canad. J. comp. Med., 33*, 72, 76.
(11) Sojka, W. J. *et al.* (1960). *Res. vet. Sci., 1*, 17.
(12) Buxton, A. & Tomlinson, J. R. (1961). *Res. vet. Sci., 2*, 73.
(13) Campbell, S. G. (1959). *Vet. Rec., 71*, 909.
(14) Roberts, H. E. & Vallely, T. F. (1959). *Vet. Rec., 71*, 846.
(15) Pan, I. C. *et al.* (1970). *Canad. J. comp. Med., 34*, 148.
(16) Sweeney, E. J. *et al.* (1960). *Res. vet. Sci., 1*, 260.
(17) Rees, T. A. (1959). *J. comp. Path., 29*, 334.
(18) Terpstra, J. I. (1958). *T. Diergeneesk., 83*, 1078.
(19) Gregory, D. W. (1960). *Amer. J. vet. Res., 21*, 88.
(20) Gouge, H. E. & Elliott, R. F. (1959). *Vet. Med., 54*, 295.
(21) Kernkamp, H. C. H. *et al.* (1965). *J. Amer. vet. med. Ass., 146*, 353.
(22) Thomlinson, J. R. and Buxton, A. (1963). *Immunology, 6*, 126.
(23) Smith, H. W. & Halls, S. (1968). *J. med. Microbiol., 1*, 45.
(24) Kurtz, H. J. *et al.* (1969). *Amer. J. vet. Res., 30*, 79.

Enteric Colibacillosis of Feeder Pigs

Outbreaks of enteritis in pigs after weaning and up to 16 weeks of age, and rarely in adults, and caused by haemolytic *E. coli* are becoming more common. The disease is readily confused with salmonellosis and swine dysentery because of the age group of pigs affected and the similarity of clinical signs. It also occurs under the same conditions of management as does gut oedema, and the prevalent serotypes of *E. coli* in both diseases are the same (1, 2, 3). Early weaning of pigs (3 weeks instead of 6 to 8 weeks) has become very popular but poor weight gains and frequent diarrhoea plague these very early weaned pigs (7). Although the development of a gut flora dominated by haemolytic *E. coli* is common in these pigs, the setback they encounter is due to their immaturity rather than to the infection.

The factors involved in the proliferation of these serotypes is unknown but they appear to be related to the variable ability of different litters to adjust to dietary change (6). The most common syndrome is one of depression, anorexia, fever (40·5°C or 105°F) and diarrhoea. There is a mild bluish discolouration of the skin. A less common syndrome observed in herds in which enteritis is evident is manifested by sudden death without prior signs of illness. In general the disease is not as acute, nor the mortality rate as high as in salmonellosis and marked purple discolouration of the skin is characteristic of the latter disease. The fever in colibacillosis is maintained for several days and this together with the absence of dysentery helps to differentiate the disease from *Vibrio coli* infections.

Affected pigs are usually in very good condition and on heavy grain feed, outbreaks commonly occurring after a sudden change in feeding or other management practices. For example heavy grain feeding in the immediate post-weaning period has been shown to increase the numbers of *E. coli* in the intestine and the incidence of diarrhoea (4). The introduction of pigs is not often a part of the history as it is in salmonellosis. At necropsy there is a moderate to severe enteritis and haemolytic *E. coli* are found in almost pure culture in the colon and caecum. A severe haemorrhagic gastro-enteritis also occurs in herds, often in association with gut oedema and is thought to develop as part of a hypersensitivity state (5).

In live pigs examination of faeces should include examination of a smear, to eliminate the possibility of vibriosis, cultural examination to identify the presence of *E. coli* or *Salmonella* spp., and determination of the drug sensitivity of the organism. Seriously affected pigs require prompt treatment parenterally and orally with an antibiotic and, in the light of the possible anaphylactic pathogenesis of the disease as described under gut oedema, with an antihistamine. Unaffected, in-contact pigs can be satisfactorily treated by medication of the drinking water or feed. Nitrofurazone and neomycin are effective in most outbreaks. Reduction of feed intake is also recommended as a prophylactic procedure. Creep feeding prior to weaning may also help to prevent outbreaks. Feeding lactic acid (8) or cultures of *Lactobacillus acidophilus* may assist in controlling the coliform population after weaning.

REFERENCES

(1) Richards, W. P. C. & Fraser, C. M. (1961). *Cornell Vet.*, *51*, 245.
(2) Roberts, H. E. & Vallely, T. F. (1959). *Vet. Rec.*, *71*, 846.
(3) Gregory, D. W. (1962). *J. Amer. vet. med. Ass.*, *141*, 947.
(4) Palmer, N. C. & Hulland, T. J. (1965). *Canad. vet. J.*, *6*, 310.
(5) Thomlinson, J. R. & Buxton, A. (1963). *Immunology*, *6*, 126.
(6) Kenworthy, R. & Allen, W. D. (1966). *J. comp. Path*, *76*, 31.
(7) Miniats, O. P. & Roe, C. K. (1968). *Canad. vet. J.*, *9*, 210.
(8) Cole, D. J. A. *et al.* (1968). *Vet. Rec.*, *83*, 459.

DISEASES CAUSED BY *SALMONELLA* Spp.

Salmonellosis

(*Paratyphoid*)

Salmonellosis is a disease of all animal species caused by a number of different species of salmonellae and manifested clinically by one of three major syndromes: a peracute septicaemia, an acute enteritis or a chronic enteritis.

Incidence

The disease occurs in most countries, and in all species, and notifications of its occurrence, particularly in cattle and sheep, have increased during the past decade due in part to its wider dissemination but due also to failure in the past to recognize the disease. The increase in the prevalence of the disease has been, to an extent, due to increased intensification of cattle-raising, especially calves and young cattle. In cattle, a seasonal distribution with the principal peak in the autumn and early winter has been recognized (1, 2). The passage of calves through dealers' yards is one of the important contamination mechanisms (3). In pigs the importance of salmonellosis has been recognized for a long time. The disease occurs only sporadically in horses and is of minor importance in that species, occurring chiefly in foals, and to a less extent in other classes of horses after transport or surgery.

Surveys of the incidence of infection with salmonellae in animals usually indicate a high rate of inapparent infections. Figures from the U.K. indicate a nine-fold increase of *S. dublin* infection in cattle during the period 1959 to 1971. A smaller but significant increase was apparent in *S. typhimurium* infection (1, 2). A New Zealand survey showed a 13 to 15 per cent infection rate in dairy cows, calves and sheep and 4 per cent in beef cattle. Data from the Netherlands show that 25 per cent of healthy pigs at abattoirs harbour salmonellae. American figures indicate a 10 to 13·6 per cent infection rate in cattle. Data from abattoir material must be accepted with caution because of the known increase in the salmonella population of the gut in animals kept in holding yards for several days.

The morbidity rate in outbreaks of salmonellosis in pigs, sheep and calves is usually high, often reaching 50 per cent or more, whereas sporadic cases are the rule in adult cattle. The mortality rate is high in all species, reaching 100 per cent in some outbreaks. On individual farms, death losses due to this disease may be serious and the animals that recover from the acute form are usually chronically debilitated and require a long period of convalescence. The disease has public health importance because salmonellosis is one of the commonest diseases of man and its principal reservoir is domestic animals (1, 4, 5). Transmission to man occurs via contamination of drinking water or consumption of contaminated milk or meat, especially sausage. Contamination of milk usually occurs after the milk leaves the cow but the organism may be excreted in the milk during the acute phase of the disease and occasionally by carrier animals.

Aetiology

Many species of salmonellae are capable of causing disease in animals (1). The following list includes only the common ones. Cattle—*Salm. typhimurium* and *Salm. dublin*: Sheep—*Salm. typhimurium* and *Salm. dublin*: Swine:—*Salm. choleraesuis* and *Salm. typhimurium*: Horses—*Salm. typhimurium*. Unusual or exotic salmonellae for each species are often derived from other species and contamination of cattle pasture, drinking water or housing by other species needs careful attention.

Salmonellae are not usually present in large numbers in the faeces of normal animals although in herd infections many normal animals may pass large numbers of organisms. Infection with salmonellae does not necessarily cause disease although young animals are more susceptible than adults and oral dosing with young cultures of *Salm. choleraesuis* causes salmonellosis consistently in young pigs. In cattle *S. dublin* infections occur about equally in adults and calves but *S. typhimurium* occurs most commonly in calves under 6 months of age. Adult animals are more likely to become clinically normal carriers unless some debilitating influence increases their susceptibility and permits the development of the disease. In pigs such debilitating influences include intercurrent virus infections, particularly hog cholera, nutritional deficiencies such as a deficiency of nicotinic acid, and changes in intestinal flora caused by sudden changes in ration or antibiotic feeding. Horses which are overfed before shipment and which receive insufficient food, water and rest during transport, and excessive food on arrival are thought to be particularly susceptible, cases appearing within one to four days after shipment. Dosing with irritant compounds, especially anthelmintics, and vaccination with living virus vaccines, e.g. rinderpest, may also precipitate attacks of the disease.

In ruminants, details of the predisposing causes are not well understood, but in adult sheep and cattle, starvation and exhaustion during transport, recent parturition and intercurrent infection are commonly associated with attacks of salmonellosis. In adult cattle the most common occurrence is in cows which have calved during the preceding week. In calves up to 3 months of age the disease is quite common; in some areas the incidence may be as high as that of colibacillosis, and no precipitating environmental causes appear to be necessary.

The common occurrence of the disease after transportation is also related to increased exposure to infection in sale barns, stock yards and transport vehicles. As a result salmonellosis may be an important disease in some cattle feedlots.

Transmission

The main source of infection is the infected animal which contaminates pasture, feed, and drinking water with faeces containing the organism. For *S. dublin* the donor animals are very likely to be sheep or cattle, for *S. typhimurium* the donor can be any domestic or wild animal (1). The donor animal may be suffering from the clinical form of the disease or be a clinically normal 'carrier'. All adult animals which recover from the disease act as 'carriers' for variable periods of time. In *S. dublin* infections most recovered adult clinical cases become carriers for indefinite periods, and this infection is derived largely from other cattle. In *S. typhimurium* infections adult cattle rarely remain infective for any length of time, new infections often deriving from other animal species (2). Calves rarely become carriers (6). The carrier state may exist for up to 67 days in sheep and in horses. Information on this point is not available for the other species.

After contamination, the infectivity of inert materials varies with environmental conditions, particularly wetness and temperature, the organism being susceptible to drying and sunlight. *Salm. typhimurium* can remain viable for periods up to 7 months in soil, water and faeces, and on pasture.

In housed cattle, particularly calves, the contamination of the intensive environment and the rapid turnover of brought-in calves provide optimum chances for persistence of the disease. In cattle running at extensive pasture contamination of stagnant drinking water is important, in contrast to pasture in intensive grazing systems. The use of 'slurry' as a means of disposal of manure from cow housing or zero-grazing areas has led to the more efficient spread of salmonella infection than occurs with more conventional manure disposal. The chances of cows becoming infected are even greater if the slurried pasture is grazed soon afterwards (7, 8). Pasture has also been contaminated by human sewage (37). If food is premixed into a liquid form for pumping to feeding stations, as is common in piggeries, storage of the liquid feed can result in gross contamination with salmonellae because of their multiplication (9). Although transmission of infection on inanimate objects and by other agents such as flies (10) does occur the important mechanism in pigs is movement of the infected animal (11). The density of housing and the increased susceptibility of the 3 to 7 months age group are the other important factors.

In sheep extensive contamination of sheepyards,

drinking water and recycled dip wash are probably the important methods of spread (12).

The portal of entry is by ingestion and the severity of an outbreak will depend on the environmental conditions which govern the viability of the bacteria and the degree of contamination of the environment. Thus, in young calves, explosive outbreaks may occur, but in cattle at pasture the disease usually spreads slowly. In pigs the disease spreads rapidly and the morbidity is high. The condition in range sheep occurs usually during drought periods when grazing is concentrated around water holes, or in holding yards when sheep drink contaminated water from puddles or troughs (13, 14). Under these circumstances, the morbidity rate is usually low (5 to 10 per cent) but the mortality rate is high (80 per cent). A high incidence of the disease in an area is unusual but the occurrence of the disease simultaneously on a large number of farms has been recorded in sheep. In one instance the infection appeared to be spread by contamination of the drinking water by birds eating carrion. In horses recently transported and exposed to a highly contaminated environment, up to 50 per cent may be affected.

Infection may be introduced on to a farm by clinically normal 'carriers' or in plant or animal products used as feedstuffs or fertilizer. Organic feedstuffs, including bone meal, have been incriminated and up to 70 per cent of specimens of bone meal in some surveys have been found to be infected with salmonellae (15). Such meals need to be heated at 82°C (180°F) for an hour to be sterilized (16). Infection of feed materials may derive from ante-mortem infection in animals used for the preparation of bone meal but is also likely to occur in offal in abattoirs or during storage. Rodents and domestic or wild birds may also be an important source of infection.

Pathogenesis

Infection with salmonellae in young animals, or adults whose resistance has been decreased by intercurrent infection, results in rapid multiplication of the bacteria in the intestine and invasion of the blood stream. The resulting septicaemia may be rapidly fatal. If the systemic invasion is sufficient to cause only a bacteraemia, acute enteritis may develop (13). Many animals survive this stage of the disease but localization of the salmonellae occurs in mesenteric lymph nodes, liver, spleen, and particularly the gall-bladder. In healthy adults there may be no clinical illness when infection first occurs but there may be localization in abdominal viscera. In either instance the animals become chronic carriers and discharge salmonellae intermittently from the gall-bladder and foci of infection in the intestinal wall into the faeces, and occasionally into the milk. For this reason they are important sources of infection for other animals and for humans. Carrier animals may also develop an acute septicaemia or enteritis if their resistance is lowered by environmental stresses or intercurrent infection. In pigs and to a less extent in cattle, ulcerative lesions may develop in the intestinal mucosa, and these may be of sufficient size to cause chronic or intermittent diarrhoea.

During the septicaemic or bacteraemic phases of the disease in pigs, localization in the lungs or meninges, causing pneumonia and meningitis, is not uncommon and adds to the complexity of the syndrome.

Clinical Findings

The disease is most satisfactorily described as four syndromes classified arbitrarily according to severity.

Septicaemia. Newborn calves and foals, and young pigs up to 4 months of age are commonly affected by this form, particularly during the early stages of an outbreak. There is depression, dullness, high fever (40·5 to 42°C or 105 to 107°F) and death within 24 to 48 hours. Calves affected by *Salm. dublin* may show signs of involvement of the nervous system including inco-ordination and nystagmus. In pigs affected by *S. choleraesuis* a dark red to purple discolouration of the skin is evident, especially on the abdomen and ears, and subcutaneous petechial haemorrhages may also be visible. Nervous signs, including tremor, weakness, paralysis and convulsions, may be prominent and occur in a large proportion of affected pigs. The mortality rate in this form is usually 100 per cent. A semi-specific entity occurring in pigs up to 4 weeks old is manifested by meningitis and clinical signs of prostration and clonic convulsions (17).

Acute enteritis. This is the common form in adult animals of all species. In all species there is a high fever (40 to 41°C or 104 to 106°F), with severe, watery diarrhoea, sometimes dysentery, and in some cases, tenesmus. The fever may disappear precipitously with the onset of diarrhoea. The faeces have a putrid smell and contain mucus, shreds of mucous membrane, and in less severe cases, casts of intestinal mucosa. In sheep they are a light grey-green colour. There is complete anorexia but great thirst may be manifested. The pulse rate is rapid, the mucosae are reddened and the respirations rapid and shallow. Pregnant animals commonly abort. The mortality rate in this form of the disease is usually 75 per cent or more.

Additional signs are characteristic of the disease in the various species. In cattle there is complete cessation of milk flow and dysentery is often severe, whole blood being voided in large clots. Abdominal pain, with kicking at the belly, rolling, crouching, groaning and looking at the flanks, is common in adult cattle. Rectal examination at this stage usually causes severe distress. In horses acute abdominal pain is characteristic and the animal's actions are often violent. Acute pneumonia is a common accompaniment of this form of the disease in swine, and nervous signs and cutaneous discolouration as described in the septicaemic form may also be present.

In all species, severe dehydration and toxaemia develop, the animal loses condition very quickly, becomes recumbent and dies in 2 to 5 days. Foals and calves which survive the acute stages may subsequently develop a painful polyarthritis.

Subacute enteritis. In adult horses on farms where the disease is enzootic many show only mild clinical signs including anorexia, fever (about 39 °C or 103 °F) for 4 to 5 days and faeces of the consistency of cow manure. *Salm. dublin* infection in ewes may cause a high proportion of abortions, some deaths in ewes after abortion and a heavy mortality due to enteritis in lambs born alive.

Chronic enteritis. This is a common syndrome in pigs and occurs occasionally in cattle. There is persistent diarrhoea, severe emaciation and intermittent fever. At intervals the faeces contain spots of blood, mucus and occasionally firm, intestinal casts. This chronic phase is often preceded by an attack of the acute enteric form of the disease.

Abortion occurs frequently in association with other forms of the disease. Thus it is a common sequel in cows that survive an attack of acute enteritis. However, infection with *S. dublin* is also a significant cause of abortion in cattle without there having been any other clinical signs (18).

In summary the occurrence of the syndromes described above in the various animal species is as follows: Cattle—the peracute form occurs in newborn calves; calves from one week of age and up to adult animals are most commonly affected by the acute enteric form with occasional cases of the chronic enteric form. Joint involvement may occur in calves, and abortion in adults. In sheep the peracute form may occur early in the outbreak, followed by the more common, acute enteric form. In horses the acute enteric form is the common syndrome in animals which have recently been transported and this may be followed by septi-caemia or bacteraemia with localization in various organs. A subacute enteric form occurs also in adult horses. In foals up to 2 days of age, a peracute septicaemia may occur but acute enteritis is more usual. In older foals acute enteritis is more common. In pigs the disease varies widely and, although all forms occur in this species, there is often a tendency for one form to be more common in any particular outbreak. In the acute form in pigs there is also a tendency for pulmonary involvement to occur, but the main feature of the disease is enteritis, with pneumonia and occasionally encephalitis present as only secondary signs.

Clinical Pathology

The ante-mortem laboratory diagnosis of salmonellosis presents many difficulties. In cattle the organisms are present in the blood stream and milk of acute cases for only a brief period before diarrhoea commences and may not appear in the faeces for up to two weeks after the commencement of illness. Agglutinins do not appear in the serum until about the same time. If the animal is examined during the acute stage of the disease, all tests may therefore be negative and it will be necessary to depend upon faecal culture and agglutination tests of in-contact animals to confirm a diagnosis of herd infection. Positive serum agglutination titres persist for variable periods. Calves do not usually remain 'carriers', the agglutination test becoming negative in 2 to 3 months. In adult cattle and pigs infection and a positive serum agglutination test persist for more than a year in about 5 per cent of animals (19).

If a diagnosis of salmonellosis on a herd basis is to be attempted, periodic faecal cultures at 15 day intervals using enriching media should be combined with serological examinations. When *Salm. typhimurium* is the causative bacteria the faeces of other species of animals on the farm should be examined, because ducks, dogs, horses, pigs, sheep and cattle may be sources of infection for each other. It is always advisable to examine the drinking water and feed for evidence of infection.

Necropsy Findings

Peracute septicaemic form. There may be an absence of gross lesions in animals which have died peracutely but there is usually evidence of septicaemia in the form of extensive submucosal and subserous petechial haemorrhages. In cases that survive for one or more days, the necropsy findings may include those of the acute form.

Acute enteric form. Gross lesions are most prominent in the large and small intestines.

Inflammation is evident and varies from a muco-enteritis with submucosal petechiation to diffuse haemorrhagic enteritis. Similar lesions may be present in the abomasum, and in *Salm. dublin* infections in calves multiple mucosal erosions and petechiation of the abomasal wall may be accompanied by gastritis. Enteritis is inconstant. The intestinal contents are watery, have a putrid odour and contain mucus, and are blood tinged or contain whole blood. In cases which have survived for longer periods, superficial necrosis may proceed to the development of an extensive diphtheritic pseudo-membrane. The mesenteric lymph nodes are enlarged, oedematous and haemorrhagic. The wall of the gall-bladder may be thickened and inflamed. Enlargement and fatty degeneration of the liver occur and the serous cavities may contain blood stained fluid. Variable degrees of subserous petechiation occur but are always present under the epicardium. In pigs the petechiae are very prominent and may give the kidney the 'turkey-egg' appearance usually associated with hog cholera. Congestion and hepatization of lung tissue may be present especially in pigs.

Skin discolouration is marked in pigs and, depending on the severity of the case, this varies from extreme erythema with haemorrhages, to plaques and circumscribed scabby lesions similar to those of swine pox.

Chronic form. In cattle the chronic form is usually manifested by discrete areas of necrosis of the wall of the caecum and colon. The wall is thickened and covered with a yellow-grey necrotic material overlying a red, granular surface. In pigs the lesion is similar but usually more diffuse. Less commonly the lesions are discrete in the form of button ulcers, occurring most commonly in the caecum around the ileocaecal valve. Button ulcers commonly occur in chronic hog cholera but there is some doubt as to whether the lesions are caused by the hog cholera virus or by secondary invasion by salmonellae. The mesenteric lymph nodes and the spleen are swollen. Chronic pneumonia may also be present.

Salmonellae are present in the heart blood, spleen, liver, bile, mesenteric lymph nodes and intestinal contents in both septicaemic and acute enteric forms. In the chronic form, the bacteria may be isolated from the intestinal lesions and less commonly from other viscera. The most satisfactory method for immediate examination is a thick smear from the lining of the gall-bladder.

Diagnosis

The diagnosis of salmonellosis presents considerable difficulty in the living animal largely because of the variety of clinical syndromes which may occur and the variations in clinical pathology outlined above. At necropsy the isolation of salmonellae from tissues and intestinal contents, although suggestive of the presence of salmonellosis, does not of itself confirm the diagnosis and care must be taken to ascertain whether other disease is present.

Cattle. The peracute form in calves resembles septicaemia due to *E. coli* so closely that differentiation is possible only by bacteriological examination. There is a strong tendency for salmonellosis to occur in calves during the second and third weeks of life rather than in the first week, a more common characteristic in colibacillosis. The acute enteric form may be confused with coccidiosis especially if the fever has subsided. The acute abdominal pain may suggest acute intestinal obstruction but profuse diarrhoea and dysentery are unlikely to occur in the latter. Winter dysentery occurs in explosive outbreaks and is self-limiting; mucosal disease is characterized by typical mucosal lesions and epizootiology; bracken fern poisoning has considerable resemblance to salmonellosis but a history of access to bracken is usually available. Other poisonings, especially arsenic and to a less extent, lead, and a number of miscellaneous weeds may cause a similar acute enteritis. Chronic cases may resemble Johne's disease or chronic molybdenum poisoning but dysentery and epithelial casts do not occur in these diseases. Massive stomach fluke infestations may also cause diarrhoea and dysentery.

Sheep. Diarrhoea caused by infections with coccidia or *Vibrio* sp., or by parasitic infestation may be confused with that caused by *Salmonella* spp. but the latter is usually more acute and more highly fatal.

Horses. The acute form in foals may resemble the acute infections caused by *E. coli* and *Act. equuli*. A history of recent transport often helps in making a diagnosis of salmonellosis in adult horses.

Pigs. Peracute salmonellosis can resemble hog cholera and pasteurellosis very closely and laboratory examination is usually necessary for identification. Acute erysipelas, in those cases where characteristic skin lesions have not appeared, is usually indicated at necropsy by the larger, subserous ecchymoses but again laboratory examination may be necessary if doubt exists. The lesions of swine dysentery are confined to the alimentary tract. Salmonella meningitis in young pigs is clinically indistinguishable from streptococcal meningitis.

Treatment

Many drugs are used successfully but in many cases recovered animals continue to excrete the organism in the faeces, and act as 'carriers' of the infection (20, 21). It is not advisable to leave affected animals untreated because of the high mortality rate; if cattle and foals (22) are treated early there should be almost no deaths, if they are not treated the mortality rate will be of the order of 100 per cent. Standard dose rates are recommended but combined oral and parenteral routes of administration are recommended for sick animals.

The choice of drugs to be used depends on a test of drug sensitivity in each case or outbreak but failing this the following generalizations can be applied. In calves for *S. dublin* infections the descending order of preference is chloramphenicol, furazolidone, sulphamethylphenazole and neomycin (23). Sulphadimidine, ampicillin (24) and framomycin are also widely used and recommended. Many veterinarians use a combination of two drugs, e.g. chloramphenicol by injection and nitrofurazone by mouth. One of the advantages of nitrofurazone is its adaptability to large scale medication via the drinking water (25).

For pigs the same list of drugs is available but treatment of individual pigs is usually by ampicillin, chloramphenicol or neomycin and mass treatment by nitrofurazone (26). Where large numbers of pigs are affected mass medication via the feed or drinking water is usually practised. Because sick pigs do not eat, water treatment is necessary and if drugs are unpalatable individual treatment is the last recourse. Drugs that dissolve readily and are palatable are therefore in demand.

Ancillary treatment, by providing demulcent and astringent preparations for oral use and fluids, either orally or parenterally, to replace lost electrolytes and fluids will help animals to survive the period of acute dehydration and toxaemia.

Control

Prevention of introduction would be ideal but it is an objective not easily achieved. The principle sources of infection are carrier animals and contaminated food-stuffs containing feeds of animal origin. A closed herd removes half the risk, but is not a practicable procedure for the types of animal producer for which salmonellosis is a major problem—the calf-rearer and the commercial pig fattener. For such people the following rules apply (27):

(*a*) Introduce the animals directly from the farm of origin. Avoid dealers' yards, sale yards and public transport, all of which are likely to be contaminated. Determine that the farm of origin is free of salmonellosis. This is not an attractive proposition to many pig and calf fatteners because the gamble with high stakes in their enterprise rests on the speculative purchase of large groups of animals where and when the local market is depressed.

(*b*) If possible purchase animals when they are older, say 6 weeks for calves, to give an opportunity for specific and non-specific immunity to develop. If these animals can come from vaccinated herds so much the better.

(*c*) Dealers premises, sale yards, and transport vehicles should be under close surveillance and the need for frequent vigorous disinfection stressed.

(*d*) Introduce only those animals determined not to be 'carriers'. Unfortunately the detection of carriers is inaccurate and expensive. To have any confidence in the results one must submit serum samples for agglutination tests and faecal samples for culture on at least three occasions.

Limitation of spread within a herd. When an outbreak occurs, procedures for limiting spread, as set out below, need to be strictly enforced, and medication of affected groups, and of susceptible groups at high risk, carried out. The drugs to be used are those listed under treatment, the choice of the individual drug depending on its efficiency and cost. In an endemic herd the procedure is the same but the tempo can be more leisurely.

(*a*) Identify the carrier animals and either cull them or isolate and treat them vigorously. Treated animals should be rechecked subsequently to determine whether a 'clean' status has been achieved. Our personal experience is that much can be achieved by this measure in well-managed herds whose individual animals are valuable, but experience in the elimination of carrier foals by the administration of nitrofurazone and neomycin, and in pigs by full doses of chloramphenicol, nitrofurazone or ampicillin, has been disappointing.

(*b*) Restrict the movement of animals around the farm and limit the infection to as small a group as possible. Pasture and permanent buildings are both important although the major source of infection in most cases is the drinking water.

(*c*) The water supply should be provided in troughs which should not be capable of faecal contamination. Infected static drinking water or pasture may remain infected for as long as six months.

(*d*) Vigorous disinfection of buildings is important. An all-in-all-out policy should be adopted and steam cleaning and chemical sterilization performed after each batch. For calves individual pens are of tremendous value but their costs of construction and maintenance probably preclude their use for other than pedigree herds. Pig houses need especially careful treatment (26). Dirt yards present a problem, especially those used for sheep and calves, but provided they can be kept dry and empty two sprayings, one month apart, with 5 per cent formalin is reputed to eliminate the infection (28).

(e) Suitable construction of housing is important. Impervious walls to stop spread from pen to pen, pen design to permit feeding without entering the pen, avoidance of any communal activity and slatted floors to provide escape routes for manure, all assist in limiting the spread of enteric diseases. Deep litter systems appear to be hazardous but have keen supporters provided they are kept very dry and plenty of bedding is available.

(f) Heat treatment of food is an effective procedure for pigs. Heating during pelleting greatly reduces the bacterial content of feed and special treatment is worthwhile because of the very high proportion of animal derived feeds which are infected (26). The availability of such feeds guaranteed to be salmonella-free would be an advantage.

(g) Disposal of infective material should be carried out with great care. Carcases should be burnt, or better still sent to an institution for diagnosis, rather than to a knackery to be converted into still more contaminated bone meal. Slurry and manure for disposal should be placed on crops rather than on pasture.

(h) All persons working on infected premises should be warned of the hazards to their own health. Other peripatetic species, especially dogs, should be kept under close restraint.

(i) Vaccination is an active subject of discussion in salmonellosis control. The reaction of research workers and field workers is mixed. If viewed in a conservative light it must be evident that it is a most valuable procedure but that it is not a complete answer to the problem on its own. If it is combined with the hygienic precautions listed above so that the immune barrier is not assaulted too heavily or too frequently, it is a valuable auxiliary weapon. Two methods are available, a killed bacterin and a live attenuated vaccine. Either can be used as prenatal vaccines to provide passive immunization of the newborn. The following generalizations apply. An autogenous bacterin, made from bacteria collected on the farm, has advantages, especially if a killed vaccine of low antigenicity is to be used. Its principal disadvantage is cost. In cattle S. dublin is the infection likely to be endemic in a herd and com-

mercial vaccine, to be effective, must have a strong S. dublin component. The vaccine Strain 51, produced in the U.K. from a rough, variant strain of this organism, has been found to be very efficient and safe and to provide good protection against S. typhimurium as well as S. dublin, by far the most important causes of salmonellosis at least in farm animals in the U.K. (29, 30, 31). It has the disadvantages of a living vaccine but calves can be vaccinated successfully at 2 to 4 weeks of age.

The autogenous bacterin, which must be precipitated on aluminium hydroxide to have any significant effect, is given as two injections two weeks apart. Good immunity is produced but calves and pigs less than 6 weeks of age are refractory, and anaphylactic reactions may cause the loss of a significant number of animals. To protect young calves the best programme is to vaccinate the cows during late pregnancy. This will give passive protection to the calves for 6 weeks, provided they take sufficient colostrum, and the calves can be vaccinated at that time if danger still exists. Reported results have not been enthusiastic (32) but if proper attention is given to the detail of the programme it has been sufficient, in our hands, to provide almost complete protection.

Because of the early age at which pigs need to be immune, it is recommended that sows be vaccinated three times at 7 to 14 day intervals. The young pigs are vaccinated at 3 weeks of age. In horses a similar regimen with a booster dose for all mares in late pregnancy, appears to be effective (33). Results in sheep have been unconvincing (34, 35). There has been a report of a commercial adjuvant vaccine containing S. bovismorbificans and S. typhimurium and of its successful use in sheep (36).

Animals being transported are a special case. They should be unloaded or exercised at least once every 24 hours and given water and food, the feed being provided first and at least two hours before watering. Hay or chopped hay is preferred to succulent feeds. All railway cars, and feeding and watering troughs should be properly cleaned and disinfected between shipments. Horses which are to be transported should be yarded and handfed on hard feed for 4 or 5 days beforehand. If the disease is likely to occur, prophylactic feeding with sulphonamides or antibiotics has been shown to decrease the incidence in all species. Ampicillin (50 mg. orally) has been shown to be effective for this purpose (34). Apart from the risk that this practice will produce resistant bacteria, there has been a suggestion that it may so change the normal bacterial flora of the gut as to encourage the proliferation of salmonellae and lead to the development of the clinical disease.

REFERENCES

(1) Sojka, W. T. & Field, H. I. (1970). *Vet. Bull.*, *40*, 515.
(2) Hughes, L. E. *et al.* (1971). *Brit. vet. J.*, *127*, 225.
(3) Stevens, A. J. *et al.* (1967). *Vet. Rec.*, *80*, 154.
(4) Anonymous (1966). *J. Amer. vet. med. Ass.*, *149*, 1079.
(5) Taylor, J. (1967). *Vet. Rec.*, *80*, 147, 154.
(6) Robinson, R. A. & Loken, K. I. (1968). *J. Hyg., Camb.*, *66*, 207.
(7) Jack, E. J. & Hepper, P. T. (1969). *Vet. Rec.*, *84*, 196.
(8) Taylor, R. J. & Burrows, M. R. (1971). *Brit. vet. J.*, *127*, 536.
(9) Linton, A. H. *et al.* (1970). *Res. vet. Sci.*, *11*, 452.
(10) Greenberg, B. *et al.* (1970). *Infect. Immun.*, *2*, 800.
(11) Linton, A. H. *et al.* (1970). *Res. vet. Sci.*, *11*, 523.
(12) Robinson, R. A. & Royal, W. A. (1971). *N.Z. J. agric. Res.*, *14*, 442.
(13) McCaughey, W. J. *et al.* (1971). *Brit. vet. J.*, *127*, 549.
(14) Stewart, D. F. (1940). *Aust. vet. J.*, *16*, 169.
(15) Gray, D. F. *et al.* (1960). *Aust. vet. J.*, *36*, 246.
(16) Gibson, E. A. (1969). *Brit. vet. J.*, *125*, 431.
(17) McErlean, B. A. (1969). *Irish vet. J.*, *23*, 10.
(18) Hinton, M. (1971). *Vet. Bull.*, *41*, 973.
(19) Zagaevskii, I. S. (1962). *Veterinariya*, *9*, 15–20.
(20) Henning, M. W. (1953). *Onderstepoort J. vet. Res.*, *26*, 3, *25*, 45.
(21) Rutquist, L. *et al.* (1961). *Nord. Vet.-Med.*, *13*, 3.
(22) Bryans, J. T. *et al.* (1965). *Vet. Med.*, *60*, 626.
(23) van der Walt, K. *et al.* (1967). *J. S. Afr. vet. med. Ass.*, *38*, 425.
(24) Larkin, P. J. & Hicks, M. (1967). *Vet. Rec.*, *81*, 231.
(25) Singh, V. K. (1968). *J. Amer. vet. med. Ass.*, *153*, 65.
(26) Heard, T. W. *et al.* (1968). *Vet. Rec.*, *82*, 92.
(27) B.V.A. (1967). *Vet. Rec.*, *80*, 357.
(28) Robinson, R. A. *et al.* (1970). *N.Z. vet. J.*, *18*, 214.
(29) Smith, H. Williams (1967). *Vet. Rec.*, *80*, 142.
(30) Pay, M. G. (1967). *Vet. Rec.*, *80*, 317.
(31) Rankin, J. D. *et al.* (1967). *Vet. Rec.*, *80*, 247, 720.
(32) Rankin, J. D. & Taylor, R. J. (1970). *Vet. Rec.*, *86*, 254.
(33) Bryans, J. T. *et al.* (1961). *Cornell Vet.*, *51*, 467.
(34) Kerr, W. J. & Brander, G. C. (1964). *Vet. Rec.*, *76*, 1105.
(35) Davis, G. B. (1969). *N.Z. vet. J.*, *17*, 62.
(36) Rudge, J. M. *et al.* (1968). *N.Z. vet. J.*, *16*, 23; *15*, 62, 66; *17*, 62.
(37) Bicknell, S. R. (1972). *J. Hyg., Camb.*, *70*, 121.

Abortion in Mares and Septicaemia in Foals Caused by *Salmonella abortivoequina*

This is a specific disease of equidae characterized by abortion in females, testicular lesions in males and septicaemia in the newborn.

Incidence

Although widely reported, the incidence of the disease appears to be decreasing and it is now one of the less common causes of either abortion or septicaemia in horses (1).

Aetiology

The infection appears to be limited to horses and donkeys (6).

Salm. abortivoequina can be isolated from affected animals and cultures of the organism are capable of causing the disease. However, in some outbreaks in which the organism is isolated from aborted material, a filterable agent capable of causing abortion is also found and the salmonellae are judged to be secondary invaders. In the absence of viral infections other predisposing causes are thought to increase the chances of infection and of abortion (4).

Transmission

Natural infection may be due to the ingestion of foodstuffs contaminated by uterine discharges from carriers or mares which have recently aborted. Transmission from the stallion at the time of service is also thought to occur. The infection may persist in the uterus and cause repeated abortion or infection of subsequent foals.

Pathogenesis

When infection occurs by ingestion, a transient bacteraemia without marked systemic signs is followed by localization in the placenta, resulting in placentitis and abortion. Foals which are carried to term probably become infected in utero or soon after birth by ingestion from the contaminated teat surface or through the umbilicus.

Clinical Findings

Abortion usually occurs about the seventh to eighth month of pregnancy. The mare may show signs of impending abortion followed by difficult parturition but other evidence of illness is usually lacking. Retention of the placenta and metritis are common sequels and may cause serious illness but subsequent sterility is unusual. A foal which is carried to term by an infected mare may develop an acute septicaemia during the first few days of life or survive to develop polyarthritis 7 to 14 days later. Polyarthritis has also been observed in foals from vaccinated mares who showed no signs of the disease (5).

Infection in the stallion has also been reported, clinical signs including fever, oedematous swelling of the prepuce and scrotum, and arthritis. Hydrocele, epididymitis and inflammation of the tunica vaginalis are followed by orchitis and testicular atrophy (2).

Clinical Pathology

The organism can be isolated from the placenta, the uterine discharge, the aborted foal and from the joints of foals with polyarthritis. A high titre of salmonella agglutinins in the mare develops about

2 weeks after abortion. Vaccinated mares will give a positive reaction for up to a year.

Necropsy Findings

The placenta of the aborted foal is oedematous and haemorrhagic and may show areas of necrosis. Acute septicaemia will be manifested in foals dying soon after birth and polyarthritis in those dying at a later stage.

Diagnosis

Abortion in mares may be caused by the viruses of equine viral rhinopneumonitis and equine viral arteritis and by *Streptococcus genitalium*. Septicaemia and polyarthritis of foals is also caused by this latter organism, and by *E. coli*, *Salm. typhimurium* and *Act. equuli*. Identification of the disease must depend upon isolation of the organism and the positive agglutination test in the mare.

Treatment

The same drugs which have been recommended in the treatment of salmonellosis should also be effective in this disease.

Control

Careful hygiene, including isolation of infected mares and disposal of aborted material, should be practised to avoid spread of the infection. Infected stallions should not be used for breeding. In the past, when this disease was much more common than it is now, great reliance was placed on vaccination as a control measure. An autogenous or commercial bacterin, composed of killed *Salm. abortivoequina* organisms, was injected on 3 occasions at weekly intervals to all mares on farms where the disease was enzootic, commencing 2 to 3 months after the close of the breeding season. A formol-killed, alum-precipitated vaccine is considered to be superior to a heat-killed, phenolized vaccine (3).

REFERENCES

(1) Winkinwerder, W. (1967). *Zbl. Bakt.*, *203*, 69.
(2) Koser, A. (1956). *Dtsch. tierärztl. Wschr.*, *63*, 275.
(3) Dhanda, M. R. *et al.* (1955). *Indian J. vet. Sci.*, *25*, 245.
(4) Muranyi, F. & Vanyi, A. (1963). *Magy. Allatorv. Lap.*, *18*, 239.
(5) Garbers, G. V. & Monteverde, J. J. (1964). *Rev. Med. vet.* (*B. Aires*), *45*, 305.
(6) Singh, I. P. *et al.* (1971). *Brit. vet. J.*, *127*, 378.

Abortion in Ewes Caused by Salmonella abortusovis

Salm. abortusovis is a relatively uncommon cause of abortion in ewes but appear to be enzootic in particular areas (1). Spread of the disease may occur after the introduction of carrier animals. Ingestion is thought to be the main mode of infection. Venereal spread has been postulated, and rams certainly become infected but all the evidence is against spread at coitus. Abortion 'storms' occur about 6 weeks before lambing, and septic metritis and peritonitis subsequently cause a few deaths among the ewes (2). Identification of the disease depends upon isolation of the organism which is present in large numbers in the foetus, placenta and uterine discharges, and the presence of a strong positive agglutination test in the ewe. The clinical and serological findings in *Salm. dublin* infections in ewes are very similar (4, 5). A strong immunity develops after an attack and an autogenous vaccine has given good results in the control of the disease (3). The results of vaccination need to be very carefully appraised because flock immunity develops readily and the disease tends to subside naturally in the second year (1). Vaccination with *S. dublin* vaccine is ineffective. *Salm. ruiru* has also been recorded as a cause of abortion in ewes, and ewes with salmonellosis caused by *Salm. typhimurium* may also lose their lambs. The administration of broad spectrum antibiotics may aid in controlling an outbreak but available reports (1) are not encouraging.

REFERENCES

(1) Jack, E. J. (1968). *Vet. Rec.*, *82*, 558.
(2) Lovell, R. (1931). *J. Path. Bact.*, *34*, 13.
(3) Endrejat, E. (1955). *Dtsch. tierärztl. Wschr.*, *62*, 233.
(4) Baker, J. R. (1971). *Vet. Rec.*, *88*, 270.
(5) Gitter, M. & Sojka, W. (1970). *Vet. Rec.*, *87*, 775.
(6) Dennis, S. M. & Armstrong, J. M. (1965). *Aust. vet. J.*, *41*, 178.

DISEASES CAUSED BY PASTEURELLA Spp.

Pasteurellae occur in many animal diseases and, although in some instances they act as primary causes, the number of conditions in which they appear to play only a secondary role is gradually increasing. This is not to say that their importance is any the less. A primary viral pneumonia may be an insignificant disease until the intervention of a secondary pasteurellosis converts it into an outbreak of pneumonia of major economic importance. The common diseases in which *Pasteurella* spp. play an important aetiological role are dealt with in this section with due regard to their possible secondary nature. Mastitis caused by *Pasteurella* spp. is dealt with in the section on mastitis. Pasteurellae may also play an important role in atrophic rhinitis of pigs and in calf pneumonia.

Other isolated instances of disease caused by *Past. multocida* are meningo-encephalitis of calves (1) and yearling cattle (2), manifested by muscle tremor, opisthotonus, rotation of the eyeballs, collapse, coma and death within a few hours, and lymphadenitis in lambs which show enlargement of the submandibular, cranial, cervical and prescapular lymph nodes (3). An epidemic of meningo-encephalitis in horses, donkeys and mules has been reported from Mexico. The causative agent was *Past. haemolytica*. Clinical findings included incoordination, paralysis of the tongue, tremor and blindness. Death occurred 1 to 7 days after the commencement of the illness (4). There is also a report of a fatal septicaemia in horses and donkeys in India in which *P. multocida* appeared to be implicated as a causative agent (10).

Past. pseudotuberculosis is a common cause of epizootic disease in birds and rodents and occasionally causes disease in domestic animals. The infection has been observed as a cause of abortion in cattle and sheep (5, 9) epididymitis-orchitis in rams (6), multiple abscess formation in sheep (7) and in pigs dying of a disease manifested by enteritis, hepatitis and nephritis (8).

REFERENCES

(1) Shand, A. & Markson, L. M. (1953). *Brit. vet. J.*, *109*, 491.
(2) Rose, W. K. & Rac, R. (1957). *Aust. vet. J.*, *33*, 124.
(3) Madeyski, S. *et al.* (1957). *Med. vet. Varsovie*, *13*, 75 cited in (1957), *Vet. Bull.*, *27*, 394.
(4) Valdes Ornelas, O. (1963). *Bull. Off. int. Épizoot.*, *60*, 1059.
(5) Mair, N. S. & Harbourne, J. F. (1963). *Vet. Rec.*, *75*, 559.
(6) Jamieson, S. & Soltys, M. A. (1947). *Vet. Rec.*, *59*, 351.
(7) Nagy, A. (1963). *Magy. Allatorv. Lap.*, *18*, 204.
(8) Reuss, U. (1962). *Berl. Münch. tierärztl. Wschr.*, *75*, 203.
(9) Langford, E. V. (1969). *Canad. vet. J.*, *10*, 208.
(10) Pavri, K. M. & Apte, V. H. (1967). *Vet. Rec.*, *80*, 437.

Pasteurellosis

The nomenclature of the diseases caused by infections with *Pasteurella* spp. in farm animals has been indefinite and confusing. A suggested nomenclature is set out below which is based on the clinical findings and on the bacteria which are commonly associated with each entity (5).

Septicaemic pasteurellosis of cattle (haemorrhagic septicaemia or barbone), commonly associated with infection by *Past. multocida* Type 1 or B, is the classical disease of southern Asia characterized by a peracute septicaemia and a high mortality rate.

Pneumonic pasteurellosis of cattle, commonly associated with infection by *Past. multocida* Type 2 or A and *Past. haemolytica*, is a common disease in Europe and the western hemisphere. It is characterized by bronchopneumonia, a longer course and a lower mortality rate than is the case in septicaemic pasteurellosis.

Pasteurellosis of swine, sheep and goats. Pasteurellosis of swine is usually associated with infection by *Past. multocida* and is mainly pneumonic in form. Pasteurellosis of sheep and goats is usually associated with infection by *Past. haemolytica* and although it is often pneumonic in form, a septicaemic form of the disease is not unusual, especially in lambs.

There are a number of immunologically distinct types of the common causative organism, *Past. multocida*. These have been classified as Types 1 (or B), 2 (or A), 3 (or C) and 4 (or D) and there is a loose relationship between the serotype and the host species (1, 2). There is also some relationship between the serotype and the disease produced. Septicaemic pasteurellosis is caused only by Type 1 (3) and as this type does not occur in the U.K. and is uncommon in North America, it is not surprising to find that this form of the disease does not occur there (4).

The position with *Past. haemolytica* is more obscure but preliminary work suggests that a number of serotypes occur and that there may be biological differences in virulence between them (6, 7).

The name 'shipping fever' is avoided because of its poor definition. In its usual context, it implies an infectious febrile disease of cattle, and to a lesser extent other species, which is usually accompanied by clinical signs of involvement of the respiratory tract or alimentary tract or both, and which occurs as outbreaks, mainly in animals which have recently been transported. Accurate clinical, clinicopathological and necropsy examinations have not always been carried out and it is often impossible to decide from recorded descriptions of the disease which of the many aetiological entities commonly occurring in cattle under these circumstances is under discussion. Pneumonic pasteurellosis, virus pneumonia of calves, salmonellosis, sporadic bovine encephalomyelitis and infectious bovine rhinotracheitis are some of the disease entities which may occur alone or in combination after shipping. However, in our experience the great majority of cases of 'shipping fever' in cattle are cases of pneumonic pasteurellosis associated with infection by *Past. multocida* or *Past. haemolytica*.

REVIEW LITERATURE
Carter, G. R. (1967). *Advanc. vet. Sci.*, *11*.

REFERENCES

(1) Roberts, R. S. (1947). *J. comp. Path.*, *57*, 261.
(2) Carter, G. R. & Rowsell, H. C. (1958). *J. Amer. vet. med. Ass.*, *132*, 187.
(3) Bain, R. V. S. (1954). *Bull. Off. int. Épizoot.*, *42*, 256.
(4) Kyaw, M. H. (1942). *Vet. J.*, *98*, 3.
(5) Carter, G. R. & Bain, R. V. S. (1960). *Vet. Rev. Annot.*, *6*, 105.
(6) Biberstein, E. L. *et al.* (1960). *Cornell Vet.*, *50*, 283.
(7) Smith, G. R. (1961). *J. comp. Path.*, *71*, 194.

Septicaemic Pasteurellosis of Cattle

(*Haemorrhagic septicaemia, barbone*)

Septicaemic pasteurellosis of cattle, yaks, camels and water buffalo and, to a much smaller extent, of pigs and horses, is recorded chiefly from southern Asia where it causes very heavy death losses, particularly in low lying areas, and when the animals are exposed to wet, chilly weather or exhausted by heavy work (1). It is also recorded in bison and cattle in the U.S.A. (7, 8) and the causative bacteria and its endotoxin have been used to produce the disease experimentally (9). Both morbidity and mortality rates vary between 50 and 100 per cent and animals that recover require a long convalescence. The disease is presumed to be a primary pasteurellosis caused by *Past. multocida* Type 1 (or B) and occasionally type 4 (D).

Septicaemic pasteurellosis occurs in outbreaks during periods of environmental stress, the causative organism in the intervening periods persisting on the tonsillar and nasopharyngeal mucosae of carrier animals. Spread occurs by the ingestion of contaminated foodstuffs, the infection originating from clinically normal carriers or clinical cases, or possibly by ticks (5) and biting insects. The saliva of affected animals contains large numbers of pasteurellae during the early stages of the disease. Although infection occurs by ingestion, the organism does not survive on pasture for more than 24 hours (1).

The disease is an acute septicaemia and clinically it is characterized by a sudden onset of fever (106 to 107°F or 41 to 42°C), profuse salivation, submucosal petechiation, severe depression and death in about 24 hours. Localization may occur in subcutaneous tissue, resulting in the development of hot, painful swellings about the throat, dewlap, brisket or perineum, and severe dyspnoea may occur if the respiration is obstructed. In the later stages of an outbreak, some affected animals develop signs of pulmonary or alimentary involvement. Pasteurellae may be isolated from the saliva and the blood stream. The disease in pigs is identical with that in cattle (3).

At necropsy the gross findings are usually limited to generalized petechial haemorrhages, particularly under the serosae, and oedema of the lungs and lymph nodes. Subcutaneous infiltrations of gelatinous fluid may be present and in a few animals there are lesions of early pneumonia and a haemorrhagic gastroenteritis. Isolation of the causative bacteria is best attempted from heart blood and spleen.

Apart from its regional distribution, septicaemic pasteurellosis presents little in the way of diagnostic, clinical and necropsy findings and it can only be differentiated from anthrax, some cases of blackleg and acute leptospirosis by bacteriological examination.

The disease occurs chiefly in areas where veterinary assistance is not readily available and no detailed reports of the efficiency of various forms of treatment have been published. Oxytetracycline has been shown to be highly effective in pigs (3) and sulfadimidine in cattle (4) and the other treatments listed under pneumonic pasteurellosis of cattle should also be effective in this disease. Vaccines have been used for many years to protect cattle during the danger periods but the method was only moderately effective until the recent introduction of a stable vaccine composed of killed organisms in an adjuvant base containing paraffin and lanolin. This vaccine has been highly effective, especially when used prophylactically, although vaccination in the face of an outbreak may also reduce losses (1). Immunity after vaccination appears to be solid for at least 12 months and the only apparent disadvantage is the development of persistent subcutaneous swellings when the vaccine is improperly administered (6). Anaphylactic shock may occur in up to 1 per cent of animals after the injection of some batches of vaccine. A satisfactory dried vaccine is also in use (2).

REFERENCES

(1) Bain, R. V. S. (1963). *Hemorrhagic Septicemia*, p. 78. Rome: F.A.O. Agricultural Studies, No. 62.
(2) Dhanda, M. R. (1960). *Bull. Off. int. Épizoot.*, *53*, 128.
(3) Murty, D. K. & Kaushik, R. K. (1965). *Vet. Rec.*, *77*, 411.
(4) Ilahi, A. & Afzal, H. (1965). *W. Pak. J. Agric. Res. 3*, No. 4, 1–18.
(5) Macadam, I. (1962). *Vet. Rec.*, *74*, 689.
(6) Thomas, J. *et al.* (1969). *Kajian Vet. Malaysia-Singapore*, *2*, 4.
(7) Heddleston, K. L. & Gallagher, J. E. (1969). *Bull. Wildl. Dis. Ass.*, *5*, 206.
(8) Kradel, D. C. *et al.* (1969). *Vet. Med. small Anim. Clin.*, *64*, 145.
(9) Rhoades, K. R. *et al.* (1967). *Canad. J. comp. Med.*, *31*, 226.

Pneumonic Pasteurellosis of Cattle

This form of pasteurellosis in cattle is usually associated with infection by *Past. multocida* Type 2 (or A), or *Past. haemolytica*. It is manifested clinically by acute bronchopneumonia.

Incidence

Pneumonic pasteurellosis is the common form of the disease in cattle in Europe, the U.K, and North America but does not appear to be of any importance in Australasia. The morbidity and mortality rates in young beef cattle approximate 17 per cent and 7·5 per cent respectively (1). In addition to death losses, there is serious loss of production in both beef and dairy cattle and the treatment of sick animals and vaccination of susceptible animals add further to the economic toll of the disease.

Pneumonic pasteurellosis in cattle has a common association with their recent transport and it forms a major part of 'shipping fever' which is an important hazard in the practice of rearing beef cattle on range country and then transporting them long distances to other centres for fattening. Although the disease occurs most commonly in young beef cattle soon after their introduction to feedlots, it is not uncommon in dairy herds, especially when introductions have been made or cattle are returned to their home farms after summer grazing on communal pastures, or exhibition at fairs.

Aetiology

Past. multocida Type 2 (or A) and *Past. haemolytica* have an aetiological association with pneumonic pasteurellosis of cattle but there is some doubt that these bacteria are the primary cause. It is generally believed that a devitalizing influence, either in the form of intercurrent infection, fatigue or other deleterious environmental change, is necessary for the development of the disease. Virus pneumonia is thought to be a common precursor of pneumonic pasteurellosis. The myxovirus para-influenza 3 or SF 4 can be isolated from many cases and although it is not capable of causing authentic cases of pneumonic pasteurellosis (2, 3, 4) its administration in combination with *Past. multocida* and *Past. haemolytica* can do so (5). On the other hand pasteurellosis is an uncommon complication in infectious bovine rhinotracheitis and the experimental introduction of IBR virus with *Past. haemolytica* causes a disease which is not of much greater severity than that caused by either agent alone (6). Among the reasons for doubting the importance of pasteurellae as primary pathogens is the difficulty encounted by many investigators in reproducing the disease with cultures of the organism and the ease with which the organism can be isolated from the upper respiratory tract of normal animals. On the other hand, the presence of large numbers of pasteurellae in the lungs is always associated with the presence of typical bronchopneumonia and affected animals show many more pasteurellae in their nasal mucus than do normal animals (7). Irrespective of the primary cause of pneumonic pasteurellosis there seems to be little doubt that *Past. multocida* and *Past. haemolytica* are capable of bringing cases of pneumonia in cattle to a severe and often fatal termination (8).

Draughty or humid and poorly ventilated barns, exposure to inclement weather, transport, fatigue and starvation are commonly followed by outbreaks of the disease in cattle. The incidence is highest in spring and autumn, particularly the latter, due in part to the extensive movement of livestock and to the sudden changes in weather which occur at these times. An increase in virulence of the infection is often evident after animal passage; at the commencement of an outbreak only those animals which have been subjected to devitalizing influences are affected but the disease may subsequently spread to other animals in the group. There is little tendency for the disease to become an area problem, sporadic outbreaks occurring with the appearance of conditions favourable to the development of the disease.

All age groups of cattle may be affected but animals in the 6 months to 2 years age group are more susceptible than young calves or adults although extensive outbreaks can occur in adults exposed to infected animals.

Transmission

Transmission of pneumonic pasteurellosis occurs by the inhalation of infected droplets coughed up or exhaled by infected animals which may be clinical cases or recovered carriers in which the infection persists in the upper respiratory tract. *Past. multocida* and *Past. haemolytica* are highly susceptible to environmental influences and it is unlikely that mediate contagion is an important factor in the spread of the disease. When conditions are optimum, particularly when cattle are closely confined in damp barns, the disease may spread very quickly and affect a high proportion of the herd within 48 hours, but in animals at pasture, the rate of spread may be much slower.

Pathogenesis

The role of pasteurellae in the aetiology of the disease and their common association with other disease-producing agents has already been discussed. Pneumonic pasteurellosis is a respiratory infection characterized by bronchopneumonia, which may be fibrinous, and pleurisy. Because of the aerogenous route of infection, the pneumonia affects primarily the ventral lobes and causes consolidation. Involvement of the bronchi results in the development of loud râles, and the pleurisy causes severe thoracic pain and the appearance of a pleuritic friction rub. Death occurs as a result of anoxia and toxaemia.

Clinical Findings

There is a sudden onset of high fever (40 to 41°C or 104 to 106°F), depression, anorexia and dyspnoea, with coughing and a slight mucopurulent nasal discharge. Auscultation reveals the presence of bronchopneumonia and pleurisy especially in the anterior and ventral parts of the lungs. If cases are seen in the early stages, there is often only a general increase in the vesicular murmur, but an increase in the rate and depth of respiration will be observed. An ocular discharge and diarrhoea may be present but these signs vary a great deal between outbreaks.

The course in the majority of animals is variable, depending upon the degree of pulmonary involvement, and deaths occur at any time up to 3 weeks after the onset of the disease. The disease responds well to treatment, and even without it some animals recover in 3 to 7 days. On an affected farm calves may be affected but very young calves may die of septicaemia without having shown previous signs of illness.

Clinical Pathology

Nasal swabs taken from clinical cases before treatment often yield an almost pure culture of pasteurellae. A test of the drug-sensitivity of the bacteria should be carried out if possible as considerable variation in resistance to the standard drugs used in treatment is often encountered. Differentiation between *Past. multocida* and *Past. haemolytica* may also be of value in prognosis as infection with the latter is thought to cause a more severe disease.

Haematological examinations are of little value, as a leucocytosis and neutrophilia occur in some animals but in others there may be a neutropenia or no significant change (9).

Necropsy Findings

Pneumonic pasteurellosis is manifested by marked hepatization involving a third or more of the lungs, and most commonly affecting the apical and cardiac lobes. The stage of pneumonia varies from area to area in the lung, commencing with congestion and passing through various stages of hepatization with accumulation of serofibrinous exudate in the interlobar spaces. A catarrhal bronchitis and bronchiolitis, and a serofibrinous pleurisy are usually present and may be accompanied by a fibrinous pericarditis. The pleurisy is characterized by the accumulation of large amounts of effusion. In chronic cases there are residual lesions of bronchopneumonia with overlying pleural adhesions.

Isolation of the organism from the affected lung may be attempted and an impression smear may be of value if a rapid diagnosis is required. Care must be taken that all bipolar-staining organisms are not taken to be pasteurellae. In chronic cases many bacteria other than pasteurellae are commonly found in residual lesions in the lung.

Diagnosis

Pneumonic pasteurellosis of cattle closely resembles contagious bovine pleuropneumonia, both clinically and at necropsy, although the latter disease spreads in plague form through a susceptible population. In young animals, virus pneumonia of calves should be considered in the differential diagnosis of this disease. In the latter, the systemic reaction is usually not so severe, nor the toxaemia so marked, and although there is consolidation of the apical and cardiac lobes, there is a marked absence of moist râles and pleuritic sounds. The response to treatment is also much less marked in the viral disease. Less common causes of acute pneumonia in calves and young cattle include infection with *Klebsiella pneumoniae*, *Streptococcus* spp., and *Sphaerophorus necrophorus*, all of which are characterized by a bronchopneumonia indistinguishable clinically from pneumonic pasteurellosis.

Acute dyspnoea is also characteristic of fog fever and anaphylaxis in cattle but the onset is usually more sudden, the dyspnoea more severe and the lungs more diffusely affected than in pneumonic pasteurellosis. Chronic emphysema and lungworm infestations may resemble chronic pasteurellosis although in the latter, dry, crepitant râles are characteristic and are usually localized to the ventral parts of the lungs.

Infectious bovine rhinotracheitis affects only the

upper respiratory tract except in cases where spread to the lungs occurs secondarily. Bovine malignant catarrh is characterized by involvement of the eyes, mucosal lesions in the mouth, terminal signs of nervous involvement and a high mortality rate. Sporadic bovine encephalomyelitis may closely resemble pneumonic pasteurellosis but the fever is prolonged, there are obvious nervous signs and the response to standard treatments for pasteurellosis is poor.

Treatment

If cases are treated early, the parenteral, or even oral, administration of sodium sulphadimidine gives excellent results. One treatment with a dose rate of 1 g. per 15 lb. body weight is usually sufficient by any route, although severely affected animals or those which relapse are best treated on three successive days with the same dose rate. Injections are usually administered intravenously or intraperitoneally as a 12 per cent or 25 per cent solution. Penicillin is less efficient but streptomycin gives results comparable to those obtained with sodium sulphadimidine and it is often given together with the latter in severe cases. Adequate doses of streptomycin (5 to 10 mg. per lb. body weight) should be used because of the tendency for drug-resistance to develop at low dosage levels. Hyperimmune serum is of little value in treatment (10).

Parenteral or oral treatment with any of the tetracyclines or chloramphenicol also gives excellent results, especially if treatment is continued for 3 days in stubborn cases. The dose rate of all these drugs by parenteral injection is 2 mg. per lb. body weight, the tetracyclines being administered by any route, chloramphenicol only by intramuscular injection (8). General supportive treatment as outlined in the treatment of pneumonia should also be implemented.

Control

Vaccines consisting of killed organisms (bacterins) are extensively used in the control of pneumonic pasteurellosis in all species but most reports suggest that their efficiency is very limited (9, 11, 12). Hyperimmune serum is similarly ineffective. One of the possible reasons for this inefficiency is that the vaccine or serum may not have been prepared from the serotype of the organism which is prevalent. In North America, Past. multocida Type A and Past. haemolytica are most commonly encountered in pneumonic pasteurellosis and logically, biological preparations used in the area should be prepared from these types. The benefits of a vaccine prepared from local strains of pasteurellae have been well shown in Kenya (13) where a concentrated, formalinized vaccine prepared from highly virulent strains confers an immunity of very high order in cattle. A high incidence of anaphylactic shock has been observed after vaccination and the administration of antiserum against pasteurellosis in cattle. Adrenaline and antihistamines are effective antidotes provided they can be administered *promptly*. This is often impossible to arrange and mortalities can be high. The use of alum-precipitated or other adjuvant vaccines would reduce this loss. In buffaloes an avianized *P. multocida* vaccine has been used with good effect (20).

As a result of the suspected association between respiratory viruses and pasteurellae in the development of the disease, vaccination against the viral infections has been recommended. In general such vaccines have not been satisfactory on their own but their use in combination with pasteurella vaccines does appear to have a beneficial effect (14).

Because of the common occurrence of pneumonic pasteurellosis at the time of shipment from range to fattening areas, much attention has been given to reducing the incidence of the disease at this time. Vaccination of cattle before shipment with a vaccine prepared from a bovine parainfluenza virus does not prevent the occurrence of pneumonic pasteurellosis (15). Vaccination with bacterins containing pasteurellae before shipping or with serum afterwards has not been successful but prophylactic injections of penicillin are widely used. The feeding of antibiotics at the fattening unit is recommended. Oxytetracycline fed at the rate of 1 to 2 mg. per lb. body weight per day for 3 to 5 days after arrival considerably reduced the incidence of the disease and the mortality rate in one trial (16).

Cattle should be on dry feed for at least 12 hours before loading. Reduction of trauma and exhaustion at shipment has been considered a desirable objective in controlling the disease. Tranquillizing drugs have been used to this end and they may have some place as a preventive if given before shipment (17, 18). Careful loading and transport are important and direct shipment without passing through sale or trucking yards is usually safest. On arrival the cattle should be housed in dry, sheltered quarters and should not be disturbed unnecessarily for the first 2 to 3 weeks in their new environment. The procedures recommended for getting cattle on feed will vary with their condition and the stress to which they have been subjected. As a general rule it is advisable to limit their roughage to predominantly grass hay for the first three weeks.

After the first 48 hours small amounts (up to 2 lb. for calves or 4 lb. for yearlings) of bulky concentrate can be provided as a starter ration. At the end of the first week, a small proportion of the regular fattening ration can be incorporated in the starter and this proportion can be gradually increased until the cattle are on full feed after about three weeks in the feedlot. The animals should be inspected frequently and any which show signs of illness should be immediately removed from the group and treated.

In general the prophylaxis of pneumonic pasteurellosis is unsatisfactory. The administration of sulphonamides and antibiotics, the provision of vitamin A and tranquillizers and careful handling and feeding may exert some influence on the incidence and severity of the disease but these measures, together with the use of vaccines and antisera, are not capable of providing a guaranteed level of protection in many circumstances (1). One of the greatest needs of the beef cattle industry in North America is the development of a cheap and satisfactory immunizing procedure against pneumonic pasteurellosis. The development of such a procedure is necessary before 'preconditioning' can develop its full potential. At present some ranchers market calves which have been conditioned to withstand the stresses of shipping and adjustment to the feedlot (19). The programme includes weaning at least three weeks before shipment, adjusting to dry feed and vaccinating against common diseases. The low antigenicity of the available pasteurella, viral and chlamydial vaccines requires that 2 injections be given, one 2 weeks and one 4 weeks before shipping. Obviously such a programme requires a significant price premium and this is the main deterrent to its general acceptance.

REFERENCES

(1) Schipper, I. A. (1963). *Vet. Med.*, *58*, 731.
(2) Carter, G. R. & Rowsell, H. C. (1958). *J. Amer. vet. med. Ass.*, *132*, 187.
(3) Heddleston, K. L. *et al.* (1962). *Amer. J. vet. Res.*, *23*, 548.
(4) Gale, C. & King, N. B. (1961). *J. Amer. vet. med. Ass.*, *138*, 235.
(5) Baldwin, D. E. *et al.* (1967). *Amer. J. vet. Res.*, *28*, 1773.
(6) Collier, J. R. *et al.* (1960). *Amer. J. vet. Res.*, *21*, 195.
(7) Thompson, R. G. *et al.* (1969). *Canad. J. comp. Med.*, *33*, 194.
(8) Collier, J. R. *et al.* (1962). *J. Amer. vet. med. Ass.*, *140*, 807.
(9) Hoerlein, A. B. & Marsh, C. L. (1957). *J. Amer. vet. med. Ass.*, *131*, 123.
(10) Kheng, C. S. & Phay, C. P. (1963). *Vet. Rec.*, *75*, 155.
(11) King, N. B. *et al.* (1958). *Vet. Med.*, *53*, 67.
(12) Rice, C. E. *et al.* (1955). *Canad. J. comp. Med.*, *19*, 329.
(13) Shirlaw, J. F. (1957). *Brit. vet. J.*, *113*, 35 & 71.
(14) Hamdy, A. H. & Trapp, A. L. (1964). *Amer. J. vet. Res.*, *25*, 1648.
(15) Woods, G. T. *et al.* (1961). *J. Amer. vet. med. Ass.*, *139*, 1208.
(16) Hawley, G. E. (1957). *Vet. Med.*, *52*, 481.
(17) Hoerlein, A. B. & Marsh, C. L. (1957). *J. Amer. vet. med. Ass.*, *131*, 227.
(18) Foley, E. J. *et al.* (1958). *Vet. Med.*, *53*, 515.
(19) Pierson, R. E. (1968). *J. Amer. vet. med. Ass.*, *152*, 920.
(20) Cerrutti, C. *et al.* (1968). *Clin. vet. (Milano)*, *91*, 71.

Pasteurellosis of Swine, Sheep and Goats

Pasteurellosis of swine, sheep and goats is usually pneumonic in form although a septicaemic form is not uncommon in lambs.

Incidence

Pasteurellosis causes heavy losses in pigs and sheep in most parts of the world, both through deaths and depression of body weight gains. Morbidity and mortality rates up to 40 per cent and 5 per cent respectively are usual in both species. In sheep at pasture, the disease tends to spread slowly and the morbidity rate is lower than in feeder lambs and pigs maintained in small areas. Death losses in feeder lambs are usually of the order of 5 per cent (1), but may be as high as 20 per cent (2). A mortality rate of 20 per cent has been recorded in goats kept in confined quarters after collection from a number of centres (3).

Aetiology

Pasteurellosis in swine is usually a complication of enzootic pneumonia of pigs, *Past. multocida* (Types A and D) acting as a secondary invader. *Past. multocida* (Type B) is a common pathogen in cattle but has been isolated only rarely in pigs (10). This infection causes haemorrhagic septicaemia rather than pneumonia.

The position in sheep is not so well-defined. An enzootic pneumonia is common and may be a frequent precursor of pasteurellosis but the evidence indicates that *Past. haemolytica* is often the primary cause of the disease in this species (4, 5). The significance of the pleuropneumonia-like organism (*Mycoplasma hyorhinis*) which is so often also present in pigs is undetermined but it is thought to have low pathogenicity (10). An attempt has been made to differentiate between strains of *Past. haemolytica* isolated from outbreaks of septicaemic pasteurellosis in lambs. On the basis of pathogenicity and antigenicity two biotypes have been identified; Type A is usually associated with enzootic pneumonia and septicaemia in very young lambs and Type T with septicaemia in older lambs (5). These biotypes differ in their geographical distribution and thus cause variations in the patterns of disease encountered (14). Very young lambs and goats are much more susceptible to *Past. haemolytica* than adults and the organism is presumed to be a primary pathogen in kids (12). *P. multocida* is an uncommon pathogen in sheep (17), and attempts to implicate *Myxovirus parainfluenza 3* as a contributing causative agent have not been successful (16).

Deleterious changes in environment, similar to those which are thought to precipitate the disease in cattle, also appear to be important in the species under discussion. Draughty or poorly ventilated barns, exposure to bad weather, transport and malnutrition are often associated with severe outbreaks of the disease. In range sheep, confinement for shearing, mating or supplementary feeding may precipitate an outbreak, and severe parasitism may also increase susceptibility.

Transmission

As in pneumonic pasteurellosis of cattle, transmission occurs probably by the inhalation or ingestion of infected material, the infection deriving from carrier animals and clinical cases rather than inanimate objects. Another method of spread of the disease is by lambs sucking ewes with mastitis caused by *Past. haemolytica*. The reverse can also happen.

Pathogenesis

The development of pasteurellosis in swine, sheep and goats is in general the same as in pneumonic pasteurellosis of cattle. An acute fibrinous bronchopneumonia is accompanied by pleurisy. An acute septicaemia occurs less commonly. Caseous lymphadenitis caused by *Past. multocida* has also been observed in lambs.

Clinical Findings

Pigs. An acute bronchopneumonia, accompanied by fever and toxaemia, causes a clinical syndrome similar to that of pneumonic pasteurellosis. There is a marked tendency for the disease to become chronic resulting in reduced weight gains and frequent relapses. A more acute disease with death occurring within 12 hours and without signs of pneumonia has been observed in baby pigs (11).

Sheep and goats. In these animals, outbreaks often commence with sudden deaths in the absence of premonitory clinical signs. In groups of lambs this occurrence of sudden death without prior illness may continue throughout the outbreak (8), but in older sheep some will show signs of respiratory embarrassment which can be accentuated by driving. As the outbreak progresses, respiratory involvement becomes more evident, signs including dyspnoea, slight frothing at the mouth, cough and nasal discharge (4, 6). Death may occur as soon as 12 hours after the first signs of illness but the course in most cases is about three days. In cases produced experimentally, arthritis, pericarditis and meningitis occur in lambs that survive the acute stages of the disease but these are not often observed in natural cases.

Clinical Pathology and Necropsy Findings

The organism can be found in very large numbers in nasal mucus and in one area a bimodal curve of nasal carriage of *P. haemolytica* in sheep has been observed with the peaks of the carrier rates in spring and autumn coinciding with the seasonal peaks of enzootic pneumonia in the area (15).

In general the findings in pneumonic pasteurellosis of cattle apply here also, except that the pleurisy in sheep is not accompanied by the effusion that occurs commonly in cattle. In lambs dying of septicaemia, pulmonary lesions may be confined to haemorrhage, oedema and congestion. Ulcerative lesions on the pharynx and larynx are common (8).

Diagnosis

Enzootic pneumonia of pigs, unless accompanied by pasteurellosis, is not manifested by a marked systemic or pulmonary involvement. Dyspnoea is a prominent sign in Glasser's disease, but there is obvious arthritis, and at necropsy the disease is characterized by arthritis, a general serositis and meningitis. The septicaemic and acute enteric forms of salmonellosis in swine are often accompanied by pulmonary involvement but these usually are overshadowed by signs of septicaemia or enteritis. Chronic pasteurellosis has to be differentiated from lungworm infestations and ascariasis.

The common enzootic pneumonia of sheep is of minor clinical importance but it may be accompanied by a secondary bacterial pneumonia which may be caused by *Past. haemolytica* or *Corynebacterium pyogenes*. Parasitic pneumonia, jaagsiekte and maedi are the common chronic pneumonias of sheep, but these should not be confused with pasteurellosis because of their longer course. When deaths occur in lambs without prior clinical illness the disease may be mistaken for septicaemia caused by *Haemophilus agni*, especially because of the necropsy findings, but in pasteurellosis the rate of spread in the flock is much slower and the flock mortality rate much less.

Treatment

The treatments prescribed for pneumonic pasteurellosis of cattle are used with similar results in swine, sheep and goats. Penicillin has also been described as a successful treatment in goats (6).

Control

The general recommendations for the control of the disease in cattle apply equally in these species. The use of a formalin-killed vaccine to prevent the disease in sheep is only partly effective. The mortality rate in lambs is reduced by two vaccinations at 2 and 5 weeks of age but the incidence of pneumonia is unaffected (3, 7, 9, 14). An autogenous vaccine may offer some advantage (18). Vaccination in swine has had limited success but the use of a concentrated, adjuvant-type vaccine as recommended for cattle may be advantageous.

REFERENCES

(1) Biberstein, E. L. & Kennedy, P. C. (1959). *Amer. J. vet. Res.*, *20*, 94.
(2) Stamp, J. T. *et al.* (1955). *J. comp. Path.*, *65*, 183.
(3) Jirina, K. (1953). *Mh. Vet.-Med.*, *8*, 271, cited in (1953). *Vet. Bull.*, *23*, 533.
(4) Smith, G. R. (1964). *J. comp. Path.*, *64*, 241.
(5) Biberstein, E. L. *et al.* (1967). *J. comp. Path.*, *77*, 181.
(6) Borgman, R. F. & Wilson, C. E. (1955). *J. Amer. vet. med. Ass.*, *126*, 198.
(7) Dolder, W. & Leuenberger, M. (1948). *Schweiz. Arch. Tierheilk.*, *90*, 656.
(8) Biberstein, E. L. *et al.* (1959). *J. Amer. vet. med. Ass.*, *135*, 61.
(9) Hamdy, A. H. *et al.* (1963). *J. Amer. vet. med. Ass.*, *142*, 379.
(10) L'Ecuyer, C. *et al.* (1961). *Amer. J. vet. Res.*, *22*, 1020.
(11) Edwards, B. L. (1959). *Vet. Rec.*, *71*, 208.
(12) Gourlay, R. V. & Barber, L. (1960). *J. comp. Path.*, *70*, 211.
(13) Murty, D. K. & Kaushik, R. K. (1965). *Vet. Rec.*, *77*, 411.
(14) Stevenson, R. G. (1969). *Vet. Bull.*, *39*, 747.
(15) Biberstein, E. L. *et al.* (1970). *J. comp. Path.*, *80*, 499.
(16) Biberstein, E. L. *et al.* (1971). *J. comp. Path.*, *81*, 339.
(17) Palit, N. & Rao, C. C. P. (1969). *Ind. vet. J.*, *46*, 459.
(18) van der Veen, R. R. & Zumpt, I. F. (1967). *J. S. Afr. vet. med. Ass.*, *38*, 415.

Tularaemia

Tularaemia is a highly contagious disease of rodents which may spread to farm animals, causing a severe septicaemia and a high mortality rate.

Incidence

Tularaemia in animals has been recorded in the U.S.A., Canada, Russia, Austria, Scandinavia and Japan. In North America the disease is most prevalent in farm animals in the north-western states of the U.S.A. and the adjoining areas of Canada. The morbidity rate in affected flocks of sheep is usually about 20 per cent but may be as high as 40 per cent and the mortality rate may reach 50 per cent especially in young animals. Man is highly susceptible and the disease is an occupational hazard to workers in the sheep industry in areas where the disease occurs. Serological surveys in this group have indicated a high incidence of positive reactors (1). Spread of the disease to man may also occur in abattoir workers who handle infected sheep carcases.

Aetiology

Past. (*Francisella*) *tularensis* is the causative organism. It is a Gram-negative organism which does not form spores, and gives partial cross-agglutination with *Brucella* spp. The organism persists for long periods in mud and water and may proliferate in these media (2). It does not appear to survive in carcases for more than 24 hours (10) unless they are frozen when persistence for 60 to 120 days has been recorded (3). The natural hosts are rodents but almost all animals and birds are susceptible (4), the disease being recorded among farm animals, most commonly in sheep and pigs and to a lesser extent in calves. Sheep and pigs of all ages are susceptible but most losses occur in lambs, and in swine clinical illness occurs only in piglets (6). There is a sharp seasonal incidence, the bulk of cases occurring during the spring months.

Transmission

Past. tularensis has remarkable invasive powers and infection in man can occur through the unbroken skin. In sheep, transmission occurs chiefly by the bites of the wood tick, *Dermacentor andersoni*, although the organism has also been isolated from the tick, *Haemaphysalis otophila*, the ticks becoming infected in the early part of their life cycle when they feed on rodents. The adult ticks infest sheep, and pastures bearing low shrubs and brush are particularly favourable to infestation. The ticks are found in greatest numbers on the sheep around the base of the ears, the top of the neck, the throat, axillae and udder. It is assumed that sheep are relatively resistant to tularaemia but become clinically affected when the infection is massive and continuous. Transmission to pigs and horses is thought to occur chiefly by tick bites.

The causative organism persists in mud and water for at least 16 months (2) and this may be the reason for the high incidence in such rodents as beaver and muskrat.

Pathogenesis

Tularaemia is an acute septicaemia but localization occurs, mainly in the parenchymatous organs, with the production of granulomatous lesions.

Clinical Findings

Sheep. The incubation period has not been determined. A heavy tick infestation is usually evident. The onset of the disease is slow with a gradually increasing stiffness of gait, dorsiflexion of the head and a hunching of the hind quarters, and affected animals lag behind the group. The pulse and respiratory rates are increased, the temperature is elevated up to 42°C (107°F) and a cough may develop. There is diarrhoea, the faeces being dark and foetid, and urination occurs frequently with the passage of small amounts of urine. Body weight is lost rapidly, and progressive weakness and recumbency develop after several days, but there is no evidence of paralysis, the animal continuing to struggle while down. Death occurs usually within a few days but a fatal course may be as long as 2 weeks. Animals that recover commonly shed part or all of the fleece but are solidly immune for long periods.

Swine. The disease is latent in adult pigs but young piglets show fever up to 42°C (107°F), accompanied by depression, profuse sweating and dyspnoea. The course of the disease is about 7 to 10 days.

Horses. In horses fever (up to 42°C or 107°F) and stiffness and oedema of the limbs occur. Foals are more seriously affected and may show dyspnoea and inco-ordination in addition to the above signs (5).

Clinical Pathology

An agglutination test is available for the diagnosis of tularaemia, a titre of 1:50 being regarded as a positive test in swine. Serum from pigs affected with brucellosis does not agglutinate tularaemia antigen but serum from pigs affected with tularaemia agglutinates brucellosis antigen. Cross-agglutination between *Past. tularensis* and *Brucella abortus* is less common in sheep and an accurate diagnosis can be made on serological grounds because of the much greater agglutination which occurs with the homologous organism. Titres of agglutinins in affected sheep range from 1:640 to 1:5000 and may persist at levels of 1:320 for up to 7 months. A titre of 1:200 is classed as positive in sheep. In horses the titres revert to normal levels in 14 to 21 days (5).

An intradermal sensitivity test using 'tularin' is suggested as being more reliable as a diagnostic aid in pigs than the agglutination test but is unreliable in sheep (6).

Necropsy Findings

Great care should be exercised when a necropsy examination is made of a suspected case because of the danger of human infection. In sheep, large numbers of ticks may be present on the hides of fresh carcases. In animals that have been dead for some time, dark red areas of congestion up to 3 cm. in diameter are found on the underneath surface of the skin and may be accompanied by local swelling or necrosis of tissues. These lesions mark the attachment sites of ticks. Enlargement and congestion of the lymph nodes draining the sites of heaviest tick infestation are often noted. Congestion and hepatization of the lung and severe pulmonary oedema are inconstant findings.

In swine the characteristic lesions are pleurisy, pneumonia and abscessation of submaxillary and parotid lymph nodes. The organisms can be isolated from lymph nodes and spleen and from infected ticks. Isolation can also be effected by experimental transmission to guinea pigs which are highly susceptible.

Diagnosis

The occurrence of a highly fatal septicaemia in sheep during spring months when the sheep are heavily infested with *Dermacentor andersoni* should suggest the possibility of tularaemia, especially if the outbreak occurs in an enzootic area. Tick paralysis, which commonly occurs in the same area, and at the same time of the year as tularaemia, is not accompanied by fever and there is marked flaccid paralysis. Recovery from tick paralysis occurs commonly if the ticks are removed. Other septicaemias of sheep in the age group in which tularaemia occurs are unusual. *Past. haemolytica*, *E. coli* and *H. agni* may cause fatal septicaemia without diagnostic lesions in very young lambs but these diseases are not associated with heavy tick infestations. Tick-borne fever has a limited and different geographical distribution and rickettsiae can be detected in the lymphocytes.

Treatment

Streptomycin, the tetracyclines and chloramphenicol are effective treatments in man. Oxytetracycline (3 to 5 mg. per lb. body weight) has been highly effective in the treatment of lambs and much more effective than penicillin and streptomycin (7).

Control

An outbreak of tularaemia in sheep can be rapidly halted by spraying or dipping with Gammexane or DDT preparations to kill the vector ticks. In areas where ticks are enzootic, sheep should be kept away from shrubby, infested pasture or sprayed regularly during the months when the tick population is greatest.

REFERENCES

(1) Jellison, W. L. & Kohls, G. M. (1955). *Publ. Hlth monogr.*, 28, 17.
(2) Parker, R. R. *et al.* (1951). *Natn. Inst. Hlth Bull.*, 193, 61.
(3) Airapetyan, V. G. *et al.* (1957). *J. Microbiol. Epidem. Immunobiol.*, 28, 21.
(4) McKeever, S. *et al.* (1958). *J. infect. Dis.*, 103, 120.
(5) Klaus, K. D. *et al.* (1959). *J. Bact.*, 78, 294.
(6) Airapetyan, V. G. *et al.* (1959). Cited in *Vet. Bull.*, 29, 420.
(7) Frank, F. W. & Meinershagen, W. A. (1961). *Vet. Med.*, 56, 374.

DISEASES CAUSED BY *BRUCELLA* Spp.

The important diseases of animals caused by *Brucella* spp. are those caused by *Br. abortus*, *suis* and *melitensis*, their host preference in order being cattle, swine and sheep and goats. Although brucella organisms have a wide host range, they are not readily transmitted from preferential to dissimilar hosts and, when this occurs, they usually localize in the mammary gland and reticuloendothelial system rather than in the uterus and foetal membranes (3). *Bordetella bronchiseptica* is not uncommonly present in the lungs of calves and pigs with chronic pneumonia. This organism is also suspected of being a primary cause of pneumonia in baby pigs (1, 2). In affected herds the incidence may be as high as 100 per cent and signs and necropsy lesions characteristic of pneumonia are observed. The pulmonary lesions are scattered areas of bronchopneumonia different in their appearance and distribution from those of enzootic pneumonia. Treatment with tetracyclines, chloramphenicol or sulphonamides is recommended. The disease is likely to persist on the premises, recurring in successive crops of baby pigs. In these circumstances the use of an autogenous bacterin in the pregnant sows is recommended.

REFERENCES

(1) L'Ecuyer, C. *et al.* (1961). *Vet. Med.*, 56, 420.
(2) Dunne, H. W. *et al.* (1961). *J. Amer. vet. med. Ass.*, 139, 897.
(3) Meyer, M. E. (1964). *Amer. J. vet. Res.*, 25, 553.

Brucellosis Caused by *Brucella abortus*

(*Bang's Disease*)

The disease of cattle caused by infection with *Br. abortus* is characterized by abortion late in pregnancy and a subsequent high rate of infertility.

Incidence

Brucellosis is widespread and of major economic importance in most countries of the world, particularly amongst dairy cattle. The incidence varies considerably between herds, between areas, and between countries, and details of the percentage of animals affected are of little value for this reason. An incidence of 15 per cent to 50 per cent in infected herds has been recorded in the United Kingdom and European countries and 16 per cent in the U.S.A. but in recent years the prevalence of the disease has been greatly reduced.

From the viewpoint of human health, the disease is important because the causative organism can cause undulant fever in man. The possibility of infection occurring by the drinking of infected milk necessitates the pasteurization of milk. However, most cases in humans are occupational and occur in farmers, veterinarians and butchers. The organism can be isolated from many organs other than the udder and uterus, and the handling of a carcase of an infected animal may represent severe exposure. The importance of the disease in humans is an important justification for its eradication.

Losses in animal production due to this disease can be of major importance, primarily because of the decreased milk production by aborting cows. This has been estimated in England to be in the region of £16 million per year (1). The common sequel of infertility increases the period between lactations and in an infected herd the average intercalving period may be prolonged by several months. In addition to the loss of milk production, there is the loss of calves and interference with the breeding programme. This is of greatest importance in beef herds where the calves represent the sole source of income. A high incidence of temporary and permanent infertility results in heavy culling of valuable cows and some deaths occur as a result of acute metritis following retention of the placenta.

Aetiology

Infections with *Br. abortus* have been recorded in most species but occur commonly only in cattle. Infection occurs in cattle of all ages but persists only in sexually mature animals. The organism can be recovered from naturally infected pigs and, although not normally pathogenic in this species, may occasionally cause abortion. The disease is not uncommon in sheep (2), usually in association with infected cattle, a fact with significant implications for brucellosis eradication (3). In horses the organism is often found in chronic bursal enlargements but is probably present as a secondary invader rather than a primary pathogen. It is commonly present with *Actinomyces bovis* in fistulous withers and poll evil.

A high incidence has been recorded in bison and elk (7), and the probability is that the disease occurs in other wild ruminants. Occasional cases occur in dogs which remain positive to the serum agglutination tests for periods exceeding one year. Their significance in the spread of brucellosis is not known (8).

Naturally infected animals and those vaccinated as adults remain positive to the serum, and other agglutination tests for long periods. Most animals vaccinated between 4 and 8 months of age return to a negative status to the test within a year. All are considered to have a relative immunity to infection. Calves from cows which are positive reactors to the test are passively immunized via the colostrum. It is possible that some calves remain immune for sufficiently long to interfere with vaccination (9).

Transmission

Br. abortus achieves its greatest concentration in the contents of the pregnant uterus, the foetus and the foetal membranes, and these must be considered as the major source of infection. The methods by which the disease is transmitted are ingestion, penetration of the intact skin and conjunctiva and contamination of the udder during milking.

Ingestion of pasture or other feedstuffs contaminated by discharges from infected cows is by far the commonest method of spread. Infected horses, especially those with fistulous withers and hygromata, may contaminate pasture by the excretion of organisms in discharges or in the faeces. In most cases, contamination is direct and, although the possibility of introduction of infection by flies, dogs, rats, ticks, infected boots, fodder and other inanimate objects exists, it is not considered to be of great importance in relation to control measures. The organism can survive on grass for variable periods depending on environmental conditions. In temperate climates, infectivity may persist for 100 days in winter and 30 days in summer. The organism is susceptible to heat, sunlight and standard disinfectants but freezing permits almost indefinite survival. In average circumstances pasture, static water and buildings should be rested for three months unless adequate disinfection of the latter is possible (10).

A cow's tail heavily contaminated with infected uterine discharges may spread infection if it comes into contact with the conjunctiva or the intact skin of other animals. In the same way as the more common forms of mastitis can be spread during milking, *Br. abortus* infection can be spread from a cow whose milk contains the organism to an uninfected cow. This may have little significance in terms of causing abortion, but it is of particular importance in its effects on agglutination tests on milk and the presence of the organism in milk used for human consumption.

Bulls do not transmit infection from infected to non-infected cows mechanically. Bulls that are themselves infected and discharge semen containing organisms are most unlikely to transmit the disease but the chance of spread from the bull is very great if the semen is used for artificial insemination (11). Some infected bulls give negative blood agglutination tests and can only be detected by the isolation of organisms from the semen or agglutination tests on seminal plasma. Excretion of *Br. abortus* in the semen of a stallion has also been observed (12).

So few infected cows ever recover completely that it is safest to consider them all as permanent carriers of infection whether or not abortion actually occurs. Excretion of the organism in the milk is usually intermittent but appears to be more common during late lactation and can continue for several years. In cattle vaccinated before infection the degree of excretion of *Br. abortus* in the milk is less than in non-vaccinated animals.

Pathogenesis

Br. abortus has a predilection for the pregnant uterus, udder, testicle and accessory male sex glands, lymph nodes, joint capsules and bursae. After the initial invasion of the body, localization occurs initially in the lymph nodes draining the area and spreads to other lymphoid tissues including the spleen and the mammary and iliac lymph nodes. In calves, infection may persist in the lymph nodes for a short while but is not usually permanent as localization does not occur in the immature udder and uterus. In the adult, non-pregnant cow, localization occurs in the udder, and the uterus, if it becomes gravid, is infected from periodic bacteraemic phases originating in the udder. Infected udders are clinically normal but they are important as a source of reinfection of the uterus, as a source of infection for calves or humans drinking the milk and because they are the basis for the agglutination tests on milk and whey. Erythritol, a substance produced by the foetus and capable of stimulating the growth of *Br. abortus*, occurs naturally in greatest concentration in the placenta and foetal fluids and is probably responsible for localization of the infection in these tissues.

When invasion of the gravid uterus occurs the initial lesion is in the wall of the uterus but spread to the lumen of the uterus soon follows, leading to a severe ulcerative endometritis of the intercotyledonary spaces. The allanto-chorion, foetal fluids and placental cotyledons are next invaded and the villi destroyed. Abortion occurs principally in the last three months of pregnancy, the incubation period being inversely proportional to the stage of development of the foetus at the time of infection.

Clinical Findings

Abortion after the fifth month of pregnancy is the cardinal clinical feature of the disease. In subsequent pregnancies the foetus is usually carried to full term although second or even third abortions may occur in the same cow. Retention of the placenta and metritis are common sequelae to abortion. Mixed infections are usually the cause of the metritis which may be acute, with septicaemia and death following, or chronic, leading to sterility.

In the bull, orchitis and epididymitis occur occasionally. One or both scrotal sacs may be affected with acute, painful swelling to twice normal size, although the testes may not be grossly enlarged. The swelling persists for a considerable time and the testis undergoes liquefaction necrosis and is eventually destroyed. The seminal vesicles may be affected and their enlargement can be detected on rectal palpation. Affected bulls are usually sterile when the orchitis is acute but may regain normal fertility if one testicle is undamaged. Such bulls are potential spreaders of the disease if they are used for artificial insemination.

Br. abortus can often be isolated from lesions of non-suppurative synovitis in cattle. Hygromatous swellings, especially of the knees, should be viewed with suspicion.

The history of the disease in a susceptible herd can usually be traced to the introduction of an infected cow. Less common sources are infected bulls or horses with fistulous withers. In the past in such a susceptible herd it was common for the infection to spread rapidly and for an abortion 'storm' to occur. The 'storm' might last for a year or more, at the end of which time most of the susceptible cows were infected and had aborted and proceeded to carry their calves to full term. Retained placentae and metritis could be expected to be common at this time. As the abortion rate subsided, the stage of 'herd resistance', in which abortion was largely restricted to first-calf heifers and introductions, followed, and might continue indefinitely. In recent years, particularly in areas where vaccination is extensively practised, there has been a tendency for the development of a more insidious form of the disease which spreads much more slowly and in which abortion is much less common.

In horses, the common association of Br. abortus is with chronic bursal enlargements of the neck and withers, but it has also been identified as a cause of abortion in a mare (4). When horses are run with infected cattle, a relatively high proportion can become infected and develop a positive reaction to the serum agglutination test. Some horses appear to suffer a generalized infection with clinical signs including general stiffness, fluctuating temperature and lethargy (6, 5).

Clinical Pathology

Laboratory tests used in the diagnosis of brucellosis include isolation of the organism, and tests for the presence of Br. abortus agglutinins in blood serum, milk, whey, vaginal mucus and seminal plasma.

Isolation of the organism by culture or guinea pig inoculation is most easily effected from the abomasum or lungs of the aborted foetus or from the placenta. If neither are available, a sample of uterine exudate may be of value because the organism is present for some time after calving. Stained smears made from placental attachments often show large numbers of brucellae and are used to make presumptive diagnoses. Isolation from milk or semen is usually attempted only in special circumstances.

Serological tests based on the detection of Br. abortus agglutinins in both blood serum and milk are available. They have been exhaustively reviewed and only the salient features are presented here (13, 14). The use of the Milk Ring Test on bulk milk samples is recommended as a screening test to select infected herds. The serum agglutination test is recommended for detecting individually affected animals but the standards used for interpretation of test need to be accurately defined in terms of the circumstances. Where problem cows or herds are identified because of low titres, or because of the probable presence of chronic carriers of Br. abortus infection or because Strain 19 vaccination has been used on adults, other supplementary tests should be used. One of these is the heat inactivation test (15) but the choice of tests is wide and the selection should be left to the laboratory. The alternative procedure of increasing the severity of judgements with the serum agglutination test results in the culling of an unnecessarily large number of cattle. The recommended criteria for use in the tube agglutination test have been specified (16). Animals with a *Brucella abortus* antibody titre of less than 30 I.U. will pass. Those with a titre of more than 67 I.U. will fail. Animals between these titres will be classed as 'inconclusive'.

Although the general recommendation is made that a standard test be used initially and supplementary tests included when problems arise there is support for the use of two tests, e.g. tube agglutination and complement fixation tests (17) from the beginning. The tests available are (13):

(*a*) On blood serum: Tube (Slow) Agglutination, Plate (Rapid) Agglutination, Complement Fixation, Heat Inactivation, Acid Plate Agglutination, Mercapto-Ethanol, Rivanol (or Acridine Dye), Blocking Antibody, Coombs, Fluorescent Antibody, Castaneda or Surface Fixation, Precipitin or Gel Diffusion Tests.

(*b*) Milk tests (18) include: Milk Ring Test (19), Whole Milk Plate Agglutination, Whey Tube Agglutination, Whey Plate (21), Coombs, and Whey Complement fixation (20) tests.

(*c*) Agglutination test on vaginal mucus, seminal plasma.

(*d*) Culture of vaginal mucus, semen, milk, aborted conceptus.

Clarification of the infection status of animals giving inconclusive or false positive reactions is of importance if valuable animals are to be retained, and in the closing stages of an eradication programme when the incidence of such reactors is likely to be relatively much higher than in the early stages. Although, as stated earlier, the decision on how to handle this situation must be made by the controlling authority, a combination of vaginal mucus agglutination and whey agglutination and milk culture is an efficient one. It has also been suggested that a cheaper, more rapid test could be used as a screening test on serum, e.g. Rose Bengal Plate Agglutination Test, sera reacting to the test going to one of the more selective tests, e.g. complement fixation test (21).

An alternative procedure which may have application where adult vaccination is practised, is the use of 42/50 vaccine to produce a reaction to the Coombs Antibovine Globulin Test, the degree of the anamnestic serological response being used to determine infected versus non-infected status (22).

Necropsy Findings

Necropsy findings in adults are of no importance in diagnosis. In some foetuses, a primary pneumonia is found. The placenta is usually oedematous, there may be leathery plaques on the external surface of the chorion and there is necrosis of the cotyledons.

Diagnosis

The diagnosis of the cause of abortion in a single animal or in a group of cattle is difficult because of the multiplicity of causes which may be involved. When an abortion problem is under investigation, the following procedure is recommended. Ascertain the age of the foetus by inspection and from the breeding records; take blood samples for serological tests for brucellosis, vibriosis, listeriosis and leptospirosis; examine uterine fluids and the contents of the foetal abomasum at the earliest opportunity for trichomonads, and subsequently by cultural methods for brucellae, vibrios, trichomonads, listeria and fungi; supplement these tests by cultural examination of foetal lungs for leptospirae, and of the placenta or uterine fluid for bacteria and fungi, especially if the foetus is not available; examine placenta fixed in formalin for evidence of placentitis. It is most important that all examinations be carried out in all cases as coincident infections with more than one agent are not uncommon.

In the early stages of the investigation, the herd history may be of value in suggesting the possible aetiological agent. For example, in brucellosis, abortion at 6 months or later is the major complaint, whereas in trichomoniasis and vibriosis, failure to conceive and prolongation of the dioestral period is the usual history. A summary of the differential diagnosis of contagious abortion in cattle is provided in the table on p. 374. Of special interest is the epizootic viral bovine abortion observed in California (23), Germany and Israel (24). The disease occurs at a very high level of incidence but only in cattle introduced to a certain area; resident cattle are unaffected. Cattle returned to the area each winter are unaffected after the first abortion. The cows are unaffected systemically. Aborted foetuses show characteristic multiple petechiae in the skin, conjunctiva and mucosae, enlargement of lymph nodes, anasarca and nodular involvement of the liver. A chlamydia has been isolated which reproduces the disease on experimental inoculation (23, 26, 25). It is thought that the geographical distribution of the disease is limited by the habitat of an as yet unidentified insect vector.

In most countries where brucellosis is well under control and artificial insemination limits the spread of vibriosis and trichomoniasis, leptospirosis may be the commonest cause of abortion in cattle. However, surveys in such countries reveal the disquieting fact that in about two-thirds of the abortions which occur no causative agent is detected. Currently under review as causes of abortion in cattle are the viruses of infectious bovine rhinotracheitis and mucosal disease and others (27).

Treatment

Treatment is not usually undertaken. Trials using bovine plasma, sulphadiazine, streptomycin and chlortetracycline given parenterally, and the latter two as udder infusions, have been unsuccessful in eliminating the infection. Horses with fistulous withers and positive serum agglutination tests are commonly treated by vaccination with *Br. abortus* Strain 19. Three injections of the vaccine are given with 10 days between injections. In the U.K. an equine brucellosis vaccine is used for this purpose (5).

Control

The control of bovine brucellosis is based on hygiene, vaccination and test and disposal of reactors. All three are of importance and neglect of any one may make the task of eradication very much more difficult. Many criticisms have been levelled at brucellosis control programmes in recent years because they have tended to rely heavily upon vaccination alone, and although the abortion rate has been markedly reduced by vaccination, the incidence of infection has not been reduced at the same rate (28). There is another side to the argument. Apart from questions of human exposure to infection, the value of brucellosis control and eradication depends on the economic gain achieved by better reproductive efficiency. Some control programmes would appear to cost a great deal more than they benefit.

Hygienic measures include the isolation or disposal of infected animals, disposal of aborted foetuses, placentae and uterine discharges, and disinfection of contaminated areas. It is particularly important that infected cows be isolated at parturition. All cattle, horses and pigs brought on to the farm should be tested, isolated for 30 days and retested. Introduced cows which are in advanced pregnancy should be kept in isolation until after parturition, since occasional infected cows may not show a positive serum reaction until after calving or abortion.

Vaccination with *Br. abortus* Strain 19 living vaccine is the most valuable aid in brucellosis control. Its main value is that it protects uninfected animals living in a contaminated environment, enabling infected animals to be disposed of gradu-

ally. This overcomes the main disadvantage of the test and disposal method of eradication in which infected animals have to be disposed of immediately to avoid spread of the infection.

Strain 19 *Br. abortus* has a low virulence and is incapable of causing abortion except in a proportion of cows vaccinated in late pregnancy, although it can cause undulant fever in man. Its two other weaknesses are its failure to completely prevent infection, especially infection of the udder, and the persistence of vaccinal titres in some animals. In addition it is possible that some calves which suffer very heavy exposure soon after birth may become infected and remain so until they are adults or they may be refractory to vaccination and become infected subsequently (29). The optimum age for vaccination is between 4 and 8 months and there is no significant difference between the immunity conferred at 4 or 8 months of age. In calves vaccinated between these ages the serum agglutination test returns to negative by the time the animals are of breeding age except in a small percentage (6 per cent) of cases. There is some evidence that the duration of the vaccination reaction can be reduced by vaccinating at 2 to 3 months of age, without reducing the efficiency of the vaccination (30) but the technique is seldom utilized. In most control programmes, vaccination is usually permitted up to 12 months of age but the proportion of persistent post-vaccinal serum and whey reactions increases with increasing age of the vaccinates. Such persistent reactors may have to be culled in an eradication programme unless the reaction can be proved to be the result of vaccination and not due to virulent infection. Vaccination of adult cattle is usually not permitted if an eradication programme is contemplated but it may be of value in reducing the effects of an abortion 'storm'. There is no evidence that vaccination of bulls has any value in protecting them against infection and vaccination has resulted in the development of orchitis and the presence of *Br. abortus* Strain 19 in the semen (31). For these reasons the vaccination of bulls should be actively discouraged. Vaccination of adult cows and males is usually restricted to adjuvant 45/20 vaccine.

Systemic reactions to vaccination with Strain 19 are common in both calves and adults, and seem to be more severe in Jersey calves than in other breeds. A local swelling occurs particularly in adult cattle and there may be a severe systemic reaction manifested by high fever (40·5 to 42 °C or 105 to 108 °F) lasting for 2 to 3 days, anorexia, listlessness and temporary slackening of the milk yield in cows. An occasional animal goes completely dry. The local

Causes of Abortion in Cattle—Diagnostic Summary

Disease	Clinical Features	Abortion Rate	Time of Abortion	Field Examination		Lab. Diagnosis	
				Placenta	Foetus	Isolation of Agent	Serology
BRUCELLOSIS (*Br. abortus*)	Abortion.	High, up to 90% in susceptible herds. *30%*	6 months + *7-9*	Necrosis of cotyledons. Leathery, opaque placenta with oedema.	May be pneumonia.	Culture of foetal stomach, placenta, uterine fluid, milk and semen.	Serum and blood agglutination test, milk ring test, whole milk plate agglutination test. Whey plate agglutination, semen plasma and vaginal mucous agglutination test.
TRICHOMONIASIS (*Tr. foetus*)	Infertility—return to heat at 4 to 5 months, abortion and pyometra.	Moderate, 5 to 30%.	2 to 4 months. *1-4*	Flocculent material and clear, serous fluid in uterine exudate.	Foetal maceration and pyometra common.	Hanging drop or culture examination of foetal stomach and uterine exudate within 24 hours of abortion.	Cervical mucous agglutination test.
VIBRIOSIS (*V. foetus*)	Infertility, irregular, moderately prolonged dioestrus.	Low, up to 5%, may be up to 20%.	5 to 6 months. *4-6 or 5-7*	Semi-opaque, little thickening. Petechiae, localized avascularity and oedema.	Flakes of pus on visceral peritoneum.	Culture of foetal stomach, placenta and uterine exudate.	Blood agglutination after abortion (at 3 weeks). Cervical mucous agglutination test at 40 days after infected service.
LEPTOSPIROSIS (*Lept. pomona*)	Abortion may occur at acute febrile stage, later or unassociated with illness.	25 to 30%.	Late, 6 months + *8-9*	Avascular placenta, atonic yellow-brown cotyledons, brown gelatinous oedema between allantois and amnion.	Foetal death common.	Isolation from pleural fluid, kidney and liver of foetus.	Positive serum agglutination test 14 to 21 days after febrile illness.
MYCOSES (Aspergillus, Absidia)	—	Unknown, 6 to 7% of all abortions encountered.	3 to 7 months. *5-7*	Necrosis of maternal cotyledon, adherence of necrotic material to chorionic cotyledon causes soft, yellow, cushion-like structure. Small yellow, raised, leathery lesions on intercotyledonary areas.	May be small, raised, grey-buff, soft lesions, or diffuse white areas on skin. Resemble ringworm.	Direct examination of cotyledon and foetal stomach for hyphae, suitable cultural examination.	—
LISTERIOSIS (*List. monocytogenes*)	May be an associated septicaemia.	Low. *5-15%*	About 7 months. *marked necrosis*		No abnormality.	Organisms in foetal stomach, placenta and uterine fluid.	Agglutination titres higher than 1:400 in contact animals classed as positive.

IBR
BVD

(handwritten marginalia: "last half", "early half", "liter lepto / like lyte", "Blood tinged fluid at Kidney", "cereb hypo", "paired serum samp", "2L. Ab")

Causes of Abortion in Cattle—Diagnostic Summary (cont.)

Disease	Clinical Features	Abortion Rate	Time of Abortion	Field Examination		Lab. Diagnosis	
				Placenta	Foetus	Isolation of Agent	Serology
EPIZOOTIC VIRAL ABORTION	Mainly winter. Herd immunity develops.	High, 30 to 40%.	6 to 8 months.	Negative.	Subcutis oedema, ascites, oeso-phageal and tracheal petechiae, degenerative lesions in liver.	Chlamydia isolated (23).	No accurate test.
NUTRITIONAL	Ingestion of excessive amounts of pre-formed oestrogens in the diet may cause abortion. There are usually accompanying signs due to increased vascularity of the udder and vulva. Possibly dietary factor in so-called 'lowlands abortion'.						
ISO-IMMUNIZA-TION OF PREGNANCY	Has not been observed to occur naturally in cattle. It has been produced experimentally by repeated intravenous injections of blood from the one bull. Intravascular haemolysis occurs in the calves.						
UNKNOWN	From 30 to 75% of most series of abortions examined are undiagnosed. The ingestion of large quantities of pine needles is suspected as a cause of abortion in range cattle in the U.S.A. (43). Infection with the viruses of infectious bovine rhinotracheitis and mucosal disease and *Mycoplasma* spp. are other causes of undetermined relative importance.						

swellings are sterile and do not rupture but a solid, fibrous mass may persist for many months. Deaths within 48 hours of vaccination have been recorded in calves after the use of lyophilized vaccine. Septicaemia due to *Br. abortus* may cause some deaths but in most cases the reaction is thought to be anaphylactic, and vaccinated calves should be kept under close observation. Immediate treatment with adrenaline hydrochloride (1 ml. of 1:1000 solution subcutaneously) or antihistamine drugs is recommended and is effective provided it can be administered in time.

Cows in advanced pregnancy may abort if vaccinated but the abortion rate is low and, although *Br. abortus* Strain 19 organisms can be recovered from the foetus and placenta, their virulence is unchanged and they do not cause further spread of infection. Vaccination with Strain 19 does not have a deleterious effect on the subsequent conception rate.

Vaccination technique is of vital importance; the vaccine is a living agent and must be handled with care if satisfactory results are to be obtained. Lyophilized vaccine is superior to liquid vaccine because of its greater stability and greater longevity but it must be kept under refrigeration at all times, be reconstituted only when required, and unused material discarded (33). It must be used in an aseptic manner to avoid its contamination with other bacteria. Intradermal and intracaudal vaccination, using 0·2 ml. and 1·0 ml. respectively, have been shown to give as good results as the standard subcutaneous injection of 3 to 5 ml. of vaccine (34). Under experimental conditions, a small (0·2 ml.) dose given subcutaneously is equally effective (21). However, none of these modifications of the standard subcutaneous technique have come into general use.

Efficiency of Strain 19 vaccine can be assessed by its effect on the incidence of abortion and the effect on the incidence of infection as determined by laboratory examination. Field tests show a marked reduction in the number of abortions which occur although the increased resistance to infection, as indicated by the presence of *Br. abortus* in milk, may be less marked. Vaccinated animals continually exposed to virulent infection may eventually become infected and act as carriers without showing clinical evidence of the disease In summary, the position is that vaccination with a single 5 ml. dose of *Br. abortus* Strain 19 vaccine given subcutaneously at about 6 months of age confers adequate immunity against abortion for five or more subsequent lactations under conditions of field exposure. Multiple or late vaccinations have no appreciable advantage and increase the incidence of post-vaccinal positive agglutination reactions. When breakdowns occur, they are due to excessive exposure to infection and not to enhanced virulence of the organism.

Other Vaccines

To overcome the disadvantages of the severe systemic reaction and the persistent agglutination titre which occurs after vaccination with Strain 19 vaccine a search is being made for a killed non-agglutinogenic vaccine. Attention is also being given, particularly in Europe, to the use of *Br. melitensis* as an immunizing agent. A killed vaccine containing strain H38 of this organism shows promise (32). The only non-agglutinogenic vaccine with any currency is Strain 45/20 in adjuvant. Because it is a dead vaccine it has obvious attractions for vaccination of adult cows and males. When used in calves of 6 months of age or over the immunity is solid. For calves up to 8 or 9 months Strain 19 is still the preferred choice. Beyond that age some consideration should be given to 45/20 in adjuvant because of the lesser tendency to produce persistent high antibody levels. The vaccine is not completely non-agglutinogenic but titres in serum rarely reach inconclusive levels (36). Complement fixation antibodies are unaffected and no agglutinins appear in the milk (37). There are difficulties with the vaccine. The official vaccine K45/20A has a standard adjuvant but the characteristics of the vaccine can vary from batch to batch and need to be checked in animals (38). Two vaccinations are necessary. It is ineffective when given before 6 months of age. It produces granulomas. It is expensive, but it has the advantage that it can be used to identify the chronic inconclusive cow as described earlier.

Eradication programmes on a herd basis vary with the incidence of the infection. Scandinavian countries were the first to complete eradication and use flexible programmes which could be modified to suit particular sets of conditions (39). The following recommendations are based on the need for flexibility.

(*a*) *During an abortion 'storm'*, test and disposal of reactors is unsatisfactory because spread occurs faster than eradication. In these circumstances, the vaccination of all non-reactors is recommended or, if testing is impracticable, vaccination of all cattle. Strain K45/20A is the logical vaccine to use and must be given in two doses. It is preferable to retest the herd before the second vaccination and to discard cows with three or more dilutions rise in agglutination titre. The subsequent handling of these herds will be in the manner described in

(*b*) below, but eventual eradication will be greatly delayed.

(*b*) *Heavily infected herds in which few abortions are occurring* do not present such an urgent problem because the stage of herd resistance has been reached. All calves should be vaccinated with Strain 19 immediately and positive reactors among the remainder should be culled as soon as possible, preferably within 3 years. Periodic (preferably 2-month, no more than 3-month, intervals) Milk Ring Tests on individual cows are supplemented by complement fixation and culture tests. One year after first herd test, retest by agglutination test and revaccinate with K45/20A.

(*c*) *Lightly infected herds* present a special problem. If they are situated in an area where infection is likely to be introduced, vaccination of the calves and immediate culling of positive reactors should be carried out. If eradication is proceeding in the area, the culling of reactors will suffice, but special market demands for vaccinated cattle may dictate a calfhood vaccination policy. When a herd is declared to be free of brucellosis on the basis of serum agglutination tests, its status can be maintained by introducing only negative-reacting animals from brucellosis-free herds, and annual blood-testing. In areas where dairying predominates, semi-annual testing by the milk tests may be substituted for blood testing.

In all of the above programmes the careful laboratory examination of all aborted foetuses is an important and necessary corollary to routine testing.

There are many difficulties in the way of achieving eradication on a herd basis (35, 40). These relate mainly to the failure of owners to realize the highly infectious nature of the disease and to co-operate fully in the details of the programme. Particularly they may fail to recognize the recently calved cow as the principal source of infection. In a herd control programme such cows should be isolated at calving and blood tested at 14 days, since prior to that time false negative reactions are not uncommon.

Eradication programmes for control of the disease in an area should conform to the general pattern of reducing the susceptibility of the cattle population until the incidence of the disease is low enough to make complete eradication by test and disposal economically practicable. It is advisable to start such a programme in self-sufficient, cattle raising areas by encouraging vaccination and hygienic practices, and where possible, eradication on a herd basis. This stage may be voluntary, with inducements, including free vaccination and blood testing, and listing as accredited herds, being offered to encourage farmers to co-operate. It is in this stage that the milk tests described above are highly suitable for screening herds or areas to give some idea of the incidence of infection. Farms with a low incidence may find it possible to engage in an eradication programme immediately provided the incidence on surrounding farms is low. Disastrous breakdowns may occur if there are accidental introductions from nearby affected farms, and in these circumstances it is hazardous to have a herd which is not completely vaccinated. When the area incidence is judged to be low enough (about 5 per cent), that replacements can be found within the area or adjoining free areas, and that immediate culling of reactors can be carried out without crippling financial loss, compulsory eradication by testing and disposal of reactors for meat purposes can be instituted. Compensation for culled animals should be provided to encourage full participation in the programme. When an area or country is freed of the disease, testing of all or part of the population need be carried out only at intervals of two or three years although annual testing of bulk milk samples and of culled beef cows in abattoirs and bacteriological examination of all aborted foetuses should be instituted as checks on the eradication status. Such a programme has achieved virtual eradication of the disease in Switzerland, Sweden, and Northern Ireland (40, 41).

In all eradication programmes some problem herds will be encountered in which testing and disposal does not eliminate the infection. Usually about 5 per cent of such herds are encountered and are best handled by a 'problem herd' programme (42). Fifty per cent of these herds have difficulty because of failure to follow directions. The other half usually contain infected animals that do not respond to standard tests. Supplementary bacteriological and serological tests as set out above allow these spreader animals to be identified and the disease to be eradicated. One other source of difficulty is the persistence of infection in young vaccinates below the normal testing age of 30 months. In problem herds in which the reason for the difficulty is not apparent the testing of younger age groups is recommended.

REFERENCES

(1) Bothwell, P. W. et al. (1962). Vet. Rec., 74, 1091.
(2) Luchsinger, D. W. & Anderson, R. K. (1967). J. Amer. vet. med. Ass., 150, 1017.
(3) Allsup, T. N. (1969). Vet. Rec., 84, 104.
(4) McCaughey, W. J. & Kerr, W. R. (1967). Vet. Rec., 80, 186.
(5) Denny, H. R. (1972). Vet. Rec., 90, 86.
(6) Cosgrove, J. S. M. (1961). Vet. Rec., 73, 1377.
(7) Corner, A. H. & Connell, R. (1958). Canad. J. comp. Med., 22, 9.
(8) Kimberling, C. V. et al. (1966). J. Amer. vet. med. Ass., 148, 900.
(9) Bisping, W. (1962). Rindertuberkulose, 11, 51.
(10) Daminova, L. F. (1967). Veterinariya, 8, 103.
(11) Rankin, J. E. F. (1965). Vet. Rec., 77, 132.
(12) Vandeplassche, M. & Devos, A. (1960). Vlaams diergeneesk. T., 29, 199.
(13) Morgan, W. J. B. (1967). Vet. Rec., 80, 612.
(14) Nicoletti, P. (1969). Amer. J. vet. Res., 30, 1811; Cornell Vet., 59, 349.
(15) Pathak, R. C. & Singh, C. M. (1969). Veterinarian, Oxford, 6, 35.
(16) Anonymous (1967). Vet. Rec., 80, May 27th Suppl., 1.
(17) van Waveren, G. M. (1965). Bull. Off. int. Épizoot., 63, 1015.
(18) Roepke, M. H. & Stiles, F. C. (1970). Amer. J. vet. Res., 31, 2145.
(19) McCaughey, W. J. (1972). Vet. Rec., 90, 6.
(20) Farrell, I. D. & Robertson, L. (1968). J. Hyg., Camb., 66, 19.
(21) Morgan, W. J. B. et al. (1969). Vet. Rec., 85, 636.
(22) Cunningham, B. & O'Connor, M. (1971). Vet. Rec., 89, 680.
(23) Storz, J. & McKercher, D. G. (1970). Cornell Vet., 60, 192.
(24) Afshar, A. (1965). Vet. Bull., 35, 673.
(25) Bassan, Y. & Ayalon, N. (1971). Amer. J. vet. Res., 32, 703.
(26) Storz, J. et al. (1971). J. comp. Path., 81, 299.
(27) Afshar, A. (1965). Vet. Bull., 35, 735.
(28) Robertson, A. (1954). Vet. Rec., 66, 567.
(29) Hignett, P. G. & Nagy, L. K. (1964). Nature (Lond.), 201, 204.
(30) Redman, D. R. et al. (1967). J. Amer. vet. med. Ass., 150, 403.
(31) Lambert, G. et al. (1964). J. Amer. vet. med. Ass., 145, 909.
(32) Valette, L. R. & Renoux, G. (1967). Rev. Immunol. (Paris), 31, 329, 341.
(33) Love, E. L. et al. (1966). J. Amer. vet. med. Ass., 149, 1177.
(34) Gregory, T. S. (1953). Aust. vet. J., 29, 117.
(35) Plenderleith, R. W. J. (1970). Vet. Rec., 87, 404.
(36) Cunningham, B. & O'Reilly, D. J. (1968). Vet. Rec., 82, 678.
(37) Cunningham, B. (1970). Vet. Rec., 86, 2.
(38) Morgan, W. J. B. & McDiarmid, A. (1968). Vet. Rec., 83, 184.
(39) Thomsen, A. (1957). Advanc. vet. Sci., 3, 197.
(40) Christie, T. E. (1969). Vet. Rec., 85, 268, 269.
(41) Christie, T. E. et al. (1968). Vet. Rec., 82, 176.
(42) Mingle, C. K. (1964). Proc. 68th ann. gen. Mtg U.S. Live Stock sanit. Ass., 115–35.
(43) Abstract (1960). J. Amer. vet. med. Ass., 137, 44 (adv.).

Brucellosis Caused by *Brucella ovis*

The disease caused by the infection of sheep with *Br. ovis* is characterized by infertility in rams due to epididymitis. In ewes abortion and neonatal mortality are thought to be caused by the infection.

Incidence

Brucellosis of sheep caused by *Br. ovis* has been reported only in relatively recent times in Australia,

New Zealand, the U.S.A., South Africa, and Europe. The incidence has been very high in some areas, and there was much economic loss at one time. In California 30 to 40 per cent of rams were thought to be affected and an annual loss of $2 million was estimated (1). In one survey of a large number of rams conducted in Australia, the incidence of clinical epididymitis was 5·3 per cent and the incidence on individual farms was as high as 50 per cent (2). If the number of affected rams in a flock is greater than about 10 per cent the fertility of the flock is appreciably decreased.

Aetiology

The causative organism has been designated as *Br. ovis*. In nature only sheep are affected and most laboratory animals are refractory to the infection. Amongst sheep Merinos show a much lower incidence of the disease than do British breeds and crossbreeds. The disease occurs more commonly in adult rams, due probably to greater exposure to infection (2). The organism can survive on pasture for several months but transmission from ram to ram via the ewe's vagina seems to be the most common method.

Transmission

Complete details of the method of spread of infection are not yet available. Experimentally rams can be infected by the intravenous, subcutaneous, intratesticular, oral, and conjunctival and preputial instillation routes. Ewes in early pregnancy can also be infected by the oral and intravenous routes. Under natural conditions, spread from ram to ram occurs during the breeding season and when the rams are run together. However, spread from rams to ewes during mating does not occur readily, and spread between ewes by ingestion of contaminated pasture has not been observed. The exact means by which the disease spreads in a flock of ewes is not understood.

The infection in ewes is short lived and persists in only a few animals but the organism is present in the placenta, vaginal discharges and milk after abortion. In most rams the active excretion of the bacteria in semen probably persists indefinitely. Lambs born from infected ewes and drinking infected milk do not become infected.

Pathogenesis

An initial bacteraemia, often with a mild systemic reaction, is followed by localization in the epididymis of the ram causing infertility (4, 22). In ewes abortion due to placentitis has been produced experimentally (5) and has been observed

in natural cases in New Zealand and suspected in Australia (3), but has not been observed in other countries. Intra-uterine infection produced experimentally also causes lesions in and death of the foetus but the significance of this in natural cases is undetermined (21). In general the evidence is that *Br. ovis* has low pathogenicity for ewes (23).

Clinical Findings

The first reaction in rams is a marked deterioration in the quality of the semen together with the presence of leucocytes and brucellae. Acute oedema and inflammation of the scrotum may follow. A systemic reaction, including fever, depression and increased respiratory rate accompanies the local reaction. Regression of the acute syndrome is followed, after a long, latent period, by the development of palpable lesions in the epididymis and tunicae of one or both testicles. Palpation of both testicles simultaneously from behind is the best method of examination. The epididymis is enlarged and hard, more commonly at the tail, the scrotal tunics are thickened and hardened and the testicles usually atrophic. The groove between the testis and epididymis may be obliterated. The abnormalities are often detectable by palpation but many affected rams show no acute inflammatory stage and others may be actively secreting brucellae and poor quality semen in the chronic stage in the absence of palpable abnormalities.

Abortion in ewes is a characteristic of the disease as it occurs in New Zealand but not elsewhere. In the ewe, abortion, or the birth of weak or stillborn lambs is accompanied by macroscopic placentitis. The placental lesion varies from a superficial purulent exudate on an intact chorion to a marked oedema of the allantois, with necrosis of the uterine surface and the foetal cotyledons.

In spite of the seminal changes in affected rams, the fertility of their flock is often relatively unimpaired provided the proportion of affected rams is less than 10 per cent.

Clinical Pathology

In the ram, semen examination is essential. Semen quality should be determined, smears made for examination of inflammatory cells and culture for the organism undertaken. Bacteriological examination of the placenta and foetus should be carried out on aborted material. Complement fixation is now used routinely to detect serum antibodies to *Br. ovis* (3) and a haemagglutination-inhibition test is also available. An allergic skin test using killed organisms as an antigen has undergone preliminary examination (2) but is unlikely to be used extensively.

Necropsy Findings

In the acute stage, there is inflammatory oedema in the loose scrotal fascia, exudate in the tunica vaginalis and early granulation tissue formation (7). In the chronic stage, the tunics of the testes become thickened and fibrous and adhesions develop between them. There are circumscribed indurations in the epididymis and these granulomata may also be present in the testicle. In advanced stages they undergo caseation necrosis. As the epididymis enlarges the testicle becomes atrophied.

The arbortus is characterized by thickening and oedema, sometimes restricted to only a part of the placenta, firm, elevated yellow-white plaques in the intercotyledonary areas and varying degrees of abnormality of the cotyledons which in the acute stages are much enlarged, firm and yellow-white in colour. When abortion occurs the organism can be isolated from the placenta and the stomach and lungs of the lamb.

Diagnosis

The diagnosis of brucellosis in rams is based on three examinations, a complement fixation test on serum, physical palpation of the contents of the scrotum and cultural examination of semen or aborted material.

Other forms of epididymitis require to be differentiated. Suppurative epididymitis of rams is a specific, transmissible disease caused by *Cor. pseudotuberculosis* or by infection with *Act. seminis* (11). Abortion in ewes may be caused by a number of infectious diseases summarized in the table on p. 384. A severe infection with Q fever in sheep is an uncommon cause of abortion (2).

Treatment

In experimentally infected rams, the combined administration of chlortetracycline (800 mg. I/V) and streptomycin (1 g. S/C), injected daily for 21 days, eliminated infection. Streptomycin alone and streptomycin plus sulphadimidine were not satisfactory (12). Treatment is economically practicable only in valuable rams and must be instituted before irreparable damage to the epididymis has occurred.

Control

The primary objective in control programmes directed against brucellosis in sheep is to prevent the spread of infection between rams. Thus the basis of any such programme is the rigid isolation of young rams from old rams which are likely to be affected and from ewe flocks which have been mated to these older rams. To further reduce the chances of spread to young rams vaccination or test and slaughter programmes are recommended.

Vaccination. Vaccination is carried out on all yearling rams at least 2 to 3 months before they are used for mating (13, 14, 15). A number of vaccines are in use. The most common one is a single injection of a combination of killed *Br. ovis* in an adjuvant base and *Br. abortus* Strain 19. Although a high level, durable immunity is produced, the vaccine has several disadvantages; if used within two months of mating the fertility of the rams is likely to be reduced; a high titre of antibodies against *Br. ovis* as detected by the tube agglutination test persists for up to 3 years (24), which may confuse diagnosis and hinder eradication; some severe outbreaks of osteomyelitis have been recorded 10 to 20 days after vaccination in which affected rams are lame and weak in one or all limbs, many become recumbent and although recovery is usual the illness is a long one and affected animals are badly stunted in growth (16). A satisfactory alternative procedure to the above method is two injections of killed *Br. ovis* 24 weeks apart (20).

In South Africa a vaccine containing living attenuated *Br. melitensis* (referred to as Elberg Rev 1) has been found to be highly effective and is generally recommended (6, 17). It too suffers from the disadvantage that vaccinated animals become positive to the complement fixation tests.

If venereal transmission is the only means by which the disease is spread, effective vaccination and control of the rams is all that should be necessary. There is no evidence that vaccination of the ewes is of value in reducing spread but where it has been carried out vaccination has increased the percentage of lambs weaned (15).

Test and slaughter. In some countries vaccination is not permitted and eradication by test and slaughter is attempted. The identification of animals to be culled must depend on laboratory testing. Culling based on physical palpation can achieve only temporary improvement in a flock. The programme of testing used has varied and depends largely on the incidence and rate of spread of the disease. In static situations where the new infection rate is low, semi-annual testing is satisfactory (18) but when the disease has been recently introduced testing at monthly intervals may be necessary (19).

In both instances the rate of spread of infection is highest during the mating season and it is not recommended that eradication should be attempted

Infectious Abortion of Ewes—Diagnostic Summary

Disease	Trans- mission	Time of Abortion	Clinical Data	Laboratory Finding		Vaccination
				Foetus	Serology	
BRUCELLOSIS (*Br. ovis*)	Probably coitus.	Late or still- births.	Epididymitis in rams. In ewes abor- tion only. Not in U.S.A.	Organisms in foetal stomach and placenta.	Complement fixation test.	Simultaneous Str. 19 *Br. abortus* and killed *Br. ovis* adjuvant vaccine.
VIBRIOSIS (*V. foetus*)	Ingestion.	2 months.	Metritis in ewes after abortion.	Vibrios in stomach.	Agglutination test—flock only.	—
ENZOOTIC VIRUS ABORTION OF EWES (8)	Ingestion.	Last 2 to 3 weeks.	Illness before. Re- tained placenta and metritis after.	Elementary bodies in foetal cotyledons. Degenerative changes in placenta.	Complement fixation test.	Killed virus adju- vant vaccine. Gives good im- munity to 30 months (9).
LISTERIOSIS (*List. monocytogenes*)	Probably ingestion, possibly coitus.	After 3 months.	Retained placenta and metritis. Septi- caemia in some ewes.	Organisms in foetal stomach.	Agglutination test of doubtful value.	—
SALMONELLOSIS (*Salm. abortus- ovis*)	Probably ingestion.	Last 6 weeks.	Metritis after abor- tion.	Organisms in foetal stomach.	Agglutination test.	—
SALMONELLOSIS (*Salm. dublin*) (10)	Ingestion.	Last month.	Abortion: Fatal metritis, neonatal mortality.	Organisms in stomach.	Agglutination test.	—
TOXOPLASMOSIS (New Zealand Type 2)	Not known.	Late or still- births.	Abortion, stillbirths and neonatal mortality.	Multiple small necrotic foci in foetal cotyledons. Toxoplasma in cells of trophoblast epithelium.	Dye tests for toxoplasmosis appear efficient.	Nil.

until after the rams are taken out of the flock. Any policy which does not permit vaccination is likely to be hazardous in areas where the disease is not under control and infected replacements are likely to be introduced.

REFERENCES

(1) Crenshaw, G. L. *et al.* (1963). *Calif. Vet.*, *17*, No. 6, 42.
(2) Hall, W. T. K. *et al.* (1955). *Aust. vet. J.*, *31*, 7, 10 & 11.
(3) Lawrence, W. E. (1961). *Brit. vet. J.*, *117*, 435.
(4) Biberstein, E. L. *et al.* (1964). *Cornell Vet.*, *54*, 27.
(5) Collier, J. R. & Molello, J. A. (1964). *Amer. J. vet. Res.*, *25*, 930.
(6) Renoux, G. (1957). *Advances in Veterinary Science*, Vol. 3, pp. 241–273. New York: Academic Press.
(7) Jebson, J. L. *et al.* (1955). *N.Z. vet. J.*, *3*, 100.
(8) Tunnicliff, E. A. (1960). *J. Amer. vet. med. Ass.*, *136*, 132.
(9) Foggie, A. (1959). *Vet. Rec.*, *71*, 741.
(10) Watson, W. A. (1960). *Vet. Rec.*, *72*, 62.
(11) Simmons, G. C. *et al.* (1966). *Aust. vet. J.*, *42*, 183.
(12) Kuppuswamy, P. B. (1954). *N.Z. vet. J.*, *2*, 110.
(13) Buddle, M. B. (1956). *Proc. 3rd int. Congr. Anim. Reprod.*, *Cambridge*, Sec. 2, pp. 37–38.
(14) Buddle, M. B. (1957). *N.Z. vet. J.*, *5*, 43.
(15) Buddle, M. B. (1958). *N.Z. vet. J.*, *6*, 41.
(16) Kater, J. C. & Hartley, W. J. (1963). *N.Z. vet. J.*, *11*, 65.
(17) Heerden, K. M. van (1964). *Bull. Off. int. Epizoot.*, *62*, 997.
(18) Clapp, K. H. *et al.* (1962). *Aust. vet. J.*, *38*, 482.
(19) Ryan, F. B. (1964). *Aust. vet. J.*, *40*, 162.
(20) Buddle, M. B. *et al.* (1963). *N.Z. vet. J.*, *11*, 90.
(21) Osburn, B. I. & Kennedy, P. C. (1966). *Path. vet.*, *3*, 110.
(22) Murray, R. M. (1969). *Aust. vet. J.*, *45*, 63.
(23) Hughes, K. L. (1972). *Aust. vet. J.*, *48*, 12, 18.
(24) Ris, D. R. (1967). *N.Z. vet. J.*, *15*, 94.

Brucellosis Caused by *Brucella suis*

Brucellosis caused by *Br. suis* is a chronic disease of pigs manifested by sterility and abortion in sows, heavy piglet mortality and orchitis in boars.

Incidence

The disease occurs in most countries but, in spite of its widespread occurrence in the U.S.A., it has not appeared in Canada (15) or Great Britain.

In an enzootic area, the proportion of herds infected is usually high (30 to 60 per cent) but the number of individual pigs infected may be quite low (5 to 10 per cent). The disease owes its economic importance to the infertility and reduction in numbers of pigs weaned per litter which occur in infected herds (7). The mortality which occurs during the first month of life may be as high as 80 per cent. The mortality rate is negligible in mature animals but sows and boars may have to be culled because of sterility, and occasional pigs because of posterior paralysis. In addition, eradication involves much financial loss if complete disposal of a registered herd is undertaken.

Br. suis presents a public health hazard particularly to abattoir workers, and to a less extent to farmers and veterinarians. *Br. abortus* and *Br. melitensis* may also be found in pig carcases and present similar hazards to public health (1). *Br. suis* may also localize in the mammary gland of cattle without causing clinical abnormality, and where cattle and pigs are run together, the hazard to humans drinking unpasteurized milk may be serious.

Aetiology

The organism *Br. suis* is more resistant to adverse environmental conditions than *Br. abortus*, although its longevity outside the body has not been fully examined. It is known to survive in faeces, urine and water for 4 to 6 weeks (14). The organism is pathogenic only for pigs and man although other species, including cattle and horses, may be infected. Isolations have also been made from wild animals including rats (13) and hares (8). Amongst pigs, susceptibility varies with age, the incidence of infection being much higher in adults than in young pigs. Although infection before weaning is uncommon, sucking pigs on infected sows may become infected, with maximum agglutinin titres appearing at 8 to 12 weeks of age but disappearing at 16 weeks. The susceptibility is much greater in the post-weaning periods and is the same for both sexes.

No durable immunity develops, and although a stage of herd resistance is apparent after an acute outbreak, the herd is again susceptible within a short time and a further outbreak may occur if infection is reintroduced. A partial immunity to the disease has been observed in some breeds of pigs (11).

Transmission

Under field conditions the disease is spread by ingestion and by coitus. Although ingestion of food contaminated by infected semen and urine and discharges from infected sows is probably the commoner method of spread, the localization of infection in the genitalia of the boar makes venereal transmission important in this disease. Introduction into a piggery is usually effected by the introduction of infected pigs. Less commonly the infection may be brought in by other species or on inanimate objects. Wild animals, including hares and rats may provide a source of infection and ticks are also suspected of transmitting the disease. Spread through a herd is rapid because of the conditions under which pigs are kept. The severe effects of the disease subside quickly as herd resistance is attained, and in herds in which replacements are reared, no further trouble may be experienced. When pigs are introduced continuously, further outbreaks are likely to occur.

Pathogenesis

As in brucellosis caused by *Br. abortus*, there is initial systemic invasion, the organism appearing in the blood stream for up to 2 months. However, infection with *Br. suis* differs from that caused by *Br. abortus* in that it shows no predilection for localization in the uterus and udder, the organism being found in all body tissues and producing a disease similar to undulant fever in man. The more common manifestations of localization are abortion and infertility due to localization in the uterus; lymphadenitis, especially of the cervical lymph nodes; arthritis and lameness due to bone and joint localization, and posterior paralysis due to osteomyelitis. In boars, involvement of testicles often leads to clinical orchitis (16). It is the widespread involvement of all body tissues which makes handling of the freshly killed carcase such a hazardous procedure and increases the risk of undulant fever in humans eating improperly cooked pork.

A characteristic of the disease is that positive agglutination titres tend to subside with time, especially in sows, although such animals may still be infected and be capable of transmitting the disease.

Clinical Findings

The clinical findings in swine brucellosis vary widely, depending upon the site of localization. As in undulant fever in man, the signs are not diagnostic and in many herds a high incidence of reactors is observed with little clinical evidence of disease.

Most prominent are signs of genital tract involvement. In the sow, infertility, which may be temporary, irregular oestrus, small litters and abortion occur. The incidence of abortion varies widely between herds but is usually low. Sows abort only once as a rule, and although abortion is most common during the third month, it may occur earlier. Affected sows usually breed normally thereafter. In boars, orchitis with swelling and necrosis of one or both testicles is followed by sterility. Lameness, inco-ordination and posterior paralysis occur fairly commonly. They are usually gradual in onset and may be caused by arthritis, or more commonly, osteomyelitis of lumbar and sacral vertebral bodies.

A heavy mortality in piglets during the first month of life is sometimes encountered. Most of the losses result from stillbirths and the death of weak piglets within a few hours of birth.

Clinical Pathology

Laboratory identification of the disease is difficult. *Isolation of the organism* should be attempted if suitable material is available. Such material for culture or guinea pig inoculation includes aborted foetuses, testicular lesions, abscesses and blood. An *agglutination test* carried out on serum is the simplest diagnostic aid but in this disease it has serious limitations. A positive titre does not arise until 8 weeks after infection and many infected pigs have a low titre. For these reasons the test can be used only as a herd test. Herds in which no pigs have titres greater than 1:100 are classified as negative but, in infected herds, any individual pig with a titre greater than 1:25 is classified as positive (2). Because of the limitations of the standard agglutination test, the Coombs test and allergic skin sensitivity tests are under investigation.

Necropsy Findings

Many organs may be involved with chronic changes being most apparent. Chronic metritis manifested by nodular inflammatory thickening and abscessation of the uterine wall is characteristic. Arthritis and necrosis of vertebral bodies in the lumbar region may be found in lame and paralysed pigs. The clinical orchitis of boars is revealed as testicular necrosis, often accompanied by lesions in the epididymis and seminal vesicles. Pronounced lymphadenopathy, due to reticulo-endothelial hyperplasia, and splenic enlargement occur in some cases. Nodular splenitis, in the absence of other lesions, justifies a presumptive diagnosis of brucellosis in pigs (10).

Diagnosis

The protean character of this disease makes it difficult to diagnose unless one is accustomed to including it in a list of diagnostic possibilities. Once this difficulty is overcome, the routine serological examinations of herds soon places the disease in its proper local perspective. It is likely to be confused with brucellosis caused by *Br. melitensis*. Individual animals with posterior paralysis present a major problem in diagnosis since there are so many causes in pigs, including hypovitaminosis A, deficiency of vitamin B complex factors, and fractures of the lumbar vertebrae in osteomalacia. Many poisonings such as organic arsenicals, mercury, rotenone and organophosphatic insecticides may cause posterior paralysis among other things. A summary of the differential diagnosis of posterior paralysis is given in the section on diseases of the spinal cord.

Abortion 'storms' are common in piggeries but in most instances the cause is not determined (9). Known causes include leptospirosis and acute infectious diseases, especially erysipelas. Other bacteria commonly isolated from aborted porcine foetuses include *List. monocytogenes*, *Staphylococcus*, *Streptococcus* and *Corynebacterium* spp., and occasionally *Salm. abortus-ovis*. Mortality in young sucking pigs is also caused by many agents and the important entities are listed under diseases of the newborn.

Treatment

Exhaustive trials of treatment with a combination of streptomycin parenterally and sulphadiazine orally for long periods failed to reduce the infection rate in pigs (3). Chlortetracycline is also ineffective (4). It is unlikely that the treatments available at present will ever be attempted on a commercial scale.

Control

No suitable vaccine is available. Strain 19 *Br. abortus*, *Br. abortus* 'M' vaccine, and phenol and ether extracts of *Br. suis* are all ineffective (5, 6). Control must be by test and disposal. In herds where the incidence of reactors is high, complete disposal of all stock as they reach marketing age is by far the best procedure because of the difficulty in detecting individual infected animals. This is most practicable in commercial pork-producing herds. Restocking the farm should be delayed for six months.

The alternative is to commence a two-herd,

segregation programme and this is recommended for pure bred herds which supply pigs for breeding purposes. Total disposal is not usually economical in these herds. Once a herd diagnosis has been established, all the breeding animals must be considered to be infected; all piglets at weaning are submitted to the serum agglutination test and, if negative, go into new quarters to start the nucleus of a free herd (7). It is probably safer to wean the pigs as young as possible and submit them to the test again at a later stage before mating. If complete protection is desired, these gilts should be allowed to farrow only in isolation, be retested and their piglets used to start the clean herd. A modified scheme based on the above method of weaning and isolating the young pigs as soon as possible but without submitting them to the serum agglutination test has been proposed but its weakness is that infections may occur and persist in young pigs. Repopulation programmes utilizing specific pathogen-free pigs should be effective in eliminating the disease.

After eradication is completed, breakdowns are most likely to occur when infected animals are introduced. All introductions should be from accredited, free herds, should be clinically healthy, and be negative to the serum agglutination test twice at intervals of 3 weeks before introduction.

Eradication of swine brucellosis from an area can only be achieved by developing a nucleus of accredited, free herds and using these as a source of replacements for herds which eradicate by total disposal. Sale of pigs from infected herds for breeding purposes must be prevented.

REFERENCES

(1) McCullough, N. B. et al. (1951). Pub. Hlth Rep. (Wash.), 66, 205.
(2) Hubbard, E. D. & Hoerlein, A. B. (1952). J. Amer. vet. med. Ass., 120, 138.
(3) Hutchings, L. M. et al. (1950). Amer. J. vet. Res., 11, 388.
(4) Bunnell, D. E. et al. (1953). Amer. J. vet. Res., 14, 160.
(5) Manthei, C. A. (1948). Amer. J. vet. Res., 9, 40.
(6) Bunnell, D. E. et al. (1953). Amer. J. vet. Res., 14, 164.
(7) Cameron, H. S. (1957). Advances in Veterinary Science, Vol. 3, pp. 275–285, New York: Academic Press.
(8) Bendtsen, H. (1960. Nord. Vet.-Med., 12, 343.
(9) Saunders, C. N. (1958). Vet. Rec., 70, 965.
(10) Anderson, W. A. & Davis, C. L. (1957). J. Amer. vet. med. Ass., 131, 141.
(11) Cameron, H. S. et al. (1943). Amer. J. vet. Res., 4, 387.
(12) Lowbeer, L. (1959). Lab. Invest., 8, 1448.
(13) Cook, I. et al. (1965). Aust. vet. J., 42, 5.
(14) Luchsinger, D. W. et al. (1965). J. Amer. vet. med. Ass., 147, 632.
(15) Malkin, K. L. et al. (1968). Canad. J. comp. Med., 32, 598.
(16) Retnasabapathy, A. & Chong, S. K. (1967). Malay vet. J., 4, 130.

Brucellosis Caused by *Brucella melitensis*

Br. melitensis causes the typical syndrome of brucellosis in goats and is the cause of classical 'Malta' or 'Mediterranean' fever of man.

Incidence

This disease was originally observed in southern Europe but has since been found in Central America, the U.S.A. and Africa, and probably occurs in most parts of the world where goats are raised except perhaps Britain and Scandinavia. The importance and distribution of this form of brucellosis in animals have not been accurately determined but it has considerable importance because of the role of the organism in the production of 'Malta' or 'Mediterranean' fever in humans drinking infected milk from goats, cattle and sheep.

Aetiology

Br. melitensis is capable of infecting most species of domestic animals. Goats are highly susceptible, sheep less so (1). The organism is capable of causing disease in cattle and has been isolated from swine. In Europe the incidence of the infection in cattle appears to be increasing and in Malta about a third of the cattle reacting positively to the brucellosis agglutination test are infected with *Br. melitensis* (7). Accurate identification of the organism can only be carried out by the use of serological tests and many identifications based on cultural and biochemical tests have been invalid (5).

Transmission

Transmission between species occurs readily and is probably by ingestion as in other forms of brucellosis. Infected does, whether they abort or kid normally, discharge large numbers of brucellae in their uterine exudates. The vaginal exudate of infected virgin or open animals may also contain the bacteria. In sheep the degree of infection of milk and uterine exudate is much less than in goats. Viable kids are infected, and in some cases the disease persists in a latent form until sexual maturity when clinical signs become evident (6). The same conditions may apply in *Br. melitensis* infection in sheep (7).

Pathogenesis

As in other forms of brucellosis, the pathogenesis depends upon localization in lymph nodes, udder and uterus after an initial bacteraemia. In goats this bacteraemia may be sufficiently severe to produce a systemic reaction, and blood culture may remain positive for a month, often with no detectable agglutinins in the serum. Localization in the placenta leads to the development of placentitis with subsequent abortion (10). After abortion, uterine infection persists for up to 5 months and the mammary gland may remain infected for years. Spontaneous recovery may occur particularly in goats which become infected while not pregnant (7). In sheep the development of the disease is very similar to that in goats (8).

Clinical Findings

Abortion during late pregnancy is the most obvious sign in goats and sheep, but as in other species there may be a 'storm' of abortions when the disease is introduced, followed by a period of flock resistance during which abortions do not occur. In experimental infections, a systemic reaction with fever, depression, loss of weight and sometimes diarrhoea occurs. These signs may also occur in acute, natural outbreaks in goats and may be accompanied by mastitis, lameness, hygroma and orchitis. Osteoarthritis, synovitis and nervous signs are not uncommon in sheep. In pigs the disease is indistinguishable clinically from brucellosis caused by *Br. suis*. In many instances, *Br. melitensis* infection reaches a high incidence in a group of animals without signs of obvious illness.

Clinical Pathology

Positive blood culture soon after the infection occurs, or isolation of the organism from the aborted foetus, vaginal mucus or the milk are the common laboratory procedures used in diagnosis. The bacteraemia persists for a month after infection, and mammary gland infection may persist for years (2). An agglutination test and a complement fixation test are available (17) but results are likely to be confusing because of the transient rise in titre in some animals. An intradermal allergic test has been described but is of limited value in control of the disease in areas where the disease is enzootic (7). Tests are also conducted on milk. They include the Milk Ring Test, the whey complement fixation tests, whey Coombs or antiglobulin test and whey agglutination tests (4). The Milk Ring Test is less specific than serum agglutination test but is good enough for a screening test. Laboratory diagnosis is not easy and for detection of the disease in individual animals a number of tests carried out on several occasions may be necessary (9).

Necropsy Findings

There are no lesions characteristic of this form of brucellosis. The causative organism can often be isolated from all tissues but the spleen is the most common site of infection.

Diagnosis

In many instances, a diagnosis of *Br. melitensis* infection in animals is made only because the infection has been diagnosed in human contacts, provoking an examination of the local animal population. The disease varies in its manifestations, and its positive diagnosis can only be made by isolation of the organism.

Treatment

Treatment is unlikely to be undertaken in animals.

Control

Control measures must include hygiene at kidding or lambing and the disposal of infected or reactor animals. Because of the possibility that kids may be infected at birth and carry the disease for life, it may be more economic to dispose of the entire flock. Living avirulent organisms are now used in a vaccine—Elberg's Rev 1 vaccine—and its use in sheep and goats has proved effective (3, 14). A high degree of immunity is produced and lasts for more than 4 years in goats (5) and $2\frac{1}{2}$ years in sheep (13). Reduction of the number of organisms in the vaccinating dose has made it less likely to cause abortion, be excreted in the milk or interfere with serological tests (15). A higher degree of immunity is claimed from a formalin killed adjuvant vaccine 53 H 38 (16). *Br. abortus* Strain 19 has also been used and appears to give protection which is as good as that achieved with the attenuated *Br. melitensis* vaccine (11, 12).

REFERENCES

(1) Renoux, G. *et al.* (1957). *Vet. Bull.*, 27, 283.
(2) Meyer, K. F. (1951). *Bol. Ofic. sanit. panamer.*, 30, 9.
(3) Alton, G. G. & Elberg, S. S. (1967). *Vet. Bull.*, 37, 793.
(4) Ebadi, A. (1971). *Brit. vet. J.*, 127, 105.
(5) Alton, G. G. (1968). *J. comp. Path.*, 78, 173.
(6) Alton, G. G. (1970). *Brit. vet. J.*, 126, 61.
(7) Renoux, G. (1957). *Advanc. vet. Sci.*, 3, 241.
(8) Paltrionieri, S. *et al.* (1956). *Ann. Fac. Med. vet. Pisa*, 9, 251.
(9) Renoux, G. (1961). *Ann. Zootech.*, 10, 233.
(10) Collier, J. R. & Molello, J. A. (1964). *Amer. J. vet. Res.*, 25, 930.
(11) Neeman, L. (1963). *Refuah vet.*, 20, 134.

(12) Jones, L. M. *et al.* (1964). *J. comp. Path.*, *74*, 17.
(13) Entessor, F. *et al.* (1967). *J. comp. Path.*, *77*, 367.
(14) Unel, S. *et al.* (1969). *Res. vet. Sci.*, *10*, 254.
(15) Alton, G. G. (1970). *Res. vet. Sci.*, *11*, 54.
(16) Ghosh, S. S. *et al.* (1968). *J. comp. Path.*, *78*, 387.
(17) Unel, S. *et al.* (1969). *J. comp. Path.*, *79*, 155.

DISEASES CAUSED BY *HAEMOPHILUS* AND *MORAXELLA* Spp.

Haemophilus suis plays an important role as a secondary bacterial invader in swine influenza and is dealt with under that heading.

An acute, highly fatal pneumonia of sheep caused by *Haem. ovis* occurs rarely. There is a sudden onset of fever, prostration, dyspnoea and cyanosis. Dysentery and the discharge of a blood stained fluid from the nostrils are less constant signs. At necropsy the characteristic lesion is bronchopneumonia affecting the anterior lobes but there are, in addition, petechial haemorrhages in many organs, intense congestion of the abdominal viscera and a yellow, friable liver (1).

An unidentified haemophilus-like organism, culturally distinct from *Haem. suis*, has been isolated from cases of pneumonia in pigs (2). Cultures of the organism injected intratracheally into pigs do not cause disease but when the injection is combined with the virus of hog cholera, a nodular pneumonia with pleurisy develops. An acute, often fatal pleuropneumonia caused by *Haem. pleuropneumoniae* is recorded from the Argentine (3). The disease is highly contagious and is easily produced by intranasal instillation of the organism; subcutaneous injection does not cause the disease but causes a solid immunity. A similar disease has been recorded in Switzerland (4) and Denmark (5) and the causative organism is identified as *Haem. parahaemolyticus*. It has been used to reproduce the disease experimentally.

REFERENCES

(1) Mitchell, C. A. (1925). *J. Amer. vet. med. Ass.*, *68*, 8.
(2) Pattison, I. H. *et al.* (1957). *J. comp. Path.*, *67*, 320.
(3) Shope, R. E. *et al.* (1964). *J. exp. Med.*, *119*, 357 & 369.
(4) Nicolet, J. *et al.* (1969). *Schweiz. Arch. Tierheilk.*, *111*, 164.
(5) Nielsen, R. (1970). *Nord. Vet.-Med.*, *22*, 240 & 246.

Infectious Keratitis of Cattle

(*Pink-eye, Blight*)

The common infectious keratitis of cattle is caused by *Moraxella* (*Haemophilus*) *bovis*.

Incidence

The disease occurs in most countries of the world and is most common in summer and autumn. The incidence varies greatly from year to year and may reach epizootic proportions in feedlots and in cattle running at pasture. Loss of milk production or bodily condition may be caused by the discomfort, failure to feed and temporary blindness. Occasionally animals become completely blind and those at pasture may die of starvation.

Aetiology

M. bovis is known to be an important factor in the development of the disease but it is doubtful that it is the only infectious agent concerned (1). The IBR virus causes a different disease, a conjunctivitis rather than a keratitis but it may also be involved with *M. bovis* in causing the more severe disease. Other unidentified rickettsiae, chlamydia and viruses have been postulated (2) and identified (3). Because the naturally occurring disease is usually much more severe than that produced experimentally factors other than infectious agents have been examined. Solar radiation has been shown to have an enhancing effect (4) and flies and dust are suspected. On the other hand, the introduction of pure cultures of *M. bovis* into the conjunctival sac of cattle cause the disease, mild though it might be, even when the conjunctiva is uninjured (5). Also the organism is not usually found in the conjunctival sacs of cattle with no history of 'pink-eye'. Both *Neisseria catarrhalis* (6) and a *Mycoplasma* sp. (7) are also suspected of being involved as aetiological agents.

Only cattle are affected, the young being most susceptible. The disease has been reproduced experimentally in mice (8).

Transmission

Because the disease is most common in summer and autumn, and reaches epizootic proportions when flies and dust are abundant and grass is long, transmission is thought to be by means of these agents contaminated by the ocular discharges of infected cattle. The face fly (*Musca autumnalis*), because of its preference for the area around the eyes, is thought to be an important vector of the infection and is known to remain infected for periods of up to 3 days (9). The conjunctiva is the probable portal of entry. Persistence of the disease from year to year is by means of infected animals which can act as carriers for periods exceeding 1 year.

Pathogenesis

A dermonecrotic endotoxin is produced by the organism and is capable of causing typical lesions in calves and rabbits when injected intracorneally (10). In natural cases the lesions are localized in the eye, the organism not reaching the blood stream of the affected animal. Serum agglutinins to *M. bovis* are detectable (3) and immunity after an attack is usually good for up to a year although recurrent attacks may occur in the one animal. The immunity may be local only and possibly due to the persistence of the organism in the conjunctival sac.

Clinical Findings

An incubation period of 2 to 3 days is usual although longer intervals, up to 3 weeks, have been observed after experimental introduction of the bacteria. Injection of the corneal vessels and oedema of the conjunctiva are the earliest signs and are accompanied by a copious, watery lacrimation, blepharospasm, photophobia and, in some cases, a slight to moderate fever with fall in milk yield and depression of appetite. In 1 to 2 days, a small opacity appears in the centre of the cornea and this may become elevated and ulcerated during the next 2 days although spontaneous recovery at this stage is quite common. This opacity becomes quite extensive and at the peak of the inflammation, about 6 days after signs first appear, it may cover the entire cornea. The colour of the opacity varies from white to deep yellow. As the acute inflammation subsides, the ocular discharge becomes purulent and the opacity begins to shrink, complete recovery occurring after a total course of 3 to 5 weeks.

One or both eyes may be affected. The degree of ulceration in the early stages can be readily determined by the infusion of a 2 per cent fluorescein solution into the conjunctival sac, the ulcerated area retaining the strain.

About 2 per cent of eyes have complete residual opacity but most heal completely with a small, white scar persisting in some. In severe cases the cornea becomes conical in shape, there is marked vascularization of the cornea, and ulceration at the tip of the swelling leads to under-running of the cornea with bright yellow pus surrounded by a zone of erythema. These eyes may rupture and result in complete blindness.

Clinical Pathology

Swabs should be taken from the conjunctival sac and the sensitivity of cultured organisms determined. *M. bovis* has rather exacting requirements in culture media and special care is needed if the organism is to be identified. Serum agglutinins (1:80 to 1:640) are present 2 to 3 weeks after clinical signs commence (4). Necropsy examinations are not usually carried out and the paucity of pathological information contributes to the poor definition of the disease.

Diagnosis

Traumatic conjunctivitis is usually easily diagnosed because of the presence of foreign matter in the eye or evidence of a physical injury. The infectious nature of keratitis caused by *M. bovis* presents difficulties in differentiation between it and the conjunctivitis of infectious bovine rhinotracheitis and the keratitis of bovine malignant catarrh. The latter two diseases have other obvious signs and their ocular lesions and development are quite different. Photosensitive keratitis and thelaziasis are other diseases requiring to be differentiated.

Treatment

Early, acute cases respond well to treatment with many preparations including sulphonamides, particularly sulphacetamide and collyria or ointments, containing chloramphenicol (0·1 to 1·0 per cent), chlortetracycline (0·25 to 0·5 per cent) and eye pellets which contain oxytetracycline (5 mg.), polymixin B sulphate (10,000 units) and tetracaine hydrochloride (1 mg.). Daily treatment with a solution of tylosin (50 mg. per ml.—0·5 ml. per eye) sprayed into affected eyes and an ointment containing 0·5 per cent ethidium bromide are also effective. Lotions, ointments and pellets are preferred to dusting powders which are easy to apply but cause initial irritation. An aerosol powder containing furazolidone has been recommended (11). The medicament should be applied at least once daily and preferably three times daily if signs have been present for a few days.

When ulceration has occurred, recovery is always protracted and more drastic measures should be combined with the treatments listed above. Cauterization of the ulcer with a silver nitrate stick may produce the desired result. The subconjunctival injection of cortisone (0·1 g.) has been recommended and may promote more rapid healing and relieve the patient's distress. The subcutaneous injection of a mixed bacterin or one containing killed *M. bovis* has been used in treatment with variable results.

Control

Eradication or prevention of the disease does not seem possible because of the method of spread.

Probably the best that can be done is to keep animals under close surveillance and isolate and treat any cattle that show excessive lacrimation and blepharospasm. The fact that affected animals are immune for up to 12 months suggests that vaccination may be efficient in control. However, commercial bacterins, although available, have given inconsistent results.

REFERENCES

(1) Wilcox, G. E. (1968). *Vet. Bull.*, *38*, 349.
(2) Pugh, G. W. *et al.* (1970). *Amer. J. vet. Res.*, *31*, 653.
(3) Wilcox, G. E. (1970). *Aust. vet. J.*, *46*, 409, 415.
(4) Hughes, D. E. & Pugh, G. W. (1970). *J. Amer. vet. med. Ass.*, *157*, 443, 452.
(5) Pugh, G. W. & Hughes, D. E. (1971). *Cornell Vet.*, *61*, 23.
(6) Wilcox, G. E. (1970). *Aust. vet. J.*, *46*, 253.
(7) Langford, E. V. & Dorward, W. J. (1969). *Canad. J. comp. Med.*, *33*, 275.
(8) Pugh, G. W. *et al.* (1968). *Amer. J. vet. Res.*, *29*, 2057.
(9) Steve, P. C. & Lilly, J. H. (1965). *J. econ. Ent.*, *58*, 444.
(10) Henson, J. B. & Grumbles, L. C. (1961). *Cornell Vet.*, *51*, 267.
(11) Vernimb, G. D. *et al.* (1969). *Vet. Med.*, *64*, 708.

Septicaemia Caused by *Haemophilus agni*

An acute, highly fatal septicaemia caused by *Haem. agni* has occurred in lambs aged 6 to 7 months (1). Depression, high fever (42°C or 107°F) and disinclination to move due to muscle stiffness are the obvious clinical signs and affected lambs may die within 12 hours of becoming ill. Lambs which survive more than 24 hours develop a severe arthritis. The method of transmission is unknown but the disease does not appear to spread by pen contact nor can it be produced by oral, nasal or conjunctival exposure to the organism. At necropsy the most striking feature is the presence of multiple haemorrhages throughout the carcase. Focal hepatic necrosis surrounded by a zone of haemorrhage is also a constant finding. Lambs which die in the early stages of the disease show minimal joint changes but those that survive for more than 24 hours develop a fibrinopurulent arthritis. A basilar meningitis also develops in the more protracted cases. Death appears to result from asphyxia due to pulmonary congestion and oedema. Histologically the disease is basically a disseminated bacterial thrombosis leading to a severe focal vasculitis. This change is most apparent in the liver and skeletal muscles.

The characteristic hepatic lesions and histology serve to identify the disease, and final diagnosis depends on isolation of the organism. A complement fixation test is available (2), detectable antibodies persisting for about 3 months. The disease is likely to be confused with acute septicaemia caused by *E. coli* or *Past. haemolytica*, and enterotoxaemia.

The morbidity rate is undetermined but the mortality rate is likely to be 100 per cent unless treatment is undertaken. Streptomycin is effective if given early. Because of the acute nature of the disease, vaccination is likely to be the only satisfactory method of control. Although a satisfactory vaccine has not been developed, immunity after a field attack seems to be solid.

A similar disease has been observed in baby pigs of 1 to 2 weeks of age and from which an organism of the *Haem. parainfluenzae* group has been isolated (3). Treatment of in-contact pigs with streptomycin after the first death prevented further losses in subsequent episodes.

REFERENCES

(1) Kennedy, P. C. *et al.* (1958). *Amer. J. vet. Res.*, *19*, 645.
(2) Biberstein, E. L. *et al.* (1959). *J. Amer. vet. med. Ass.*, *135*, 61.
(3) Thomson, R. G. & Ruhnke, H. L. (1963). *Canad. vet. J.*, *4*, 271.

Thromboembolic Meningo-encephalitis

(*Sleeper Syndrome*)

An infectious meningo-encephalitis has been observed in feedlot cattle in the U.S.A. (1) and Canada (2) and has reached a sufficient incidence to arouse concern. The causative organism has been classified as one closely resembling *Haem. agni* and *Act. actinoides*. The morbidity rate is usually low but may reach 10 per cent and the mortality rate is about 95 per cent. Older cattle of 800 to 1000 lb. body weight, and which have been on feed for 1 to 4 months are the group principally affected.

The earliest signs of illness are stiffness and reluctance to move accompanied by a high fever (42°C or 107°F). A characteristic sign is holding of the head up and forward. Subsequent stupor, opisthotonus, ataxia, weakness and paralysis occur. Other, inconstant nervous signs include circling, nystagmus, strabismus and blindness. The course of the disease is very short and death commonly occurs within 6 hours of the first signs of illness. Clonic convulsions are not uncommon in the terminal stages.

At necropsy the conspicuous lesions are haemorrhagic infarcts in any part of the brain. These are often multiple and vary in colour from bright red to brown and in diameter from 1 to 4 cm. Opalescence of the meninges may be apparent in the vicinity of the lesions. Haemorrhages may also be present in the myocardium, skeletal muscles and kidneys and there is excess fluid in the pericardial sac and joint capsules.

This disease is reported to be only one of a series of syndromes caused by this infection (3). In addition to the peracute neurological form described there are in addition an acute respiratory form and a subacute–chronic form manifest as an arthritis. In the respiratory form there is a harsh, dry cough, a temperature of 41 °C (106 °F) and other signs of respiratory distress. In the chronic form there is arthritis with stiffness and lameness. Some involvement of the cervical intervertebral joints occurs, causing stiffness of the neck. The Pandy globulin test on CSF is usually strongly positive (4).

Treatment with streptomycin or broad spectrum antibiotics in the very early stages is highly effective but animals with advanced signs respond poorly to parenteral treatment. In these cases withdrawal of excess cerebro-spinal fluid and injection of an antibiotic may be of value. Satisfactory control measures have not been developed although application of the usual sanitary procedures is recommended. In persistent outbreaks dispersal of confined cattle to pasture may be indicated.

REFERENCES

(1) Kennedy, P. C. *et al.* (1960). *Amer. J. vet. Res.*, *21*, 403.
(2) van Dreumel, A. A. *et al.* (1970). *Canad. vet. J.*, *11*, 125.
(3) Panciera, J. R. *et al.* (1968). *Path. vet.*, *5*, 212.
(4) Little, P. B. & Sorenson, D. K. (1969). *J. Amer. vet. med. Ass.*, *155*, 1892.

Infectious Polyarthritis

(*Glasser's Disease, Porcine Polyserositis*)

This disease of young pigs caused by *Haemophilus suis* occurs in outbreaks and is manifested by acute polyarthritis, pleurisy, pericarditis and peritonitis.

Incidence

Reports of this disease have come mainly from Europe (4), but it has also been observed in Australia (1), the U.S.A. (2) and Canada (3).

Outbreaks usually occur in 2- to 4-months-old pigs which have been recently chilled or transported. Although it seems to occur in most countries, there are few records of the disease. Usually a number of pigs in each group is affected and the mortality rate is high if the pigs are not treated.

Aetiology

Haem. suis has been identified as the cause of the disease (4, 9) but similar syndromes have been attributed to other causative agents. A Gramnegative coccoid to coccobacillary organism which cannot be cultivated on ordinary media but can be propagated in the yolk sac of 5- to 7-day chick embryos has been isolated (2). Pleuropneumonialike organisms isolated from pigs (3) and goats (5) have also been used to produce a disease indistinguishable from infectious polyarthritis and these organisms may combine with *Haem. suis* to produce Glasser's disease. A polyserositis is not uncommon in enzootic pneumonia of pigs and is probably caused by the agent of that disease. Another unidentified, filterable agent has also been described as a cause (6).

Certain circumstances, particularly transport, chilling and parasitism, appear to precipitate attacks of the disease.

Transmission and Pathogenesis

Little is known of the method of transmission or the pathogenesis of the disease. The disease cannot be accurately described as contagious because of its sporadic nature and its close association with devitalizing influences. It has been suggested that the causative bacteria is common in most herds and that the disease arises only when pigs from uninfected herds are introduced to a contaminated environment, especially if they have been exposed to environmental stress during transport (7).

Clinical Findings

The onset is sudden with a moderate to high fever (40 to 42 °C or 104 to 107 °F), complete anorexia, an unusual, rapid, shallow dyspnoea with an anxious expression, extension of the head, and mouth breathing. Coughing may occur. The animals are very lame, stand up on their toes and move with a short, shuffling gait. All the joints are swollen and painful on palpation. A red to blue discolouration of the skin appears near death. Most cases die 2 to 5 days after the onset of illness. Animals which survive the acute stage of the disease may develop chronic arthritis and some cases of intestinal obstruction caused by peritoneal adhesions occur. Meningitis occurs in some pigs and is manifested by muscle tremor, paralysis and convulsions (8). Although Glasser's disease can occur in pigs of any age, weanling pigs are most commonly and most seriously affected.

Clinical Pathology

Few details are available but the organism should be recoverable from joint fluid and pleural exudate. The disease can be diagnosed serologically on the presence of precipitins in the serum of recovered pigs (4).

Necropsy Findings

A fibrinous pleurisy, pericarditis and peritonitis are constantly present. Pneumonia may also be apparent. The joint fluid is turbid, there is inflammation and oedema of the periarticular tissues and the joint cavities contain flattened, discoid deposits of yellowish green fibrin. A fibrinopurulent meningitis is common and often extends to involve the superficial layers of the brain. *Haem. suis* is most readily isolated from the cerebrospinal fluid.

Diagnosis

As a rule the unusual combination of arthritis, fibrinous serositis and meningitis is sufficient to make a diagnosis of Glasser's disease, but differentiation from the many similar disease entities apparently caused by other agents can only be confirmed by bacteriological examination (4).

The disease may be confused with erysipelas, mycoplasmal arthritis and streptococcal arthritis on clinical examination. Mycoplasmosis is a much milder disease and is manifested principally by the presence of a few unthrifty or lame pigs in the litter just before weaning, rather than an acute outbreak with a high mortality (10). Differentiation between cases of Glasser's disease with meningitis and the other diseases of the nervous system in young pigs, especially streptococcal meningitis and Teschen disease may not be possible without necropsy examination.

Treatment

Sulphadimidine and streptomycin appear to be highly effective in clinical cases provided they are given early in the course of the disease, but the tetracyclines, either by injection or administration in drinking water, are preferred.

Control

Avoidance of undue exposure to adverse environmental conditions at weaning is recommended. Prophylactic dosing at the time of shipping or medication of feed or drinking water on arrival with the above mentioned drugs may be of value in preventing outbreaks.

REFERENCES

(1) Sutherland, A. K. & Simmons, G. C. (1947). *Aust. vet. J.*, *23*, 91.
(2) Willigan, D. A. & Beamer, P. D. (1955). *J. Amer. vet. med. Ass.*, *126*, 118.
(3) Carter, G. R. & Schroder, J. D. (1956). *Cornell Vet.*, *46*, 344.
(4) Hjarre, A. (1958). *Advanc. vet. Sci.*, *4*, 235.
(5) Cordy, D. R. *et al.* (1958). *Cornell Vet.*, *48*, 25.
(6) McNutt, S. H. *et al.* (1945). *Amer. J. vet. Res.*, *6*, 247.
(7) Leece, G. (1960). *J. Amer. vet. med. Ass.*, *137*, 345.
(8) Radostits, O. M. *et al.* (1963). *Canad. vet. J.*, *4*, 265.
(9) Neil, D. H. *et al.* (1969). *Canad. J. comp. Med.*, *33*, 187.
(10) King, S. J. (1968). *Aust. vet. J.*, *44*, 227.

18

Diseases Caused by Bacteria—IV

DISEASES CAUSED BY *MYCOBACTERIUM* Spp.

TUBERCULOSIS, Johne's disease and skin tuberculosis are described in this section. Mastitis due to *Mycobacterium lacticola* is described in the section on mastitis.

Tuberculosis Caused by *Mycobacterium bovis*

The disease caused by *Myco. bovis* is characterized by the progressive development of tubercles in any of the organs in most species.

Incidence

Tuberculosis occurs in every country of the world and is of major importance in dairy cattle. The disease can occur in all species including man and is of importance for public health reasons as well as for its detrimental effects on animal production. The relative importance of environment in the causation of the disease is suggested by the high incidence in those countries in which animals are housed indoors during the winter months. In spite of the low overall incidence in countries where cattle are at pasture all the year round, individual herds with 60 to 70 per cent incidence may be encountered. Amongst beef cattle the degree of infection is usually much lower because of the open range conditions under which they are kept. However, individual beef herds may suffer a high morbidity if infected animals are introduced and large numbers of animals have to drink from stagnant water holes, especially during dry seasons (1). It is difficult to assess the economic importance of the disease in cattle. Apart from actual deaths, it is estimated that infected animals lose 10 to 25 per cent of their productive efficiency.

In pigs the incidence is usually much lower but reflects the incidence in the local cattle population from which the infection derives either by the ingestion of dairy products or by grazing over the same pasture as cattle. The lower relative incidence in pigs is due to a number of factors, particularly the tendency of the disease to remain localized in this species and the early age of slaughter. The incidence is higher in older pigs. When the disease is common among dairy cattle in an area, 10 to 20 per cent of the local pigs are likely to be infected. Because the disease is relatively benign in pigs, major financial loss does not occur. Some losses are experienced due to the rejection of carcases or parts at the abattoir.

In horses and sheep the disease occurs rarely, largely due to limited exposure to infection but natural resistance also appears to play a part. In goats the disease is uncommon but natural resistance is not as high as in horses and sheep, and if heavy exposure to *Myco. bovis* does occur, a high morbidity rate may be encountered.

Spread of tuberculosis from animals to man makes this an important zoonosis. Infection in man occurs largely through consumption of infected milk by children but spread can also occur by inhalation. Transmission to man can be almost completely eliminated by pasteurization of milk but only complete eradication of the disease can protect the farmer and his family.

Aetiology

All species and age groups are susceptible to *Myco. bovis*, with cattle, goats and pigs most susceptible and sheep and horses showing a high natural resistance (2). Zebu (Brahman) type cattle are much more resistant to tuberculosis than European cattle and the effects on the animal are much less severe (1). Goats are quite susceptible and if they are maintained in association with infected herds of cattle the incidence may be as high as 28 per cent. Tuberculosis may also be encountered in camels, deer, bison and other wild fauna and birds and these animals may act as a source of infection for cattle.

Myco. bovis is the common cause of tuberculosis in cattle. In the other animal species, *Myco. avium* may account for a considerable proportion of cases of tuberculosis especially in pigs kept in close association with infected birds (4, 3). In these circumstances many of the infections are caused by *M. avium*-like bacteria rather than *M. avium*. Infection seems to occur via the alimentary tract and there is a great tendency for self-cure of gross lesions to occur. The subject is discussed elsewhere under the heading of tuberculosis caused by atypical mycobacteria (p. 405). The human strain (*Myco. tuberculosis*) may account for a small proportion of cases in animals.

Although the organism does not form spores, it is moderately resistant to heat, desiccation and many disinfectants. It is readily destroyed by direct sunlight unless it is in a moist environment. In warm, moist, protected positions, it may remain viable for very long periods.

Transmission

Although mediate contagion can occur, the infected animal is the main source of infection. Organisms are excreted in the exhaled air, in sputum, faeces (from both intestinal lesions and swallowed sputum from pulmonary lesions), milk, urine, vaginal and uterine discharges and discharges from open peripheral lymph nodes. Commonly entry is effected by inhalation or ingestion. Inhalation is more probable when animals are housed. On the other hand, ingestion is the more common route of infection when animals are at pasture and contaminate the feed and communal drinking water and feed troughs. Under natural conditions, stagnant drinking water may cause infection up to 18 days after its last use by a tuberculous animal, whereas a running stream does not represent an important source of infection to cattle in downstream fields. It is difficult to give details of the persistence of infectivity of pasture and other inanimate objects because of the varying conditions under which experiments have been carried out. Viable *Myco. tuberculosis* can be isolated from the faeces of infected cattle and from ground in contact with the faeces for 6 to 8 weeks after the faeces are dropped but the duration of the infectivity of the pasture to susceptible cattle varies widely. The period may be as short as one week if the weather is dry and pastures are harrowed but will be much longer in wet weather. Separation of infected and susceptible animals by a fence provides practical protection against spread of the disease.

The drinking of infected milk by young animals is one of the commonest methods by which tuberculosis is spread. Less common routes of infection include intra-uterine infection at coitus, by the use of infected semen or of infected insemination or uterine pipettes, and intramammary infection by the use of contaminated teat siphons or by way of infected cups of milking machines. The feeding of tuberculous cattle carcases to pigs has also caused a severe outbreak of the disease. Unusual sources of infection are infected cats, goats or even human caretakers.

Pathogenesis

Tuberculosis spreads in the body by two stages, the primary complex and postprimary dissemination. The primary complex consists of the lesion at the point of entry and in the local lymph node. A lesion at the point of entry is common when infection is by inhalation. When infection occurs via the alimentary tract, a lesion at the site of entry is unusual although tonsillar and intestinal ulcers may occur. More commonly the only observable lesion is in the pharyngeal or mesenteric lymph nodes.

Post-primary dissemination from the primary complex varies considerably in rate and route. It may take the form of acute miliary tuberculosis, discrete nodular lesions in various organs, or chronic organ tuberculosis caused by endogenous or exogenous re-infection of tissues rendered allergic to tuberculoprotein. In the latter case there may be no involvement of the local lymph node. Depending upon the sites of localization of infection, clinical signs vary but there is the constant underlying toxaemia which causes weakness, debility and the eventual death of the animal.

In cattle, horses, sheep and goats, the disease is a progressive one and, although generalized tuberculosis is not uncommon in pigs, localization as non-progressive abscesses in the lymph nodes of the head and neck is the most common finding.

Clinical Findings

Cattle. Although signs referable to localization in a particular organ usually attract attention to the possible occurrence of tuberculosis, some general signs are also evident. Some cows with extensive miliary tubercular lesions are clinically normal but progressive emaciation unassociated with other signs should always arouse suspicion of tuberculosis. A capricious appetite and fluctuating temperature are also commonly associated with the disease. The condition of the hair-coat is variable; it may be rough or sleek. Affected animals tend to become more docile and sluggish but the eyes remain bright and alert. These general signs often become more pronounced after calving.

Pulmonary involvement is characterized by a chronic cough due to bronchopneumonia. The cough is never loud or paroxysmal, occurring only once or twice at a time and is low, suppressed and moist. It is easily stimulated by squeezing the pharynx or by exercise and is most common in the morning or in cold weather. In the advanced stages when much lung has been destroyed, dyspnoea with increased rate and depth of respiration becomes apparent. At this stage, abnormalities may be detected by auscultation and percussion of the chest. Areas with no breath sounds and dullness on percussion are accompanied by areas in which squeaky râles are audible. Tuberculous pleurisy may occur but is usually symptomless and there is no effusion. Involvement of the bronchial lymph nodes may cause dyspnoea because of constriction of air passages, and enlargement of the mediastinal lymph node is commonly associated with recurrent and then persistent ruminal tympany.

The most common signs of alimentary involvement are caused by pressure of enlarged lymph nodes on surrounding organs. Rarely tuberculous ulcers of the small intestine cause diarrhoea. Retropharyngeal lymph node enlargement causes dysphagia and noisy breathing due to pharyngeal obstruction. Such lymph node enlargements may be part of a primary complex or be due to post-primary dissemination. Pharyngeal palpation with the aid of a speculum reveals a large, firm, rounded swelling in the dorsum of the pharynx.

Chronic, painless swelling of the submaxillary, prescapular, precrural and supramammary lymph nodes is relatively rare. Uterine tuberculosis is uncommon with bovine strains except in advanced cases. It may occur as a result of coitus or the use of contaminated uterine catheters, or by contiguity from tuberculous peritonitis, but in most cases results from generalized haemotogenous spread. In the case of spread by contiguity from peritonitis, bursitis and salpingitis are common, the lesions in the salpinx taking the form of small enlargements containing a few drops of yellow fluid. Similar lesions may occur by upward spread from the uterus to the peritoneum. In tuberculous metritis, there may be interference with conception, or conception may be followed by recurrent abortion late in pregnancy, or a live calf is produced which in most cases dies quickly of generalized tuberculosis. Lesions similar to those of brucellosis occur on the placenta. In cows which fail to conceive, there may be a chronic purulent discharge heavily infected with the organism and the condition is very resistant to treatment. A number of cows will have an associated tuberculous vaginitis affecting chiefly the ducts of Gärtner. Rare cases of tuberculous orchitis are characterized by the development of large, indurated, painless testicles.

Tuberculous mastitis is of major importance because of the danger to public health, and of spread of the disease to calves and the difficulty of differentiating it from other forms of mastitis. Its characteristic feature is a marked induration and hypertrophy which usually develops first in the upper part of the udder, particularly in the rear quarters. Palpation of the supramammary lymph nodes is essential in all cases of suspected tuberculous mastitis. Enlargement of the nodes with fibrosis of the quarter does not necessarily indicate tuberculosis but enlargement without udder induration suggests either tuberculosis or lymphomatosis. In the early stages, the milk is not macroscopically abnormal but later very fine floccules appear which settle after the milk stands leaving a clear, amber fluid. Later still the secretion may be an amber fluid only.

Pigs. Tuberculous lesions in cervical lymph nodes usually cause no clinical abnormality unless they rupture to the exterior. Generalized cases present a syndrome similar to that seen in cattle although tuberculous involvement of the meninges and joints is rather more common.

Horses. The commonest syndrome in horses is caused by involvement of the cervical vertebrae in which a painful osteomyelitis causes stiffness of the neck and inability to eat off the ground (5). Less common signs include polyuria, coughing due to pulmonary lesions, lymph node enlargement, nasal discharge and a fluctuating temperature.

Sheep and goats. Bronchopneumonia is the commonest form of the disease in these species and is manifested by cough and terminal respiratory embarrassment. In some goats intestinal ulceration, with diarrhoea, and enlargement of the lymph nodes of the alimentary tract occurs. In both species the disease is only slowly progressive, and in affected flocks many more reactors and necropsy-positive cases are often found than would be expected from the clinical cases which are evident. In kids the disease may be more rapidly progressive and cause early death.

Clinical Pathology

Because of the universal dependence on the tuberculin test for diagnosis and the policy of slaughtering all positive reactors whether they are open cases or not, few clinico-pathological tests are now carried out. Sputum or discharges may be examined by inoculation into guinea pigs with necropsy of the guinea pigs at 6 to 7 weeks. An alternative procedure is to use a tuberculin test on the experimental animals 19 to 21 days after inoculation.

The basis of all tuberculosis eradication schemes is the tuberculin test and a knowledge of the various tests used, their deficiencies and advantages is essential. It should be remembered, however, that clinical examination is still of value particularly in seeking out the occasional advanced cases which do not give a positive reaction to a tuberculin test. Much attention is being directed to devising tests to detect such animals but the eye of an observant clinician can still be the most important factor in problem herds where positive reactors keep recurring. The application of control measures based on a knowledge of the epidemiology of the disease is too often neglected when such measures may considerably reduce the time necessary to eradicate the disease from a herd.

Single intradermal test. (SID test). This test is applied by the intradermal injection of 0·05 ml. of tuberculin into an anal fold. The tuberculin is prepared from cultures of *Myco. tuberculosis* or *Myco. bovis* grown on synthetic media. The former is more potent than the latter, particularly when used on poorly sensitized animals. The reaction is read between 72 and 96 hours after injection and a positive reaction constitutes a diffuse swelling at the injection site. Comparison with the opposite fold by palpation and inspection is desirable when making a decision. In the U.S.A., an additional injection is made into the lip of the vulva at the mucocutaneous junction.

In England the injection is made into the skin of the neck and measurement of the injection site with calipers gives more accuracy in determining reactions. The skin of the neck area is much more sensitive than that of the tail area but the test suffers from the necessity to restrain each animal and measure all reactions carefully. Varying dose rates of tuberculin have been recommended and, with increasing demands for standardization of the test to increase its accuracy, the exact dose for the particular tuberculin should be strictly adhered to when the cervical skin test is used. In the U.S.A., 0·1 ml. is recommended for herds of unknown status and 0·2 ml. in known infected herds when cases with low sensitivity are to be carefully sought. The method of injection of tuberculin also has some importance when the cervical site is used. A careful intradermal injection produces the largest swelling and a quick thrust the least. Variations in technique appear to have little effect on the size of reaction when the caudal fold is used.

The main disadvantage of the SID test is its lack of specificity and the number of no-visible-lesion reactors (NVLs) which occur. Mammalian tuberculin is not sufficiently specific to differentiate between reactions due to infection with *Myco. bovis* and infection with *Myco. avium*, *Myco. tuberculosis*, *Myco. paratuberculosis* (including vaccination) or *Nocardia farcinicus*. The maximum permissible rate of NVL reactors is 10 per cent and when this rate is exceeded, tests other than the SID test should be used. Other disadvantages of the SID test include failure to detect cases of minimal sensitivity such as may occur in the early or late stages of the disease, in old cows and in cows which have recently calved. This failure to detect tuberculous animals can be of considerable importance and must receive close attention when reactors are detected at an initial test. Serological tests to detect these cases of minimal sensitivity have been devised but are not sufficiently accurate for use in individual animals. The available tests devised to overcome these deficiencies of the SID test are the Short Thermal, Stormont and comparative tests. The use of diluted tuberculins does not increase the specificity of the tuberculin test (6).

Short thermal test. Intradermal tuberculin (4 ml.) is injected subcutaneously into the neck of cattle with a rectal temperature of not more than 39 °C (102 °F) at the time of injection and for 2 hours later. If the temperature at 4, 6 and 8 hours after injection rises above 40 °C (104 °F), the animal is classed as a positive reactor. The temperature peak is usually at 6 to 8 hours. Preliminary evidence indicates a high efficiency of the test in detecting 'spreader' cases giving negative intradermal tests. Occasional deaths due to anaphylaxis occur at the peak of the reaction, and there is one report of recumbency, which responded to intravenous therapy with calcium salts, in a large number of tuberculous cows submitted to this test.

Intravenous tuberculin test. Such a test has been used experimentally but requires a special research tuberculin (7). As in the previous test a positive reaction is a febrile one at 4 to 6 hours after injection, continuing for at least 8 hours and the elevation of temperature to exceed 1·7 °C. There is difficulty in interpreting the test and haematological changes may have to be considered to avoid false negative tests (8).

Stormont test. This test has been devised to select those animals which are poorly sensitized for any reason. The test is performed similarly to the single intradermal test in the neck with a further injection at the same site 7 days later. An increase in skin thickness of 5 mm. or more, 24 hours after this second injection is a positive result. The increased sensitivity is thought to be due to the attraction of antibodies to the site by the first injection. The increased sensitivity begins at the fifth day, is at its peak at the seventh and ends on the twelfth day after the injection. Preliminary trials indicate very high efficiency in detecting the poorly sensitized animal but extensive field trials have not as yet been reported. Cattle infected with *Myco. avium* do not give a positive reaction but 'skin tuberculosis' cases do. It is more accurate than the single intradermal test and has been adopted as the official test in Northern Ireland. A practical difficulty is the necessity for three visits to the farm. Special purified protein derivative (PPD) tuberculin of a specified potency must be used to fulfil the requirements of the test.

The comparative test. Where the presence of Johne's disease or avian tuberculosis is suspected or 'skin tuberculosis' is apparent, non-specific sensitization must be considered, and a comparative test used. Transitory sensitization may occur in cattle due to the presence of human tuberculosis in their attendants but the comparative test will not differentiate the sensitivity from that due to bovine strain infection.

The comparative test depends on the greater sensitivity to homologous tuberculin. Avian and mammalian tuberculin are injected simultaneously into two separate sites on the same side of the neck, 12 cm. apart and one above the other, and the test is read 72 hours later. Care must be taken in placing the injections as sensitivity varies from place to place in the skin. The greater of the two reactions indicates the organism responsible for the sensitization. The test is not generally intended for primary use in detecting reactors but only to follow up known reactors to determine the infecting organism. However, the single intradermal comparative test has been used in the highly successful eradication programme in Great Britain. Its use as a primary test is recommended when a high incidence of avian tuberculosis or Johne's disease is anticipated, or when vaccination against Johne's disease has been carried out. The comparative test is adequate to differentiate between vaccination against Johne's disease and tuberculosis and the distinction is easier the longer ago the vaccination was performed (9).

Special Aspects of Sensitivity to Tuberculin

Site of injection. Sensitivity to tuberculin injected intradermally varies considerably from site to site on the body. In cattle the relative sensitivities of different areas to tuberculin and to johnin have been determined as follows: Back—1, Upper Side—$1\frac{3}{4}$, Lower Side—$2\frac{1}{2}$, Neck—$2\frac{3}{4}$–3. The cervical area is also much more sensitive than the anal fold, and has the advantages that reactions are more pronounced, animals can be retested immediately and the area is more sanitary. Its disadvantages are that restraint of each animal is necessary and the proportion of NVL reactors increases.

Potency of tuberculins. In the search for more specific and potent allergens, bovine and human types have been used to prepare tuberculins for comparison, the latter being the more potent. PPD tuberculins are in general use because of the greater ease with which they are standardized and their greater specificity.

Desensitization during tuberculin testing. When a suspicious reactor is encountered, the question of when to retest is complicated by the phenomenon of desensitization. When tuberculin is absorbed into the body, desensitization occurs and its degree increases in general terms with the amount of tuberculin and the amount of other foreign proteins absorbed. Thus desensitization is more marked and of longer duration after a subcutaneous than after an intradermal injection. One of the characteristics of the allergic reaction is the variation in differential white cell count of the blood which occurs. Polymorphonuclear cells increase and lymphocytes decrease and there is a suggestion that the greater the variation in cell count the longer the duration of desensitization. After a single intradermal injection, the leucocytic reaction is of a minor degree and is not a very reliable guide to the diagnosis of tuberculosis. Moreover the period of desensitization is short and the animal can be retested within a few days. However, after a Stormont test the leucocyte reaction is very marked in sensitive animals and is of diagnostic significance. Although the period of desensitization after this test is not definitely known, it is of relatively long duration although not more than 6 months. The diagnostic value of this leucocyte reaction is vitiated to some extent by the variation in the time at which it occurs (6 to 24 hours) and by the fact that other factors such as parturition, injection of adrenal cortical hormone and infective processes produce a similar reaction.

One further aspect of the desensitization phenomenon is that use can be made of it to obscure a positive reaction. If tuberculin is injected so that the test is made in the desensitized period, no reaction will occur in infected animals.

Post-parturient desensitization. Tuberculous cattle go through a period of desensitization immediately before and after calving and as many as 30 per cent give false negative reactions returning to a positive status 4 to 6 weeks later. The loss of sensitivity is probably due to the removal of fixed cell antibodies from the skin into the general circulation and subsequent drainage into the colostrum. Calves drinking this colostrum give positive reactions for up to 3 weeks after birth even though they are not infected.

Summary of testing procedures in cattle. In summary it is usual to use the single intradermal test as a routine procedure but the test is not completely accurate and the following deficiencies may occur.

False positive reactions (no gross lesion reactors) may be given by:

(i) Animals sensitized to other mycobacterial allergens. These may include animals infected with human or avian tuberculosis or with Johne's disease. Animals with minimal local lesions caused by relatively non-pathogenic mycobacteria, e.g. skin tuberculosis, also react to tuberculin. It is also possible that animals infected with, or which perhaps only ingest (10), non-pathogenic mycobacteria can also become sensitized and react to the test. For example atypical mycobacteria in permanent waters inhabited by birds are thought to be the cause of the very high incidence of non-specific reactors in Kenyan cattle. Stagnant water is one of the most potent sources of saprophytic mycobacteria and some attention

should be given to it when non-specific reactors occur. Another source is poultry litter fed to cattle when the birds are infected with *M. avium* (4).

(ii) Animals sensitized to other allergens which may be bacterial, e.g. *N. farcinicus* in bovine farcy (11), or not.

False negative reactions may be given by:

(i) Advanced cases of tuberculosis.

(ii) Early cases until 6 weeks after infection.

(iii) Cows which have calved within the preceding 6 weeks.

(iv) Animals desensitized by tuberculin administration during the preceding 8 to 60 days.

(v) Old cattle.

A summary of the tests available and their recommended use is set out in the table below. A field comparison of the methods has been conducted in New Zealand (12) which concludes that a repeat of the SID test in the caudal fold is the most effective way of differentiating between specific and non-specific tuberculin sensitivity. The best results were obtained by rigid definition of the permissible levels of reactions and their measurement by instrument.

Reactors which are thought to be non-specific should be retested by the comparative test in the cervical region 1 to 2 months after the initial test (13). For greater accuracy sensitins prepared from

Tuberculin Tests and When to Use Them

Circumstances	Tests to be Used	Comments
Initial test in unknown herd	1. S.I.D.	Preferred because only two visits required and period of desensitization short. Considerable error with non-specific reactors and animals with reduced sensitivity, e.g. recent calving, advanced cases.
	2. Stormont.	Three trips required and long period of desensitization preventing frequent retests.
Probable advanced cases in heavily infected herd	1. Stormont. 2. Short Thermal.	Accurate. Too time-consuming for ordinary circumstances.
Cows calved within preceding 6 weeks	Stormont.	Accuracy of Short Thermal test unknown in this group.
Suspicious reactors	1. Stormont.	S.I.D. easily converted to Stormont with two more visits and answer obtained quickly.
	2. Isolate and retest with S.I.D. in 1 month.	Long wait for answer.
	3. Immediate S.I.D. in other fold.	During desensitization period and animal may not react.
In herds where avian T.B. or Johne's disease suspected	1. S.I.D. comparative. 2. Stormont.	Relative merits uncertain. Stormont does not react with Johne's or avian T.B.
Introduction to free herd or recently assembled herd	S.I.D. and repeat in 1 or 2 months.	Stormont would prevent quick retest and early cases may be missed for too long.

other mycobacteria, e.g. the poorly pathogenic Runyon IV (4), can be included in the test agents (14).

Tuberculin testing in pigs. The most generally used method is the SID test, injecting 0·1 ml. of standard potency mammalian tuberculin into a fold of skin at the base of the ear, but the test is relatively inaccurate in this species (2, 15). The test is read 24 to 48 hours later and an increase in skin thickness of 5 mm. or more constitutes a positive reaction. In positive animals the reactions are quite marked, the skin thickening often exceeding 10 mm. and showing superficial necrosis and sloughing. If the animal is infected with *Myco. avium*, the maximum skin thickening may not occur until 48 hours after injection. When no attempt is being made to determine the type of infection, mixed avian and mammalian tuberculins may be used and the test read at 24 or 48 hours. If avian tuberculin alone is used, the test should be read at 48 to 72 hours and an increase in skin thickness of 4 mm. is classed as positive.

Many suspicious reactions occur in pigs because of the tendency of lesions to regress and the sensitivity to tuberculin to diminish, maximum sensitivity occurring 3 to 9 weeks after infection. A retest in 6 to 8 weeks should determine whether or not the disease is progressing. Although positive reactors may in time revert to a negative status, there may be macroscopic lesions in these animals at necropsy. However, viable organisms are not usually recoverable from the lesion, the infection apparently having been overcome.

The Stormont test is unlikely to have any application in pigs because there is no local increase in skin sensitivity after one injection. Some decrease in skin sensitivity after parturition occurs in sows affected with *Myco. bovis* but may not occur when the infection is caused by *Myco. avium*. Comparative tests work efficiently in this species with little or no reaction to heterologous tuberculin. Haematological changes in pigs during the period of reaction to tuberculin are comparable to those which occur in cattle.

Tuberculin testing in other species. In the horse the results obtained with subcutaneous and intradermal tuberculin tests are very erratic and must be assessed with caution especially when the test is positive as many false positives occur (16, 17). The horse appears to be much more sensitive than cattle to tuberculin and much smaller doses of standardized tuberculin are required than in cattle (2, 16). As little as 0·1 ml. of PPD tuberculin is sufficient to elicit a positive reaction and a normal dose may provoke an anaphylactic reaction. No safe recommendations can be made on tests in this species because of lack of detailed information, but the occurrence of a systemic reaction with a positive cutaneous test can be accepted as indicating the presence of infection.

The single intradermal test has been used in sheep and goats but is relatively inaccurate, some tuberculous animals giving negative reactions (2). The test injection is usually given in the caudal fold as in cattle and an increase in thickness of 5 mm. in the fold constitutes a positive reaction.

Serological Tests for Diagnosis of Tuberculosis

Serological tests including complement fixation (18), fluorescent antibody (27), direct bacterial agglutination, precipitin and haemagglutination tests are under review but seem to have little potential value for the diagnosis of tuberculosis (19), except for the observed marked rise in haemagglutination antibodies which occurs in many infected cattle one week after an injection of tuberculin (20). The fluorescent antibody test can detect sensitivity to *M. avium* in calves, but is unable to distinguish between that antigen and *M. paratuberculosis*. The complement fixation test reponse to both antigens is poor (19).

Necropsy Findings

Cattle, sheep and goats show identical lesions with a standard distribution. Tuberculous granulomas may be found in any of the lymph nodes, but particularly in bronchial and mediastinal nodes, and many organs. In the lung, miliary abscesses may extend to cause a suppurative bronchopneumonia. The pus has a characteristic cream to orange colour and varies in consistency from thick cream to thick, crumbly cheese. Small nodules may appear on the pleura and peritoneum. These also contain tuberculous pus but are not accompanied by effusion.

All localized lesions of tuberculosis tend to stimulate an enveloping fibrous capsule but the degree of encapsulation varies with the rate of development of the lesion. Apart from the value of a necropsy examination in making a diagnosis, a close study of the lesions may indicate the importance of the subject animal as a spreader of the disease to others. Active or 'open' cases are the dangerous spreaders and these are denoted by the presence of miliary tuberculosis with small, transparent, shot-like lesions in many organs, or by pulmonary lesions which are not well encapsulated and caseated. The presence of bronchopneumonia or hyperaemia around pulmonary lesions is highly suggestive of active disease. Cases with tuberculous mastitis or discharging tuberculous metritis must also be considered as open cases.

'Closed' lesions are characteristically discrete and nodular and contain thick, yellow to orange, caseous material, often calcified and surrounded by a thick, fibrous capsule. Although such lesions are less likely to cause heavy contamination of the environment than open lesions, affected animals may still be important as sources of infection.

Pigs. Some cases of generalized tuberculosis, with miliary tubercles in most organs, are found in pigs. The common finding is localization in the tonsils, submaxillary, cervical, hepatic, bronchial, mediastinal and mesenteric lymph nodes. The nodes are markedly enlarged and consist of masses of white, caseous, sometimes calcified, material, surrounded by a strong, fibrous capsule and interlaced by strands of fibrous tissue. Because of the regressive nature of the disease in pigs, these lesions are often negative on culture and guinea pig inoculation.

Horses. Although the lesions in horses have a characteristic distribution in the intestinal wall, mesenteric lymph nodes and spleen, the lesions themselves have a distinctive appearance which is peculiar to this species. Chronic lesions are firm to the touch and on cutting have an appearance similar to that of neoplastic tissue. In the horse, too, there is a tendency for lesions to develop in the skeleton, particularly the cervical vertebrae.

Diagnosis

Because of the chronic nature of the disease and the multiplicity of signs caused by the variable localization of the infection, tuberculosis is difficult to diagnose on clinical examination. If the disease occurs in an area, it must be considered in the differential diagnosis of many diseases of cattle. In pigs the disease is usually so benign that cases do not present themselves as clinical problems and are found only at necropsy. The rarity of the disease in horses, sheep and goats makes it an unlikely diagnostic risk except in groups which have had abnormally high exposure to infected cattle.

In cattle other chronic pulmonary diseases which may be confused with tuberculous pneumonia are lung abscess due to aspiration pneumonia, pleurisy and pericarditis following traumatic reticulitis and chronic contagious bovine pleuropneumonia. A few animals survive the acute stages of aspiration pneumonia, and show emaciation, chronic cough and changes at auscultation and percussion identical with those of tuberculosis. A history of previous parturient paresis or inefficient drenching are the only points short of tuberculin testing on which to base a differentiation. Sequelae of traumatic reticulitis can produce a clinical picture indistinguishable from tuberculosis but there is usually a history of a severe attack of illness some time previously with gradual but incomplete recovery. Chronic contagious bovine pleuropneumonia is to be suspected in an enzootic area and the complement fixation test provides a suitable diagnostic method. Simultaneous infection with both diseases is not uncommon.

Snoring respiration is relatively common in cattle and some differentiation of the cause is necessary and practicable. In true 'snoring' due to pharyngeal obstruction, the noise produced is guttural and nasal airflow is unobstructed. Enlarged pharyngeal lymph nodes and granulomatous lesions can be detected on internal palpation of the pharynx. Lymph node enlargement may be due to tuberculosis or actinobacillosis but granulomatous lesions are usually caused by the latter. A tuberculin test is usually necessary to differentiate between these diseases.

Nasal snoring is more common and is a higher pitched, wheezing noise often audible from a distance. It is usually accompanied by nasal discharge and partial or complete obstruction to nasal airflow. Pharyngeal palpation is negative and mouth breathing may be evident. The common causes of nasal obstruction in cattle are allergic rhinitis, mucous polyps in the posterior nares and nodular thickening of the nasal mucosa.

In tuberculous mastitis, fibrosis begins at the base of the gland instead of about the cistern as in most other forms of mastitis, and abnormal milk commonly comes at the end of milking instead of the first few streams and is not marked until the late stages of the disease. Avian tuberculosis may localize in the udder on rare occasions. Tuberculous metritis is characterized by the continued discharge of large quantities of yellow pus. The pus has the appearance of curdled milk and is unlike that in any other form of metritis.

Peripheral lymph node enlargements should be suspected of having a tuberculous origin, but abscesses caused by mixed infections or infection with *Actinobacillus lignieresi* of the lymph nodes of the head are much more common. Bacteriological examination of pus obtained by needle puncture is a simple method of differentiation. Lymphomatosis may be confused with tuberculous lymphadenitis but it is usually characterized by simultaneous, bilateral enlargement of several lymph nodes. The enlarged nodes are softer and smoother than tuberculous nodes and do not usually contain pus.

At necropsy the lesions of tuberculosis in cattle are characteristic but differentiation from lesions caused by actinobacillus, *Corynebacterium pyogenes* infection, coccidioidomycosis and mucormycosis requires some care. Accurate identification may necessitate laboratory examination. In horses, tuberculous lesions closely resemble neoplastic tissue and in pigs, confusion with a number of other diseases is likely to occur. In meat inspection surveys, as many as 50 per cent of suspected tuberculous lesions in pigs are non-tuberculous (15). Opinions differ on the ease with which infections with *Cor. equi* can be distinguished from those caused by mycobacteria on macroscopic or histological grounds (21). Lesions caused by *Myco. avium* are characterized by an absence of necrosis, the lesions being firm and homogeneous with rare foci of calcification.

Treatment

Because of the progress being made in the treatment of human tuberculosis with such drugs as isoniazid, combinations of streptomycin and para-aminosalicylic and other acids, the treatment of animals with tuberculosis has undergone some examination and claims have been made for the efficiency of long term oral medication with isoniazid both as treatment and as prophylaxis (22, 23, 24).

Control

Eradication of bovine tuberculosis has been virtually achieved in many countries. The methods used have depended on a number of factors but ultimately the test and slaughter policy has been the only one by which effective eradication has been achieved.

Control on a herd basis. Control in a herd rests on removal of the infected animals, prevention of spread of infection and avoidance of further introduction of the disease. All three points are of equal importance and neglect of one may result in breakdown of the eradication programme.

Detection of infected animals depends largely upon the use of the tuberculin test. The single intradermal test is widely used but other tests are available (see table on p. 399) and should be used where they are indicated. All animals over three months of age should be tested and positive reactors disposed of according to local legislation. Suspicious reactors may be dealt with in several ways as indicated in the table on p. 399. At the

initial test, a careful clinical examination should be conducted on all animals to ensure that there are no advanced clinical cases which will give negative reactions to the test. Doubtful cases and animals likely to have reduced sensitivity, particularly old cows and those that have calved within the previous six weeks, may be tested by one of the special tests described above or retested subsequently. The comparative test should be used where infection with *Myco. paratuberculosis* or *Myco. avium* is anticipated or where a high incidence of reactors occurs in a herd not showing clinical evidence of the disease.

If the incidence of reactors is high at the first test or if 'open' lesions are found at necropsy in culled animals, emphasis must be placed on repeat testing at short intervals or the spread of the disease may overtake the culling rate. Tests should be conducted at 2-monthly intervals if the incidence is high. Other herds may be retested at 3-monthly intervals until a negative test is obtained. A further test is conducted 6 months later and if the herd is again negative, it may be classed as free of the disease. Subsequent check tests should be carried out annually.

Hygienic measures to prevent the spread of infection should be instituted as soon as the first group of reactors is removed. Feed troughs should be cleaned and thoroughly disinfected with hot, 5 per cent phenol or equivalent cresol disinfectant. Water troughs and drinking cups should be emptied and similarly disinfected. Suspicious reactors being held for retesting should be isolated from the remainder of the herd. If a number of reactors are culled, attention must be given to the possibility of infection being reintroduced with replacements which should come from accredited herds. Failing this, the animals should be tested immediately, isolated and retested in 60 days.

It is most important that calves being reared as herd replacements be fed on tuberculosis-free milk, either from known free animals or pasteurized. Rearing calves on skim milk from a communal source is a particularly dangerous practice unless the skim milk is properly sterilized. All other classes of livestock on the farm should be examined for evidence of tuberculosis. Farm attendants should be checked as they may provide a source of *Myco. tuberculosis* infection, resulting in transient positive reactions in the cattle. Humans may also act as a source of *Myco. bovis* infection.

Steps should be taken to ensure that reinfection does not occur by testing all introductions, preventing communal use of watering facilities or pasture, and maintaining adequate boundary fences. A special problem is created when tuberculosis occurs in cattle run on extensive range country with little manpower and few fences. It is inadvisable to attempt a control programme until it can be guaranteed that all animals can be gathered, identified, tested and segregated. In some areas it is uneconomic to do this.

Control on an area basis. The method used to eradicate bovine tuberculosis from large areas will depend on the incidence of the disease, methods of husbandry, attitude of the farming community and the economic capacity of the country to stand losses from a test and slaughter programme.

An essential first step in the inauguration of an eradication programme is the prior education of the farming community. Livestock owners must be apprised of the economic and public health significance of the disease, its manifestations and the necessity for the various steps in the eradication programme. Eradication must also be compulsory since voluntary schemes have never achieved more than limited control and always leave foci of infection. Adequate compensation must be paid to encourage full co-operation. This may take the form of compensation for animals destroyed or bonuses for disease free herds or their milk or beef.

It is essential at the beginning of a programme to determine the incidence and distribution of the disease by tuberculin testing of samples of the cattle population and a meat inspection service. Information collected in this way indicates the herds and areas which are free of tuberculosis or which have a low incidence. The disease can be readily eradicated from these latter areas, thus providing a nucleus of tuberculosis-free cattle which can supply replacements for further areas as they are brought into the eradication scheme. Finally, the eradication programme can be extended to the residual area.

When the incidence of tuberculosis is high, a routine test and slaughter programme may be economically impossible. Two herd schemes have been used in Europe and elsewhere but are now of historical interest only. Ostertag's method was based on separation of the cattle into two herds on the basis of clinical examination. Bang's method utilized the tuberculin test to separate the infected and uninfected animals into two herds. The most attractive alternative to an immediate test and slaughter programme is to gradually free farms and areas and allow reactors to go into other farms or areas so that fewer cattle are continually being exposed to infection. The infected animals live out their economic lives before they are discarded. Whichever preparatory method of reducing an initial high incidence of the disease is used, compulsory testing of residual units is advised when 70 to 90 per cent of herds are free. In Denmark the general preparatory approach was along the lines proposed by Bang, and the disease has now been eradicated in that country. In the United Kingdom, voluntary testing was permitted for two years in an eradication area before compulsory testing was introduced, but all reactors were slaughtered.

Vaccination may be considered under certain circumstances, particularly when an eradication programme cannot be instituted for some time but it is desired to reduce the incidence of the disease in preparation for eradication. BCG vaccination is the only method available for field use, the vole acid-fast vaccine varying too much in virulence. BCG vaccine has many disadvantages. Vaccination is carried out by the subcutaneous injection of 50 to 100 ml. vaccine and large and unsightly lumps appear at the injection site. Injection by the alternative intravenous route is attended by risk of severe systemic reactions. Vaccination must be repeated annually and the vaccinated animal remains positive to the tuberculin test. Calves must be vaccinated as soon after birth as possible and do not achieve immunity for 6 weeks. The immunity is not strong and vaccinated animals must not be submitted to severe exposure.

When the overall incidence of tuberculosis is 5 per cent or less, compulsory testing and the slaughter of reactors is the only satisfactory method of eradication. A combination of lines of attack is usually employed. Accredited areas are set up by legislation, and all cattle within these areas are tested and reactors removed. Voluntary accreditation of individual herds is encouraged outside these areas. In some countries, focal points of extensive infection outside accredited areas have been attacked under special legislation. The usual method of encouraging herd accreditation and then introducing compulsory eradication has resulted in the virtual eradication of the disease in the U.S.A. When an area or country has been freed from the disease, quarantine barriers must be set up to avoid its reintroduction. Within the area, the recurrent cost of testing can be lessened by gradually increasing the inter-test period to 2 and then to 3 or even 6 years as the amount of residual infection diminishes. Meat inspection services provide a good observation point should any increase in incidence of the disease occur. Amongst range beef cattle it is usual to check samples of animals at intervals rather than the entire cattle population.

Problems in Tuberculosis Eradication

Complete eradication of tuberculosis has not really been achieved in any country. In many a state of virtual eradication has been in existence for years but minor recrudescences occur. The major problems which arise are as follows.

In the final stages of an eradication programme a number of problems achieve much greater importance than in the early stages of the campaign (25). The percentage of no gross lesion reactors which occurs rises steeply and creates administrative and public relations difficulties. Individual herds which have been accredited after a number of free tests are found to have the disease again, often with a very high incidence. Another major problem is that of 'traceback' of infected animals at packing plants to their herds of origin—even with major effort it is often impossible to determine the origin of more than 50 per cent of affected carcases. The answer to the first problem must await the definition of a test or tests which will differentiate between tuberculosis and sensitivity to other agents, particularly other mycobacteria. There is as yet no highly reliable test to detect the poorly sensitized animals in the early or late stages of the disease which are the usual cause of recrudescence in herds which have been classified as being free of the disease. 'Traceback' becomes the principal source of information on the location of infected herds in the final stages of a programme and a major advance would be a suitable method of identifying individual animals which could be utilized up to the killing floor (25).

Control of Tuberculosis in Pigs

In pigs, because of the non-progressive nature of the disease, transmission from pig to pig is unlikely to occur to a significant extent except perhaps in breeding animals. Pigs serve mostly as a repository for tuberculosis from other species and elimination of the source of infection is usually sufficient to eradicate the disease from previously affected groups. When tuberculosis is positively diagnosed, every effort should be made to type the organism as this gives some indication of the species from which the infection has been derived. Human type (*Myco. tuberculosis*) infections are usually the result of feeding offal from a tubercular household or contact with a tuberculous attendant. Avian type (*Myco. avium*) infections occur when tuberculous chickens are allowed to run freely with the pigs. *Myco. bovis* infection in pigs usually results from the feeding of infected milk, skim milk or whey to pigs or allowing cattle and pigs to graze the same pasture. The first step in the control of tuberculosis in a pig herd is to remove the source of infection, and then to test and remove the reacting animals. This second step is made less efficient by the relative inaccuracy of the tuberculin test in this species (26).

REFERENCES

(1) Clay, A. L. (1971). *Aust. vet. J.*, *47*, 409.
(2) Luke, D. (1958). *Vet. Rec.*, *70*, 529.
(3) Kleeberg, H. H. *et al.* (1969). *J. S. Afr. vet. med. Ass.*, *40*, 33, 253, 259.
(4) Carriere, J. A. J. *et al.* (1968). *Canad. vet. J.*, *9*, 178.
(5) Nielsen, S. W. & Spratling, F. R. (1968). *Brit. vet. J.*, *124*, 503.
(6) Lesslie, I. W. & Hebert, C. N. (1965). *Brit. vet. J.*, *121*, 427.
(7) Kopecky, K. E. *et al.* (1968). *Amer. J. vet. Res.*, *29*, 31.
(8) Kopecky, K. E. *et al.* (1971). *Amer. J. vet. Res.*, *32*, 1343.
(9) Larsen, A. B. *et al.* (1969). *Amer. J. vet. Res.*, *30*, 2167.
(10) Ray, J. A. *et al.* (1963). *Proc. 67th ann. gen. Mtg U.S. Live Stock sanit. Ass.*, 438.
(11) Awad, F. I. (1963). *Proc. 17th World vet. Congr., Hanover*, *1*, 465.
(12) Jong, H. de & Ekdahl, M. D. (1969). *N.Z. vet. J.*, *17*, 213.
(13) Rushford, B. H. (1966). *Aust. vet. J.*, *42*, 70.
(14) Worthington, R. W. & Kleeberg, H. H. (1965). *J. S. Afr. vet. med. Ass.*, *36*, 191, 395.
(15) Pullar, E. M. & Rushford, B. H. (1954). *Aust. vet. J.*, *30*, 221.
(16) Richter, W. (1967). *Arch. exp. Vet.-Med.*, *21*, 1235.
(17) Konhya, L. D. & Kreier, J. P. (1971). *Rev. resp. Dis.*, *103*, 91.
(18) Vardoman, T. H. & Larsen, A. R. (1966). *Amer. J. vet. Res.*, *27*, 545.
(19) Thurton, J. R. (1964). *Proc. 68th ann. gen. Mtg U.S. Live Stock sanit. Ass.*, 314.
(20) Towar, D. R. (1964). *Proc. 68th ann. gen. Mtg U.S. Live Stock sanit. Ass.*, 320.
(21) Lesslie, I. W. *et al.* (1968). *Vet. Rec.*, *83*, 647.
(22) Kleeberg, H. H. *et al.* (1966). *J. S. Afr. vet. med. Ass.*, *37*, 219.
(23) Rotov, V. I. (1965). *Bull. Off. int. Épizoot.*, *63*, 1513.
(24) Straka, J. (1968). *Vet. Med. (Praha)*, *13*, 545.
(25) Ranney, A. F. (1970). *Proc. 70th ann. gen. Mtg U.S. Live Stock sanit. Ass.*, 194.
(26) Mallinan, W. L. *et al.* (1962). *Proc. 66th ann. gen. Mtg U.S. Live Stock sanit. Ass.*, 180, 184.
(27) Gilmour, N. J. L. *et al.* (1970). *J. comp. Path.*, *80*, 181.

Tuberculosis Caused by *Mycobacterium avium*

Tuberculosis caused by the avian tubercle bacillus is not a major disease problem in cattle but can cause much difficulty in tuberculosis eradication programmes in cattle and pigs since infected animals are sensitive to mammalian tuberculin and many valuable animals may be slaughtered as positive reactors. In the U.K. where the situation has been carefully examined it is apparent that in recent years the proportion of positive reactors to tuberculin in pigs which are due to *M. avium* has increased to the point where 80 to 90 per cent of cases are caused by *M. avium* (1, 7). Infected cattle and pigs are now considered to be sources of infection for the increasing number of *M. avium* infections in man. Although the infection is commonly contracted from domestic poultry (2), there is the possibility that infection is transmitted between mammals, especially pigs (3). The use of a comparative tuberculin test to differentiate between infections with the two bacterial species has already been discussed.

In cattle, sensitivity to tuberculin may disappear soon after they are removed from contact with infected birds. Local lesions may persist in the mesenteric lymph nodes, the meninges and in the uterus and udder, and occasional cases of open pulmonary tuberculosis, caused by *Myco. avium*, have been observed. The uterus is a common predilection site for avian tuberculosis and recurrent abortion may occur. Mammary localization is common and induration and involvement of lymph nodes, as in infection with *Myco. bovis*, do occur (4). Generalized tuberculosis can occur in up to 50 per cent of cases (5).

In pigs the disease is non-progressive and usually restricted to the lymph nodes of the head and neck. Occasional generalized cases occur. The lesions are characteristically free of suppuration and resemble neoplastic tissue rather than tuberculous lesions (6). Horses are resistant to infection with *Myco. avium*, although rare, generalized cases of avian tuberculosis have been recorded in this species (8). Goats and sheep appear to have a strong natural resistance to infection with *Myco. avium* but their relative freedom from the disease may be due to lack of contact with infected birds. A high incidence of avian tuberculosis has been observed in a flock of goats (9) and although the disease progresses slowly in this species goats may act as spreaders for other species. Infection in wild deer has been observed and it is postulated that deer may serve as a source of infection for carrion eating birds (10).

REVIEW LITERATURE

Boughton, E. (1969). *Vet. Bull.*, *39*, 757.

REFERENCES

(1) Lesslie, I. W. & Birn, K. J. (1970). *Tubercle, Lond.*, *51*, 446.
(2) Vasilenko, K. F. (1964). *Veterinariya*, *41*, 26.
(3) Gwatkin, R. & Mitchell, C. A. (1952). *Canad. J. comp. Med.*, *16*, 345.
(4) Cassidy, D. R. *et al.* (1968). *Amer. J. vet. Res.*, *29*, 405.
(5) Lesslie, I. W. & Birn, K. J. (1967). *Vet. Rec.*, *80*, 559.
(6) Luke, D. (1958). *Vet. Rec.*, *70*, 529.
(7) Lesslie, I. W. *et al.* (1968). *Vet. Rec.*, *83*, 647.
(8) Lesslie, I. W. & Davies, D. R. T. (1958). *Vet. Rec.*, *79*, 82.
(9) Lesslie, I. W. (1960). *Vet. Rec.*, *72*, 25.
(10) Hopkinson, F. & McDiarmid, A. (1964). *Vet. Rec.*, *76*, 1521.

Tuberculosis caused by Atypical Mycobacteria

An extensive literature has grown up in the past five years about the subject of infections, especially of pigs, caused by the atypical group of mycobacteria. This includes *M. intracellulare*, *M. kansasii*, *M. fortuitum*, *M. aquae* and *M. scrofulaceum* (10). It is not intended to completely review that literature but it is necessary to point out that these infections can cause macroscopic lesions visible at necropsy examination and cause false positive reactions to the tuberculin test especially when the single intradermal test is used. The comparative tuberculin test is becoming more widely used because of the growing importance of these infections (1, 7).

The use of peat as bedding for cattle has led to infection with atypical mycobacteria, the peat being contaminated before use (6).

In pigs the use of deep litter, rather than bare concrete, enhances the prospects of infection with *M. intracellulare* and the development of macroscopic lymphadenitis in the majority of the pigs (3, 8). The lesions are essentially non-progressive and become calcified. Although not clinically ill, human workers have been found to be infected on farms when the disease occurred in pigs (4). Drinking water is also commonly identified as a source of infection of atypical mycobacteria (5). Vaccination with BCG vaccine does not protect pigs against infection with *M. cellulare* (9).

There is an important zoonotic aspect of these diseases. Infections with atypical mycobacteria are not uncommon in man and their differential diagnosis can present difficulties. It is likely that infections in man and animals on the one farm come from the one source, but it is also possible that spread from animals to man occurs (10).

REFERENCES

(1) Worthington, R. W. (1967). *Onderstepoort J. vet. Res.*, *34*, 345.
(2) Reznikov, M. *et al.* (1971). *Aust. vet. J.*, *46*, 239; *47*, 622.
(3) Tammemmagi, L. & Simmons, G. C. (1971). *Aust. vet. J.*, *47*, 337.
(4) Reznikov, M. & Robinson, E. (1971). *Aust. vet. J.*, *46*, 606.
(5) Kazda, J. (1967). *Zbl. Bakt.*, *203*, 190.
(6) Martma, O. V. (1967). *Veterinariya*, *6*, 35.
(7) Waddington, F. G. (1967). *Part 2 FAO/EPTA*, Report No. TA 2011, p. 37.
(8) Brooks, O. H. (1971). *Aust. vet. J.*, *47*, 424.
(9) Tammemmagi, L. (1970). *Aust. vet. J.*, *46*, 284.
(10) Oudar, J. *et al.* (1966). *Rev. Path. comp.*, *66*, 477.

Tuberculosis Caused by
Mycobacterium tuberculosis

Most cases of tuberculosis in animals caused by *Myco. tuberculosis* of human origin are transitory and without lesions. Removal of tuberculous humans from the environment usually results in the disappearance of positive reactors in cattle. In cattle herds the reactors and necropsy lesions are most common in the young stock (1). Many reactors have no visible lesions: those which do occur are small and confined to the lymph nodes of the digestive and respiratory systems. Pigs may develop minor lesions in lymph nodes, but sheep, goats and horses appear to be resistant. A high incidence of sensitivity to tuberculin due to exposure of cattle to tuberculous attendants has been recorded in Kenya (2).

REFERENCES

(1) Lesslie, I. W. (1960). *Vet. Rec.*, 72, 218.
(2) Waddington, F. G. (1965). *Brit. vet. J.*, *121*, 319.

'Skin Tuberculosis'

Chronic indurative lesions of the skin in cattle, occurring usually on the lower limbs, are called 'skin tuberculosis' because they frequently sensitize affected animals to tuberculin. They are not caused by pathogenic mycobacteria.

Incidence

The disease occurs in most countries of the world, particularly where animals are housed. The lesions cause little inconvenience but they are unsightly and affected animals may give a suspicious or positive reaction to the tuberculin test when they are in fact free of tuberculosis. This becomes important when herds and areas are undergoing eradication and attention is focused on any condition which complicates the tuberculin test.

Aetiology

Acid fast organisms can often be found in the lesions in small numbers. They have not been identified and are probably not true pathogens (1). Iatrogenic lesions appear to have been caused by the use of aluminium adsorbed vaccines. These produced subcutaneous granuloma which were colonized by acid-fast bacteria (3).

Transmission

The frequent occurrence of lesions on the lower extremities suggests cutaneous abrasions as the probable portal of entry of the causative organism.

Pathogenesis

Tuberculoid granulomas occur at the site of infection with spread along local lymphatics but without involvement of lymph nodes.

Clinical Findings

Small (1 to 2 cm. diameter) lumps appear under the skin. The lower limbs are the most common site, particularly the fore limbs, and spread to the thighs and forearms and even to the shoulder and abdomen may occur. The lesions may be single or multiple and often occur in chains connected by thin, radiating cords of tissue. The nodules are attached to the skin, may rupture and discharge thick, cream to yellow pus. Ulcers do not persist. Individual lesions may disappear but complete recovery to the point of disappearance of all lesions is unlikely if the lesions are large and multiple.

Clinical Pathology

Affected animals may react to the tuberculin test. Bacteriological examination of smears of pus may reveal the presence of acid fast bacteria.

Necropsy Findings

The lesions comprise much fibrous tissue, usually containing foci of pasty or inspissated pus, and are sometimes calcified.

Diagnosis

The lesions of cattle farcy and ulcerative lymphangitis have a similar distribution but chronic ulcers and lymph node involvement occur. Bacteriological examination may be necessary to confirm the diagnosis. In herds with tuberculosis, reactors which have lesions of skin tuberculosis are disposed of in the usual way. In herds free of tuberculosis a positive reaction to the tuberculin test in animals with skin tuberculosis is usually taken to be non-specific and the affected animal is retained provided it is negative on retest (2).

Treatment and Control

Treatment or control measures are not usually instituted although surgical removal may be undertaken for cosmetic reasons.

REFERENCES

(1) Thomann, H. (1949). *Schweiz. Arch. Tierheilk.*, *91*, 237.
(2) Anonymous (1948). *So-called Skin Tuberculosis of Bovines and its Relation to the Tuberculin Test*, p. 16, National Vet. Med. Ass. Gr. Brit. & Ire.
(3) Lami, G. *et al.* (1970). *Magy. Állatorv. Lap.*, *25*, 151.

Johne's Disease

(Paratuberculosis)

Johne's disease is a specific, infectious enteritis of cattle, sheep and goats. It is characterized by progressive emaciation in all species affected and in cattle by chronic diarrhoea and a thickening and corrugation of the wall of the intestine.

Incidence

Johne's disease is widespread in cattle in Europe and has been carried to many countries by the export of purebred stock. The disease is common in sheep, particularly in Iceland where it was introduced by a small shipment of stud rams from Germany. It is of major importance in cattle and sheep in temperate climates and some humid, tropical areas. The incidence is greatest in animals kept intensively under suitable climatic and husbandry conditions. The morbidity rate is difficult to estimate because of the uncertainty of diagnosis, but the annual mortality rate in infected flocks and herds may be as high as 10 per cent.

Although death losses are not high, when these are added to the losses occasioned by long periods of ill-health and reduced productivity, the disease may cause severe economic embarrassment in affected herds. The reclamation value of clinically affected animals is usually negligible because of severe emaciation. Johne's disease is not a dramatic disease, the slow spread and chronic course resulting in a recurrent rather than an acute economic loss.

Johne's disease is most common in cattle and to a lesser extent in sheep and goats. When the disease becomes established in goat flocks it can cause losses and immunization may be advisable (2). The main importance of sheep is as carriers of infection for cattle. They are easily infected experimentally (1) and discharge large numbers of M. paratuberculosis but usually show spontaneous recovery. In some instances the disease can cause significant financial losses to the sheep farmer (3). It also occurs in water buffalo, in captive wild ruminants including deer, reindeer, antelopes, camels, llamas and yaks. Mice and hamsters are susceptible and are used extensively in experimental work (4). Pigs running with infected cattle may develop enlargement of the mesenteric lymph nodes suggestive of tuberculosis and from which the causative organism can be isolated (5). Pigs infected experimentally develop granulomatous enteritis and lymphadenitis (6, 7), as do horses (24).

Aetiology

Mycobacterium paratuberculosis, the causative bacteria of Johne's disease, persists in pasture for long periods without multiplication and such pastures are infective for up to a year. It is relatively susceptible to sunlight and drying, to a high calcium content and high pH of the soil and continuous contact with urine and faeces reduce the longevity of the bacteria (8). The alkalinity of the soil may also influence the severity of the clinical signs. Herds raised on alkaline soils, particularly in limestone areas, may have a high incidence of infection but little clinical disease. Adult cattle from these herds often develop severe fatal Johne's disease when they are moved to areas where the soil is acid. This observation may have some practical value in the control of the disease but it is probable that factors other than the dietary intake of calcium or the pH of the soil will also influence susceptibility to the infection. Experimental work in goats did not reveal any significant difference in susceptibility between goats on normal and calcium deficient rations.

Three strains of Myco. paratuberculosis are capable of causing the disease in cattle; the usual bovine strain and two sheep strains. The two sheep strains include the one which causes Johne's disease of sheep in Iceland and a highly pigmented strain which occurs only in the United Kingdom. A pigmented variant which causes orange coloured lesions in the intestines and mesenteric lymph nodes of an experimentally infected calf has been reported (9).

The disease can be reproduced experimentally by oral dosing or intravenous injection of the organism in all ruminant species but the incubation period is shorter and the clinical course more acute than in natural cases.

Young animals seem to be more susceptible, most infections occurring early in life and in most cases developing to the clinical stage after 2 years of age. Exact details of the effect of exposure to infection in adults are not available but it is probable that some animals exposed for the first time as adults do develop the clinical disease while others only develop a sensitivity to johnin for short periods although they may become carriers of the disease without manifesting clinical signs. Stress, including parturition, transport and nutritional deficiencies or excesses may influence the development of clinical signs. Field observations indicate a much higher incidence in Channel Island and beef Shorthorn cattle, but this may be related to increased exposure rather than to increased susceptibility. Nevertheless there is evidence of differences in susceptibility between strains of mice and this may also be true in farm animals. The possibility that there may be some cross protection between tuberculosis and Johne's disease has given rise to the suggestion that eradication of tuberculosis may make the cattle population generally more susceptible to Johne's disease but this is not borne out by North American field experience.

Transmission

Under field conditions the disease is transmitted by the ingestion of food and water contaminated by the faeces of infected animals. Because of the long incubation period, infected animals may excrete organisms in the faeces for 15 to 18 months before clinical signs appear. Also, animals reared in an infected environment may become permanent or temporary carriers of the disease without becoming clinically affected. The organism has been isolated from the genitalia and the semen of infected bulls, survives antibiotic addition and freezing (10), and as a result intra-uterine infection occurs commonly but its importance in the transmission of the disease is unknown. Although *Myco. paratuberculosis* can occasionally be found in the milk of clinical cases, it is unlikely that this represents an important source of infection.

Pathogenesis

In an infected environment most calves are infected. Some recover spontaneously within a few months. The remainder become carriers with *Myco. paratuberculosis* persisting in the intestinal wall. From among these latter animals clinical cases arise. The causative bacteria localize and multiply in the mucosa of the small intestine, its associated lymph nodes and, to a less extent, in the tonsils and suprapharyngeal lymph nodes. The post-primary dissemination of the lesions is more widespread in adult animals than in calves and the early lesions are more severe in the former but the organisms do not persist. In calves *Myco. paratuberculosis* proliferate slowly, particularly in the small intestinal site, and set up the massive cellular infiltration of the intestinal submucosa which results in hypermotility, decreased absorption, chronic diarrhoea and a resulting malabsorption (11). In adult cows infection may penetrate to the foetus and cause prenatal infection. Uterine infection occurs more frequently than is commonly thought, and often in animals that are clinically normal themselves (12). From experimental observations in sheep and calves it appears that vaccination against Johne's disease does not prevent infection but restricts the cellular response to the intestinal wall and thus prevents the onset of clinical disease (4).

Important features of the natural history of Johne's disease are the long incubation period of 2 years or more and the development of sensitization to johnin and to mammalian and avian tuberculin. This sensitivity develops in the preclinical stage but has disappeared in most cases by the time clinical signs are evident. On the other hand, complement fixing antibodies appear late in the disease and in general increase with increasing severity of the lesions. This suggests that two independent antibodies are involved in the two reactions.

Clinical Findings

In cattle, clinical signs do not appear before 2 years of age and are commonest in the 2 to 6 years age group. Emaciation is the most obvious abnormality and is usually accompanied by submandibular oedema which has a tendency to disappear as diarrhoea develops. A fall in milk yield and absence of fever and toxaemia are apparent. The animal eats well throughout but thirst is excessive. The faeces are soft and thin, like thick pea soup, homogeneous and without offensive odour. There is marked absence of blood, epithelial debris and mucus. Diarrhoea may be continuous or intermittent with a marked tendency to improve in late pregnancy only to reappear in a severe form soon after parturition. A temporary improvement may also occur when animals are taken off pasture and placed on dry feed. The course of the disease varies from weeks to months but always terminates in severe dehydration, emaciation and weakness necessitating destruction. Cases occur only sporadically because of the slow rate of spread of the disease.

In sheep and goats the disease is manifested only by emaciation although shedding of wool may occur in sheep. Diarrhoea is not severe although the faeces may be sufficiently soft to lose their usual pelleted form.

Clinical Pathology

The following tests used in the diagnosis of Johne's disease can be used in all species but must be applied at a suitable time during the development of the disease. In the early stages, tests based on skin sensitivity should be applied but these are of little value once clinical signs appear. Culture of faeces has been recommended as the most accurate diagnostic method at this stage but has obvious disadvantages in that several months are required before the colonies can be identified (13). Simple smear examination is much too inaccurate and gives many false positives. In the later stages, microscopic examination of the faeces and serological tests are of greatest value.

Sensitivity test. All three available tests suffer from the deficiencies that preclinical and advanced cases have minimal skin sensitivity and animals with bovine or avian tuberculosis and animals vaccinated against Johne's disease may give suspicious or positive reactions. The latter problem may be overcome by the use of a comparative tuberculin test but in general terms the tests are of value only as herd tests. There is little to choose in efficiency between the single intradermal johnin, the double intradermal avian tuberculin and the intravenous avian tuberculin tests, although severe systemic reaction may occur after the intravenous injection of avian tuberculin into infected cattle. The single intradermal johnin test is most popular and is reasonably accurate although not sufficiently so as to be a dependable diagnostic method in individual animals because of the poor sensitivity which the infection produces. The test is performed by injecting 0·2 ml. of johnin or its PPD fraction intradermally in the cervical area. This area is more sensitive than the caudal fold which also suffers from its lack of availability if further tests are to be performed. For a period of over 3 months after an injection of johnin there is local desensitization of the skin at the site of injection and if further tests are required, the neck offers a greater choice of sites than the caudal fold. The test should be read at 48 hours as most significant reactions occur at that time. The development of an appreciable oedematous swelling signifies a positive reaction. In the U.S.A. the official criterion of a positive reaction is an increase of skin thickness of 3 mm. or more. Failure to pick out early clinical cases can be overcome by repeated testing. The intradermal avian tuberculin test is carried out in the same way as a double intradermal tuberculin test.

The intravenous test using avian tuberculin is performed by injecting 10 ml. of avian tuberculin intravenously. A rise in temperature of 1 °C (2 °F) at 5 to 8 hours after injection is a positive reaction. A systemic reaction, including anorexia, depression, dyspnoea, erection of the hair coat and severe scouring may accompany the temperature rise. An intravenous johnin test has also been devised (14). A temperature rise to over 39·5 °C (103·2 °F) (an elevation of over 1 °C) within 3 and 7½ hours after the intravenous injection of 2 to 4 ml. johnin is considered to be a positive reaction.

Bacteriological examination of the faeces. Cultural examination of the faeces is a valuable diagnostic tool but is very severely limited in its application because of the poor growth of the organism. Direct examination of stained faecal smears is the best method of examination when diarrhoea is present but it may be necessary to examine smears on several occasions to obtain a positive result. Clumps of acid-fast bacteria in epithelial cells are diagnostic and are more likely to be observed during a diarrhoeic phase than in a period when faeces are normal, as epithelial cells are more likely to be shed at the former time. Scrapings of rectal mucosa are of no great advantage compared to faecal smears as it is probably only in the late stages that the rectal mucosa is invaded.

Serological tests. Complement fixation and micro-complement fixation tests are available for use in cattle and small stock. The test reflects the severity of the lesions rather than the severity of the clinical abnormality, but early cases and non-clinical carriers fail to give positive reactions and a number of non-specific, transient, positive reactions do occur. The test is probably about 90 per cent accurate in clinically affected animals and 25 per cent accurate in infected but clinically unaffected animals (15). Because positive reactions are given by tuberculous animals, the test is limited to use in tuberculosis-free herds. The parallel use of both complement fixation and intradermal test has value in early cases. Repeated use of the complement fixation test on several occasions at 2 to 3 week intervals is also recommended to identify a rising titre and the probability of early infection (17). A fluorescent antibody test is available but is unable to distinguish between the antigens of *M. avium* and *M. paratuberculosis* (16).

Necropsy Findings

Lesions are confined to the posterior part of the alimentary tract and its associated lymph nodes. The terminal part of the small intestine, the caecum and the first part of the colon are usually affected. In advanced cases the lesions may reach from the rectum to the duodenum. Thickening of the intestinal wall up to three or four times normal thickness, with corrugation of the mucosa, is characteristic. The ileocaecal valve is always involved, the lesion varying from reddening of the lips of the valve in the early stages to oedema with gross thickening and corrugation later. A high incidence of arteriosclerosis has been observed in advanced cases of Johne's disease, with a distinct correlation between the vascular lesions and macroscopic changes in the intestine. In sheep there may be a deep yellow pigmentation of the intestinal wall and, although corrugation of the mucosa is not a common finding, the wall may be thickened. No ulceration or discontinuity of the mucosal surface occurs. The mesenteric and ileocaecal lymph nodes are enlarged and oedematous in cattle, and in sheep there may be necrosis, caseation and calcification in these nodes. Gross necropsy lesions are often minimal in animals that showed severe clinical signs during life. In these animals the presence of lymphadenitis of the intestinal lymph vessels and characteristic histological findings provide satisfactory confirmation of the diagnosis. No lesions occur in an infected foetus but the organism can be isolated from its viscera and from the placenta and uterus.

Diagnosis

Difficulty is often encountered in the diagnosis of Johne's disease in individual animals because of the lack of dependability of the available tests. Herd testing may provide valuable supporting information. The chronic nature of the disease is usually sufficient to differentiate it from the other common enteritides of cattle. Salmonellosis, coccidiosis and parasitism are usually acute and the latter two occur principally in young animals and are distinguishable on faecal examination for oocysts and helminth eggs. Chronic molybdenum poisoning is likely to be confused with Johne's disease in cattle but is usually an area problem affecting large numbers of animals and responds well to the administration of copper.

Parasitism in sheep can be confused with Johne's disease although diarrhoea is much more common in the former. Wasting due to cobalt deficiency may be difficult to differentiate from Johne's disease in sheep.

Treatment

Myco. paratuberculosis is more resistant to chemotherapeutic agents in vitro than *Myco. tuberculosis* so that prospects for suitable treatment are poor. Streptomycin has most activity against the organism but treatment of affected cattle with daily doses of 25 mg. per lb. body weight causes only a transient improvement in clinical signs. Isoniazid has a minor degree of activity against the organism but has failed to cure clinical cases of Johne's disease. A rimino phenazine, B663, shows some activity against early infection in sheep (18).

Control

The lack of accurate tests and the long incubation period of the disease combine to make Johne's disease difficult to control. Because of the in-

accuracy of the diagnostic tests available it is impossible to eradicate the disease, other than by completely clearing a farm and then restocking, and to prevent the subsequent reintroduction of infected animals (19).

Control on a herd basis depends upon eradication of infected animals, hygiene to prevent further spread and, in some instances, vaccination to increase the resistance of the residual population.

The conservative method of eradication depends upon the identification of carrier animals by the tests described above, and their immediate sale for slaughter. The farm is quarantined and residual animals are retested at 6-month intervals until two consecutive negative herd tests are achieved. Unfortunately the method rarely succeeds in eradicating the disease. If the individual animals are of such value that complete disposal of all stock is impracticable, the above method may keep losses at a low level. An alternative method is to maintain infected and non-infected herds as determined by the johnin test, and to transfer all calves from the infected to the non-infected herd at birth. Although the disease can be eliminated by disposal of all cattle and leaving the farm unstocked for 1 to 3 years, this method can seldom be implemented.

If one has to live with the disease, a number of hygienic precautions can be taken to limit the spread of infection. Avoidance of faecal pollution of drinking water and feed by providing troughs in high positions, fencing of marshes and ponds, and closing up of contaminated pastures for up to 3 years are worth-while measures. Strip grazing should be avoided as faecal contamination of pasture is likely to be intense. Frequent harrowing of pasture fields to disseminate dung pats facilitates destruction of the bacteria by exposing them to sun and drying. Yard and barn manure should be spread only on cultivated fields. Although congenital infection may occur, it is still advisable to rear calves away from infected cows, and if possible in individual pens to prevent spread among the calves (20). Calves from cows which are clinically affected should not be reared as herd replacements. Sucking on dams and nurse cows should not be permitted. Milk for bucket feeding should be collected hygienically and rearing on milk substitutes should be encouraged. In infected herds, any animal which shows mild signs suggestive of the disease should be isolated until its status has been determined. Adoption of these hygienic precautions has been shown to greatly reduce the prevalence of the disease, down to a third, and of sensitivity to johnin, reduced by 90 per cent (21).

Provided local legislation permits it, vaccination

will reduce the rate of spread in a herd and has been shown to be capable of eradicating the disease. Vallée's vaccine of live *Myco. paratuberculosis* organisms in a paraffin oil—pumice stone vehicle, or the Sigurdsson vaccine which contains killed organisms, are the vaccines in common use, although a microvaccine prepared by grinding the bacteria in a ball mill and suspending them in a paraffin oil vehicle has been used in sheep. There is less local reaction than with the usual ovine vaccine of live or killed organisms in oil, but the resulting antibody titre, and probably the immunity, wanes more quickly than with the other vaccines.

In cattle vaccination is carried out only in calves less than one month of age. Contrary to previous recommendations revaccination is not carried out because the degree of protection appears to diminish as a result and because of the unsightly nodules which sometimes develop. The vaccine is of no benefit to infected animals, but it is incapable of causing the disease or of producing carriers (22). A major complication is that vaccinated animals are positive to the johnin test and to the tuberculin test, using both avian and mammalian tuberculin, but the reaction is much less to the mammalian tuberculin (23). In general terms, vaccination can be recommended in heavily infected, tuberculosis free herds but only in areas where tuberculosis eradication is neither under way nor projected. It is possible that the vaccine gives some protection against tuberculosis.

In sheep, vaccination with Sigurdsson vaccine of heat-killed *Myco. paratuberculosis* in mineral oil has given excellent results, reducing the disease to negligible proportions. The use of vaccination in sheep is not impeded by interference with tuberculin testing.

Control on an area basis. Eradication on an area basis has seldom been attempted because of the lack of dependability of available diagnostic tests and the relative unimportance of Johne's disease in the past. Two general lines of approach to the eradication problem can be followed. If the incidence is sufficiently low, a test and slaughter programme on a herd basis could be instituted with all cattle being cleared from infected farms and the farms being left unoccupied by ruminants for at least one year. A great deal of public support would be necessary for such a programme to succeed. If the incidence is high and tuberculosis eradication has been completed or is not projected, vaccination may be advisable, and is at present undergoing trials in European countries. If the disease is eradicated, the prevention of re-infection becomes a problem. The tests used to detect infected animals are not sufficiently accurate and quarantine of introductions is impossible because of the long incubation period. A guarantee of freedom from disease in the place of origin is the best recommendation but is still subject to error.

At the present time, in most countries the incidence of Johne's disease is not sufficiently high to necessitate an intensive area eradication programme, nor are the available diagnostic tests sufficiently accurate to form the basis for such a programme. In these circumstances, the owners of affected farms should be encouraged to adopt the general procedures outlined under herd control, preferably with technical and financial assistance from government authorities.

REFERENCES

(1) Kluge, J. P. *et al.* (1968). *Amer. J. vet. Res.*, 29, 953.
(2) Yakin, N. & des Francs, E. (1970). *Rec. Méd. vét.*, 146, 807.
(3) Davidson, R. M. (1970). *N.Z. vet. J.*, 18, 28.
(4) Gilmour, N. J. L. (1965). *Vet. Rec.*, 77, 1322.
(5) Ringdal, G. (1963). *Nord. Vet.-Med.*, 15, 217.
(6) Larsen, A. B. *et al.* (1971). *Amer. J. vet. Res.*, 32, 539.
(7) Jorgensen, J. B. (1969). *Acta vet. scand.*, 10, 275.
(8) Larsen, A. B. *et al.* (1956). *Amer. J. vet. Res.*, 17, 549.
(9) Stuart, P. (1965). *Brit. vet. J.*, 121, 332.
(10) Larsen, A. B. & Kopecky, K. E. (1970). *Amer. J. vet. Res.*, 31, 255.
(11) Patterson, D. S. P. & Berrett, S. (1969). *J. med. Microbiol.*, 2, 327.
(12) Kopecky, K. E. *et al.* (1967). *Amer. J. vet. Res.*, 28, 1043.
(13) Merkal, R. S. *et al.* (1968). *Amer. J. vet. Res.*, 29, 1533.
(14) Larsen, A. B. & Kopecky, K. E. (1965). *Amer. J. vet. Res.*, 26, 673.
(15) Larsen, A. B. *et al.* (1965). *Amer. J. vet. Res.*, 26, 254.
(16) Gilmour, N. J. L. *et al.* (1970). *J. comp. Path.*, 79, 71; 80, 181.
(17) Pearson, J. K. L. (1967). *Brit. vet. J.*, 123, 31.
(18) Gilmour, N. J. L. (1968). *Brit. vet. J.*, 124, 492.
(19) Larsen, A. B. (1964). *Proc. 68th ann. gen. Mtg U.S. Live Stock sanit. Ass.*, 342.
(20) Ovdienko, N. P. (1971). *Veterinariya*, 4, 49.
(21) Larsen, A. B. & Merkal, R. S. (1968). *J. Amer. vet. med. Ass.*, 152, 1771.
(22) Doyle, T. M. (1964). *Vet. Rec.*, 76, 73.
(23) Huitema, H. (1967). *Bull. Off. int. Épizoot.*, 68, 743.
(24) Larsen, A. B. *et al.* (1972). *Amer. J. vet. Res.*, 33, 2185.

DISEASES CAUSED BY *ACTINOMYCES BOVIS, ACTINOBACILLUS* Spp., *NOCARDIA* Spp. AND *DERMATOPHILUS* Spp.

This group of infectious diseases includes actinomycosis, actinobacillosis, mycotic dermatitis, strawberry footrot of sheep, bovine farcy, glanders and shigellosis of foals. Nocardial mastitis in cattle has been dealt with in the chapter on mastitis.

Less common occurrences of infection with this group of organisms include *Act. actinoides* as a secondary bacterial invader in enzootic pneumonia of calves and seminal vesiculitis in bulls (3), *A. bovis* in a large proportion of unopened lesions of fistulous withers and poll evil (1), and *Actinomyces* spp. in an abscess in a mandibular lymph node in a horse (2). A septicaemic disease of swine has been attributed to *Act. suis*, a variant of *Act. lignieresi*. *A. seminus* has been isolated from the joints of lambs affected by purulent polyarthritis (4) and from the semen of rams with epididymitis (5).

REFERENCES

(1) Kimball, A. & Frank, E. R. (1945). *Amer. J. vet. Res.*, 6, 39.
(2) Burns, R. H. G. & Simmons, G. C. (1952). *Aust. vet. J.*, 28, 34.
(3) Jones, T. H. *et al.* (1964). *Vet. Rec.*, 76, 24.
(4) Watt, D. A. *et al.* (1970). *Aust. vet. J.*, 46, 515.
(5) Baynes, J. D. & Simmons, G. C. (1968). *Aust. vet. J.*, 44, 339.

Actinomycosis

(*Lumpy Jaw*)

The most common manifestation of this disease in cattle is a rarefying osteomyelitis of the bones of the head, particularly the mandible and maxilla. On rare occasions it involves soft tissues, particularly the alimentary tract.

Incidence

Although actinomycosis occurs only sporadically in affected herds, it is of importance because of its widespread occurrence and poor response to treatment. It is recorded from most countries of the world.

Aetiology

Act. bovis is the primary cause but other bacteria may be present in extensive lesions. The disease is common only in cattle where a tendency towards inherited susceptibility has been observed (10). Occasional cases occur in pigs and horses (9).

Transmission

Act. bovis is a common inhabitant of the bovine mouth and infection is presumed to occur through wounds to the buccal mucosa caused by sharp pieces of feed or foreign material. Infection may also occur through dental alveoli, and may account for the more common occurrence of the disease in young cattle when the teeth are erupting. Infection of the alimentary tract wall is probably related to laceration by sharp foreign bodies.

Pathogenesis

In the jawbones a rarefying osteomyelitis is produced. The lesion is characteristically granulomatous both in this site and where visceral involvement occurs. The effects on the animal are purely physical. Involvement of the jaw causes interference with prehension and mastication, and when the alimentary tract is involved there is physical interference with ruminal movement and digestion, both resulting in partial starvation. Rarely localization occurs in other organs, caused apparently by haematogenous spread from these primary lesions.

Clinical Findings

Cattle. Actinomycosis of the jaw commences as a painless, bony swelling which appears on the mandible or maxilla, usually at the level of the central molar teeth. The enlargement may be diffuse or discrete and in the case of the mandible may appear only as a thickening of the lower edge of the bone with most of the enlargement in the intermandibular space. Such lesions are often not detected until they are too extensive for treatment to be effective. The more common, discrete lesions on the lateral surfaces of the bones are more readily observed. Some lesions enlarge rapidly within a few weeks, others slowly over a period of months. The swellings are very hard, are immovable and, in the later stages, painful to the touch. They usually break through the skin and discharge through one or more openings. The discharge of pus is small in amount and consists of sticky, honey-like fluid containing minute, hard, yellow-white granules. There is a tendency for the sinuses to heal and for fresh ones to develop periodically. Teeth embedded in the affected bone become malaligned and painful and cause difficult mastication with consequent loss of condition. In severe cases, spread to contiguous soft tissues may be extensive and involve the muscles and fascia of the throat. Excessive swelling of the maxilla may cause dyspnoea. Involvement of the local lymph nodes does not occur. Eventually the animal becomes so emaciated that destruction is necessary although the time required to reach this stage varies from several months to a year or more. The most common form of actinomycosis of soft tissues is involvement of the oesophageal groove region, with spread to the lower oesophagus and the anterior wall of the reticulum. The syndrome is one of impaired digestion (1, 2). There is periodic diarrhoea with the passage of undigested food material, chronic bloat and allotriophagia. Less common lesions of soft tissue include orchitis in bulls (3) and abscess in the brain (4, 5, 6) or lungs (7).

Pigs. Rare cases of wasting occur due to visceral actinomycosis (8) but extensive granulomatous lesions on the skin, particularly over the udder, are more common.

Clinical Pathology

Smears of the discharging pus stained with Gram's stain provide an effective simple method of confirming the diagnosis. Gram-positive filaments of the organism are most readily found in the centres of the crushed granules.

Necropsy Findings

Rarefaction of the bone and the presence of loculi and sinuses containing thin, whey-like pus with small, gritty granules is usual. An extensive fibrous tissue reaction around the lesion is constant, and there may be contiguous spread to surrounding soft tissues. The presence of 'club' colonies containing the typical, thread-like bacteria is characteristic of the disease. These formations may be seen on microscopic examination of smears made from crushed granules in pus or on histological examination of sections. Granulomatous lesions containing pockets of pus may be found in the oesophageal groove, the lower oesophagus and the anterior wall of the reticulum. Spread from these lesions may cause a chronic, local peritonitis. There may be evidence of deranged digestion with the rumen contents sloppier than usual, an empty abomasum and a mild abomasitis and enteritis. Involvement of local lymph nodes does not occur, irrespective of the site of the primary lesion.

Diagnosis

Abscesses of the cheek muscles and throat region are quite common when spiny grass-awns occur in the diet. They are characterized by their movability and localization in soft tissues compared to the immovability of an actinomycotic lesion. Needle puncture reveals the presence of pus, which may be thin and foetid or caseous depending on the duration of the abscess. Prompt recovery follows opening and drainage. Foreign bodies or accumulations of dry feed jammed between the teeth and cheek commonly cause a clinical picture which resembles that caused by actinomycosis and the inside of the mouth should be inspected if the enlargement has occurred suddenly.

The syndrome of indigestion caused by visceral actinomycotic lesions resembles that caused by chronic peritonitis.

Cutaneous and mammary lesions in sows closely resemble necrotic ulcers caused by *Borrelia suilla*.

Treatment and Control

The treatment and control of actinomycosis is dealt with under actinobacillosis.

REFERENCES

(1) Bruere, A. N. (1955). *N.Z. vet. J.*, *3*, 121.
(2) Begg, H. (1950). *Vet. Rec.*, *62*, 797.
(3) Kimball, A. *et al.* (1954). *Amer. J. vet. Res.*, *15*, 551.
(4) Trevisan, G. (1957). *Veterinaria (Milano)*, *6*, 122.
(5) Fankhauser, R. (1950). *Schweiz. Arch. Tierheilk.*, *92*, 82.
(6) Ryff, J. F. (1953). *J. Amer. vet. med. Ass.*, *122*, 78.
(7) Bellazi, D. (1954). *Riv. Med. vet. (Parma)*, *6*, 147.
(8) Vawter, L. R. (1946). *J. Amer. vet. med. Ass.*, *109*, 198.
(9) Tritschler, L. G. & Romach, F. E. (1965). *Vet. Med.*, *60*, 605.
(10) Becker, R. B. *et al.* (1964). *Bull. Florida agric. Exp. Sta. No. 670*, pp. 24.

Actinobacillosis

(*Wooden Tongue*)

Actinobacillosis is a specific infectious disease, and in cattle it is characterized by inflammation of the tongue, less commonly the pharyngeal lymph nodes and oesophageal groove. In sheep the lesions are restricted to the soft tissues of the head and neck and occasionally the nasal cavities. Involvement of the tongue does not usually occur.

Incidence

The disease in cattle is world wide in distribution and, like actinomycosis, it is usually of sporadic occurrence on particular farms. However, it is amenable to treatment and causes only minor losses. In sheep the disease is common in Scotland (1) and is recorded in most sheep-raising countries (2, 3, 11). In most instances, only occasional cases occur but in some flocks a morbidity rate of up to 25 per cent may be encountered.

Aetiology

Actinobacillus lignieresi may be recovered in pure culture from the lesions but other pyogenic organisms may also be present. The organism is susceptible to ordinary environmental influences and lives for not more than 5 days on hay or straw (12).

Transmission

Infected discharges are the source of the infection and transmission is effected by the ingestion of contaminated pasture or feed. As in actinomycosis, injury to the buccal mucosa permits easy entry of the infection and a high incidence is recorded in cattle grazing 'burnt-over' peat pastures in New

Zealand (4). These pastures contain much gravel and ash likely to cause oral injury. A similar high incidence has been observed in sheep fed prickly pear (*Opuntia* spp.).

Pathogenesis

Local infection by the organism causes an acute inflammatory reaction and the subsequent development of granulomatous lesions in which necrosis and suppuration occur, often with the discharge of pus to the exterior. Spread to regional lymph nodes is usual. Lingual involvement in cattle causes interference with prehension and mastication due to acute inflammation in the early stages and distortion of the tongue at a later stage. Visceral involvement is recorded and is identical with that described under actinomycosis.

Clinical Findings

Cattle. The onset of lingual actinobacillosis is usually acute, the affected animal being unable to eat for a period of about 48 hours. There is excessive salivation and gentle chewing of the tongue as though a foreign body were present in the mouth. On examination the tongue is swollen and hard, particularly at the base, the tip often appearing to be normal. Manipulation of the tongue causes pain and resentment. Nodules and ulcers are present on the sides of the tongue and there may be an ulcer at the anterior edge of the dorsum. In the later stages when the acute inflammation is replaced by fibrous tissue, the tongue becomes shrunken and immobile and there is considerable interference with prehension. Lymphadenitis is common and is often independent of lesions in the tongue. There may be visible and palpable enlargement of the submaxillary and parotid nodes. Local, firm swellings develop and often rupture with the discharge of thin, non-odorous pus. Healing is slow and relapse is common. Enlargement of the retropharyngeal nodes causes interference with swallowing and loud snoring respiration.

An unusual occurrence of cutaneous actinobacillosis has been recorded in cattle (13). Lesions occurred in the mouth, but not on the tongue, on the head, chest wall, flanks and thighs and were in the form of large ulcers which exuded yellow pus, or nodules of various shapes and sizes (up to 15 cm.) often obviously on lymphatics. Local lymph nodes were always involved but were firm, cold and painless. *Act. lignieresi* was isolated and although treatment with chloramphenicol or streptomycin was effective, spontaneous recovery occurred in other animals which were not treated.

Sheep. In sheep the tongue is not usually affected.

Lesions, up to 8 cm. in diameter, occur on the lower jaw, face and nose, or in the skin folds from the lower jaw to the sternum. They may be superficial or deep and usually extend to the cranial or cervical lymph nodes. Viscid, yellow-green pus containing granules is discharged through a number of small openings. Extensive lesions cause the formation of much fibrous tissue which may physically impede prehension or respiration. Thickening and scabbiness of the lips may also be observed. Involvement of the nasal cavities may cause persistent bilateral nasal discharge. Affected sheep have difficulty in eating and many die of starvation. *Act. lignieresi* has been incriminated as an occasional cause of mastitis in ewes (15).

Clinical Pathology

Examination of smears or culture of pus for the presence of *Act. lignieresi* is advisable.

Necropsy Findings

Necropsy examination is not usually carried out in cattle affected by the disease. In sheep, lymphangitis and abscesses containing thick, tenacious, yellow-green pus occur around the local lesion. Typical club colonies are visible on staining sections of affected tissue. Culture of material from lesions usually detects the presence of *Act. lignieresi*.

Diagnosis

The salivation, chewing and anorexia of the lingual form in cattle may resemble early rabies or foreign bodies in the mouth, particularly bones jammed between the molars. Enlargement of the lymph nodes, particularly when the tongue is unaffected, requires careful consideration. A tuberculin test may be necessary to differentiate this form of the disease from tuberculosis. Treatment with iodine effects considerable reduction in the size of the nodes in both diseases. Lymphomatosis usually affects multiple nodes. Abscesses of the throat region of cattle may be caused by a number of non-specific pyogenic infections following trauma. They usually consist of a single cavity containing thin pus and heal readily after draining.

In sheep, mandibular abscesses caused by grass seed penetration of alveoli causes large, bony swellings on the mandible. The lesion is usually on the anterior part of the mandible, causing displacement of the incisor teeth. It is an osteomyelitis and greyish, fluid, foul-smelling pus is present (5). Actinobacillosis of the nasal cavities bears some resemblance to melioidosis in this species.

Treatment

Iodides are still a standard treatment for both actinomycosis and actinobacillosis. In the former, the results are relatively inefficient but in actinobacillosis, response is usually dramatic and permanent. Laboratory studies suggest that iodides have little bactericidal effect against *Act. lignieresi* and that the sulphonamides are of greater value (6). It is probable that iodides exert their effect by reducing the severity of the fibrous tissue reaction. The sulphonamides, penicillin, streptomycin and the broad spectrum antibiotics are now in general use for both diseases. In vitro, sensitivity tests of a large series of strains have shown the organism to be sensitive to streptomycin, the tetracyclines, chloramphenicol and erythromycin but not to other antibiotics (12). Treatment of any sort is more likely to be of value in actinobacillosis than in actinomycosis and surgical treatment may be necessary in the latter. Roentgenological treatment has been used extensively but is of doubtful permanent value.

Oral or intravenous dosing of iodides may be used. Potassium iodide, 6 to 10 g. per day for 7 to 10 days, given orally as a drench to cattle, is a time-consuming treatment but effective. Organic iodide salts are more palatable and can be given in the feed. Treatment may be continued until iodism develops. Lacrimation, anorexia, coughing and the appearance of dandruff indicate that maximum systemic levels of iodine have been reached. Sodium iodide (1 g. per 25 to 30 lb. body weight) can be given intravenously as a 10 per cent solution in one dose to both cattle and sheep. One course of potassium iodide or one injection of sodium iodide is usually sufficient for soft tissue lesions, the acute signs in actinobacillosis disappearing in 24 to 48 hours after treatment. At least one or preferably two further treatments at 10- to 14-day intervals are required for bony lesions.

The most that can be expected with bony lesions is the arrest of further development. With time, the lesion may subside but rarely disappears completely. Occasional animals show distress, including restlessness, dyspnoea, tachycardia and staggering during injections of sodium iodide. Although abortion has been recorded in heavily pregnant cows after injection (7), this does not appear to be a common occurrence. Subcutaneous injections of sodium iodide have also been recommended (8). The injection causes severe irritation and local swelling immediately. The irritation disappears within an hour or two but the swelling persists for some days. Subcutaneous injection is the standard route of administration for sheep, the dose rate of sodium iodide being 20 ml. of a 10 per cent solution weekly for 4 to 5 weeks.

Sulphanilamide, sulphapyridine and sulphathiazole effect rapid cures in human actinomycosis and have been used in the disease in cattle. One g. per 15 lb. body weight per day for 4 to 5 days is suggested as a course of treatment.

Penicillin has been reported to be of value in actinomycosis (9). If possible, systemic treatment should be accompanied by injection into the substance of the lesion. Streptomycin, given by intramuscular injection (5 g. per day for 3 days) and repeated if necessary, has given good results in actinomycosis in cattle when combined with iodides and local surgical treatment (10). Isoniazid has been used as a treatment for actinomycotic infections in man and it has been reported on favourably as an adjunct to antibiotic or iodide therapy in cattle. The daily dose rate recommended is 3 to 5 mg. per lb. body weight, orally or intramuscularly, continued for 2 or 3 weeks (14). Surgical treatment usually consists of the opening of the bony tumour to provide drainage, and packing, usually with gauze soaked in tincture of iodine.

Control

Restriction of the spread of both diseases is best implemented by quick treatment of affected animals and the prevention of contamination of pasture and feed troughs. Isolation or disposal of animals with discharging lesions is essential, although the disease does not spread readily unless predisposing environmental factors cause a high incidence of oral lacerations.

REFERENCES

(1) Taylor, A. W. (1944). *J. comp. Path., 54*, 228.
(2) Hayston, J. T. (1948). *Aust. vet. J., 24*, 64.
(3) Johnston, K. G. (1954). *Aust. vet. J., 30*, 105.
(4) Gerring, J. C. (1947). *Aust. vet. J., 23*, 122.
(5) Edgar, G. (1935). *Aust. vet. J., 11*, 19.
(6) Smith, H. W. (1951). *Vet. Rec., 63*, 674.
(7) Farquharson, J. (1937). *J. Amer. vet. med. Ass., 91*, 551.
(8) Linton, F. A. (1946). *N.Z. J. Agric., 73*, 25.
(9) Lewis, E. F. (1947). *Vet. Rec., 59*, 435.
(10) Kingman, H. E. & Palen, J. S. (1951). *J. Amer. vet. med. Ass., 118*, 28.
(11) Marsh, H. & Wilkins, H. W. (1939). *J. Amer. vet. med. Ass., 94*, 363.
(12) Till, D. H. & Palmer, F. P. (1960). *Vet. Rec., 72*, 527.
(13) Hebeler, H. F. *et al.* (1961). *Vet. Rec., 73*, 517.
(14) Koger, L. M. (1963). *Mod. vet. Pract., 44*, 56.
(15) Laws, L. & Elder, J. K. (1969). *Aust. vet. J., 45*, 401.

Glanders

Glanders is a contagious disease of solipeds, occurring in either acute or chronic form, and is characterized by nodules or ulcers in the respiratory tract and on the skin. The disease is highly fatal and of major importance in any affected horse population.

Incidence

Glanders is restricted geographically to Eastern Europe, Asia Minor, Asia and North Africa. It has been virtually eradicated from North America. Since the elimination of large concentrations of horses in cities, the disease is of major importance only when there is extensive movement of horses. In such circumstances, heavy mortality rates occur and in the few animals that recover, there is a long convalescence with the frequent development of the 'carrier' state. Rarely animals make a complete recovery. Carnivores may be infected by eating infected meat, and infections have been observed in sheep and goats.

Aetiology

Actinobacillus (Malleomyces) mallei is the causative organism. It is readily destroyed by light, heat and the usual disinfectants and is unlikely to survive in a contaminated environment for more than 6 weeks. Horses, mules and donkeys are the species usually affected. Horses tend to develop the chronic form, mules and donkeys the acute form. Man is susceptible and the infection is usually fatal. Cases usually occur in persons working with the organism in the laboratory or in close contact with affected animals (3). Animals which are badly fed and kept in a poor environment are more susceptible.

Transmission

Infected animals or carriers that have made an apparent recovery from the disease are the important sources of infection. Spread to other animals occurs mostly by ingestion, the infection spreading on fodder and utensils, particularly communal watering troughs, contaminated by nasal discharge or sputum. Rarely the cutaneous form appears to arise through contamination of skin abrasions by direct contact or from harness or grooming tools. Spread by inhalation can also occur but this mode of infection is probably rare under natural conditions.

Pathogenesis

Invasion occurs mostly through the intestinal wall and a septicaemia (acute form) or bacteraemia (chronic form) is set up. Localization always occurs in the lungs but the skin and nasal mucosa are also common sites. Other viscera may become the site of the typical nodules. Terminal signs are in the main those of a bronchopneumonia, and deaths in typical cases are caused by anoxic anoxia.

Clinical Findings

In the acute form there is a high fever, cough and nasal discharge with rapidly spreading ulcers appearing on the nasal mucosa, and nodules on the skin of the lower limbs or abdomen. Death due to septicaemia occurs in a few days. In the chronic form, the signs may be related to the lesions which occur in one or more of the predilection sites. When the localization is chiefly pulmonary, there is a chronic cough, frequent epistaxis and laboured respiration. The chronic nasal and skin forms commonly occur together. Nasal lesions appear on the lower parts of the turbinates and the cartilaginous nasal septum. They commence as nodules (1 cm. in diameter) which ulcerate and may become confluent. In the early stages there is a serous nasal discharge which may be unilateral and which later becomes purulent and blood stained. Enlargement of the submaxillary lymph nodes is a common accompaniment. On healing, the ulcers are replaced by a characteristic stellate scar. The skin form is characterized by the appearance of subcutaneous nodules (1 to 2 cm. in diameter) which soon ulcerate and discharge pus of the colour and consistency of dark honey. In some cases the lesions are more deeply situated and discharge through fistulous tracts. Thickened fibrous lymph vessels radiate from the lesions and connect one to the other. Lymph nodes draining the area become involved and may discharge to the exterior. The predilection site for cutaneous lesions is the medial aspect of the hock but they can occur on any part of the body. Animals affected with the chronic form are usually ill for some months, frequently showing improvement but eventually either dying or making an apparent recovery to persist as occult cases.

Clinical Pathology

The principal tests used in the diagnosis of glanders are the mallein test, the complement fixation test on serum, and the injection of pus from lesions into guinea pigs. Other tests used are an indirect haemagglutination test using mallein as the antigen (4) and the conglutinin complement absorption test (6).

Mallein test. The intradermopalpebral test has largely displaced the ophthalmic and subcutaneous tests. Mallein (0·1 ml.) is injected intradermally into the lower eyelid with a tuberculin syringe. The test is read at 48 hours, a positive reaction comprising marked oedema of the lid with blepharospasm and a severe, purulent conjunctivitis.

Complement fixation test. This is the most accurate of the serological tests available but some strains of *Act. mallei* give cross reactions with *Pseudomonas pseudomallei*. If pus is available, either from open ulcers or necropsy material, the organism can be cultured or the pus injected intraperitoneally into male guinea pigs to attempt to elicit the 'Strauss' reaction. This is a severe orchitis and inflammation of the scrotal sac but it is not highly specific for *Act. mallei*.

Necropsy Findings

In the acute form there are multiple petechial haemorrhages throughout the body and a severe catarrhal bronchopneumonia with enlargement of the bronchial lymph nodes. In the more common chronic form, the lesions in the lungs take the form of miliary nodules, similar to those of miliary tuberculosis, scattered throughout the lung tissue. Ulcers are present on the mucosa of the upper respiratory tract, especially the nasal mucosa and to a lesser extent that of the larynx, trachea and bronchi. Nodules and ulcers may be present in the skin and subcutis of the limbs which may be greatly enlarged. Local lymph nodes receiving drainage from affected parts usually contain foci of pus and the lymphatic vessels have similar lesions. Necrotic foci may also be present in other internal organs.

Diagnosis

In advanced clinical cases, the typical lymphangitis in the cutaneous form and the nasal ulcers in the pneumonic form immediately attract attention. Epizootic lymphangitis is very similar, especially as it occurs in outbreaks like glanders. However, the lesions on the nasal mucosa derive from nibbling of the leg lesions and do not penetrate into the nasal cavity to the septum, nor is pneumonia present as in glanders. Gram-positive, double-walled spores are present in the pus. Other forms of lymphangitis and skin ulceration, e.g. sporotrichosis and ulcerative lymphangitis, occur sporadically only, and there is no lymph node or systemic involvement. A horse with an infected tooth may show a unilateral nasal discharge but the discharge is odorous and no ulceration of the mucous membrane occurs. The acute pneumonic form may be confused with other pneumonias of the horse, particularly infectious equine pneumonia and severe strangles. Clinically they may be difficult to distinguish, and the area in which the disease occurs and necropsy and cultural findings may have to be considered in making a definite diagnosis. The mallein or complement fixation tests must be used to detect the occult, carrier cases which are the chief problem in the control of the disease.

Treatment

Penicillin and streptomycin have no detectable effect on the progress of the disease but sodium sulphadiazine has been highly effective in the treatment of experimental glanders and melioidosis in hamsters (1). Treatment for a period of 20 days was necessary to effect 100 per cent recovery. Combinations of a formolized preparation of *Malleomyces mallei* and sulphadiazine, or mallein and sulphadimidine are reported to be effective in the treatment of affected horses (2).

Control

Although clinical and serological recovery from glanders occurs occasionally, it has been observed that recovered animals are not solidly immune and attempts to produce artificial immunity have been uniformly unsuccessful.

Complete quarantine of affected premises is necessary. Clinical cases should be destroyed and the remainder subjected to the mallein test at intervals of 3 weeks until all reactors have been removed. A vigorous disinfection programme for food and water troughs and premises generally should be instituted to prevent spread while eradication is being carried out. Restriction of the movement of horses should be instituted and the mallein test carried out in horses which may have had contact with the infected group (5).

REFERENCES

(1) Miller, W. R. *et al.* (1948). *Amer. J. Hyg.*, *47*, 205.
(2) Fathi, R. *et al.* (1953). *Arch. Inst. Hessarek*, *7*, 22–26.
(3) McGilvray, C. D. (1944). *J. Amer. vet. med. Ass.*, *104*, 255.
(4) Gangulee, P. C. *et al.* (1966). *Ind. vet. J.*, *43*, 386.
(5) Hickman, J. (1970). *Equ. vet. J.*, *2*, 153.
(6) Sen, G. P. *et al.* (1968). *Ind. vet. J.*, *45*, 286.

Bovine Farcy

(*Mycotic Lymphangitis, Bovine Nocardiosis*)

This disease of cattle occurs principally in tropical countries and is caused by *Nocardia farcinicus* (4). It is characterized by purulent lymphangitis and lymphadenitis, and the common occurrence of lesions on the lower limbs suggests that the causative organisms are soil-borne and gain entry through minor injuries. Initially there is a chronic, painless, localized subcutaneous cellulitis which spreads along lymphatics to involve local lymph nodes. Further spread to the lungs may occur.

Typical lesions include chronic, indurated, subcutaneous swellings, and enlargement and thickening of local lymphatics and lymph nodes. Discrete swellings develop along the affected lymphatic vessels and these may rupture and discharge pus through sinuses or from indolent ulcers. The general health of affected animals is not impaired unless the lesions are extensive or pulmonary involvement occurs. The lesions may occur at the prescapular, precrural or head lymph nodes, in front of the shoulder joint, along the lymphatics in all four legs, at the base of the ear, in the cheeks or on the mandible or in the parotid area (7). Farcy nodules may also be present at favoured points of tick attachment, on the perineum, in the axilla or the crutch. The lesions may rupture to discharge odourless thick grey or yellow pus which is often granular or cheesy. Healing and redischarging is common. The causative organism can be isolated from the purulent discharges by the examination of smears or by culture. In fatal cases there are usually multiple, small nodules throughout the lungs.

The disease may be confused with 'skin tuberculosis' but ulcers and sinuses do not usually develop in the latter. Ulcerative lymphangitis caused by *Cor. paratuberculosis* is a rare occurrence in cattle but is manifested by involvement of local lymph nodes and lymphatics as well as cutaneous lesions. Cases of bovine farcy with pulmonary involvement bear some clinical and pathological resemblance to tuberculosis and may give transient positive reactions to the tuberculin test (1, 6). Although smears from pus may be sufficient to establish a diagnosis (2) inoculation of material into guinea pigs may be necessary in some cases (3). An antigen prepared from *N. asteroides* has been used to detect cutaneous hypersensitivity and the presence of complement-fixing antibodies in the serum of affected animals. The resulting tests have diagnostic value (5).

The parenteral administration of sodium iodide is recommended as a treatment. Early disinfection of cutaneous abrasions in cattle on affected farms is recommended to reduce the incidence of the disease.

REFERENCES

(1) Awad, F. I. (1958). *J. comp. Path.*, 68, 324.
(2) El Nasri, M. (1961). *Vet. Rec.*, 73, 370.
(3) Awad, F. I. (1961). *Vet. Rec.*, 73, 515 (corresp.).
(4) Moustafa, E. I. (1966). *Vet. Bull.*, 36, 189.
(5) Pier, A. C. *et al.* (1968). *Amer. J. vet. Res.*, 29, 397.
(6) Mostafa, I. E. (1967). *Vet. Rec.*, 81, 74.
(7) Mostafa, I. E. (1967). *J. comp. Path.*, 77, 223, 231.

Mycotic Dermatitis

(*Cutaneous Streptothricosis, Senkobo Disease of Cattle; Lumpy Wool of Sheep; Cutaneous Actinomycosis*)

This is a dermatitis occurring in all species and is caused by infection with organisms of the genus, *Dermatophilus* Van Saceghem. It has been suggested that the disease in cattle be called cutaneous streptothricosis and the disease in sheep, mycotic dermatitis.

Incidence

Mycotic dermatitis has been recorded in cattle, sheep, goats and horses. The disease appears to be most common under warm, moist climatic conditions but has been reported as far north as Canada, northern U.S.A. and Great Britain (1). Large numbers of animals may become affected. In sheep, damage to the fleece causes severe losses and may be so extensive in lambs that spring lambing has to be abandoned. Other losses in sheep are caused by interference with shearing and a very great increase in susceptibility to blow fly infestation. In tropical Africa the disease in cattle causes great losses and many deaths (2, 3). In temperate climates deaths are uncommon but cows that fail to respond to treatment and have to be culled are not infrequent.

Aetiology

The nomenclature of the causative organisms has not been finalized and we have used that suggested by Roberts (4). The previous nomenclature of *D. congolensis* in cattle, *D. dermatonomus* and *D. pedis* in sheep has been discarded and *D. congolensis* is the officially approved name. The *Dermatophilus* spp. infecting horses has also been identified as *D. congolensis* (5). Animals of all ages are susceptible, including sucklings a few weeks old. In these young animals, infection commences on the muzzle, probably from contact with the infected udder or because of scalding by milk in bucket-fed calves. Cool, wet weather conditions predispose to the disease. From observations on fleece rot of sheep it seems probable that continued wetting of the skin causes softening and swelling of the cornified epithelium leading to a mild dermatitis and increasing the chances of infection. Increased environmental humidity, as distinct from wetting of the skin, does not appear to promote the development of lesions. The introduction of infection into the skin through cuts made at shearing time is thought to be an important portal of entry. The coccal form of the causative organism is relatively resistant and may be the form by which the infection persists from year to year. Although the infection is capable of persisting in soil for more than 4 months the usual source of infection is thought to be active cases or inapparent carriers in sheep. Mycotic dermatitis has been observed in deer in the U.S.A. (6) taking the form of a chronic dermatitis on the lower parts of the legs, flanks, back, neck and around the nostrils. The disease spread to four persons who handled the deer. The organism isolated closely resembled *D. congolensis*. The disease in cattle and horses has not been observed to infect man in spite of ample opportunity (7).

Transmission

Contact with infected animals leads to spread of the disease. In beef cattle there is a particular tendency for lesions to occur on the rump in young males and females probably due to the introduction of the infection through minor skin abrasions caused by mounting. In cattle the role of ticks in transmission may be important in some areas (8) and under these conditions tick control reduces the incidence of the disease. In horses biting flies (*Stomoxys calcitrans*) are thought to act as mechanical vectors of the infection (5) and the house fly (*Musca domestica*) has also been shown to act as a carrier (9). In sheep the infection appears to exist in a mild form in many animals and is manifested by a few, small scabs on the hair-covered face and ears. In these animals the disease spreads to the wool-covered areas under the influence of climatic factors. Between sheep the disease is spread by contact for periods as short as 15 seconds, especially in wet conditions. Thus dipping, showering or yarding wet sheep are conducive to spread (10). Dipping fluids may become contaminated and further aid spread (11).

Pathogenesis

The organism invades cutaneous abrasions and sets up a bacterial dermatitis. Exudate, epithelial debris and the mycelial forms of the organism produce characteristic crusts not unlike those of ringworm. Secondary bacterial invasion may occur and gives rise to extensive suppuration and severe toxaemia. In most cases the lesion appears to be self-limiting and the scab separates from the healed lesion but is still held loosely in place by hair or wool fibres. There are three stages in development of the lesions (7). At first the hair is erect and in tufts with greasy exudate forming crumbly crusts which are hard to remove. Next come dirty yellow scabs which are greasy and fissure at flexion points. In the third stage the scabs are hard, horny and confluent and there is alopecia. In some animals the disease is acute, developing quickly, responding well to treatment or disappearing spontaneously in a matter of weeks. In others the disease is chronic and persists for months, resisting all efforts to completely cure it.

The natural skin and wool waxes act as effective barriers to infection and coarse-woolled sheep and Merino lambs, being deficient in wax, are most susceptible to the disease. Factors such as continuous wetting of the face or injury by shearing blades predispose to infection. In cattle, the extension of lesions on the body appears to be largely through the agency of ectoparasites (5).

Clinical Findings

In cattle, lesions occur on the neck, body, or back of the udder and may extend over the sides and down the legs and the ventral surface of the body (13). Commonly they commence along the back from the withers to the rump and extend halfway down the rib cages. In some animals the only site affected is the flexor aspect of the limb joints. In calves lesions usually commence on the muzzle and spread over the head and neck. In goats lesions appear first on the lips and muzzle and then spread, possibly by biting, to the feet and scrotum. In sheep the distribution of lesions is chiefly over the dorsal parts of the body, spreading laterally and ventrally. The muzzle, face and ears may also be involved. Lesions in horses may appear on the head, beginning at the muzzle and spreading up the face to the eyes, and if sufficiently extensive they may be accompanied by lacrimation and a profuse, mucopurulent nasal discharge. In other horses the lesions are confined to the lower limbs, with a few on the belly. In very bad environmental conditions the lesions may be widespread and cover virtually the whole of the back and sides (12). The lesions on lower limbs are most common behind the pastern, around the coronet and on the anterior aspect of the hind cannon bones. This variable distribution of lesions may depend upon the origin of the cutaneous wounds which act as portals of entry.

No itching or irritation is apparent although in horses the sores are tender to the touch. In adult cattle the characteristic lesions are thick, horny crusts, varying in colour from cream to brown. They are 2 to 5 cm. in diameter and are often in such close apposition that they give the appearance of a mosaic. In the early stages the crusts are very tenacious and attempts to lift them cause pain. Beneath the crusts there is granulation tissue and some pus. In the later stages, the dermatitis heals and the crusts separate from the skin but are held in place by penetrating hairs or wool fibres and are easily removed. In young calves plaque and crust formation does not occur. There is extensive hair loss with tufting of the fibres, heavy dandruff and thickening and folding of the skin in later stages. Vesicular and pustular lesions 1 cm. in diameter have also been described in the early stages of the disease (14).

The crusts are often pyramidal in a sheep fleece because of the spread of the lesion as the crust is formed. In this animal, too, the crusts are much thicker, up to 3 cm., roughly circular and often pigmented. The value of an affected fleece is much reduced. Part of the damage is the secondary discoloration which is commonly present. These bacterial discolorations of wool have been reviewed (15).

Heavy mortalities can occur in very young lambs but in general the health of the animal is unaffected unless the lesions are wide-spread. Such animals are covered with scabs and are in poor condition and may die. In occasional cases a secondary pneumonia due to the organism may cause the death of the animal. In the average case, healing of skin lesions occurs in about 3 weeks.

Clinical Pathology

The causative organism may be isolated from scrapings or a biopsy section and is much easier to isolate from an acute case than a chronic one (7). An impression smear, made directly from the ventral surface of a thick scab and pressed firmly on to a slide, may also be of value, suitable staining techniques demonstrating the presence of typical branching organisms. Because of the motility of the zoospores in water the technique of chopping up a scab and making a suspension in water before examining the material is recommended (4). Fluorescent antibody techniques have also been used.

Necropsy Findings

In the occasional animals that die, there is extensive dermatitis, sometimes a secondary pneumonia, and often evidence of intercurrent disease.

Diagnosis

Diagnosis depends upon the detection of the mycelia-like organisms in scrapings or biopsy sections, and culture of suspected tissues. In the early stages, the disease may be confused with photosensitization because of the dorsal distribution of the lesions but they are not selectively distributed on unpigmented areas. Fleece rot is a very similar condition and occurs under the same circumstances, but the thick scabs of mycotic dermatitis are absent. In calves, involvement of the muzzle and face may arouse suspicion of bovine malignant catarrh or mucosal disease. The thick scabs of mycotic dermatitis are characteristic and there is no diarrhoea or stomatitis. Congenital ichthyosis of calves is present at birth but the mosaic of scabs may resemble that of mycotic dermatitis.

Treatment

There is no completely satisfactory treatment for cases which show very extensive involvement, or those being constantly reinfected or exposed to predisposing causes. Parenterally administered antibiotics are the only rational treatment and have been found to be effective. Tetracyclines (2 mg. per lb. body weight) repeated weekly as required is recommended. Penicillin and streptomycin at very heavy dose rates (70 mg. streptomycin and procaine penicillin G 70,000 units per kg. body weight) is recommended as being 100 per cent effective in heavily infected sheep.

In general terms better results are obtained during dry hot weather and in dry climates. In tropical Africa treatments which are reasonably effective elsewhere are of little or no value (2). Topical applications are not generally recommended because of the impossibility of introducing them into infected layers of skin. If these are applied to acute cases where spontaneous recovery is about to occur the recovery rate will be attractive. From that point of view the following treatments recommended for sheep may be used for cattle.

Affected sheep should be shorn as soon as the scabs lift sufficiently. For large numbers it is best to treat immediately by dipping or spraying with 0·2 to 0·5 per cent zinc sulphate. A solution containing 0·2 per cent copper sulphate has also been used but causes staining of the wool. Its use should be limited to hand application to individual lesions. For this purpose quaternary ammonium compounds in a 1 in 200 dilution have been reported to be even more effective. In vitro studies indicate that a dilute solution of alum (potassium aluminium sulfate) should be highly effective and significant improvement has been observed in natural and artificial cases in sheep. The alum was administered as a 1 per cent dip or 57 per cent dust in an inert carrier (16). Dipping fluids may become contaminated and act as carriers of infection. This can be prevented by the use of alum zinc sulfate or magnesium fluosilicate in the dip solution (10). The removal of scabs and exudate prior to topical treatment is recommended when practicable.

It should be remembered that one could not expect a dramatic response to the treatment of establishing or established cases with the above topical applications if weather conditions are suitable for spread of the disease (11).

To overcome the problem of shearing infected sheep chemical defleecing has been used and is reported to be highly effective (17). Cyclophosphamide administered orally at a dose rate of 25 mg. per kg. body weight alone was an effective treatment in 77 per cent of cases. Severely affected sheep were not cured. When the treatment was combined with parenteral penicillin and streptomycin the cure rate was raised to 93 per cent.

Although horses generally respond well, in bad weather even they can be recalcitrant to treatment. Topical applications are of limited value but are preferred when horses are racing. Parenteral treatment with penicillin with or without streptomycin is the recommended treatment in bad cases (12).

Control

The disease usually disappears in dry weather. Isolation of infected animals and avoidance of contact with infected materials such as grooming tools appears desirable. In tropical areas, tick control is thought to be of considerable importance. A satisfactory control measure in sheep is spraying or dipping in 0·2 to 0·5 per cent solution of zinc sulphate or a solution of magnesium fluosilicate (18). The prophylactic use of alum as set out under treatment is recommended after shearing as a means of controlling the disease without eradication (12). Attempts at prophylaxis by vaccination have been unsuccessful (4).

REFERENCES

(1) Hart, C. B. (1967). *Vet. Rec.*, *81*, 36.
(2) Coleman, C. H. (1967). *Vet. Rec.*, *81*, 251.
(3) Oduye, O. O. & Lloyd, D. H. (1971). *Brit. vet. J.*, *127*, 505.
(4) Roberts, D. S. (1967). *Vet. Bull.*, *37*, 513.
(5) Macadam, I. (1964). *Vet. Rec.*, *76*, 194, 354, 420.
(6) Dean, D. J. (1961). *N.Y. St. J. Med.*, *61*, 1283.
(7) Searcy, G. P. & Hulland, T. J. (1967). *Canad. vet. J.*, *9*, 7, 16.
(8) Lloyd, D. H. (1971). *Brit. vet. J.*, *127*, 572.
(9) Richard, J. L. & Pier, A. C. (1966). *Amer. J. vet. Res.*, *27*, 419.
(10) Le Riche, P. D. (1968). *Aust. vet. J.*, *44*, 64.
(11) Le Riche, P. D. (1967). *Aust. vet. J.*, *43*, 265.
(12) Pascoe, R. R. (1971). *Aust. vet. J.*, *47*, 112; *48*, 32.
(13) Pier, A. C. *et al.* (1963). *J. Amer. vet. med. Ass.*, *142*, 995.
(14) Thorold, P. W. (1964). *J. S. Afr. vet. med. Ass.*, *35*, 549.
(15) Mulcock, A. P. (1965). *N.Z. vet. J.*, *13*, 87.
(16) Hart, C. B. & Tyszkiewicz, K. (1968). *Vet. Rec.*, *82*, 272.
(17) McIntosh, G. H. *et al.* (1971). *Aust. vet. J.*, *47*, 542.

Strawberry Footrot
(*Proliferative Dermatitis*)

This is a proliferative dermatitis of the lower limbs of sheep.

Incidence

The disease is recorded only from the United Kingdom (1) and occurs extensively in some parts of Scotland. It is not fatal but severely affected animals do not make normal weight gains. Up to 100 per cent of affected flocks may show the clinical disease.

Aetiology

The causative agent is *Dermatophilus pedis* (2). All ages and breeds appear susceptible but under natural conditions, lambs are more commonly affected. Most outbreaks occur during the summer months and lesions tend to disappear in cold weather. Although the disease is recorded naturally only in sheep, it can be transmitted experimentally to man, goats, guinea pigs and to rabbits. Complete immunity does not develop after an attack and there is no cross-immunity against sheep pox (3), although sheep recently recovered from contagious ecthyma may show a transient resistance (4).

Transmission

The natural method of transmission is unknown but the frequency of occurrence of lesions at the knee and coronet suggests infection from the ground through cutaneous injuries. Dried crusts containing the causative agent are infective for long periods and ground contamination by infected animals is the probable source of infection.

Pathogenesis

Histologically the lesions are those of a superficial epidermitis similar to that of contagious ecthyma.

Clinical Findings

Most cases appear 2 to 4 weeks after sheep have been moved on to affected pasture but incubation periods of 3 to 4 months have been observed. Small heaped-up scabs appear on the leg from the coronet to the knee or hock. These enlarge to 3 to 5 cm. in diameter and become thick and wart-like. The hair is lost and the lesions may coalesce. Removal of the scabs reveals a bleeding, fleshy mass resembling a fresh strawberry, surrounded by a shallow ulcer. In later stages the ulcer is deep and pus is present.

There is no itching or lameness unless lesions occur in the interdigital space. Most lesions heal in 5 to 6 weeks but chronic cases may persist for 6 months.

Clinical Pathology

Swabs and scrapings should be examined carefully for the causative organism.

Diagnosis

Lesions of strawberry footrot closely resemble those of contagious ecthyma but are restricted in their distribution to the lower limbs whereas lesions of contagious ecthyma occur mostly on the face and rarely on the legs. Sheep which have recovered from the disease are still susceptible. The absence of a systemic reaction and the wart-like character of the lesions differentiate it from sheep pox. A final diagnosis must depend on the isolation of the organism or the experimental transmission of the disease.

Treatment

No specific treatment is available but iodides by mouth or parenterally may be of value.

Control

In the light of present knowledge, isolation of infected sheep and the resting of infected fields are the only measures which can be recommended.

REFERENCES

(1) Harriss, S. T. (1948). *J. comp. Path.*, *58*, 314.
(2) Austwick, P. K. C. (1948). *Vet. Rev. Annot.*, *4*, 33.
(3) Horgan, E. S. & Haseeb, M. A. (1948). *J. comp. Path.*, *58*, 329.
(4) Abdussalam, M. & Blakemore, F. (1948). *J. comp. Path.*, *58*, 333.

Shigellosis of Foals

(Sleepy Foal Disease)

Shigellosis is an acute, highly fatal septicaemia of newborn foals. Foals that survive for a few days show evidence of localization in various organs.

Incidence

Shigellosis is an important cause of neonatal deaths in foals in most countries of the world and may represent as high a proportion as 25 per cent of all infections in newborn foals (1, 2, 3, 4, 5, 6). Successive foals on a particular farm may be affected with a mortality rate approaching 100 per cent.

Aetiology

The causative organism, *Actinobacillus equuli* (*Shigella equirulis*), is often found in the intestine and tissues of normal horses. Shigellosis is limited to horses and although newborn foals are the most susceptible age group, there have been reports of the septicaemic form·of the disease in older animals (8, 9) especially when their resistance is lowered by concurrent infection.

Transmission

Although foals may become infected in utero, it is probable that postnatal infection, usually via the navel, is more frequent. The mare is not clinically affected and the organism does not persist in the uterus for long periods. The method of spread between mares is unknown but intrauterine infection appears to occur in the same mare in successive years, possibly from a focus in some other organ.

Pathogenesis

In foals the disease is an acute septicaemia, in many cases causing death before specific lesions are produced. In such cases adrenal cortical deficiency may be a major factor in causing death (11). Foals which survive the illness for more than 24 hours develop suppurative lesions in the renal cortex, in joints and intestines. In older animals it has been postulated that the infection may be carried to various organs by migrating strongyle larvae.

Clinical Findings

The foal may be sick at birth or show signs from within a few hours of birth up to 3 days of age. There is a sudden onset of fever, prostration, diarrhoea, occasionally dysentery and rapid respiration, and the foal ceases to suck. Foals which are sleepy or comatose at birth or soon afterwards occur commonly. These so-called sleepers may be aroused but quickly revert to a comatose state. Death within 24 hours is usual. Occasional foals show severe abdominal pain in the early stages of the disease. Foals that survive the acute, febrile phase develop arthritis with swollen joints and lameness within 1 or 2 days. Death usually occurs in these more protracted cases during the period between the second and seventh days.

Clinical Pathology

Cervical swabs from the mare should be examined bacteriologically for the presence of the organism.

Necropsy Findings

Foals that die within 24 hours of the onset of illness show septicaemia and severe enteritis but there may be no pin point abscesses in the kidney. The adrenals are enlarged and dark red in colour (11). Foals dying after a longer interval show tendosynovitis and arthritis. In the early stages the synovial fluids are sanguineous and turbid but soon become purulent. In these foals it is also usual to find the diagnostic pin point abscesses in the renal cortices. Shigella are recoverable from the blood stream in acute cases and from joints and other organs in cases of longer duration.

Diagnosis

The presence of minute abscesses in the renal cortices and *Act. equuli* in the foetal tissues is diagnostic. Other than the high proportion of sleeper foals in shigellosis, there is little to go on in the differentiation of this disease from septicaemias caused by *Escherichia coli*, *Salmonella typhimurium* and *Salm. abortivoequina*. Other conditions to be considered in arriving at a diagnosis include congenital heart anomalies, ruptured bladder, and iso-immune haemolytic anaemia.

Treatment

In foals, streptomycin gives excellent results when administered parenterally, early and in sufficiently large and frequent doses (1 g. 6-hourly). Chlortetracycline (5 mg. per lb. body weight) given intravenously for 5 days gives good results also, although in vitro tests of blood levels reached with this drug suggest that the dose rate should be 10 mg. per lb. body weight once daily (7). Chloramphenicol (10 mg. per lb. body weight intramuscularly daily) is also highly effective and can be supplemented by oral administration of the same drug at the same dose rate (10). Supportive treatment by blood transfusions is also of value and is described in diseases of the newborn.

Control

Control of the disease depends upon elimination of the infection by culling or treating infected mares, preventing spread by hygienic precautions at foaling time, and by treating susceptible foals prophylactically at birth with one of the drugs prescribed for treatment.

REFERENCES

(1) Gunning, O. V. (1947). *Vet. J.*, *103*, 47.
(2) Cottew, G. S. & Ryley, J. W. (1952). *Aust. vet. J.*, *28*, 302.
(3) Dimock, W. W. *et al.* (1947). *Cornell Vet.*, 37, 89.
(4) Flatla, J. L. (1942). *Norsk. vet. Tidskr.*, *54*, 249 & 322.
(5) Harms, F. (1942). *Dtsch. tierärztl. Wschr.*, *50*, 408.
(6) Leader, G. H. (1952). *Vet. Rec.*, *64*, 241.
(7) McCollum, W. H. & Doll, E. R. (1951). *Vet. Med.*, *46*, 84.
(8) Stricker, F. & Gouvert, Z. (1956). *Vet. Čas.*, *5*, 260.
(9) Hirato, K. (1941). *Jap. J. vet. Sci.*, *3*, 482.
(10) Littlejohn, A. (1959). *J. S. Afr. vet. med. Ass.*, *30*, 143.
(11) Du Plessis, J. L. (1963). *J. S. Afr. vet. med. Ass.*, *34*, 25.

Shigellosis of Piglets

A high incidence of fatal enteritis in pigs 10 to 14 days old and caused by *Shigella dysenteriae* has been reported (1). Sows suckling affected pigs showed little abnormality but profuse yellow diarrhoea and vomiting followed by many deaths characterized the illness in the piglets. Treatment with neopolymixin was effective.

REFERENCE

(1) Baker, W. L. (1960). *Vet. Med.*, *55*, 36.

19

Diseases Caused by Bacteria—V

DISEASES CAUSED BY *FUSIFORMIS* Spp.

INFECTION BY *Fusiformis* spp., especially *F. necrophorus*, is common in all species of farm animals. In many instances the organism is present as a secondary invader rather than as a primary cause of disease. The specific diseases dealt with here as being caused by primary infection with *Fusiformis* spp. are footrot of cattle, oral necrobacillosis, footrot of sheep and pigs and foot abscess of sheep. In footrot of sheep the causative organism (*F. nodosus*) occurs in association with *Spirochaeta penortha* and in footrot of pigs a species of Sphaerophorus and spirochaetal organisms are commonly found together.

Some of the common conditions in which *Fusiformis* spp. are found as secondary invaders are navel ill and hepatic necrobacillosis in sheep and cattle, in pneumonia of calves and in the secondary infections of covering epithelium. These include necrotic enteritis caused by *Salmonella* spp. in pigs, necrotic rhinitis and atrophic rhinitis of pigs, most diseases in which vesicular eruption and erosive lesions of the buccal mucosa and coronary skin of cattle and sheep occur, and in vulvitis, vaginitis and metritis.

An unusual outbreak of necrobacillosis of the brain and meninges has been recorded in a flock of sheep in which about 5 per cent showed varying degrees of inco-ordination (1).

REFERENCE
(1) Horter, R. (1957). *Dtsch. tierärztl. Wschr.*, *64*, 420.

Necrobacillosis of the Liver

This disease of lambs and cattle is caused by localization in the liver of an infection originating in the navel or rumen. In many cases the animal's health is unaffected and the abscesses are discovered only at necropsy. There may be acute, fatal toxaemia or chronic ill-health without localizing signs.

Incidence

The disease is of greatest importance in feeder cattle where it occurs secondarily to rumenitis. In these animals there is considerable financial loss due to condemnation of livers in abattoirs. An incidence of 22 per cent has been observed in 'barley beef' cattle in the U.K. (7) and about 5 per cent of bovine livers in the U.S.A. are rejected because of hepatic abscess. In lambs, occasional losses are recorded in housed and range flocks.

Aetiology

Fusiformis (*Sphaerophorus*) *necrophorus* is commonly found in pure culture in hepatic abscesses in ruminants. The disease can be produced experimentally in cattle and sheep by the intraportal injection of cultures of the organism (1). *Corynebacterium pyogenes* and streptococci are also often present in the lesions (6).

Transmission

The organism is a common inhabitant of the environment of farm animals and the existence of a predisposing injury may be all that is required for the disease to occur. In lambs infection usually occurs through the navel at birth or through ruminal ulcers, the infection originating from infected bedding grounds or barns (2, 3). *F. necrophorus* is not capable of prolonged survival outside the animal body, one month being the probable maximum period under favourable conditions, and constant reinfection is probably necessary to render soil or surroundings highly infective (8). The organism is a common inhabitant of the intestine and rumen in normal cattle.

Pathogenesis

Vascular drainage from the primary lesion, omphalitis or rumenitis, leads to localization in the liver. It is commonly held that in cattle the sudden change from pasture to high grain diets causes rumenitis due to the development of acidity in the rumen, and *F. necrophorus* invades the erosive lesion produced (1). Doubt has been thrown on this as being the only pathogenesis by the absence of ruminal lesions in cattle on heavy grain diets that show a very high incidence of hepatic abscess (7). If there is sufficient hepatic involvement a toxaemia develops from the bacterial infection causing a chronic or acute illness. However in most instances the lesions are too small to produce clinical signs. Haematogenous spread from hepatic lesions, including rupture into the caudal vena cava, may result in multiple lesions in many organs and a rapidly fatal termination.

Clinical Findings

In acute cases there is fever, anorexia, depression, fall in milk production and weakness. Abdominal pain is evidenced on percussion over the posterior ribs on the right side and affected cattle show arching of the back, and reluctance to move or lie down. The liver may be so enlarged that it is readily palpable behind the costal arch. The abdominal pain may be sufficiently severe to cause grunting with each breath. In chronic cases there are no localizing signs but anorexia, emaciation and intermittent diarrhoea and constipation occur. Animals affected at birth show signs at about 7 days of age and omphalophlebitis is usually present.

Clinical Pathology

A marked increase in total leucocytes and neutrophils can be anticipated in acute cases.

Necropsy Findings

In rumenitis in cattle the anterior, ventral sac is most commonly affected. There are local or diffuse lesions of rumenitis with thickening of the wall, superficial necrosis and the subsequent development of ulcers. Multiple hepatic abscesses are present, and in lambs there may be lesions at the cardial end of the oesophagus. The hepatic lesions may be deep in the parenchyma or under the capsule, especially on the diaphragmatic surface. Extension to the diaphragm or perirenal tissues is not unusual.

Diagnosis

The diagnosis of non-specific liver abscess is discussed elsewhere. Bacillary haemoglobinuria is characterized clinically by fever, jaundice and haemoglobinuria and at necropsy by hepatic infarcts instead of abscesses. Acute cases in cattle resemble cases of traumatic reticuloperitonitis and differentiation can only be made on localization of the pain and by exploratory rumenotomy. The latter is essential if traumatic hepatitis is a possible diagnosis.

Treatment

A course of sulphadimidine or tetracyclines causes a transitory response but relapse is common because of incomplete control of the localized infection.

Control

The high incidence of hepatic abscesses in feedlot cattle can be reduced by the feeding of a lower proportion of grain in the ration and by a gradual change-over from pasture to fattening rations when the animals first come into the lot (1). Feeding chlortetracycline (75 mg. per day) throughout the fattening period may reduce the number of hepatic abscesses which occur but the incidence may still be as high as 70 per cent (4, 5). In sheep the disease can be controlled by disinfection of the navel at birth and providing clean bedding or bedding grounds.

REFERENCES

(1) Jensen, R. *et al.* (1954). *Amer. J. vet. Res.*, *15*, 5, 202 & 425.
(2) Marsh, H. (1944). *J. Amer. vet. med. Ass.*, *104*, 23.
(3) Harris, A. N. A. (1947). *Aust. vet. J.*, *23*, 152.
(4) Flint, J. C. & Jensen, R. (1958). *Amer. J. vet. Res.*, *19*, 830.
(5) Avery, R. J. (1962). *Canad. vet. J.*, *3*, 15.
(6) Rubarth, S. (1960). *Acta vet. scand.*, *1*, 363.
(7) Rowland, A. C. (1966). *Vet. Rec.*, *78*, 713.
(8) Smith, L. D. S. (1963). *Bull. Off. int. Épiz.*, *59*, 1517.

Infectious Footrot of Cattle
(*Infectious Pododermatitis, Foul in the Foot, Fouls*)

This is an infectious disease of cattle characterized by inflammation of the sensitive tissues of the feet and severe lameness.

Incidence

The disease is common in most countries. It is of greatest economic importance in dairy cattle, in which it reaches the highest level of incidence, because of the intensive conditions under which they are kept. In beef cattle at range the incidence is usually low but many cases may occur in purebred herds and in feedlot cattle. Loss of production occurs in affected cattle and an occasional animal may suffer a serious involvement of the joint and other deep structures of the foot necessitating amputation of a claw. Under favourable conditions as many as 25 per cent of a group may be affected at one time but the usual picture is for the disease to occur sporadically on affected farms. The disease is not fatal but some cases may have to be slaughtered because of joint involvement.

Aetiology

Footrot is usually described as being caused by *Fusiformis* (*Sphaerophorus*) *necrophorus* but there is lack of conclusive evidence on this point (1). A Gram negative bacillus which resembles *F. nodosus* and unidentified spirochaetes are also thought to have aetiological significance (10). The disease appears to be contagious and the incidence is much higher during wet humid weather or when conditions are wet underfoot. Stony ground, lanes filled with sharp gravel and pasturing on coarse stubble also predispose to the condition. The observation that the disease is common on some farms and does not occur at all on others suggests that there may be factors which limit the persistence of infectivity in certain soils. Introduction of the infection to a farm by transient cattle is often observed but again the disease may not develop on some farms in spite of the introduction of the infection. *Chorioptes bovis* infestation has been advanced as a possible precipitating cause of footrot (8), but this mite is often not present on farms where footrot is common. Cattle of all ages, including young calves, may be affected but the disease is much more common in adults.

Transmission

Discharges from the feet of infected animals are the probable source of infection. Duration of the infectivity of pasture or bedding is unknown. Infection gains entrance through abrasions to the skin on the lower part of the foot. Abrasions are more likely to occur when the skin is swollen and soft due to continual wetting. The increased incidence in wet summer and autumn months may be so explained in part although wet conditions may also favour persistence of the infection in pasture.

Pathogenesis

The morbid anatomy of the disease has been described (1) but the mode of development has not.

Clinical Findings

Severe foot lameness appears suddenly, usually in one limb only and may be accompanied by a moderate systemic reaction with a fever of 39 to 40°C (103 to 104°F). There is temporary depression of milk yield in cows and affected bulls may show temporary infertility. The animal puts little weight on the leg although the limb is carried only when severe joint involvement occurs. Swelling of the coronet and spreading of the claws are obvious.

The typical lesion occurs in the skin at the top of the interdigital cleft and takes the form of a fissure with swollen, protruding edges which may extend along the length of the cleft or be confined to the anterior part or that part between the heel bulbs. Pus is never present in large amounts but the edges of the fissure are covered with necrotic material and the lesion has a characteristic odour. Occasionally in early cases no external lesion may be visible but there is lameness and swelling of the coronet. Such cases are usually designated 'blind fouls' and respond well to parenteral treatment.

Spontaneous recovery is not uncommon but if the disease is left untreated the lameness usually persists for several weeks with adverse effects on milk production and condition. The incidence of complications is also higher if treatment is delayed and some animals may have to be destroyed because of local involvement of joints and tendon sheaths. In such cases the lameness is severe, the leg usually being carried and the animal strongly resenting handling of the foot. Swelling is usually more obvious and extends up the back of the leg. There is poor response to medical treatment and surgical measures are necessary to permit drainage. Radiological examination may be of value in determining the exact degree of involvement of bony tissue. Long continued irritation may result in the development of a wart-like mass of fibrous tissue, the interdigital fibroma, in the anterior part of the cleft and chronic mild lameness. Interdigital fibroma occurs commonly without the intervention of footrot, the important cause being inherited defects in foot conformation in heavy animals.

Clinical Pathology

Bacteriological examination is not usually necessary for diagnosis but it may help in confirmation and is of interest in view of the uncertain aetiology of the condition.

Necropsy Findings

Necropsy examinations are rarely carried out in cases of footrot but details of the pathology are available (1). Dermatitis is followed by necrosis of the skin and subcutaneous tissues. In complicated cases there may be suppuration in joints and tendon sheaths.

Diagnosis

The characteristic site, nature and smell of the lesion, the pattern of the disease in the group and the season and climate are usually sufficient to indicate the presence of true footrot. Traumatic injury to bones and joints, puncture by foreign bodies, bruising of the heels and gross overgrowth of the hoof can usually be distinguished by careful examination of the foot. Laminitis may cause lameness but there are no local foot lesions.

Stable footrot is a disease which occurs commonly in cattle which are housed for long periods.

Although the condition occurs most commonly when the cattle are kept under insanitary conditions it is also seen in well-managed herds. The causative agent has not been established but *F. nodosus* has been isolated in outbreaks which were clinically and pathologically similar (12, 13). The initial lesion is an outpouring of sebaceous exudate at the skin-horn junction, particularly at the bulbs of the heel. There is a penetrating foul odour, the lesion is painful to touch but there is little swelling and no systemic reaction. More than one foot is commonly affected. In long-standing cases there is separation of the horn at the heel-bulb and this is followed by secondary bacterial infection of the sensitive structures of the foot. Often there is a purulent dermatitis of the interdigital space (11). Stable footrot does not respond satisfactorily to the standard parenteral treatments used in footrot but local treatments as set out below are effective.

Treatment

Local treatment is often laborious and in recent years has been largely replaced by parenteral treatment with comparable results (2). For best results local and parenteral treatment should be combined. Sodium sulphadimidine (1 g. per 15 lb. body weight) solution given by intravenous or intraperitoneal injection is highly effective. Penicillin (3000 units per lb body weight) intramuscularly is also used (3) as are other parenterally administered antibiotics. When a high incidence of footrot is experienced in a herd treatment of all animals simultaneously has been carried out (9). Sulphabromomethazine at the rate of 1 oz. per day in 2 lb. grain was given for 2 consecutive days to calves weighing 300 lb. and results were excellent.

Local treatment necessitates casting, or slinging the affected leg to an overhead beam. The foot is scrubbed, all necrotic tissue curetted away and a local dressing applied under a pad or bandage. Any antibacterial, and preferably astringent, dressing appears to be satisfactory. A wet pack of 5 per cent copper sulphate solution is cheap and effective. Ointment preparations are usually easier to apply. The main advantage of local treatment is that the foot is cleaned and kept clean. If conditions underfoot are wet the animal should be kept stabled in a dry stall. In animals running at pasture, local treatment may be omitted provided the disease is in the early stage and the animal can be prevented from gaining access to wet, muddy areas.

In cases where the lesion has remained superficial but has become chronic with separation of the horn from the coronary band, the horn should be trimmed back and the area cleaned and painted daily with a 5 per cent copper sulphate solution or less frequently with a mixture of 10 per cent copper sulphate in wood tar. When there is spread of infection to the deep structures of the foot, surgery may sometimes be avoided by the parenteral administration of a broad-spectrum antibiotic together with an enzyme (100,000 units of streptokinase and 75,000 units of streptodornase combined with human plasminogen). Repeated treatments for 2 to 4 days are usually necessary (4). In refractory cases shoeing or even surgical removal of the affected claw may be necessary.

Control

Prevention of foot injuries by filling in muddy and stony patches in barnyards and lanes will reduce the incidence of the disease. Provision of a footbath containing a 5 to 10 per cent solution of copper sulphate, in a doorway so that cows have to walk through it twice daily, will practically eliminate the disease on dairy farms. A mixture of 10 per cent copper sulphate in slaked lime is often used in the same manner. Similar measures can be adopted for small groups of beef animals. Feeding chlortetracycline to feedlot cattle (500 mg. per day per head for 28 days, followed by 75 mg. per day throughout the fattening period) has reduced the incidence of footrot considerably (5). The feeding of organic iodides (200 to 400 mg. of ethylenediamine dihydriodide daily in feed) has also been recommended as a preventive in feedlot cattle (6). Although extravagant claims are not made to support the use of vaccines some commercial products appear to exert a beneficial preventive effect (7).

REFERENCES

(1) Flint, J. C. & Jensen, R. (1951). *Amer. J. vet. Res.*, *12*, 5.
(2) Roberts, S. J. *et al.* (1948). *Cornell Vet.*, *38*, 122.
(3) Chambers, E. E. (1951). *N. Amer. Vet.*, *32*, 479.
(4) Leventhal, A. A. & Easterbrooks, H. L. (1956). *J. Amer. vet. med. Ass.*, *129*, 422.
(5) Johnson, W. P. *et al.* (1957). *Vet. Med.*, *52*, 375.
(6) Burch, G. R. (1957). *Allied Vet.*, *28*, 9.
(7) Gilder, R. P. (1960). *Aust. vet. J.*, *36*, 151.
(8) Monlux, W. S. *et al.* (1961). *J. Amer. vet. med. Ass.*, *138*, 379.
(9) Breen, H. & Ryff, J. F. (1961). *J. Amer. vet. med. Ass.*, *138*, 548.
(10) Gupta, R. B. *et al.* (1964). *Cornell Vet.*, *54*, 66.
(11) Smedegaard, H. H. (1964). *Veterinarian (Oxford)*, *2*, 299.
(12) Egerton J, R. & Parsonson, I. M. (1966). *Aust. vet. J.*, *42*, 425.
(13) Raven, E. T. & Cornelisse, J. L. (1971). *Vet. med. Rev.* No. 2/3, 223.

Infectious Footrot of Sheep

Infectious footrot is a disease of sheep characterized by inflammation of the skin at the skin-horn junction, under-running of the horn and inflammation of the sensitive laminae of the foot, and severe lameness.

Incidence

Footrot of sheep is common in most countries where there are large numbers of sheep except that it does not occur in arid and semi-arid areas. The incidence is highest on good, improved pastures during warm, moist periods. In these circumstances as many as 75 per cent of a flock may be affected at one time and lameness be so severe that many sheep are forced to walk on their knees. In such circumstances loss of bodily condition is extreme and this, combined with a moderate mortality rate and the expense of labour and materials to treat the disease adequately, makes footrot one of the most costly of sheep diseases. Little quantitative pathology has been done so that an accurate estimate of wastage is impossible. One experiment in sheep on pasture does show an improvement in body weight of infected over control sheep (1).

Aetiology

The lesions of footrot are caused by infection by *Fusiformis* (*Sphaerophorus*) *nodosus*. Although two other bacteria, *Spirochaeta* (*Treponema*) *penortha* and a motile fusiform bacillus, are commonly present and were thought to have aetiological importance, the disease can occur in their absence (2). Infection can persist for years in the feet of sheep but dies out within a few days in pasture, a point of great importance in the control of the disease. Sheep and goats are the species principally affected and they are susceptible at all ages over 2 months. Sheep of the Merino type are most susceptible. British breeds, particularly Romney Marsh, are less susceptible and suffer from a milder form of the disease. Immunity does not develop and repeated attacks can occur in the one animal. The infection has also been identified as a herd problem in pastured cattle (3).

The great variation in the incidence of the disease is due principally to variations in climate, particularly moistness of pasture, and environmental temperature. Most serious outbreaks in sheep at pasture occur in the spring when the weather is warm and wet and the wetness has to be of considerable duration; short, heavy rainfalls are not significant, persistent rain over several months is (4). The climate must provide continued free water on the ground for transmission to occur. But free surface water in winter exerts no effect on footrot— the daily mean temperature must be above 10°C. Housed sheep are also more commonly affected when conditions underfoot are wet. Any factor which concentrates sheep in small areas will favour spread of the disease. Improved pasture, especially when irrigated, is particularly conducive to a high incidence of footrot. The feet of the sheep become soft and the bacteria are protected in a moist, warm environment. Skin penetration by larvae of the nematode *Strongyloides* spp. may also be a predisposing cause (2).

Transmission

Discharge from infected feet is the source of infection. Many affected sheep recover spontaneously but about 10 per cent persist as nonclinical, chronic 'carriers' for several years. Conditions of wetness and warmth favour persistence of the bacteria in pasture and increase susceptibility of the feet to injury and dermatitis, thus facilitating spread of the disease from carrier sheep. Hot, dry conditions aid healing of the feet and are inimical to persistence of the bacteria on pasture. Spread of footrot occurs for very short periods but the infection rate may be very high so that a lot of acute cases occur together creating 'outbreak' conditions. Infected cattle may on occasions serve as a source of infection for sheep (13).

Pathogenesis

An initial local dermatitis, caused by infection with *F. necrophorus* at the skin–horn junction, may progress no further (5) or it may be complicated by invasion with *F. nodosus* and the development of clinical footrot, or by extension of the original infection into the bulbar soft tissues of the heel (6). At least part of the capacity of *F. nodosus* to invade horny tissue lies in its characteristic of producing keratolytic enzymes which digest horn.

Clinical Findings

The earliest sign of acute footrot is swelling and moistness of the skin of the interdigital cleft. This inflammation is accompanied by slight lameness which increases as necrosis under-runs the horn in the cleft. When extensive under-running has occurred lameness is severe, the animal may carry the leg, and if more than one foot is affected, may walk on its knees or remain recumbent. At this stage there is a foul smelling discharge, which is always small in amount. The detached horn can be lifted up and pared off in large pieces. Abscessation does not occur. A systemic reaction, manifested by anorexia and fever, may occur in severe cases. Recumbent animals become emaciated and may die of starvation. Secondary bacterial invasion may result in the spread of inflammation up the legs and in severe cases the hoof may slough off. Rams appear to be more severely affected than ewes or wethers, possibly because of their greater weight.

Symptomless 'carriers' may be affected for periods of up to 3 years. Most such animals have a misshapen foot and a pocket of infection beneath under-run horn can be found if the foot is pared. A less common form of the chronic disease is an area of moist skin between the claws without involvement of the claw. With either form acute footrot may develop when warm, moist climatic conditions occur.

Clinical Pathology and Necropsy Findings

No clinico-pathological tests are usually performed although bacteriological examination of swabs of pus is necessary for accurate identification of the disease. With the identification of benign footrot and ovine interdigital dermatitis the prognosis in a flock with foot lesions depends largely on the identity of the organisms isolated and particularly the proteolytic/keratolytic index of any *F. nodosus* present (7). Because of the non-fatal nature of footrot necropsy examinations are not usually performed. Details of the pathology are available (8).

Diagnosis

There are a number of conditions which may be confused with footrot, especially when they occur in the same environmental conditions. Foot abscess, affecting usually only one foot, is not so highly contagious and is characterized by extensive suppuration. Cases of contagious ecthyma and blue-tongue may have foot lesions but typical lesions are always present around the mouth.

Benign footrot (9), or footscald, is very similar to early footrot and like it occurs under very wet conditions but it often occurs on farms where footrot is not known to occur and where there is no history of the recent introduction of sheep. The interdigital skin becomes inflamed and covered by a thin film of moist necrotic material; the horn is pitted and blanched. Maceration and necrosis occur at the skin–horn junction and although there is an odour, it lacks the rancidity of footrot. There is separation of the horn at the heel but the dermis is normal and there is no suppuration. Under-running of the horn is limited to the heel. The extensive under-running of the horn of the wall and sole and the accumulation of foul smelling exudate which are characteristic of footrot do not occur in footscald. Benign footrot is caused by infection with strains of *F. nodosus* which are less virulent, due to their low keratolytic capacity, than those which cause virulent footrot (9). Clinically it is indistinguishable

from interdigital dermatitis caused by *F. necrophorus* and, like it, is capable of being converted to virulent footrot by the introduction of virulent strains of *F. nodosus*.

Laminitis, after engorgement on grain, may cause lameness and recumbency, but, although the feet may be hot and painful, there are no superficial lesions. Suppurative cellulitis, caused by *F. necrophorus*, commences as an ulcerative dermatitis of the pastern above the bulb of the heel, and extends up the leg to the knee or the hock and more deeply into subcutaneous tissues. Separation of the wall of the foot (shelly hoof) occurs commonly in Merino sheep on improved pasture. The abaxial wall of the hoof separates from the sole near the toe and the crevice formed becomes packed with mud and manure. The hoof in the region is dry and crumbly.

Treatment

The methods of treatment of footrot in sheep have undergone extensive examination in recent years. Until recently it was believed that only topical applications could be effective. It is now known that up to 96 per cent recovery can be achieved by a single intramuscular injection of penicillin and streptomycin (70,000 units procaine penicillin G and 70 mg. streptomycin per kg. body weight) without paring the feet (11). As with most other treatments for footrot the treatment is much more effective in dry weather (10). In wet conditions the concentration of antibiotic at the tissue level is much reduced. Treatment can be carried out in wet weather but treated sheep should be kept indoors for 24 hours after treatment. The method is expensive but reduces labour costs and removes the need for ruthless, severe hoof paring.

Although parenteral treatment alone may be sufficient, the results can be significantly improved by trimming, not paring, the feet and foot bathing in 5 per cent formalin. The following comments apply to that circumstance and to these circumstances in which only local treatment is used. Because of the labour required for topical treatments an intensive search has been carried out to determine the most satisfactory treatment based on the proportion of permanent cures, keeping in mind the varying environmental circumstances in which the disease occurs. This is most important during wet weather when topical applications are likely to be washed off the feet. Irrespective of the local medicament used one principle of treatment is inescapable. All under-run horn must be carefully removed so that the antibacterial agent to be applied can come into contact with infective material. This necessitates painstaking and careful examination and paring of all feet. When only a few sheep are affected, bandaging heavily pared feet may hasten recovery. Very sharp instruments including a knife and hoof secateurs are necessary to do the job properly and they should be disinfected after each use. The parings should be collected and burnt.

The local preparation to be used will depend on a number of factors. Some of the less efficient may be adequate in dry seasons when natural recovery is likely to occur. They may be applied by brush, by spray or aerosol or in a foot bath. Preparations suitable for foot baths include 5 per cent formalin, which does not deteriorate with pollution, and 5 per cent copper sulphate solution which does, and has the added disadvantage of colouring the wool. The local application of formalin to normal feet after all treatments and examinations for footrot reduces the chance of spread of infection by material left on the hooves. Regardless of the agent used, it is recommended that the sheep be kept standing on concrete or dry ground for a few hours after treatment.

The relative merits and disadvantages of the various preparations used are: copper sulphate solution (5 per cent) colours the wool, deteriorates with pollution and may cause excessive contamination of the environment with copper; formalin solution (5 per cent) must be applied weekly for 4 weeks and delayed relapses are likely to occur about 3 weeks later. This is a major disadvantage as sheep may be classified as cured and subsequently become active spreaders of the disease. The use of solutions containing more than 5 per cent formalin or dipping at intervals of less than 1 week may cause irritation of the skin. Local applications include chloramphenicol (10 per cent tincture in methylated spirits or propylene glycol), oxytetracycline (5 per cent tincture in methylated spirits) and cetylrimethyl ammonium bromide or Cetavlon (20 per cent alcoholic tincture); dichlorophen as a 10 per cent solution in diacetone alcohol or ethyl alcohol give comparable results with single treatments. Chloramphenicol is expensive but efficient, provided the 10 per cent tincture is used, and is probably as good as any other preparation under both wet and dry conditions. Oxytetracycline must be used as a 5 per cent tincture for optimum results and is not as efficient as chloramphenicol under wet conditions but gives excellent results when the weather is dry. Delayed relapses occur with this drug as well as with formalin. Cetavlon is a relatively cheap product and appears to be as effective as chloramphenicol

under all conditions. It is possible that in different countries with different climates and environmental conditions the efficiency of particular treatments will vary. Thus, English experience is that about the same results are achieved by the use of a 10 per cent formalin foot bath as by the application of a 10 per cent tincture of chloramphenicol or oxytetracycline, whereas under Australian conditions treatment with antibiotics is much superior.

With all of these treatments the treated feet must be examined subsequently and feet showing inflammation re-treated. In dry summer months 90 to 100 per cent cures can be anticipated with one treatment but in wet seasons 75 per cent is the maximum rate of cure with one treatment. Animals showing persistent inflammation should be treated until cured or culled.

Control

The eradication of footrot in sheep can be accomplished with relative ease in many areas, but where rainfall is heavy and the ground moist most of the year, much greater difficulty may be encountered (12). Control programmes are based on the fact that the causative bacteria do not usually persist in pasture for long periods and if fields are kept free of sheep for 14 days they can be considered to be clean. Thus if all infected animals are culled or cured and infection removed from the pasture eradication is achieved. The programme must take into account the fact that *F. nodosus* can be carried on the feet of cattle (3, 13).

Eradication of the disease should be undertaken during a dry summer season. All feet of sheep are examined and affected or suspicious sheep are segregated. Clean sheep are run through a foot bath (5 per cent formalin) and put into fresh fields, while the affected are isolated and treated, either parenterally with antibiotics, or locally with one of the preparations described above. Local treatments must be repeated weekly. Sheep which do not respond must be culled. If the incidence of carriers is high the clean flock should be re-examined one month later. When examinations are carried out during dry weather the feet are likely to be hard and the disease at a quiescent stage. In such circumstances minor lesions may be missed, necessitating an extremely careful trimming and examination of all feet. Most breakdowns in eradication occur because of inefficient examination and treatment or the introduction of affected sheep without first ensuring that they are free from the disease. In areas where flocks are small and there are insufficient fields to carry out this programme completely, it has been found to be sufficient to treat all affected sheep weekly but to put all affected sheep back in the flock and the flock back onto the infective pasture.

During a major outbreak new infections are occurring too rapidly to make eradication practicable at that time. The objective should be to limit the spread as much as possible so that the mess to be cleared up later is manageable. Foot bathing and isolation of infected flocks are the two important procedures at this time.

The whole subject of footrot control is now back in the melting pot because of the advent of an apparently successful vaccination procedure (14, 15, 16). The vaccine is effective in curing the disease as well as preventing it and has the virtue of longevity. Just what part vaccination will play in footrot control remains to be seen. Preliminary field experiments look most promising (16).

REFERENCES

(1) Littlejohn, A. I. & Hebert, C. N. (1968). *Vet. Rec.*, *82*, 690.
(2) Beveridge, W. I. B. (1934). *Aust. vet. J.*, *10*, 43.
(3) Egerton, J. R. & Parsonson, I. M. (1966). *Aust. vet. J.*, *42*, 425.
(4) Graham, N. P. H. & Egerton, J. R. (1968). *Aust. vet. J.*, *44*, 235.
(5) Parsonson, I. M. *et al.* (1967). *J. comp. Path.*, *77*, 309; *79*, 207, 217.
(6) Egerton, J. R. *et al.* (1966). *Aust. vet. J.*, *42*, 440.
(7) Morgan, I. R. *et al.* (1972). *Aust. vet. J.*, *48*, 23.
(8) Thomas, J. H. (1964). *Aust. J. agric. Res.*, *15*, 1001.
(9) Egerton, J. R. & Parsonson, I. M. (1969). *Aust. vet. J.*, *45*, 345.
(10) Egerton, J. R. *et al.* (1968). *Aust. vet. J.*, *44*, 275.
(11) Egerton, J. R. & Parsonson, I. M. (1966). *Aust. vet. J.*, *42*, 97.
(12) Beveridge, W. I. B. (1963). *Bull. Off. int. Épizoot.*, *59*, 1537.
(13) Wilkinson, F. C. *et al.* (1970). *Aust. vet. J.*, *46*, 382.
(14) Egerton, J. R. & Roberts, D. S. (1971). *J. comp. Path.*, *81*, 179.
(15) Egerton, J. R. (1970). *Aust. vet. J.*, *46*, 114, 517.
(16) Egerton, J. R. & Morgan, I. R. (1972). *Vet. Rec.*, *91*, 447, 453.

Foot Abscess of Sheep

Foot abscess occurs most commonly during very wet seasons as does footrot but the former is limited largely to adult sheep, especially ewes heavy in lamb, or rams (1) and does not cause such a high morbidity as footrot. Usually only one foot and one claw is involved, although in severe outbreaks all four feet may become affected (2). *F. necrophorus* is the cause of the disease although *Cor. pyogenes* and *Escherichia coli* are commonly found in chronic lesions. 'Foot abscess' really includes two diseases (3). Toe abscess is a lamellar suppuration with purulent under-running of the horn, particularly at the toe. There is severe lame-

ness, swelling of the coronet with pain and heat apparent, and usually rupture and purulent discharge at the coronet between the toes. Penetration to deeper structures may also occur.

The other common lesion is 'heel abscess' or infectious bulbar necrosis. It results as an extension from ovine interdigital dermatitis into the soft tissues of the heel and is therefore caused by *F. necrophorus* and *Corynebacterium pyogenes* (3, 4). When the phalangeal joints are involved there is severe swelling at the back of the feet. Rupture of the swellings is followed by a profuse discharge of pus which does not occur in footrot. Treatment by surgical drainage, parenteral treatment with sodium sulphadimidine solution (1 g. per 15 lb. body weight) and the application of a local dressing, is usually adequate (1). Sulphonamide therapy may need to be continued for several days.

REFERENCES

(1) Thomas, J. H. (1962). *Aust. vet. J.*, *38*, 159.
(2) Goodner, D. E. (1961). *N.Z. vet. J.*, *9*, 59.
(3) Roberts, D. S. *et al.* (1968). *J. comp. Path.*, *78*, 1.
(4) Roberts, D. S. (1969). *J. infect. Dis.*, *120*, 720.

Footrot of Pigs

Footrot in pigs bears some clinical resemblance to footrot in other species and is included here for this reason although the cause of the disease has not been determined.

Incidence

The disease has been reported from several countries but in most instances it is relatively uncommon as a clinical condition. An abattoir survey conducted in England showed that about 65 per cent of slaughter pigs showed lesions of the disease. The extent to which weight gains were affected is unknown. It is recognized that severely affected animals lose weight but with average minor lesions food conversion and growth rate are not significantly affected and fatalities are rare (5). The morbidity rate may reach 20 to 50 per cent of pigs in the susceptible age group on an infected farm.

Aetiology

The disease has been produced experimentally by confining pigs on abrasive concrete floors (4) but only moderately severe lesions developed on excessively rough floors. This does suggest the possibility of an additional causative agent. Dietary deficiency, particularly a deficiency of biotin, has been suggested as a contributory cause in some instances.

Unidentified spirochaetes and Gram negative

fusiform organisms are present in large numbers in the lesions but other bacteria are also found. There is a close correlation between the incidence of foot-rot and of ulcerative granuloma. Young pigs, 3 to 6 months of age, are most commonly affected but cases occur in adults. The disease occurs only in pigs housed on concrete floors, and the highest incidence is during summer months. The disease tends to recur on infected farms.

Transmission

Infection of foot wounds by material from infected feet of other pigs is suggested as the method of spread.

Pathogenesis

The disease appears to be a local infection of the feet which gains entrance through a separation between the wall and the sole caused by excessive wearing on the lateral edge of the hoof on abrasive concrete floors. Infection works its way up to the coronet and discharges to the exterior.

Clinical Findings

Where the disease is due to abrasion of the horn by rough concrete surfaces a number of characteristic lesions occur. These include erosion of the sole, either at the toe or the heel, so as to produce a lesion at the white line or a false sand crack. Bruising of the heel or the heel–sole junction is a common early finding (4).

Severe lameness is apparent. In most cases only the lateral digit on one foot is affected. Swelling at the coronet continues into the hoof and a crack is always present between the wall and the sole on the lateral edge. Necrosis extends up between the sole and sensitive laminae and may discharge at the coronet causing the development of a granulomatous lesion, or it may extend to deeper structures of the foot with multiple sinuses discharging to the exterior. Very little pus is present. The recovery rate is satisfactory with treatment although a permanently deformed foot may result and destruction may be necessary in severe cases.

Clinical Pathology

Bacteriological examination of discharges from the lesions may aid in deciding the treatment to be used.

Necropsy Findings

Necrosis of the laminar tissue with indications of progression from an infected sole are the usual findings.

Diagnosis

Most other causes of lameness in pigs are not manifested by foot lesions. In adult pigs housed indoors an overgrowth of the hoof may occur and be followed by under-running of the sole, necrosis and the protrusion of granulation tissue causing severe lameness and often persistent recumbency (3). The general appearance of these feet is not unlike that of canker in horses. Swelling of the hoof is caused by an extensive fibrous tissue reaction. Vesicular exanthema and foot-and-mouth disease are characterized by the presence of vesicular lesions on the coronets and snout.

Treatment

Parenteral injection of sodium salts of sulphonamides (1), or penicillin (2), have given inconsistent results and topical applications of copper sulphate or formalin (5 to 10 per cent) have been more successful.

Control

Prevention of excessive wear of the feet by the use of adequate bedding and less abrasive flooring in pig pens is suggested as a reasonable control measure. The use of a footbath containing 5 to 10 per cent formalin, or twice weekly use of one containing 10 per cent copper sulphate, delays but does not prevent the development of lesions (4). Any existing dietary deficiency should be corrected.

REFERENCES

(1) Bishop, W. H. (1948). *Aust. vet. J., 24*, 256.
(2) Osborne, H. G. & Ensor, C. R. (1953). *N.Z. vet. J., 3*, 91.
(3) Hogg, A. H. (1952). *Vet. Rec., 64*, 39.
(4) Wright, A. I. *et al.* (1972). *Vet. Rec., 90*, 93.
(5) Penny, R. H. C. *et al.* (1963). *Vet. Rec., 75*, 1225.

Oral Necrobacillosis

The term oral necrobacillosis is applied to infections of the mouth and larynx with *Fusiformis necrophorus*. It includes calf diphtheria in which the lesions are largely confined to the larynx and pharynx, and necrotic stomatitis in which the lesions are restricted to the oral cavity. They are considered together because the essential lesion and infection are the same in both instances.

Incidence

The disease has no geographical limitations but is more common in countries where animals are housed in winter or maintained in feedlots. In the U.S.A. infections involving the pharynx and larynx appear to be more prevalent in the western states than in other sections of the country. There is also a difference in age incidence, necrotic stomatitis occurring mainly in calves 2 weeks to 3 months of age while laryngeal infections commonly affect older calves and yearlings. Although the disease is more common in housed or penned animals it can occur in animals running at pasture (1, 2, 3, 4).

Aetiology

F. necrophorus is present in large numbers in the lesions and is considered to be the causative agent, probably aided by prior injury to the mucosa. Oral infection occurs principally in calves less than 3 months old whereas laryngeal involvement is more common in older calves up to 18 months of age. The disease is seen commonly only in cattle but has been observed in sheep (6). Animals suffering from intercurrent disease or nutritional deficiency are most susceptible and the incidence is highest in groups kept in confined quarters under insanitary conditions.

Transmission

The causative bacterium is a common inhabitant of the environment of cattle and under insanitary conditions the infection may be spread on dirty milk pails and feeding troughs. Entry through the mucosa is probably effected through abrasions caused by rough feed and erupting teeth. The difficulty of reproducing the disease and the irregularity of its occurrence even when *F. necrophorus* is known to be present suggests the possibility of aetiological factors presently unknown.

Clinical Findings

In describing the clinical findings a distinction must be drawn between calf diphtheria characterized by involvement of the throat and the more common necrotic stomatitis. In the former a moist painful cough, accompanied by severe inspiratory dyspnoea, salivation, painful swallowing movements, complete anorexia and severe depression are the characteristic signs. The temperature is high (41°C or 106°F), the pharyngeal region may be swollen and is painful on external palpation and there is salivation and nasal discharge. The breath has a most foul rancid smell. Death is likely to occur from toxaemia or obstruction to the respiratory passages on the second to seventh day. Most affected calves die without treatment but only a small proportion of calves in a group are usually affected. Spread to the lungs may cause a severe, suppurative bronchopneumonia.

In calves affected with necrotic stomatitis there is usually a moderate increase in temperature (39·5 to 40°C or 103 to 104°F), depression and anorexia.

The breath is foul and saliva, often mixed with straw, hangs from the mouth. A characteristic swelling of the cheeks may be observed posterior to the lip commissures. On opening the mouth this is found to be due to a deep ulcer in the mucosa of the cheek. The ulcer is usually filled with a mixture of necrotic material and food particles. An ulcer may also be present on the adjacent side of the tongue. In severe cases the lesions may spread to the tissues of the face and throat and into the orbital cavity. Similar lesions may be present on the vulva and around the coronets, and spread to the lungs may cause fatal pneumonia. In other cases death appears to be due to toxaemia.

Clinical Pathology

Bacteriological examination of swabs from lesions may assist in confirming the diagnosis.

Necropsy Findings

Severe swelling, due to oedema and inflammation of the tissues surrounding the ulcer, is accompanied by the presence of large masses of cheesy, purulent material. Similar lesions to those in the mouth, pharynx and larynx may be found in the lungs and in the abomasum.

Treatment

Regardless of the site of the lesion a favourable response can be expected following sulphonamide therapy. Sodium sulphadimidine (1 g. per 15 lb. body weight) repeated daily for 2 to 3 days is effective (5). Parenteral administration may be necessary if the animal is unable to swallow. Because in many cases the animals do not drink well care should be taken that adequate fluids are administered during sulphonamide therapy. Penicillin, streptomycin, the tetracyclines and chloramphenicol are also effective. Local treatment with antiseptics, including tincture of iodine, is often instituted but probably has little effect on the course of the disease unless systemic antibacterial treatment is also employed. Tracheotomy may occasionally be necessary to relieve dyspnoea. The prognosis is favourable if treatment is begun early but less so if the ulceration has been extensive or if secondary pneumonia or abomasitis has developed.

Control

Proper hygienic precautions in calf pens or feeding and drinking places together with avoidance of rough feed should prevent the spread of the disease. When the incidence is high prophylactic antibiotic feeding may keep the disease in check.

REFERENCES

(1) Farquharson, J. (1942). *J. Amer. vet. med. Ass.*, *101*, 88.
(2) Kingman, H. E. & Stansbury, W. M. (1944). *N. Amer. Vet.*, *25*, 671.
(3) Lovell, R. (1945). *Vet. Rec.*, *57*, 179.
(4) Sutherland, A. K. (1950). *Aust. vet. J.*, *26*, 238.
(5) Hayes, A. F. & Wright, G. M. (1949). *J. Amer. vet. med. Ass.*, *114*, 80.
(6) Diplock, P. T. (1958). *Vet. Insp. N.S.W.*, pp. 51 and 53.

Necrotic Rhinitis

(*Bullnose*)

Necrotic rhinitis is often confused with atrophic rhinitis. It occurs in young growing pigs and may occur in herds where atrophic rhinitis is present and even in the same pig but there appears to be no relationship between the two diseases. The common occurrence of *Fusiformis necrophorus* in the lesions suggest that any injury to the face, or nasal or oral cavities may lead to invasion especially if the environment is dirty and heavily contaminated. The incidence of the disease has diminished in recent years, due probably to a general improvement in hygiene in piggeries.

The lesions develop as a necrotic cellulitis of the soft tissues of the nose and face but may spread to involve bone. Local swelling is obvious and extensive lesions may interfere with respiration and mastication. Depression of food intake and toxaemia result in poor growth and some deaths. Treatment by the local application of antibacterial drugs and the oral administration of sulphonamides is satisfactory in early cases. Oral dosing with sulphadimidine has been effective in young pigs (1). Improvement of sanitation, elimination of injuries and disinfection of pens usually result in a reduction of incidence.

The disease differs from atrophic rhinitis by the presence of oral and facial lesions. Necrotic ulcer of pigs may involve the mouth and face but the lesions are erosive rather than necrotic.

REFERENCE

(1) Eieland, E. & Faanes, T. (1950). *Nord. Vet.-Med.*, *2*, 204.

DISEASES CAUSED BY *PSEUDOMONAS* Spp.

Occasional cases of generalized infection with *Pseudomonas aeruginosa* have been described, usually following an attack of mastitis caused by this organism (1, 2). Systemic invasion is manifested by fibrinous pericarditis and pleurisy and chronic pyelonephritis. An acute, fatal pneumonia has also been recorded in pigs in contact with infected cows (3) and in calves (4). Infections with *Pseudomonas* spp. are notoriously difficult to treat. There has been a recent introduction of an antibiotic carbenicillin (Pyopen) which on its own, or in combination with gentamicin, is effective against these bacteria (5).

REFERENCES

(1) Winter, H. & O'Connor, R. F. (1957). *Aust. vet. J.*, *33*, 83.
(2) Gardiner, M. R. & Craig, J. (1961). *Vet. Rec.*, *73*, 372.
(3) Baker, W. L. (1962). *Vet. Med.*, *57*, 232.
(4) Prasad, B. M. *et al.* (1967). *Acta vet. Hung.*, *17*, 363.
(5) Rolinson, G. N. & Sutherland, R. (1968). *Antimicrob. Agents Chemother.*, 609.

Melioidosis

Melioidosis is primarily a disease of rodents with an occasional case occurring in humans but the disease has recently been observed in farm animals. Clinical and necropsy findings are similar to those of glanders in the horse.

Incidence

Amongst rodents and humans, the disease occurs almost exclusively in tropical countries. In domestic animals the disease has occurred in outbreak form in pigs, goats and sheep in Australia (1, 2, 3), in the Caribbean area (4) and in Cambodia (10), in horses in Malaya (5) and Iran (14), and in pigs and cattle in Papua, New Guinea (11). Most cases occur during the wet season and in low-lying swampy areas. Its chief importance in farm animals has been in sheep in which heavy mortalities have occurred. The fatal nature of this disease in man makes melioidosis an important zoonosis.

Aetiology

Pseudomonas (*Malleomyces*) *pseudomallei* is relatively susceptible to environmental influences and disinfectants although it can survive in water at room temperature for up to 8 weeks and in muddy water for up to 7 months (9). In tropical and subtropical areas water-borne infection is probably an important source of infection. Cases have occurred in rodents, humans, animals in zoological gardens, dogs, cats, horses, cattle, pigs, sheep and goats. The disease can also be produced experimentally in rats, mice and hamsters. Varying degrees of virulence are observed in different strains of the organism but starvation or other conditions of stress appear to increase the susceptibility of experimental animals to infection (7).

Transmission

The source of infection is infected animals which pass the organism in their faeces. The disease in rodents runs a protracted course, making these animals important reservoirs of infection for man and possibly other species. Infection can be spread by ingestion of contaminated food or water, by insect bites, cutaneous abrasions and possibly by inhalation.

Pathogenesis

The development of the disease is presumed to be the same as in glanders with an initial septicaemia or bacteraemia and subsequent localization in various organs.

Clinical Findings

In humans the disease is highly fatal, an acute septicaemia terminating after an illness of about 10 days. Melioidosis in rodents is also highly fatal and is characterized by weakness, fever and ocular and nasal discharge. In these animals the course may be as long as 2 to 3 months. Signs in sheep consist mainly of weakness and recumbency with death occurring in 1 to 7 days. In experimentally infected sheep, a severe febrile reaction occurs and is accompanied by anorexia, lameness and a thick, yellow exudate from the nose and eyes. Some animals show evidence of central nervous system involvement including abnormal gait, deviation of the head and walking in circles, nystagmus, blindness, hyperaesthesia and mild tetanic convulsions. The disease is usually fatal. Skin involvement is not recorded. In horses the syndrome is one of an acute metastatic pneumonia with high fever and a short course. Cough and nasal discharge are minimal and there is a lack of response to treatment with most drugs. In goats the syndrome may resemble the acute form as seen in sheep but more commonly runs a chronic course (6). The disease in pigs is usually chronic and manifested by cervical lymphadenitis but in some outbreaks there are signs similar to those in other species. In such outbreaks slight posterior paresis, mild fever, coughing, nasal and ocular discharge, anorexia, abortion and some deaths may occur (10).

Clinical Pathology

The organism is easily cultured and may be isolated from nasal discharges. Injection into guinea pigs and rabbits produces the typical disease. An allergic skin test using melioidin as an antigen (2), a complement fixation test (15), and an indirect haemagglutination test (12) are available but have not had extensive trials. Affected horses may give a positive reaction to the mallein test (8).

Necropsy Findings

Multiple abscesses in most organs, particularly in the lungs, spleen and liver, but also in the subcutis and the associated lymph nodes, are characteristic of the disease in all species. In sheep these abscesses contain thick or caseous, green-tinged pus similar to that found in *Corynebacterium pseudotuberculosis* lesions. Lesions in the nasal mucosa proceed to rupture with the development of ragged ulcers. An acute polyarthritis, with distension of the joint capsules by fluid containing large masses of greenish pus, and an acute meningo-encephalitis have been observed in experimental cases.

Diagnosis

The fatal nature of the disease and the multiple abscessation in various organs serve to differentiate it from caseous lymphadenitis in sheep. The lesions of nasal actinobacillosis of sheep may also resemble those of melioidosis but this disease is relatively non-fatal and isolation of the organism provides a positive diagnosis. In horses the disease may be confused with strangles or glanders, but there is no enlargement of lymph nodes or involvement of the nasal mucosae or skin.

Treatment

Little information is available on satisfactory treatments of melioidosis. Penicillin, streptomycin, chlortetracycline and polymyxin are ineffective but in vitro tests suggest that terramycin, novobiocin, chloramphenicol and sulfadiazine (13) are most likely to be valuable with terramycin preferred. Treatment is unlikely to be undertaken because of the nature of the disease and the risk of exposure to humans.

Control

The elimination of infected animals and the disinfection of premises should be the basis of control procedures.

REFERENCES

(1) Cottew, G. S. *et al.* (1952). *Aust. vet. J., 28*, 113.
(2) Olds, R. J. & Lewis, F. A. (1954). *Aust. vet. J., 30*, 253.
(3) Olds, R. J. & Lewis, F. A. (1955). *Aust. vet. J., 31*, 273.
(4) Sutmoller, P. *et al.* (1957). *J. Amer. vet. med. Ass., 130*, 415.
(5) Davie, J. & Wells, C. W. (1952). *Brit. vet. J., 108*, 161.
(6) Cottew, G. S. (1955). *Aust. vet. J., 31*, 155.
(7) Dannenberg, A. M. & Scott, E. M. (1958). *Amer. J. Path., 34*, 1099.
(8) McLennan, I. S. (1953). *J. roy. Army vet. Cps, 24*, 130.
(9) Laws, L. & Hall, W. T. K. (1964). *Aust. vet. J., 40*, 309.
(10) Omar, A. R. *et al.* (1962). *Brit. vet. J., 118*, 421.
(11) Rampling, A. (1964). *Aust. vet. J., 40*, 241.
(12) Ileri, S. Z. (1965). *Brit. vet. J., 121*, 164.

(13) Eickhoff, T. C. *et al.* (1970). *J. infect. Dis.*, *121*, 95.
(14) Baharsefat, M. & Amjadi, A. R. (1970). *Arch. Inst. Razi.*, *22*, 209.
(15) Laws, L. (1967). *Qd J. agric. Anim. Sci.*, *24*, 207.

DISEASES CAUSED BY *VIBRIO* Spp.

Winter Dysentery of Cattle

Winter dysentery is a highly contagious disease of cattle characterized by a brief attack of severe diarrhoea and sometimes dysentery.

Incidence

Under the name winter dysentery, vibrionic diarrhoea occurs commonly in cattle in North America, and possibly in Britain (6), Sweden (5) and Australia (1). Its similarity to other diseases, particularly mucosal disease, makes its positive identification difficult to establish. The disease is a serious one in dairy herds because, although few animals die, there may be serious loss of condition and milk flow. From 10 to 100 per cent of the herd may show clinical signs. There is one record of diarrhoea due to infection with a vibrio in sheep (2) but the incidence of the disease is unknown.

Aetiology

In cattle *Vibrio jejuni* has been identified as the causative agent but there is a strong possibility that this organism plays a secondary role in the disease. Considerable difficulty is experienced in transmitting the disease from some outbreaks but not from others. This suggests that a precipitating cause, either environmental or infectious, may operate or that cattle used in transmission experiments have been immune as a result of previous attacks (3). The possibility of a primary virus infection being the precipitating cause is suggested by work in Canada (4) and Israel (8), but the probability is that two clinically similar diseases exist. A similar disease has been described in Sweden in which no vibrios were detected in the faeces (5) and in Australia a disease similar to winter dysentery has been observed as a large-scale epidemic (7). At least winter dysentery and mucosal disease of cattle are not the same disease (3).

The vibrio organisms isolated from sheep with dysentery have not been identified but closely resemble *V. foetus*.

Winter dysentery in cattle is most serious in adult milking cows, particularly those which have recently calved. Young stock may be affected but show only mild clinical signs. The disease is most common in cattle when they are housed. A moderate immunity, which persists for about 6 months, develops after a natural attack, and recurrent attacks in the one animal or herd seldom occur in less than 2 to 3 years.

Transmission

Faeces from clinical cases, or clinically normal carriers, are the source of infection, and contamination of feed or drinking water is the method of spread. The disease is highly contagious and appears to be brought on to farms by human visitors, carrier animals and on inert objects. Details of the viability of the organisms are not available but oral ingestion is the method by which infection occurs.

Pathogenesis

The disease appears to be a simple enteritis affecting chiefly the small intestine.

Clinical Findings

Cattle. After an incubation period of 3 to 7 days, there is an explosive herd outbreak of diarrhoea which, in the course of the next 4 to 7 days, affects the majority of adult cattle. Young stock in the group may show mild signs of the disease. A transient febrile period (39·5 to 40·5°C or 103 to 105°F) may precede the attack of diarrhoea but when clinical signs are evident, the temperature is usually normal. At this time there is a precipitate fall in milk yield which lasts for about a week, anorexia of short duration, and some loss of condition. The faeces are very thin, watery and homogeneous without much odour and with no mucous or epithelial shreds, and are dark green to almost black in colour. They are often passed with little warning and with considerable velocity. A harsh cough occurs in some outbreaks and may be accompanied by the explosive expulsion of faeces. In most animals the course is short and the faeces return to normal consistency in 2 to 3 days. In occasional cases the syndrome is more severe, dehydration and weakness are apparent, and dysentery, either with faeces flecked with blood or the passage of whole blood, occurs. The disease in the herd usually subsides in 1 to 2 weeks.

Sheep. Little information is available but scouring and emaciation have been reported (2).

Clinical Pathology

A smear of faeces from a clinical case usually shows the presence of many vibrios, particularly in epithelial shreds.

Necropsy Findings

Necropsy material is not usually available but in experimentally infected cattle the changes are limited to the alimentary canal and comprise hyperaemia of the abomasal mucosa and a mild catarrhal inflammation of the small intestine. There may be some hyperaemia of the caecal and colonic mucosae. More severe changes have been recorded in some outbreaks of a disease which resembles winter dysentery in cattle but which has some similarity also to mucosal disease (4).

Diagnosis

The disease in cattle is characterized by the explosive nature of the outbreaks that occur. Similar outbreaks may occur in mucosal disease but lesions of the oral mucosa are evident and the clinical signs are more severe. Individual cases of winter dysentery may resemble coccidiosis or salmonellosis but both of these diseases are more severe and usually affect only one or two animals at a time. Final differentiation depends upon examination of faecal material for the causative agent. A variety of toxic agents may also cause outbreaks of diarrhoea in cattle. The more common of these are listed under the aetiology of enteritis.

Treatment

The treatment of winter dysentery of cattle is of dubious value (3), most animals recovering spontaneously. Alimentary tract disinfectants, including 30 ml. of a mixture of equal parts pine oil and creolin twice daily or 30 ml. of 5 per cent copper sulphate solution twice daily, are most popular. Because of their efficiency in the treatment of swine dysentery it might be supposed that nitrofurazone, tylosin or an arsenical would be of value, particularly for prophylactic dosing of in-contact animals. Replacement of fluids lost by diarrhoea is probably the most effective method of relieving the dehydration and hastening recovery. One gallon of electrolyte solution administered parenterally each day is an effective supportive treatment in severe cases.

Control

Because of the explosive nature of the disease and the lack of information on possible precipitating causes, effective control measures cannot be recommended. Every effort must be made to avoid the spread of infection on inanimate objects such as boots, feeding utensils and bedding but even the greatest care does not appear to prevent the spread of the disease within a herd.

REFERENCES

(1) Hutchins, D. R. (1958). *Aust. vet. J.*, *34*, 300.
(2) Russell, R. R. (1955). *N.Z. vet. J.*, *3*, 60.
(3) Kahrs, R. F. (1965). *Cornell Vet.*, *55*, 505.
(4) McPherson, L. W. (1957). *Canad. J. comp. Med.*, *21*, 184.
(5) Hedstrom, H. & Isaacson, A. (1951). *Cornell Vet.*, *41*, 251.
(6) Rollinson, D. H. L. (1948). *Vet. Rec.*, *60*, 191.
(7) Edwards, M. J. & Sier, A. M. (1960). *Aust. vet. J.*, *36*, 402.
(8) Komarov, A. *et al.* (1959). *Refuah Vet.*, *16*, 111.

Swine Dysentery

Swine dysentery is a specific, contagious enteritis of pigs caused by *Vibrio coli*.

Incidence

Swine dysentery is widely distributed throughout the world, and it may cause a heavy mortality in young weaned pigs. The disease is particularly prevalent in pigs which have passed through sale barns. A morbidity rate of 30 to 40 per cent and a mortality rate of 60 to 70 per cent are usual. The occurrence of a chronic form of the disease suggests that there may be more subtle losses. The effect of outbreaks on production efficiency can be significant. An average drop in weaning weight of 6·5 lb. and an increase in age at marketing of 22 days is recorded (1) but it is possible to maintain productivity in the face of this disease (2).

Aetiology

Largely by default *Vibrio coli* is presently accepted as the cause of the disease but it has been necessary to postulate variations in pathogenicity of several types, based on cultural differences, to explain the very variable results of transmission experiments (3, 4). Infection with *Vibrio coli* is easily established in gnotobiotic and conventional pigs (5) but the clinical disease is regularly reproducible only with minced gut. The general dissatisfaction with *V. coli* as the primary cause has led to a widespread search for other agents. A 'borrelia-like' spirochaete appears to be the favoured candidate at present (6, 7), and the disease has been reproduced by feeding cultures of this organism. The disease is primarily one of young pigs of 8 to 12 weeks of age in the early post-weaning period although adult pigs may develop a mild form of the disease. Baby pigs as young as 3 days of age may also be affected. No immunity appears to develop and the disease may pass from pen to pen in a piggery and then recur in the first pen in a week or two. No antibodies are detectable in the serum of recovered pigs (4).

Transmission

The disease appears to spread by the ingestion of feed contaminated by the faeces of infected pigs. There is often a history of recent introductions and these animals may act as carriers. However, many outbreaks occur when no such introductions have been made. Once the disease appears in a piggery it tends to become established there and all subsequent batches of weaned pigs become affected. Experimentally infected pigs are known to excrete *V. coli* for five or six months after recovery. Since outbreaks often follow recent introductions, it is assumed that asymptomatic carriers may be responsible.

Pathogenesis

Swine dysentery is an enteritis without systemic invasion by the causative bacteria. Death appears to be due to dehydration and bacterial toxaemia.

Clinical Findings

After an incubation period of 4 to 21 days, there is an acute onset of severe diarrhoea, with anorexia and inconstantly a mild fever (up to 40 °C or 104 °F). The faeces are very thin and watery and are passed in a continuous stream without straining. They are usually bright yellow in colour but within 1 to 2 days they may become black or blood-tinged or contain whole clots of blood. Shreds of epithelium are often present and the faeces have a putrid odour. There is severe depression and dehydration and there may be evidence of pain on palpation of the abdomen. The temperature falls as the diarrhoea develops and may be subnormal in the late stages. In severe cases, death may occur within 24 hours of the first signs of illness but the course is usually longer, recovery or death occurring in 2 to 4 days and in some cases up to several weeks. As indicated above, there is no apparent immunity and the disease may recur in a pen within 1 to 2 weeks of its disappearance. During these secondary attacks, the clinical signs may be just as severe as in the original attack and the morbidity and mortality rates are likely to be as high. A chronic form of the disease, with persistent diarrhoea and failure to grow, may follow the acute form in some pigs, or may be the only syndrome observed.

Uncommonly outbreaks of the disease occur in adult pigs, especially sows on the point of farrowing or, less commonly, in mid lactation (2).

Clinical Pathology

Examination of a smear of faeces often reveals the presence of very large numbers of vibrios and this finding is of particular significance when the organisms are present in epithelial cells. Culture of the faeces often reveals *V. coli* in almost pure culture.

Necropsy Findings

In the early stages of the disease, there is a severe haemorrhagic enterocolitis with congestion, haemorrhage and an increased secretion of mucus, and a great increase in size of the goblet cells in the large bowel. The mesenteric lymph nodes are swollen and juicy. There may be a mild gastritis but the small intestine is usually normal. Later, a diffuse, diphtheritic pseudomembrane develops throughout the lower bowel and extends into the lower part of the intestine. Severe hydropic degeneration of the hepatic cells around large portal tracts may be apparent in acute cases and be visible macroscopically as elevations of paler than normal liver tissue surrounding portal vessels.

Diagnosis

Swine dysentery always presents a problem in diagnosis because of its similarity to the acute form of salmonellosis (8). Diarrhoea and dysentery occur in both but are usually more severe in swine dysentery. Pigs affected with salmonellosis usually show marked skin discolouration and frequently signs of pneumonia and nervous system involvement. The septicaemic nature of salmonellosis, compared to the largely local effects in vibrionic dysentery, is also evident at necropsy. In some outbreaks of enteritis in pigs after weaning, the cause is a haemolytic *E. coli* but this is a more common finding in younger pigs. Transmissible gastroenteritis is another disease with predominantly alimentary tract signs which occurs in younger pigs. The 'haemorrhagic bowel syndrome' differs in its pathological and epidemiological features.

Treatment

Organic arsenical preparations give excellent results in clinical cases of swine dysentery when given by injection (neoarsphenamine 0·5 to 1·0 g. intravenously or intramuscularly). The larger dose rate is given to adults and the smaller dose to pigs of 3 to 5 months of age (4). Acetarsone N.F. (Stovarsol) given by mouth in single 0·5 g. doses to weaner or older pigs, also gives excellent results. Usually deaths stop immediately and seriously affected pigs recover quickly. Because the outbreak is likely to spread rapidly, it is safest to dose all pigs in a group as soon as the first case appears. Only one dose of these arsenical preparations is ordinarily required.

Because of the difficulty encountered in the oral dosing of individual pigs, medication in the feed or drinking water is preferred when large numbers of pigs have to be handled. Provided the pigs are restricted to the medicated water or feed either arsanilates or nitrofurazone are effective, and there appears to be little difference in the efficiency of these two groups of drugs. The arsanilates (arsanilic acid or sodium arsanilate) are usually preferred because of their lower cost, nitrofurazone being used when evidence of resistance to the arsenical preparation appears. The recommended dose rates for the arsenical preparations are 175 ppm of sodium arsanilate in the drinking water or 250 ppm (250 to 500 g. per ton of feed) of arsanalic acid in the feed (9). The higher concentration is administered for 1 week, the lower concentration for 3 weeks. Because of the ease of administration and the variation of intake of water with changes in environmental temperature, administration in the feed is preferred. The usual recommendation with either method is to restrict administration to periods of one week with intervals of at least 1 week between them. However, where the disease is a major problem continuous administration through the fattening period is practised. If this is done a careful watch for signs of arsenical poisoning—incoordination and blindness—should be kept. Such signs have been observed in pigs on a continuous intake as low as 200 ppm of arsanilic acid in the feed. Nitrofurazone (15 g. per 40 gallons of water for 4 to 7 days) is effective (10). Streptomycin (0·5 to 2·0 g. per pig per day), bacitracin (100,000 units per pig per day) and chlortetracycline (20 mg. per lb. body weight per day) for several days can be used in the same manner, and these antibiotics can also be used parenterally for the treatment of individual sick pigs.

Tylosin has also given excellent results. Recommended levels of administration are 1 to 2 g. per gallon of all drinking water consumed or 40 to 100 g. per ton of feed (11). Individual pigs can be treated by an intramuscular injection of 200 mg. of tylosin. All of the above treatments are satisfactory in that they prevent losses from further deaths but they do not prevent the disease from spreading unless they are given over a period of time in the drinking water. Differences in efficiency between the above treatments in terms of removal of carriers and of rapidity of weight gain after recovery probably exist and should be investigated further. Bacitracin appears to have some advantage over other drugs in this regard.

Spiromycin is an efficient remedy and is to be used at the rate recommended for tylosin. Erythromycin is effective but is unsuitable for mass medication.

Dimetridazole is reported to be effective as treatment (12, 13). It can be administered in drinking water and the dose rate suggested is 20 mg. per kg. for 4–5 days.

Carbadox [methyl 3-(2-quinoxalinyl-methylene) carbazate N', $N4$ dioxide] at the rate of 50 g. per ton of feed, is also an effective preventive (14).

Control

Vibrionic dysentery is such a common disease of swine and occurs so readily in pigs exposed to the stress of transport and sale through yards that the purchase of store pigs should be restricted to private sales. Such purchases should be made only from farms known to be free of diarrhoea. If purchases are made from a number of farms the groups should be kept separately if possible. Small groups of about 25 pigs are optimal and the groups should be housed in the one pen from introduction to sale. Pens should be constructed so that the need to enter them is minimized and suitable hygienic precautions should be taken when moving from pen to pen (11).

The prophylactic medication of feed or water as described in treatment is used extensively to reduce the spread and severity of the disease but should be restricted to herds in which the disease is present. If an outbreak occurs all pigs on the farm are put on to an antibiotic supplement in the feed, rigid hygiene is enforced and energetic disinfection of the pen is carried out as soon as it is vacated.

REFERENCES

(1) Ducasse, F. B. W. & Nixon, R. C. (1967). *J. S. Afr. vet. med. Ass.*, 38, 205.
(2) Alexander, T. J. L. & Taylor, D. J. (1969). *Vet. Rec.*, 85, 89.
(3) Hurvell, B. & Reiland, S. (1970). *Nord. Vet. Med.*, 22, 456.
(4) Roberts, D. S. (1956). *Aust. vet. J.*, 32, 27, 114.
(5) Andress, C. E. *et al.* (1968). *Canad. J. comp. med.*, 32, 522, 529.
(6) Ritchie, A. E. & Brown, L. N. (1971). *Vet. Rec.*, 89, 608.
(7) Taylor, D. J. & Alexander, T. J. L. (1971). *Brit. vet. J.*, 127, viii.
(8) Sweeney, E. J. (1966). *Vet. Rec.*, 78, 372.
(9) Smith, I. D. (1961). *J. Anim. Sci.*, 20, 768.
(10) Roe, C. K. & Drennan, W. G. (1958). *Canad. J. comp. Med.*, 22, 97.
(11) Curtis, R. A. (1962). *Canad. vet. J.*, 3, 285.
(12) Cottereau, P. (1971). *Rev. Med. vet.*, 122, 361.
(13) Griffin, R. M. (1972). *Vet. Rec.*, 91, 349.
(14) Davies, J. W. *et al.* (1968). *J. Amer. vet. med. Ass.*, 153, 1181.

DISEASES CAUSED BY *LEPTOSPIRA* Spp.

Leptospirosis

There are no clinical signs which are diagnostic of infection by any of the leptospiral species except perhaps that the disease caused by *Leptospira icterohaemorrhagiae* is almost always septicaemic. The acute septicaemic and associated subacute syndrome and the 'abortion' form occur in most domestic species except that the 'abortion' form is not known to occur in sheep and goats. Equine periodic ophthalmia may be a sequel to leptospiral infection.

Incidence

Leptospirosis in the large domestic animals has come into prominence only during relatively recent years and details of its incidence are only now becoming available. The disease appears to be world wide in its distribution. In general terms the disease is most common in areas or seasons when the climate is warm and humid, soils are alkaline and there is an abundance of surface water.

Cattle. Although the mortality rate is low (5 per cent) in this species, the morbidity rate is usually high as determined clinically and serologically and may approach 100 per cent of in-contact animals. In calves the mortality rate is much higher than in adult cattle. A high rate of abortions (up to 30 per cent) and loss of milk production are the major causes of loss but deaths in calves may also be significant.

Pigs. In infected herds the incidence of positive reactors to serological tests is high, and in large affected pig populations averages about 20 per cent. Economic losses are about equally divided between abortions and deaths of weak and unthrifty newborn pigs.

Sheep and goats. The disease in sheep has been reported from many countries and the disease in goats from Israel. Deaths of animals and loss of condition in mildly affected animals are the main causes of loss. Although few outbreaks are recorded, a morbidity rate of 100 per cent is not uncommon in sheep and mortality rates usually average about 20 per cent in this species and up to 45 per cent in goats.

Horses. The disease is relatively mild in horses, and losses, except for blindness due to associated periodic ophthalmia, are negligible. When groups of horses are known to be infected, an average of up to 30 per cent of the adult horses can be expected to give positive serological tests.

One of the important features of leptospirosis is its transmissibility to man and it represents an occupational hazard to butchers, farmers and veterinarians. The incidence of positive agglutination tests in humans in contact with infected cattle is surprisingly low and clinical cases in man in which the infection is acquired from animals are not common. Human infection is most likely to occur by contamination with infected urine or uterine contents. Although leptospirae may be present in the milk for a few days at the peak of fever in an acute case the bacteria does not survive for long in the milk and does not withstand pasteurization.

Aetiology

As in some other important areas the microbiologists are having difficulty in making up their minds on leptospiral nomenclature (1). For convenience now, and on the assumption that in the future the nominative turmoil will be resolved, the prior system will be retained. *L. pomona* is the commonest infection in all animals. Its survival in the environment depends largely upon variations in soil and water conditions in the contaminated area; it is particularly susceptible to drying, and to changes in pH away from neutrality or mild alkalinity. A pH lower than 6·0 or greater than 8·0 is inhibitory. Temperatures lower than 7 to 10 °C or higher than 34 to 36 °C are detrimental to its survival. Moisture is the most important factor governing the persistence of the organism in bedding or soil: it can persist for as long as 183 days in water-saturated soil but survives for only 30 minutes when the soil is air dried. The organism survives in free, surface water for very long periods, the survival period being longer in stagnant than in flowing water although persistence in the latter for as long as 15 days has been recorded.

L. pomona infection has been recorded in cattle, pigs, horses and the ovine infection has been provisionally identified as *L. pomona*, and the disease has been produced experimentally in this latter species by injection of bovine and porcine strains of the organism. *L. canicola* infection has been recorded in cattle and in pigs and specific antibodies have been detected in horses. *L. icterohaemorrhagiae* is a rare isolation in large animals but has been reported in cattle and pigs, and serological evidence of infection has been found in the horse. *L. hyos* (*L. mitis*) has been isolated from cattle and pigs, *L. grippotyphosa* from cattle and goats, and positive serological tests have been obtained in horses. *L. sejroe*, *L. hebdomadis* and *L. hardjo* infection have been observed in cattle, and the experimental disease produced by the latter has been described (2). A much more detailed and extensive list is provided by Michna (1).

Calves and lambs are highly susceptible and are likely to develop the septicaemic form of the disease. Strong immunity after an attack may occur and a reduced susceptibility has been observed in pigs which is probably sufficient to produce a state of herd immunity. Passive transfer of antibodies to newborn calves occurs via the colostrum and the antibodies persist in the calves for 2 to 6 months (3).

Transmission

The source of infection is usually an infected animal which contaminates pasture, drinking water and feed by infected urine, aborted foetuses and infected uterine discharges. All of the leptospiral types are transmitted in this way and can pass between the animal species although the importance of sheep and horses in the epizootiology of leptospirosis is uncertain. The semen of an infected bull may carry leptospirae and transmission from such a bull to heifers by coitus and artificial insemination has been observed. In rams the semen is likely to be infective for only a few days during the period of leptospiraemia (4) and in boars there is no evidence of coital transmission.

Because of the rapidly accumulating evidence of a high rate of infection with *Leptospira* spp. in wild life these animals are suspected of playing a significant role in the spread of the disease to domestic animals. For example, feral pigs have been shown to have a high incidence of infection, rats are known to be a source of *L. icterohaemorhagiae*, *L. canicola* is known to spread from domestic dogs and jackals to cattle and, when hygiene is poor, even from humans to cattle. Although surveys of the incidence of leptospirosis in wildlife have been conducted in North America (5) and Great Britain (6) and the pathogenic effects of *L. pomona* on some species, particularly deer (37), have been determined, the real significance of feral leptospirosis as a source of infection for domestic animals has not been determined. There seems little doubt, from experimental evidence and from observations on field outbreaks, that many wild species do act as carriers of the disease.

Entrance of the organism into the body occurs most probably through cutaneous or mucosal abrasions. Transplacental transmission is not common but neonatal infection, probably contracted in utero, has been recorded. Oral dosing is an unsatisfactory method for experimental transmission as compared to injection and installation into the nasal cavities, conjunctival sac and vagina. Contamination of the environment and capacity of the organism to survive for long periods under favourable conditions of dampness lead to a high incidence of the disease on heavily irrigated pastures, in areas with high rainfall and temperate climate, in fields with drinking water supplies in the form of easily contaminated surface ponds, and in marshy fields and muddy paddocks or feedlots. Because of the importance of water as a means of spreading

infection new cases are most likely to occur in wet seasons and low lying areas, especially when contamination and susceptibility are high.

Urine is the chief source of contamination because animals, particularly pigs, even after clinical recovery, may pass leptospirae in the urine for long periods. For example, young pigs may act as carriers for a year and adult sows for 2 months. (7). Cattle have been shown to have leptospiruria for a mean period of 36 days (10 to 118 days) with the highest excretion rate in the first half of this period (8). Sheep do not appear to be a ready source of infection for other species, probably because of their intermittent and low-grade leptospiruria, although this may persist for 9 months in natural cases of the disease (9). Horses are also a dubious source of infection because the leptospiruria is of slight degree although it may persist for up to 4 months. In goats, leptospiruria persists for at least a month after infection (10). The leptospirae may persist in the kidney for much longer periods than they can be recovered from the urine by routine laboratory methods. It is probable that apparently recovered animals intermittently pass the organisms in the urine and thus act as 'carriers'.

Pathogenesis

After penetration of the skin or mucosa the organisms multiply rapidly in the blood stream and can be isolated from peripheral blood for several days until the fever subsides, at which time antibodies appear in the blood stream and organisms in the urine. Persistence of leptospires in renal lesions leads to prolonged leptospiruria.

A haemolysin has been isolated from *L. pomona* which causes marked haemolysis and hepatic and renal tubular necrosis in cattle and sheep. In pregnant animals of these species there was also marked necrosis of the placenta, due apparently to anoxia of tissue resulting from the haemolytic anaemia. The erythrocytes of pigs are resistant to the haemolysin (10).

Acute leptospirosis is a severe septicaemia with haemolytic anaemia which may be fatal. In animals that survive, there is localization of the organism in the liver and kidneys. This syndrome is characteristic of *L. icterohaemorrhagiae* infections in calves and piglets and of *L. pomona* in calves and lambs. Localization of the organism in nervous tissue is common in sheep and goats and may result in the appearance of signs of encephalitis. In the subacute form, the pathogenesis is similar to that of the acute septicaemic form except that the reaction is less severe. It occurs in all species but is the common one in adult cattle and horses.

Experimental production of leptospirosis with *L. pomona* in calves (11) causes a febrile reaction, accompanied by leptospiraemia, after a 4 to 9 day incubation period. The disappearance of organisms from the blood stream 2 to 4 days later coincides with a fall in temperature and is followed by leptospiruria and albuminuria coinciding with active infection of the kidney. During the febrile period, there is a leucocytosis, and transitory anaemia, haemoglobinuria and jaundice due to intravascular haemolysis. Although focal interstitial nephritis and hepatic necrosis occur during the experimental disease, no biochemical indications of renal or hepatic insufficiency have been observed. Experimental production of leptospirosis with *L. canicola* produces a similar syndrome except that there is no haemoglobinuria or jaundice (36) and there is no significant renal or hepatic impairment. There is a mild anaemia.

Leptospirosis produced experimentally in pigs is manifested by practically no clinical illness other than a slight fever, and in pregnant sows abortion or stillbirths. Maximum leptospiruria occurs 20 to 30 days after exposure and, although the urine is virtually clear of infection in most pigs 3 weeks later, the leptospiruria may persist for much longer. The most severe lesion is an interstitial nephritis and the leptospirae persist longer in the kidney (more than 45 days) than in any other organ. In sheep the experimental disease usually assumes the acute form with a clinical syndrome similar to that seen in calves. Although the leptospires appear to be able to penetrate the placental barrier abortion does not appear to be a common sequel.

In sheep the experimental disease is manifested by high fever, and significant pathological changes in the uterine endometrium (12). Although abortion may not be a common field sequel of leptospiral infection in sheep it can be produced experimentally, the pathogenesis consisting of foetal death (13) with a degree of autolysis of the foetus and placenta preceding abortion. Experimental leptospirosis in goats causes no apparent illness. The experimental disease in horses is similar to that seen in calves except that haemoglobinuria is exceptional. A moderate fever occurs on the 7th to 10th day after exposure at which time leptospirae can be cultured from the blood. Leptospirae subsequently appear in the urine and may persist for up to 120 days. Agglutinating antibodies appear at 9 days after exposure and ocular lesions of periodic ophthalmia are present in most horses up to 15 months later (14).

After both the acute and subacute forms, abortion commonly occurs in cattle and horses but abortion without prior clinical illness is also common. This is particularly the case in sows and occurs to a less extent in cows and mares, and may be due to degenerative changes in the placental epithelium. Leptospirae are rarely present in the aborted foetuses. Occult cases with no clinical illness but with rising antibody titres are common in all animals.

Although final proof is lacking that there is a direct causal relationship between leptospiral infection and periodic ophthalmia in the horse, there is strong presumptive evidence linking the two (15). There is a much higher incidence of positive reactors to serum agglutination tests for leptospiral antibodies in groups of horses affected with periodic ophthalmia than in normal animals. Agglutinins are present in the aqueous humor in greater concentration than in the serum. The absence of leptospirae from affected eyes and the fact that ophthalmia may not occur for 1 to 2 years after systemic infection has given rise to the suggestion that the ophthalmia may be due to an allergic reaction to spirochaetal protein. Many other factors including a nutritional deficiency of riboflavin and invasion of the eye by microfilariae of *Onchocerca cervicalis* (16) have been considered as causes of the disease.

Clinical Findings

The clinical findings in leptospirosis are quite similar in each animal species and do not vary greatly with the species of leptospira except that infection with *L. icterohaemorrhagiae* usually causes a severe septicaemia. For convenience the various forms of the disease are described as they occur in cattle, and comparisons are drawn with the disease in other species. In all animals the incubation period is from 3 to 7 days.

Cattle. Leptospirosis in cattle may appear as acute, subacute or chronic forms.

Acute leptospirosis, to which calves up to a month old are most susceptible, is manifested by septicaemia, with high fever (40·5 to 41·5°C or 105 to 107°F), anorexia, petechiation of mucosae, depression, and by acute haemolytic anaemia with haemolytic anaemia with haemoglobinuria, jaundice and pallor of the mucosae. Because of the anaemia there is a marked increase in heart rate, an increase in the absolute intensity of the heart sounds and a more readily palpable apex beat. Dyspnoea is also prominent. The mortality rate is high and if recovery occurs, convalescence is prolonged. Abortion, due to the systemic reaction, is likely to occur at the acute stage of the disease. Additional signs in cattle are related to the udder and milk flow. Milk flow almost ceases and the secretion is red-coloured or contains blood clots, and the udder is limp and soft. Mastitis, as part of leptospirosis, has often been described in cattle (17, 18) and the presence of many leucocytes in the grossly abnormal milk does suggest this diagnosis but these changes are due to a general vascular lesion rather than local injury to mammary tissue. Severe lameness due to synovitis is recorded in some animals and a necrotic dermatitis, probably due to photosensitization, in others.

Subacute leptospirosis differs from the acute form only in degree, approximately the same signs being observed in a number of affected animals but not all of the signs necessarily being present in the one animal. Fever is milder (39 to 40·5°C or 102 to 105°F), depression, anorexia, dyspnoea and a degree of haemoglobinuria are constant but jaundice may or may not be present. Abortion may occur 3 to 4 weeks later. In addition, one of the characteristic signs is the fall in the milk yield and the appearance of blood stained or yellow-orange, thick milk in all four quarters without apparent physical change in the udder.

Chronic leptospirosis is manifested by mild clinical signs which may be restricted to abortion. Severe 'storms' of abortions occur most commonly in groups of cattle which are at the same stage of pregnancy when exposed to infection. The abortions usually occur during the last third of pregnancy. Apart from the production of abortion there appears to be no significant depression of reproductive efficiency in cattle affected by leptospirosis. Many animals in the group develop positive agglutination titres without clinical illness.

There are occasional reports of leptospiral meningitis in cattle. Inco-ordination, excessive salivation, conjunctivitis and muscular rigidity are the common signs.

Pigs. Chronic leptospirosis is the commonest form of the disease in pigs and is characterized by the occurrence of abortion and a high incidence of stillbirths (19). Infertility is not usually observed in leptospirosis but has been reported in infections with *L. canicola.* In an infected herd the rearing rate may fall as low as 10 to 30 per cent. An abortion 'storm' may occur when the disease first appears in a herd but abortions diminish as herd immunity develops. Most abortions occur 2 to 4 weeks before term. Piglets produced at term may be dead or weak and die soon after birth.

Rarely the acute form as it occurs in calves also occurs in piglets in both natural field outbreaks and in experimentally produced cases (19). *L. ictero-haemorrhagiae* infection causes septicaemic leptospirosis with a high mortality rate.

Sheep and goats. Good descriptions of the naturally occurring disease in sheep and goats are lacking, most affected animals being found dead apparently from septicaemia. Affected animals snuffle, hang their heads down, a proportion show jaundice and most die within 12 hours. Lambs, especially those in poor condition, are most susceptible. The chronic form may occur and is manifested by loss of bodily condition but abortion seems to be almost entirely a manifestation of the acute form. The experimentally produced disease assumed the acute form accompanied in some cases by diarrhoea and, rarely, jaundice.

Horses. The subacute form as described for cattle occurs commonly but the illness is mild and short-lived (20). Icterus and a degree of depression are common signs. Abortion and periodic ophthalmia may follow. The chronic form, with abortion at the seventh to tenth month of pregnancy, has also been reported. Periodic ophthalmia is characterized clinically by recurrent attacks of ocular signs including photophobia, lacrimation, conjunctivitis, keratitis, a pericorneal corona of blood vessels, hypopyon and iridocyclitis. Recurrent attacks usually terminate in blindness in both eyes (21, 14, 15). The disease has been produced experimentally by producing infection with *L. pomona* (22).

Clinical Pathology

Laboratory procedures are most important in the diagnosis of the disease and include isolation of the organism, and examination for the presence of agglutinins in serum. The pathogenesis of the disease dictates that examinations be carried out at particular times in the development of the disease. During the septicaemic stage, leptospirae are present only in the blood. There is also anaemia and increased erythrocyte fragility and in some cases, haemoglobinuria. A leucopenia has been observed in cattle while in other species there is a mild leucocytosis. However, the only positive diagnostic measure at this stage is examination of blood for the presence of leptospirae. If abortion occurs, the kidney, lung and pleural fluid of the aborted foetuses should be examined for the presence of leptospirae.

In the stage immediately after the subsidence of the fever, the leptospirae disappear from the blood and appear in the urine. The leptospiruria is accompanied by albuminuria of varying degrees and persists for varying lengths of time in the different animal species. Detectable agglutinins appear in the serum 2 to 3 weeks after the infection has become generalized and are at their peak at about 4 weeks, subsiding thereafter but remaining at appreciable levels for over 3 months in sheep, for over a year in cattle and pigs, and longer still in horses. A presumptive diagnosis is often made on the basis of a rising titre of antibodies in paired sera taken 10 to 14 days apart.

Isolation of leptospirae is best carried out by the immediate intraperitoneal injection of blood, milk or urine into guinea pigs, or by culture on special media. Material sent to a laboratory for examination should have 1 drop of commercial formalin added to each 20 ml. of urine to prevent overgrowth by other bacteria. Examination of urine by darkground illumination may reveal the presence of viable leptospirae but the examination must be carried out as soon as the urine is collected. Of these tests the culture of blood or urine, depending on the stage of the disease, is preferred (23).

Serological tests include a haemagglutination-lysis, or more properly a microscopic agglutination (MA), test, a complement fixation test, and tube and plate agglutination tests. The haemagglutination-lysis test is most accurate and is in general use. Titres of 1:500 in cattle and 1:200 in pigs are considered to be positive in the agglutination test. Many animals in infected groups show titres greater than 1:200 without having shown any clinical abnormality. Antibodies also appear in urine and milk and their measurement may have some significance in special circumstances.

Necropsy Findings

In the acute form, anaemia, jaundice, haemoglobinuria and subserous and submucosal haemorrhages are constant. There may be ulcers and haemorrhages in the abomasal mucosa in cattle and if haemoglobinuria has been severe, there may be associated pulmonary oedema and emphysema. Histologically there is focal or diffuse interstitial nephritis and centrilobular hepatic necrosis and in some cases vascular lesions in the meninges and brain. Leptospirae may be visible in sections and attempts should be made to isolate them from the kidney.

In the later stages the characteristic finding is a progressive interstitial nephritis manifested by small, white, raised areas in the renal cortex.

A characteristic focal hepatitis has been observed in aborted piglets. The necrotic foci are 1 to 4 mm. in diameter, irregular in outline and are found in the liver in 40 per cent of aborted foetuses. The foetal membranes are thick, oedematous, brown and necrotic.

Diagnosis

Positive diagnosis of leptospirosis in individual animals is often difficult because of the variation in the nature of the disease, the rapidity with which the organism dies in specimens once they are collected and their transient appearance in various tissues. Transmission by blood or urine should be attempted on the farm, injecting the material directly into the peritoneal cavity of several guinea pigs.

Cattle. The acute and subacute forms in this species need to be differentiated from babesiasis, anaplasmosis, rape and kale poisoning, post-parturient haemoglobinuria, bacillary haemoglobinuria, and the acute haemolytic anaemia which occurs in calves after drinking large quantities of water. The discolouration or presence of blood in the milk is the principal abnormality which differentiates leptospirosis clinically from the other infectious haemolytic diseases, which as a group are differentiated from the non-infectious group by the occurrence of fever. The absence of swelling of the udder is sufficient to differentiate this abnormality from mastitis. The chronic form can be differentiated from abortion due to other causes by laboratory examination.

Pigs. Abortion is the common manifestation of leptospirosis in pigs and can be distinguished from brucellosis only by laboratory examination, although hepatic necrosis in foetuses aborted due to leptospiral infection may help in presumptive diagnosis. The herd history of brucellosis, with infertility, orchitis in the boar and high neonatal mortality, may also give a general idea of the causative infection. Severe systemic reactions caused by many bacterial infections including erysipelas may also cause abortion in sows. It is not possible to describe in detail here the differential diagnosis of the causes of abortion and stillbirths in pigs but this has been summarized recently (24). *L. icterohaemorrhagiae* infection may be confused with eperythrozoonosis because of the severe haemolytic anaemia which is common to both diseases. Examination of blood smears reveals the presence of protozoa in erythrocytes in the latter.

Sheep and goats. Chronic copper poisoning and poisoning caused by rape in sheep may present a clinical picture similar to that in leptospirosis but there will be no febrile reaction. Anaplasmosis caused by *Anaplasma ovis* may be accompanied by fever and haemoglobinuria but is more commonly a chronic, emaciating disease.

Horses. Leptospirosis does not appear to occur commonly in newborn foals so that iso-immunization haemolytic anaemia in this group is a much more likely cause of acute haemolytic disease. Infectious equine anaemia, especially the peracute form, has clinical similarity to leptospirosis except that the latter is much milder and unlikely to be fatal. The myoglobinuria of azoturia must not be mistaken for the haemoglobinuria of leptospirosis. Abortion in mares is an important problem and although leptospirosis may be a cause, infection with the viruses of equine viral rhinopneumonitis and equine viral arteritis and with *Streptococcus genitalium* and *Salmonella abortus-equi* are more common. Periodic ophthalmia is characterized by periodic attacks of panophthalmitis and blindness. Hypopyon due to other causes, for example, in foal septicaemia due to *Str. genitalium*, is restricted to the anterior chamber. Conjunctivitis, keratitis and hypopyon may also occur in equine viral arteritis.

Treatment

The primary aim of treatment in all leptospiral infections is to control the infection before irreparable damage to the liver and kidneys occurs. This is best effected by treatment with streptomycin or one of the tetracyclines as soon as possible after signs appear. The results of treatment are often disappointing because in most instances animals are presented for treatment only when the septicaemia has subsided. The secondary aim of treatment is to control the leptospiruria of 'carrier' animals and render them safe to remain in the group. In this instance the shedding of leptospirae in the urine can be controlled but the agglutination-lysin titre is not affected.

Penicillin and erythromycin are reasonably effective in preventing deaths due to septicaemia but do not prevent the development of chronic renal lesions nor eliminate leptospiruria.

Streptomycin (5 mg. per lb. body weight twice daily for 3 days) injected intramuscularly or oxytetracycline or chlortetracycline (2·5 mg. per lb. body weight daily for 5 days) given parenterally are effective both in the treatment of the systemic infection and in the elimination of leptospiruria. For the elimination of leptospiruria in pigs and cattle a single injection of streptomycin (25 mg. per kg.) is recommended (25, 26). Eradication of the disease from pig herds has been achieved largely through the application of this technique (27). In groups of pigs, the feeding of antibiotics provides a much simpler method of treatment than individual dosing. The feeding of oxytetracycline (800 g. per short ton of feed for 8 to 11 days) is claimed to eliminate carriers (28). Antibiotic feeding should begin 1 month before farrowing to avoid the occurrence of abortion. Other experimental trials using tetracyclines by injection or in the feed have been inconclusive (29) and the use of mass feeding techniques as control programmes should not be recommended lightly. Antibiotic feeding has also been suggested as a preventive measure in calves. The feeding of small amounts of tetracyclines (0·5 mg. per lb. body weight per day) for 7 days before and 14 days after exposure prevents the appearance of clinical signs but not infection as measured by the agglutination-lysis reaction.

The treatment of periodic ophthalmia has undergone many changes in recent years and most recommended treatments have little effect on the course of the disease. A course of a suitable antibiotic and the administration of cortisone, either subconjunctivally, intraocularly or parenterally, is most likely to be satisfactory.

Control

The control of leptospirosis depends upon the elimination of carrier animals, appropriate hygienic measures to control the spread of infection and vaccination of susceptible animals.

Detection and elimination of carrier animals presents some difficulties. Positive reactors to the agglutination-lysis test may not void infected urine but to determine their status as carriers necessitates repeated examination of their urine by culture and guinea pig inoculation. For practical purposes, suspicious and positive reactors to the serum test should be considered as carriers and be culled or treated as described above unless examination of the urine can be carried out. In groups of pigs, it is probably advisable to consider the infection to be herd-wide and to treat all pigs as though they were carriers. In these circumstances the feeding of antibiotics, as described above, provides some protection although it is not guaranteed to eliminate the carrier state from the herd. Although bulls infected with leptospirosis should not be used for artificial insemination the chances of spread of infection by artificial insemination are negligible if standard concentrations of penicillin and streptomycin are used in the semen diluent (30).

If the mediate source of infection is recognized, in the form of yards, marshes and damp calf pens, every attempt must be made to avoid animal contact with the infected surroundings. Damp areas should be drained or fenced and pens disinfected after use by infected animals. The possibility that rats and other wild animals may act as a source of infection suggests that contact between them and farm animals should be controlled.

Vaccination against leptospirosis is now in general use. A killed bacterin, which may be alum precipitated, is used in cattle, pigs and horses and appears to be a safe procedure except that, in horses, moderate local swellings are likely to occur. A similar vaccine has provided complete protection in sheep. In cattle, challenge experiments have shown that protection does result but that the efficiency of the immunity wanes quickly and protection against infection may last for only 6 months. However, a degree of immunity against the disease, in that only mild signs appear and few kidney infections leading to development of carrier animals occur, persists for about 18 months. Similar results have been obtained in pigs and for effective prevention in both species, revaccination at 6-month intervals is recommended.

Egg-attenuated living vaccines are in use and although they produce a stronger immunity this is accompanied by a high persistent antibody titre which may interfere with control programmes (31). The titre produced by a killed bacterin is quite low (1 : 10 to 1 : 25) and is unlikely to confuse the results of a serological test (32). A different attenuated vaccine, produced by cultivation on a synthetic medium, has given good immunity in pigs and cattle (33).

Vaccination of animals less than 3 months of age is unlikely to be effective and is not recommended but vaccination of cows in late pregnancy gives effective immunity to their calves. This procedure appears to be less effective in sows although moderately good results are possible with an adjuvant vaccine (35).

The question of whether or not to vaccinate depends largely upon the cost of the procedure relative to the losses which can be anticipated. If the disease is spreading rapidly, as evidenced by the frequent appearance of clinical cases, a high range of titres or rising titres in a number of animals, all clinical cases and positive reactors should be treated, the negative animals vaccinated and the herd moved on the first day of treatment to a clean field. Retesting a group to determine the rate of spread would be an informative procedure but active measures must usually be commenced before this information is available. Another circumstance in which vaccination is recommended, and has been shown to be very effective, is in the protection of animals continuously exposed to infection from

wild-life (34), other domestic species, and particularly rodents.

If only sporadic cases occur, it might be more profitable to attempt to dispose of reactors or treat them to ensure that they no longer act as carriers. A degree of immunity is likely to occur in pigs after natural infection, and when the disease is enzootic, 'herd immunity' may significantly decrease the ravages of the disease. This must be taken into account when assessing the results of vaccination.

When the disease has been eliminated, introduced animals should be required to pass a serological test on two occasions at least 2 weeks apart before allowing them to enter the herd. Urine examination for leptospirae should be carried out if practicable.

REVIEW LITERATURE

Alston, J. M. & Bloom, J. C. (1958). *Leptospirosis in Man and Animals*, Edinburgh: E. & S. Livingstone.
van der Hoeden, J. (1958). *Advances in Veterinary Science*, Vol. 4, pp. 278–341, New York: Academic Press.

REFERENCES

(1) Michna, S. W. (1970). *Vet. Rec.*, 86, 484.
(2) Sullivan, N. D. (1970). *Aust. vet. J.*, 46, 121, 123, 125.
(3) Hanson, L. E. *et al.* (1964). *Proc. 68th ann. gen. Mtg U.S. Live Stock sanit. Ass.*, 136.
(4) Smith, R. E. *et al.* (1965). *Cornell Vet.*, 55, 412.
(5) McGowan, J. E. & Karstad, L. (1965). *Canad. vet. J.*, 6, 243.
(6) McDiarmid, A. (1961). *Vet. Rec.*, 73, 1329.
(7) Ryley, J. W. (1956). *Aust. vet. J.*, 32, 4.
(8) Doherty, P. C. (1967). *Qd J. agric. anim. Sci.*, 24, 329.
(9) Lindquist, K. J. *et al.* (1958). *Cornell Vet.*, 48, 277.
(10) Sleight, S. D. & Langham, R. F. (1962). *J. infect. Dis.*, 111, 63.
(11) Spradbrow, P. B. & Seawright, A. A. (1963). *Aust. vet. J.*, 39, 423.
(12) Dozsa, L. & Sahu, S. (1970). *Cornell Vet.*, 60, 254.
(13) Smith, R. E. *et al.* (1970). *Cornell Vet.*, 60, 40.
(14) Morter, R. L. *et al.* (1964). *Proc. 68th Ann. gen. Mtg U.S. Live Stock sanit. Ass.*, 147.
(15) Twigg, G. I. & Hughes, D. M. (1971). *Equ. vet. J.*, 3, 52.
(16) Cross, R. S. N. (1966). *Vet. Rec.*, 78, 8.
(17) Sullivan, N. D. & Callan, D. P. (1970). *Aust. vet. J.*, 46, 537.
(18) Howell, D. *et al.* (1969). *Vet. Rec.*, 84, 122.
(19) Michna, S. W. (1965). *Vet. Rec.*, 77, 559, 802.
(20) Roberts, S. J. *et al.* (1952). *J. Amer. vet. med. Ass.*, 133, 189.
(21) Jones, T. C. (1942). *Amer. J. vet. Res.*, 3, 45.
(22) Mooter, R. G. *et al.* (1969). *Fed. Proc.*, 28, 621.
(23) Blenden, D. C. (1964). *Proc. 101st ann. Mtg Amer. vet. med. Ass., Chicago*, 219.
(24) Dunne, H. W. & Hokanson, J. F. (1963). *Proc. 100th ann. Mtg Amer. vet. med. Ass.*, New York, 54.
(25) Stalheim, O. H. V. (1969). *Amer. J. vet. Res.*, 30, 1317.
(26) Doherty, P. C. (1967). *Aust. vet. J.*, 43, 135.
(27) Dobson, K. J. (1971). *Aust. vet. J.*, 47, 186.
(28) Stalheim, O. H. V. (1967). *Amer. J. vet. Res.*, 28, 161.
(29) Doherty, P. C. & Baynes, I. D. (1967). *Aust. vet. J.*, 43, 135.
(30) Sleight, S. D. (1965). *Amer. J. vet. Res.*, 26, 365.
(31) Kenzy, S. G. *et al.* (1963). *Proc. 66th ann. gen. Mtg U.S. Live Stock sanit. Ass.*, 146.

(32) Kiesel, G. K. & Dacres, W. G. (1959). *Cornell Vet.*, *49*, 332.
(33) Stalheim, O. H. V. (1968). *Amer. J. vet. Res.*, *29*, 1463.
(34) Killinger, A. H. *et al.* (1969). *Bull. Wildl. Dis. Ass.*, *5*, 182.
(35) Chaudhary, R. K. *et al.* (1966). *Canad. vet. J.*, *7*, 106, 121.
(36) Imbabi, S. E. *et al.* (1967). *Amer. J. vet. Res.*, *28*, 413.
(37) Andrews, R. D. (1969). *Bull. Wildl. Dis. Ass.*, *5*, 174.

Ulcerative Granuloma

(Necrotic Ulcer)

Ulcerative granuloma is an infectious disease of pigs caused by the spirochaete, *Borrelia suilla* (1), and characterized by the development of chronic ulcers of the skin and subcutaneous tissues.

It occurs most commonly under conditions of poor hygiene in Australia and New Zealand and is recorded in the U.K. (2).

Lesions occur on the central abdomen of sows and on the face of sucking pigs, suggesting infection of cutaneous or mucosal abrasions as the portal of entry.

Initially the lesions are small, hard, fibrous swellings which ulcerate in 2 to 3 weeks to form a persistent ulcer with raised edges and a centre of excessive granulation tissue covered with sticky, grey pus. The lesions expand, often to 20 to 30 cm. in diameter, on the belly of the sow. They are usually single or in small numbers. In young pigs, whole litters may be affected. The lesions commence about the lips and erode the cheeks, sometimes the jawbone, and often cause shedding of the teeth.

In adult animals there is considerable inconvenience if the lesions are permitted to develop. In young pigs there may be heavy losses due to severe damage to the face.

Necrotic ulcers on the udders of sows may be mistaken for lesions of actinomycosis and swabs should be taken from the ulcers for bacteriological examination. A course of potassium iodide given orally, or a single injection of penicillin provide the best methods of treatment. Dusting with sulphanilamide, arsenic trioxide or tartar emetic have also been recommended. The injection of 0·2 ml. of a 5 per cent solution of sodium arsenite into the substance of the lesion is reported to give good results. Improvement in hygiene and disinfection of skin wounds should reduce the incidence in affected piggeries.

REFERENCES

(1) Hindmarsh, W. L. (1937). *N.S.W. Dept. Agric. Vet. Res. Rpt. 7*, pp. 64–70.
(2) Blandford, T. B. *et al.* (1972). *Vet. Rec.*, *90*, 15.

DISEASES CAUSED BY *MYCOPLASMA* Spp.

Diseases in which *Mycoplasma* spp. appear to have aetiological significance are being identified with increasing frequency. Bovine mastitis caused by these organisms is described in the section on mastitis. Mycoplasma have been identified from the bovine genital tract and have been proposed as a cause of granular vulvovaginitis and unexplained infertility in cattle (1, 6).

Mycoplasma (*M. hyorhinis*, *M. hyosynoviae* and *M. granulare*) are associated with arthritis and polyserositis in pigs (3, 4, 5, 9), and the disease is reproducible experimentally (2). The disease is endemic in some herds and may cause arthritis in up to 15 per cent of pigs. Clinically there is a short episode of fever, lameness and joint swelling. Most cases recover in a few days. Tylosin is an effective treatment but stunting persists in most cases. The mortality rate is low and never exceeds 10 per cent. Mycoplasma have also been observed to cause a fibrinous or fibrinopurulent arthritis in calves (7, 8). Many joints are affected, particularly the stifle, and a local tendonitis may occur. The joints are swollen and the affected calves are lame. Contracture of the joints occurs in long-standing cases.

Mycoplasma have also achieved prominence as the cause of enzootic pneumonia of swine, and are dealt with under that heading. They are also found in the lungs of calves affected with pneumonia.

REFERENCES

(1) Afshar, A. (1967). *Vet. Bull.*, *37*, 879.
(2) Davenport, P. G. *et al.* (1970). *N.Z. vet. J.*, *18*, 165.
(3) Moore, R. W. *et al.* (1966). *Amer. J. vet. Res.*, *27*, 1649.
(4) Ross, R. F. *et al.* (1968). *Arthr. Rheum.*, *11*, 507.
(5) Switzer, W. P. (1967). *J. Amer. vet. med. Ass.*, *151*, 1656.
(6) Jasper, D. E. (1967). *J. Amer. vet. med. Ass.*, *151*, 1650.
(7) Simmons, G. C. & Johnston, L. A. Y. (1963). *Aust. vet. J.*, *39*, 11.
(8) Hughes, K. L. *et al.* (1966). *Vet. Rec.*, *78*, 276.
(9) Ross, R. F. *et al.* (1971). *Amer. J. vet. Res.*, *32*, 1743.

Contagious Bovine Pleuropneumonia

Contagious bovine pleuropneumonia is a highly infectious septicaemia characterized by localization in the lungs and pleura. It is one of the major plagues in cattle causing heavy losses in many parts of the world.

Incidence

Contagious bovine pleuropneumonia is still enzootic in many large areas throughout eastern Europe, Asia, Africa, and the Iberian Peninsula. Australia has been plagued with the disease for many years but it is now under control and although not yet eradicated it is at a very low level of incidence and should be eradicated within a decade (1, 2). The disease was eradicated from the U.S.A. in 1892 and from South Africa in 1916. In the affected countries enormous losses are experienced each year from the deaths of animals and the loss of production during convalescence. The highly fatal nature of the disease, the ease of spread and the difficulty of detecting carriers also mean that close restriction must be placed on the movement of animals from enzootic areas. For example, in Australia many feeder cattle are reared on range country where the disease is enzootic and it is necessary to move these animals for fattening into more closely settled areas which are free of the disease. In spite of strict quarantine measures to prevent the movement of infected animals, periodic outbreaks occur in these free areas with heavy losses of cattle and major expense for eradication programmes. In groups of susceptible cattle the morbidity rate approaches 100 per cent and the mortality rate may be as high as 50 per cent.

Aetiology

Mycoplasma mycoides var. *mycoides* is the cause of the disease in cattle. The causative organisms of contagious pleuropneumonia in cattle and in goats are very similar culturally and antigenically but infection does not spread between the two species (1). It is extremely pleomorphic and some of its forms are filterable. The organisms are sensitive to all environmental influences, including disinfectants, heat and drying and do not survive outside the animal body for more than a few hours, although they can be maintained readily in special culture media and in embryonated hens' eggs. The disease occurs commonly only in cattle although rare natural cases have been observed in buffaloes, yak, bison, reindeer and antelopes. The disease has been produced experimentally in captive African buffaloes (3) but was not detectable in 8 species of wildlife (4). A local cellulitis without pulmonary involvement occurs in sheep and goats after injection of cultures. A strong immunity develops after an attack of the natural disease in cattle and vaccination plays an important part in control.

Transmission

Spread of the disease occurs only directly from the infected animal by the inhalation of infected droplets. Mediate infection by contamination of inanimate objects does not occur. Because of the method of spread, outbreaks tend to be more extensive in housed animals and in those in transit by train or on foot. The focus of infection is often provided by recovered 'carrier' animals in which a pulmonary sequestrum preserves a potential source of organisms for periods as long as 3 years. Under conditions of stress due to starvation, exhaustion

or intercurrent disease, the sequestrum breaks down and the animal becomes an active case. Droplet infection is usually associated with a donor lesion in the lungs. Renal lesions are not uncommon in this disease and the organism *M. mycoides* has been identified in urine leading to the suggestion that the inhalation of urine droplets may be a route of infection (5).

A low incidence can be anticipated in arid regions because of the rapid destruction of the organism in exhaled droplets. Although 6 metres is usually considered to be sufficient separation between animals, transmission over distances as great as 45 metres has been suspected to occur. Spread of the disease may also occur by discharges from local tail lesions resulting from vaccination with virulent culture. Cattle may be exposed to infection for periods of up to 8 months before the disease becomes established and this necessitates a long period of quarantine before a herd can be declared to be free of the disease.

Pathogenesis

Contagious bovine pleuropneumonia is an acute lobar pneumonia and pleurisy developing by localization from an initial septicaemia. Death results from anoxia and presumably from toxaemia. Transplacental transmission appears to occur and foeti become infected when the disease is produced experimentally in cattle (6). Under natural conditions a number of animals in a group do not become infected, either because of a natural immunity or because they are not exposed to a sufficiently large infective dose. These animals may show a transient positive reaction to the complement fixation test. Approximately 50 per cent of the animals that do become infected go through a mild form of the disease and are often not recognized as clinical cases.

Clinical Findings

After an incubation period of 3 to 6 weeks (in occasional instances up to 6 months) there is a sudden onset of high fever (40°C or 105°F), a fall in milk yield, anorexia and cessation of rumination. There is severe depression and the animals stand apart or lag behind a travelling group. Coughing, at first only on exercise, and chest pain are evident, affected animals being disinclined to move, standing with the elbows out, the back arched and the head extended. Respirations are shallow, rapid and accompanied by expiratory grunting. Pain is evidenced on percussion of the chest. Auscultation reveals pleuritic friction sounds in the early stages of acute inflammation, and dullness, fluid sounds and moist gurgling râles in the later stages of effusion. Dullness of areas of the lung may be detectable on percussion. Inconstantly oedematous swellings of the throat and dewlap occur.

Recovered animals may be clinically normal but in some an inactive sequestrum forms in the lung, with a necrotic centre of sufficient size to produce a toxaemia causing unthriftiness and mild respiratory distress on exercise. These sequestra commonly break down when the animal is exposed to environmental stress and cause an acute attack of the disease. A chronic cough is also common. Approximately 50 per cent of the affected animals die acutely and 25 per cent remain as recovered carriers with or without clinical signs. In fatal cases death occurs after a variable course of from several days to 3 weeks.

Clinical Pathology

The complement-fixation (CF) test on serum is the most useful method of detecting infection. In a small proportion of animals the results may be deceptive. Early cases may give a negative reaction and some positive reactors show no lesions on necropsy. The test is particularly effective in detecting carriers. Animals recovering from the disease gradually become negative and vaccinated animals give a positive reaction for about 6 weeks although this period may be much longer if severe vaccination reactions occur (7). A slide flocculation test and a rapid slide agglutination test (8) have been used but their sensitivity is lower than that of the complement fixation test and they are recommended for herd diagnosis rather than for use in individual animals (8). However, the plate agglutination test has been very accurate and efficient in Australia and has made virtual eradication of the disease a possibility (9). A modified complement-fixation test, the 'plate CF test', has been introduced recently (10). It is more accurate than the standard CF test and is much more economical of time and equipment. With all of these tests there is a progressive loss of reliability if testing is delayed for very long after the clinical disease has passed (11).

Necropsy Findings

Lesions are confined to the chest cavity. There is thickening and inflammation of the pleura often with heavy deposits of fibrin and large amounts of clear, serous effusion containing shreds of fibrin. One or both lungs may be completely or partially affected with marked consolidation. Affected lobules show various stages of grey and red hepatization and the interlobular septa are greatly distended with serofibrinous exudate—the classical 'marbled' lung of this disease. In recovered cases careful section of the lung tissue is necessary to detect the presence of foci of necrotic tissue surrounded by a fibrous capsule—the sequestra of carrier cases. Adhesions between pleural surfaces are also a constant finding in such cases. The postmortem diagnosis can be confirmed by examination of freshly collected effusion fluid for the presence of the organism or by culture from lung or fluid. In a few cases only oedematous lesions may be found in the lymph nodes of the chest or in the tonsillar tissue.

Diagnosis

A diagnosis based on a history of contact with infected animals, clinical findings, a complement fixation test, necropsy findings and cultural examination leaves little room for error. Pneumonic pasteurellosis may be very similar clinically and at necropsy but is differentiated bacteriologically by the presence of pasteurellae in the tissues and by the complement fixation test. Other severe pulmonary disorders of cattle include fog fever and enzootic and parasitic pneumonia of calves.

Treatment

Treatment is usually undertaken only in areas where the disease is enzootic, eradication being the more logical practice when the disease breaks out in a new area. Sulphadimidine and organic arsenicals are used extensively and appear to reduce the mortality rate. Penicillin is of little value, streptomycin has some curative effect, and oxytetracycline and chloramphenicol have some value. Tylosin is highly effective in the control of excessive vaccination reactions and should be of value in the treatment of clinical cases (12). The dose rate of tylosin tartrate recommended for intramuscular injection is 2 to 5 mg. per lb. body weight every 12 hours for 6 injections. Daily injections are not effective. Erythromycin is effective against some mycoplasmas.

Control

On a herd basis. When the disease becomes established in a herd the following measures may be adopted to prevent its spread.

Hygiene. Any procedure which brings the animals together should be avoided if possible, especially in the early stages of the disease. Passage through the milking shed, collecting for inspection, bleeding and vaccination all facilitate the spread of the disease. It should be remembered that droplet infection is more likely to occur in humid conditions. Strict quarantine of the infected and in-contact herds must be maintained until all residual infection has been eliminated. Usually 12 weeks after the removal of the last reactor and/or clinical case is sufficient time. Animals in quarantine should be kept under constant surveillance so that clinical cases may be observed.

Removal of sources of infection. Infected animals should be removed from the herd as soon as possible. The CF test is adequate to identify the infected animals and if possible it should be carried out in conjunction with clinical examination. Because animals in the incubative and early stages of the disease may give negative reactions it is necessary to have two completely negative tests 2 months apart before the herd can be classified as clean. After vaccination a positive reaction occurs but it usually disappears within 2 months although in rare cases it may persist for as long as 5 months. All positive and suspicious reactors and clinical cases are destroyed or transported under close control to abattoirs. Where this cannot be done without a chance of spread to animals along the route destruction on the property is necessary. Animals which are eventually to go to abattoirs should be kept under quarantine until slaughter, irrespective of their status.

In circumstances where a minimum of handling is desired the herd may be blood tested and examined for clinical signs, and vaccinated all in the one visit. Animals which react to the test are then destroyed even though they have been vaccinated. The only difficulty that arises with this method is that cattle in the incubative stages of the disease may give a negative reaction to the test and because of the serological reaction resulting from vaccination retesting cannot be performed until 2 months later.

Vaccination. Vaccination is an effective procedure in the control of bovine pleuropneumonia but its application is usually controlled by local legislation. All the vaccines in use are living preparations, and their use is always subject to the suspicion that they may spread the disease. When tail vaccination with organisms of reduced virulence is practised the possibility of spreading the disease is remote but, because the possibility exists, vaccination is usually only permitted in herds or areas where the disease is known to be present. The value of calfhood vaccination is limited because although calves give sufficient serological reactions arthritis, myocarditis and valvular endocarditis occur 3 to 4 weeks after vaccination of calves less than 2 months old. Vaccination of calves after this age is

recommended because it avoids the occasional deaths which occur after vaccination of adults.

The vaccines available include pleural exudate from natural cases (natural lymph), cultured organisms of reduced virulence, and an avianized vaccine of low virulence. Vaccination is usually carried out by injection into the tough connective tissue at the tip of the tail with a high-pressure syringe. 'Natural lymph' is unsatisfactory because of the possibility of spreading this and other diseases and because of the severe lesions which commonly result. Severe reactions with this type of vaccine may cause sloughing of the tail and extensive cellulitis of the hindquarters necessitating destruction or causing death of the animal.

In general, vaccines made from *M. mycoides* grown in broth-culture produced less severe reactions but a correspondingly briefer immunity of about 6 to 10 months and required annual revaccination (22). Avianized vaccines were developed which overcame the brevity of the immunity, increasing its duration to 3 to 4 years (13). These vaccines are the major ones in use now and are capable of great variation in their virulence. In spite of increasing the attenuation the use of these vaccines was followed on occasions by severe local reactions and pulmonary lesions. This led to an investigation of the KH3J strain which is less virulent than the standard V5 strain (14, 1) and the production of a vaccine attenuated by egg culture but grown in its last passage in broth (15). This latter procedure eliminated the egg proteins from the vaccine which were thought to produce some of the local reactions. However, the more virulent vaccines are still in use and, provided tylosin is available to control undesirably severe reactions, are generally preferred (16, 17, 2).

Difficulty has been experienced in the preparation of a dried vaccine for field use. A dried vaccine is available but it must be reconstituted in agar and used within 2 hours (18). It has the advantage of requiring a very small dose and of retaining its potency for well over a year (19). Another vaccine containing a virulent strain KH3J plus 20 per cent brain suspension is an efficient immunizing agent and is stable and freeze dries easily (20). All vaccines against CBPP are susceptible to light and should be kept in a dark place.

On an area basis. The prevention of entry of contagious bovine pleuropneumonia into a free area is a difficult task. Only the following classes of cattle should be permitted to enter: (i) Cattle which have not been in an infected area nor in contact with infected animals for at least 6 months. This may be relaxed to permit entry of cattle going to immediate slaughter after a clinical examination and a period of 1 month in a free area. (ii) Cattle which have given negative reactions to the complement fixation test on two occasions within the preceding 2 months and have not been in contact with infected animals during this period. These animals may or may not have been vaccinated. Less rigid measures than these will permit introduction of the disease.

When the disease is already present in an area two methods of control are possible, vaccination, and eradication by test and slaughter of reactors. The method chosen will depend largely on the economy of the cattle industry in the affected area. A vaccination programme may be the first step to reduce the incidence of the disease to the point where eradication becomes possible.

In areas where properties are large, fencing is poor and the collection of every animal cannot be guaranteed, eradication of the disease by test and slaughter is impractical. Vaccination with culture vaccine can be practised whenever the cattle are brought together. Animals moving from infected areas or into infected areas, and groups of cattle which contain active cases, must be vaccinated. Moving cattle which develop the disease should be halted, clinical cases slaughtered and the remainder vaccinated. Results are usually good provided the vaccination is carried out carefully but some further cases due to prevaccination infection are to be expected. Extensive vaccination in Australia has reduced the incidence of the disease to an extremely low level and complete eradication of the disease is anticipated within a short time (21, 2). The residual problems are largely geographical and an annoying but low proportion of false positive reactors to the CF test. Eradication has been greatly facilitated by the use of the Huddart plate test in a mobile laboratory and autopsy of reactors 24 hours later. Of great help also was the appointment of special meat inspectors to local abattoirs during the eradication programme.

When outbreaks occur in small areas where herds can be adequately controlled complete eradication should be attempted by periodic testing and the destruction of reactors, and in-contact animals should be vaccinated. To avoid unnecessary contact between cattle, retesting is delayed until 5 to 6 months after the first test when vaccination reactions have usually subsided. Under most circumstances all non-reactors should be vaccinated. This practice is particularly applicable in feeder cattle which will be slaughtered subsequently and when extensive outbreaks occur in closely settled areas where the chances of spread are great. Simple test and slaughter in these latter circumstances will be too slow to control the rate of spread. In either case the herd should not be released from quarantine until two tests at an interval of more than 2 months are completely negative.

REVIEW LITERATURE

Hudson, J. R. (1971). F.A.O. Agricultural Series No. 86.

REFERENCES

(1) Hudson, J. R. & Leaver, D. D. (1965). *Aust. vet. J.*, *41*, 29, 36, 43.
(2) Pierce, A. E. (1969). *Bull. Off. int. Épizoot.*, *71*, 1313, 1329.
(3) Shifrine, M. *et al.* (1970). *Bull. epizoot. Dis. Afr.*, *18*, 201.
(4) Shifrine, M. & Domermuth, C. H. (1967). *Bull. epizoot. Dis. Afr.*, *15*, 319.
(5) Masiga, W. N. *et al.* (1972). *Vet. Rec.*, *90*, 247.
(6) Stone, S. S. *et al.* (1969). *Res. vet. Sci.*, *10*, 368.
(7) Campbell, A. D. & Turner, A. W. (1953). *Aust. vet. J.*, *29*, 154.
(8) Adler, H. E. & Etheridge, J. R. (1964). *Aust. vet. J.*, *40*, 38.
(9) Ladds, P. W. (1969). *Aust. vet. J.*, *45*, 1.
(10) Karst, D. (1970). *Bull. epizoot. Dis. Afr.*, *18*, 5.
(11) Stone, S. S. & Bygrave, A. C. (1969). *Bull. epizoot. Dis. Afr.*, *17*, 11.
(12) Hudson, J. R. & Etheridge, J. R. (1965). *Aust. vet. J.*, *41*, 130.
(13) Hyslop, N. St. G. (1956). *Brit. vet. J.*, *112*, 519.
(14) Hudson, J. R. & Turner, A. W. (1963). *Aust. vet. J.*, *39*, 373.
(15) Davies, G. *et al.* (1968). *Vet. Rec.*, *83*, 239.
(16) Hyslop, N. St. G. (1968). *Bull. Off. int. Épizoot.*, *69*, 695.
(17) Hudson, J. R. (1968). *Aust. vet. J.*, *44*, 83, 123.
(18) Webster, W. (1945). *Aust. vet. J.*, *21*, 64.
(19) Priestley, F. W. & Dafalla, E. N. (1957). *Bull. epizoot. Dis. Afr.*, *5*, 177.
(20) Hudson, J. R. (1968). *Bull. epizoot. Dis. Afr.*, *16*, 165.
(21) Lloyd, L. C. (1969). *Aust. vet. J.*, *45*, 147.
(22) Gilbert, F. R. *et al.* 1(970). *Vet. Rec.*, *86*, 29.

Serositis-Arthritis, Pleuropneumonia and Agalactia of Goats and Sheep

The diseases of goats and sheep caused by *Myco-plasma* spp. are not accurately identified. Two specific organisms are involved, *Myco. agalactia*, and *Myco. mycoides* var. *capri* (1). There are many reports of diseases in sheep and goats caused by pleuropneumonia-like organisms (PPLO) in which the identity of the organism has not been established. There are three main clinical syndromes recorded, serositis-arthritis, pleuropneumonia and agalactia—but many records exist of diseases caused by PPLOs in which the signs and lesions of more than one of these diseases occur in the one animal. Thus mastitis and pleuropneumonia have occurred together in sheep and goats and pleuropneumonia and arthritis have also been observed to occur concurrently. It would appear that generalized infections can occur with both *Myco. mycoides* var. *capri* and *Myco. agalactia* but that the former is more likely to localize in the lungs and the latter in the udder.

SEROSITIS-ARTHRITIS

A disease observed in California and Australia in goats is characterized by a diffuse, fibrinous peritonitis, pleurisy, pericarditis and arthritis, and in some cases a leptomeningitis. An unnamed mycoplasma, antigenically unrelated to *Myco. mycoides* var. *capri* or *Myco. agalactiae*, has been identified as the cause of the disease. There is high fever, pain and swelling of limb joints and suppression of lactation. Neither mammary nor pulmonary involvement has been observed. Although the organism can be isolated from pneumonic lungs it is not capable of causing a primary pneumonia (2). In California the disease has been found to occur most commonly in very young kids and yearling does at parturition and weaning time (3). Cellulitis occurs after local inoculation of the organism and secondary eye involvement may occur if the eye is injured. The disease is transmissible experimentally to goats, sheep and pigs but not to calves, and the organism is present in the faeces and urine of infected animals. Complement fixation antibodies to *Myco. mycoides* are present in the serum 15 days after experimental inoculation (4). In vitro the organism is only slightly susceptible to streptomycin and chloramphenicol but highly sensitive to oxytetracycline and erythromycin. Sensitivity to organic arsenicals and other tetracyclines is variable (4).

CONTAGIOUS PLEUROPNEUMONIA OF GOATS AND SHEEP

The disease in sheep and goats is very similar clinically to contagious bovine pleuropneumonia but the infection is not transmissible from sheep and goats to cattle. The causative bacteria is *Myco. mycoides* var. *capri*. Under adverse climatic conditions the disease may occur in a septicaemic form with little clinical or post-mortem evidence of pneumonia.

The disease is highly fatal in sheep and goats and mortality rates of 60 to 100 per cent are not unusual. It is transmitted readily by inoculation and inhalation but the organism does not persist for long outside the animal body. An outbreak of the disease associated with heavy nasal bot (*Oestrus ovis*) infestation has led to the suggestion that the pleuropneumonia may be secondary to the bot infestation. Reports of the disease come most commonly from North Africa, Spain and the Mediterranean littoral, Asia Minor and India. The disease 'Abu Nini' described in the Sudan (5) is probably identical with CCPP but may be complicated by the presence of other infections. Although CCPP has not been observed in Australia a non-fatal respiratory disease of goats characterized by coughing, fever and extensive pleurisy and pneumonia has occurred (6). The suspected causative organism was closely related to *Myco. agalactiae*. A mycoplasmal pneumonia has also been recorded in lambs in Australia. The disease occurs naturally and has been reproduced experimentally (7). It is a slowly developing interstitial pneumonia with lesions similar to those of enzootic pneumonia in pigs. Clinically the disease is characterized by poor growth, intolerance to exercise, dry pulmonary rales and a moderate mortality.

Treatment with organic arsenicals, chloramphenicol, oxytetracycline and tylosin has been highly successful (8) and vaccination with an aluminium hydroxideterpene vaccine has given good results (10).

CONTAGIOUS AGALACTIA OF GOATS AND SHEEP

The disease has approximately the same geographical distribution as contagious pleuropneumonia of goats and sheep. There is usually an acute onset of mastitis, ophthalmitis and arthritis with painful swelling of affected joints. The mortality rate is high (10 to 30 per cent) and the udder is permanently damaged. Kids are more seriously affected than adults. Abortion occurs commonly and there is a long period of illness of from one to several months (9).

Herd diagnosis is possible by the isolation of the organism (*Myco. agalactiae*) from the blood stream and mammary tissue and by a complement fixation test which becomes positive soon after a clinical attack. If recovery occurs a solid immunity persists (10). Three types of causative organism have been identified (11). One is non-pathogenic, another causes most outbreaks of the disease, but the third is associated with severe udder oedema and a high mortality in goats.

Vaccination of sheep and goats with either an attenuated live vaccine or a killed adjuvant vaccine gives mixed results; in late pregnant ewes the former being rather too virulent, and the latter insufficiently so (9); in ewes before mating good efficiency was observed (12). Treatment of affected goats with tylosin was found to be effective in 80 per cent of cases provided treatment was given early (13). Oxytetracycline was thought to limit the severity of the disease without reducing the excretion of mycoplasma in the milk (11). The extensive use of a live, attenuated vaccine and a killed, adjuvant vaccine over a period of 13 years has resulted in almost complete disappearance of the disease from Roumania (14).

REFERENCES

(1) Adler, H. E. (1965). *Advanc. vet. Sci.*, *10*, 205.
(2) Boidin, A. G. *et al.* (1958). *Cornell Vet.*, *48*, 410.
(3) Cordy, D. R. *et al.* (1955). *Cornell Vet.*, *45*, 50.
(4) Laws, L. (1956). *Aust. vet. J.*, *32*, 326.
(5) Ottee, E. (1960). *Vet. Rec.*, *72*, 140, 353.
(6) Cottew, G. S. & Lloyd, L. C. (1965). *J. comp. Path.*, *73*, 363.
(7) St. George, T. D. *et al.* (1971). *Aust. vet. J.*, *47*, 382.
(8) Sharma, G. L. & Bhalla, N. P. (1962). *Indian J. vet. Sci.*, *32*, 119.
(9) Foggie, A. *et al.* (1971). *J. comp. Path.*, *81*, 165.
(10) Ceocarelli, A. & Fontanelli, E. (1950). *Zooprofilassi*, *5*, 409, 489.
(11) Arisoy, F. *et al.* (1967). *Türk. vet. Hekim. dern. Derg.*, *37*, 11.
(12) Foggie, A. *et al.* (1971). *J. comp. Path.*, *81*, 393.
(13) Spais, A. G. *et al.* (1970). *Hellen. Kten. Thessaloniki*, *13*, 113.
(14) Popovici, I. & de Simon, M. (1966). *Arch. vet.*, *1*, 21.

Enzootic Pneumonia of Pigs

(*Viral Pneumonia of Pigs, VPP*)

This is a highly contagious disease of pigs manifested clinically by a pneumonia of moderate severity and failure to grow at a normal rate.

Incidence

The disease has been identified, at least provisionally, in most countries. The incidence appears to be high in all countries in which pig raising is a major industry; in fact it is unusual to find large herds which are not affected. It is not uncommon to find 50 per cent of market hogs at abattoirs with active or inactive lesions. Economic losses are tremendous, the annual loss from this disease in Britain being estimated at over £2,000,000 sterling. In affected herds chronic low-grade pneumonia results in failure to make weight gains, a result often ascribed to other causes. It seems probable that most of this effect of reducing productivity may be due to complication of the disease by secondary bacterial invaders. At least there is good evidence that this is so and that good management can greatly reduce the losses (1). However on average performance the loss per pig in infected herds is estimated to be £0·90 sterling. This sort of loss can be recouped by repopulation in one year (18).

As a rule the morbidity rate is high and the mortality rate is negligible. However, on some occasions, particularly when the disease is first introduced into piggeries where the husbandry is poor, the mortality rate in young pigs may reach as high as 50 per cent.

Aetiology

The search for the causative agent in this disease was prolonged and exhaustive (1). It is now known to be *Mycoplasma hyopneumoniae* (19), but it is possible that a combined infection with an adenovirus might produce a still more severe disease (20). It is also possible that many other agents can supplement or replace *M. hyopneumoniae* (24) but field experience suggests that the disease should be handled as though caused by one significant agent.

Secondary invasion of pneumonic lesions by pasteurellae, streptococci, mycoplasma, *Bord. bronchiseptica* and *Klebsiella pneumoniae* is very common and largely influences the outcome of the disease in individual pigs. Of some incidental interest is the observation that ovine pneumonia virus is capable of causing pneumonia in pigs (16).

Pigs are the only species affected and, although all age groups are susceptible, young pigs are most severely affected. Environmental conditions undoubtedly influence the spread of the disease but their main importance is their effect on its severity. Pigs kept in insanitary, draughty housing exposed to inclement weather and poorly fed, are more likely to suffer from the acute form of the disease than pigs that are well cared for. Signs and lesions tend to be less severe under conditions of high temperature and humidity (17). Pigs infested with lungworms (*Metastrongylus* spp.) develop more extensive lesions of enzootic pneumonia than pigs with pneumonia alone (2).

Transmission

The enzootic nature of the disease is due to the persistence of the causative agent in clinically normal pigs which have recovered from the disease. Infection is probably transmitted from generation to generation in each piggery. Airborne transmission has been demonstrated (3). Infection in young, susceptible pigs occurs through contact with the dam or after weaning when litters are brought together. Introduction into a herd is usually by infected feeder pigs or chronic carriers among breeding animals.

Pathogenesis

The causative agent exists in pulmonary lesions and the regional lymph nodes for long periods. The lesions are persistent and show little tendency to regress. A delicate balance seems to be set up between the host and the pulmonary infection so that pigs kept under good husbandry conditions seem to suffer little, whereas pigs exposed to any devitalizing influence may be severely affected. In many cases post mortem lesions are minor and fail to account for the severity of the unthriftiness. It is possible that some other factor is responsible for the unthriftiness and may be a predisposing cause that increases susceptibility to enzootic pneumonia.

The distribution of lesions has aroused comment. They occur in the right cardiac lobe, the right apical and left cardiac lobes, the left apical and the diaphragmatic lobes in that order of frequence. It has been suggested that this distribution is in part due to the more vertical disposition of the bronchi in the more commonly affected lobes (4).

Clinical Findings

A natural incubation period of 10 to 16 days is shortened to 5 to 12 days by experimental transmission. Two forms of the disease are described. In the relatively rare acute form a severe outbreak may occur in a susceptible herd when the infection is first introduced. In such herds pigs of all ages are susceptible and a morbidity of 100 per cent may be experienced. Suckers 10 days old have been infected. The mortality rate is often high and deaths are due to the virus without the participation of secondary bacteria. Acute respiratory distress with or without fever is characteristic.

The chronic form of the disease is much more common and causes the greatest economic loss. Young piglets may become infected when they are 3 to 10 weeks old, the disease commencing with transient diarrhoea and a dry cough. In sucking pigs a short period of sneezing may be observed in the early stages. Coughing is most severe in the morning and after exercise, and may disappear after 2 to 3 weeks or persist indefinitely. Respiratory embarrassment is rare. Although appetite is maintained, retardation of growth occurs. In a single litter there may be a number of stunted pigs, with the remainder of normal size. Some pigs affected with the chronic form of the disease may later develop acute pneumonia due to secondary invasion with pasteurellae or other organisms.

Clinical Pathology

Now that the aetiological agent can be isolated there have been big advances in the development of diagnostic laboratory tests (1). Complement fixation tests are available but the tests are complex and need refinement before they can be used to diagnose the presence of the infection in an individual animal (22). Experimental fluorescent antibody techniques (23) and an indirect haemagglutination test (25) are also available.

Necropsy Findings

Lesions are confined almost entirely to the apical and cardiac lobes and are clearly demarcated from the normal lung tissue. The lesions are commonly more severe in the right than in the left lung. Plum-coloured or greyish areas of consolidation resembling lymphoid tissue are scattered along the ventral borders of the lobes. Liquefaction of the pneumonic tissue, pericarditis and pleurisy are unusual in the pure infection. Enlarged oedematous bronchial lymph nodes are characteristic. In acute cases there is intense oedema and congestion of the lung and frothy exudate in the bronchi. When secondary invasion occurs, pleurisy and pericarditis are common and there may be severe hepatization and congestion with necrotizing bronchopneumonia.

Diagnosis

Enzootic pneumonia of pigs, with or without secondary bacterial invasion, is the commonest respiratory infection in this species. An acute outbreak may be confused with swine influenza, but this disease is much less common and is characterized by a short course in which sneezing and muscle pain are prominent and the signs are in general more indicative of an upper respiratory infection than of pneumonia. In swine influenza *Haem. suis* is always present and lungworm infestation is an integral part of the disease. Uncomplicated lungworm (*Metastrongylus* spp.) infestation may also cause respiratory signs in pigs. However, at necropsy, patchy bronchopneumonia is most marked in the dorsal part of the diaphragmatic lobes and worms can be demonstrated. Contagious pleuropneumonia of pigs caused by *Haem. pleuropneumoniae* is a much more acute and highly fatal disease.

Ascaris lumbricoides infestations are commonly cited as a cause of chronic swine pneumonia, but experimental ascariasis produces mainly hepatic damage by migrating larvae. In the lungs some haemorrhage occurs and there may be a mild febrile reaction and a soft moist cough lasting for up to 5 days during the stage of larval migration, but the respiratory signs do not persist. Occasional fatal cases of pulmonary ascariasis occur. Under field conditions coughing is never marked in ascariasis, while it is the major sign in enzootic pneumonia (5).

A positive diagnosis of enzootic pneumonia depends upon the necropsy findings and culture of the mycoplasma, a difficult procedure.

Treatment

The disease is moderately susceptible to chlortetracycline but not to sulphonamides, penicillin or streptomycin. Herd treatment with tetracycline in clinical trials has reduced the severity of the pneumonia but the pigs are not sterilized and are still infective. Tylosin, furaltodone and erythromycin were ineffective (1, 6). Antibiotic therapy may be advisable in some outbreaks to control secondary bacterial invaders. This can be effectively managed by feeding the antibiotic as a feed additive, or by including it in the drinking water if the pigs are not eating well. Acutely affected pigs should be given individual parenteral treatment with a broad-spectrum antibiotic, but the response is only moderately good.

Control

There are two levels at which control can be practised: complete eradication, which is most desirable for breeding herds, and keeping the disease at a low level, which is the most that can be hoped for in commercial fattening units.

Control in commercial fattening units. When pigs are continually being brought into a herd, infection will be brought in also. In these circumstances control measures include vaccination, good management and possibly the use of antibiotic feeding. No specific vaccine is available but vaccines are under test (25). Killed vaccine containing Types A and D, *Past. multocida* may be useful in restricting secondary bacterial pneumonia (7). It is advisable to avoid the introduction of affected pigs if this is possible. Pigs purchased in sale yards or on farms should be inspected for evidence of coughing or unthriftiness. Litters of uneven size are particularly suspect. Good housing, nutrition and hygiene are most important to keep the effects of the disease to the lowest possible level.

Attempts at controlling the disease by the use of antibiotics have given conflicting results. Sulpha-dimidine, penicillin, streptomycin and chloram-phenicol are ineffective. Chlortetracycline or oxytetracycline injected at the rate of 1 mg. per kg. body weight per day prevent infection, but the method is unsatisfactory for commercial use. Feeding tetracyclines or oxytetracycline at 11 to 22 mg. per kg. body weight per day prevents infection but chlortetracycline at 33 mg. per kg. body weight per day is only partly effective (8, 9). The feeding of antibiotics is particularly suitable for droves of young pigs brought together for commercial fattening.

Eradication in breeding herds. Complete eradication should be attempted in breeding herds and this has proved to be practicable provided close veterinary supervision is available. Two techniques are used: repopulation with *Specific Pathogen Free* (SPF) pigs and the *Isolated Farrowing Programme*.

Repopulation with SPF pigs is aimed primarily at the eradication of enzootic pneumonia and atrophic rhinitis, but may also assist in the control of many other diseases. The technique has spread extensively in North America and Great Britain during the past 15 years and its general efficiency has been described by many authors (10, 11, 12). Briefly the method is to remove baby pigs at term from sows from approved farms by Caesarean section or by hysterectomy. The baby pigs are reared artificially by the unit preparing the pigs and are used to repopulate existing farms where all pigs are removed 30 days before arrival of the SPF pigs. This is a practical proposition in the hands of a good farmer but significant losses are to be expected before pigs reach 90 kg. weight (13).

The Isolated Farrowing Programme is based on removal of infected adults and isolation of litters from non-infective sows. Hygiene must be good, and lack of understanding or coordination on the part of the farmer can easily lead to failure. Individual sows are farrowed in strict isolation so that any infection that occurs in the piglets must have come from the dam. The dam is checked clinically and a proportion of each litter by necropsy. Affected litters and their dams are eliminated. Replacement sows are kept only from those litters in which all findings are negative.

New breeding stock can be added to the herd from known virus-free herds or by the purchase of pregnant sows from apparently clean herds. The litters are reared in isolation and tested for freedom from the disease by slaughter and examination of 2 or 3 pigs from each litter. Old sows are less dangerous as potential sources of infection than young gilts (14).

Under temperate climatic conditions in Australia it has been found a relatively simple matter to eradicate the disease from piggeries by isolation of each unit (sow and litter) so that there is at least 3 m. of air space between units (15). The units are then checked by necropsy examination, using the farrows and cull sows as test animals. Because it is necessary to separate the units in a pig house by leaving every alternate pen empty, a big reduction in pig numbers is necessary to begin with. Every opportunity must be provided for the disease to spread within each unit so that infected units will be detected when a selection of the pigs is necropsied. On the other hand, once a unit is known to be infected, it should be discarded as soon as possible to avoid unnecessary risks to the quarantine barrier. When a unit is discarded, a pen or yard should be cleaned and disinfected before re-use, although these measures need not be heroic, as the disease is spread mainly by direct contact. The replacement unit should be one of the residual progeny of a known free unit. Careful selection of sows at the commencement of the programme is necessary to avoid undue wastage of units at a later date. Introduced sows should go through a similar testing procedure as the home reared sows. Boars present a rather difficult problem. They may be purchased from known free farms, used by artificial insemination or run with known free pigs which are subsequently examined at slaughter as a test for infectivity of the boar. The alternative method is to purchase boar and sow replacements in utero, remove them at birth and rear them artificially as a group and, if necessary, test by slaughter of some of the group.

Eradication of enzootic pneumonia has been achieved by the Isolated Farrowing method, usually within a year, in areas where pigs run outdoors or in well ventilated, semi-open pig houses, but the method has obvious limitations in countries with a long hard winter where pigs are housed in completely enclosed barns. In these areas repopulation with SPF pigs is the method of choice. The latter method has the advantages in any country of being quicker, more certain and more likely to be effective against other diseases, particularly atrophic rhinitis.

One of the important corollaries of area control of enzootic pneumonia is the necessity to provide pigs free of the disease as replacements for herds attempting eradication. It is not sufficient to purchase pigs from a commercial supplier of SPF pigs, nor from second generation farms which have undertaken repopulation and are ostensibly free of the disease. There is need for a programme of certification of freedom from enzootic pneumonia (15). This can be done only by a governmental agency, and the need for accuracy is obvious. No laboratory test is available and the only practicable method is the examination of lungs grossly and, if lesions are present, microscopically, for evidence of enzootic pneumonia. The pigs examined should be chosen from average or slow growing groups—the ones most likely to be affected. Usually pigs going to slaughter in the normal course of events are picked out and their lungs retained at the abattoir. For most breeding herds 10 pigs should be examined each year (10). The presence of enzootic pneumonia lesions in any pig disqualifies the herd from the classification of 'pneumonia-free'.

After a great deal of experience in controlling the disease, Goodwin (21) feels that eradication cannot proceed beyond voluntary participation by individual farms because of the relatively high risk of reinfection and the difficulty of differentiating the disease from other chronic pneumonias.

REFERENCES

(1) Huhn, R. G. (1970). *Vet. Bull.*, *40*, 249.
(2) Mackenzie, A. (1963). *Vet. Rec.*, *75*, 114.
(3) Betts, A. O. (1952). *Vet. Rec.*, *64*, 283.
(4) Pullar, E. M. (1949). *Aust. vet. J.*, *25*, 262.
(5) Betts, A. O. (1954). *Vet. Rec.*, *66*, 749.
(6) Huhn, R. G. (1971). *Canad. J. comp. Med.*, *35*, 77.
(7) Carter, G. R. (1957). *Vet. Med.*, *52*, 308.
(8) Betts, A. O. & Campbell, R. C. (1956). *J. comp. Path.*, *66*, 89.
(9) Lannek, N. & Boronfors, S. (1956). *Vet. Rec.*, *68*, 53.
(10) Young, G. A. & Underdahl, N. R. (1960). *J. Amer. vet. med. Ass.*, *137*, 185.
(11) Caldwell, J. D. *et al.* (1961). *J. Amer. vet. med. Ass.*, *138*, 141; *139*, 342.
(12) Betts, A. D. & Luke, D. (1961). *Vet. Rec.*, *73*, 283, 295, 1349.
(13) Alexander, T. J. L. & Roe, C. K. (1962). *Canad. vet. J.*, *3*, 299.
(14) Goodwin, R. F. W. (1965). *Vet. Rec.*, *77*, 383.
(15) McDermid, K. A. (1964). *Canad. vet. J.*, *5*, 95.
(16) Pan, I. C. & Cordy, D. R. (1962). *Bull. Int. Zool. Acad. Sinica, Taiwan*, *1*, 29.
(17) Gordon, W. A. M. (1963). *Brit. vet. J.*, *119*, 307.
(18) Goodwin, R. F. W. (1971). *Vet. Rec.*, *89*, 77.
(19) Hodges, R. T. *et al.* (1969). *Vet. Rec.*, *84*, 268.
(20) Kasza, L. *et al.* (1969). *Vet. Rec.*, *84*, 262.
(21) Goodwin, R. F. W. (1967). *Vet. Rec.*, *81*, 643.
(22) Roberts, D. H. & Little, T. W. A. (1970). *J. comp. Path.*, *80*, 211.
(23) L'Ecuyer, C. & Boulanger, P. (1970). *Canad. J. comp. Med.*, *34*, 38.
(24) Jericho, K. (1968). *Vet. Rec.*, *82*, 507, 520.
(25) Lam, K. M. & Switzer, W. P. (1971). *Amer. J. vet. Res.*, *32*, 1731, 1737.

Diseases Caused by Viruses and Chlamydia—I

VIRAL DISEASES WITH MANIFESTATIONS OF SEPTICAEMIA

Hog Cholera

(*Swine Fever*)

HOG CHOLERA is a highly infectious, viral septi-caemia affecting only pigs. Its former character-ization as an acute, fatal disease with a clinical and post-mortem picture of septicaemia and haemor-rhage has been expanded to include a chronic illness, recovery when supportive treatment is given to older pigs, and the appearance of newborn pigs with congenital defects (1). This expansive definition has led to the suggestion that the disease should be defined as 'any disease associated with a swine fever virus' (2).

Incidence

Although hog cholera appears to have originated in the United States it is now virtually world wide in distribution. In the past the important free areas have been Canada, Australia, New Zealand and South Africa, which has not experienced the disease since it was eradicated in 1918. Swine fever was eradicated from the U.K. during the period 1963–7 (2, 3). Outbreaks have occurred in these countries from time to time but have been quickly controlled by a rigorous policy of slaughter and quarantine. Usually the disease occurs in severe outbreak form, often with a morbidity of 100 per cent and a mortality rate approaching this. How-ever, in recent years outbreaks of a relatively slowly spreading, mild form of the disease have caused great concern in many countries (4). Hog cholera is undoubtedly the most costly disease affecting swine. Losses due to the death of pigs are aggravated by the high cost of vaccination pro-grammes in enzootic areas. Recovered or partially recovered pigs are very susceptible to secondary infections, and exacerbation of existing chronic infections such as virus pneumonia are likely to occur during the convalescent period.

Aetiology

It is probable that a number of strains of the causative virus occur and have varying degrees of pathogenicity. The main importance of so-called 'variant' strains is that they appear to be a com-mon cause of failure of vaccination. The 'neuro-tropic' strain is the commonest variant. It has been a commonly held view that an association exists between hog cholera and salmonellosis. This belief does not deny the independent existence of the two diseases but suggests that the two causa-tive agents may be a dangerous combination. This is supported by the increased ease of transmission of hog cholera when the virus is administered to-gether with small doses of *Salmonella choleraesuis*. However the synergism does not appear to be sufficiently strong to overcome the immunity of pigs vaccinated with commercial vaccines nor to interfere with the development of the immunity (5). As described under the heading of mucosal disease, a strong antigenic relationship appears to exist between the agents of mucosal disease and hog cholera.

The virus of hog cholera is destroyed by boiling, by 5 per cent cresol, and by sunlight but it persists in meat which is preserved by salting, smoking and particularly by freezing. Survival for 1 month in the meat, and 2 months in the bone marrow of salt-cured pork is recorded. Persistence in frozen meat has been observed after $4\frac{1}{2}$ years. The virus persists for 3 to 4 days in decomposing organs and for 15 days in decomposing blood and bone marrow.

All ages of pigs are affected. Suckling white mice are the most suitable laboratory animals for transmission of the virus but it can be grown in tissue culture. The virus can be passaged through sheep and rabbits and serial passage through the latter has been used to prepare a modified virus suitable for use as a vaccine. Recovery from natural infection with the hog cholera virus results in the development of a lasting immunity and use has been made of this in the production of effective vaccines. The immunity is transmitted passively in the colostrum, the degree of protection resulting in the piglets being dependent upon the immune status of the dam. Thus sows vaccinated with live virus and serum provide protection for their piglets for 10 or more weeks, while those vaccinated with attenuated virus vaccines provide immunity only for about 4 weeks. Although recovered or vaccinated adult pigs do not appear to harbour the virus and act as 'carriers' the foetus and the newborn pig, because of their state of immune tolerance, can support a viraemia for long periods (6).

Transmission

The resistance and high infectivity of the virus make spread of the disease by inert materials, especially uncooked meat, a major problem. The source of virus is always an infected pig and its products and the infection is usually acquired by ingestion but inhalation is also a possible portal. The survival period in poorly ventilated buildings may be as long as two years but outside pens lose their infectivity in 1 to 2 days in warm weather. Survival periods in meat are given above. All excretions, secretions and body tissues of affected pigs contain the virus and it is excreted in the urine for some days before clinical illness appears and for 2 to 3 weeks after clinical recovery.

In areas free of the disease introduction is usually effected by the importation of infected pigs or the feeding of garbage containing uncooked pork scraps. Birds and humans may also act as physical carriers for the virus. In enzootic areas transmission to new farms can occur in feeder pigs purchased for fattening, or indirectly by flies or on bedding, feed, boots, automobile tyres or transport vehicles. Persistence of infection in clinically normal 'carrier' pigs is unlikely but persistence of the virus in piglets has been observed when their vaccinated dams are infected or are vaccinated during pregnancy. There is no evidence that the sows continue to carry the virus but surviving piglets appear to be able to harbour it for up to 56 days (7) and may be the source of new outbreaks. A similar 'carrier' state has been observed in young pigs from non-immune sows, the young pigs having been vaccinated with attenuated virus vaccine.

When the disease is introduced into a susceptible population an epidemic usually develops rapidly because of the resistance of the virus and the short incubation period. In recent years outbreaks have been observed in which the rate of spread is much reduced and this has delayed field diagnosis (4).

Pathogenesis

Passage of the virus through the mucosa of the upper part of the digestive or respiratory tracts is followed by septicaemia and invasion of vascular endothelium. Most of the lesions are produced by hydropic degeneration and proliferation of vascular endothelium which results in the occlusion of blood vessels. Atrophy of the thymus, depletion of lymphocytes and germinal follicles in peripheral lymphoid tissues, renal glomerular changes and splenitis are characteristic (8). In many cases secondary bacterial infection occurs and plays an important part in the development of lesions and clinical signs.

The experimental disease is characterized by a biphasic temperature elevation at the second and sixth day after inoculation, a profound leucopenia and an appreciable anaemia 24 hours after inoculation, diarrhoea at the seventh day, and anorexia and death on the fourth to fifteenth day (9).

Clinical Findings

Clinical signs usually appear 5 to 10 days after infection, although longer incubation periods of 35 days or more are recorded. At the beginning of an outbreak young pigs may die peracutely without clinical signs having been evident. Acute cases are the most common. Affected pigs are depressed, do not eat, and stand in a drooped attitude with the tail hanging. They are disinclined to move, and when forced, do so with a swaying movement of the hindquarters. They tend to lie down and burrow into the bedding, often piled one on top of the other. Prior to the appearance of other signs a high temperature (40·5 to 41·5°C or 105 to 107°F) is usual. Other early signs include constipation followed by diarrhoea and vomiting. Later a diffuse purplish discolouration of the abdominal skin occurs. Small areas of necrosis are sometimes seen on the edges of the ears, on the tail, and lips of the vulva. A degree of conjunctivitis is usual and in some pigs the eyelids are stuck together by dried, purulent exudate. Nervous signs are often observed even in the early stages of illness. Circling, incoordination, muscle tremor and convulsions are the commonest manifestations. Death can be expected 5 to 7 days after the commencement of illness.

A form of the disease in which nervous signs predominate has been described and attributed to a variant strain of the virus. The incubation period is often shorter and the course of the disease more acute than usual. Pigs in lateral recumbency show a tetanic convulsion for 10 to 15 seconds followed by a clonic convulsion of 30 to 40 seconds. The convulsion may be accompanied by loud squealing and may occur constantly or at intervals of several hours, often being followed by a period of terminal coma. In some cases convulsions do not occur but nervous involvement is manifested by coarse tremor of the body and limb muscles. Apparent blindness, stumbling and allotriophagia have also been observed.

A chronic form occurs rarely in field outbreaks and occasionally after serum-virus, simultaneous vaccination (9). The incubation period is longer than normal and there is emaciation and the appearance of characteristic skin lesions including alopecia, dermatitis, blotching of the ears and a terminal, deep purple colouration of the abdominal skin.

Lesser forms of the disease occur and include foetal resorptions, mummified foetuses, stillbirths and anomalies when sows are vaccinated with attenuated virus in early pregnancy, and congenital trembling, stillbirths and a high incidence of weakling piglets in vaccinated sows exposed to natural infection in early pregnancy (7). One of the common anomalies in the latter group is cerebellar hypoplasia which has been produced experimentally by infecting sows in early pregnancy with a virus isolated from piglets with the same disease (16). Only 1 of 31 outbreaks of cerebellar hypoplasia was not associated with swine fever infection in the dam.

Clinical Pathology

A valuable ante-mortem laboratory examination is the total and differential white cell count. Pigs in the early stages of hog cholera show a pronounced leucopenia, the total white cell count falling from a normal range of 14,000 to 24,000 per cmm. to 4000 to 9000 per cmm. In the late stages of hog cholera a leucocytosis, due to secondary bacterial invasion, may develop. Baby pigs less than 5 weeks old normally have low leucocyte counts. Where possible, transmission experiments using blood taken at the height of the fever and injected into susceptible pigs should be attempted. Negative cultural examinations of faeces may help to eliminate other diseases as diagnostic possibilities.

With the advent of comparatively mild forms of the disease a great deal of attention has been focused on the development of suitable serological methods of identifying the presence of the hog cholera virus. A gel diffusion test for the presence of precipitins in pig tissues, particularly pancreas, appears to be of value provided the pig has been clinically affected for at least 5 days (17, 18). A modified CF test has been devised which is reasonably accurate provided material from a pig at the height of the disease is used. It is considered suitable as a herd test (19). Examination of serum by a virus neutralization test is also used as a diagnostic procedure (4). Fluorescent antibody tests, both direct on tissue and indirect on tissue culture virus, are being used increasingly, especially the fluorescent antibody-tissue culture test (10, 11, 12). The FA test applied to frozen sections of tonsillar tissue has great advantages (15). An indirect test, Taylor's iodine reduction test, is based on the reduction of amylolytic activity in pancreas of infected animals. It appears to have some merit as a screening test (13). A modern problem in the serological diagnosis of swine fever is the capacity of some strains of bovine mucosal disease virus to give false positive serological reactions to swine fever (14).

Necropsy Findings

In peracute cases there may be no gross changes at necropsy. In the common, acute form there are many submucosal and subserosal petechial haemorrhages but these are inconstant and to find them it may be necessary to examine two or more cadavers from an outbreak. The haemorrhages are most noticeable under the capsule of the kidney, about the ileocaecal valve, in the cortical sinuses of the lymph nodes and in the bladder and larynx. The haemorrhages are usually petechial and rarely ecchymotic. Enlargement of the lymph nodes is constant and the spleen may contain marginal infarcts. Infarction in the mucosa of the gallbladder is a common but not constant finding and appears to be an almost pathognomonic lesion. There is congestion of the liver and bone marrow and often of the lungs. Circular, raised button ulcers in the colonic mucosa are often seen. Although these gross necropsy findings are fairly general in cases of hog cholera, they cannot be considered as diagnostic unless accompanied by the clinical and epizootological evidence of the disease. They can occur in other diseases, particularly salmonellosis.

There are characteristic, microscopic lesions of a non-suppurative encephalitis in most cases and a presumptive diagnosis of hog cholera can be made if they are present. Histologically, the main site of tissue injury in hog cholera is the reticuloendothelial system where hydropic degeneration and proliferation of the vascular endothelium cause occlusion of blood vessels (4). The more virulent 'neurotropic' strains produce lesions of similar nature but greater severity. Material for laboratory examination should include brain stem and lymph node in 10 per cent formalin.

In the chronic form of the disease, necrotic ulceration of the mucosa of the large intestine is usual and histologically there is transverse calcification of the distal portion of the rib. Secondary pneumonia and enteritis commonly accompany the primary lesions of hog cholera. Virus can be isolated from infected pigs by filtration of macerated tissues, especially spleen, and the disease can be produced by the injection of filtrates into susceptible pigs.

Diagnosis

A positive diagnosis of hog cholera is always difficult to make without evidence from transmission tests. This is particularly true of the chronic, less dramatic forms of the disease. A highly infectious, fatal disease of pigs with a course of 5 to 7 days in a group of unvaccinated animals should arouse suspicion of hog cholera, especially if there are no signs indicative of localization in particular organs. Nervous signs are probably the one exception. The gross necropsy findings are also non-specific and apart from transmission experiments most reliance must be placed on the leucopenia in the early stages and the non-suppurative encephalitis visible on histological examination. Both of these features may be obscured if a coincident bacterial infection, particularly salmonellosis, is present.

A definitive diagnosis depends upon the production of the disease by experimental transmission to susceptible pigs and preferably by failure to transmit to immune pigs. Because of the emergence of strains of the virus which are of low virulence attention must be given to the occurrence of fever and leucopenia as the only evidence of satisfactory transmission. Such pigs should be challenged with virulent virus subsequently. Again because of the possibility of strains of low virulence more and more attention is being paid to tissue culture neutralization and gel diffusion precipitin tests as herd diagnostic procedures (4). Because of the strong antigenic relationship between the viruses of mucosal disease and hog cholera the presence of the former disease in local cattle is a possible confounding factor in diagnosis by serological means and has been postulated as a cause of low mortality and slow spread in some outbreaks. However, the possibility of interspecies spread of mucosal disease seems unlikely.

The major diseases which resemble hog cholera include salmonellosis which is usually accompanied by enteritis and dyspnoea, acute erysipelas in which the subserous haemorrhages are likely to be ecchymotic rather than petechial, and acute pasteurellosis. In all of these diseases extensive skin discolouration occurs but it is often patchy or discrete and is usually accompanied by oedema and haemorrhage. Other encephalitides, particularly viral encephalomyelitis and salmonellosis produce similar nervous signs. African swine fever, apart from its greater severity, is almost impossible to differentiate from hog cholera without serological tests.

Treatment

Hyperimmune serum is the only available treatment and may be of value in the very early stages of the illness if given in doses of 50 to 150 ml. It has more general use in the protection of in-contact animals. A concentrated serum permitting the use of much smaller doses is now available.

Control

The methods used in the control of the disease include eradication and control by vaccination. General control procedures are dealt with first and are followed by a description of the immunizing products available.

Outbreak control in hog cholera free areas. In areas where the disease does not normally occur complete eradication by slaughter of all in-contact and infected pigs is possible and should be practised. The pigs are slaughtered and disposed of, preferably by burning. All piggeries in the area should be quarantined and no movement of pigs permitted unless for immediate slaughter. Hyperimmune hog cholera antiserum may be used to protect pigs on farms in the quarantine area but this method is expensive. All vehicles used for the transport of pigs, all pens and premises and utensils must be disinfected with strong chemical disinfectant such as 5 per cent cresylic acid. Contaminated clothing should be boiled. Entry to and departure from infected premises must be carefully controlled to avoid spread of the disease on footwear, clothes and automobile tyres. Legislation commanding the boiling of all garbage before feeding must be enforced. This eradication procedure has controlled outbreaks which have occurred in Canada and Australia and has served to maintain these countries free from the disease.

Control where Hog Cholera is Enzootic

Area control. In enzootic areas control is largely a problem of choosing the best vaccine and using it intelligently. Much can also be done to keep the incidence of the disease low by the education of farmers whose co-operation can be best assured by a demonstration that eradication is both desirable and practicable. Once farmer enthusiasm is aroused the greatest stumbling block to control, failure to notify outbreaks, is eliminated. Education of the farmer should emphasize the highly infectious nature of the disease and the ease with which it can be spread by the feeding of uncooked garbage and the purchase and sale of infected or in-contact pigs. The common practice of sending pigs to market as soon as illness appears in a group is one of the major methods by which hog cholera is spread.

Of the vaccines available those containing killed or attenuated virus are to be preferred. Live, virulent virus vaccines produce a more solid immunity but are capable of introducing the infection and of actually causing the disease when vaccination 'breaks' occur. The reaction to live virus vaccine may be severe and the susceptibility of pigs to other diseases may be increased. Eradication of the disease is impossible while the use of this type of vaccine is permitted.

Herd control. When an outbreak occurs in a herd the immediate need is to prevent infection from spreading further. This can be best achieved by removing the source of infection and increasing the resistance of in-contact animals by the injection of hyperimmune serum or one of the available vaccines. Removal of the source of infection necessitates isolation of infected animals, suitable hygienic precautions to prevent the spread of infections on boots, clothing and utensils, disposal of carcases by burning and disinfection of pens. The pens should be scraped, hosed and sprayed with 5 per cent cresylic acid solution or other suitable disinfectant. The choice of serum or vaccine may depend on local legislation and will depend upon circumstances. Pigs in the affected pen should receive serum (20 to 75 ml. depending on size) and pigs in unaffected pens should be vaccinated. Pigs receiving only serum will require active vaccination at a later date if a strong immunity is to be achieved.

Hog cholera eradication. The elimination of hog cholera from a country where it is well established presents a formidable problem. Before the final stage of eradication can be attempted, the incidence of the disease must be reduced to a low level by widespread use of vaccination and the enforcement of garbage cooking regulations. The position in the United States at the present time is that the incidence has been drastically reduced in a number of states, so much so that final, drastic stamping out procedures, including the prohibition of vaccination of any kind, have now been implemented (20).

One of the most important problems encountered in eradication programmes is the clinically normal 'carrier' animal (7, 21) and steps need to be taken to avoid the sale of all pigs from infected premises. A procedure which has been particularly effective in the control of this and other diseases of pigs is the complete prohibition of all community sales of feeder pigs. There are obvious political difficulties in such a prohibition but, despite their usefulness as marketing agencies, community sales continue to be a major source of swine infections. Further necessary steps include the immediate prohibition of virulent virus as an immunizing agent, the use of attenuated virus only in special circumstances and for a limited period, and a radical policy in handling outbreaks as described above.

The eradication of swine fever in the United Kingdom during a 4-year campaign ending in 1966 has been a very important achievement and the salient features of the campaign have been recorded (2, 3). Control was radical in that all herds in which the disease was diagnosed were slaughtered and all carcases burned or buried to avoid missing atypical cases and recurrence through the swill cycle. The two focal points which became apparent were the need to avoid vaccination and the need to diagnose accurately. Vaccination was not permitted because it was not completely effective, because it produced 'carriers', and because it encouraged the development of mild and chronic forms of the disease. The need to diagnose accurately led to changes in diagnostic procedure as the campaign progressed. As the proportion of textbook outbreaks lessened there was increasing dependence on immunodiffusion in agar gel and neuropathology. These tests eliminated certain strains of infection but the diagnostic programme was reinforced with fluorescent antibody techniques and serological tests. Transmission tests were used infrequently because of the need to use SPF pigs as recipients. The reporting of all outbreaks of congenital tremor and cerebellar hypoplasia detected a large number of infected herds.

Immunization Methods

Very few pigs possess natural immunity to hog cholera and, until the introduction of the serum-virus method of vaccination, an outbreak of the disease in a herd meant virtually that the herd would be eliminated. The situation changed rapidly thereafter and it can be safely claimed that the development of the swine industry in the United States would have been impossible without the protection which serum and virus afforded. On the other hand, the dangers inherent in the use of fully virulent virus have led to a constant search for new and safer methods of immunization. In recent years several vaccines, both killed and attenuated, have been developed and the practitioner can now choose a vaccination programme to fit the circumstances of the herd and area. Attenuated vaccines are not without disadvantages. Their use in very young or stressed pigs may be followed by some deaths, and they may interfere with the serological or histological diagnosis of the disease. A killed vaccine, preferably crystal violet vaccine administered twice at monthly intervals, is most favoured (22).

Serum-virus vaccination produces an immediate, solid and lasting immunity when properly administered to healthy swine. The virus, produced by collecting blood 6 to 7 days after artificial infection, is injected subcutaneously in 2 ml. doses followed immediately by serum in doses graduated to the size of the pigs and varying from 20 ml. for suckling pigs to 75 ml. for adults. Overdosing with serum will not prevent the development of immunity. Vaccination is performed at any age after 4 weeks.

Attenuated vaccines include a tissue vaccine, a tissue culture vaccine and a lapinized virus vaccine. The *tissue vaccine*, prepared by the treatment of infected tissue with eucalyptol, is slow in producing immunity (3 weeks) which is of short duration (6 months). *Tissue culture vaccines* prepared by serial passage through tissue culture need to be administered simultaneously with serum but produce satisfactory immunity. *Lapinized virus vaccines* have been produced by attenuating the virus through rabbit passage or by alternate swine and rabbit passage. Some lapinized vaccines show virtually no pathogenicity for swine and their use is recommended without serum while others require the simultaneous administration of small doses of serum. These vaccines have the advantage of producing immunity within a few days, even when administered without serum, and they can therefore be used during the course of an outbreak, although the use of serum in such circumstances is recommended. At least some lapinized strains produce solid immunity for 2 years or more. These vaccines have the disadvantage of being rather unstable in their degree of attenuation. A modification

of lapinized virus by attenuation in tissue culture appears to improve its safety (22).

It is possible that a virus which is non-pathogenic for pigs but is capable of protecting them against hog cholera, such as that described under mucosal disease of cattle, may be of some importance in the control of this disease (28). Experience with mucosal disease virus has shown that the protection provided by it varies from 0 to 100 per cent depending on the strain of hog cholera virus used as a challenge (23).

Crystal violet vaccine stores well, does not lose or vary in its potency and the infection is not transmitted to in-contact pigs. Immunity persists for about 12 months and when given to pregnant sows the vaccine confers a passive immunity on the piglets by passage of antibodies in the colostrum but the piglets must still be vaccinated at 6 to 8 weeks of age. A disadvantage is that immunity after vaccination does not develop until about the twelfth day. The administration of serum around the time of vaccination should be practised with caution as it may interfere with the degree of immunity produced. It is claimed that this interference does not occur provided the serum is administered outside the period of 5 days before to 5 days after vaccination. Within this period the degree of interference depends on the potency of the serum. The dose rates for the vaccine recommended are 5 ml. for pigs less than 70 lb. and 10 ml. for heavier pigs. The disadvantages of this type of vaccine are that immunity is of short duration only, pigs may be rendered more susceptible to erysipelas, and the production of immune antibodies may cause a high incidence of iso-immune haemolytic anaemia in some breeds of pigs. Its use during an outbreak is limited by the fact that immunity does not develop for 12 days after vaccination.

Breakdowns in vaccination programmes occur, regardless of the type of vaccine used (24). When such breakdowns occur following the use of serum and fully virulent virus, it is customary to classify them as 'serum breaks' or 'virus breaks', depending largely on when they occur in relation to the time of vaccination. 'Serum breaks' occur within a few days after vaccination and are due to the failure of the serum to counteract effectively the administered virus. 'Virus breaks' occur some time later and are due to failure of the virus to activate a sufficient degree of immunity to protect against subsequent infection. This may be the result of prior dosage or overdosage with serum at vaccination, vaccination of pigs with passive immunity from the dam or immunity after previous exposure. The commonest cause of failure is probably the administration of the vaccine between 1 and 7 days after passive immunization with serum, a circumstance likely to arise when pigs are purchased through saleyards. In most cases, 'serum breaks' result from faulty vaccination technique, vaccination of debilitated pigs or those in the early stage of the disease and cannot be charged to defective serum. Vaccination of pigs in poor condition should be avoided if possible but, if it is thought necessary, the dose rate of serum should be doubled. Variant strains may cause breaks resulting in 100 per cent mortality or the development of chronic hog cholera. These may be either serum or virus breaks depending on whether the variant was the administered virus or the virus to which the pigs were later exposed. In general, 'virus breaks' are due to improper handling of the virus before use or to the vaccination with serum and virus of pigs which are already passively immune.

While breakdowns are more likely to occur following serum and virus vaccination, they may occur in other vaccination programmes but the classification into 'serum and virus breaks' is hardly applicable and a more general classification of 'long term breaks' (when hog cholera appears 2 to 4 weeks after vaccination) and 'short term breaks' (when the disease develops within 10 days of vaccination) has been suggested. Vaccination of anaemic pigs may produce an anaphylactic-type shock.

A major difficulty in vaccinating against hog cholera is the protection of baby pigs in enzootic areas. This has been a particular problem in garbage-fed herds but the increase in the cooking of garbage in recent years has reduced its importance. Sows in enzootic areas or herds will normally be immune because of vaccination. The piglets are passively immunized by absorption of antibodies from colostrum and cannot be actively immunized by vaccination (25). Effective passive immunity persists for about 4 weeks, the time varying with the amount of antibody ingested in the colostrum. In high risk herds, serum can be administered at that time and again at 8 weeks followed by active immunization at 12 weeks. When sucking pigs under 7 weeks old and from immune sows are vaccinated with serum and virus the dose of both should be increased by about 50 per cent. The use of lapinized virus without serum, or vaccination with crystal violet vaccine at 4 weeks of age are also suggested in sucking pigs from immune sows. Those vaccinated with crystal violet vaccine should probably be vaccinated again after weaning.

Vaccination of sows during the first third of pregnancy should be avoided because of the risk of producing congenital defects in the piglets and a high incidence of foetal resorptions (27). Included in the congenital defects are anasarca and deformed noses and kidneys. Their incidence is highest when the sows are vaccinated between the 15th and 25th days of pregnancy. Cerebellar hypoplasia, hypomyelinogenesis (26) and mycoclonia congenita or congenital trembling is also recorded in piglets born from sows vaccinated during early pregnancy.

REFERENCES

(1) Carbrey, E. A. et al. (1966). J. Amer. vet. med. Ass., 149, 1720.
(2) Done, J. T. (1969). Brit. vet. J., 125, 349.
(3) Beynon, A. G. (1969). Vet. Rec., 84, 623.
(4) Keast, J. C. & Golding, N. K. (1964). Aust. vet. J., 40, 137.
(5) Rodabaugh, D. E. et al. (1964). J. Amer. vet. med. Ass., 145, 252.
(6) Carbrey, E. A. et al. (1966). J. Amer. vet. med. Ass., 149, 23.
(7) Huck, R. A. & Aston, F. W. (1964). Vet. Rec., 76, 1151.
(8) Cheville, N. F. & Mengeling, W. L. (1969). Lab. Invest., 20, 261.
(9) Mengeling, W. L. & Packer, R. A. (1969). Amer. J. vet. Res., 30, 409.
(10) Hoorens, J. et al. (1969). Bull. Off. int. Épizoot., 72, 789.
(11) Solozarno, R. F. et al. (1966). J. Amer. vet. med. Ass., 149, 31.
(12) Mengeling, W. L. & Torrey, J. P. (1967). Amer. J. vet. Res., 28, 1653.
(13) O'Neill, P. A. F. (1971). Vet. Rec., 88, 468.
(14) Snowdon, W. A. & French, E. L. (1968). Aust. vet. J., 44, 179.
(15) Meyling, A. & Scherning-Thiesen, K. (1968). Acta vet. scand., 9, 50.
(16) Done, J. T. & Harding, J. D. J. (1966). Proc. roy. Soc. Med., 59, 1083.
(17) Mansi, W. I. & King, A. A. (1963). Vet. Rec., 75, 933.
(18) Matthaeus, W. & Korn, G. (1970). Zbl. vet. Med., 17B, 1010.
(19) Boulanger, P. et al. (1965). Canad. J. comp. Med., 29, 201.
(20) Tillery, M. J. (1971). Proc. 74th ann. Mtg U.S. Animal Health Ass., 1970, Maryland, U.S.A.
(21) Dunne, H. W. (1963). Vet. Med., 53, 222.
(22) Keeble, S. A. et al. (1966). Brit. vet. J., 122, 190.
(23) Langer, P. H. (1964). Proc. 67th ann. gen. Mtg U.S. Live Stock sanit. Ass., 358.
(24) Torrey, J. P. et al. (1956). Proc. 59th ann. gen. Mtg U.S. Live Stock sanit. Ass., 1955, 343.
(25) Aiken, J. M. & Blore, I. C. (1964). J. Amer. vet. med. Ass., 25, 1134.
(26) Emerson, J. L. & Delez, A. L. (1965). J. Amer. vet. med. Ass., 147, 47.
(27) Dunne, H. W. & Clark, C. D. (1968). Amer. J. vet. Res., 29, 787.
(28) Baker, J. A. et al. (1969). J. Amer. vet. med. Ass., 155, 1866.

African Swine Fever

(African Pig Disease, Wart Hog Disease)

African swine fever is a peracute, highly fatal, highly contagious disease of pigs caused by a virus which is antigenically distinct from that of hog cholera. Clinically and at necropsy the disease resembles hog cholera closely but is even more severe.

Incidence

Until 1957 African swine fever had not occurred outside the African continent where it causes serious losses in the pig population and in some areas precludes the raising of swine. To the rest of the world it represented the most formidable of the exotic diseases of swine, a disease which had to be kept within its existing boundaries at all costs. In domestic pigs the disease is almost always fatal, the morbidity rate approaches 100 per cent, and no effective method of vaccination is available. However, African swine fever broke out of Africa, appearing in Portugal in 1957 and Spain in 1960, resulting in the death and slaughter of thousands of pigs. Subsequently the disease has appeared in France, apparently due to the importation of infected pigs from Spain. During 1960 losses in Spain due to the disease were estimated to be about $9 million.

Until recent years the occurrence of African swine fever in Africa was limited to explosive outbreaks in European pigs which came in contact with indigenous African pigs. These outbreaks tended to be self-limiting because all pigs in affected herds died or were destroyed, but after a number of years the disease became enzootic in domestic herds. The virus which was introduced to Europe in 1957 was quite capable of persisting in European pigs and after a period of several years in which the disease was epizootic a change to an enzootic character occurred (1, 2).

Aetiology

A specific myxovirus, antigenically distinct from that of hog cholera, is the cause of the disease. Pigs artificially immunized against hog cholera are still fully susceptible to the virus of African swine fever. Only pigs are affected, domestic pigs of all ages and breeds being highly susceptible, but the virus can be passaged in tissue cultures, rabbits and embryonated hen eggs. Hippopotami, which might be expected to be susceptible, do not appear to carry the virus (3). The virus is highly resistant to putrefaction, heat and dryness and survives in chilled carcases for up to 6 months (1). Several antigenic strains of varying virulence occur but little is known of the immunity produced or the antigenic relations between strains because of the high mortality rate in infected pigs. Resistance to infection does occur after recovery and may be due in some pigs to persistence of the virus in the body or to the production of interferon (1). Protective antibodies do not appear to be produced.

Transmission

In Africa the disease is a transmissible infection of warthogs and bush pigs but produces no clinical disease in these animals. Contact with domesticated pigs is a common cause of fresh outbreaks. Direct contact with infected animals is the most important means of spread but indirect contact via infected pens, which remain infective for more than 3 months after occupation, and the ingestion of contaminated water and feed, including uncooked garbage, is reputed to be capable of causing infection but oral feeding with the virus has been shown to be variably effective (4, 5), and long-term cohabitation with warthogs known to be carrying the virus has not always resulted in infection in domestic pigs (6). The observation that spread of the disease from infected pigs to non-infected pigs does not occur if the groups are separated by a pig-proof fence indicates that airborne transmission does not occur. Spread by insect vectors has, in the past, been considered to be unlikely because of the large size of the virus. However, there is now a great deal of evidence that the infection can be, and is, transmitted by the argasid tick, *Ornithodoros moubata*, in which transovarian transmission occurs (4). Ticks can remain infected for as long as eight months.

The virus is present in large quantities in all secretions and excretions and in all organs of acutely ill pigs and, once the disease is established in a herd, it spreads extremely rapidly. Although the infective medium responsible for spread of the disease from warthogs to domestic pigs has not been identified, the seasonal incidence of spread appears to be related to the farrowing season of the warthog and suggests that the foetus and uterine fluids may be the source of virus. Warthogs and recovered domestic pigs are likely to remain as inapparent carriers for long periods. The virus may persist in the latter for up to 15 months.

Pathogenesis

As in hog cholera the main reaction of tissues to the virus of African swine fever is in the vascular endothelium. Damage to the endothelial lining of small vessels results in the development of haemorrhages, serous exudates, infarction, local oedema and engorgement of tissues. The lymphopenia is largely due to the massive destruction of lymphocytes, a characteristic result of infection with the virus of African swine fever.

When the disease is produced experimentally in

susceptible pigs (5, 8) generalization of the infection is demonstrable at 72 hours. Much of the virus becomes localized to erythrocytes and in the lymph nodes of the neck. Infectivity and contact transmission did not develop until after more than 72 hours.

Clinical Findings

The incubation period after contact exposure varies from 5 to 15 days. A high fever (40·5°C or 105°F) appears abruptly and persists, without other apparent signs, for about 4 days. The fever then subsides and the pigs show marked cyanotic blotching of the skin, depression, anorexia, huddling together, disinclination to move, weakness and inco-ordination. Extreme weakness of the hindquarters with difficulty in walking is an early and characteristic sign. Co-ordination remains in the front legs and affected pigs may walk on them, dragging the hind legs. A rapid pulse rate, and serous to mucopurulent nasal and ocular discharges occur and dyspnoea and cough are present in some pigs. Diarrhoea, sometimes dysentery, and vomiting occur in some outbreaks and pregnant sows usually abort. Purple discolouration of the skin may be present on the limbs, snout, abdomen and ears. Death usually occurs within a day or two after the appearance of obvious signs of illness, and is often preceded by convulsions.

Although African swine fever is a highly fatal disease some subacute and chronic cases occur and persist as carriers for up to 15 months (9). Chronic cases are intermittently febrile, become emaciated and develop soft oedematous swellings over limb joints and under the mandible. In recent years there has been a progressive increase in the number of outbreaks of a mild form of the disease (2).

Clinical Pathology

As in hog cholera there is a fall in the total leucocyte count down to about 40 to 50 per cent of normal by the fourth day of fever. There is a pronounced lymphopenia and an increase in immature neutrophils.

The fluorescent antibody technique, the modified direct complement fixation test and the agar double diffusion precipitation tests used in swine fever have been successfully adapted for use in African swine fever (2, 10). Diagnosis is now possible 24 hours after the first signs of fever.

Pig leucocyte tissue cultures have been useful in confirming field diagnosis but confirmation of the diagnosis depends on the detection and identification of the virus. The injection of infective material into two groups of pigs, one of which has been actively or passively immunized against hog cholera, is a suitable method (1).

Necropsy Findings

Gross changes at necropsy resemble closely those found in hog cholera except that in the acute cases the lesions are more severe. In chronic cases the lesions are essentially the same but there are, in addition, pericarditis, interstitial pneumonia and lymphadenitis (11). Petechial haemorrhages are present under all serous surfaces and in lymph nodes, and under the epicardium and endocardium, and there is severe, submucosal congestion in the colon and oedema and congestion of the lungs. Button ulcers in the caecum and colon and splenic infarcts and the petechial haemorrhages in the renal cortex and bladder are less common than in hog cholera. Histologically the lesions are more diagnostic. There is severe damage to vascular endothelium and marked karyorrhexis of lymphocytes in both normal lymphoid deposits and in infiltrations in parenchymatous organs. An encephalitis comparable in type to that of hog cholera is present.

Diagnosis

The disease is easily confused with hog cholera and very careful examination is required to differentiate the two. Clinically the illness is much shorter (2 days as against 7 days) than in hog cholera. Gross necropsy changes are similar to but more severe than those of hog cholera. The marked karyorrhexis of lymphocytes characteristic of African swine fever is not observed in hog cholera. The best available method of differentiation entails the injection of infective material into hog cholera-immune pigs.

Treatment and Control

No effective treatment has been described. Prevention of introduction of the disease to free countries is based on the prohibition of importation of live pigs or pig products from countries where African swine fever occurs. Strict application of the prohibition has prevented the spread of the disease from enzootic areas to South Africa. If a breakdown does occur control must consist of prevention of spread by quarantine, slaughter of infected and contact animals and suitable hygienic precautions. The need for close contact between pigs for the disease to spread and the ease with which this can be prevented by the erection of pig-proof fences facilitates control. Conversely the disease is virtually uncontrollable when pigs from a number of farms have access to communal grazing. The virus is highly resistant to external influences including chemical agents and the most practicable disinfectant to use against the virus is a strong solution of caustic soda. Contaminated sties can remain infective for periods exceeding 3 months. These factors and the persistance of the virus in recovered pigs probably contributed to the difficulties encountered in the eradication programme in Portugal where the disease was stamped out but reappeared in 1960 (12). However the most important factor appears to have been the indiscriminate use of attenuated vaccines which fostered the development of carrier pigs.

Several vaccines have been used including an ineffective killed virus vaccine (7) and vaccines composed of virus attenuated by passage through eggs, räbbits and tissue culture (13). Although the latter have some protective properties, results following their use have been neither satisfactory nor safe and they have the two disadvantages of confounding laboratory tests and producing 'carrier' pigs. A multiplicity of virus strains in an area makes the production of a suitable vaccine extremely difficult. There is a report of an apparent transfer of passive immunity from hyper-immunized sows to their offspring (14).

REFERENCES

(1) Scott, G. R. (1965). *Vet. Rec.*, 77, 1421.
(2) Sanchez Botija, C. *et al.* (1970). *Rev. Patron. Biol. anim.*, 14, 133.
(3) Stone, S. S. & Heuschele, W. P. (1965). *Bull. epizoot. Dis. Afr.*, 13, 23, 157.
(4) Plowright, W. *et al.* (1969). *Vet. Rec.*, 85, 668.
(5) Colgrove, G. S. *et al.* (1969). *Amer. J. vet. Res.*, 30, 1343.
(6) Heuschele, W. P. & Coggins, L. (1969). *Bull. epizoot. Dis. Afr.*, 17, 179.
(7) Stone, S. S. & Hess, W. R. (1967). *Amer. J. vet. Res.*, 28, 475.
(8) Plowright, W. *et al.* (1968). *J. Hyg. Camb.*, 66, 117.
(9) de Tray, D. E. (1963). *Advanc. vet. Sci.*, 8, 299.
(10) Boulanger, P. *et al.* (1966). *Bull. Off. int. Épizoot.*, 66, 723.
(11) Moulton, J. & Coggins, L. (1968). *Cornell Vet.*, 58, 364.
(12) Ribiero, M. J. & Azevedo, R. J. (1961). *Bull. Off. int. Épizoot.*, 55, 88.
(13) Coggins, L. *et al.* (1968). *Cornell Vet.*, 58, 525.
(14) Coelho, M. A. T. (1967). *Rev. Estud. ger. Univ. Moçambique, Ser. 4, Ciene vet*, 4, 317.

Equine Infectious Anaemia
(*Swamp Fever*)

Equine infectious anaemia is a contagious disease of horses caused by a virus, and characterized by a long, chronic illness after an initial acute attack.

Incidence

The disease has been diagnosed on all continents (1). In Europe it is most prevalent in the northern and central regions. It has appeared in most of the states of the U.S.A. and the provinces of Canada but the principal enzootic areas are the Gulf Coast region and the northern wooded sections of Canada. Diagnosis of the disease was made in Australia in 1959 but how long the disease has been present there and its distribution have not been determined. Although statistics of incidence of the disease are unreliable because of failure to diagnose and report the disease it is of major importance and appears to be increasing in incidence. The morbidity varies considerably and may approach 100 per cent in some areas and the mortality rate is usually about 50 per cent although true recovery in the sense that the animal no longer carries the virus seldom, if ever, occurs. The difficulty of diagnosis and the persistence of the 'carrier' state for periods of many years have resulted in embargoes on the introduction of horses into free countries, resulting in recent years not so much in economic embarrassment as in interference with sporting events. Large-scale movements of horses during wartime have been responsible for extensive dissemination of the disease.

Aetiology

A specific virus, presently unclassified but resembling an oncorna virus, is the cause of equine infectious anaemia. The disease occurs only in Equidae although possible experimental transmission to pigs (2) and sheep has been recorded. All breeds and age groups of Equidae are equally susceptible. One case has been reported in humans with anaemia as the principal manifestation. Successful passage of the virus has been reported in mice and hen eggs but results in rabbits have been inconclusive. The virus has been grown in cultures of equine leucocytes and passed back into horses and into tissue culture (3, 4). The virus is relatively resistant to most environmental influences such as boiling for up to 15 minutes and disinfectants but is destroyed by sunlight. It persists for several months at room temperature in urine, faeces, dried blood and serum. The virus persists for long periods in clinically recovered animals and most of such animals are resistant to reinfection. Whether or not true immunity to EIA develops is uncertain. It appears probable that there are marked differences in virulence between different strains of the virus.

There is a marked seasonal incidence of the disease, most cases occurring in the summer and autumn. It has been associated with low lying and newly settled bush areas due to the greater number of insect vectors in such areas. Undernourished, parasitized and debilitated animals are most susceptible.

A number of bacteria, particularly *Salmonella* and *Shigella* spp. have been isolated from horses dying of EIA and it is probable that in some instances secondary bacterial infections contribute to the clinical picture.

Transmission

The virus is present in all tissues, secretions and excretions and may persist in the body for up to 18 years preventing reinfection but providing a source of infection for most of the animal's life. Clinically normal 'carriers' are the usual means by which the disease is introduced into clean areas, although its failure to become established permanently after introduction to some areas is a feature of EIA. Short term contact is usually insufficient to cause spread but continued, close association with susceptible animals usually results in infection. Spread within a group is slow although occasionally fairly rapid spread is observed in large groups of horses assembled at race tracks or army depots.

The disease can be readily transmitted by the injection of small quantities of infected blood intravenously, subcutaneously, intramuscularly or intracerebrally. Biting flies, particularly *Tabanidae*, and mosquitoes can transmit the infection and this, together with the observation that the disease spreads most actively in summer and in marshy or wooded areas, suggests that bites by insects may be the most important method of spread. Intra-uterine infection can take place (17) and foals have become infected through the milk of infected dams, but relatively large amounts of virus must be ingested to cause infection and the digestive tract is not a major portal of entry. Transmission via migrating strongyle larvae has been mooted because of the isolation of the virus from the worm. However, the virus has not been found in the worm eggs (5).

Infection can be readily achieved by the use of contaminated surgical instruments or needles or by the injection of minute quantities of virus, and the use of a common needle when injecting groups of horses may cause a serious outbreak of the disease (2). The increasing use of injections by non-veterinarians, particularly at race tracks, increases the chance of spread of the disease because of the frequent neglect of asepsis. In enzootic areas outbreaks have been caused by the use of untreated biologics of equine origin. In such circumstances all biological preparations produced in horses can be sterilized by the addition of 0·5 per cent phenol and storage for 3 months before use.

The virus is also capable of invasion through intact oral and nasal mucosae, wounds and even unbroken skin, but these portals are probably of minor importance in field outbreaks. Transmission of infection from horse to horse seems possible via swabbing instruments used in collecting saliva for doping tests.

Pathogenesis

The virus is present in the blood 2 to 5 days after experimental inoculation but a febrile reaction does not occur until the 10th to 29th day. The virus localizes in many organs, especially spleen, liver, kidney and lymph nodes (6) and can be detected there in greatest quantity when a severe clinical attack is evident. It disappears from tissues during periods between attacks (7). Damage to the intima of the small blood vessels, reticulo-endothelial involvement, and excessive destruction of erythrocytes follow invasion by the virus. Damage to the vascular endothelium is followed by inflammatory changes in the parenchymatous organs, particularly the liver. There is good evidence that the vascular lesions and the erythrocyte fragility are part of an immune reaction. Immunoglobulin and a fraction of complement are deposited in the lesions in EIA (8). The haemolysis, which is intravascular and extravascular, is characterized by shorter life spans of erythrocytes, e.g. horses with acute EIA have life spans for erythrocytes of 28 to 87 days, compared to 89 to 113 days for subacute cases and 119 to 153 days in normals (9).

Clinical Findings

An incubation period of 2 to 4 weeks is usual in natural outbreaks of equine infectious anaemia. Outbreaks usually follow a pattern of slow spread to susceptible horses after the introduction of an infected animal. On first exposure to infection, horses manifest signs of varying degree, classified as acute or subacute. Occasionally the initial attack is mild and may be followed by rapid clinical recovery. As a rule there is initial depression, profound weakness to the point of inco-ordination, and loss of condition. There is intermittent fever (up to 41 °C or 106 °F) which may rise and fall rapidly, sometimes varying as much as 1 °C within one hour. Jaundice, oedema of the ventral abdomen, the prepuce and legs, and petechial haemorrhages in the mucosae, especially under the tongue and in the conjunctivae, may be observed. Pallor of the mucosae does not occur in this early stage. There is a characteristic increase in rate and intensity of the heart sounds which are greatly exacerbated by moderate exercise. Myocarditis, manifested by tachycardia and arrhythmia, is described as being diagnostic (10). Respiratory signs are not marked, there is no dyspnoea until the terminal stages, but there may be a thin serosanguineous nasal discharge. There is considerable enlargement of the spleen which may rarely be palpable per rectum. Pregnant mares may abort. Many animals show temporary recovery from this acute stage, after a course of 3 days to 3 weeks. Others become progressively weak, recumbent and die after a course of 10 to 14 days of illness.

Animals showing temporary recovery may appear normal for 2 to 3 weeks and then relapse with similar but usually less severe signs although death may occur during such a relapse. Relapses continue to occur often coinciding with periods of stress, and are characterized by recurrent febrile episodes, increasing emaciation, weakness and cardiac insufficiency and the development of pallor of the mucosae, a late sign of this disease. In this chronic stage the appetite is usually good although allotriophagia may be observed. Some affected animals appear to make a complete recovery although they may remain infected and suffer relapses in later years.

Alimentary involvement is not commonly recorded in equine infectious anaemia but a foetid, watery diarrhoea has been observed as a prominent sign. In such cases secondary infection is probably involved.

Clinical Pathology

The marked fall in erythrocytes which is characteristic of the disease is not usually seen during the initial attack. When it occurs during subsequent episodes its degree varies with the severity of the signs. Normoblasts and other immature red cells are absent. Usually there is a slight leucopenia at the time of the attack with relative lymphocytosis or mononucleosis. The sedimentation rate is usually increased to about 50 per cent in 15 minutes. A single haematological examination is of less value in diagnosis than serial tests matched with a temperature curve because the blood picture gradually returns to near normal between attacks. Unfortunately definitive tests for the presence of the virus are lacking. The precipitin test has been reported as 90 per cent accurate provided 2 tests are carried out 1 week apart but is unlikely to detect infected horses during periods when the disease is quiescent (11). A CF test shows some promise, there being a measurable titre for as long as 2 or 3 months after an attack with the titre peak occurring within 10 to 20 days (2, 12). Albuminuria is usually present during clinical episodes. Experimental transmission of the disease to susceptible horses by the subcutaneous injection of 20 ml.

whole blood or Seitz-filtered plasma is also used as a diagnostic test and is a valuable, although expensive, supplement to other tests. The donor blood should be collected during a febrile episode when the viraemia is most pronounced. The recipient animals are checked for increases in body temperature twice daily. Liver biopsy has been used in diagnosis but is unreliable. Some significance is attached to changes in the albumin-globulin ratio of affected horses. The presence of siderocytes in the blood in excess of 4 to 7 per 10,000 leucocytes is also used as evidence of infection (9) although their presence is not diagnostic in itself.

At the present time an agar gel immunodiffusion test, based on virus collected from the spleen of infected horses, is in most general use as a diagnostic tool (13). It has proved to be very accurate and may be suitable as a basis for an eradication programme. A Japanese modification of the test uses a tissue culture virus as the antigen (14). Indirect immunofluorescence is also being used to detect the presence of the virus in tissues (15). Complement fixation and serum neutralization tests are available but have severe limitations as diagnostic tools.

Necropsy Findings

In the acute stages there may be subcutaneous oedema, jaundice and petechial or ecchymotic subserous haemorrhages. There is considerable enlargement, with swelling of the edges, of the liver and spleen and their local lymph nodes. In the chronic stages emaciation and pallor of tissues are the only gross findings. Histological examination is helpful in diagnosis. Characteristic lesions include extensive proliferation of the reticuloendothelial system and vascular intima, perivascular round cell infiltrations, especially in the liver, and haemosiderosis. Virus is present in greatest concentration in the spleen, liver, bone marrow and abdominal lymph nodes.

Diagnosis

Laboratory diagnosis is now satisfactorily provided for with an agar gel immunodiffusion test—the Coggins test. Clinical diagnosis is still difficult irrespective of whether the disease is in the acute or chronic stage. Continuous observations are necessary, particularly as recurrent fever and haemolytic crises are important features of the disease. Transmission experiments are still relevant and should always be carried out when the disease is suspected in a new area. The identification of the transmitted disease depends upon the clinical, clinico-pathological and necropsy findings listed above. In individual animals the disease may be confused with purpura haemorrhagica, babesiasis, ehrlichiosis, leptospirosis, severe strongylosis or fascioliasis, and with anaemia caused by suppression of haemopoiesis by chronic suppurative processes. Leptospirosis is a much milder disease and affected horses usually recover spontaneously within a few days.

Treatment

No specific treatment is available. Supportive treatment including blood transfusions, and haematinic drugs may facilitate clinical recovery.

Control

Because animals recovering from the disease remain as carriers they should be destroyed. Other horses on the farm should be examined daily for elevations of body temperature. If the disease continues to occur for more than 2 years in spite of the above measures, serious consideration should be given to disposal of all horses from the farm, or the institution of a permanent quarantine. The introduction of horses from enzootic to clean areas is attended by great risk and should be avoided. If suspect horses are to be introduced they should be kept under close surveillance for at least 6 months before entry.

Draining of marshy areas and the control of biting insects may aid in limiting spread of the disease. A degree of protection may be obtained by the use of insect repellents and by stabling in screened stables. Great care must be taken to avoid transmission of the disease on surgical instruments and hypodermic needles which can only be satisfactorily sterilized by boiling for 15 minutes or by autoclaving at 15 lb. (6·6 kg.) pressure for a similar period. Although the immune response in recovered animals is poor and there seems to be little possibility of producing a satisfactory vaccine, the practicability of this approach is being explored (1, 16). It is possible to attenuate the virus with modern culture methods.

REVIEW LITERATURE

Henson, J. B., McGuire, T. C., Koboyashi, K., Banks, K. L., Davis, W. C. & Gorham, J. R. (1969). *Proc. 2nd int. Conf. equine infect. Dis.*, Paris, pp. 178–99.
Ishitani, R. (1970). *Natn. Inst. anim. Hlth Qt. Tokyo*, 10, 1.

REFERENCES

(1) Hyslop, N. St G. (1966). *Vet. Rec.*, 78, 858.
(2) Boulanger, P. *et al.* (1969). *Canad. J. comp. Med.*, 33, 148.
(3) Kono, Y. & Yokomizo, Y. (1968). *Natn. Inst. anim. Hlth Qt. Tokyo*, 8, 182.
(4) Moore, R. W. *et al.* (1970). *Amer. J. vet. Res.*, 31, 1569.
(5) Ohshima, K. *et al.* (1970). *Res. vet. Sci.*, 11, 4, 405.
(6) McGuire, T. C. *et al.* (1971). *Amer. J. Path.*, 62, 283.
(7) Kono, Y. *et al.* (1971). *Natn. Inst. anim. Hlth Qt. Tokyo*, 11, 11.
(8) Perryman, L. E. *et al.* (1971). *J. Immun.*, 106, 1074.
(9) McGuire, T. C. *et al.* (1969). *Amer. J. vet. Res.*, 30, 2091.
(10) Goret, P. *et al.* (1969). *Proc. 2nd int. Conf. equine infect. Dis.*, Paris, 166.
(11) Russell, L. H., jun. (1965). *Diss. Abst.*, 26, 319.
(12) Kono, Y. & Koboyashi, K. (1966). *Natn. Inst. anim. Hlth Qt. Tokyo*, 6, 194, 204.
(13) Coggins, L. & Norcross, N. L. (1970). *Cornell Vet.*, 60, 330.
(14) Nakajima, H. & Ushimi, C. (1971). *Infect. Immun.*, 3, 373.
(15) Ushimi, C. *et al.* (1970). *Natn. Inst. anim. Hlth Qt. Tokyo*, 10, 90.
(16) Kono, Y. *et al.* (1970). *Natn. Inst. anim. Hlth Qt. Tokyo*, 10, 106, 113.
(17) Kemen, M. J., jun. & Coggins, L. (1972). *J. Amer. vet. med. Ass.*, 161, 496.

Ephemeral Fever

Ephemeral fever is an infectious disease of cattle characterized by inflammation of mesodermal tissues as evidenced by muscular shivering, stiffness, lameness and enlargement of the peripheral lymph nodes. The disease is caused by a virus which is transmitted by insect vectors.

Incidence

Ephemeral fever occurs enzootically on the African continent, in most of Asia and the East Indies (4). It has occurred sporadically in Australia (1, 2, 8). Although it is of minor importance, considerable loss occurs in dairy herds due to the depression of milk flow. Occasional animals die of intercurrent infection or prolonged recumbency. The morbidity rate in outbreaks is usually about 35 per cent, but if the population is highly susceptible and environmental conditions favour the spread of the disease, the morbidity rate may reach 100 per cent. In enzootic areas only 5 to 10 per cent will be affected.

Aetiology

The causative virus is closely associated with the leucocyte-platelet fraction of the blood. Artificially the disease can be transmitted only by the injection of whole blood or the leucocyte fraction. Cyclic development of the virus in insect vectors is suspected. After experimental infection there is solid immunity against homologous strains for up to two years. Immunity against heterologous strains is much less durable which probably accounts for the apparent variations in immunity following field exposure. Among domestic animals, only cattle are known to be affected and although all age groups are susceptible the disease is more common in adults (3). Experimental animals are in general not susceptible but the infection is transmissible to unweaned hamsters and mice (4). The virus has also been adapted to tissue culture (6, 10).

Transmission

The source of infection is the animal affected with the clinical disease. Spread occurs via insect vectors of which the sandfly, *Ceratopogonidae* sp., is probably the most important. A great deal of work in recent years has not clearly defined the vector list (11). Spread is largely independent of cattle movement and transmission does not occur through contact with infected animals or their saliva or ocular discharge. Spread of the disease depends largely on the insect vector population and the force and direction of prevailing winds. When strong winds prevail the vectors may be carried over large tracts of land or water (5). The disease tends to disappear for long periods to return in epizootic form when the resistance of the population is diminished. Recurrence depends primarily on suitable environmental conditions for increase and dissemination of the insect vector.

Pàthogenesis

After an incubation period of from 2 to 10 days a viral septicaemia develops with localization and inflammation in mesodermal tissues particularly joints, lymph nodes and muscles. A febrile reaction, limb stiffness and pain are characteristic of the disease.

Clinical Findings

Calves are least affected, those less than 6 months of age showing no clinical signs. Fat cows and bulls are worst affected.

In most cases the disease is acute. There is a sudden onset of fever (40·5 to 41°C or 105 to 106°F), sometimes with morning remissions. Anorexia and a sharp fall in milk yield occur. There is severe constipation in some animals and diarrhoea in others. Respiratory and cardiac rates are increased and stringy, nasal and watery ocular discharges are evident. The animals shake their heads constantly and muscle shivering and weakness are observed. There may be swellings about the shoulders, neck and back. Muscular signs become more evident on the second day with severe stiffness, clonic muscle movements and weakness in one or more limbs. A posture similar to that of acute laminitis is often adopted. About the third day the animal begins eating and ruminating, and the febrile reaction disappears, but lameness and weakness may persist for 2 or 3 more days. Some animals remain standing during the acute stages but the majority go down and assume a position reminiscent of parturient paresis with the hind legs sticking out and the head turned into the flank.

Occasional animals adopt a posture of lateral recumbency. In most cases recovery is rapid and complete after an illness of 3 to 5 days unless there is exposure to severe weather, or unless aspiration of a misdirected drench, or ruminal contents occurs. Occasional cases show persistent recumbency and have to be destroyed. Milder cases may occur at the end of an epizootic with signs restricted to pyrexia and lack of appetite.

Clinical Pathology

A leucocytosis with a relative increase in neutrophils occurs during the acute stage of the disease. Serological tests are being developed (2, 4). A complement fixation test, and serum neutralization tests are under scrutiny. Their use has made it possible to demonstrate that the virus of ephemeral fever does persist in Australian cattle between major outbreaks but it is thought that the persisting virus has low pathogenicity (9). A fluorescent antibody test has been developed and is reported to be simple, sensitive and dependable as a diagnostic aid (12).

Necropsy Findings

Post-mortem lesions are not dramatic. All lymph nodes are usually enlarged and oedematous and the serous membranes show patchy congestion with some effusion and occasionally petechiation. Congestion of the abomasal mucosa is usual and may also be apparent in the nasal cavities, the small intestine and the kidneys. In experimentally produced cases a serofibrinous polysynovitis, tendovaginitis and periarthritis were obvious lesions (7).

Diagnosis

The diagnosis of ephemeral fever in a cattle population is not difficult on the basis of its transient nature and its rapidity of spread. It may present a problem in individual animals in which it may resemble traumatic reticulitis, acute laminitis, or parturient paresis. In the first case differentiation is almost impossible unless a metal detector test is negative or a rumenotomy is performed. Laminitis is accompanied by local pain in the feet and usually occurs after overfeeding. The response to injected calcium solutions is a good diagnostic test to differentiate the disease from parturient paresis. The diagnosis can be confirmed only by the inoculation of blood from an animal in the acute stages of the disease into a susceptible animal.

Treatment

Palliative treatment with salicylates or buta-zolidine may benefit the muscle stiffness but drenching should be avoided because of the risk of aspiration pneumonia. Proper nursing of the re-cumbent animal is all that is required.

Control

Control of the vectors is not possible. Because of the immunity that develops after the natural disease and because the virus becomes attenuated by pas-sage through mice and hamsters strong efforts have been made to produce vaccines. However, there are difficulties and no field vaccine is available at this time.

REFERENCES

(1) Seddon, H. R. (1938). *Aust. vet. J.*, *14*, 90.
(2) MacKerras, I. M. *et al.* (1940). *Coun. sci. industr. Res., Aust., Bull. No. 136*, p. 116.
(3) Mulhearn, C. R. (1937). *Aust. vet. J.*, *13*, 186.
(4) Burgess, G. W. (1971). *Vet. Bull.*, *41*, 887.
(5) Murray, M. D. (1970). *Aust. vet. J.*, *46*, 77.
(6) Snowdon, W. A. (1970). *Aust. vet. J.*, *46*, 258.
(7) Basson, P. A. *et al.* (1970). *J. S. Afr. vet. med. Ass.*, *40*, 385.
(8) Newton, L. G. & Wheatley, C. H. (1970). *Aust. vet. J.*, *46*, 561.
(9) Snowdon, W. A. (1971). *Aust. vet. J.*, *47*, 312.
(10) Matumoto, M. *et al.* (1970). *Jap. J. Microbiol.*, *14*, 413.
(11) Standfast, H. A. & Dyce, A. L. (1972). *Aust. vet. J.*, *48*, 77, 81.
(12) Theodoris, A. (1969). *Onderspoort J. vet. Res.*, *36*, 87.

African Horse Sickness

African horse sickness is a highly fatal, infec-tious disease of horses, mules and donkeys. It is caused by a number of strains of a virus spread by insect vectors. Acute, subacute and mild forms of the disease occur. Its recent spread from the African continent presents a major problem to the horse industry in countries of the western world.

Incidence

African horse sickness was confined to the Afri-can continent until the Second World War when serious outbreaks occurred in the Middle East (6). The disease came into prominence again in 1959 when it spread to Iran and Pakistan (6). In 1960 further spread occurred, in the east to India and to the west through the Middle East, including Turkey, to the eastern Mediterranean and Cyprus. Spread of the disease to Spain has recently occurred. It continues as an enzootic disease in Africa, recurring annually in most of southern, equatorial and eastern Africa, south of the Sahara. In enzootic areas it is virtually impossible to raise horses. In areas where outbreaks occur the morbidity rate varies with the number of insect vectors present; the mortality rate in susceptible horses is about 90 per cent. Mules (50 per cent) and donkeys do not suffer such a high mortality rate but the disease is a crippling one in these species because of gross debility.

The serious nature of the disease itself is com-pounded by the tremendous problem of eradica-tion. Vaccination reduces the ravages of horse sickness but even when practised on a wide scale cannot eradicate it because the infection is insect borne, and uncontrolled hosts provide a reservoir of infection.

Aetiology

Horse sickness is caused by a viscerotrophic arbovirus present in all body fluids and tissues of affected animals from the onset of fever until recovery. The virus is moderately resistant to external environmental influences such as drying and heating and it can survive in putrid blood for 2 years.

A number of antigenic strains of the virus exist (42 at present) and although there is evidence of some cross-immunity between strains it is essen-tial in large-scale vaccination programmes to in-clude a number of strains in the vaccine. The vaccine currently in use contains 7 strains and is effective in most areas (1). The strain in the current Middle East outbreak is not related to known African strains (5).

Natural infection occurs only in the equine species, the most severe disease occurring in horses, with mules and donkeys showing lesser degrees of susceptibility in that order. Zebras are highly resistant and there is one record of the disease in dogs (3). Dogs, goats, ferrets, mice, guinea pigs and rats can be infected experimentally and the virus can be grown in tissue culture (8, 10), chick embryos and the brains of mice. Rabbits are not susceptible. Vaccines which are at present in use are prepared by attenuation of the virus by serial intracerebral passages (62 to 72 passages) in mice (2) and tissue culture vaccines are on trial (12). Immunity after natural infection or vaccination by an homologous strain is solid but can be over-come by strong challenge by another strain. The development of immunity is slow and may require 3 weeks to be appreciable: titres may continue to rise for 6 months after infection. Foals from im-mune dams appear to derive passive immunity from the colostrum and are immune until 5 to 6 months of age.

The incidence of the disease is often seasonal be-cause of the seasonal variations in the number of

Culicoides spp. present. New cases of the disease do not appear more than 10 days after a killing frost causes disappearance of the insects, and extensive outbreaks are always preceded by a period of heavy rain. Even in Africa the disease has a geographical distribution, the areas most severely affected being low lying and swampy and most cases occur after midsummer.

Transmission

The disease is spread by the passive transfer of very small quantities of blood by biting insects. Spread does not occur between animals in direct contact unless the requisite insect vectors are present. Biting midges or gnats, *Culicoides* spp., are the most probable vectors and climatic conditions which govern the breeding status and movement of these insects also govern the spread and morbidity rate of horse sickness. These insects have almost world wide distribution. Many other biting insects have been named as vectors but there is a lack of satisfactory evidence in many reports. The mosquitoes *Aedes aegypti*, *Anopheles stephensi* and *Culex pipiens* have been shown to be true biological carriers (9).

Although clinically affected equidae are the major source of virus during an outbreak the current view is that in enzootic areas there must be a silent, non-equine reservoir host which perpetuates the virus between seasons when no insects are present. It is possible that dogs may act as silent hosts. It has been shown that they can be infected naturally by the ingestion of infected meat (3). However, in some countries the disease has been introduced but has died out in the succeeding winter, presumably because no reservoir hosts were available. In those new countries to which the disease has now been introduced, presumably in aircraft, a silent host is not necessary because the mild winters permit the persistence of the insects and the constant infection of fresh horses.

Artificially the disease is readily transmitted by the intravenous injection of very small amounts of blood. Transmission can also be effected by subcutaneous injection or oral dosing but larger amounts of blood are required, particularly with oral dosing.

In areas where the disease is enzootic outbreaks still occur, often cyclically at intervals of 10 to 20 years. This is a common enough pattern in diseases carried by insects and is caused by periodic elevations in immunity, seasonal and yearly variations in the vector population and periodic redistribution of new strains of the virus.

Pathogenesis

The virus is present in the blood stream from the first day of clinical illness and persists for about 30 days and up to 90 days. It can be recovered from defibrinated blood by intracerebral inoculation into infant mice.

Clinical Findings

The incubation period in natural infections is about 5 to 7 days; in artificially produced infections it varies from 2 to 21 days. Three clinical forms of the disease occur, an acute or pulmonary form, a cardiac or subacute form and a mild form known as horse sickness fever. An intermittent fever of 40 to 41 °C (105 to 106 °F) is characteristic of all forms.

Acute (pulmonary) horse sickness. This is the most common form in acute outbreaks in susceptible animals. Initially there is fever followed by very laboured breathing and severe paroxysms of coughing. There is a profuse nasal discharge of yellowish serous fluid and froth. Profuse sweating commences and the horse becomes very weak, develops a staggery gait and becomes recumbent. At this time the nasal discharge is usually voluminous. The appetite may be good until the breathing becomes so laboured that the animal is unable to eat. Death follows within a few hours after a total course of 4 to 5 days. In the few animals which recover severe dyspnoea persists for many weeks. This is the form of the disease which has been reported as occurring naturally in dogs.

Subacute (cardiac) horse sickness. This form is more common in horses in enzootic areas. The incubation period may be longer, up to 3 weeks in length, and the fever develops more slowly and persists for longer than in the acute disease. The most obvious sign is oedema in the head region, particularly in the temporal fossa, the eyelids and the lips, and this may spread to the chest. This may not develop until the horse has been febrile for a week. The oral mucosa is bluish in colour and petechiae may develop under the tongue. Restlessness and mild abdominal pain are often evident. Auscultation of the heart and lungs reveals evidence of hydropericardium, endocarditis and pulmonary oedema. Paralysis of the oesophagus with inability to swallow and regurgitation of food and water through the nose is not uncommon. The mortality rate is not as high as in the acute disease but recovery is prolonged. A fatal course may be as long as 2 weeks.

A mixed form is described in which both pulmonary and cardiac signs appear. A horse with an initial subacute cardiac syndrome may suddenly develop acute pulmonary signs; a primary pulmonary syndrome may subside but cardiac involvement causes death. This mixed form is not common in field outbreaks.

Horse sickness fever presents no diagnostic signs and may go unrecognized except that it usually occurs in areas in which the disease is enzootic. It occurs most commonly as an immunization reaction or when an existing immunity is partially overcome and it is the only form of the disease which can be produced artificially in donkeys and Angora goats. The temperature rises to 40·5°C (105°F) over a period of 1 to 3 days but returns to normal about 3 days later. The appetite is poor, there is slight conjunctivitis and moderate dyspnoea.

Clinical Pathology

A complement fixation test is available but requires convalescent serum and the test is suitable only for rough diagnosis. A fluorescent antibody test shows promise (15). For accurate detection of the virus strain, neutralization in the mouse of the suspected viral material by known horse sickness immune serum is recommended.

Necropsy Findings

Gross findings in acute cases include severe hydrothorax and pulmonary oedema and moderate ascites. The liver is acutely congested and there is oedema of the bowel wall. The pharynx, trachea and bronchi are filled with yellow serous fluid and froth. In cases of cardiac horse sickness there is marked hydropericardium, endocardial haemorrhage, myocardial degeneration and anasarca, especially of the supraorbital fossa.

Diagnosis

The possibility that this disease may spread to and become permanently established in very large areas which have been free hitherto makes accurate diagnosis of great importance. The complement fixation and serum neutralization tests are adequate for this purpose, the latter being necessary for strain identification (7).

Pulmonary horse sickness resembles equine infectious pneumonia, but the latter is rare nowadays and is restricted in its occurrence almost entirely to large groups of horses in confined quarters and under poor hygienic and management conditions. Cardiac horse sickness has much in common with equine infectious anaemia, babesiasis and purpura haemorrhagica. Equine viral arteritis also has a passing resemblance to this form of the disease. The paucity of diagnostic signs in horse sickness fever would make it difficult to differentiate from many mild, sporadic diseases were it not for the rare occurrence of the disease separate from obvious clinical cases of the other forms of horse sickness.

Treatment

No treatment has been shown to have any effect on the course of the disease but careful nursing and symptomatic treatment is not without value.

Control

This disease can be introduced into new areas by the spread of infected *Culicoides* spp. either blown by strong winds or carried in fast-moving air transport. Provided the carrier insects can persist in the environment the disease is then permanently established. It is possible that infected horses may introduce the disease, again especially if they are shipped by air. This eventuality can be prevented by restricting the importation of horses from countries known to have the disease, by vaccinating and quarantining horses at the point of embarkation, by quarantining them in insectproof enclosures at the point of entry, and by vaccinating all horses within a 10 mile radius of where horses are permitted to enter from abroad. At the present time there is a 30 day quarantine period for horses brought into the U.S.A. from Asia, Africa and the Mediterranean countries.

To prevent the spread of the disease across large land masses vaccination of all equidae in a wide buffer zone is the only effective measure. Vaccination of horses in the infected area with polyvalent virus attenuated by adaptation to mouse brain tissue (neurotropic virus) should be instituted, but the individual protection obtained is not absolute and this measure alone will not prevent spread. Some of the vaccine 'breaks' observed in enzootic areas are attributed to the poor antigenicity of some of the component viruses used in the vaccines (11). The vaccine in use in the Middle East and India is the one developed by African workers. It contains seven strains of attenuated virus and has proved to be effective in the 1960 outbreak (4). Immunity after vaccination is solid for at least a year but annual revaccination of all horses, mules and donkeys is recommended. Vaccination of foals from immune mares is without effect and should be delayed until they are at least 8 months old. Live tissue culture, formalized tissue culture and egg-attenuated vaccines are also produced (13). The formalin-killed aluminium precipitated vaccine, injected twice one month apart, gave protection for at least 6 months (14).

In enzootic areas the vector insect cannot be controlled but some protection of horses against being bitten can be obtained by stabling indoors in insectproof stables, not permitting horses outside except in broad daylight, using fly repellents when risk is high and by keeping horses and stables on high, insectfree ground as much as possible. None of these measures is more than mildly effective.

Complete eradication appears at the moment to be impossible. A completely effective vaccine and the elimination of uncontrolled reservoirs could lead to eradication. Attempts at control by slaughter without the use of vaccination have had disastrous results (5).

REFERENCES

(1) McIntosh, B. M. (1958). *Onderstepoort J. vet. Res.*, *27*, 465.
(2) Rafyi, A. (1961). *Bull. Off. int. Épiz.*, *56*, 216.
(3) Piercy, S. E. (1951). *E. Afr. agric. J.*, *17*, 1.
(4) Maurer, F. D. (1960). *J. Amer. vet. med. Ass.*, *138*, 15.
(5) Howell, P. G. (1960). *J. S. Afr. vet. med. Ass.*, *31*, 329.
(6) Reid, N. R. (1961). *Brit. vet. J.*, *118*, 137.
(7) Maurer, F. D. & McCully, R. M. (1963). *Amer. J. vet. Res.*, *24*, 235.
(8) Mirchamsy, H. & Taslimi, H. (1962). *C. R. Acad. Sci. (Paris)*, *255*, 424.
(9) Ozawa, Y. *et al.* (1970). *Arch. Inst. Razi*, *22*, 113.
(10) Erasmus, B. J. (1963). *Nature, Lond.*, *200*, 716.
(11) Howell, P. G. & Erasmus, B. J. (1963). *Bull. Off. int. Épiz.*, *60*, 883.
(12) Ozawa, Y. *et al.* (1966). *Amer. J. vet. Res.*, *26*, 154.
(13) Rweyemamu, M. M. (1970). *Vet. Bull.*, *40*, 73.
(14) Mirchamsy, H. *et al.* (1970). *Arch. Inst. Razi*, *22*, 11, 103; (1970). *Proc. 2nd int. Conf. equine infect. Dis., Paris, 1969*, pp. 212–21.
(15) Tessler, J. (1972). *Canad. J. comp. Med.*, *36*, 167.

Rift Valley Fever

Rift Valley fever is an acute, febrile disease of cattle, sheep and man characterized in lambs and calves by hepatitis and high mortality, in adult sheep and in cattle by abortion and in man by an influenza-like disease. Transmission of the infection between animals is by biting insects, chiefly mosquitoes.

Incidence

Although Rift Valley fever is still confined to the African continent it has great potential for spread to other countries (2). The main occurrence of the disease is in epizootics observed in southern and central Africa, the first thoroughly investigated epizootic being in 1930 (1). Losses are due mainly to deaths in young lambs and calves although there may be a high incidence of abortions, and some deaths, in adult sheep and cattle. A particular point of interest is the ability of the virus to infect humans. The groups exposed to greatest risk are laboratory workers handling the virus and those working amongst infected animals or their products.

Aetiology

The causative arbovirus, of which there appears to be only one strain, can be grown on embryonating hen eggs and tissue culture and can be attenuated by serial passage through mouse brains. Cattle, sheep, monkeys, man, mice, rats, ferrets and hamsters are highly susceptible and goats moderately so, but horses, pigs, rabbits, guinea pigs and poultry are not (4). Mice and other rodents may provide a means of supporting the virus during periods between epidemics.

Transmission

A pronounced viraemia occurs for about a week and facilitates the spread of the disease by biting insects. Other than milk and aborted foetuses no body secretions or excretions contain the virus. The incidence of the disease varies with the size of the vector population and is greatest in warm, moist seasons. Eight species of mosquitoes have been identified as vectors, and other bloodsucking insects are likely to be implicated (7). Experimental transmission can be effected by most routes including the inhalation of aerosols. In man infection is most likely to occur via skin abrasions in persons handling infective material (3).

Pathogenesis

The disease appears to be an acute hepatic insufficiency caused by destruction of liver cells by the rapidly multiplying virus (5).

Clinical Findings

In lambs and calves after an incubation period of about 12 hours there is a sudden onset of high fever and inco-ordination followed by collapse and sudden death within 36 hours in 95 to 100 per cent of affected lambs and 70 per cent of young calves (4).

In adult sheep and cattle abortion is the outstanding sign but the mortality rate in adult sheep may be as high as 20 to 30 per cent and 10 per cent in cattle. In fatal cases sudden death is preceded by a high fever for 1 to 2 days. Goats show a febrile reaction but few other clinical signs.

In man there is an abrupt onset of anorexia,

chills, fever, headache and muscular and joint pains. Deaths from the disease are rare, but some patients suffer temporary or permanent impairment of vision due to retinal haemorrhage.

Clinical Pathology

Severe leucopenia is a common finding. Antibodies appear in the serum about one week after infection and persist for long periods. Efficient serum-neutralization and CF tests are available and a fluorescent antibody technique has been developed (9). Transmission tests to White Swiss mice and sheep are also used.

Necropsy Findings

Extensive hepatic necrosis is the characteristic lesion in Rift Valley fever. Other non-specific lesions include venous congestion and petechiation in the heart, lymph nodes and alimentary tract. Microscopically there is focal or diffuse necrosis of the liver and in young lambs there are usually acidophilic inclusion bodies in hepatic cells.

Diagnosis

Rift Valley fever is unlikely to be confused with other diseases because of its characteristic hepatic lesions. Its seasonal limitation may lead to confusion with bluetongue in sheep and ephemeral fever in cattle and its capacity to kill large numbers of lambs quickly may suggest a diagnosis of enterotoxaemia. In adult animals other causes of abortion, including Wesselbron disease in sheep, would need to be considered. A tentative diagnosis can be based on the clinical, epidemiological and necropsy findings but a definitive diagnosis must depend on the laboratory tests listed above.

Treatment

Little attention has been given to this aspect of the disease and there is no known treatment which is of any value.

Control

To prevent introduction of Rift Valley fever into countries free of the disease the importation of all susceptible species from Africa should be prohibited and all necessary steps to prevent the introduction of infective insects and infected biological materials should be taken. The possibility of human beings carrying the infection from country to country is a very real one and international travellers should be made aware of the clinical symptoms of the disease and of the importance of the disease to other humans and to domestic animals.

Although control of insect vectors has been attempted it is expensive and, to a large extent impractical; and in an enzootic area control depends on the use of attenuated vaccines. In man a vaccine prepared from a formalin-killed, tissue culture virus is used effectively and a safe vaccine for sheep comprises a virus attenuated by passage through mouse brain—the so-called neurotropic virus. The vaccine can be used safely on day old lambs from susceptible ewes but vaccination of pregnant ewes is not recommended because of pre- and post-partum deaths of lambs (6). The vaccine has also provided good protection for cattle which lasted for at least 28 months (8).

REFERENCES

(1) Daubney, R. et al. (1931). J. Path. Bact., 34, 545.
(2) Murphy, L. C. & Easterday, B. C. (1962). J. Amer. vet. med. Ass., 141, 960.
(3) Kaschula, V. R. (1957). J. Amer. vet. med. Ass., 131, 219.
(4) Easterday, B. C. et al. (1962). Amer. J. vet. Res., 23, 1224.
(5) Easterday, B. C. et al. (1962). Amer. J. vet. Res., 23, 470.
(6) Weiss, K. E. (1962). Onderstepoort J. vet. Res., 29, 3.
(7) Easterday, B. C. (1965). Advances in Veterinary Science, Vol. 10, New York: Academic Press.
(8) Coackley, W. et al. (1967). Res. vet. Sci., 8, 399, 406.
(9) Pini, A. et al. (1970). Res. vet. Sci., 11, 82.

VIRAL DISEASES CHARACTERIZED BY ALIMENTARY TRACT SIGNS

Foot-and-Mouth Disease

Foot-and-mouth disease is an extremely contagious, acute disease of all cloven-footed animals, caused by a virus and characterized by fever and a vesicular eruption in the mouth and on the feet.

Incidence

Foot-and-mouth disease is enzootic in Africa, Europe, Asia, Japan, the Philippines and South America. Of recent years the most important new territories invaded by the disease have been Mexico, where it followed the introduction of cattle from Brazil, and Canada, where the virus was apparently introduced in the baggage of a European immigrant. In both instances the disease was promptly controlled and eradicated but the movement of cattle and cattle products between the affected countries and the U.S.A. was brought to a standstill. Outbreaks also occur from time to time in Britain and in the Channel Islands due to the introduction of infection from Europe and South America. Australia and New Zealand have never experienced the disease and the U.S.A. has not had an outbreak since 1929.

Losses due to the disease occur in many ways

although loss of production, the expense of eradication and the interference with movement of livestock and meat between countries are the most important economic effects. Although the disease is not a killing one (the mortality rate in adults is only 2 per cent and in young stock 20 per cent) animals are so severely affected during the acute stages of the disease and the period of convalescence is so prolonged that production, both of meat and milk, is seriously impaired. When the disease breaks out in susceptible cattle it spreads very rapidly and the morbidity rate approximates 100 per cent. Although the mortality rate is usually low severe outbreaks of a more violent form sometimes occur with a mortality rate of up to 50 per cent. During the severe outbreak in Europe in 1951–2 the estimated direct losses were $400 million and annual losses in Argentina due to foot-and-mouth disease are estimated at $150 million (1).

Aetiology

Three major strains of the causative enterovirus occur—A, O and C—but there is evidence of substrains with different serological and immunological characteristics and with different degrees of virulence within these strains. Three additional strains, SAT1, SAT2 and SAT3, have been isolated in Africa and a further strain, ASIA–1, from the Far East. Unfortunately the virus seems to be capable of infinite mutation so that new, antigenically different, subtypes are constantly appearing (2). The difficulties presented to vaccination programmes are obvious—not only may there be great changes in antigenicity between developing strains, but the virulence may change dramatically also (3).

Of the three standard strains O appears to be the most common and C the least common. There is no cross-immunity between strains and substrains.

The virus is resistant to external influences including common disinfectants and the usual storage practices of the meat trade. It may persist for over a year in infected premises, for 10 to 12 weeks on clothing and feed, and up to a month on hair. It is particularly susceptible to changes in pH away from neutral. Sunlight destroys the virus quickly but it may persist on pasture for long periods at low temperatures. Boiling effectively destroys the virus if it is free of tissue but autoclaving under pressure is the safest procedure when heat disinfection is used. The virus can survive for at least a month in bull semen frozen to $-79\,°C$. In general, the virus is relatively susceptible to heat and insensitive to cold. Most common disinfectants exert practically no effect but sodium hydroxide or formalin (1 to 2 per cent) or sodium carbonate (4 per cent) destroy the virus within a few minutes.

Hedgehogs, coypu, many rodents and wild ruminants are susceptible and may provide reservoirs of infection for domestic animals (4). Of 39 wild animal species in Africa examined for FMD specific antibodies, 16 were positive and all were cloven-footed (35). The disease in wild ungulates in Africa may be present without obvious signs and the disease is perpetuated independently in each group with cross infection between them from time to time (36). The disease is most important in cattle but pigs, goats and sheep are also affected, some strains of the virus being limited in their infectivity to particular species (3). The importance of these small stock is largely as carriers of the disease to cattle. Sheep may remain as carriers for up to 5 months, maintaining a continuous low-level multiplication of virus, principally in the pharyngeal area (5). Immature animals and those in good condition are relatively more susceptible, and hereditary differences in susceptibility have also been observed. The typical disease occurs rarely in man.

In enzootic areas periodic outbreaks occur which sweep through the animal populations and then subside. This is probably due to the disappearance of immunity which develops during an epizootic and the sudden flaring up from small foci of infection when the population becomes susceptible again. In cattle the immunity which develops after natural infection varies between one year and more than four years (6). In pigs the duration of this immunity is about 30 weeks (7). When outbreaks follow each other in quick succession the presence of more than one strain of the virus should be suspected.

Transmission

The common method of transmission is by the ingestion of feedstuffs containing the virus. However, aerogenous dissemination can occur (8), and may result in spread of the disease over distances as great as 60 km. (9). The force and direction of the prevailing wind, the amount and duration of rainfall affect spread. There are peaks of spread at dawn and dusk. It seems probable that the portal of infection with aerogenous spread is the respiratory tract (10). The quantitative aspects of foot-and-mouth disease virus, the yield of virus, its movement and the infective dose required, have been examined and throw light on the probable relative importance of each mode of transmission (11).

Virus appears in the blood and milk soon after

infection and in the saliva before the appearance of vesicles in the mouth. All excretions including the urine, milk, faeces and semen may be infective before the animal is clinically ill and for a short period after signs have disappeared. However, the period of maximum infectivity is when vesicles in the mouth and on the feet are discharging, the vesicular fluid containing the virus in maximum concentration. Pigs are known to excrete the most virus followed by cattle and sheep (12). There are variations too between the various sub-types of the virus. Although it is generally conceded that affected animals are seldom infective for more than 4 days after the rupture of vesicles, except in so far as the virus may persist on the skin or hair, the possibility exists that some animals may remain as carriers for very long periods, and the intermittent passage of small amounts of virus may lead to the establishment of new outbreaks. Mammary gland is one of the tissues in which persistence can take place, the virus living in this tissue for 3 to 7 weeks (13). Wild fauna may also serve as a reservoir of the disease, as may ticks. Man may also be a vehicle for transmission of FMD virus (14). It has been recovered from the nasal mucosa of persons working with infected cattle for up to 28 hours after contact. Nose blowing did not eliminate the virus nor cotton face-masks prevent the infection.

All meat tissues, including bone, are likely to remain infective for long periods, especially if quick frozen and to a less extent meat chilled or frozen by a slow process. The survival of the virus is closely associated with the pH of the medium. The development of acidity in rigor mortis inactivates the virus but quick freezing suspends acid formation and the virus is likely to survive. However, on thawing, the suspended acid formation recommences and the virus may be destroyed. Prolonged survival is more likely in viscera, bone marrow and in blood vessels and lymph nodes where acid production is not so great. Meat pickled in brine, or salted by dry methods may also remain infective. Fomites, including bedding, mangers, clothing, motor tyres, harness, feedstuffs and hides may also remain a source of infection for long periods (15).

The disease is spread from herd to herd either directly by the movement of infected animals, or possibly even infected humans, or indirectly by the transportation of the virus on inanimate objects, particularly uncooked and unprocessed meat products and animal products other than meat. Milk is now recognized as an important vehicle by which the virus may be spread (16). The pH and the temperature of the milk significantly affect survival which may be as long as 18 hours (17). Introduction of the disease into a herd or country as a result of the use of infected semen for artificial insemination is possible (18). The virus can pass unchanged through the alimentary tracts of birds which may thus act as carriers and transport infection for long distances and over natural topographical barriers such as mountain ranges and sea.

Epizootics in free areas occur intermittently and from a number of sources. In England it is estimated that outbreaks arise in the following manner—transportation by birds 16 per cent, by meat products used as pig food 40 per cent, contact with meat and bones other than swill 9 per cent, unknown causes probably swill 7 per cent and completely obscure 28 per cent (19). The greatest danger appears to be from uncooked meat scraps fed to pigs. However, more unusual methods of introduction must not be disregarded. Infected smallpox vaccine has been the cause of some outbreaks. With modern methods of transport it is possible that farm workers may carry the virus long distances in their clothing and that frozen bull semen could be a source of infection.

During the latter months of 1967 the United Kingdom experienced a very bad outbreak of foot-and-mouth disease (20). Control measures which had been effective in many hundreds of outbreaks for many years failed to halt the spread of the disease. As a result a great deal of investigational work was carried out, especially with respect to methods of spread. A committee, the Northumberland Committee, considered the control programmes being used and made recommendations about future policies (26). The most important decision was that a basic choice existed—either introduce vaccination and admit the disease was endemic in the U.K., or prevent the importation of meat and offal from countries in which foot-and-mouth disease exists. The decision was for the latter option. The outbreak is thought to have originated in frozen Argentine lamb fed to pigs (22).

Pathogenesis

Irrespective of the portal of entry, once infection gains access to the blood stream the virus shows a predilection for the epithelium of the mouth and feet and, to a less extent, the teats. Characteristic lesions develop at these sites after an incubation period of 1 to 21 (usually 3 to 8) days. Predilection for lesions to occur on the oral mucosa is attributed to the hyperplastic state of the epithelium caused by persistent local irritation. The initial phase of viral septicaemia is often unnoticed and it is only when localization in the mouth and on the feet occurs that the animal is found to be clinically abnormal. The experimental disease in sheep is characterized by an incubation period of 4 to 9 days after contact. After inoculation the period is 1 to 3 days, viraemia occurs at 17 to 74 hours, hyperthermia from the 17th to 96th hour. Clinical signs are serous nasal discharge, salivation and buccal lesions in 75 per cent and foot lesions in 25 per cent of cases (23).

Clinical Findings

In typical field cases in cattle there is an initial period of high fever (40 to 41 °C or 104 to 106 °F), accompanied by severe dejection, and anorexia, followed by the appearance of an acute painful stomatitis. At this stage the temperature reaction is subsiding. There is abundant salivation, the saliva hanging in long, ropy strings, a characteristic smacking of the lips, and the animal chews carefully. Vesicles and bullae (1 to 2 cm. in diameter) appear on the buccal mucosa, and on the dental pad and the tongue. These rupture within 24 hours leaving a raw painful surface which heals in about a week. The vesicles are thinwalled, easily ruptured and contain a thin, straw-coloured fluid. Concurrently with the oral lesions, vesicles appear on the feet particularly in the clefts and on the coronet. Rupture of the vesicles causes acute discomfort and the animal is grossly lame, often recumbent, with a marked, painful swelling of the coronet. Secondary bacterial invasion of the lesions may interfere with healing and lead to severe involvement of the deep structures of the foot. Vesicles may occur on the teats and when the teat orifice is involved severe mastitis often follows. Abortion and subsequent infertility are common sequels. Very rapid loss of condition and fall in milk yield occur during the acute period and these signs are much more severe than would be anticipated from the extent of the lesions. Eating is resumed in 2 or 3 days as the lesions heal but the period of convalescence may be as long as six months. Young calves are rather more susceptible than adults and heavy mortality may occur during an outbreak without typical lesions being present.

In most outbreaks of foot-and-mouth disease the rate of spread is high and the clinical signs are as described above but there is a great deal of variation in the virulence of the infection and this may lead to difficulty in field diagnosis. For example there is a malignant form of the disease in which acute myocardial failure occurs. There is a typical course initially but a sudden relapse occurs

on the fifth to sixth day with dyspnoea, a weak and irregular heart action, and death during convulsions. Occasional cases show localization in the alimentary tract with dysentery or diarrhoea indicating the presence of enteritis. Ascending posterior paralysis may also occur.

A sequel to foot-and-mouth disease in cattle, due probably to endocrine damage, is a chronic syndrome of dyspnoea, anaemia, overgrowth of hair and lack of heat tolerance described colloquially as 'panting'. Diabetes mellitus has also been observed as a sequel in cattle.

In sheep, goats and pigs the disease is usually mild and is important mainly because of the danger of transmission of the disease to cattle. As a rule affected animals show only occasional, small lesions in the mouth but all four feet may be badly affected with severe lameness resulting. Sucking pigs may suffer a heavy mortality usually associated with a severe gastroenteritis and very young lambs may die in large numbers with myocarditis, the common necropsy finding Rarely an acute syndrome occurs in pigs or goats which causes only mild signs on transmission to cattle.

Although FMD in sheep is usually inapparent clinically and is detectable only by demonstration of lesions at a careful necropsy examination, it can be an extremely crippling disease (24). Vesicular or necrotic lesions can be found on the tongue, dental pad, gums, cheeks, on the feet at the coronets and in the interdigital and heel areas. The teats, prepuce, vulva and ruminal mucosa may also be involved. In young lambs there may be myocardial and skeletal muscle necrosis and a short, fatal course.

Clinical Pathology

Exhaustive laboratory studies are needed for diagnosis, for determination of the strain of virus involved and to differentiate the disease from vesicular stomatitis and vesicular exanthema. The major methods available are tissue culture, the complement fixation test and experimental transmission in test animals.

Tissue culture. The FMD virus is cultivable on tissue culture and in hen eggs, and use is made of this in the preparation of live, attenuated vaccines. In diagnosis neutralization of virus by known antisera is highly efficient.

Complement-fixation test. Type specific and strain specific complement fixing antisera can be prepared which permit the typing of strains in an outbreak. Diagnostic antisera can also be prepared for differentiation from vesicular stomatitis. The test can take the place of large animal inoculation for the differentiation of the two diseases but large animal inoculation is still necessary to determine the presence of a mixed infection.

Experimental transmission in unweaned white mice. The propagation of the virus in unweaned white mice can be used to detect the presence of virus in suspect material, the presence of antibodies in serum and for investigations into the transmission of immunity and the pathogenesis of the disease.

Guinea pig inoculation. The presence of virus in suspected material can be detected by the intradermal injection of fresh vesicular fluid into the plantar pads of guinea pigs. Vesicles appear on the pads in 1 to 7 days and secondary vesicles in the mouth 1 to 2 days later.

Large animal inoculation may be used for the differentiation of foot-and-mouth disease, vesicular stomatitis and vesicular exanthema based on the different species susceptibilities to the three viruses.

Necropsy Findings

The lesions of foot-and-mouth disease are relatively mild except for those in the mouth and on the feet and udder. These lesions may be extensive if secondary bacterial infection has occurred. In some cases the vesicles may extend to the pharynx, oesophagus, forestomachs and intestines. The trachea and bronchi may also be involved. In the malignant form of the disease there is extensive myocarditis. If the animal survives there is replacement fibrosis and the heart is enlarged and flabby. On section the heart muscle appears streaked with patches of yellow tissue interspersed with apparently normal myocardium.

Diagnosis

The need to identify foot-and-mouth disease is of paramount importance in all countries even in those countries where it occurs enzootically. It is of particular importance in those countries which do not experience the disease because of the need to introduce control measures quickly. The field veterinarian must be able to recognize suspicious cases and laboratory facilities must be available to confirm the diagnosis. In countries where the other vesicular diseases do not occur suspicions will be readily aroused, but in North America the presence of vesicular stomatitis and vesicular exanthema may result in misdiagnosis. Vesicular stomatitis of horses, cattle and swine and vesicular exanthema of swine resemble foot-and-mouth disease closely. Bluetongue of sheep may also present a problem in differentiation. Details of these diseases are provided separately but a summary of the differential points is given in the table below.

Differentiation of Acute Vesicular Diseases (14, 15)

Animal Species, etc.	NATURAL INFECTION				EXPERIMENTAL TRANSMISSION				
	Foot and Mouth	Ves. Stom.	Ves. Exanth.	Blue-tongue	Route of Inoculation	Foot and Mouth	Ves. Stom.	Ves. Exanth.	Blue-tongue
Cattle	+	+	−	+ rarely	I/D tongue, gum and lips.	+	+	−	
					I/musc.	+	−	−	+
Pig	+	+	+	−	I/D snout, lips.	+	+	+	
					I/ven.	+	+	+	
					I/musc.	+	−	−	
Sheep and Goat	+	±	−	+	Various.	+	+	−	+
Horse	−	+	−	−	I/D tongue.	−	+	+ some strains.	
					I/musc.			+ some strains.	
G. Pig					I/D foot-pad.	+	+	−	−
U.W.W. Mice						+	+	−	+ (hamsters also).
Adult Chicken					I/D tongue.	+	+	−	
Embryonated Hen Egg	+	+	−	+		±	+	−	+
Tissue Culture	+	−	+	+		+	+	+	
Complement Fixation Test	+	+	+	+					

A syndrome in pigs has been identified in Italy (21) and more recently in the U.K. which is clinically similar to foot-and-mouth disease but is caused by an enterovirus.

Mucosal-type diseases and rinderpest are easily differentiated by the lesions which develop in the mucosa and sometimes on the feet. The lesions are never vesicular, commencing as superficial erosions and proceeding to the development of ulcers.

Treatment

Other than mild disinfectant and protective dressings to inflamed areas to prevent secondary infection no treatment is recommended.

Control

Many factors govern the control procedure in a given area. The procedures commonly used are control by eradication and control by vaccination or a combination of the two. In countries where the disease is enzootic, eradication is seldom practicable. In areas where the disease occurs only as occasional epizootics, slaughter of all infected and in-contact animals is usually carried out. It must be remembered that vaccination is costly and sometimes ineffective and that eradication is the logical objective in all countries. It seems evident that this is not achievable in countries in large continents such as Europe, unless international cooperation is achieved (2).

Control by eradication. The success of an eradication programme depends on the thoroughness with which it is applied. As soon as the diagnosis is established all cloven footed animals in the exposed groups should be immediately slaughtered and burned or buried. No reclamation of meat should be permitted and milk must be regarded as infected. Inert materials which may be contaminated must not leave infected premises without proper disinfection. This applies particularly to human clothing, motor vehicles and farm machinery. Bedding, feed, feeding utensils, animal products and other articles which cannot be adequately disinfected must be burned. Barns and small yards must be cleaned and disinfected with 1 to 2 per cent sodium hydroxide or formalin or 4 per cent sodium carbonate solution. Acids and alkalis are the best inactivators of foot-and-mouth disease virus and their activity is greatly enhanced by the presence of a detergent. The effective pH at a disinfection surface may be grossly altered by the presence of organic matter and needs to be adequately maintained (25). When all possible sources of infection are destroyed the farm should be left unstocked for six months and restocking permitted only when 'sentinel' test animals are introduced and remain uninfected. Recommendations for outdoor sites are difficult to make. Observations in Argentina suggest that contaminated pastures and unsheltered yards are clear of infection if left unstocked for 8 to 10 days. Human movement to and from infected premises must be reduced to a minimum. Persons working on the farm should wear waterproof clothing which can be easily disinfected by spraying and subsequently removed as the person leaves the farm. Clothing not suitable for chemical disinfection must be boiled. Because of the rapidity with which the disease may spread immediate quarantine must be imposed on all farms within a radius of 10 to 15 miles of the outbreak. No animal movement can be permitted and human and motor traffic must be reduced to a minimum.

Although the eradication method of control is favoured when the incidence is low, it imposes severe losses on the cattle industry in affected areas and is economically impracticable in many countries. However, it must be regarded as the final stage in any control programme when vaccination has reduced the incidence of the disease to a suitably low level. Containment of an outbreak in a country free of foot-and-mouth disease is a difficult task with high rewards. The U.K. has had a great deal of experience in this field and recommended procedures have been developed (26).

Vaccination. Killed trivalent (containing O, A and C strains) vaccines are in general use but because of the increasing occurrence of antigenically dissimilar substrains the production of vaccines from locally isolated virus is becoming a more common practice. The virus is obtained from infected tongue tissue, a tissue culture of bovine tongue epithelium or other tissue culture (27). The virus is killed either with crystal violet or saponin, or with formalin and adsorbed on aluminium hydroxide. Serviceable immunity after a single vaccination can be relied on for only 6 to 8 months, vaccines produced from 'natural' virus giving longer immunity than those produced from 'culture' virus. To ensure a full year's protection two injections of a killed vaccine, 3 to 4 months apart, are recommended. In practice only one injection is usually given in countries where the disease is enzootic and all animals over 4 months of age are vaccinated each spring and results have been excellent. Immunity is present 7 to 20 days after vaccination, the time interval varying with the antigenicity of the vaccine. To avoid the dangers inherent in the use of living vaccines there have been many attempts to improve efficiency of killed vaccines. The variations introduced have included the use of tissue culture virus, its inactivation with special agents and the use of adjuvants (28).

Because of the short duration of the immunity produced by killed vaccines, attention is now focused on the production of an attenuated living virus vaccine. The major difficulty encountered so far has been the narrow margin between loss of virulence and loss of immunogenicity. Attenuated vaccines have been produced by passage through white mice, embryonated hen eggs, rabbits and tissue culture (4, 29). Spread of the infection from vaccinated to unvaccinated cattle does not appear to occur. In spite of the deaths in calves which occur after vaccination with attenuated viruses their use, particularly of the mouse-adapted virus, is becoming more general especially when massive epizootics threaten. Their use in South Africa has contributed to the eradication of the disease and in Venezuela has proved effective where killed virus vaccines failed to stem a major outbreak. Provided constant surveillance can be maintained over vaccinated animals, their value in such circumstances cannot be denied. In spite of the uncertain stability of the lapinized virus, control of the disease in Russia has been reported after the use of a rabbit-passaged vaccine.

General vaccination as a means of control is fraught with many difficulties. The following disadvantages are suggested by the U.K. Departmental Committee on Foot-and-Mouth Disease (19). (a) To be effective the programme should consist of vaccination against a number of strains three times yearly. More frequent vaccination may be necessary in the face of outbreaks during optimum conditions for spread. (b) Vaccination of sheep and pigs does not provide adequate protection in these animals but there is current activity in the field of pig vaccination. A trivalent, inactivated, adjuvant vaccine gives strong immunity for 6 months and some resistance for 12. A local reaction lasts for 12 months (30). In sheep monovalent or trivalent vaccines give immunity for 5 to 6 months but the sheep may act as inapparent carriers (33). (c) Inapparent infections may occur in animals whose susceptibility has been reduced by vaccination permitting the existence of 'carrier' foci. It has become generally recognized that the number of carrier animals produced by vaccination is very much greater than previously thought. Apart from the fact that these animals are a potent method of spreading the disease, they also provide an excellent medium for the mutation of existing virus strains, because the hosts are immune (31). The carrier state in vaccinated and unvaccinated cattle may persist for as long as 6 months and be capable of causing new outbreaks in all species (32). (d) Importation of vaccinated animals is often prohibited. An additional disadvantage is the production of sensitivity resulting in a very high incidence of anaphylaxis in cattle vaccinated repeatedly, especially when the vaccines contain antibiotics or the vaccine contains foreign protein not associated with the antigen, or the virus has been killed with formalin which has also denatured the protein in the vaccine. Oedema, urticaria, dermatitis, abortion and fatal anaphylaxis all occur (34). Calves from immune cows are passively immunized by antibodies passed to them by the colostrum and do not respond to vaccination.

Alternatives to general vaccination are modified programmes including 'ring' vaccination to contain outbreaks, 'frontier' vaccination to produce a buffer area between infected and free countries and vaccination of selected herds on a voluntary basis when an outbreak is threatened. It is generally conceded that vaccination of an entire population may be necessary when eradication is incapable of preventing the spread of the disease.

Prevention of entry of the disease into free areas is an ever increasing problem because of modern developments in communications. The following prohibitions are necessary if the disease is to be excluded. (i) There must be a complete embargo on the importation of animals and animal products from countries where the disease is enzootic. The embargo should include hay, straw and vegetables. Where the disease occurs only as occasional outbreaks the importation of animals can be permitted provided they are subjected to a satisfactory period of quarantine. (ii) Particular attention should be given to preventing the entry of uncooked meats from ships, aeroplanes and other forms of transport and in parcels originating in infected areas. In danger areas all swill fed to pigs must be cooked and all food waste satisfactorily disposed of. (iii) The personal clothing and other effects of people arriving from infected areas should be suitably disinfected.

REVIEW LITERATURE

Brooksby, J. B. (1969). *The Veterinary Annual*, pp. 1–11. Bristol: Wright.

Hyslop, N. St G. (1970). 'The epizootiology and epidemiology of foot and mouth disease.' *Advanc. vet. Sci.*, *14*, 262.

Graham, A. M. (1967). *Vet. Rec., Info. Suppl.* 7, pp. 25–30.

REFERENCES

(1) Henderson, W. M. (1960). *Advanc. vet. Sci.*, *6*, 19.
(2) Henderson, W. M. (1970). *Brit. vet. J.*, *126*, 115.
(3) Brooksby, J. B. (1967). *Nature (Lond.)*, *213*, 120.
(4) Capel-Edwards, M. (1971). *Vet. Bull.*, *41*, 815.

(5) Burrows, R. (1968). *J. Hyg. Camb.*, *66*, 633.
(6) Cunliffe, H. R. (1964). *Cornell Vet.*, *54*, 501.
(7) Bauer, K. *et al.* (1969). *Bull. Off. int. Épizoot.*, *71*, 519.
(8) Sellers, R. F. & Parker, J. (1969). *J. Hyg. Camb.*, *67*, 671.
(9) Hugh-Jones, M. E. & Wright, P. B. (1970). *J. Hyg. Camb.*, *68*, 253.
(10) Norris, K. P. & Harper, G. J. (1970). *Nature (Lond.)*, *225*, 98.
(11) Sellers, R. F. (1971). *Vet. Bull.*, *41*, 431.
(12) Donaldson, A. I. *et al.* (1970). *J. Hyg. Camb.*, *68*, 557.
(13) Burrows, R. *et al.* (1971). *J. Hyg. Camb.*, *69*, 307.
(14) Sellers, R. F. *et al.* (1970). *J. Hyg. Camb.*, *68*, 565.
(15) Cottral, G. E. (1969). *Bull. Off. int. Épizoot.*, *71*, 549.
(16) Dawson, P. S. (1970). *Vet. Rec.*, *87*, 543.
(17) Sellers, R. F. (1969). *Brit. vet. J.*, *125*, 163.
(18) Cottral, G. E. *et al.* (1968). *Arch. ges. Virusforsch.*, *23*, 362.
(19) Report of the U.K. Departmental Committee on Foot-and-Mouth Disease (1954). *Vet. Rec.*, *66*, 483.
(20) Anonymous (1968). *J. Amer. vet. med. Ass.*, *152*, 213.
(21) Nardelli, L. *et al.* (1968). *Nature (Lond.)*, *219*, 1275.
(22) Reid, J. (1968). *Vet. Rec.*, *82*, 286, 288.
(23) Rivara, L. R. *et al.* (1969). *Gac. vet. (B. Aires)*, *31*, 223.
(24) Geering, W. A. (1967). *Aust. vet. J.*, *43*, 485.
(25) Sellers, R. F. (1968). *Vet. Rec.*, *83*, 504.
(26) Northumberland Committee Report (1970). *Vet. Rec.*, *86*, 11.
(27) Rweyemamu, M. M. (1970). *Vet. Bull.*, *40*, 73.
(28) Callis, J. J. *et al.* (1968). *J. Amer. vet. med. Ass.*, *153*, 1798.
(29) Martin, W. B. *et al.* (1965). *Res. vet. Sci.*, *6*, 196.
(30) McKercher, P. D. & Gailiunas, P. (1969). *Arch. ges. Virusforsch.*, *28*, 165.
(31) Sutmoller, P. *et al.* (1967). *Proc. 71st ann. gen. Mtg U.S. Live Stock sanit. Ass.*, pp. 386–95.
(32) Sutmoller, P. *et al.* (1967). *Amer. J. vet. Res.*, *28*, 101.
(33) Fontaine, J. *et al.* (1969). *Bull. Off. int. Épizoot.*, *71*, 421.
(34) Mayr, A. *et al.* (1969). *Zbl. vet. Med.*, *163*, 487.
(35) Condy, J. B. *et al.* (1969). *J. comp. Path.*, *79*, 27.
(36) Brooksby, J. B. (1969). *Symp. zool. Soc., London, 1968*, *24*, 3.

Swine Vesicular Disease

The diagnosis of foot-and-mouth disease has been made more difficult by the recent appearance of swine vesicular disease in the U.K. (1, 2). The lesions of this disease are indistinguishable from those of foot-and-mouth disease in pigs. Differentiation of the diseases is possible only in the laboratory by the use of the complement fixation test and by culture of the virus.

The epidemiological behaviour differs from that in foot-and-mouth disease. The evidence suggests that the virus is excreted in volume only via the vesicular fluid and because most of the lesions are on the feet the principal source of infection is the ground. Thus the disease tends to be spread between herds via the movement of pigs and the spread within herds is almost completely devoid of lateral spread from pen to pen. However introduction into the U.K. and some transmission between herds appears to have occurred via swill. The morbidity in affected pens may be 90 per cent and on an entire farm as high as 65 per cent.

The acute form of the disease greatly resembles FMD. Typical vesicular lesions occur on the coronary bands, especially on the lateral aspect of the foot. Rupture of the vesicles produces shallow ulcers. Lameness is common but not inevitable. There is a high fever (40·5°C) for a day or two. In only 5 to 10 per cent of affected pigs are there vesicles on the snout or in the mouth.

Problems occur in the clinical diagnosis of a subacute form of the disease in which there may be only one vesicle on a pig and where the morbidity rate is very low. Chronic foot lesions of any sort in pigs should be viewed with suspicion in any environment where swine vesicular disease occurs, especially if there is evidence of separation of the horn at the coronary band.

The virus appears to be capable of survival for some time on inanimate objects such as lorry floors. A complete list of effective disinfectant agents is available (2).

REFERENCES

(1) Anonymous (1972). *Vet. Rec.*, *91*, 681.
(2) Anonymous (1973). *Vet. Rec.*, *92*, 234.

Vesicular Stomatitis

Vesicular stomatitis is an infectious disease caused by a virus and characterized clinically by the development of vesicles on the mouth and feet. While primarily a disease of horses it has come to assume major importance as a disease of cattle and pigs.

Incidence

Geographically the disease is limited to the Western Hemisphere and is enzootic in parts of North, Central and South America. The first major occurrence of the disease was in military horses in the U.S.A. during the 1914–18 war but in recent years it has come to assume greater importance in cattle and pig herds. The disease itself causes little harm apart from inconvenience and temporary inability to feed. The morbidity rate varies considerably (5 to 10 per cent is usual but in dairy herds it may be as high as 80 per cent) and there is usually no mortality. Outbreaks are not usually extensive but the disease closely resembles foot-and-mouth disease and has achieved considerable importance for this reason. Occasional human infections give the disease some public health significance.

Aetiology

Three antigenically distinct strains of the causative virus, the Indiana, New Jersey and Cocal (Trinidad) strains, have been isolated. The New Jersey strain is the most virulent and the one most commonly found. The virus is much less resistant to environmental influences than the virus of foot-and-mouth disease and it is more readily destroyed by boiling.

Horses, donkeys, cattle and pigs are susceptible but sheep are resistant. Outbreaks of the disease are most common in cattle and to a less extent in pigs. Calves are much more resistant to infection than adult cattle. Humans are susceptible, infection causing an influenza-like disease. The disease occurs in man, and the development of high antibody titres in man often accompanies outbreaks in cattle (1, 2). Experimentally the disease can be produced in swine by intradermal injection in the snout and by intravenous injection but not by intramuscular injection. In horses and cattle transmission can also be effected by intradermal and intramucosal injection but not by intramuscular injection. Guinea pigs can be infected by intradermal injection in the foot pads or by intralingual injection. The susceptibility of rabbits varies depending upon the strain of virus used. Passage can also be effected in unweaned white mice and embryonated hen eggs. There is considerable evidence that natural infection in deer, raccoon and feral swine can occur. The importance of these animals in the epidemiology of the disease is doubtful except that deer, because of their liberation of large quantities of virus from oral vesicles, can act as an amplifier host (3). Immunity after a natural attack is solid but lasts for only about six months (4).

Transmission

The saliva and vesicular fluid from clinically affected animals are highly infective but infectivity diminishes rapidly and may be lost within a week after the vesicles rupture. Although mediate or immediate contagion can occur by ingestion of contaminated materials the disease is not readily spread in this way and skin abrasions or insect bites appear to be necessary for infection to occur. The method of transmission of this disease is not completely clear. It can be carried by insects but it seems certain that the ingestion of contaminated pasture is also a method of infection (5). Spread within dairy herds appears to be aided by milking procedures (6). There is a marked seasonal incidence of the disease, cases decreasing sharply with the onset of cold weather. This together with the commonly observed high incidence in low lying areas has given rise to the view that insects, including biting flies and mosquitoes, play a large part in the spread of the disease both locally and from infected to clean areas. The virus has been isolated from *Phlebotomus* spp. sandflies (1) and from *Aedes* spp. mosquitoes (7) and has been shown to multiply in the mosquito *Aedes aegypti* and it is therefore a true arthropod-borne virus. The phlebotomine sandfly *Lutzomyia trapidoi* is also a true vector of the virus (8). It is thought that biting insects carry infection in from Mexico, where the disease is enzootic, to the United States, giving rise to periodic outbreaks (4, 6). Native fauna may similarly provide a reservoir of infection and by their uncontrolled movement act as a means of spread of the disease. It has also been suggested that the infection may persist from year to year in cold-blooded animals such as frogs. Although the causative virus is resistant to environmental influences, its infectivity is not high and outbreaks are not so extensive as in foot-and-mouth disease. For the same reason control of the disease is readily achieved by standard hygienic precautions.

Pathogenesis

As in foot-and-mouth disease there is a primary viraemia with subsequent localization in the mucous membrane of the mouth and the skin around the mouth and coronets. The frequent absence of classical vesicles on the oral mucosa of affected animals in field outbreaks has led to careful examination of the pathogenesis of the mucosal lesions. Even in experimentally produced cases only 30 per cent of lesions develop as vesicles, the remainder dehydrating by seepage during development and terminating by eroding as a dry necrotic lesion.

Clinical Findings

In cattle after a short incubation period of several days there is a sudden appearance of mild fever and the development of vesicles on the dorsum of the tongue, dental pad, lips and the buccal mucosa. The vesicles rupture quickly and the resultant irritation causes profuse, ropy salivation and anorexia. Confusion often arises in field outbreaks of the disease because of failure to find vesicles. In some outbreaks with thousands of cattle affected, vesicles have been almost completely absent. They are most likely to be found on the cheeks and tongue where soft tissues are abraded by the teeth. At other sites there is an erosive, necrotic lesion. In milking cows there is a marked decrease in milk yield. Lesions on the feet and udder occur only rarely except in milking cows where teat lesions may be extensive and lead to the development of mastitis. Recovery is rapid, affected animals being clinically normal in 3 to 4 days, and secondary complications are relatively rare. In horses the signs are broadly similar but not infrequently the lesions are limited to the dorsum of the tongue or the lips. Other less common sites include the udder of the mare and the prepuce of males. In pigs vesicles develop on or behind the snout or on the feet and lameness is more frequent than in other animals.

Clinical Pathology

Animal transmission experiments and culture on embryonated hen eggs as set out in the table on p. 468 may be attempted using fluid collected from unruptured vesicles. Typical vesicles develop after inoculation. A complement fixation test is available which is capable of differentiating the virus from that of foot-and-mouth disease and between the two strains of vesicular stomatitis virus. A resin agglutination inhibition and a serum neutralization test are also used in diagnosis, titres to the latter persisting for much longer than the CF test, often well beyond the point at which the animal has again become susceptible to experimental challenge (9).

Necropsy Findings

Necropsy examinations are not usually undertaken for diagnostic purposes but the pathology of the disease has been adequately described.

Diagnosis

Because of its similarity to foot-and-mouth disease, prompt and accurate diagnosis of the disease is essential. Foot-and-mouth disease does not occur in horses and vesicular exanthema occurs naturally only in pigs. Apart from these species susceptibilities, differentiation on clinical and epizootiological grounds is hazardous. To ensure accurate diagnosis material must be sent to a laboratory for examination as set out in the table on p. 479. Other forms of stomatitis in which lesions occur on the feet, including mucosal disease and bovine malignant catarrh are not characterized by vesicle formation and can be differentiated on this and other clinical grounds. The frequent absence of vesicles in vesicular stomatitis has already been pointed out. Failure to recognize this feature of the disease may unnecessarily delay a correct diagnosis. Similar necrotic lesions occur in necrotic glossitis of steers but this disease can be differentiated serologically from vesicular stomatitis.

Treatment

Treatment is seldom undertaken but mild antiseptic mouth washes may contribute to the comfort of the animal and the rapidity of recovery.

Control

Hygienic and quarantine precautions to contain the infection within a herd are sufficient control, the disease usually dying out of its own accord. Immunity after an attack appears to be of very short duration, probably not more than 6 months. Inactivated virus vaccines have been studied but are not available for field use (10). A live virus vaccination procedure appears to have given good results (11).

REFERENCES

(1) Shelokov, A. & Peralta, P. H. (1967). *Amer. J. Epidem.*, 86, 149.
(2) Fields, B. N. & Hawkins, K. (1967). *New Engl. J. Med.*, 277, 989.
(3) Karstad, L. H. (1963). *Proc. 1st int. Conf. Wildlife Dis.*, New York, 1962, pp. 298–309.
(4) Hanson, R. P. (1952). *Bact. Rev.*, 16, 179.
(5) Hanson, R. P. (1968). *Amer. J. Epidem.*, 87, 264.
(6) Acree, J. A. et al. (1965). *Proc. 68th ann. gen. Mtg U.S. Live Stock sanit. Ass.*, 375.
(7) Sudia, W. D. et al. (1967). *Amer. J. Epidem.*, 86, 598.
(8) Tesh, R. B. et al. (1972). *Science, N.Y.*, 175, 1477.
(9) Geleta, J. N. & Holbrook, A. A. (1961). *Amer. J. vet. Res.*, 22, 713.
(10) Correa, W. M. (1964). *Amer. J. vet. Res.*, 25, 1300.
(11) Lauerman, L. H. & Hanson, R. P. (1964). *Proc. 67th ann. gen. Mtg U.S. Live Stock sanit. Ass.*, 473, 483.

Vesicular Exanthema

Vesicular exanthema is an acute, febrile, infectious disease of swine caused by a virus. It is indistinguishable clinically from foot-and-mouth disease in swine.

Incidence

Except for isolated outbreaks in Hawaii and Iceland the disease has occurred only in the U.S.A. It is important because of its direct effect and because of the confusion it causes in the diagnosis of foot-and-mouth disease. Although vesicular exanthema is a mild disease with a low mortality rate (usually less than 5 per cent although there may be many deaths in unweaned pigs) affected animals may suffer a severe loss of body weight and convalescence may require several weeks. Pregnant sows may abort and lactating sows may go dry with resultant heavy losses in baby pigs. The disease was eradicated from the U.S.A. in 1959, 27 years after its initial apperance (1).

Aetiology

Eleven antigenic strains of the causative virus have been isolated (2, 3). There is some variation in virulence between the strains. Only pigs are susceptible although experimental transmission to horses can be effected with some strains of the virus. No experimental animals are susceptible but the virus can be grown in tissue culture. All ages and breeds of pigs are susceptible to infection. The virus is resistant to environmental influences and persists in frozen and chilled meats. It is readily destroyed by a 2 per cent solution of sodium hydroxide (4). A good immunity develops after an attack and persists for about 20 months. There is no appreciable cross-immunity between the strains of the virus and a series of outbreaks, each caused by a different strain of the virus, may occur in the one herd of pigs.

Transmission

The sources of infection are infected live pigs and infected pork. Infected pigs excrete the virus in saliva and faeces but not in the urine for 12 hours before vesicles develop and for 1 to 5 days afterwards. Raw garbage containing infected pork scraps is the most common medium of spread from farm to farm. On infected premises the disease is spread by direct contact and, although the virus is resistant to environmental influences, spread by indirect means does not occur readily (1). Pigs frequently become infected, as evidenced by the development of immunity, without showing clinical signs of the disease. Ingestion of infected material is sufficient to produce infection.

Pathogenesis

As in other vesicular diseases there is a viraemia, lasting for 72 to 84 hours and commencing 48 hours before vesication, with localization occurring in the buccal mucosa and the skin above the hooves.

Clinical Findings

The incubation period varies with the virulence of the causative strain of virus but is usually 1 to 3 days. There is an initial high fever (40·5 to 41°C or 105 to 106°F) followed by the development of vesicles in the mouth, on the snout, on the teats and udder and on the coronary skin, the sole, the heel bulbs and between the claws, and accompanied by extreme lassitude and complete anorexia. The initial lesion is a blanched area which soon develops into a vesicle full of clear fluid. The vesicles rupture easily leaving raw, eroded areas. This usually occurs about 24 to 48 hours after they appear and is accompanied by a rapid fall of temperature. Secondary crops of vesicles often follow and may cause local swelling of the face and tongue. Lesions on the feet may predominate in some outbreaks whereas in others they may be of little significance. The affected feet are very sensitive and there is severe lameness. Healing of the oral vesicles occurs rapidly although secondary bacterial infection often exacerbates the lesions on the feet. Recovery in uncomplicated cases is usually complete in one to two weeks. When sows become infected late in pregnancy abortion frequently occurs and lactating sows may go dry.

Clinical Pathology

Fluid from the vesicles is used in transmission experiments and for tissue culture. Blood serum is used for the complement fixation, viral neutralization in cell culture and gel diffusion precipitin tests (1).

Necropsy Findings

Post-mortem examinations are not of much value in the diagnosis of vesicular exanthema but the pathology of the disease has been defined (4).

Diagnosis

Vesicular exanthema in pigs cannot be differentiated from foot-and-mouth disease or vesicular stomatitis by clinical or necropsy examination and a definite diagnosis can only be made on transmission experiments or by use of the serological tests as tabulated on p. 479. A similar disease, caused by an enterovirus, has been reported from Italy (6) and the U.K. All cases of lameness in pigs in which a number of animals are affected should be examined for the presence of vesicular lesions. Footrot of pigs is readily distinguishable by the absence of vesicles and by the typical under-running of the hoof wall.

Treatment

No treatment appears to be of value but hyper-immune sera against strains A and B appear to have prophylactic efficiency even in pigs exposed to infection 24 hours previously. This may be of some value in preventing infection in pigs during shipment or in preventing heavy losses which commonly occur in groups of unweaned pigs.

Control

Eradication of the disease should be attempted whenever practicable. The first step is to quarantine infected premises and restrict movement of pigs in the area. Infected animals should be slaughtered but the carcases may be salvaged for human consumption provided the meat undergoes special treatment to ensure destruction of the virus. Normal freezing and chilling procedures are not sufficient to destroy it. All garbage fed to pigs must be boiled. Infected premises should be thoroughly cleaned and disinfected with a 2 per cent sodium hydroxide solution before restocking. The implementation of these measures was eminently successful in eradicating the disease from the U.S.A. (5).

Active immunization may be practicable if the disease reappears and other control measures fail. A formalin-killed virus preparation produces an immunity lasting for at least 6 months but commercial production of a vaccine is limited by the expense of producing the virus in pigs and the necessity of providing a multivalent vaccine (4).

REFERENCES

(1) Bankowski, R. A. (1965). Advanc. vet. Sci., 10, 23.
(2) Bankowski, R. A. et al. (1957). Proc. 60th ann. gen. Mtg U.S. Live Stock sanit. Ass., 302.
(3) Shahan, M. S. (1960). Canad. vet. J., 1, 427.
(4) Madin, S. H. & Traum, J. (1955). Bact. Rev., 19, 6.
(5) Henderson, W. M. (1960). Advanc. vet. Sci., 6, 19.
(6) Nardelli, L. et al. (1968). Nature (Lond.), 219, 1275.

Rinderpest

Rinderpest is an acute, highly contagious disease of ruminants and swine caused by a virus and characterized by high fever and focal, erosive lesions confined largely to the mucosa of the alimentary tract. The disease occurs in plague form and is highly fatal.

Incidence

Historically rinderpest (cattle plague) has been among the most devastating of cattle diseases. It still occurs enzootically in equatorial and northeast Africa and in parts of Asia and epizootics of major importance occur from time to time in free countries, such as Eastern Europe, when diseased cattle are introduced. The disease has never appeared in North America but there have been single outbreaks which were quickly eradicated in South America and Australia. Rinderpest still has more influence on the world's food supply than any other animal disease and has tremendous destructive potential in such high-risk areas as central and southern Africa (6).

When epizootics occur in highly susceptible populations the morbidity and mortality rates are high and large numbers of in-contact animals must be destroyed if eradication is undertaken. In enzootic areas most of the cattle population have some degree of immunity and major outbreaks are rare although subacute cases are common. In outbreaks which occur as a result of spread from these areas to areas with highly susceptible populations morbidity rates approximating 100 per cent and mortality rates of 50 per cent (25 to 90 per cent) are to be anticipated.

Aetiology

The causative myxovirus occurs as many strains with considerable variation in virulence between them but all are immunologically identical. The virus seems to have some antigenic relationship to the viruses of distemper (1) and measles and to a virus of sheep and goats which appears to be a strain of rinderpest virus which has become adapted to these species but which has lost its ability to infect cattle by contact (2). The virus of this disease PPR (peste de petits ruminants) is antigenically related to rinderpest virus, but the virus of Kata, a rinderpest-like disease of Nigerian dwarf goats, is unrelated. These diseases present a formidable barrier to rinderpest eradication in Africa (3). It is very sensitive to environmental influences and is readily destroyed by heat, drying and most disinfectants. It is relatively resistant to cold and may survive for as long as a month in blood kept under refrigeration. It survives in premises for a few days only.

All ruminants and pigs are susceptible to infection with rinderpest virus but natural infection occurs commonly only in cattle and buffaloes. Indian buffaloes develop typical signs of the disease and are protected against infection by vaccination with tissue-culture vaccine (4). European pigs are susceptible to infection but a mild transient fever is the only clinical sign. Pigs indigenous to Thailand and Malaysia are highly susceptible and natural spread of the clinical disease occurs commonly. Goats and sheep in India, Ceylon and Africa contract the disease in the field although they are relatively resistant to infection. Egyptian sheep and goats develop antibodies when inoculated with virulent virus but show no clinical signs and are not a source of infection for other animals (5). Wild ruminants are a common source of infection and are a very great hindrance to an eradication programme (6). Amongst the races of cattle the Zebus are most resistant. Rabbits can be artificially infected and this is made use of in the production of lapinized virus. One-humped camels become infected, but show no clinical signs and are considered not to be a source of infection for other animals (7).

Some strains of the virus can be cultivated on the chorio-allantoic membranes of embryonated hens' eggs and the virus can now be grown successfully on cell cultures. The technique promises to be of value in diagnosis and has provided tremendous impetus to the development of a suitably attenuated virus for use as a vaccine (2). Immunity after a natural infection is long but does not always persist for life. Immunity after vaccination varies in duration, generally in proportion to the severity of the clinical response obtained.

Transmission

The virus is present in the blood, tissues, secretions and excretions of infected animals, reaching its peak of concentration at about the height of the temperature reaction and subsiding gradually to disappear about a week after the temperature returns to normal in those animals that recover. The virus is very susceptible to external influences and does not persist outside the animal body for more than a few hours at normal temperatures and dies in cadavers within 24 hours. Close contact between infected and non-infected animals is usually necessary for spread of the disease to occur. Although the precise site of entry of field strains of the virus in natural infections is not known the bulk of evidence indicates that infection occurs principally by inhalation (2, 8). Ingestion of food contaminated by the discharges of clinical cases or animals in the incubation stage, or animals with subclinical infections, may also be an important mode of infection, especially in pigs. Insects, many of which have been shown to contain the virus, are unlikely to act as vectors. Other species including European breeds of pigs in particular, and sheep, goats, camels and wild ruminants may serve as a source of the virus for cattle. Although there may be rare exceptions (9), it is doubtful that recovered animals act as carriers for more than a few days. Because of the failure of the virus to persist outside the body rinderpest is relatively easy to control provided wild animals do not serve as a reservoir of infection.

Pathogenesis

The virus of rinderpest has a high degree of affinity for lymphoid tissue and alimentary mucosa. There is a striking destruction of lymphocytes in tissues and although this has little or no effect on the clinical or gross necropsy findings it is the cause of the leucopenia which occurs. The virus is intimately associated with the leucocytes, only a small proportion being free in the plasma and thus filterable. The focal, necrotic stomatitis and enteritis which are characteristic of the disease are the direct result of the viral infection (9).

Clinical Findings

The following descriptions present the principal clinical signs of rinderpest but it must be remembered that an almost unlimited series of variations in syndromes may be encountered depending upon the virulence of the strain of virus, the susceptibility of the host and the presence of other diseases which may occur concurrently or be aggravated by the occurrence of the clinical illness of rinderpest.

An incubation period of 6 to 9 days is usual in field cases but it may be only 2 to 3 days after experimental administration of the virus. The first stage of the disease is a period of several days in which there is high fever (40·5 to 41·5°C or 105 to 107°F), without localizing signs. Anorexia, a fall in milk yield, lacrimation and a harsh, staring coat accompany the fever. Inflammation of the buccal and nasal mucosae and the conjunctivae follows and there may be hyperaemia of the vaginal mucosa and swelling of the vulva. The lacrimation becomes more profuse and then purulent and is accompanied by blepharospasm. Bubbly salivation of clear blood-stained saliva is followed by purulent saliva as mouth lesions develop. A serous nasal discharge similarly becomes purulent. Discrete, necrotic lesions (1 to 5 mm. in diameter) develop, appearing in the first instance on the inside of the lower lip and the adjacent gum, on the cheek mucosa at the commissures and the lower surface of the tongue. Later they become general in the mouth, including the dorsum of the tongue, and may become so extensive that they coalesce. Similar lesions are common on the nasal, vulval and vaginal mucosae. The lesions are greyish in colour, slightly raised and obviously necrotic. The necrotic material sloughs leaving a raw, red area with sharp edges. Vesicles are not present at any stage. Skin lesions affecting the perineum, scrotum, flanks, the inner aspects of the thighs and the neck occur in some cases. The skin becomes moist and reddened and later covered with scabs. Severe diarrhoea, and sometimes dysentery with tenesmus, appear as lesions develop in the abomasum and intestines.

After a period of illness lasting from 3 to 5 days there is a sudden fall in temperature accompanied by exacerbation of the mucosal lesions, dyspnoea, cough, severe dehydration and sometimes abdominal pain. Prostration and a further fall in body temperature to subnormal occur on the sixth to twelfth day after which death usually occurs within 24 hours.

In enzootic areas where resistance to the infection is high a subacute form and a skin form occur. In the subacute form the temperature reaction is mild and the accompanying anorexia and malaise are not marked. The inflammation of the mucosae is catarrhal only and there is no dysentery. Ulcers may develop in the abomasum without causing clinical signs. In the skin form the systemic reaction is absent and small pustules develop on the neck and over the withers, inside the thighs and on the scrotum. It is possible that these cases are dual infections of rinderpest and cutaneous streptothricosis.

Signs and lesions similar to those which occur in cattle develop in sheep and goats but the disease does not appear to spread readily from these species to cattle. European pigs are susceptible but the disease is clinically inapparent, whereas Asian pigs develop the typical clinical disease and suffer a high mortality. Spread from pigs to cattle occurs sufficiently frequently to make them a dangerous source of infection for cattle. In some areas rinderpest is featured by pneumonia, the disease closely resembling contagious pleuropneumonia.

Clinical Pathology

A marked leucopenia occurs at the height of the infection and after vaccination in cattle and in experimentally infected sheep and pigs even though these animals may show minimal clinical illness. The total count usually falls to below 4000 per cmm. with a marked neutrophilia a few days later.

A complement fixation test suitable for diagnostic purposes on a herd basis is available (10). Antibodies in serum reach peak levels about 14 days after the development of the clinical disease (9). In animals which have recovered for longer periods the antibody level may be so low that the test is unsatisfactory and the serum neutralization test is used (5). The test is unlikely to be used in countries where outbreaks occur for the first time. In these circumstances material is likely to be submitted for examination at earlier stages of the disease and the following techniques of virus recovery and identification are more applicable. Confirmation by the experimental transmission of the disease is expensive and dangerous unless isolation facilities with maximum security are available. The recipient group should include one or more animals immune to rinderpest, an unlikely facility in a country free of the disease. The intravenous injection of 5 ml. of blood from an affected animal at the height of the disease into susceptible cattle is followed by the development of signs in 3 to 10 days. Sheep can be used as recipients but there may be only a mild febrile reaction and erosions may not appear.

A technique suitable for laboratory use is the agar gel diffusion technique using needle biopsy samples of lymph node as antigen. Provided samples are taken at the optimum time, 3 to 5 days after fever commences, a high proportion of correct diagnoses is obtained. The proportion of positive reactors to the test falls sharply after diarrhoea commences. The isolation of the virus and its identification is now practicable in tissue culture. Irrespective of the method used, the optimum tissue for the detection of antigen or the isolation of virus is fresh lymph node and the optimum time of collection is the 3rd to 6th day of fever (9).

Necropsy Findings

The important necropsy findings are observed in the alimentary tract (11). Small, discrete, necrotic areas develop on the mucosa and separation of the necrotic material leaves sharply walled, deep erosions with a red floor which may coalesce to form large erosions. They are present in the mouth, pharynx and first third of the oesophagus and may extend into the nasal cavities. Similar lesions are present on the mucosa of the abomasum which is characteristically red and swollen and shows multiple small, submucosal haemorrhages. These changes are most marked in the pyloric region. There are no lesions in the forestomachs. In severe cases the lesions extend into the first and last parts of the small intestine and into the large intestines particularly at the caecocolic junction. Zones of haemorrhage and erythema running transversely across the colonic mucosa produce a characteristic striped appearance. Congestion, swelling and erosion of the vulval and vaginal mucosae may occur. The histology of rinderpest is characterized by the massive destruction of lymphocytes, particularly noticeable in lymph nodes and material sent for laboratory examination should include fixed sections of lymph node and alimentary tract lesions as well as fresh spleen, blood and alimentary tract for transmission experiments.

Diagnosis

Rinderpest should be suspected when a number of animals are affected by a febrile, fatal, highly infectious disease characterized by erosion and inflammation of the alimentary tract mucosa and by diarrhoea. Salivation, nasal discharge and lacrimation are also characteristic. Confirmation of the diagnosis requires transmission experiments or suitable laboratory tests. Because the disease spreads so rapidly and because animals are capable of discharging infective virus before signs appear an early provisional diagnosis is essential.

Foot-and-mouth disease and haemorrhagic septicaemia are other diseases which occur in epizootics but are sufficiently dissimilar to present no difficulty in differentiation. The mucosal type diseases, including bovine malignant catarrh, mucosal disease, ulcerative stomatitis and muzzle disease present the major difficulty in diagnosis. Bovine malignant catarrh rarely affects many animals in one herd and is characterized by specific eye lesions and nervous signs. Mucosal disease either occurs in explosive outbreaks like rinderpest but the mortality rate is low, or it occurs sporadically, but is uniformly fatal. Ulcerative stomatitis is not accompanied by signs of intestinal involvement and has a low mortality rate. Muzzle disease is characterized by oral and foot lesions, diarrhoea is not usually present and the death rate is low. In sheep and goats bluetongue and sheep and goat pox may present problems in differentiation.

Treatment

Treatment is ineffective and should not be undertaken because of the danger of disseminating the disease. Caprinized vaccine is of no value in treatment and animals in the incubation stage or infected up to 48 hours after vaccination are not protected by use of the vaccine.

Control

Rinderpest is a simple disease and easy to eradicate. Its complete elimination awaits only the development of sufficient veterinary personnel and suitable facilities and the control of free-living animals of susceptible species. These are unfortunately long-term goals and the following outline of control measures will probably apply for many more years.

Although the introduction of rinderpest to a previously uninfected country is most likely to occur by the importation of infected animals, particularly to zoological gardens, the possibility does exist that carcase meat infected with the virus could be a portal of entry. Uncooked, infected garbage has been shown to be capable of infecting pigs which subsequently spread the infection to other pigs and to cattle. Prevention of the introduction of ruminants and pigs from known infected areas is routinely practised in countries which do not have the disease. Countries with land borders to enzootic areas can usually be adequately protected by satisfactory quarantine at the border and the erection of immune barrier zones.

When epizootics occur in normally free areas it is necessary to prevent movement of both living animals and fresh animal products. All susceptible animals in infected and in-contact groups must be slaughtered and disposed of on the respective farms. All ruminants and pigs must be considered susceptible and special attention should be given to native fauna. Infected premises should be disinfected as an additional precaution. When outbreaks are threatened or when an outbreak is extensive and likely to get out of control, all ruminants and pigs in the danger area should be vaccinated with an attenuated virus vaccine.

In enzootic areas control depends upon the use of an efficient vaccination procedure. Periodic vaccination of all susceptible livestock, especially yearling cattle, is generally practised. When outbreaks occur all affected and in-contact animals are vaccinated. Suitable legal and administrative powers are necessary for the proper use of control by vaccination. The choice of vaccine depends upon the availability of livestock for repeated vaccinations, a necessary step if attenuated vaccines are used. Failing this, lapinized virus is preferred. Eradication can be contemplated in an enzootic area if wild ruminants can be eliminated as a source of infection and if the incidence in domestic species can be reduced to a suitable level by vaccination. The greatest problem in a vaccination programme is the selection of a vaccine which will produce adequate immunity without causing a severe reaction in the vaccinated animals. Susceptibility to the rinderpest virus varies greatly between different classes of stock. In general young animals and British breeds of cattle are much more susceptible than indigenous native stock although some local African breeds are highly susceptible. A standard vaccine capable of producing an immune reaction in susceptible cattle may fail to produce a satisfactory immune response in native cattle. Conversely a standard vaccine capable of producing immunity in native cattle often produces severe reactions in susceptible cattle. The ideal vaccine is one which can be produced with varying degrees of attenuation suitable for safe and effective vaccination of cattle with different levels of susceptibility.

The second most important problem associated with rinderpest vaccination is the activation of existing latent infections in vaccinated animals. In general the problem is greater after the use of less attenuated vaccines. Although protozoal infections present the greatest risk, bacterial and viral diseases may also be activated (2). Vaccination of cattle with ears heavily infested with the tick *Rhiphicephalus appendiculatus* should be avoided. Calves present a special problem. If they receive no antibodies in the colostrum they can be successfully vaccinated at 1 day of age, but if they are from immune cows the vaccination will be ineffective if carried out before about 9 months of age (12). Correspondingly colostrum fed calves from immune cows are passively immune for periods of 4 to 8 months, the duration depending upon the immune status of the dam. A number of vaccination procedures is available (2). Preparation of the vaccines is simplified by the common antigenicity of all known strains of the rinderpest virus. Thus a vaccine prepared from one strain will protect against all other strains. The simultaneous serum-virus vaccine has been virtually discarded because of the danger of spreading the disease. An inactivated virus vaccine has been used but produces immunity for short periods only unless multiple vaccination is practised. An adjuvant vaccine containing formalinized, rinderpest-infected bovine spleen in a mixture of mineral oil and freeze-dried, heat-killed mycobacteria is an effective immunizing agent but is not practicable because of the severe local reaction produced. Although the rinderpest virus has no serological similarity to that of mucosal disease, immunity to the latter provides some protection against infection with the former (13).

The following attenuated viruses are in general use.

Goat-adapted virus produces lifelong immunity and is satisfactory for use in Zebu-type cattle and in some areas where a degree of natural immunity is to be anticipated. It is still sufficiently virulent to cause undesirably severe reactions in susceptible animals, particularly calves, buffaloes and British breeds of cattle. Pyrexia, severe gastroenteritis and agalactia result. The reaction can be prevented by the use of hyperimmune serum but this is too costly for general use.

Rabbit-adapted virus. Lapinized virus vaccine can be sufficiently attenuated to avoid severe reactions in susceptible animals but it is then too attenuated for use in Zebu-type animals. There is doubt also as to the stability of the attenuation of vaccine. The immunity produced is solid for about two years. A particular advantage claimed for the lapinized virus is that it can be transported and maintained in rabbits where no refrigeration facilities are available.

Chicken embryo-adapted virus. Adaptation of the rinderpest virus to grow on hen eggs is achieved with some difficulty but the vaccine produced is cheap, stable, and capable of varying degrees of attenuation so as to be safe for highly susceptible and partially resistant cattle. The vaccine has not undergone extensive field trials and its efficiency is variable (14). Until the vaccine has been proved under all field conditions it is unlikely to supplant the goat-adapted virus which is in general use in enzootic areas. The immunity produced persists for at least 16 months.

Cell culture vaccine. The adaptation of the rinderpest virus to tissue culture has led to the development of cell culture vaccines (15, 16). These are now undergoing extensive field tests. It is already apparent that they have enormous advantages and are likely extensively to supplement, if not totally supplant, the other attenuated viruses. They are easy and cheap to produce, are capable of varying degrees of attenuation, and are thus safer in all situations, and appear to produce an immunity of sufficient duration. The attenuated virus does not spread from vaccinated to in-contact cattle (8).

Measles vaccine protects calves against rinderpest at an age when ordinary rinderpest vaccines are ineffective. It is also an efficient vaccine for use in adult cattle (17).

REFERENCES

(1) Delay, P. D. *et al.* (1965). *Amer. J. vet. Res.*, *26*, 1359.
(2) Scott, G. R. (1964). *Advanc. vet. Sci.*, *9*, 114.
(3) Johnson, R. H. & Ritchie, J. S. D. (1968). *Bull. epizoot. Dis. Afr.*, *16*, 411.
(4) Singh, K. V. *et al.* (1967). *Cornell Vet.*, *57*, 638.
(5) Ata, F. A. & Singh, K. V. (1967). *Bull. epizoot. Dis. Afr.*, *15*, 213.
(6) Branagan, D. & Hammond, J. A. (1965). *Bull. epizoot. Dis. Afr.*, *13*, 225.
(7) Taylor, W. P. (1968). *Bull. epizoot. Dis. Afr.*, *16*, 405.
(8) Taylor, W. P. & Plowright, W. (1965). *J. Hyg. Camb.*, *63*, 263, 497.
(9) Plowright, W. (1965). *Vet. Rec.*, *77*, 1431.
(10) Nakamura, J. & Macleod, A. J. (1959). *J. comp. Path.*, *69*, 11.
(11) Maurer, F. D. *et al.* (1955). *J. Amer. vet. med. Ass.*, *127*, 512.
(12) Smith, V. W. (1966). *J. comp. Path.*, *76*, 217.
(13) Delay, P. D. & Kniazeff, A. J. (1966). *Amer. J. vet. Res.*, *27*, 117.
(14) Provost, A. *et al.* (1961). *Rev. Élev.*, *14*, 375, 385.
(15) Barber, T. L. & de Boer, C. J. (1965). *Cornell Vet.*, *55*, 590.
(16) Plowright, W. *et al.* (1971). *Res. vet. Sci.*, *12*, 40.
(17) Provost, A. *et al.* (1968). *Rev. Élev.*, *21*, 145.

Bovine Malignant Catarrh

(Malignant Head Catarrh, Malignant Catarrhal Fever)

Bovine malignant catarrh (BMC) is an acute, highly fatal, infectious disease of cattle caused by a virus. It is characterized by the development of a catarrhal inflammation of the upper respiratory and alimentary epithelia, keratoconjunctivitis, encephalitis, cutaneous exanthema and lymph node enlargement. It may occur sporadically or in explosive outbreaks.

Incidence

Bovine malignant catarrh occurs in most countries but is probably of most importance in Africa. The disease has also been recorded in the United States, Canada, Australia, New Zealand, Europe, Scandinavia and the East Indies. The disease is almost invariably fatal, although a recovery rate of 38 per cent is recorded (1). The morbidity rate varies. In most instances the disease occurs as an isolated case in individual herds but a high morbidity (up to 50 per cent in a herd) occurs occasionally in North America (2) and Scandinavia (1) and even higher morbidity rates have been observed in Africa.

Aetiology

The causative herpes virus is difficult to isolate from the blood because of its close association with either red or white blood cells, particularly the latter. Amongst domestic animals the clinical disease occurs only in cattle and buffalo, but sheep, goats and wild ruminants develop inapparent infections. The causative virus has been isolated from clinically normal blue wildebeeste in Africa and from clinically affected Père David's deer in a British zoo. All ages, races and breeds of cattle are equally susceptible but field cases are most common in adults. The disease shows the greatest incidence in late winter, spring and summer months. The virus of BMC is very fragile and the usual methods of storage, including freezing, destroy it quickly. Material collected for transmission experiments must be used within 24 hours.

There appear to be a number of strains of the virus which may be antigenically different. Some strains can be transmitted with difficulty by intracerebral inoculation in rabbits (3) and, in general, the European and American virus is difficult to transmit experimentally to cattle. On the other hand the African virus can be readily transmitted by several routes. The virus has been adapted to grow on egg yolk-sac and transmission to rabbits, to yolk-sac, to cattle has been achieved (4). BMC virus isolated from blue wildebeeste has been cultivated successfully in tissue culture (6).

Transmission

Transmission can be effected experimentally at the height of the febrile reaction by the transfusion of uncoagulated blood but the difficulty of obtaining infective blood causes many failures in transmission. The use of lymph node inoculated into lymph node is a more satisfactory technique.

The method by which BMC spreads naturally is uncertain. Spread by direct contact between cattle does not seem to occur. The slow rate of spread in most instances and the seasonal incidence in the warmer months suggests spread by an insect vector of an infection that is available from the donor for a short period only. However, the occurrence of outbreaks in which large numbers of cattle become affected within a short period and during the winter months suggests that infection can occur by other routes.

Most records show a close association between outbreaks of BMC and communal raising of cattle and sheep (1). This is particularly true in Europe and North America where affected cattle usually have a history of close contact with sheep and there is no doubt that sheep and probably goats can carry the virus as an inapparent infection. Cattle to sheep to cattle transmission has been effected on a number of occasions. In North America outbreaks of BMC most commonly occur when cattle are housed with the sheep, the outbreak usually occurring soon after lambing (2). This supports the view that congenital infection can occur and may be an important method of transmission, especially in carrier species. A report is on record of a cow giving birth to four infected calves during an 80 month period following an inapparent infection (5). In Africa outbreaks in cattle occur commonly where they have access to wild ruminants, particularly blue wildebeeste and transmission from this species to cattle has been observed when they are housed together. A continuous viraemia of up to 10 weeks duration, during which they are infective to cattle, makes the young blue wildebeeste an important source of infection (6). Viraemia does not occur in wildebeeste calves over thirteen months old.

The persistence of the infection in a particular feedlot, or on a particular farm, from year to year when no contact with these carrier species exists, is unexplained. Persistence of the virus on inanimate fomites has been suggested but the virus is a most fragile one and this seems unlikely. The observation that some recovered cattle show a persistent viraemia for many months suggests that carrier animals may be the source of these carry-over infections (7). A reservoir of infection in wild rabbits has also been suggested.

Pathogenesis

Bovine malignant catarrh is a generalized infection of primitive mesenchyme in which the virus causes necrosis and proliferation, involvement of the vascular adventitia accounting for the development of gross lesions, including the epithelial erosions and keratoconjunctivitis. The lymph node enlargement is due to atypical proliferation of sinusoidal cells, and the cerebromeningeal changes, usually referred to as encephalitis, are in fact a form of vasculitis.

Clinical Findings

The incubation period in natural infection varies from 3 to 8 weeks, and after artificial infection averages 22 days (14 to 37 days). BMC is described as occurring in a number of forms, the peracute, the alimentary tract form, the common 'head and eye' form and the mild form, but these are all gradations, cases being classified on the predominant clinical signs. In serial transmissions with one strain of the virus all of these forms may be produced.

In the 'head and eye' form there is a sudden onset of extreme dejection, anorexia, agalactia, high fever (41 to 41·5°C or 106 to 107°F), rapid pulse rate (100 to 120 per minute), a profuse mucopurulent nasal discharge, severe dyspnoea with stertor, ocular discharge with variable degrees of oedema of the eyelids, blepharospasm, and congestion of scleral vessels. Superficial necrosis is evident in the anterior nasal mucosa and on the buccal mucosa. The necrosis may be present in small discrete areas or be diffuse. In the mouth it is most evident inside the lips and on the adjacent gums and in the commissures of the mouth. The skin of the muzzle is often extensively involved commencing with discrete patches of necrosis at the nostrils which soon coalesce causing the entire muzzle to be covered by tenacious scabs. Similar lesions may occur at the skin-horn junction of the feet. The skin of the teats in acute cases may slough off entirely on touching or become covered with dry, tenacious scabs. Nervous signs, particularly weakness in one leg, inco-ordination, a demented appearance and muscle tremor may develop very early, and with nystagmus are common in the late stages. Head pushing, paralysis and convulsions may occur in the final stages. The superficial lymph nodes are often visible and usually palpably enlarged.

The consistency of the faeces varies from constipation to profuse diarrhoea with dysentery. In some cases there is gross haematuria with the red colouration most marked at the end of urination. Opacity of the cornea is always present in some degree, commencing as a narrow, grey ring at the corneoscleral junction and spreading centripetally. Hypopyon is observed in some cases. The ocular discharge and the nasal discharge may become profuse and purulent if the animal survives for more than a few days. With the development of oral lesions, continual chewing movements and bubbly salivation occur. In cases of longer duration, skin changes, including local papule formation with clumping of the hair into tufts over the loins and withers, may occur and eczematous weeping may result in crust formation particularly on the perineum, around the prepuce, in the axillae and inside the thighs. Infection of the cranial sinuses may occur with pain on percussion over the area. The horns and rarely the hooves may be shed. Persistence of the fever is a characteristic of bovine malignant catarrh, even cases that persist for several weeks having a fluctuating temperature, usually exceeding 39·5°C (103°F).

During some outbreaks an occasional animal makes an apparent recovery but usually dies 7 to 10 days later of acute encephalitis. In the more typical cases the illness lasts for 3 to 7 and rarely up to 14 days.

In the peracute form the disease runs a short course of 1 to 3 days and characteristic signs and lesions of the 'head and eye' form do not appear. There is usually a high fever, dyspnoea and an acute gastroenteritis. The alimentary tract form resembles the 'head and eye' form except that there is marked diarrhoea and only minor eye changes consisting of conjunctivitis rather than ophthalmia. The mild form occurs most commonly in experimental animals. There is a transient fever and mild erosions appear on the oral and nasal mucosae. Recovery is usual.

Clinical Pathology

A leucopenia, commencing at first illness and progressing to a level of 3000 to 6000 per cmm. has been recorded but is not a general observation. The leucopenia recorded was due mainly to an agranulocytosis. In our experience a moderate leucocytosis is more common. Material for transmission experiments should include whole blood (500 ml.), nasal swabs or washings and preferably lymph node collected by biopsy, and should be used immediately after collection (3).

Necropsy Findings

Lesions in the mouth, nasal cavities and pharynx vary from minor degrees of haemorrhage and erythema, through extensive, severe inflammation to discrete erosions. These may be shallow and almost imperceptible or deeper and covered by cheesy diphtheritic deposits. Erosion of the tips of the cheek papillae, especially at the commissures, is common. Longitudinal, shallow erosions are present in the oesophagus. The mucosa of the forestomachs is not grossly abnormal. There may be some erythema, or sparse haemorrhages or erosions. Similar lesions occur in the abomasum and are more marked than in the forestomachs. Catarrhal enteritis of moderate degree and swelling and ulceration of the Peyer's patches are constant. The faeces may be loose and blood-stained.

Similar lesions to those in the mouth and nasal cavities are present in the trachea and sometimes in the bronchi but the lungs are not usually involved except for occasional emphysema or secondary pneumonia. The liver is swollen and shows evidence of degeneration. All lymph nodes are swollen, oedematous and often haemorrhagic. The ocular lesions are as described clinically. Petechial haemorrhages may be visible in brain and meninges as well as congestion and cloudiness of the meninges especially over the cerebellum and occipital poles.

Histologically BMC is characterized by perivascular, mononuclear cell cuffing in most organs and by degeneration and erosion of affected epithelium. Acidophilic, intracytoplasmic inclusion bodies in neurones have been described by one author (1) but the identity of these as viral inclusions has not been established. Inclusion bodies have been recorded in nasal epithelium by some authors but others regard these as being degenerate cytoplasmic droplets. Large numbers of inclusion bodies have been observed in the tissues of artificially infected rabbits (9). Material for histological examination should include brain, lymph node, alimentary tract mucosa, liver, adrenal gland and kidney.

Diagnosis

Clinically, a presumptive diagnosis of BMC can be made when the nasal, oral and ocular lesions are observed, with a persistent high temperature, enlargement of the peripheral lymph nodes and terminal encephalitis. The histological findings of perivascular, mononuclear cell aggregations in most organs can be accepted as confirmatory evidence. Difficulties involved in isolating the virus have so far prevented the use of serological tests.

Mucosal disease, rinderpest, muzzle disease and the infectious stomatitides are not accompanied by typical ocular lesions, lymph-node enlargement or encephalitis and they each have a distinctive histopathology. Infectious bovine rhinotracheitis is not usually fatal, recovery is rapid, the lesions are restricted to the upper respiratory tract and the disease is readily transmitted. Rinderpest may resemble BMC but there is primarily inflammation of the alimentary tract, rapid spread of the disease, a high mortality rate and karyorrhexis of lymphocytes visible on histological examination. Pneumonic pasteurellosis is not accompanied by oral, nasal or ocular lesions and responds well to treatment. In younger animals, calf diphtheria may show many of the characteristics of bovine malignant catarrh but there is no involvement of the eye and the buccal ulcers are usually much deeper, have a strong smell and are covered by thick, caseous pus. The poor response to treatment in chronic cases of calf diphtheria may arouse suspicion of BMC.

The other important viral encephalitis of cattle is sporadic bovine encephalomyelitis in which there are no epithelial lesions. Mycotic dermatitis may cause lesions on the muzzle, particularly in sucking animals but extensive cutaneous lesions are usually present and there are no oral lesions. Photosensitive dermatitis causes skin lesions with a similar distribution to those of BMC but again there is no spread of lesions to the mucosae.

Treatment

Treatment of affected animals is unlikely to influence the course of the disease. Most antibiotics, including oxytetracycline, have been used without effect.

Control

Isolation of affected cattle is usually recommended but its value is questioned because of the slow rate of spread and the uncertainty regarding the mode of transmission. Because of the field observation that sheep are important in the spread of the disease, separation of cattle and sheep herds is recommended and has resulted in the disappearance of the disease in some instances. The introduction of sheep from areas where the disease has occurred should be avoided.

Recovered animals are immune to further infection with an homologous strain for 4 to 8 months.

A formalin-killed vaccine has been used and appeared to halt an outbreak of the disease but vaccinated animals did not withstand experimental challenge (8). Attempts to produce a vaccine have not been extensive because of the limited immunity following natural infection and the generally sporadic nature of the disease.

REFERENCES

(1) Stenius, P. I. (1952). *Bovine Malignant Catarrh*. Helsinki, Finland: Institute of Pathology, Veterinary College.
(2) Murray, R. B. & Blood, D. C. (1961). *Canad. vet. J.*, *2*, 277, 319.
(3) Piercy, S. E. (1955). *Brit. vet. J.*, *111*, 484; *109*, 59.
(4) Danskin, D. (1955). *Nature (Lond.)*, *176*, 518.
(5) Plowright, W. *et al.* (1972). *Res. vet. Sci.*, *13*, 37.
(6) Plowright, W. (1968). *J. Amer. vet. med. Ass.*, *152*, 795.
(7) Plowright, W. *et al.* (1960). *Nature (Lond.)*, *188*, 1167.
(8) Piercy, S. E. (1954). *Brit. vet. J.*, *110*, 87.

Mucosal Disease

(*Virus Diarrhoea*)

Mucosal disease is an infectious disease of cattle caused by a virus and manifested clinically by erosions of the alimentary mucosa and by diarrhoea. Until recent years two disease entities, virus diarrhoea with a high morbidity but low mortality rate, and mucosal disease characterized by a low morbidity but a high mortality rate, were recognized. The common identity of the two diseases on aetiological grounds now appears to be established and it is proposed to refer to the disease as mucosal disease.

Incidence

Mucosal disease was first recorded in the U.S.A. as virus diarrhoea (1) and has since been observed in most countries (2).

The morbidity and mortality rates vary widely and were the basis of the original distinction drawn between virus diarrhoea and mucosal disease. Although many variations occur there are in general two patterns of incidence. In one, referred to as the epidemic form, the morbidity rate approximates to 100 per cent, but the mortality rate is of the order of 4 to 8 per cent, although it may be much higher in calves. In the sporadic form the morbidity rate is usually 2 to 5 (but up to 20) per cent, but the mortality rate is usually greater than 90 per cent. Serological surveys have highlighted the widespread infection rate which occurs in many cattle populations in spite of a low rate of apparent clinical disease and the disease is now considered to be one of the commonest infectious diseases of cattle in the U.S.A. (2). In the U.K. 50 per cent of cattle are serologically positive and in Australia 89 per cent, varying from 91 per cent in tropical areas to 54 per cent in temperate areas (3). In Kenya 19 per cent of native cattle and 47 per cent of grade cattle are serologically positive (4). The strains are antigenically identical to strains found in U.S.A. and Germany (5).

An important feature of the disease is its resemblance to rinderpest, and other virus diseases causing erosive lesions in the alimentary tract.

Aetiology

A virus capable of causing the disease has been isolated and can be passaged through rabbits and grown on tissue culture. The common identity of the two diseases described originally as virus diarrhoea and 'mucosal disease' has been established but the widely divergent epidemiological patterns of the two extreme forms of the disease—the epidemic and the sporadic—suggest varying pathogenicities of strains of the causative virus. The alternative possibility is that the same virus has different clinical and epidemiological manifestations under different systems of management or with differences in nutrition, climate or heredity.

Immunologically the causative virus is distinct from the virus of rinderpest but is related to the virus of hog cholera. Experimental inoculation of pigs with the virus causes no observable illness in pigs but confers a degree of immunity against subsequent challenge with hog cholera virus (6). In cattle immunity after an attack appears to be solid and persists for an indefinite period.

All ages of cattle are susceptible although young calves, cows in late pregnancy and cattle in the 8 months to 2 years age group are most susceptible, the bulk of sporadic cases occurring in the latter age group. An unusual occurrence of a disease resembling mucosal disease has been recorded in newborn calves with deaths occurring at 18 to 96 hours after birth (7). There was no apparent illness in the dams and transmission experiments were unsuccessful. The typical disease usually appears on a farm and then disappears without recurrence in subsequent years, suggesting the development of a herd immunity. There is an apparent high seasonal incidence in winter, and cases occur in both housed and range animals. The disease appears to be more common in beef than in dairy cattle.

Cattle are the only species affected, although a disease with some similarity to mucosal disease has been observed in deer and buffalo and inapparent infection in sheep is suggested by transmission experiments and by serological surveys. Australian sheep have an overall incidence of 8 per cent of animals serologically positive (8). Some strains of mucosal disease virus, when injected experimentally into pigs, cause false positive reactions to tests for swine fever antibodies and protect against subsequent challenge with swine fever virus (9). The importance of these and other species as a source of infection for cattle is unknown.

Transmission

Mucosal disease is readily transmitted by oral dosing or injection of material from infected animals. Under field conditions spread occurs readily by direct and indirect contact and visitors are a common means of spread between farms. Spread through a herd in the epidemic form is very rapid, most of the animals showing clinical signs within a period of 2 to 3 days. In the sporadic form the rate of spread of infection may be as rapid, but the disease appears to be sporadic because only a few animals show clinical signs. British workers have described the appearance of a widespread, mild syndrome characterized by a sharp attack of diarrhoea in most of the herd, followed 1 to 2 months later by a few severe cases of typical mucosal disease.

Although the major method of spread is probably ingestion of faecal contaminated food the disease has been shown to be transmitted via infected urine and via nasal instillation (10, 11).

Pathogenesis

After infection an initial viraemia occurs and the virus can be found in the blood at the height of the fever. Localization in the alimentary mucosa follows and the local lesions and mucosal oedema which develop produce the clinical syndrome of stomatitis and enteritis.

The gross lesions are confined to the alimentary tract and are primarily erosive. There is shrinkage of lymphoid tissue and an absence of leucocytic aggregation about lesions. The primary development of intestinal lesions on Peyer's patches and the destruction of lymphoid tissue are strikingly similar to the pathogenesis of rinderpest. A leucopenia develops in this disease also. The basic lesion in mucosal disease is a small vesicle-ulcer, which affects only epithelial cells and heals rapidly. If secondary bacterial invasion occurs, the ulcers penetrate more deeply and granulating or diphtheritic changes may follow. Death due to dehydration may occur when only a few small ulcers are present in the mouth.

The experimental production of the disease in colostrum-free calves is characterized by necrosis of circulating lymphocytes followed by destruction of lymphoid tissue in spleen, Peyer's patches, and lymph nodes. Oral hyperaemia and erosions occur on the 6th to 7th day. Virus was present in blood and urine for 14 days, and the lower respiratory tract for 56 days (12). Because fatal enteritis can be produced in newborn calves with mucosal disease virus, this has led to the suggestion that it may be a significant cause of neonatal calf enteritis (13). It has also been observed that infection of pregnant cows can lead to the production of offspring with high titres of mucosal disease antibodies and lesions characteristic of the disease (14). Of even greater interest is the observation of the relationship between infection during early pregnancy with the mucosal disease virus and the subsequent development of congenital defects in calves. In experiments with cattle injection of the virus has been followed by the appearance of mummified foetuses, abortions and stillbirths (15, 16). In naturally occurring infections in cows in early pregnancy abortion and mummification are common findings but cerebellar hypoplasia has also been observed (17, 18). The calves have mucosal disease antibodies at birth and before colostrum is taken. Calves with a series of congenital defects including cleft palate (19) and arthrogryposis are also reported to have had mucosal disease. Other abnormalities in newborn calves from cows infected with mucosal disease in early pregnancy are retinal atrophy, optic neuritis and cataract, microphthalmia and retinal dysplasia (20). An enzootic disease of Australian lambs characterized by muscle tremors, hairy birth coat and poor viability and with some similarity to 'border disease' has been linked with mucosal disease infection in the dams (21). Experimental injection of the virus into pregnant ewes caused the appearance of mummified foetuses, one lamb with hydrocephalus and one with cerebellar hypoplasia, hydrocephalus and hind limb deformity (22).

Clinical Findings

In *Epidemic mucosal disease* there is an incubation period of 1 to 3 weeks in field cases but signs appear 4 to 10 days after experimental infection. In the experimental disease a moderate rise in temperature occurs accompanied by a fall in the leucocyte count by about 50 per cent. This is followed on the seventh to eighth day by a secondary temperature rise to 40·5 to 41°C (105 to 106°F). The greatest concentration of the virus in the blood stream occurs in the period between the fever peaks. This diphasic temperature curve has not been observed in field cases in which a sudden fall in milk yield, severe depression, anorexia and a high fever (106°F or 41°C) appear together. The pulse rate is rapid and the faeces are profuse, foul smelling, watery and may contain blood or mucus. Polypnoea and a harsh dry cough are also common in some herds. Additional signs include excessive, stringy salivation and a muco-purulent nasal discharge associated with the appearance of discrete necrotic erosive lesions on the mucosa of the mouth and pharynx and some-times on the skin of the nose. Although these erosive lesions are highly significant in the identi-fication of the disease they may be absent in up to 20 per cent of affected animals, particularly in the latter part of an outbreak. Lacrimation and cor-neal opacity are sometimes observed. The ruminal movements are always poor and moderate bloat may occur. Pregnant cows commonly abort as a result of the infection, usually after the acute stage has passed and sometimes as long as 3 months after apparent recovery. As a rule the illness lasts only a few days, the diarrhoea persisting for about 5 days (2 to 20 days). In some cases recurrent attacks of diarrhoea occur for 2 to 3 months. Such animals remain thin and stunted, have a rough hair coat and bloat readily.

Lameness is common in some areas. The lame-ness appears to be due to a laminitis and inter-digital dermatitis and coronitis and hoof deformi-ties may follow. Lymph node enlargement does not occur but dermatitis of the perineum and be-tween the thighs is fairly constant. Occasional animals show signs of encephalitis, particularly convulsions, but whether this is caused by the virus is unknown.

The erosive lesions on the buccal mucosa are usually discrete, shallow ulcers from which necrotic mucosa has been separated. They occur inside the lips, on the gums and dental pad, on the posterior part of the hard palate, at the commissures of the mouth and on the tongue. Similar lesions occur on the muzzle and may become confluent and covered with scabs and debris. In animals that recover rapidly the lesions on the mucosa heal quickly but in chronic cases new crops of ulcers may develop and secondary bacterial infection is likely to occur. Infection by corynebacteria and sphaero-phorus organisms is common and extension from these lesions may cause pneumonia or other serious complications. Very mild or subclinical cases are by far the most common and are mani-fested by a leucopenia and fever with or without diarrhoea.

In *sporadic mucosal disease* anorexia is accom-panied by a high fever (41°C or 106°F) in the early stages but the fever subsides in 2 to 3 days. Superficial discrete areas of necrosis appear on the buccal mucosa, including the dorsum of the tongue, on the muzzle and in the anterior nares. The lesions are very superficial and, if the necrotic material is wiped off, the erosions are shallow and difficult to identify. The appearance of the lesions is accompanied by the onset of profuse salivation, a purulent nasal discharge and watery diarrhoea, sometimes dysentery. Straining at defaecation is often marked. Complete anorexia persists and dehydration and emaciation develop. There are no nervous signs. Lameness develops in about 10 per cent of cases. Shallow erosive lesions covered with scabs can be found on the perineum, around the scrotum, between the legs and at the skin-horn junction around the dew claws, in the interdigital cleft and at the heels, and there may be extensive scaliness of the skin. In long-standing cases separa-tion of the hoof from the underlying tissues occurs especially at the heels. Skin lesions are more com-mon in those cases that persist for some time and may be present around the preputial orifice and the vulva. Some ocular discharge also occurs in a small percentage of cases and corneal opacity originating in the centre of the cornea and extend-ing centrifugally has been recorded in a few cases. In the late stages the faeces contain a large quan-tity of mucus. Death usually occurs in 4 to 15 days, but occasional cases may linger on for a month or so.

A *subacute* or *chronic* form of sporadic mucosal disease has also been described (23). It is charac-terized by a very long course of up to 17 months, comparative rarity of mucosal erosions in the oral cavity and of diarrhoea and fever. In most other respects it conforms to the more typical picture.

Clinical Pathology

Serological methods of identification, including an agar gel diffusion technique (2), are available and viral neutralization tests in cell culture are also of diagnostic value (24).

A severe leucopenia is characteristic of the disease and is present in the very early stages when the temperature rises but before other clinical signs are evident. The fall is commonly to below 50 per cent of normal and total leucocyte counts of 1000 to 4000 per cmm. are usual. The leuco-penia and an accompanying anaemia persist for some weeks.

Transmission experiments may be conducted with filtrates of infective blood collected at the height of the fever and injected intravenously and intramuscularly. Intraperitoneal injections of whole blood or splenic suspensions, or oral dosing with faeces from clinical cases have also been used to transmit the disease. Additional routes sometimes used are the intravenous, intraperitoneal and intraepithelial (tongue and lips) injection of cell-free filtrates of blood and faeces. Temperatures of the injected animals should be checked several times daily with particular attention to the 7th to 9th days. Care should be exercised in selecting test animals since inapparent infections may have created widespread immunity.

Necropsy Findings

The lesions found at necropsy are in general the same for most recorded forms of the disease. The gross abnormalities are confined to the alimentary tract. Characteristic shallow erosions with very little inflammation around them and with a raw, red base are present on the muzzle, in the mouth, to a less extent in the pharynx, larynx and posterior nares, but in large numbers in the oesophagus where they are linear in shape and lie in the direction of the folds of the oesophageal mucosa. Similar lesions may be present in the forestomachs but are usually confined to the pillars of the rumen and the leaves of the omasum. Erosion may be numerous in the abomasum and caecum but are less common in the small intestine where they usually occur in the Peyer's patches. In the abomasum there is a marked erythema of the mucosa accompanied by multiple submucous haemorrhages and gross oedema of the wall. These changes are present to a less degree in the small intestine but are marked in the colon and caecum, the discolouration being particularly marked on the mucosal folds giving the mucosa a striped appearance similar to that seen in rinderpest. Histologically there is a pronounced absence of inflammatory cells around the local lesions.

In cases which run a chronic course the necrotic epithelium may not be eroded by alimentary movements but instead remain *in situ* as slightly elevated, yellow, friable plaques, especially between the villi on the tongue and in the rumen. Subacute cases with a very prolonged course may show very few lesions in the mouth, some in the oesophagus and none in the stomachs and intestines.

Diagnosis

The differentiation of the diseases causing erosive lesions of the buccal mucosa is extremely difficult, both clinically and at necropsy (25). The similarity between them is the more important because rinderpest and foot-and-mouth disease are major plague diseases. The situation is so dangerous that, if there is any doubt as to the identity of the disease under examination, it should be submitted for laboratory tests.

Differentiation from rinderpest depends on the low morbidity but high mortality rate. The same comment applies generally to sporadic mucosal disease. The epidemic form of the disease is not so highly fatal as rinderpest. Neither of these comments may apply in areas where rinderpest is enzootic and the clinical severity of mucosal disease may be very much less in areas where it is enzootic. In an individual animal it may be impossible to differentiate between the three diseases without laboratory assistance and this should always be sought when doubt exists. Bovine malignant catarrh bears some resemblance to this disease but the ocular lesions, terminal encephalitis and high mortality common to BMC serve to differentiate the two. In infectious ulcerative stomatitis and muzzle disease erosions do not extend beyond the mouth and diarrhoea does not occur. Winter dysentery occurs in explosive outbreaks but there are no erosive lesions as in mucosal disease. Serological investigations (26) suggest that there is no relationship between the two diseases. An as yet unidentified disease with some resemblance to mucosal disease has been observed in Canada, Sweden and Australia (27). The diseases are not necessarily identical but have in common a tendency to very rapid spread, restriction of incidence to adults, absence of erosive lesions of the buccal mucosa and a high morbidity but very low mortality. Described as 'epizootic diarrhoea' and 'epizootic enteritis' of cattle the aetiology of these diseases has not been defined, although a virus was isolated from the Canadian disease and there was some evidence that a virus was the causative agent in the Australian disease (28).

There are no large vesicles in mucosal disease as there are in foot-and-mouth disease and the other vesicular diseases. Necrotic glossitis of steers is manifested only by lingual lesions. Infectious bovine rhinotracheitis is a disease with signs restricted to the upper respiratory tract rather than the alimentary tract and should not be difficult to differentiate. Other causes of chronic diarrhoea including parasitism, Johne's disease and molybdenum poisoning, can be differentiated from mucosal disease by the absence of oral lesions.

Treatment

No specific treatment has been reported but supportive treatment with alimentary tract astringents and parenteral electrolyte solutions may reduce the convalescent period and limit the losses.

Control

Apart from the introduction of the disease in an infected animal the disease appears to spread very readily from farm to farm on inanimate objects such as automobile tyres, boots and containers, and hygienic precautions should be taken to limit this spread. Although the isolation of clinically affected animals is warranted, little can be done to prevent spread on the farm.

The virus passaged through rabbits loses its virulence for cattle and is capable of producing immunity in them as does the virus attenuated by passage through tissue culture (29). Attenuation of the virus by either method is now used in the production of vaccines which are used extensively in the field. One of the major difficulties with vaccination is its use in large groups of young animals entering feedlots. Such animals are likely to have lowered resistance, because of exposure, transport and change of feed. Vaccination of such animals with attenuated virus diarrhoea (mucosal disease) vaccine may result in the appearance of the clinical disease in some vaccinates (30). The use of a combined vaccine in such animals is not recommended because of the risk of vaccine 'breaks'. In addition the possibility exists that a few cattle have a unique inability to form antibodies against the virus and these will have vaccination 'breaks' 10 to 20 days after vaccination (31).

Ordinarily natural exposure to infection results in immunity for life. In the herd the overall immunity will wane and the herd will become susceptible again, if not reinfected, at about five years and vaccination should be carried out at that time. If the status of the herd with relation to the presence of antibodies is unknown it is difficult to decide on a vaccination programme. If the herd antibody levels are high early vaccination of the calves is not likely to have much effect because they will be passively immune from colostral antibodies. If the herd immunity is low postponement of calf vaccination may leave the calves unprotected for a dangerously long period (32). In general the situation is appropriately covered if calves are vaccinated at or soon after 60 days of age (33).

REFERENCES

(1) Olafson, P. *et al.* (1946). *Cornell Vet.*, *36*, 205; *37*, 104, 107.
(2) Pritchard, W. R. (1963). *Advanc. vet. Sci.*, 2.
(3) St George, T. D. *et al.* (1967). *Aust. vet. J.*, *43*, 549.
(4) Taylor, W. P. & Rampton, C. S. (1968). *Vet. Rec.*, *83*, 121.
(5) Provost, A. *et al.* (1969). *Ann. Inst. Pasteur*, *117*, 133.
(6) Beckenhauer, W. H. *et al.* (1861). *Vet. Med.*, *56*, 108.
(7). Schipper, I. A. & Eveleth, D. F. (1957). *Vet. Med.*, *52*, 73, 91.
(8) St George, T. D. (1971). *Aust. vet. J.*, *47*, 370, 428.
(9) Snowdon, W. A. & French, E. L. (1968). *Aust. vet. J.*, *44*, 179.
(10) Mills, J. H. L. *et al.* (1968). *Res. vet. Sci.*, *9*, 500.
(11) Mills, J. H. L. & Luginbuhl, R. E. (1968). *Amer. J. vet. Res.*, *29*, 1367.
(12) Mills, J. H. L. (1967). *Diss. Abstr.*, *27B*, 4003.
(13) Lambert, G. & Fernelius, A. L. (1968). *Canad. J. comp. Med.*, *32*, 440.
(14) Ward, G. M. (1969). *Cornell Vet.*, *59*, 525, 570.
(15) Kendrick, J. W. (1971). *Amer. J. vet. Res.*, *32*, 533.
(16) Casaro, A. P. E. *et al.* (1971). *Amer. J. vet. Res.*, *32*, 1543.
(17) Kahrs, R. F. *et al.* (1970). *J. Amer. vet. med. Ass.*, *156*, 851.
(18) Ward, G. M. (1971). *Cornell Vet.*, *61*, 224.
(19) Leipold, H. W. *et al.* (1970). *Amer. J. vet. Res.*, *31*, 1367.
(20) Bistner, S. I. *et al.* (1970). *Path. vet.*, *7*, 272.
(21) Acland, H. M. *et al.* (1972). *Aust. vet. J.*, *48*, 70.
(22) Ward, G. M. (1971). *Cornell Vet.*, *61*, 179.
(23) French, E. L. & Snowdon, W. A. (1964). *Aust. vet. J.*, *40*, 99.
(24) Darbyshire, J. H. (1967). *J. comp. Path.*, *77*, 107.
(25) Blood, D. C. (1967). *Aust. vet. J.*, *43*, 501.
(26) Kahrs, R. F. (1965). *Cornell Vet.*, *55*, 505.
(27) Hutchins, D. R. *et al.* (1958). *Aust. vet. J.*, *34*, 300.
(28) Johnston, K. G. (1959). *Aust. vet. J.*, *35*, 101.
(29) Coggins, L. *et al.* (1961). *Cornell Vet.*, *51*, 539.
(30) McKercher, D. G. *et al.* (1968). *J. Amer. vet. med. Ass.*, *152*, 1621.
(31) Peter, C. P. *et al.* (1967). *J. Amer. vet. med. Ass.*, *150*, 46.
(32) Kahrs, R. F. *et al.* (1966). *Proc. 70th ann. gen. Mtg U.S. Live Stock sanit. Ass.*, Buffalo, 1966, p. 145.
(33) Smith, P. E. & Mitchell, F. E. (1968). *Vet. Med.*, *63*, 457.

Infectious Ulcerative Stomatitis of Cattle

Infectious ulcerative stomatitis of cattle is caused by a virus and has certain similarities to other virus diseases in which erosive and ulcerative lesions occur on the buccal mucosa (1). Clinically there is anorexia, marked loss of body weight and erosions and ulcers in and around the mouth. The lesions commence as roughly circular, reddened, superficial erosions of about 1 cm. diameter and these enlarge to about 2 cm. in diameter and 1 cm. deep. They are present on the dorsal and ventral surfaces of the tongue, the lips, palate, muzzle, nostrils and anterior turbinates and the skin around the mouth. The soreness in the mouth prevents eating but there is no fever nor change in white cell count. The morbidity rate approximates 100 per cent but no deaths occur. The lesions heal spontaneously in 2 to 3 weeks and in a herd the disease runs a course of about 6 weeks.

The disease has been transmitted experimentally by the inoculation of scrapings of lesions and filtrates of lesion suspensions, into scarifications in the mouth. Immunity develops after an attack but calves immunized against mucosal disease are still susceptible.

Histologically the lesions in this disease are very

similar to those of mucosal disease but the absence of lesions elsewhere in the alimentary tract and the absence of clinical signs of enteritis indicate that this is a separate entity. Ulcerative stomatitis has been differentiated from vesicular stomatitis by laboratory methods. Lesions occur on other parts of the body in muzzle disease (mycotic stomatitis) but not in infectious ulcerative stomatitis. The erosions of ulcerative stomatitis differ from the proliferative lesions of proliferative stomatitis. Clinically it has many features in common with erosive stomatitis recorded in South Africa (2), parotidostomatitis recorded in India (3) and papular stomatitis (4).

REFERENCES

(1) Pritchard, W. R. *et al.* (1958). *J. Amer. vet. med. Ass., 132,* 273.
(2) Mason, J. H. & Neitz, W. O. (1940). *Onderstepoort J. vet. Sci., 15,* 159.
(3) Pande, P. G. & Krishnamurty, D. (1956). *J. infect. Dis., 98,* 142.
(4) Jansen, J. *et al.* (1955). *T. Diergeneesk., 80,* 853.

Bovine Papular Stomatitis

A disease of little importance in its own right, although it may cause mild illness and serve as a portal of entry for secondary bacterial infection, bovine papular stomatitis is of importance chiefly because of the confusion it may cause in the diagnosis of those diseases of cattle in which erosive and vesicular lesions of the mouth are an important diagnostic feature. Bovine papular stomatitis has been known for very many years but has only achieved importance in recent years because of increased interest in viral diseases of the bovine alimentary tract. It has been reported in Africa, the U.S.A., Australia, New Zealand, Canada, Great Britain and Europe.

The causative ungulate pox virus has many of the characteristics of the pox group and is classed as a 'para vaccinia virus'. There is good evidence that the papular stomatitis and the pseudo cowpox virus are identical (1, 2). It occurs in several closely related strains and can be grown on tissue culture. Clinical cases are encountered in young animals from 2 weeks up to 2 years of age and in a group the morbidity often approximates 100 per cent. There may be transient anorexia and a slight fever (39·5°C or 103°F) but in most instances the disease goes unnoticed unless a careful examination of the mouth is made. Lesions are confined to the muzzle, just inside the nostrils and on the buccal mucosa. They commence as small (0·5 to 1 cm.) papules which become dark red in colour, develop a roughening of the surface and expand peripher-

ally so that the lesions are always round or nearly so. Confluence of several lesions may cause the development of a large irregularly shaped area. As the lesion expands the periphery becomes reddened and the centre depressed, grey-brown in colour and rough on the surface, and eventually covered with necrotic tissue, or on external lesions by a scab. Those on the muzzle may be difficult to see if the area is pigmented. In the mouth the lesions occur on all mucosal surfaces except the dorsum of the tongue, and are most common inside the lips and in close proximity to the teeth. Individual lesions heal quickly, sometimes in as short a time as 4 to 7 days, but evidence of healed lesions, in the form of circular areas of dark pink mucosa, usually surrounded by a slightly paler raised zone, may persist for weeks. In the one animal there may be successive crops of lesions so that they can be found continuously or intermittently over a period of months. It is suggested that no immunity occurs and the virus may only cause lesions when intercurrent disease causes lowering of the animal's resistance (3).

Histological examination shows a characteristic ballooning degeneration and the presence of cytoplasmic inclusions in affected cells. The disease can be transmitted by the inoculation of scrapings from lesions into the oral mucosa of susceptible calves and by submucosal inoculation of undiluted tissue culture virus.

Bovine papular stomatitis resembles endemic erosive stomatitis of cattle recorded in Africa (4), proliferative stomatitis, described below, and muzzle disease. There is some similarity between papular and ulcerative stomatitis (described above), but in the latter lesions commonly occur on the dorsal surface of the tongue and the histopathology is quite different. Spread of the disease from calves to man (5) and from man to calves (6) is recorded.

REFERENCES

(1) Nagington, J. *et al.* (1967). *Vet. Rec., 81,* 306.
(2) Liebermann, H. (1967). *Arch. exp. Vet.-Med., 21,* 1337, 1353, 1391, 1399.
(3) Plowright, W. & Ferris, R. D. (1959). *Vet. Rec.,71,*718, 828.
(4) Schaaf, J. (1955). *Arch. exp. Vet.-Med., 9,* 194.
(5) Carson, C. A. & Kerr, K. M. (1967). *J. Amer. vet. med. Ass., 151,* 183.
(6) Carson, C. A. *et al.* (1968). *Amer. J. vet. Res., 29,* 1783.

Proliferative Stomatitis of Cattle

Proliferative stomatitis of cattle is a transmissible disease caused by a virus and first came under notice when it occurred in association with hyperkeratosis. During experiments with this disease the oral lesions were found to occur only irregularly, and during transmission experiments it was observed that the stomatitis could be transferred but not the other lesions of hyperkeratosis.

Very young calves, up to a month old, are susceptible without any prior preparation but older calves require conditioning with a hyperkeratosis-producing diet (1). Horses and pigs are refractory to the virus but accidental infection has occurred in man. The causative virus is distinct from that of papillomatosis. Immunity develops after a natural or experimental attack of the disease.

Initially there is a raised congested area of mucosa which later ulcerates and often develops a proliferative reaction. The lesions occur anywhere in the mouth and subsequently spread to the skin around the mouth, the muzzle and the nostrils. There is no systemic disturbance but there may be anorexia due to the painful condition of the mouth.

REFERENCE

(1) Olson, C. & Palionis, T. (1953). *J. Amer. vet. med. Ass.*, *123*, 419.

Transmissible Gastroenteritis of Pigs

Transmissible gastroenteritis is a highly infectious disease of pigs caused by a virus and is manifested clinically by vomiting, diarrhoea, dehydration and a high mortality rate in very young pigs.

Incidence

The disease occurs generally throughout the United States. It has been identified in the U.K., Japan and recently in Europe (1). The morbidity rate on infected farms is very high, most pigs becoming infected although pigs past weaning age may have the disease in a mild form. Losses are due mainly to the very heavy mortality rate in pigs up to 14 days old. The mortality rate is 40 to 60 per cent in three-week-old pigs, is much lower in weaned pigs and deaths are rare in adults. Although the disease is highly infectious and tends to spread rapidly both within the infected group and to neighbouring farms, outbreaks may occur sporadically and remain localized. In an individual herd the disease tends to occur as an explosive outbreak and then disappear if there is a sufficient time interval between farrowings to prevent carry-over of infection to new groups of susceptible pigs. The disease tends to recur in herds at intervals of several years as herd immunity disappears and the sow population is replaced.

Although oral inoculation of dogs and foxes with infective material does not cause clinical disease in these animals they may continue to shed virus for 2 weeks (2) and antibodies are detectable in serum (3). They may therefore play some part in the spread of the disease.

Aetiology

The causative virus is host specific and so far all laboratory animals have proved to be resistant. It occurs in all tissues of infected pigs with the greatest concentration in intestinal mucosa. American, Japanese, and British isolates are very similar serologically. The virus is capable of causing the disease when administered orally as filtrates of kidney tissue or intestinal mucosa but not when the same material is injected parenterally. Cultivation in tissue culture with some attenuation of the virus, has been reported (4). Attempts to grow the virus in chick embryos have so far been unsuccessful.

Details of the resistance of the virus are incomplete but it does not persist in infected premises for more than a few weeks and is readily destroyed by standard solutions of phenol and formalin, by boiling and by drying. It is not destroyed by freezing. The virus is photosensitive and this may account for the more frequent occurrence of the disease during the winter and spring months (5). All ages of pigs are affected but the syndrome is severe only in baby pigs up to about 14 days old. The disease is seasonal in that most outbreaks occur during the winter months (2). The greatest incidence occurs when the winter months and the farrowing season coincide.

Transmission

New outbreaks commonly follow the introduction of infected pigs which may appear clinically normal. Visitors, vehicles and even birds are suspected of carrying the infection to new locations. The disease can be transmitted experimentally by both oral dosing and nasal instillation of the virus but in field infections it is probable that ingestion is the principal mode of transmission. The virus is excreted in the faeces for as long as 8 weeks after clinical illness and there is ample opportunity for contamination of the environment, particularly during the active phase of the disease. Aerial spread of the virus for distances up to 1 mile have been demonstrated. Affected animals do not become permanent carriers which probably accounts for the usual failure of the infection to persist in an environment for long periods and greatly facilitates control of the disease (6).

Pathogenesis

In the U.K. the experimental disease was produced in pigs up to 11 days of age but piglets which were 19 days old were not susceptible (7).

In the U.S.A. the experimental disease in 4-month-old pigs was characterized by profuse diarrhoea 1 to 6 days after infection in some pigs. No vomiting or anorexia occurred. There was a marked leucopenia for 4 days after infection. At necropsy there were minimal gross lesions other than changes suggestive of paralytic ileus (8). One of the most interesting aspects of the disease is the way in which piglets nursing an immune sow are themselves immune, but lose their resistance in a matter of hours after ceasing to suck the sow. Antibodies must be present in the gut if the animal is to be protected (9). The cellular pathology of TGE is well documented (10), and the disease is essentially a malabsorption syndrome related to the villous atrophy caused by the virus (11).

Clinical Findings

After an incubation period of 12 to 48 hours there is a sudden onset of vomiting and diarrhoea but some affected piglets may continue to suck to within a few hours of death. The diarrhoea is profuse and violent, the faeces being watery and usually yellow-green in colour. There may be a transitory fever but in most cases the temperature is normal. Depression and dehydration are pronounced, the hair coat is ruffled, and weakness and emaciation progress with death occurring on the second to fifth day. Affected piglets which survive are severely emaciated and gain weight slowly. The illness may commence as soon as 24 hours after birth. It is not uncommon on an individual farm for the disease to become less severe and to spread more slowly with the passage of time.

In older pigs there may be signs similar to those which occur in piglets but many animals become infected without showing clinical abnormality. In clinically affected older pigs recovery is much more likely to occur, the illness lasting for up to 10 days. Sows nursing the affected litters may or may not show the typical signs of the disease. Agalactia is a common complication in sows showing clinical illness.

Clinical Pathology

In the early stages there may be a mild leucopenia but a leucocytosis develops during the recovery period. There is no marked tendency to hypoglycaemia but a moderate uraemia develops. Antibodies are detectable in the serum of recovered animals (4) and immunofluorescent techniques are available for identification of the virus in tissues and in tissue culture (12). Neutralizing antibodies appear in the serum as soon as 7 to 8 days after infection and persist for at least 18 months (9). Biochemical changes in the gut have been well documented (18).

Necropsy Findings

Except for pallor of the renal cortex and congestion of the renal medullary rays, the major necropsy lesions are confined to the intestine and stomach. In many field outbreaks and in the experimental disease the lesions may be minor but in others there is severe inflammation of the small intestine, particularly the distal portion of the ileum. Similar but less severe lesions may also be present in the stomach and large intestine. In older pigs, and in pigs where the course of the disease is fairly long, there are areas of necrosis in the intestinal wall. Loss of tone of the intestinal wall and resulting distension of the intestine with fluid ingesta is a characteristic finding. Little haemorrhage occurs in the lumen of the gut. In the stomach there may be engorgement of vessels, and necrosis of the epithelium deep in mucosal crypts. No inclusion bodies are detectable. The important histopathological change is villous atrophy with failure of epithelial cell differentiation in the small intestine. The atrophy is evident 24 hours after infection and regeneration occurs 5 to 7 days later (19). In chronic cases a thickening of the intestinal wall identical with that seen in terminal (regional) ileitis has been described.

The disease, as it occurs in Europe, is characterized by more severe intestinal lesions, often to the point of diphtheresis of the mucosa. There is also degeneration of heart muscle and, in some cases, of the skeletal muscle.

Diagnosis

The epizootiological and clinical characteristics of transmissible gastroenteritis (TGE) should make possible a presumptive diagnosis but confirmation must depend upon positive serological tests, transmission experiments and serum neutralization tests. Hog cholera in its early stages may present a similar clinical picture to that of TGE but its severity in pigs of all ages is an important point of difference. Vomiting and wasting disease has much in common with TGE in the manner in which it occurs and the age groups affected but diarrhoea is less common and transmission of the disease is not easily effected. Non-specific diarrhoea of young pigs due to faulty feeding responds satisfactorily to treatment. Enteritis due to *Escherichia coli* is a common disease, especially in very young pigs in which it may cause a very high mortality, but it is usually enzootic in a piggery, there is no vomiting and the causative bacteria can easily be isolated from the gut and the mesenteric lymph nodes and there is usually good response to treatment.

Treatment

The sulphonamides and antibiotics have been used in the treatment of TGE without demonstrable effect. Because dehydration is severe and hypoglycaemia likely to occur the intraperitoneal injection of solutions containing electrolytes and glucose is advisable if the value of the pig warrants it.

Control

The extreme infectivity of the disease makes the immediate control of an outbreak in a herd difficult and often impossible. Because it is spread by airborne and direct contact very strict hygienic precautions are necessary and where it is practicable individual isolation of pregnant sows should be attempted and farrowing pens should be carefully disinfected. Since it is probable that the highly susceptible piglets serve as the main reservoir of infection it is recommended that the breeding programme be arranged so that there is a break of at least 2 months before the next series of farrowings.

Artificial infection of the sows by feeding infective material during late pregnancy has been recommended as a method of control. The piglets from sows thus treated appear to derive an appreciable immunity from the sow's colostrum (13) but this immunity does not extend to the following litter unless the sow is re-exposed. Good results in preventing deaths during an outbreak are recorded after the administration of 10 ml. of whole citrated blood from a recovered sow. The blood was administered by mouth at birth and repeated three days later. Some success is also claimed for the method when used in the treatment of affected pigs (14). The administration of hyper-immune serum is useless as prophylaxis if it is given parenterally; it may be of use given orally.

An inactivated tissue culture vaccine administered to sows 2 or 10 weeks prior to farrowing has markedly reduced losses in newborn pigs in endemic areas (4, 15). Excellent results appear to be obtained when the inactivated vaccine is administered to the sows by intramammary infusion on several occasions 2 to 5 weeks before farrowing.

The colostrom and milk from the sows carry protective antibodies (16, 17).

REVIEW LITERATURE

Woode, G. N. (1969). Transmissible gastro-enteritis of swine. *Vet. Bull.*, *39*, 239.

REFERENCES

(1) Kretzschmar, C. (1970). *Mh. Vet. Med.*, *25*, 629.
(2) McClurkin, A. W. *et al.* (1970). *Canad. J. comp. Med.*, *34*, 347.
(3) Norman, J. O. *et al.* (1970). *Canad. J. comp. Med.*, *34*, 115.
(4) Fuller, D. A. (1971). *Vet. Med.*, *66*, 1206.
(5) Cartwright, S. F. *et al.* (1964). *Vet. Rec.*, *76*, 1332.
(6) Derbyshire, J. B. (1969). *J. comp. Path.*, *79*, 445.
(7) Chandler, R. L. *et al.* (1969). *Res. vet. Sci.*, *10*, 435.
(8) Olson, L. D. (1971). *Amer. J. vet. Res.*, *32*, 411.
(9) Cartwright, S. F. (1969). *Brit. vet. J.*, *125*, 410.
(10) Pensaert, M. *et al.* (1970). *Arch. ges. Virusforsch.*, *31*, 321, 335.
(11) Thake, D. C. (1968). *Amer. J. Path.*, *53*, 149.
(12) Black, J. W. (1972). *Proc. 75th ann. Mtg U.S. Anim. Hlth Ass.*, 492.
(13) Haelterman, E. O. (1963). *Proc. 17th World vet. Congr.*, *Hanover*, *1*, 615.
(14) Noble, W. A. (1964). *Vet. Rec.*, *76*, 1497.
(15) Welter, C. J. *et al.* (1966). *J. Amer. vet. med. Ass.*, *149*, 1587.
(16) Djurickovic, S. & Thorsen, J. (1970). *Vet. Rec.*, *87*, 62.
(17) Thorsen, J. & Djurickovic, S. (1971). *Canad. J. comp. Med.*, *35*, 99.
(18) Cross, R. F. & Bohl, E. H. (1969). *J. Amer. vet. med. Ass.*, *154*, 266.
(19) Hooker, B. E. & Haelterman, E. O. (1969). *Canad. J. comp. Med.*, *33*, 29.

Vomiting and Wasting Disease of Sucking Pigs

This disease of sucking pigs was reported from Canada in 1958 (1) and has since been reported from the U.K. (2) and West Germany (3, 4). It bears some resemblance to transmissible gastro-enteritis but is not easily transmitted experimentally and diarrhoea is not prominent. Sucking pigs, usually in the 2- to 6-weeks age group, are the only ones affected although transient anorexia and vomiting have occurred in some sows at the commencement of outbreaks.

The available evidence indicates that this disease is a manifestation of infection with haemagglutinating encephalomyelitis virus (HEV). Why this virus should cause encephalomyelitis in some pigs and vomiting and wasting in others may be related to the age at which infection occurs or to the particular strain of virus (2, 5).

The disease occurs in outbreaks often affecting a number of litters in the same piggery within a few days, the morbidity in affected litters varying from 50 to 100 per cent, although not all affected pigs show signs at the same time. Vomiting of yellow-green vomitus is the first sign and is accompanied by anorexia and thirst. Ineffective attempts to drink are characteristic. The temperature is usually normal or slightly elevated except for transient febrile reactions (up to 40·5°C or 105°F) for 24 hours in the early stages in some pigs, and the faeces are usually hard and dry. Diarrhoea may occur but is not severe and occurs mostly in the older piglets. Vomiting may continue for some days but, in all affected pigs, there is severe, rapid emaciation and dehydration. They may continue in this state for some weeks and eventually die, apparently of starvation. Most affected pigs die and heavy losses occur in individual piggeries. Necropsy findings are negative except for moderate gastro-enteritis in some acute cases. The disease appears to occur as an outbreak and then disappears from the herd.

Neither antibacterial treatments nor general supportive treatment with parenterally administered fluids and electrolytes have had an appreciable effect on the course of the disease.

The control of the disease must depend on prior exposure of sows to infection at least 10 days before farrowing. The piglets will be protected by colostral antibodies.

REVIEW LITERATURE
Cartwright, S. F. (1969). *Vet. Ann.*, p. 196. Bristol: Wright.

REFERENCES
(1) Roe, C. K. & Alexander, T. J. L. (1958). *Canad. J. comp. Med.*, *22*, 305.
(2) Cartwright, S. F. & Lucas, M. (1970). *Vet. Rec.*, *86*, 278.
(3) Schlenstedt, D. *et al.* (1969). *Dtsch. tierärztl. Wschr.*, *76*, 694, 697.
(4) Tuch, K. (1971). *Dtsch. tierärztl. Wschr.*, *78*, 496.
(5) Greig, A. S. (1969). *Vet. Rec.*, *85*, 99.

Viral Enteritis of Calves

A virus has been isolated from babies with diarrhoea which is capable of causing scours in calves (1). Natural outbreaks of the disease have not been recorded. The disease was transmissible by intranasal instillation, inoculation of whole blood or by contact, to calves 2 days to 2 months old. After an incubation period of 2 to 5 days, diarrhoea with much mucus and some blood appeared. A slight systemic reaction accompanied the diarrhoea. The disease lasted 5 to 8 days and 13 per cent of affected calves died. Affected calves were immune on recovery. At necropsy hyperaemia of the large and small intestinal mucosa and hyperaemia and enlargement of the mesenteric lymph nodes were observed.

A catarrhal enteritis associated with pneumonia occurs in calves and is caused by a virus. This 'pneumo-enteritis' has been recorded in the United States and in Britain, and is described in the section on viral pneumonia of calves (p. 517).

REFERENCE
(1) Light, J. S. & Hodes, H. L. (1943). *Amer. J. publ. Hlth*, *33*, 1451.

Bluetongue

Bluetongue is an infectious disease of sheep and occasionally cattle, caused by a virus and transmitted by insect vectors. It is characterized by catarrhal stomatitis, rhinitis and enteritis and lameness due to inflammation of the coronary bands and sensitive laminae of the feet.

Incidence

The disease is widespread on the African continent and has occurred in Cyprus, Pakistan, Japan, Israel, Turkey, the United States and Portugal and Spain. Bluetongue has been diagnosed in many states in the U.S.A. and appears to have spread widely since its first identification in 1952. The morbidity rate varies with the size of the insect population and in bad years may reach as high as 30 per cent. Although the mortality rate is low in adult sheep, severe losses may occur in young sheep. Usually from 5 to 30 per cent of affected animals die but in the Spanish outbreak the mortality rate was 60 to 80 per cent. However, as in foot-and-mouth disease in cattle, the indirect losses are of greatest importance. Adults either lose their fleece or develop a break in the staple and pregnant ewes commonly abort. There is a severe loss of condition and convalescence is prolonged, particularly in lambs.

Aetiology

A preliminary antigenic classification of strains of bluetongue virus indicates that there are probably at least sixteen antigenic strains (1, 2).

Outbreaks caused by different strains may follow one another in quick succession. The strains vary considerably in pathogenicity. The virus is stable and resistant to decomposition and it is assumed that it persists for very long periods in meat and offal. It is resistant to some commonly used virucidal agents including sodium carbonate. It is susceptible to 3 per cent sodium hydroxide solution and to Wescodyne, a complex organic iodide. All ruminants are susceptible to experimental infection and the virus will infect hamsters, unweaned white mice and developing chick embryos. It has also been grown in tissue culture and after suitable attenuation is capable of immunizing sheep without producing ill effects. After a clinical attack of the disease sheep have a solid immunity to the particular strain of virus involved but there is no cross-immunity to other strains. Infected cattle do not appear to develop a significant immunity.

The disease under natural conditions is confined almost entirely to sheep although elk (3), white-tailed deer (4) and other ruminants (5) have also been found infected. Amongst sheep, sucking lambs are relatively resistant, and if the ewes are resistant, solid passive immunity, lasting for about 2 months, is transmitted via the colostrum. Young sheep about a year old are most susceptible and British breeds and Merinos are more susceptible than native African sheep. Bluetongue virus is infective for cattle and has been isolated from this species as long as 81 days after infection. Clinical illness is not common in cattle, but it does occur naturally and may cause fatalities among a highly susceptible population (14). Exposure to solar irradiation appears to increase the severity of the disease and other forms of environmental stress are likely to be contributory. Such factors may account for the difficulty encountered in producing the clinical disease in cattle kept under experimental conditions as distinct from the occasional clinical case observed in cattle in the field. Goats and wild ruminants react to the infection in the same way as do cattle.

Transmission

Although the disease is readily transmitted experimentally by the inoculation of infective blood into susceptible sheep, under natural conditions it appears to be spread entirely by the bites of sandflies (*Culicoides* spp.) (6). Culicoid flies do not become infective until about 10 days after ingesting infective blood (7). The sheep ked (*Melophagus ovinus*) ingests the virus when sucking the blood of infected sheep and can transmit the disease in a mechanical manner (8). It is not spread by contact and there is a marked seasonal incidence, most cases occurring in the late summer and early autumn when the vector population is highest. The disease is most prevalent in wet seasons and in low-lying areas, conditions which favour insect multiplication.

The reason for the persistence of the disease from season to season has not been found. Virus has been isolated from recovered sheep 4 months after an attack of bluetongue and in some cases for longer periods. The infection may thus persist in carrier animals which may be cattle or wild ruminants. There is also the possibility of the virus overwintering in the insect vector. Cattle appear to be much more attractive to *Culicoides* spp. and this may enhance the importance of cattle as carriers (9). The disease may be spread to new areas by the transport of infected vectors or more frequently by the introduction of infected sheep or cattle. The duration of infectivity in cattle is uncertain although it may be as long as 49 days (10). To prevent the introduction of bluetongue very stringent regulations preventing the importation of ruminants from infected areas have been adopted in Australia and New Zealand.

Pathogenesis

A viraemia occurs in the early stages of the disease and localization, probably in endothelium, produces the characteristic epithelial lesions of bluetongue. After experimental inoculation in cattle a viraemia occurs with a peak about 7 days later and a positive reaction to the gel diffusion test after the 21st day (11). The congenital defects of the nervous system, which occur with the natural virus, and the attenuated vaccine virus, have been reproduced experimentally (12).

Clinical Findings

In sheep after an incubation period of less than a week (2 to 4 days experimentally), a severe febrile reaction with a maximum temperature of 40·5 to 41°C (105 to 106°F) is usual, although afebrile cases may occur. The fever continues for 5 or 6 days. About 48 hours after the temperature rise, nasal discharge and salivation, with reddening of the buccal and nasal mucosae are apparent. The nasal discharge is mucopurulent and often blood-stained and the saliva is frothy. Swelling and oedema of the lips, gums, dental pad and tongue occur and there may be involuntary movement of the lips. Excoriation of the buccal mucosa follows and the saliva becomes blood-stained and the mouth has an offensive odour. Lenticular, necrotic ulcers develop, particularly on the lateral aspects of the tongue, which is swollen and purple in colour. Swallowing is often difficult. Respiration is obstructed and stertorous and is increased in rate up to 100 per minute. Diarrhoea and dysentery may occur. Foot lesions, including laminitis and coronitis and manifested by lameness and recumbency, appear only in some animals, usually when the mouth lesions begin to heal. The appearance of a dark red to purple band in the skin just above the coronet, due to coronitis, is an important diagnostic sign. Wry-neck, with twisting of the head and neck to one side, occurs in a few cases appearing suddenly about the twelfth day. This is apparently due to the direct action of the virus on muscle tissue as is the pronounced muscle stiffness and weakness which is severe enough to prevent eating. There is a marked, rapid loss of condition. The lower parts of the face, the ears and jaws are oedematous and hyperaemia of the woolless skin may be present. Some affected sheep show severe conjunctivitis, accompanied by profuse lacrymation. A break occurs in the staple of the fleece. Vomiting and secondary aspiration pneumonia may also occur. Death in most fatal cases occurs about 6 days after the appearance of signs.

In animals that recover there is a long convalescence and a return to normal bodily condition may take several months. Partial or complete loss of the fleece is common and causes great financial loss. Other signs during convalescence include separation or cracking of the hooves and wrinkling and cracking of the skin around the lips and muzzle.

Two variants of this acute syndrome are described. In the abortive type the temperature reaction is not followed by local lesions. In the subacute type the local lesions are minimal, but emaciation, weakness and extended convalescence are severe. A similar syndrome occurs in lambs which become infected when colostral immunity is on the wane.

In cattle most infections are inapparent although a few animals may develop a clinical syndrome not unlike that seen in severely affected sheep (13). Authenticated clinical signs which have been recorded include fever (40 to 41 °C), stiffness and laminitis in all four limbs, excessive salivation, oedema of the lips, inappetence, nasal discharge and foetid breath (18). Some affected cattle also have ulcerative lesions on the tongue, dental pad, and muzzle. A severe coronitis, sometimes with sloughing of the hoof, may occur. Serosanguineous exudate may appear in the nostrils and a discharge from the eyes. Contraction of the infection during early pregnancy may cause abortion or congenital deformities (14, 25).

Clinical Pathology

Diagnosis can be confirmed by inoculation of blood into susceptible sheep, unweaned white mice or hamsters or culture in developing chick embryos. It is recommended that blood be subinoculated from the first to a second recipient sheep when even a slight fever peak occurs in the first 14 days in the first sheep (2). A complement fixation test has also been developed (13) but is not suitable for diagnostic purposes in cattle. A virus neutralization test is used to identify the strain or strains

of virus present. A fluorescent antibody technique has been introduced (24) and a micro-gel diffusion test is now available but is not highly accurate during the viraemic stage of the disease (15, 16). The skeletal myopathy which occurs in this disease is reflected by a rise in serum enzymes including creatinine phosphokinase (17). The slight leucocytosis which occurs in the early stages of the disease is commonly followed by a marked leucopenia, due largely to a depression of lymphocyte numbers (18). Infected cattle show a similar leucopenia.

Necropsy Findings

The mucosal and skin lesions have already been described. Other consistent lesions include generalized oedema, hyperaemia and haemorrhage and necrosis of skeletal and cardiac muscles and aspiration pneumonia (18). There is a most distinctive haemorrhage at the base of the pulmonary artery. Hyperaemia and oedema of the abomasal mucosa are sometimes accompanied by ecchymoses and ulceration. Muscle lesions include haemorrhages and hyaline degeneration (2).

Diagnosis

In both cattle and sheep the disease is likely to be confused with foot-and-mouth disease although the spread of the disease is usually much slower. Bluetongue has a seasonal incidence, disappearing when the insect vectors diminish. The serological tests make diagnosis certain in sheep but in cattle the only satisfactory test is the inoculation of blood from suspected beasts into susceptible sheep. A positive test depends on the appearance of diagnostic clinical signs and resistance to subsequent challenge with bluetongue virus, or a significant increase in virus-neutralizing antibodies in the recipient sheep (10). Contagious ecthyma and ulcerative dermatosis have characteristic lesions, and sheep pox is a highly fatal disease with typical pox lesions. An epizootic disease of cattle, Ibaraki disease, resembling 'bluetongue' has been identified in Japan. The causative virus is antigenically different from that of bluetongue (19). Epizootic haemorrhagic disease of white-tailed deer has much in common with bluetongue in that species (20). Because of the great variations in epidemiology and symptomatology of the disease, diagnosis, except in the classical severe form of the disease, can be greatly delayed by failure to recognize the possibility of bluetongue at a field examination.

Treatment

Local irrigations with mild disinfectant solutions may afford some relief. Affected sheep should be housed and protected from weather, particularly hot sun. Treatment with tetracyclines has been shown to be ineffective (21).

Control

Prevention of entry of the disease into a country which has effective natural barriers against uncontrolled livestock entry depends on quarantine measures to prevent the introduction of any ruminant animals from countries where the disease occurs and adequate treatment of aircraft to prevent the accidental introduction of infective insects. Because of resentment by livestock owners to the complete prohibition of international movement of ruminants, several procedures aimed at permitting limited movement are being examined. The introduction of bovine semen from low-risk areas after suitable tests of donors and a prolonged storage period is already in limited use. The importation of live cattle which have passed a test of not causing serological reactions to bluetongue in sheep after repeated blood transfusions is projected in some countries. Although these procedures provide minimum risks, the drastic consequences of an introduction of bluetongue make their use inadvisable unless there is very great need for the introduction of new genetic material.

In enzootic areas any measure which prevents exposure to nightflying insect vectors will reduce spread. Spraying with repellents, housing at night, and avoidance of low, marshy areas are recommended prophylactic measures. Vaccination is the only satisfactory control procedure once the disease has been introduced into an area. Periodic revaccination of all sheep is now practised in such areas and although the practice will not eradicate the disease it has been highly successful in keeping losses to a very low level provided immunity to all local strains of the virus is attained.

An egg-attenuated living virus is in current use in South Africa as a vaccine. The vaccine is polyvalent and contains a number of strains of virus with wide antigenicity. Reactions to vaccination are slight but ewes should not be vaccinated within 3 weeks of mating as anoestrus often results. Annual revaccination 1 month before the expected occurrence of the disease is recommended. Immunity is present 10 days after vaccination so that early vaccination during an outbreak may substantially reduce losses. Lambs from immune mothers may be able to neutralize the attenuated virus and fail to be immunized, whereas field strains may overcome their passive immunity. In enzootic

areas it may therefore be necessary to postpone lambing until major danger from the disease is passed and lambs should not be vaccinated until 2 weeks after weaning. A modified live virus vaccine has also given good results in the U.S.A. with a strong immunity lasting for 30 months.

American workers have reported that vaccination of pregnant ewes is attended by risk of deformity in the lambs. The danger period is between the fourth and eighth weeks of pregnancy with the greatest incidence of deformities occurring when vaccination is carried out in ewes pregnant for 5 to 6 weeks. The incidence of deformities may be as high as 13 per cent, with an average of 5 per cent. Abortions do not occur although some lambs are stillborn. The deformities include spasticity and oedema of the limbs and a 'dummy' syndrome. At necropsy there is no evidence of bacterial or viral infection. The cranial cavity is filled with fluid and the brain is hypoplastic with evident degenerative changes (22). Presumptive evidence exists that similar lesions may occur in calves as a result of natural infection with virulent virus (23).

REFERENCES

(1) Howell, P. G. (1970). *J. S. Afr. vet. med. Ass.*, *41*, 215.
(2) Jansen, B. C. (1966). *Aust. vet. J.*, *42*, 471.
(3) Murray, J. O. & Trainer, D. O. (1970). *Wildl. Dis.*, *6*, 144.
(4) Stair, E. L. *et al.* (1968). *Path. Vet.*, *5*, 164.
(5) Trainer, D. O. & Jochim, M. M. (1969). *Amer. J. vet. Res.*, 2007.
(6) Luedke, A. J. *et al.* (1967). *Amer. J. vet. Res.*, *28*, 457.
(7) Foster, N. M. *et al.* (1968). *Amer. J. vet. Res.*, *29*, 275.
(8) Luedke, A. J. *et al.* (1965). *Canad. J. comp. Med.*, *29*, 229.
(9) Luedke, A. J. *et al.* (1970). *J. Amer. vet. med. Ass.*, *156*, 187.
(10) Bowne, J. G. *et al.* (1966). *J. Amer. vet. med. Ass.*, *148*, 1177.
(11) Luedke, A. J. *et al.* (1969). *Amer. J. vet. Res.*, *30*, 51.
(12) Richards, W. P. C. & Cordy, D. R. (1967). *Science, N.Y.*, *156*, 530.
(13) Cox, H. R. (1954). *Bact. Rev.*, *18*, 239.
(14) Bowne, J. G. *et al.* (1968). *J. Amer. vet. med. Ass.*, *153*, 662.
(15) Metcalf, H. E. & Jochim, M. M. (1970). *Amer. J. vet. Res.*, *31*, 1743.
(16) Jochim, M. M. & Chow, T. L. (1969). *Amer. J. vet. Res.*, *30*, 33.
(17) Clark, R. & Wagner, A. M. (1967). *J. S. Afr. vet. med. Ass.*, *38*, 221.
(18) Luedke, A. J. *et al.* (1964). *Amer. J. vet. Res.*, *25*, 963.
(19) Matumoto, M. *et al.* (1970). *Jap. J. Microbiol.*, *14*, 99, 351.
(20) Fletch, A. H. & Karstad, L. H. (1971). *Canad. J. comp. Med.*, *35*, 224.
(21) Shimshoni, A. (1964). *Refuah vet.*, *21*, 163.
(22) Young, S. & Cordy, D. R. (1964). *J. Neuropath. exp. Neurol.*, *23*, 635.
(23) Richards, W. P. C. *et al.* (1971). *Cornell Vet.*, *61*, 336.
(24) Gleiser, C. A. *et al.* (1969). *Amer. J. vet. Res.*, *30*, 981.
(25) Luedke, A. J. *et al.* (1971). *J. Amer. vet. med. Ass.*, *156*, 1871.

21

Diseases Caused by Viruses and Chlamydia—II

VIRAL DISEASES CHARACTERIZED BY RESPIRATORY SIGNS

THE VIRAL INFECTIONS OF THE UPPER RESPIRATORY TRACT OF HORSES

UNTIL relatively recent years the infectious diseases of the respiratory tract of horses, apart from strangles, were differentiated largely on clinical grounds and the specific causative agents were unknown. The picture is still confused, but the identification of a number of viruses including those of equine viral arteritis, equine rhinopneumonitis and equine influenza and the definition of the syndromes they produce has done much to reduce the confusion (7). It is now known that 'virus abortion' has no separate existence but that outbreaks so described are caused by one of these viruses.

The specific diseases dealt with in detail below are equine viral rhinopneumonitis, equine viral arteritis and equine influenza. Infectious equine pneumonia is described as a clinical entity although the relationship of the causative agent to others in the group remains unclear.

There remain a number of viral infections of the upper respiratory tract of horses which are assuming some importance at the present time. They include infection with a myxovirus parainfluenza 3 virus recorded at a high level of incidence in Canada (1). Clinically there is mild fever, marked sero-purulent nasal discharge, conjunctivitis, anorexia, dyspnoea and adenitis of the submaxillary lymph nodes. Normally recovery occurs spontaneously in about 7 days, but bronchitis and a purulent rhinitis may persist for several weeks. Infection with a rhinovirus has also been reported (2).

It is characterized by an incubation period of 3 to 8 days, fever, pharyngitis, pharyngeal lymphadenitis and a variable nasal discharge. The uncomplicated disease is mild and self-limiting. Transmission of infection to in-contact humans has been reported (3). Epizootic cough or 'Hop-pengarten' cough is a disease with a long history in Germany, but its aetiology is still not determined. It is manifested by transient fever, serous nasal discharge, lacrimation, pharyngeal lymphadenitis and a persistent dry, painful cough (4).

An equine herpes virus which is not the rhinopneumonitis virus, has also been identified as a cause of mild respiratory disease of horses (5, 6).

The clinical and epidemiological features of all of the diseases in this section, and of strangles, which is dealt with elsewhere, are sufficiently similar to make differential diagnosis between them in the field virtually impossible. A positive diagnosis can be made only by isolation and identification of the virus concerned, although serological examination of paired—acute and convalescent phase—sera is often used for presumptive identification before virus isolation is attempted.

Fortunately most of the respiratory viruses can be isolated from nasal swabs or washings, preferably collected in the early stages of the disease and presented to the laboratory in a frozen state. When pharyngitis is a prominent clinical sign, as in infections with the parainfluenza viruses and rhinovirus, swabs of the pharyngeal area are superior to nasal swabs (4). It is also of importance in comparative medical studies to record the occurrence of upper respiratory tract infections in stable attendants and to submit specimens from affected persons. The position with respect to transmissibility of influenza viruses and rhinoviruses between the two species requires further clarification.

REFERENCES

(1) Ditchfield, J. *et al.* (1963). *Canad. vet. J.*, *4*, 175.
(2) Burrows, R. (1970). *Proc. 2nd int. Conf. equine infect. Dis.*, *Paris*, 1969, pp. 154–64.
(3) Plummer, G. & Kerry, J. B. (1962). *Vet. Rec.*, 74, 967.
(4) Erasmus, B. J. (1965). *J. S. Afr. med. Ass.*, *36*, 209.
(5) Studdert, M. J. (1971). *Aust. vet. J.*, *47*, 434.
(6) Studdert, M. J. *et al.* (1970). *Aust. vet. J.*, *46*, 83, 90, 583.
(7) Lewis, P. F. (1969). *Aust. vet. J.*, *45*, 231.

Equine Viral Rhinopneumonitis (EVR)

This is a mild disease of the upper respiratory tract of horses caused by a specific virus which also commonly causes abortion.

Incidence

Mild infections of the respiratory tract of horses, characterized by coughing and nasal discharge, are of widespread occurrence particularly when horses are congregated in the colder months. While it appears probable that some 'colds' are due to infection with the equine viral rhinopneumonitis (EVR) virus, the extent to which this infection occurs is unknown. The initial identification of the virus was made in the United States and its presence is now known or suspected in most countries. The association between virus abortion and upper respiratory tract infection was originally suggested by European observers. It seems clearly established that EVR is mild in character and fatalities in uncomplicated cases are unlikely. Affected animals are unable to work, racehorses have to break their training, and 'storms' of abortions occur in bands of brood mares. The infection is widespread. A recent survey of Australian horses showed that 83 per cent had been exposed to infection (1).

Aetiology

EVR is caused by a herpes virus, probably the same as that of the original 'virus abortion', antigenically distinct from the virus of equine viral arteritis (EVA) and unrelated to the viruses of the influenzas of man and swine. It can be grown in tissue culture (2) and has been adapted to embryonated eggs and to hamsters, producing lesions different from those caused by the influenza group of viruses. Unlike the latter it does not cause haemagglutination. A disease which is clinically indistinguishable from EVR but caused by an antigenically distinct virus has been recorded in the U.K. A nomenclature of equine herpes virus 1 for the EVR virus and equine herpes virus 2 for the new virus has been suggested (3).

Although horses of all ages become infected, signs of upper respiratory tract disease are usually limited to young horses. On breeding farms outbreaks occur in foals, the mares showing only abortion. Most outbreaks of abortion are associated directly with outbreaks of the respiratory disease in foals and yearlings several weeks earlier. These latter outbreaks occur most commonly in autumn and winter months. Recovery is followed by an immunity lasting for 6 to 12 months. The virus does not appear to persist in the environment for more than 7 to 14 days, although when dried on horse hairs, it may survive for up to 6 weeks.

Transmission

Transmission probably occurs by the inhalation of infected droplets or by the ingestion of material contaminated by nasal discharges or aborted foetuses. Mediate infection may occur, although the virus appears to be short lived away from its host. The duration of the infectivity of animals is unknown, but is probably some weeks and possibly longer because carrier animals seem to be necessary for persistence of the disease from year to year.

Pathogenesis

Initially there is a phase of rapid proliferation of the virus in the nasal mucosa, resulting in rhinitis, pyrexia and other clinical respiratory signs. This is followed by a systemic, viraemic phase in which the virus can be isolated from the leucocytes. It is from this vantage point that invasion of lungs, nervous tissue, and foetus occur. Damage to the foetus is more extensive than to the dam, although death of the foetus rarely occurs before the act of abortion.

Clinical Findings

There is an incubation period of 2 to 20 days. Fever, conjunctivitis, coughing and mild catarrh of the upper respiratory tract are the cardinal manifestations of the disease, but inapparent infection is common. The temperature varies from 39 to 40·5°C (102·5 to 105·5°F). In most clinical cases there is only limited involvement of the respiratory system and the appetite is unimpaired. There may be slight enlargement of the lymph nodes of the throat. These signs are more likely to occur in young horses or when horses are assembled in sale barns. Oedema of the limbs and diarrhoea occur rarely. The length of the illness is usually 2 to 5 days, although the nasal discharge and cough may persist for 1 to 3 weeks. Secondary bacterial invasion, usually streptococcal, may result in pneumonia. Young foals may develop primary pneumonia.

A heavy outbreak of abortions (up to 90 per cent) in mares may occur up to 4 months after the respiratory phase, and in many instances the latter is so mild that it is not observed. Abortion occurs without premonitory signs and the placenta is not retained. The incidence of abortion is highest in the last third of pregnancy—particularly in the 8 to 10 months period—but can occur as early as the fifth month. Infection is not always associated with abortion; the infection is quite widespread in Australia (6, 7) but abortion is relatively uncommon.

The rhinopneumonitis virus has also been isolated from the spinal cord of a stallion with severe lumbar paralysis (8). There are other reports (9, 10) of transient ataxia up to extensive paralysis in horses one week after the development of a rhinopneumonitis infection.

An unexpected, severe outbreak of encephalomyelitis has occurred in mares after the experimental injection of rhinopneumonitis virus (11). Clinical signs were paresis or paralysis and one mare died. There were pathological changes in the spinal cord and brain.

Clinical Pathology

Haematological findings include a pronounced leucopenia, due largely to depression of neutrophils. Complement-fixing antibody is present, appearing on the 10th to 12th day after experimental infection but persists for only a limited period. However, the virus-neutralizing antibodies persist for over a year and testing for them is a more reliable means of determining that previous infection with the virus has occurred. A fluorescent antibody technique is also available. The virus can be isolated in tissue culture, chick embryos and hamsters, from either nasal washings or aborted foetuses. Bacteriological examination of nasal discharges and aborted foetuses is negative unless secondary bacterial invasion has occurred. *Streptococcus equi* and *Salmonella abortivoequina* are the common secondary invaders in the respective sites.

Necropsy Findings

Histological descriptions of the lesions are available (4). The major manifestations are rhinitis and pneumonitis. Aborted foetuses show severe pulmonary congestion and focal hepatic necroses with acidophilic intranuclear inclusion bodies in the bronchial and alveolar epithelium and in hepatic parenchyma. The focal necroses in the liver appear grossly as greyish-white, subcapsular spots up to 5 mm. in diameter, and there is slight icterus. Petechial and ecchymotic haemorrhages are common especially beneath the respiratory mucosae of aborted foetuses and there is often excess fluid in the pleural cavity.

Diagnosis

The clinical picture of a mild upper respiratory infection in young and adult horses, with a high incidence of abortions in convalescent mares, and characteristic lesions in the aborted foetuses are virtually diagnostic of equine viral rhinopneumonitis. As an upper respiratory tract infection it must be differentiated from strangles, with its catarrhal rhinitis and lymph node abscessation,

from the more severe equine viral arteritis in which there are no lesions in aborted foetuses, and from infectious equine pneumonia and equine influenza. It must also be differentiated from infection with myxovirus parainfluenzae 3 shown to cause upper respiratory tract disease in young horses. The diseases are very similar, although one significant difference is the marked inflammation of the submaxillary lymph nodes in the latter. It may also be confused with purpura haemorrhagica in which subcutaneous oedema of the legs is severe. Acute leptospirosis is usually accompanied by jaundice, but the general picture of a mild febrile reaction with subsequent abortions may cause confusion in the diagnosis of the two diseases.

Experimentally the rhinopneumonitis virus has been shown to cause vaginitis in mares (5). This is not to be confused with coital vesicular exanthema which is also caused by a closely related herpes virus (13).

Confirmation of the diagnosis requires isolation of the virus in chick embryos or hamsters, the demonstration of the pathognomonic lesions in the aborted foetuses and production of the disease by injection into susceptible horses. The complement-fixation tests are of value in detecting previous infection, but should not be used to determine the cause of abortion. The occurrence of a rise in antibody titre in paired sera collected several weeks apart is of more value, but isolation of the virus from the aborted foetus is the only definitive diagnostic procedure.

Treatment

No specific treatment is likely to modify the action of the virus, but it is usual to provide antibiotics to horses with EVR to prevent and treat infection with secondary bacterial invaders. The treatment should be continued over a period of 4 to 6 days. Warm, draught free, isolated quarters should be provided if possible, with laxative foods and a constant supply of fresh drinking water.

Control

Standard hygienic procedures should be adopted to avoid spread of the disease, with particular attention being given to the isolation of introduced horses and brood mares. This may be impossible in boarding studs where mares are brought in from many places for breeding. Mares which abort should be rigidly isolated and the contaminated area thoroughly cleaned and disinfected.

A short-term immunity of 6 to 12 months occurs after natural infection and can be produced by the intradermal inoculation of suspensions of live virus prepared from the liver, lung and spleen of aborted foetuses into mares during early pregnancy. This method of vaccination can be repeated annually and may be of value in studs where the mare population is not constantly changing. Post-vaccinal hepatitis may occur in a proportion of mares as a result of the vaccination. Care must be taken to ensure that the inoculum is not contaminated, especially by the virus of equine infectious anaemia. Preliminary field tests of a neurotropic strain of the virus, produced by adaptation of the field virus to growth in hamster brain, suggests that a satisfactory field vaccine could be prepared by adaptation of the virus. Hamster tissue vaccine itself produces a too severe reaction for general use. The recommended procedure at the present time is vaccination with a virus slightly modified by passage through hamsters, or with fully virulent virus (12). For maximum immunity the vaccine is sprayed into the nasopharynx with a special tube. The duration of the immunity produced is short and the vaccine has to be administered at selected times. Young foals are vaccinated during the first month of life and again at 3 and 12 months of age. Brood mares known to be pregnant are vaccinated twice during the first third of pregnancy—at the same times as the first two vaccinations are given to the foals. European workers have developed their own tissue-culture attenuated vaccine (14). In all countries it is generally accepted that the vaccines available are of such dubious advantage that they are recommended only when a serious problem exists.

REVIEW LITERATURE

Bagust, T. J. (1971). The equine herpesviruses. Vet. Bull., 41, 79.
McGee, W. R. (1970). Proc. 2nd int. Conf. equine infect. Dis., Paris, 1969, pp. 13–17 et seq.

REFERENCES

(1) Bagust, T. J. et al. (1972). Aust. vet. J., 48, 47.
(2) McCollum, W. H. et al. (1962). Cornell Vet., 52, 164.
(3) Plummer, G. & Waterson, A. P. (1963). Virology, 19, 412.
(4) Jones, T. C. & Maurer, F. D. (1943). Amer. J. vet. Res., 4, 15.
(5) Turner, A. J. et al. (1970). Aust. vet. J., 46, 90.
(6) Duxbury, A. E. & Oxer, D. T. (1968). Aust. vet. J., 44, 58.
(7) Studdert, M. J. et al. (1970). Aust. vet. J., 46, 83, 90.
(8) Saxegaard, F. (1966). Nord. Vet.-Med., 18, 504.
(9) Bitsch, V. & Dam, A. (1971). Acta vet. scand., 12, 134.
(10) Dalsgaard, H. (1970). Medlemsbl. danske Dyrlægeforen., 53, 71.
(11) Jackson, T. A. & Kendrick, J. W. (1971). J. Amer. vet. med. Ass., 158, 1351.
(12) Bryans, J. T. (1964). Proc. 101st ann. gen. Mtg Amer. vet. med. Ass., pp. 112–21.
(13) Petzoldt, K. (1970). Dtsch. tierärztl. Wschr., 77, 162.
(14) Mayr, A. et al. (1968). Zbl. vet. Med., 15B, 406; (1970). Proc. 2nd int. Conf. equine infect. Dis., Paris, 1969, pp. 41–5.

Equine Viral Arteritis (EVA)

This disease of horses is caused by a specific virus and is manifested clinically by an acute, upper respiratory tract infection and by abortion in mares. It is characterized by specific lesions in the small arteries.

Incidence

Although information about equine viral arteritis comes largely from the U.S.A., the disease appears to be widespread. In natural outbreaks it occurs most commonly in mares in breeding studs and, although the illness is a severe one, the mortality rate is low, the chief cause of loss being the high rate of abortions (1).

Although the mortality rate is very low in natural outbreaks, it may be as high as 33 per cent in the experimental disease. The abortion rate is commonly 50 per cent in natural and experimental cases. Horses of all age groups are susceptible. The disease spreads rapidly in a group of susceptible horses, and although the course is short, an outbreak in a group of horses may persist for a number of weeks.

The proportion of the cases diagnosed clinically as 'influenza' in horses which are caused by the EVA virus is unknown, although equine viral rhinopneumonitis appears to be the more common cause of both upper respiratory tract infection and of abortion in mares.

Aetiology

A herpes virus is the cause of the disease. It is not inactivated by penicillin or streptomycin and cannot be grown on egg embryos or be propagated in experimental animals, nor does it cause haemagglutination. It can be attenuated by serial passage through tissue culture and the resulting virus is capable of causing strong immunity in vaccinated horses. The virus resists freezing but not heat. It has no relationship to human or porcine influenza viruses and only one antigenic type of the virus is known to occur.

Transmission

Details of transmission in field outbreaks are not available, but it is presumed that infection occurs by ingestion of contaminated material or by inhalation of droplets derived from infected horses, either from nasal exudate or aborted material. The disease is usually spread by direct contact, the infected animal remaining infective for about 8 to 10 days. The tissues and fluids of infected aborted foetuses contain large quantities of virus.

Pathogenesis

The necropsy findings suggest that this is a viral septicaemia causing severe vascular damage, especially in the small arteries and in the intestinal tract, the visceral lymph nodes, and the adrenals (4). A haemorrhagic enteritis results and causes diarrhoea and abdominal pain. Pulmonary oedema and pleural effusion occur and are manifested by severe dyspnoea. Petechiation of the mucosae and the conjunctiva, and oedema of the limbs also occur. Death, when it occurs, is due to a combination of dehydration and anoxia (5).

Clinical Findings

An incubation period of 1 to 6 days is followed by the appearance of fever (39 to 41°C or 102 to 106°F), a serious nasal discharge which may become purulent and be accompanied in some horses by congestion and petechiation of the nasal mucosa, conjunctivitis, excessive lacrimation developing to purulent discharge, keratitis, palpebral oedema and blepharospasm. Opacity of the aqueous humour and petechiation of the conjunctiva may also occur. Cough and dyspnoea develop and the latter is extreme in severely affected animals in which pulmonary oedema and congestion occur. The appetite is reduced or absent and in severe cases abdominal pain and diarrhoea occur due to enteritis. In these animals there may be jaundice. Oedema of the limbs is common and more marked in stabled horses than those at pasture. Depression is usual and varies in degree with the severity of the syndrome. The disease is acute and severe and deaths may occur without secondary bacterial invasion. In these cases dehydration, muscle weakness and prostration develop quickly. The course in nonfatal cases is usually within the range of 3 to 8 days. Secondary bacterial invasion is usually manifested by a catarrhal rhinitis and infection of the respiratory tract. In stallions there is often oedema of the prepuce and scrotum. Abortion occurs within a few days of the onset of clinical illness, as distinct from the much later abortions which occur in EVR, and is recorded between the 160th and 300th day of pregnancy and 12 to 30 days after exposure. The abortion is not foreshadowed by premonitory signs, and the placenta is not retained.

Clinical Pathology

Complement fixation and serum neutralization tests are available for serological diagnosis and tissue culture techniques are available for isolation of the virus (3).

There is a pronounced leucopenia due to depression of the lymphocytes and to a less extent of the neutrophils, occurring usually 1 to 3 days after the onset of fever. The virus is present in the blood during the febrile period and the disease can be transmitted to susceptible horses.

Necropsy Findings

Gross lesions include oedema of the eyelids, congestion and petechiation of the upper respiratory tract, oedema of the lungs and mediastinum, pleural and peritoneal effusion, petechiae on the serous surfaces, oedema of viscera, catarrhal and haemorrhagic inflammation of the intestinal mucosa, haemorrhage and infarction in the spleen and degeneration in the liver and kidneys. There are characteristic histological changes in the small arteries.

The virus can be isolated from the lung and spleen of aborted foetuses and from the spleen of dead animals, but there are no inclusion bodies or specific lesions in the foetus.

Diagnosis

The disease is much more severe than equine viral rhinopneumonitis and equine influenza, but in individual animals differentiation may be difficult except by laboratory examination using complement-fixation or serum protection tests. The histological lesion of arteritis is characteristic of this disease and serves to differentiate it from equine infectious anaemia, which is also accompanied by petechiation of the mucosae and jaundice in acute cases. Leptospirosis may present a rather similar clinical picture also. In purpura haemorrhagica the subcutaneous effusions contain blood and serum, are not confined to the limbs, and histologically there are septic thrombi in local veins. Clinical signs and lesions are similar to African horse sickness but the diseases have not occurred in the same area and can be distinguished serologically.

As a cause of equine abortion it can be diagnosed only by isolation of the virus. The known bacterial causes of equine abortion, *Salm. abortivoequina* and *Str. genitalium* should be eliminated by cultural examination and EVR should be eliminated as far as is possible by histological examination of the foetus and isolation of the virus.

Treatment and Control

The same general principles of treatment and control as apply to EVR can be applied in this disease. An effective, live, attenuated vaccine is available commercially and is regarded as being without risk. One vaccination protects indefinitely (2).

REFERENCES

(1) Bryans, J. T. (1964). *Proc. 101st ann. gen. Mtg Amer. vet. med. Ass.*, pp. 112–21.
(2) McCollum, W. H. (1970). *Proc. 2nd int. Conf. equine infect. Dis., Paris*, 1969, pp. 143–51 *et prec.*
(3) Burki, F. (1970). *Proc. 2nd int. Conf. equine infect. Dis., Paris*, 1969, pp. 125–29 *et seq.*
(4) Crawford, T. B. (1969). *Fed. Proc.*, *28*, 685.
(5) Estes, P. C. & Cheville, N. F. (1970). *Amer. J. Path.*, *58*, 235.

Equine Influenza

(*Infectious Equine Bronchitis, Laryngotracheobronchitis, Newmarket Cough, Hoppengarten Cough, Infectious Equine Cough*).

This is an infectious respiratory disease caused by a virus and characterized by mild fever and a severe, persistent cough. The name equine influenza is now restricted to those respiratory infections of horses caused by viruses belonging to the influenza family. Whether it will include all the clinically similar diseases which are recorded, and listed as alternate names in this section, is undecided.

Incidence

The disease is reported from most countries and, although it is not serious in itself, it causes much inconvenience in racing stables because affected horses have to break training. One of the more annoying aspects of the disease is its poor response to most forms of treatment.

Although clinically similar diseases have occurred as explosive outbreaks in most countries, for many years equine influenza was not recognized as a specific disease entity until the mid-1950s. In 1963 major epidemics of respiratory disease, affecting 50 to 90 per cent of horses in some areas, occurred in the United Kingdom and the U.S.A. The causative viruses were identified as myxovirus influenza A/Equi 1 (IA/E1) in the U.K. and this virus and influenza A/Equi 2 (IA/E2) in the U.S.A. (4, 8). At the time investigations failed to reveal the presence of IA/E2 in the U.K., but in 1965 a new outbreak due to this virus did occur (1). A major outbreak due to an unidentified virus occurred in Germany in 1961 (6) and positive serological evidence of infection with influenza virus was obtained in France and Poland in 1963 (7, 9). The magnitude of these outbreaks might have suggested that the equine population in which they occurred were being exposed to a new virus for the first time. However, outbreaks of a clinically similar disease have occurred at intervals in the preceding years and antibodies to the viruses have been detected in the sera of horses collected 15 years earlier (3). Both influenza viruses are known to have infected horses in the U.S.A. for many years. Nowadays most cases of the disease occur in 2 year old or younger horses, probably because horses of 3 years of age or older are immune (20). It is probable that the outbreaks occur as a result of a natural accumulation of young animals which have not been previously exposed (10). There appears to be a high incidence of infection without clinical signs (12).

Aetiology

The two identified causative myxoviruses, IA/E1 and IA/E2, are serologically distinct and there is some difference between the two diseases which result, that caused by IA/E2 being rather more severe especially with respect to pulmonary involvement in the form of a non-bacterial pneumonitis (18). All age groups of horses, including new-born foals are susceptible. There is some evidence that human strains of influenza virus can infect horses (11) and an influenza-like illness and related antibody responses have occurred in humans infected experimentally with IA/E2 virus (5, 14). Experimental infections have been produced in horses with the human Hong-Kong variant of the human influenza virus (15). In horses the mortality rate, in the absence of complications, is nil. After infection immunity to the homologous subtype of the virus is present, and may persist for up to 2 years (22).

By analogy with the human disease the transmission of equine influenza is expected to occur by droplet inhalation over short distances, but spread via infected fomites may also occur. In aerosol form the equine influenza virus survives longer (24 to 36 hours) than human or porcine strains (15 hours) (13). The duration of infectivity of affected horses is unknown. Most outbreaks occur during the summer months and this may be related to the greater movement of horses at this time.

Clinical Findings

Clinically the disease is ushered in by fever (38·5 to 41 °C or 101 to 106 °F) after an incubation period of 2 to 3 days. The dominating sign is cough, which is dry and hacking in the beginning and moist later, and which commences soon after the temperature rise and lasts for 1 to 3 weeks. Nasal discharge is not a prominent sign and, if it occurs, is watery only. There is no marked swelling of the submaxillary lymph nodes but they may be painful on palpation in the early stages of the disease. Lassitude, immobility and anorexia are inconstant accompaniments and stiffness and difficulty or clumsiness in rising or lying also occur. Horses that are protected against environmental stress pursue an uncomplicated course, but horses that are worked or transported or exposed to adverse climatic conditions may experience a worsening of the cough, and severe bronchitis, pneumonia and oedema of the legs may develop. Young foals, especially those which are foaled while the mare is clinically affected, may develop a severe bronchopneumonia with streptococci and *Escherichia coli* present in the lungs at necropsy. The foal is normal until the 4th to 5th day and then develops a high fever (40·5°C or 105°F), severe dyspnoea with signs of bronchopneumonia on auscultation, and a respiratory rate of 80 to 90 per minute. Death is usual after a course of about 4 days (2).

Clinical Pathology

Isolation of the virus is desirable for a definitive diagnosis, but a rise in antibody titre in paired sera collected three weeks apart is acceptable as evidence of infection. The serological tests available include the complement fixation test, the haemagglutination-inhibition test, and the serum neutralization test (19). A test using a fluorescent antibody technique is available and isolation of the virus in chick embryo is a good diagnostic aid (21).

Necropsy Findings

The characteristic lesion is a bronchiolitis which is accompanied by a profuse serous discharge which later becomes mucoid and tends to accumulate in bronchioles.

Diagnosis

Equine influenza resembles equine viral rhinopneumonitis and equine viral arteritis sufficiently to require laboratory assistance in diagnosis. Laboratory examination is also necessary to ensure that any vaccines used in control programmes contain the local virus.

Treatment and Control

Little information is available on methods of treatment. Hyperimmune serum appears to have some therapeutic efficiency and may also be of value in prophylaxis, especially in foals which are unlikely to have received passive immunity via their dam's colostrum. Heavy doses of broad-spectrum antibiotics seem logical as prophylaxis against secondary bacterial infections in foals.

Hygienic precautions can be of value in limiting the spread of the disease. Vehicles used for the transport of horses are thought to play a large part in transmission and should be thoroughly disinfected between shipments (2). The massive movement of horses from place to place for many purposes encourages the rapid spread of the disease, and the isolation of introduced animals is an essential precaution, especially when an outbreak is in progress. The degree of isolation required cannot be specified because of lack of basic information, but it is suggested that droplet infection can occur over a distance of 32 metres and that maximum security with regard to clothing, utensils and personnel must be practised (2).

Vaccination with killed viruses produces high levels of antibodies and this procedure has been utilized to develop a satisfactory vaccination programme (10). The aim of the programme is to immunize the young horses before they go to training establishments. This is done by vaccinating young horses twice at intervals of 6 to 12 weeks. Subsequent annual booster shots are recommended because of the much higher antibody levels obtained at the second year (16). On breeding farms all horses should be vaccinated similarly in the first instance; in subsequent years only the foals are vaccinated just before weaning. The vaccine should contain the virus or viruses which occur in the area as cross-immunity between the sero-types does not occur.

Some consideration is being given to the importance of inducing nasal antibody production by parenteral vaccination. Inactivated vaccines are poor in this respect but the inclusion of sufficient antigen and a suitable adjuvant, such as sodium alginate, in the vaccine makes it possible to produce significant levels of nasal antibody (17).

REVIEW LITERATURE

McQueen, J. L. *et al.* (1968). *Advanc. vet. Sci.*, *12*, 285. Academic Press, Inc., New York.

REFERENCES

(1) Beveridge, W. B. (1965). *Vet. Rec.*, 77, 427.
(2) Miller, W. M. (1965). *Vet. Rec.*, 77, 455.
(3) Beveridge, W. I. B. *et al.* (1965). *Vet. Rec.*, 77, 57.
(4) Wilson, J. C. (1965). *Amer. J. vet. Res.*, 26, 1466.
(5) Couch, R. B. *et al.* (1969). *Nature (Lond.)*, 224, 512.
(6) Bohm, H. O. & Straub, O. C. (1963). *Proc. 17th World vet. Congr., Hanover*, 1, 451.
(7) Cateigne, G. *et al.* (1963). *Bull. Acad. vét. Fr.*, 36, 399.
(8) Scholtens, R. G. *et al.* (1964). *Publ. Hlth Rep., Wash.*, 79, 393, 398.

(9) Woyciechowska, A. & Grzelakowa, A. (1963). *Proc. 17th World vet. Congr., Hanover*, *1*, 545.

(10) Bryans, J. T. (1966). *J. Amer. vet. med. Ass.*, *148*, 413.

(11) Kasel, J. A. *et al.* (1968). *Nature (Lond.)*, *219*, 968.

(12) Lief, F. S. & Cohen, D. (1965). *Amer. J. Epidem.*, *82*, 225.

(13) Mitchell, C. A. & Guerin, L. F. (1972). *Canad. J. comp. Med.*, *36*, 9.

(14) Kasel, J. A. & Couch, R. B. (1969). *Bull. Wld Hlth Org.*, *41*, 447.

(15) Todd, J. D. *et al.* (1970). *Amer. J. Epidem.*, *92*, 330.

(16) Pressler, K. (1970). *Zbl. vet. Med.*, *17B*, 1003.

(17) Rouse, B. T. (1971). *Aust. vet. J.*, *47*, 146.

(18) Gerber, H. (1970). *Proc. 2nd int. Conf. equine infect. Dis., Paris*, 1969, pp. 63–80 *et seq.*

(19) Fontaine, M. P. *et al.* (1970). *Proc. 2nd int. Conf. equine infect. Dis., Paris*, 1969, pp. 99–104.

(20) Bryans, J. T. *et al.* (1967). *Amer. J. vet. Res.*, *28*, 9.

(21) Masurel, N. *et al.* (1968). *Tr. Diergeneesk.*, *93*, 1019.

(22) Beveridge, W. I. B. & Rose, M. A. (1967). *Brit. vet. J.*, *123*, 8.

Infectious Equine Pneumonia (IEP)

Infectious equine pneumonia is a highly fatal disease characterized by severe lobar pneumonia, high fever and septicaemia.

Incidence

The disease is now rare but used to be a fairly common occurrence when large numbers of animals were brought together from various sources and kept under poor conditions of nutrition or housing. It was particularly likely to occur in horses on board ship, especially when they were purchased and brought together just prior to embarkation.

The mortality rate in individual horses or horses kept in small groups is low, but in large groups kept under unfavourable conditions, 20 per cent of affected animals may die. Although the disease is infectious, the rate of spread is slow at first and it may take several weeks for the outbreak to build up to serious proportions.

Aetiology

The primary cause is a virus but the serious nature of the disease appears to be due largely to secondary bacterial invaders including streptococci, staphylococci, pasteurellae and pseudomonads. The relationship of the causative virus to those known to cause upper respiratory infection in horses is not clear, but the same clinical disease occurs in complicated cases of equine influenza (1). Exposure, fatigue, poor nutrition and overcrowding are recognized as important predisposing causes.

Transmission

Spread of the disease is presumed to be largely by inhalation of infected droplets and possibly by ingestion.

Pathogenesis

There appears to be a preliminary viral septicaemia with a mild systemic reaction, followed by the development of an acute lobar pneumonia and pleurisy with severe respiratory signs. Death is due to a combination of toxaemia and anoxia.

Clinical Findings

After a long incubation period of up to 30 days there is a primary fever with increased pulse rate but little change in respiration. In the early stages the clinical picture is so mild that affected horses may not be noticed and be subjected to exposure or overwork during this period, enhancing the possibility that serious pneumonia will develop. After several days severe respiratory signs, including a painful moist cough, dyspnoea and a thin, red-stained, serous, nasal discharge, appear. The temperature rises, the horse is depressed and anorexia is complete. Auscultation of the chest reveals the development of congestion followed by exudation and finally consolidation. Initially there is an increased vesicular murmur which is replaced by moist râles and finally by absence of breath sounds except for harsh bronchial tones. A pleuritic friction rub may be present in the early stages. The presence of an extremely foetid breath indicates the development of pulmonary gangrene.

With adequate treatment recovery is complete in 7 to 10 days, but the prognosis is grave in severe cases and those in which gangrene develops. Animals returned to work before recovery is complete are likely to develop severe complications.

Clinical Pathology

The most useful laboratory examination comprises culture from a nasal swab to determine the presence of secondary bacterial invaders and their susceptibility to the common antibacterial drugs.

Necropsy Findings

The lungs may show acute congestion, consolidation or gangrene, depending upon the stage at which the animal dies. Distribution of the pneumonia is lobar and involves particularly the diaphragmatic lobes. The pleura is thickened and covered with fibrin and the pleural cavity contains large quantities of reddish, turbid fluid. Degenerative changes in the kidney and liver and widespread petechial haemorrhages are common accompaniments of the pulmonary lesions. The virus can be isolated from the lungs only in the early stages of the disease.

Diagnosis

Because the disease exists only as a clinical entity a positive diagnosis is impossible. When an infectious pneumonia appears in a group of horses this diagnosis is the logical one, but it should be remembered that the primary cause may be one of the upper respiratory tract viruses. Strangles may be complicated by the occurrence of pneumonia in some animals, but the characteristic signs of purulent nasal discharge and lymph node abscessation usually make clinical differentiation easy.

Treatment

The general treatment and nursing care for animals affected with pneumonia will apply. Specific treatment must be guided by the sensitivity of the bacteria which cause the serious complications. Penicillin is usually adequate, as most bacterial infections in horses are streptococcal or staphylococcal. When valuable animals are involved, a broad spectrum antibiotic to control the less common organisms is probably advisable. Parenteral treatment with sulphonamide drugs still has a place in the treatment of this disease and has given comparable or better results than the antibiotics (2).

Control

Hygiene, including isolation of infected animals, disinfection of premises and the treatment of early cases, is the only available control measure. Correction of defects in housing, nutrition and general management will do much to reduce the ravages of the disease.

REFERENCES

(1) Maurer, F. D. & Jones, T. C. (1943). *Amer. J. vet. Res., 4,* 257.
(2) Rogers, A. C. (1947). *Vet. Med., 42,* 363.

Arabian Foal Pneumonia

A highly fatal disease which appears to be limited to Arabian foals has been reported from Australia (1) and the United States (2).

The morbidity rate among exposed foals is relatively low but the mortality rate approaches 100 per cent. The disease begins with upper respiratory signs progressing to pneumonia which does not respond to the usual therapy. Diarrhoea occurs frequently and there may be shallow ulcers in the mouth. Lymphopenia is a constant finding.

There are characteristic inclusion bodies in epithelial cells and an adenovirus has been isolated frequently from affected foals along with secondary bacterial invaders. However, a recent report associating this disease with a defective thymus and hypogammaglobulinaemia points to the probability of a primary immunodeficiency disorder being involved (3). The pattern of incidence of the disease, combined with the relatively narrow genetic base of the Arabian breed, lends support to the theory that the immunodeficiency may be genetically mediated.

REFERENCES

(1) Johnston, K. G. & Hutchins, D. R. (1967). *Aust. vet. J., 43,* 600.
(2) McChesney, A. E. *et al.* (1970). *Path. Vet., 7,* 547.
(3) McGuire, T. S. & Poppie, M. J. (1973). *W.S.U. Animal Health Notes, 13,* No. 1.

Swine Influenza

Swine influenza is a specific, highly contagious disease of pigs characterized clinically by fever and signs of respiratory involvement. The disease is not usually fatal.

Incidence

Swine influenza first appeared in the U.S.A. immediately following the 1918 pandemic of human influenza, and it was generally believed that it was caused by adaptation of the human influenza virus to swine. The disease still occurs in the U.S.A., but apparently with decreasing frequency. It has also been reported from the U.K., and a number of European countries as ferkelgrippe, although in the latter instance the virus has not been identified as identical with that causing swine influenza in the U.S.A. (1).

The disease occurs in the form of explosive outbreaks with a high morbidity rate but with a low mortality rate of less than 4 per cent. Loss of condition is marked and ordinarily this is the principal cause of financial loss, although on occasions death losses may be extensive if the pigs are kept under bad husbandry conditions or if secondary bacterial infections develop. Abortions and deaths of new-born pigs have also been reported as causes of loss in this disease.

Aetiology

The disease is caused by concurrent infection with two agents, an influenza virus and *Haemo-*

philus suis. By itself the virus produces only a mild illness and *Haem. suis* is a common inhabitant of the upper respiratory tract of normal swine. Together, under favourable climatic conditions, these agents are capable of producing swine influenza. Although pigs of all ages may be affected, the disease is often confined to young pigs. Outbreaks occur mainly during the cold months of the year, commencing in the late autumn or early winter and terminating with a few outbreaks in early spring. Several days of inclement weather often precede an outbreak. The virus is cultivable in tissue culture (2).

Concurrent heavy infestation with migrating *Ascaris suum* larvae or *Metastrongylus* spp. (3) greatly exacerbates the severity of an influenza attack and it is probable that other parasites or infectious agents provoke a similar response.

Transmission

When an outbreak occurs, most of the pigs in the herd are affected within a few days, which suggests that all animals are previously infected and the interference of some external factor, probably inclement weather, precipitates the outbreak. The very rapid spread of infection from pig to pig is via the inhalation of infected droplets. The virus may be carried over from year to year in swine lungworm (*Metastrongylus* spp.) (4) and the bacterium persists in the respiratory tract of recovered swine.

Pathogenesis

Swine influenza is primarily a disease of the upper respiratory tract, the trachea and bronchi being particularly involved, but secondary lesions may develop in the lung because of the drainage of copious exudate from the bronchi. These lesions disappear rapidly, leaving little or no residual damage. This is in contradistinction to the lesions of enzootic pneumonia of pigs which persist for very long periods. Secondary pneumonia, usually due to infection with *Pasteurella multocida*, occurs in some cases and is the cause of most fatalities.

Clinical Findings

After an incubation period of 2 to 7 days the disease appears suddenly with a high proportion of the herd showing fever (up to 41·5°C or 107°F), anorexia and severe prostration. The animal is disinclined to move or to rise because of muscle stiffness and pain. Laboured, jerky breathing ('thumps') is accompanied by sneezing and a deep, painful cough which often occurs in paroxysms. There is congestion of the conjunctivae with a watery ocular and nasal discharge. In general the severity of the illness appears greater than in fact it is and after a course of 4 to 6 days signs disappear rapidly depending, in part, on the level of colostral antibody (7). However, there is much loss of weight which is slowly regained. Clonic convulsions are common in the terminal stages in fatal cases.

Clinical Pathology

A moderate leucopenia develops in the early stages and recovered animals can be identified by a virus-neutralization and a haemagglutination-inhibition test.

Necropsy Findings

The outstanding lesions are in the upper respiratory tract. Swelling and marked oedema of cervical and mediastinal lymph nodes are evident. There is congestion of the mucosae of the pharynx, larynx, trachea and bronchi, and much tenacious, colourless, frothy exudate is present in the air passages. Copious exudate in the bronchi is accompanied by collapse of the ventral parts of the lungs. This atelectasis is extensive and often irregularly distributed, although the apical and cardiac lobes are most affected, and the right lung more so than the left. The lesions are clearly demarcated, dark red to purple in colour and leathery in consistency. Surrounding the atelectatic areas the lung is often emphysematous and may show many petechial haemorrhages. The gross pulmonary lesions are very similar to those of enzootic pneumonia of pigs, but there is a great deal of difference in the histological lesions in the two diseases. There is often moderate to severe engorgement of the spleen and severe hyperaemia of the gastric mucosa, especially along the greater curvature. Patchy congestion and mild catarrhal exudation occurs in the large intestine, but there are no erosions of the mucosa.

Diagnosis

The explosive appearance of an upper respiratory syndrome, including conjunctivitis, sneezing and coughing with a low mortality rate, serves to differentiate swine influenza from the other common respiratory diseases of swine. Of these enzootic pneumonia of pigs is most commonly confused with swine influenza, but it is more insidious in its onset and chronic in its course. Hog cholera is manifested by less respiratory involvement and a high mortality rate. Outbreaks of inclusion body rhinitis in piglets may resemble swine influenza quite closely, but atrophic rhinitis has a much longer course and is accompanied by characteristic distortion of the facial bones.

Treatment

No specific treatment is available. Treatment with penicillin, sulphadimidine, or preferably a wide spectrum antibiotic, may be of value in controlling possible secondary invaders. The provision of comfortable, well-bedded quarters, free from dust, is of major importance. Clean drinking water should be available, but feed should be limited during the first few days of convalescence.

Control

Control is difficult because of the intervention of lungworms as intermediate hosts. Good housing and protection from inclement weather help to prevent the occurrence of severe outbreaks. Once the disease has appeared little can be done to prevent spread to other pigs. Recovered animals are immune to subsequent infection for up to 3 months (7). An inactivated, formalized, avianized vaccine with adjuvant has been produced (5). A method of eradication similar to that used in the control of enzootic pneumonia and atrophic rhinitis has been recorded as giving good results in the eradication of swine influenza (6).

REVIEW LITERATURE

McQueen, J. L. (1968). *Advanc. vet. Sci.*, *12*, 305.

REFERENCES

(1) Hjärre, A. (1958). *Advanc. vet. Sci.*, *4*, 235.
(2) Nakamura, R. M. & Easterday, B. C. (1970). *Cornell Vet.*, *60*, 27.
(3) Nayak, D. P. *et al.* (1964). *Cornell Vet.*, *54*, 160.
(4) Shope, R. E. (1955). *J. exp. Med.*, *102*, 567.
(5) Rweyemamu, M. M. (1970). *Vet. Bull.*, *40*, 73.
(6) Kubin, G. (1953). *Wein. tierärztl. Mschr.*, *40*, 332.
(7) Easterday, B. C. (1972). *J. Amer. vet. med. Ass.*, *160*, 645.

Inclusion Body Rhinitis of Swine

Inclusion body rhinitis is a viral disease of young pigs which has been identified in most countries (1, 2, 3, 4). The infection has been suggested as a precursor to atrophic rhinitis but is not a necessary precursor. In infected herds the morbidity and the mortality rates are high and may reach 100 and 50 per cent respectively.

Clinically there is a sudden onset of sneezing, dyspnoea, and a purulent nasal discharge. The pigs do not eat and rotation of the head occurs in some. When the infection is first introduced into a herd, animals of all ages may be affected, but only young pigs and pregnant sows show signs of severe illness (5).

Inclusion bodies are present in the epithelial cells of the nasal mucosa, and examination of nasal swabs from living animals or tissues from dead ones is an important part of the diagnosis of the disease (6). From living animals swabs are taken from the ventral nasal meatus, smears made as soon as possible and stained. The inclusion bodies disappear about 2 weeks after infection and swabs need to be taken early in the course of the disease, preferably on day 18 after infection (8).

The disease is probably identical with 'cytomegalic inclusion body disease' (7), and some growth of the causative virus is obtainable on tissue culture (8). No treatment is attempted and no satisfactory control programme has been developed. The difficulty in preventing the introduction of the disease into a country is illustrated by its introduction into Britain. Outbreaks may not commence until 6 months after pigs are introduced and a prolonged period of quarantine is essential (5).

REFERENCES

(1) Done, J. T. (1955). *Vet. Rec.*, *67*, 525.
(2) Harding, J. D. J. (1958). *Amer. J. vet. Res.*, *19*, 907.
(3) Mitchell, D. & Corner, A. H. (1958). *Canad. J. comp. Med.*, *22*, 199.
(4) Cohrs, P. (1959). *Dtsch. tierärztl. Wschr.*, *66*, 605.
(5) Cameron-Stephens, I. D. (1961). *Aust. vet. J.*, *37*, 87 & 91.
(6) Done, J. T. (1958). *Vet. Rec.*, *70*, 877.
(7) Corner, A. H. *et al.* (1964). *J. comp. Path.*, *74*, 192.
(8) Booth, J. C. *et al.* (1967). *Res. vet. Sci.*, *7*, 338, 346.

Viral Pneumonia of Calves

Viral pneumonia of calves is a highly infectious, mild disease commonly converted to a more serious disease by secondary bacterial invasion of the lungs.

Incidence

Pneumonia of calves is much more common in countries where animals are housed during the winter months, but it occurs at varying levels of incidence in most countries. The disease may be enzootic on particular farms or occur as epizootics, and the morbidity and mortality rates vary considerably with the conditions of housing, the general care of the calves and the types of bacteria which occur as secondary invaders. An incidence of 25 per cent has been recorded in an enzootic area. The morbidity rate may reach 100 per cent and mortality rate 50 per cent in severe outbreaks. Virus pneumonia is in itself a relatively mild disease and its main importance is its role as producer of primary pneumonia, permitting serious bacterial pneumonia to develop.

Aetiology

Viruses isolated from pneumonic lungs of calves and capable of causing pneumonia have been reported from many countries (1). The virus isolated most commonly from the lungs of calves with viral pneumonia in most countries is parainfluenza 3 (PI3) or SF4 (shipping fever 4) myxovirus (2) and this virus is capable of causing typical lesions and clinical signs in young calves and Indian buffaloes (3). The respiratory disease caused by PI3 virus is severe only if the calf is exposed to stress, but secondary bacterial pneumonia is common. There is a rise of specific antibody level during the course of the disease and colostral antibody titres disappear at 3 to 8 months, the optimum time for vaccination (4, 5). Surveys to determine how widespread the infection is have indicated exposure to infection in up to 80 per cent of some cattle populations (6, 7, 8). The infection is also common in sheep and is transmissible between the two species.

Other viruses known to be capable of causing pneumonia in calves are adenoviruses and a reovirus (9, 10). Adenoviruses, bovine types 1 and 2, cause gross lesions with minimal clinical signs of nasal and ocular discharge and moderate diarrhoea. Inclusion bodies are present in bronchial and alveolar epithelium (11). A rhinovirus has also been used to cause pneumonia experimentally (12), and a reovirus of bovine and human origin can cause extensive pneumonia in calves (13) but these probably act as facilitators or exacerbators rather than primary agents. Combined with *Bedsonia* spp. they produce a more severe disease (14). There are many reports of *Bedsonia/Chlamydia* spp. as causes of calf pneumonia (15, 16). Most reports are of gross lesions without clinical signs (17, 18). Diagnosis is possible by a complement fixation test (19). Mixed infections of virus and chlamydia or of PI3 virus, IBR virus and mucosal disease virus are not uncommon in young cattle which are shipped to feed-lots. In most of the diseases referred to above there is an enteritis as well as the pneumonia, but the role of the virus in the production of calf scours is uncertain. Certainly many sporadic cases and severe outbreaks of calf pneumonia occur without scouring being present as a major part of the syndrome.

The widespread occurrence of viral pneumonia and the multiplicity of bacteria found in calf pneumonia suggest that the greater majority of cases may be primarily due to the virus infection.

It has been suggested that a viral pneumonia is the predisposing cause of most cases of shipping fever caused by *Past. multocida* in North America. *Past. multocida* is the common bacterial infection encountered in pneumonia in young cattle but *Mycoplasma* spp., are being observed more and more frequently and are thought to have aetiological significance in many outbreaks. *Cor. pyogenes*, *Sphaerophorus necrophorus*, *Staph. aureus*, *Actinobacillus actinoides*, *E. coli*, *Haem.* spp., *Bord. bronchiseptica* and pleuropneumonia-like organisms are also found. A proportion of cases are bacteriologically sterile.

Many predisposing causes are considered to be important in the development of calf pneumonia. Overcrowding in barns, especially when the humidity is high or the barn is draughty, exposure to bad weather when the calf is not accustomed to it, transport in draughty vehicles, chilling due to any cause, debilitation due to other diseases, particularly scours, and raising calves in large groups are considered to be most important. The disease also occurs in calves raised outdoors and in these circumstances is most severe when the calves are reared in overcrowded, unhygienic surroundings. It is rarely if ever seen in cattle raised under extensive, ranching conditions. Most cases occur in calves which are 1 to 4 months old, but the disease can occur during the first week of life. Calves recovered from virus pneumonia are resistant to reinfection and those over 6 months of age also appear to be highly resistant.

Transmission

Experimentally the disease can be transmitted with bacteria-free filtrates by intravenous injection and intranasal instillation. Transmission also occurs by contact, and serial passage of the virus has been effected with blood taken at the height of the fever. American workers have found the virus in the lungs of healthy, adult cattle, which probably act as carriers. They also observed a high concentration of protective substances in the colostrum and found a marked increase in the resistance of calves to the virus by the second to third day of life. Inhalation appears to be the obvious portal of entry.

Pathogenesis

Viral pneumonia typically affects the anterior lobes of the lung with a mainly interstitial pneumonia resulting. This pneumonia of itself is usually of minor importance and causes only slight clinical signs, although in some cases the pneumonic changes may be extensive enough to produce severe clinical pneumonia. In this instance there is often a marked absence of toxaemia compared with a bacterial pneumonia. After the primary viral pneumonia is established, bacterial invasion may occur and the resulting pneumonia will vary with the species of bacteria which are present. Secondary bacterial pneumonias usually respond to treatment, although relapses are common if the viral pneumonia is extensive. In animals where there is an uncomplicated viral pneumonia with very extensive lesions there may be minimal clinical signs and almost complete resolution.

Clinical Findings

Irrespective of the identity of the causative virus the clinical picture in all viral pneumonias of calves is very similar (1). In the experimental disease a febrile reaction, accompanied by constipation, occurs about the 5th day and is followed by the appearance of rhinitis, pneumonia and diarrhoea. The fever is moderate only (40 to 40·5°C or 104 to 105°F). A harsh, hacking cough, easily stimulated by pinching the trachea, is characteristic.

In field cases the clinical picture is much the same, although the temperature tends to be higher. This may be due to bacterial invasion in the very early stages. The nasal discharge is only moderate in amount and is mucopurulent. On auscultation of the chest the major abnormalities can be detected over the ventral aspects of the apical and cardiac lobes. The breath sounds are loud and harsh and represent bronchial tones transmitted through consolidated lung. The heart beat may be audible more clearly than usual because of shrinkage of lung tissue in the cardiac area. Some peracute cases of uncomplicated viral pneumonia die within a few hours, although cases of average severity usually recover in 4 to 7 days.

When secondary bacterial invasion occurs, the reaction, including the temperature rise, the dyspnoea and the toxaemia, is usually more severe. When secondary infection with *Past. multocida* occurs the temperature rises to 41 to 41·5°C (106 to 107°F), the area of lung affected is much increased, and increased breath sounds due to congestion are followed by loud râles and a pleuritic friction rub. These cases usually respond rapidly to adequate treatment. When *Cor. pyogenes* is the secondary invader, consolidation is marked, there is a profound toxaemia and an absence of moist râles. In cases where *Sph. necrophorus* is present the clinical findings are similar and pulmonary abscesses are likely to develop. Necrotic lesions are often present in the mouth and pharynx in these cases and the pulmonary infec-

tion probably originates from here. With both of these latter infections there may be some response to antibiotic treatment, but there is a predisposition to relapse soon after treatment is terminated. Coughing, dyspnoea, anorexia and emaciation continue and the animal eventually has to be destroyed.

Clinical Pathology

Nasal swabs should be taken to determine the bacteria present and their sensitivity to various drugs, particularly when a number of calves are involved in an outbreak. A haemagglutination inhibition test is in general use for the identification of infection with parainfluenza 3 virus. The presence of a rising titre in H.1 antibodies to P13 virus is considered to be positive evidence of recent infection. A fluorescent antibody technique has been reported as a diagnostic aid (20) and tissue culture is available (21).

Necropsy Findings

In uncomplicated viral pneumonia, irrespective of the specific cause, there are areas of collapse with little bronchiolar reaction, accompanied by emphysema in the apical lobes and to a less extent in the cardiac lobes, and with little involvement of the diaphragmatic lobes. In the later stages a dark red consolidation with little or no fluid present in the lung and a hobnail appearance of the pleural surface affects most of the ventral portions of the apical and cardiac lobes. The lesions are always bilateral. Histologically there is interstitial pneumonia. The remainder of the lungs show congestion and occasionally a few haemorrhages. Acute inflammation of the nasal mucosa, particularly on the turbinate and ethmoid bones, is usually accompanied by a marked, mucopurulent exudation. A catarrhal enteritis is present occasionally and myocarditis has also been observed. In the PI3 infection intracytoplasmic inclusion bodies are widespread in the lungs; and after experimental infection, are present on the 5th day, but have disappeared by the 7th day after infection (22).

When bacterial invasion has occurred the lesions vary with the bacteria present. Extensive hepatization with mottled red and grey lobules and considerable interlobular aggregations of serofibrinous fluid, and often accompanied by a fibrinous pleurisy, is characteristic of *Past. multocida* infection. Extensive consolidation and suppuration occur with *Cor. pyogenes* and *Sph. necrophorus* infections. In the latter case there may be necrotic lesions in the mouth and upper respiratory tract.

Diagnosis

The diagnosis of pneumonia is not difficult to make, but a successful prognosis depends upon detection of the secondary bacterial invaders and their drug sensitivities. Most difficulty arises in differentiation from lungworm infestations and fog fever. Lungworm infestations occur usually in young calves at pasture, and dyspnoea, cough and nasal discharge may suggest pneumonia. There is often a mild fever because of a secondary pneumonia, but abnormalities on auscultation are limited to the dorsal and posterior parts of the lung. There is usually a good deal of emphysematous crackling and loud, moist râles. In fog fever the dyspnoea is extreme and is accompanied by a marked expiratory effort. The crackling of emphysema and a dry, pleuritic friction rub are usually audible on auscultation. Calf diphtheria may resemble pneumonia, but careful examination of the mouth usually reveals the typical, cheesy, necrotic ulcers. Bovine malignant catarrh is unusual in young animals and has characteristic mucosal involvement, and the lesions of infectious bovine rhinotracheitis are restricted to the upper respiratory tract.

Chronic cases may be confused with congenital cardiac defects and subacute enzootic muscular dystrophy, but in both cases pulmonary changes are absent and in the former there are abnormal sounds on auscultation of the heart. Acute myocardial dystrophy is accompanied by severe pulmonary oedema but is afebrile, while weakness and an absence of pulmonary changes characterize those cases in which there is extensive involvement of skeletal muscle. Non-specific pneumonias due to aspiration, and occasionally pulmonary invasion by *Dermatophilus congolense* in cases of mycotic dermatitis may also be confusing. In areas where tuberculosis occurs, prenatal infection with *Myco. tuberculosis* should be considered. An acute pneumonia of calves caused by *Kleb. pneumoniae* has been recorded in association with mastitis caused by this organism, and European workers have described a high incidence of pneumonia caused by *Str. pneumoniae*.

Treatment

Uncomplicated viral pneumonia is unlikely to respond to treatment but antibacterial treatment is essential because of the probability of secondary invasion. A broad spectrum drug should be used. Sulphadimidine (sulphamethazine) (1 g. per 15 lb. body weight) parenterally or orally gives good results. A mixture of penicillin and streptomycin is often adequate and has the virtue of being cheap and easy to administer when large numbers of uncontrolled, young animals have to be treated. Because of the wide range of bacteria likely to be encountered valuable animals are probably best treated with tetracyclines or chloramphenicol (5 mg. per lb. body weight). In some cases it may be sufficient to treat animals once only, but a proportion of cases are likely to relapse after an initial response. Such cases require repeated treatments for 3 to 5 days. If the number of relapses in an area or on a farm is excessive, all cases should receive multiple treatment and the possibility of producing an autogenous vaccine should be considered. Lung abscess should be treated by antibiotic therapy combined with parenteral enzyme treatment.

Control

Control of the disease is largely a question of hygiene and good husbandry. Overcrowding, draughty or unventilated housing, exposure to inclement weather, and sudden changes in environmental temperatures all predispose calves to the disease and should be avoided if possible. Newly purchased calves should be isolated for several weeks before being introduced to the group. Calves should be reared outdoors with open sheds for shelter where climatic conditions are suitable. Calf crates with elevated, wire mesh floors in maternity barns tend to reduce the incidence in very young calves. Infected calves should be isolated from the remainder of the group.

Calves recovered from virus pneumonia are immune and their serum can be used to provide passive immunity to other calves (23). Vaccines prepared from the parainfluenza 3 (SF4) virus have produced variable results in the prevention of pneumonia in calves (24).

Tissue culture, inactivated vaccines in adjuvant and attenuated, live, tissue culture vaccines have been produced (25). Because of the number of viruses capable of causing respiratory disease in calves a multivalent vaccine seems desirable (10). Parenteral vaccination with a killed PI3 vaccine appears to be of little value, whether in adjuvant or not (26, 27) and live virus vaccines have been similarly disappointing (28). Intranasal vaccination has given excellent preliminary results (27, 29). The level of antibodies in nasal secretions and the degree of protection against infection with PI3 virus is increased by aerosol exposure to the virus, when compared to parenteral exposure (31). A killed bovine adenovirus vaccine in adjuvant gives a good antibody response but has not been field tested (30).

REVIEW LITERATURE

Ide, P. (1970). *Canad. vet. J.*, *11*, 194.

REFERENCES

(1) Omar, A. R. (1966). *Vet. Bull.*, *36*, 259.
(2) Dawson, P. S. (1964). *Res. vet. Sci.*, *5*, 81.
(3) Singh, K. V. & Baz, T. I. (1966). *Nature (Lond.)*, *210*, 656.
(4) Sweat, R. L. (1968). *Amer. J. vet. Res.*, *153*, 1639.
(5) Dawson, P. S. (1966). *J. comp. Path.*, *76*, 373.
(6) Kramer, L. L. *et al.* (1963). *J. Amer. vet. med. Ass.*, *142*, 375.
(7) Dawson, P. S. & Darbyshire, J. H. (1964). *Vet. Rec.*, *76*, 111.
(8) St. George, T. D. (1969). *Aust. vet. J.*, *45*, 315, 321.
(9) Trainor, P. D. *et al.* (1966). *Amer. J. Epidem.*, *83*, 217.
(10) Phillip, J. I. H. (1970). *Vet. Rec.*, *86*, 280.
(11) Darbyshire, J. H. *et al.* (1969). *Res. vet. Sci.*, *10*, 39.
(12) Mohanty, S. B. *et al.* (1969). *Amer. J. vet. Res.*, *30*, 1105.
(13) Lamont, P. H. *et al.* (1968). *J. comp. Path.*, *78*, 23.
(14) Phillip, J. I. H. (1968). *Vet. Rec.*, *82*, Clin. Suppl. No. 14.
(15) White, G. (1965). *Vet. Rec.*, *77*, 1124.
(16) Winter, J. *et al.* (1970). *Arch. exp. Vet. Med.*, *24*, 1347.
(17) Wilson, M. R. & Thompson, R. G. (1968). *Res. vet. Sci.*, *9*, 467.
(18) Phillip, J. I. H. *et al.* (1968). *J. comp. Path.*, *78*, 89.
(19) White, G. *et al.* (1970). *Vet. Rec.*, *87*, 790.
(20) Stevenson, R. G. (1969). *J. comp. Path.*, *79*, 483.
(21) Maaten, Van Der M. J. (1969). *Canad. J. comp. Med.*, *33*, 134, 141.
(22) Betts, A. O. *et al.* (1964). *Vet. Rec.*, *76*, 382.
(23) Schoop, G. & Wachendorfer, G. (1962). *Dtsch. tierärztl. Wschr.*, *69*, 416.
(24) Mohanty, S. B. & Lillie, M. G. (1964). *Amer. J. vet. Res.*, *25*, 109.
(25) Rweyemamu, M. M. (1970). *Vet. Bull.*, *40*, 73.
(26) Woods, G. T. *et al.* (1967). *Amer. Rev. resp. Dis.*, *95*, 278.
(27) Gutekunst, D. E. *et al.* (1969). *J. Amer. vet. med. Ass.*, *155*, 1879.
(28) Woods, G. T. *et al.* (1968). *J. Amer. vet. med. Ass.*, *29*, 1349.
(29) Steves, F. E. & Baker, J. D. (1970). *Vet. Med.*, *65*, 333.
(30) Tribe, G. W. *et al.* (1969). *Vet. Rec.*, *84*, 299.
(31) Marshall, R. G. & Frank, G. H. (1971). *Amer. J. vet. Res.*, *32*, 11, 1699, 1707.

Infectious Bovine Rhinotracheitis

(*Rednose*)

Intectious bovine rhinotracheitis (IBR) is a highly infectious disease caused by a virus. The commonest syndrome is one which includes fever, nasal and ocular discharge, abortion, a relatively short course and a high recovery rate. The causative virus is identical with that which causes infectious pustular vulvovaginitis (IPV) of cattle.

Incidence

IBR has been identified in the United States, Canada, New Zealand, Australia, the United Kingdom, South Africa, and Europe, and occurs most commonly in large groups of cattle in feed-lots and large dairy farms. A serological survey of cattle in Australia and New Guinea has shown that 74 per cent of herds and 30 per cent of cattle carry significant titres against IBR virus (1). The disease is not highly fatal and losses are due largely to abortion and reduction of body condition and milk yield. In large milking herds losses can run from $25 to $50 per cow (2, 3). Morbidity and mortality rates vary considerably and are lower in dairy cattle (8 per cent morbidity, 3 per cent mortality) than in beef cattle in feedlots, in which the morbidity rate is usually 20 to 30 per cent (rarely up to 100 per cent) and the mortality rate is usually 6 to 12 per cent (4). The morbidity and mortality rates tend to remain at these higher levels in large feedlots because of the frequent introduction of susceptible animals. A morbidity rate of 30 per cent and a mortality rate of 90 per cent have been recorded in an outbreak of the encephalitic form of the disease in an area in which IPV and the respiratory form of IBR did not occur (5). The disease, the causative virus and antibodies to the virus have been observed in range cattle but the disease appears to have little or no importance in cattle run under these conditions.

Aetiology

A herpes virus has been isolated from infected animals and is capable of growing on tissue culture and of producing the respiratory disease (5), abortion, and conjunctivitis and, after intracerebral inoculation, encephalitis (6). The virus cannot be transmitted to goats, guinea pigs, white mice or embryonated hen eggs. Mule deer and goats are susceptible to infection and may act as a source of infection for cattle. Although seldom reported the disease can affect swine naturally in both the respiratory and genital form (33).

All ages and breeds of cattle are susceptible on experimental challenge, but the disease occurs naturally mostly in animals over 6 months of age, probably because of their greater exposure. There is no seasonal variation in incidence, except possibly a higher occurrence in feedlot cattle in the autumn when large numbers of susceptible animals are assembled. Recovery from an attack results in a solid immunity lasting for at least 3 months. The virus of IBR is identical with that of infectious pustular vulvovaginitis (IPV) of cows and penoposthitis of bulls (7) but the two diseases do not commonly occur together.

The observation that the IBR–IPV virus is identical with a European virus which also causes vaginitis poses a problem in epidemiology. It has been suggested that the virus was carried to North

America from Europe in infected cattle but continued to cause only lesions in the genital tract until its introduction into dense populations of cattle in feedlots encouraged rapid passage through many hosts and thus encouraged adaptation to the respiratory tract (8). The subsequent appearance of encephalitis and abortion as diseases caused by the virus, diseases which did not occur in the first decade of IBR's existence, suggests that the virus is still undergoing adaptation.

Transmission

Experimental infection has been effected by intramuscular injection and by introduction into the respiratory tract and conjunctiva of nasal washings from infected cattle and virus grown on tissue culture.

Since the virus appears to be in greatest concentration in the respiratory tract, nasal exudate and coughed up droplets must be considered to be the main source of infection. Introduction of animals into a group often precedes an outbreak of the disease. However, it can arise simultaneously in a number of dairy farms in an area and spread from these to adjacent farms until the entire area is affected. The same pattern of occurrence simultaneously in a number of foci is seen in feedlots, and from these foci infection spreads to other pens in the lot. An outbreak usually reaches its peak in the second or third week and ends by the fourth to sixth week. The virus does not appear to persist for long periods in recovered animals, but intermittent discharge of virus from the nasal mucosa for 17 months after experimental infection of a heifer has been recorded (9). Transmission by infected semen has been shown to occur (11).

Pathogenesis

Systemic invasion by the virus occurs and there is a transient viraemia (10), the resulting localization in various organs giving rise to encephalitis (4) and abortion (12). The disease of the genital tract produced by this virus has been reviewed (13).

Experimental inoculation of calves with the virus produced predictable results (14, 15). Fever, and after intranasal or conjunctival inoculation, intense conjunctivitis with lacrimation develops. Pneumonitis is gross; rhinitis, bronchitis and cholecystitis occur. There is slight non-purulent encephalitis in some. Parenteral inoculation in cows causes foetal necrosis and abortion but no other clinical signs in the cow (16, 17, 18).

Clinical Findings

After experimental infection there is an incubation period of 3 to 7 days (5), but in infected feedlots the disease occurs 10 to 20 days after the introduction of susceptible cattle. A longer incubation period has been recorded by some authors.

There is a sudden onset of severe signs including anorexia, fever (up to 42 °C or 108 °F), severe hyperaemia of the nasal mucosa, a serous discharge from the eyes and nose, increased salivation and a degree of hyperexcitability. A drastic fall in milk yield may be the earliest sign in dairy cattle. The respirations are increased in rate and are shallow, but the lungs are normal on auscultation. Respiratory distress is evident on exercise. A short, explosive cough has been characteristic of some outbreaks but is not recorded in others. Sudden death within 24 hours after first signs appear can result from extensive obstructive bronchiolitis (19).

In dairy cattle, in which the disease assumes its mildest form, signs may not increase beyond this stage, the temperature returning to normal in a day or two and recovery being complete in 10 to 14 days. In feeder cattle the illness is often more prolonged, the febrile period is longer, the nasal discharge becomes more profuse and purulent, and the convalescent period is longer. Some deaths may occur in the acute febrile period, but most fatalities are due to a secondary bronchopneumonia and occur after a prolonged illness of up to 4 months in which severe dyspnoea, complete anorexia and final recumbency are obvious signs. Some recovered cows have a persistent snoring respiration and a grossly thickened, rough nasal mucosa accompanied by nasal discharge (20).

Conjunctivitis is a common but not constant sign and, in some outbreaks of IBR, is the only sign of abnormality (21). It may affect one or both eyes and is easily mistaken for infectious keratoconjunctivitis caused by *Moraxella bovis*. However, the lesions are confined to the conjunctiva and there is no invasion of the cornea. Thus, the conjunctiva is red and swollen, there is profuse, primarily serous, ocular discharge but no corneal ulceration. Calves less than six months of age may develop encephalitis, which is marked by incoordination, excitement alternating with depression and a high mortality rate. Salivation, bellowing, convulsions and blindness are also recorded (5, 22).

Abortion is a common sequel and occurs some weeks after the clinical illness, or vaccination. It is most common in cows which are 6 to 8 months pregnant. Retention of the placenta often follows, but residual infertility is unimportant. However endometritis, poor conception and short oestrus can occur after insemination with infected semen (23). The IBR virus has been isolated from semen 12 months after storage (11).

Clinical Pathology

No changes in white cell counts occur. In prolonged cases bacteriological examination of nasal swabs is advisable to determine the types of secondary bacterial invaders present. Isolation of the virus from nasal swabs by tissue culture, and its identification by cross-protection tests and serum neutralization tests (24) is essential for positive diagnosis of the disease. The serum neutralization test is specific both for detecting antibodies by the use of known antigens and for identifying viral isolates by means of known antibodies (25). Fluorescent antibody techniques are available (26) and may be of use in identifying the presence of virus in nasal secretions and impressions of uterine cotyledons, or in tissues of aborted foetuses (27). The technique is most valuable in the diagnosis of IBR as a cause of abortion in cattle.

Necropsy Findings

Gross lesions are restricted to the muzzle, nasal cavities, pharynx, larynx and trachea, and terminate in the large bronchi. There may be pulmonary emphysema or secondary bronchopneumonia, but for the most part the lungs are normal. In the upper respiratory tract there are variable degrees of inflammation, but the lesions are essentially the same in all anatomical regions. In mild cases there is swelling and congestion of the mucosae, petechiae may be present and there is a moderate amount of catarrhal exudate. In severe cases the inflammation is more severe and the exudate is profuse and fibrinopurulent. When the exudate is removed, the mucosa is intact except for small numbers of necrotic foci in the nasal mucosa and diffuse denudation of epithelium in the upper part of the trachea. Lymph nodes in the throat and neck region are usually swollen and oedematous. Histologically there is acute, catarrhal inflammation of the mucosa. Inclusion bodies are not recorded in natural cases but do occur transiently in respiratory epithelial cells in experimentally infected animals. Secondary bacterial invasion will cause a more severe necrotic reaction which is usually followed by the development of bronchopneumonia. In very young calves a severe epithelial necrosis has been observed in the oesophagus and rumen, the adherent necrotic epithelium having the pultaceous quality of milk curd. Inclu-

sion bodies were evident in many surviving epithelial cells (28).

Aborted foetuses show moderately severe autolysis and focal necrotizing hepatitis (5, 22). The encephalitis is characterized by typical viral lesions located particularly in the cerebral cortex and the internal capsule (5).

Diagnosis

The occurrence of an infectious, non-fatal disease affecting only the upper respiratory tract of cattle should suggest the diagnosis of infectious bovine rhinotracheitis. Calf diphtheria may resemble IBR but there are typical oral lesions, a profound toxaemia, a low morbidity and high mortality rate with a long period of illness. In viral pneumonia of calves and shipping fever there is obvious pulmonary involvement, while in bovine malignant catarrh and the mucosal diseases lesions in the digestive tract are evident.

The greatest difficulty encountered in an outbreak of IBR is to differentiate it from acute allergic rhinitis. The latter does not usually occur so explosively, nor is the febrile response so marked. The possibility that IBR may be a precursor to nasal granuloma has been pointed out (20).

Treatment

Although they are unlikely to have any effect on the virus, broad spectrum antibiotics should be administered to avoid losses caused by secondary bacterial invaders. Parenteral enzyme therapy has been recommended in the treatment of severe cases with marked dyspnoea caused by obstruction of the respiratory tract.

Control

Sick animals should be isolated as soon as signs appear, as close contact seems to be necessary for spread of the disease. A vaccine has been produced by modification of the virus on passage through tissue culture. Intramuscular injection of 2 ml. of the vaccine into the gluteal muscles results in satisfactory immunity in about 14 days. The vaccine has proved to be an adequate control measure in feedlots and, although reports vary, appears to have some efficiency in preventing the occurrence of pustular vulvovaginitis (30). Abortion occurs sufficiently commonly after vaccination to warrant the recommendation that pregnant cows be not vaccinated. Heifers should be vaccinated after 6 months of age to avoid colostral immunity but preferably at least 30 days before breeding.

Administration of the vaccine should be carried

out before animals come in contact with an infected environment, but immediate vaccination may be of some value in the face of an outbreak. A formalin-killed virus vaccine does not provoke as great an antibody reaction as the tissue culture vaccine but appears to stimulate sufficient immunity to the infection. An intranasal vaccine is apparently effective (31, 32) but an advantage for this route of administration has not been clearly demonstrated.

REVIEW LITERATURE

Curtis, R. A. *et al.* (1966). *Canad. vet. J.*, *7*, 161.
Rosner, S. F. (1968). *J. Amer. vet. med. Ass.*, *153*, 1631.

REFERENCES

(1) St George, T. D. *et al.* (1967). *Aust. vet. J.*, *43*, 549.
(2) Pierson, R. E. & Vair, C. A. (1965). *J. Amer. vet. med. Ass.*, *147*, 350.
(3) Townley, M. M. (1971). *Mod. vet. Pract.*, *52*, 72.
(4) Barenfus, M. *et al.* (1965). *J. Amer. vet. med. Ass.*, *143*, 725.
(5) Gardiner, M. R. *et al.* (1964). *Aust. vet. J.*, *40*, 225.
(6) Straub, O. C. & Bohm, H. O. (1965). *Dtsch. tierärztl. Wschr.*, *72*, 124.
(7) Huck, R. A. *et al.* (1971). *Vet. Rec.*, *88*, 292.
(8) McKercher, D. G. (1963). *Amer. J. vet. Res.*, *24*, 501.
(9) Snowdon, W. A. (1965). *Aust. vet. J.*, *41*, 135.
(10) Chow, T. L. *et al.* (1956). *Proc. 59th ann. gen. Mtg U.S. Live Stock sanit. Ass.*, 1955, p. 168.
(11) Spradbrow, P. B. (1968). *Aust. vet. J.*, *44*, 410.
(12) Kendrick, J. W. *et al.* (1971). *Amer. J. vet. Res.*, *32*, 1045.
(13) Saxegaard, F. (1970). *Vet. Bull.*, *40*, 605.
(14) McKercher, D. G. *et al.* (1970). *J. Amer. vet. med. Ass.*, *156*, 1460.
(15) Markson, L. M. & Darbyshire, J. H. (1966). *Brit. vet. J.*, *122*, 522.
(16) Kendrick, J. (1967). *Amer. J. vet. Res.*, *28*, 1269.
(17) Owen, N. V. *et al.* (1968). *Amer. J. vet. Res.*, *29*, 1959.
(18) Sattar, S. A. *et al.* (1967). *Cornell Vet.*, *57*, 438.
(19) Curtis, R. A. *et al.* (1966). *Canad. vet. J.*, *7*, 208.
(20) Snowdon, W. A. (1964). *Aust. vet. J.*, *40*, 277.
(21) Timoney, P. J. & O'Connor, P. J. (1971). *Vet. Rec.*, *89*, 370.
(22) Bartha, A. *et al.* (1969). *Acta vet. Acad. Sci. hung.*, *19*, 145.
(23) Kendrick, J. W. & McEntee, K. (1967). *Cornell Vet.*, *57*, 3.
(24) Greig, A. S. (1969). *Canad. J. comp. Med.*, *33*, 85.
(25) McKercher, D. G. & Saito, J. K. (1965). *Proc. 68th ann. gen. Mtg U.S. Live Stock sanit. Ass.*, pp. 518–24.
(26) Schipper, I. A. & Chow, T. L. (1968). *Canad. J. comp. Med.*, *32*, 412.
(27) Reed, D. E. *et al.* (1971). *Amer. J. vet. Res.*, *32*, 1423.
(28) Thomson, R. G. & Savan, M. (1963). *Canad. vet. J.*, *4*, 249.
(29) Kennedy, P. C. & Richards, W. P. C. (1964). *Path. Vet.*, *1*, 7.
(30) Fastier, L. G. & Smith, B. F. (1962). *N.Z. vet. J.*, *10*, 11.
(31) McKercher, D. G. & Crenshaw, G. L. (1971). *J. Amer. vet. med. Ass.*, *159*, 1362.
(32) Todd, J. D. *et al.* (1971). *J. Amer. vet. med. Ass.*, *159*, 1370.
(33) Nelson, D. R. *et al.* (1972). *Amer. J. vet. Res.*, *33*, 1209.

Chlamydial Pneumonia of Sheep

This disease is probably more common in sheep than is generally recognized but its status as a cause of loss is unsure (4). Its occurrence has been recognized in the United States (1), Australia and Europe (2) and presumptive identification has been made in Egypt and New Zealand. The disease resembles the enzootic pneumonias of pigs and calves and may be the starting point of some of the bacterial pneumonias of sheep. A case in point is the severe pneumonia affecting lambs brought on to irrigated pasture in California for fattening (3). A high incidence occurs in lambs imported from certain areas, and cases occur 1 to 3 weeks after shipment. *Cor. pyogenes* is commonly present in the lungs of affected lambs.

Attempts to produce pneumonia in lambs experimentally by the administration of the chlamydia, of *Past. multocida*, or of the mycoplasma often associated with pneumonia in lambs, are unsuccessful unless the lambs are also exposed to environmental stress. The chlamydia does cause extensive lesions when injected intratracheally or by nebulization but there is little clinical evidence of illness. Experimentally produced chlamydial pneumonia in newborn lambs is manifested by fever, dyspnoea and anorexia (5). Macroscopic lesions of pneumonia are evident. It has been suggested that the chlamydia may be related to the causal agent of enzootic abortion of ewes (2, 6). Chlamydia isolated from pneumonia of varying degrees of severity may be identical, the response varying with the status of the animal with respect to specific and nonspecific immunity.

Pneumonia caused by parainfluenza 3 virus also occurs in sheep (4) and is widespread in the U.K. The disease is mild clinically and marked by the presence of interstitial pneumonia (7). Vaccination with an adjuvant virus is claimed to prevent infection (8). A serological survey in Australia has indicated a very high level of exposure to the infection (9).

REFERENCES

(1) Dungworth, D. L. (1964). *Proc. 67th ann. gen. Mtg U.S. Live Stock sanit. Ass.*, 1963, pp. 301–4.
(2) Charton, A. *et al.* (1964). *Bull. Acad. vét. Fr.*, *37*, 269.
(3) Shultz, G. (1963). *Proc. 66th ann. gen. Mtg U.S. Live Stock sanit. Ass.*, 1962, pp. 271–3.
(4) Stevenson, R. G. (1969). *Vet. Bull.*, *39*, 747.
(5) Stevenson, R. G. & Robinson, G. (1970). *Res. vet. Sci.*, *11*, 469.
(6) Dungworth, D. L. (1963). *J. comp. Path.*, *73*, 68.
(7) Hore, D. E. & Stevenson, R. G. (1969). *Res. vet. Sci.*, *10*, 342.
(8) Gilmour, N. J. L. (1968). *J. comp. Path.*, *78*, 463.
(9) St George, T. D. (1971). *Aust. vet. J.*, *47*, 370, 428.

Progressive Interstitial Pneumonia
(Maedi)

Maedi is a chronic pneumonia of sheep which is caused by a virus. 'Maedi' is Icelandic for dyspnoea. There is a very long incubation period, a chronic progressive pneumonia and a characteristic increase in weight of the lungs.

Incidence

Maedi occurs in Iceland, where it is believed to have been introduced in sheep imported from Germany together with pulmonary adenomatosis and Johne's disease, although maedi is not known to occur in that country. At one time maedi was enzootic in Iceland and approximately 150,000 sheep are believed to have died of the disease during a 13 year period. A high morbidity rate and a mortality rate of 10 to 20 per cent per year occurred and complete destruction of all sheep in the area was necessary to eradicate the disease, which has since reappeared in sporadic form (1). A very similar disease has been reported in Kenya (2), Germany (3) and India (4). Montana progressive pneumonia appears to be identical to maedi (11) although some cases reported under this heading may have been jaagsiekte or other disease entities.

Aetiology

A virus has been isolated from typically affected animals and is considered to be the causative agent of maedi (5). It is closely related to the visna virus and bears some serological relationship to the agents involved in progressive interstitial pneumonia in Holland and in Montana, U.S.A. (6). Among sheep only those 2 years old or over are affected. The clinical disease is likely to appear after prolonged physical exertion or exposure to bad weather. The disease occurs principally in sheep but has been observed also in goats.

Transmission

Transmission experiments have been inconclusive. The natural mode of spread is not known, but from field observations direct contact between affected and unaffected sheep seems to be necessary.

Pathogenesis

There is a gradual development of an interstitial pneumonia without any evidence of healing, nor shrinkage of tissue, so that the lungs continue to increase in size and weight. The alveolar spaces are gradually filled so that anoxia develops.

Clinical Findings

There is a very long incubation period of at least 2 years. Early signs of the disease include a slow advance of listlessness, emaciation and dyspnoea. There is no evidence of excess fluid in the lungs. The respiratory rate is increased to 80 to 120 per minute at rest. There may be coughing and some nasal discharge. The body temperature is in the high normal range. Clinical illness lasts for 3 to 6 months in most cases but may persist for several years.

Clinical Pathology

The virus can be isolated (7) and complement fixation and virus neutralizing antibodies are measurable. Together with histopathological examination these tests make the diagnosis of the disease possible (8).

There is a progressive, moderate hypochromic anaemia, with haemoglobin levels falling from 12 to 14 g. per cent down to 7 to 8 g. per cent, and some depression of the red cell count. There is a tendency to leucocytosis, and in experimental cases this is observed to be quite marked in the period between exposure and the onset of clinical disease, but the count returns to normal when signs appear.

Necropsy Findings

Gross and microscopic abnormalities are confined to the chest. The lungs are larger and 2 to 4 times as heavy as normal lungs. They collapse much less than normal when the chest is open and are grey-blue to grey-yellow in colour. There is a diffuse thickening of the entire bulk of both lungs and the abnormal colour and consistency are generalized and unvarying in all lobes. Enlargement of the bronchial and mediastinal lymph nodes is constant. Histopathological changes are characteristic of a chronic interstitial pneumonia and the bulk of the alveolar space is replaced by thickened alveolar walls. The air passages are unaffected. There is a complete absence of healing, suggesting that the disease is a progressive one and never reaches a healing stage.

Diagnosis

There are several chronic pneumonias which require to be differentiated from maedi, including jaagsiekte, in which the histological picture is quite different, profuse nasal discharge is a common sign and there is a shorter course. Epizootic adenomatosis appears to be identical with jaagsiekte. Parasitic pneumonia causes a persistent chronic cough and dyspnoea, but there are pronounced bronchial râles on auscultation over the diaphragmatic lobes. It does not run a course as prolonged as in maedi but is more chronic than pateurella pneumonia. The morbidity rate is usually higher than in either of these diseases. Melioidosis may resemble maedi clinically, but there are typical abscesses in lung tissue at necropsy. 'Laikipia' lung disease of sheep in Kenya is a progressive enzootic pneumonia resembling maedi and jaagsiekte and may, indeed, include both. One form is caused by a virus capable of producing the disease in lambs after an incubation period of 4 to 6 months, and which can be grown on eggs. A vaccine composed of formalin-killed virus is highly effective in preventing the disease. Zwoegerziekte is a progressive pulmonary disease of sheep in the Netherlands (9); Graaff-Reinet disease is another South African progressive pneumonia and Bouhite a chronic respiratory disease of sheep in France (10). All these diseases are essentially similar to maedi but local terminology frequently groups a number of diseases under a single name.

Treatment

No treatment has been successful.

Control

Eradication of the disease appears to necessitate complete destruction of all sheep in the infected area and subsequent restocking.

REFERENCES

(1) Thormar, H. (1965). *Res. vet. Sci.*, *6*, 117.
(2) Wandera, J. G. (1970). *Vet. Rec.*, *86*, 434.
(3) Weiland, F. & Behrens, H. (1970). *Dtsch. tierärztl. Wschr.*, *77*, 273.
(4) Chauhan, H. V. S. & Singh, C. M. (1970). *Brit. vet. J.*, *126*, 364.
(5) Sigurdardottir, B. & Thormar, H. (1965). *J. infect. Dis.*, *114*, 55.
(6) Thormar, H. (1966). *Lung Tumours of Animals*, pp. 393–402, Italy: University of Perugia.
(7) Kennedy, R. C. *et al.* (1968). *Virology*, *35*, 483.
(8) Gudnadottir, M. *et al.* (1968). *Res. vet. Sci.*, *9*, 65.
(9) de Boer, G. F. (1970). *Tr. Diergeneesk.*, *95*, 725.
(10) Stevenson, R. G. (1969). *Vet. Bull.*, *39*, 747.
(11) Eklund, C. M. & Hadlow, W. J. (1969). *J. Amer. vet. med. Ass.*, *155*, 2094.

Pulmonary Adenomatosis

(*Jaagsiekte*)

Jaagsiekte is Afrikaans for 'driving disease' because of the tendency for affected sheep to show clinical signs when driven. The disease is a chronic, progressive pneumonia, with the development of typical adenomatous ingrowths of the alveolar walls.

Incidence

The disease is recorded from Europe, South Africa, Asia, Britain, Iceland and Israel. There have been no confirmed reports of the disease in North America although its presence has been suspected. In Britain, Scotland appears to be the focus of infection from which other outbreaks arise. European and English figures quote an annual flock mortality rate of about 2 to 8 per cent, but a high morbidity rate has been observed in Iceland. The disease is uniformly fatal. Because of the method of spread the disease is likely to assume more importance as sheep husbandry becomes intensified. Jaagsiekte is a disease of sheep, but has also been observed in goats (1).

Aetiology

The causative virus has been cultured in tissue culture and grows best on macrophage cultures (7) although a *mycoplasma* is also commonly encountered in affected sheep and may play an aetiological role (2, 3). Close housing during the winter is a potent predisposing cause and probably accounts for the occurrence of the disease in epizootic form in Iceland. However, the disease occurs commonly in range sheep in other countries. There is no seasonal variation in incidence and only mature sheep are affected. A genetic susceptibility to the disease has been suggested.

Transmission

Experimental transmission has been effected by pulmonary or intravenous injection or by insufflation of infected lung material (2, 4). The disease has also been transmitted by inhalation of infected droplets when sheep are kept in close contact, and it is assumed that this is the natural mode of transmission.

Pathogenesis

The adenomatous ingrowths of alveolar epithelium encroach gradually upon alveolar air space so that anoxic anoxia occurs. There is no inflammation and no toxaemia. The frequent occurrence of metastases in regional lymph nodes has given rise to the commonly voiced view that the disease is a transmissible neoplasm (8). The lesions produced by experimental inoculation are identical with those of the naturally occurring disease (4).

Clinical Findings

A long incubation period of about 6 months is usual. Occasional coughing and some panting after exercise are the earliest signs. Emaciation, dyspnoea, lacrimation and a profuse watery discharge from the nose follow. Death occurs 6 weeks to 4 months later. A diagnostic test in this disease is to hold the sheep up by the hind legs: in affected animals a quantity of watery mucus (up to about 200 ml.) runs from the nostrils. Moist râles are audible over the affected lung areas and may be heard at a distance so that a group of affected animals are said to produce a sound like slowly boiling porridge. There is no elevation of body temperature and the appetite is normal.

Clinical Pathology

A complement-fixation test has shown some promise (5). Nasal exudate from affected animals may show clusters of epithelial cells with the hyperplastic adenomatous epithelium typical of pulmonary lesions (6). There is hypergammaglobulinaemia and the iodine agglutination test may have diagnostic value (9).

Necropsy Findings

Lesions are restricted to the thoracic cavity. As in maedi the lungs are grossly increased in size and in weight (up to three times normal). Extensive areas of consolidation, particularly of the ventral parts of the apical lobes and excess frothy fluid in the bronchi, are characteristic. Secondary pulmonary abscesses and pleurisy may develop. Histologically there are characteristic adenomatous ingrowths of alveolar epithelium into the alveolar spaces.

Diagnosis

Other chronic pneumonias in sheep are described under Maedi (p. 525).

Treatment

No treatment has been attempted.

Control

In Iceland, where the disease assumed epizootic proportions, eradication was effected by complete slaughter of all sheep in the affected areas. In areas where the incidence is lower the disease can be satisfactorily controlled by slaughter of the clinically affected sheep. A formalized vaccine prepared from the lungs of diseased sheep has undergone an extensive trial in Kenya and appears to have greatly reduced the incidence of the disease.

REVIEW LITERATURE

Wandera, J. G. (1971). Sheep pulmonary adenomatosis (jaagsiekte), *Advanc. vet. Sci.*, *15*, 251.

REFERENCES

(1) Rajya, B. S. & Singh, C. M. (1964). *Amer. J. vet. Res.*, *25*, 61.
(2) Markson, L. M. & Terlecki, S. (1964). *Path. Vet.*, *1*, 269.
(3) Mackay, J. M. K. & Nisbet, D. I. (1966). *Vet. Rec.*, *78*, 18.
(4) Wandera, J. C. (1970). *Brit. vet. J.*, *126*, 185.
(5) Enchev, S. & Khristoforov, L. (1963). *Vet. med. Nauki, Sofia*, *8*, 35.
(6) Nobel, T. A. *et al.* (1970). *Ztbl. vet. Med.*, *17B*, 958.
(7) Mackay, J. M. K. (1969). *J. comp. Path.*, *79*, 141, 147.
(8) Nobel, T. A. *et al.* (1968). *Refuah Vet.*, *25*, 5.
(9) Nobel, T. A. *et al.* (1971). *Zbl. vet. Med.*, *18B*, 9.

VIRUS DISEASES CHARACTERIZED BY NERVOUS SIGNS

Viral Encephalomyelitis of Horses

Viral encephalomyelitis is an infectious disease affecting horses and characterized clinically by signs of deranged consciousness, motor irritation and paralysis.

Incidence

The disease is restricted to the Americas; the United States, Canada, Venezuela, Brazil and Argentina all record its occurrence. Most states of the U.S.A. have experienced the disease and, although the incidence has fallen considerably in late years (2·36 per cent in 1938 to 0·19 per cent in 1955), an appreciable number of horses are fatally affected each year. The susceptibility of man to the causative virus gives the disease some public health importance. Morbidity rates vary widely depending upon seasonal conditions and the prevalence of insect vectors; and cases may occur sporadically or in the form of severe outbreaks affecting 20 per cent or more of a group. The incidence of infections as judged by serological examination is much higher than the clinical morbidity. The mortality rate differs with the strain of the virus; in infections with the Western strain it is usually 20 to 30 per cent and with the Eastern and Venezuelan strains up to about 90 per cent.

Aetiology

Viral encephalomyelitis is primarily an infection of birds and feral animals, and infection in other species is accidental.

Three known strains of the arbovirus exist, the Eastern, Western and Venezuelan strains. They are immunologically distinct and vary in their virulence, although the clinical disease produced is similar in each case. The Western strain is the least virulent for horses, man and experimental animals and occurs chiefly in the western states of the U.S.A. and western Canada, extending eastwards to the Appalachian mountain region. The Eastern strain is more virulent for all species and, in the U.S.A., occurs chiefly in the eastern and southern states but overlaps the Western strain to some extent extending as far west as the mid-western states. It has also been recognized in Jamaica and Brazil. Both strains occur in Argentina. The Venezuelan strain (VEE) was originally observed in Venezuela and has since occurred in Trinidad, Argentina and Florida (1). An outbreak of VEE occurred in Guatemala in 1969 (2) and in 1971 an extensive outbreak occurred in the southern U.S.A., Mexico, and Costa Rica (3). The virus has spread its geographical range greatly and has also changed its character from being chiefly a disease of horses to one in which severe infections, with many deaths, occur in man (4). It bears some antigenic relationship to the Eastern strain of the virus.

Under natural conditions the disease occurs in horses, mules, donkeys, man and possibly monkeys. Many species of wild and captive birds become infected and, although many escape any serious effects, a fatal encephalitis occurs in others. The natural disease has been observed in turkey poults. Experimentally the disease can be produced by intracerebral inoculation in calves, dogs, white mice, guinea pigs and many species of birds (5). Snakes are highly susceptible to experimental infection. Pigs have a high natural susceptibility and may carry high levels of neutralizing antibodies, but the disease has been considered non-clinical (6). The recent recording of the Eastern strain of the virus from a suckling pig with a nervous disturbance, and the subsequent transmission of the disease, may lead to a revision of this opinion (16). The virus can be grown on embryonated hen eggs and in tissue culture. It is extremely fragile and disappears from infected tissues within a few hours of death.

The disease has a marked seasonal incidence, with the great majority of cases occurring in mid and late summer when the insect population is highest. In warm climates the seasonal variation may be less evident. Young horses are most susceptible. Immunity after natural infection persists for about 2 years.

Transmission

Wild birds are the principal source of the virus and infection in horses and man is accidental. Spread occurs by insect bite, chiefly from mosquitoes, but also from ticks, bloodsucking bugs, and chicken mites and lice. Mosquitoes of the *Aedes*, *Culex* and *Mansonia* genera have been identified as vectors, the virus persisting in them for a number of generations and passing through all stages of their life cycles. Spread may occur occasionally from horse to horse by direct contact or by insect transmission, but the major route of spread appears to be from birds through insects to horses and man. The wild bird population acts as a reservoir of infection in an area and probably serves to maintain the persistence of the virus from summer to summer and may be a factor in the spread of the disease to new areas. Under experimental conditions snakes and turtles have been shown to act as overwintering reservoirs (7) and there is evidence that the infection occurs naturally in snakes and frogs (8), but the importance of these species in maintaining the infection over long, insect-free periods is undetermined. The VEE virus can be spread through horses by contact; the virus is shed by infected horses and visceral and neuronal lesions are produced (9). The VEE virus has many hosts including mammals, especially the cotton rat, reptiles and birds. Mosquitoes, especially *Culex* spp., are thought to be the principal vectors (10).

Pathogenesis

A transitory viraemia occurs at the height of the fever in the North American disease but the viraemia persists throughout the course of the Venezuelan disease and the blood thus provides a source of infection for biting insects. The virus is present in saliva and nasal discharge, and this material can be used to transmit the disease experimentally by intranasal instillation. Penetration of the virus into the brain does not occur in all cases and the infection does not produce signs, other than fever, unless involvement of the central nervous system occurs, although antibodies to the virus do appear in the blood. The lesions produced in nervous tissue are typical of a viral infection and are localized particularly in the grey matter of the cerebral cortex, thalamus and hypothalamus, with minor involvement of the medulla and spinal cord. It is this distribution of lesions which is responsible for the characteristic signs of mental derangement followed at a later stage by paralysis. The early apparent blindness and failure to eat or drink appear to be cortical in origin. True blindness and pharyngeal paralysis occur only in the late stages. Much has been written of the pathogenesis of this disease in mice but the extent to which this information can be extrapolated to the horse is problematical (11, 12).

Clinical Findings

The incubation period is from 1 to 3 weeks. In the initial viraemic stage there is fever which may be accompanied by anorexia and depression, but the reaction is usually so mild that it goes unobserved. In the experimental disease the temperature may reach 41°C (106°F) persisting for only 24 to 48 hours, with nervous signs appearing at the peak of the fever. Animals that have shown nervous signs for more than 24 hours may then have a temperature within the normal range.

Early nervous signs include hypersensitivity to sound and touch and in some cases transient periods of excitement and restlessness with apparent blindness. Affected horses may walk blindly into objects or walk in circles. Involuntary muscle movements occur, especially tremor of shoulder and facial muscles and erection of the penis. A stage of severe mental depression follows. Affected horses stand with the head hung low; they appear to be asleep and may have a half-chewed mouthful of feed hanging from the lips. At this stage the horse may eat and drink if food is placed in its mouth. The pupillary light reflex is still present. The animal can be aroused but soon relapses into a state of somnolence.

A stage of paralysis follows. There is inability to hold up the head, and it is often rested on a solid support. The lower lip is pendulous and the tongue may hang out. Unnatural postures are adopted, the horse often standing with the weight balanced on the forelegs or with the legs crossed. Head-pressing or leaning back on a halter are often seen. On walking there is obvious inco-ordination, particularly in the hind-legs, and circling is common. Defaecation and urination are suppressed and the horse is unable to swallow. Complete paralysis is the terminal stage. The horse goes down, is unable to rise and usually dies within 2 to 4 days from the first signs of illness. A proportion of affected horses do not develop paralysis and survive but are often deficient mentally and are of little use because of their inability to respond satisfactorily to stimuli.

Clinical Pathology

Blood should be collected in the early febrile stages for transmission experiments. The intracerebral injection of guinea pigs is the favoured method of testing suspected material. The presence of neutralizing, or haemagglutination-inhibiting, or complement-fixing antibodies in the serum of recovered or in-contact animals may be of value in detecting the presence of the virus in the group or in the area. Identification of the Western strain of the virus has been achieved by the use of a complement fixation test on virus grown on chick embryos.

Necropsy Findings

There are no gross changes. Histological examination of brain reveals perivascular accumulations of leucocytes and damage to neurones (13). No inclusion bodies are present. Sections for histological examination should be taken from the cerebral cortex and mid-brain. Transmission experiments after death are carried out using brain as a source of virus. The brain should be removed within an hour of death or preferably after euthanasia when the animal is in extremis.

Diagnosis

Confirmatory diagnosis can be made by transmission of the disease to guinea pigs. The strain of the virus can be determined by neutralization tests in which the virus and known strain-specific antisera are injected intracerebrally into guinea pigs. Only the homologous antiserum will protect the guinea pig against infection.

The geographical distribution of Borna disease (p. 531) is quite different and the incubation period and the course are considerably longer. Inclusion bodies occur constantly in Borna disease but not in infectious equine encephalomyelitis (IEE). The seasonal occurrence of infectious equine encephalomyelitis is a diagnostic feature. The dumb form of rabies may be mistaken for IEE, but cases are relatively rare. Encephalitis due to the Japanese B encephalitis virus has been recorded in horses in the Orient, and can only be differentiated from IEE by laboratory tests.

Nervous signs resembling those of an encephalomyelitis occur in a number of poisonings in horses. Botulism is rare in this species and the syndrome is specifically one of paralysis. There is no derangement of consciousness and signs of motor irritation are absent. At necropsy there is no histological evidence of encephalitis. Poisoning caused by *Crotalaria* spp., *Senecio* spp., and *Amsinckia* spp., produces a syndrome with all the signs of an encephalomyelitis except fever. Histologically there is no encephalitis and gross abnormality of the liver is a prominent feature. These diseases are of course not transmissible. Poisoning by yellow star thistle and mouldy corn cause an encephalomalacia. Sporadic cases of brain tumour, hydrocephalus and cholesteatoma usually run a long course, often with intermittent periods of normal behaviour. There is no fever and there are often localizing signs.

Several other exotic encephalomyelites occur in horses. One recorded in Egypt and Syria affects equidae, ruminants and wild birds and one in Slovakia occurs only in horses. The former is now thought to be Borna disease; the cause of the latter has not been identified.

Treatment

Hyperimmune serum is the only specific treatment and may be beneficial if given in large doses (500 ml.) in the early stages of the disease. Many other empirical treatments have been recommended from time to time, but it is difficult to assess their efficiency when no control animals are kept.

Supportive treatment should be undertaken, as it may enable the animal to survive the danger period. Horses able to bear some weight should be supported in stocks and fed a nutritious, laxative diet, if necessary by nasal tube. All horses should be kept in the shade and protected from the flies and heat. Recumbent animals should be provided with ample bedding and turned frequently.

Control

Little can be done to control the insect population. Housing of horses indoors at night, especially in fly-proofed stables, and the use of insect repellents may restrain the spread of the virus. Complete eradication appears to be impossible because of the method of spread and the high incidence of the infection in wild birds.

Hyperimmune serum may be of prophylactic value in an outbreak, but the passive immunity is of short duration and the serum is not available commercially. A vaccine prepared from a virus which has been attenuated by passage through chicken embryos or tissue culture when injected intradermally and repeated in 1 week gives adequate protection for 1 year. Vaccination is carried out annually before the expected danger period. Immunity does not develop for 15 days and thus delay in vaccination until cases occur may result in losses. Vaccination against both strains of the virus is advisable in areas where the strain has not been identified or where both strains exist. Subcutaneous injections of vaccine are effective, but undesirable local reactions may occur. These are avoided by the intradermal administration of the attenuated virus. A permanently attenuated naturally occurring strain of the Western virus has been shown to be a safe and effective immunizing agent (14). Colostral antibody can be detected in the blood of foals from vaccinated mares for 6 or 7 months. It is recommended that foals vaccinated during the first 8 months of life be revaccinated at one year. When outbreaks occur, vaccination of the human population should be considered. A postvaccinal hepatitis has been recorded in horses after vaccination.

During the outbreak in 1971 in the U.S.A. an attempt was made to throw a barrier of vaccinated horses across the southern U.S.A. This was augmented by aerial spraying to reduce vector population. The vaccine was prepared from an attenuated virus produced as a 'biological incapacitating agent' for biological human warfare (15). It was an effective agent but produced high fever in some horses and was suspected of causing abortion.

REVIEW LITERATURE

Kissling, R. E. & Chamberlain, R. W. (1967). *Advanc. vet. Sci.*, *11*, 65.

REFERENCES

(1) Chamberlain, R. W. *et al.* (1964). *Science, N.Y.*, *145*, 272.
(2) Sudia, W. D. *et al.* (1971). *Amer. J. Epidem.*, *93*, 137.
(3) McConnell, S. (1971). *SWest. Vet.*, *24*, 259.
(4) Sidwell, R. W. (1967). *Bact. Rev.*, *31*, 65.
(5) Bivin, W. S. *et al.* (1967). *Amer. J. trop. Med. Hyg.*, *16*, 544.
(6) Karstad, L. & Hanson, R. P. (1959). *J. infect. Dis.*, *105*, 293.
(7) Hayes, R. O. *et al.* (1964). *Amer. J. trop. Med. Hyg.*, *13*, 595.
(8) Spalatin, J. *et al.* (1964). *Canad. J. comp. Med.*, *28*, 131.
(9) Spradbrow, P. (1966). *Vet. Bull.*, *36*, 55.
(10) Galindo, P. & Grayson, M. A. (1971). *Science, N.Y.*, *172*, 594.
(11) Liu, C. *et al.* (1970). *J. infect. Dis.*, *122*, 53.
(12) Aguilar, M. J. (1970). *Infect. Immun.*, *2*, 533.
(13) Roberts, E. D. *et al.* (1970). *Amer. J. vet. Res.*, *31*, 1223.
(14) Hughes, J. P. & Johnson, H. M. (1967). *J. Amer. vet. Med. Ass.*, *150*, 167.
(15) Gilette, R. (1971). *Science, N.Y.*, *173*, 405.
(16) Pursell, A. R. *et al.* (1972). *J. Amer. vet. med. Ass.*, *161*, 1143.

Japanese B Encephalitis

Japanese B encephalitis is primarily a disease of humans who provide the source of infection for animals in most instances. Sporadic cases of encephalitis in racehorses have been observed in Malaya (1) and serum-neutralization tests have indicated the presence of Japanese B encephalitis arbovirus in affected horses. Horses imported into Malaya from Australia have also been observed to carry antibodies against Murray Valley encephalitis of humans, but this virus does not cause clinical illness in horses.

The clinical manifestations of the disease vary

widely in severity. Mild cases show fever up to 39·5°C (103°F), anorexia, sluggish movements and sometimes jaundice for 2 or 3 days only. More severe cases show pronounced lethargy, mild fever and somnolence. Jaundice and petechiation of the nasal mucosa are usual. There is difficulty in swallowing, inco-ordination, and staggering and falling, although little difficulty may be experienced in getting up. Transient signs which persist for about 36 hours include neck rigidity, radial and labial paralysis, and blindness. In the most severe cases there is high fever (40·5 to 41·5°C or 105 to 107°F), hyperexcitability, profuse sweating and muscular tremor. Violent, uncontrollable activity may occur for a short period. This severe type of the disease is uncommon, representing only about 5 per cent of the total cases, but is more likely to terminate fatally. In most cases complete recovery follows an illness lasting from 4 to 9 days.

Transmission can be effected by the subcutaneous injection of whole blood from a clinically affected to a normal horse. Natural transmission by mosquitoes has been observed. The disease can be differentiated from viral encephalomyelitis of horses by serological and by virus neutralization tests (2).

The disease in cattle, sheep and goats is largely symptomless (4), and of little overall significance. Widespread losses, however, have been reported in swine, particularly in Japan, and these animals are thought to be a major natural source of the virus. The disease occurs as a non-suppurative encephalitis in pigs under 6 months of age. Sows abort or produce dead pigs at term. Formolized vaccines afford excellent protection against the encephalitis produced experimentally or occurring naturally, but are not effective in preventing stillbirths (3).

REFERENCES

(1) Kheng, C. S. et al. (1968). Aust. vet. J., 44, 23.
(2) Gould, D. J. et al. (1964). Amer. J. trop. Med. Hyg., 13, 742.
(3) Kawakubo, A. et al. (1971). J. Jap. vet. Med. Ass., 24, 237.
(4) Spradbrow, P. (1966). Vet. Bull., 36, 55.

Borna Disease

Borna disease is an infectious encephalomyelitis of horses first recorded in Germany. It is caused by a virus which is more resistant to environmental influences than other equine encephalomyelitis viruses. The disease and the virus are indistinguishable from Near Eastern Equine Encephalomyelitis (NEEE) (5). The method of transmission is unknown, but it is thought to be by inhalation or ingestion (1), both sheep and horses being susceptible to intranasal infection (3). Insect vectors appear to play no part in transmitting the disease. The morbidity rate is not high, but most affected animals die. As a rule only horses are susceptible, but occasional cases occur in sheep (2), and goats are susceptible to experimental infection. Rabbits can be infected by all routes, but other experimental animals are less susceptible. Continued passage of the virus through rabbits causes its attenuation, and a lapinized vaccine has been used to give satisfactory immunity to horses.

In field outbreaks the incubation period is about 4 weeks. There is moderate fever, pharyngeal paralysis, muscle tremor and hyperaesthesia. Lethargy and flaccid paralysis are seen in the terminal stages and death occurs 1 to 3 weeks after the first appearance of clinical signs. Infection without detectable clinical signs is thought to be common on infected premises (4). Clinico-pathological identification is possible with a complement fixation test. At necropsy there are no gross findings, but histologically there is a typical viral encephalitis, affecting chiefly the brainstem, and a lesser degree of myelitis. Diagnostic intranuclear inclusion bodies are present in nerve cells of the hippocampus and olfactory lobes of the cerebral cortex.

REFERENCES

(1) Matthias, D. (1955). Arch. exp. vet. Med., 9, 824.
(2) Ihlenberg, H. (1957). Arch. exp. vet. Med., 11, 835.
(3) Heinig, A. (1964). Arch. exp. vet. Med., 18, 753.
(4) Ihlenberg, H. & Brehmer, H. (1964). Mh. Vet.-Med., 19, 463.
(5) Daubney, R. (1967). Res. vet. Sci., 8, 419.

Rabies

Rabies is a highly fatal viral infection of the central nervous system, which occurs in all warm-blooded animals, and is transmitted by the bites of affected animals. It is manifested by motor irritation with clinical signs of mania and an attack complex, and by an ascending paralysis.

Incidence

Rabies occurs in most countries of the world except the island countries which are able to exclude it by rigid quarantine measures or prohibition of the entry of dogs. Australia and New Zealand have never had the disease, and Britain, Hawaii and Scandinavia are currently free. Britain had two minor outbreaks each involving one dog in 1969/70 but the disease was controlled successfully on each occasion (1). The disease is enzootic in much of the U.S.A., particularly the eastern and southern states. It has become an important problem in Canada only in recent years, being carried down from the north to the populated areas largely by the migration of foxes, and has recently been diagnosed for the first time in dogs and foxes in Greenland. Silvatic rabies is now the major problem in much of Europe. The disease is still spreading from a focal point which developed in Poland in the mid-30's. The disease has spread westward to East and West Germany, Denmark, Belgium, Czechoslovakia, Austria, Switzerland and France (23), and spread continues at the rate of about 30 to 60 km. per year and the threat to the U.K. increases each year (1). Foxes are the principal vectors and, as in Canada, cattle are the principal receptors. In Canada skunks are the common vectors (4). Rabies occurs in most countries in the African continent, but the reported incidence is surprisingly low for an area with such a high population of wild carnivores. Rabies is not of major economic importance in farm animals, although individual herds and flocks may suffer many fatalities. The disease is always fatal. The prime importance of rabies is its transmissibility to humans.

Aetiology

The myxovirus of rabies is truly neurotropic and causes lesions only in nervous tissue. It is one of the larger viruses and is relatively fragile. It is susceptible to most standard disinfectants and dies in dried saliva in a few hours. The virus can be propagated in tissue culture and chick embryos. All warm-blooded animals, with the possible exception of opossums, are susceptible, and there is no variation in susceptibility with age, pigs 1 day old having contracted the disease. The question of immunity after natural infection does not arise, but immunity can be produced artificially by vaccination. Although there appears to be a variation in pathogenicity in strains of rabies virus isolated from different species, all strains tested have been serologically indistinguishable (5).

Because of rapid developments in virological techniques, especially serological screening of animal populations to obtain presumptive diagnoses of the presence of a virus in the population, the question of latent infection and inapparent carriers of rabies has assumed some importance. The presence of rabies antibodies in animals in a supposed rabies-free area is likely to arouse concern. Inapparent carriers do occur in bats and there is some evidence that latent infections can occur in other species (6).

Transmission

The source of infection is always an infected animal, and the method of spread is almost always by the bite of an infected animal, although contamination of skin wounds by fresh saliva may result in infection. Because of the natural occurrence of rabies in animals in caves inhabited by infected insectivorous bats, inhalation as a route of infection has come under suspicion. There is some experimental evidence to support this. It is still probable that inter-bat spread is by bite and that bats transmit to other species mainly by biting (7). Apart from inhalation there has also been re-examination of ingestion as a portal of infection. In mice 4 of 5 strains tested were infective by this route and infection was shown to occur through the bucal mucosa, the lung, and intestine. One strain resisted the action of digestive juices for several hours (8, 9).

Traditionally, the dog, and to a minor extent the cat, have been considered to be the main source animals. However, native fauna, including foxes, skunks, wolves, vampire, insectivorous and fruit-eating bats, raccoons, and squirrels may provide the major source of infection in countries where domestic carnivora are well controlled. Bats are the only species in which symptomless carriers are known to occur. Multiplication of the virus without invasion of the nervous system is known to occur in fatty tissues in bats and may be the basis of the 'reservoiring' mechanism known to occur in this species. Violent behaviour is rare in rabid animals of this species, but has been observed. They represent a serious threat of spread of rabies because of their migratory habits.

Domestic livestock are rarely a source of infection although chance transmission to man may occur if the mouth of a rabid animal is manipulated during treatment or examination. The virus may be present in the saliva for periods up to 5 days before signs are evident.

Spread of the disease is quite often seasonal with the highest incidence in the late summer and autumn because of large-scale movements of wild animals at mating time and in pursuit of food. In general, foxes are less dangerous than dogs, foxes tending to bite only one or two animals in a group, while dogs will often bite a large proportion of a herd or flock. Not all bites from rabid animals result in infection because the virus is not always present in the saliva and moreover may not gain entrance to the wound if the saliva is wiped from the teeth by clothing or the coat of the animal. The virus may appear in the milk of affected animals but spread by this means is unlikely as infection through ingestion is not known to occur.

Pathogenesis

It is possible that a viraemia occurs after infection. This is suggested by the possible occurrence of the virus in milk, in some organs and in foetuses, but the virus cannot be demonstrated in the blood at any time. The only lesions produced are in the central nervous system, and spread from the site of infection occurs only by way of the peripheral nerves. This method of spread accounts for the extremely variable incubation period which varies to a large extent with the site of the bite. Bites on the head usually result in a shorter incubation period than bites on the extremities. The severity and the site of the lesions will govern to a large extent whether the clinical picture is primarily one of irritative or paralytic phenomena. The two extremes of the paralytic or dumb form and the furious form are accompanied by many cases which lie somewhere between the two. It might be expected that when irritation phenomena do occur they will be followed by paralysis as the stimulated nerve cells are subsequently destroyed. This is not always the case. Gradually ascending paralysis of the hindquarters may be followed by quite severe signs of mania which persist almost until death. In these cases it is probable that destruction of spinal neurones results in paralysis, but when the virus invades the brain, irritation of higher centres produces mania, excitement and convulsions. Death is usually due to respiratory paralysis. The clinical signs of salivation, indigestion and pica, paralysis of bladder and anus and increased libido all suggest involvement of the autonomic nervous system, including endocrine glands (11).

Variations in the major manifestation as mania or paralysis may depend in part upon the source of the virus. Virus from vampire bats almost always causes the paralytic form of the disease. Certainly, 'fixed' virus which has been modified by serial intracerebral passage causes ascending paralysis in contrast to 'street' virus, which more commonly causes the furious form of the disease. The site of infection and the size of the inoculum may also influence the clinical course.

Clinical Findings

Among farm animals, cattle are most commonly affected. The incubation period is usually about 3 weeks, but varies from 2 weeks to several months in most species, although incubation periods of 5 and 6 months have been observed in cattle and

dogs. In one large-scale outbreak in sheep deaths occurred 17 to 111 days after exposure (12).

In the mild or paralytic form knuckling of the hind fetlocks, sagging and swaying of the hindquarters while walking, often deviation or flaccidity of the tail to one side, are common early signs. Decreased sensation always accompanies this weakness and is one of the best diagnostic criteria in the detection of rabies. It is most evident over the hindquarters. Tenesmus, with paralysis of the anus, resulting in the sucking in and blowing out of air usually occurs late in the inco-ordination stages just before the animal goes down. This again is a characteristic sign but it may be transient or absent. Drooling of saliva is one of the most constant signs. The so-called yawning movements are more accurately described as voiceless attempts to bellow. Paralysis follows, the animal goes down and is unable to rise. Bulls in this stage often have paralysis of the penis. Death usually occurs 48 hours after recumbency develops and after a total course of 6 to 7 days.

In furious rabies the animal has a tense, alert appearance, is hypersensitive to sounds and movement and is attracted by them so that it may look intently or approach as though about to attack. In some cases they will violently attack other animals or inanimate objects. These attacks are often badly directed and are impeded by the inco-ordination of gait. Frequent, loud bellowing is usual at this stage. The sound is characteristically hoarse and the actions are exaggerated. Sexual excitement is also common, bulls often attempting to mount inanimate objects. Multiple collections of semen for artificial insemination have been made during very short periods from bulls which later proved to be rabid. With this violent form of the disease the termination is characteristically sudden. Severe signs may be evident for 24 to 48 hours and the animal then collapses suddenly in a paralysed state, dying usually within a few hours.

There is no constant pattern either in the development or range of signs. Body temperatures are usually normal but may be elevated to 39·5 to 40·5°C (103 to 105°F) in the early stages by muscular activity. Appetite varies also. Some animals do not eat or drink, although they take food into the mouth. There is apparent inability to swallow. Others eat normally until the terminal stages. The course may vary from 1 to 6 days. So great is the variation in clinical picture that any animal known to be exposed and showing signs of spinal cord or brain involvement, should be considered rabid until proved otherwise.

In sheep, rabies often occurs in a number of

animals at one time due to the ease with which a number can be bitten by a dog or fox. Clinically the picture is very similar to that seen in cattle. Sexual excitement, attacking humans or each other, vigorous wool pulling, sudden falling after violent exertion, muscle tremor and salivation are characteristic. Excessive bleating does not occur. Horses usually show excitement and mania. Their uncontrolled actions are often violent and dangerous and include blind charges, sudden falling and rolling and, in many cases, chewing of the skin. Paralysis and death ensue as in cattle. Pigs also show excitement and a tendency to attack, or dullness and inco-ordination (13). Affected sows show twitching of the nose, rapid chewing movements, excessive salivation and clonic convulsions (14). They may walk backwards. Terminally there is paralysis and death occurs 12 to 48 hours after the onset of signs.

Clinical Pathology

No ante-mortem laboratory examination has proved to be of diagnostic value, but tests for lead on blood, urine and faeces may help to eliminate lead poisoning as a possible diagnosis. Serum neutralization tests are available, but the presence of neutralizing antibodies is not necessarily diagnostic of rabies.

Necropsy Findings

There are no gross abnormalities. Histologically, Negri bodies are detectable in the Gasserian ganglion, hippocampus, medulla oblongata or cerebellum in a high proportion of cases. Because of the absence of Negri bodies, in some cases injection of macerated fresh brain intracerebrally into mice may be undertaken. Death occurs in 7 to 24 days. Negri bodies develop and may be looked for as soon as clinical signs appear. Dogs suspected of having rabies because of abnormal behaviour should be kept in isolation for 10 days and can be classified as non-rabid if alive and well at the end of this time. Routine laboratory procedure includes the immediate examination of material from the hippocampus by impression smear or histological examination, followed in negative samples by injection of macerated hippocampal tissue into mice. The incubation period of rabies in Swiss mice is 4 to 18 (average 11 to 12) days. Examination of mouse brains is conducted as for natural materials. Fluorescent antibody techniques are also being increasingly used for the examination of natural material and inoculated mouse brains (5). In the latter case it is possible to get a positive diagnosis

as soon as 3 to 4 days after inoculation of the mice. It is still necessary to wait the full 3 weeks before making a negative diagnosis (15).

Diagnosis

The diagnosis of rabies is one of the most difficult and important duties that a veterinarian is called upon to perform. Since in most cases there is a probability of human exposure, failure to recognize the disease may place human life in jeopardy. It is not even sufficient to say that if rabies occurs in the area one will classify every animal showing nervous signs as rabid, because nervous signs may not be evident for some days after the illness commences. In addition, many animals suffering from other diseases will be left untreated. The safest attitude to adopt is to handle all suspect animals with extreme care but continue to treat them for other diseases if such treatment appears to be indicated. If the animal is rabid, it will die and the diagnosis can then be confirmed by laboratory examination.

There are a large number of diseases which are manifested by signs of motor irritation or paralysis or a combination of both. In cattle acute and subacute lead poisoning produce clinical syndromes which are very similar to those of furious and dumb rabies. In lead poisoning there is complete absence of anaesthesia, bellowing and tenesmus, and blindness is usually present. Champing of the jaws may be accompanied by frothing of the mouth but the drooling of large quantities of saliva does not occur. Lactation tetany and avitaminosis A are more convulsive than maniacal in form and the characteristic signs of rabies do not occur. Polioencephalomalacia is accompanied by obvious cerebral involvement including blindness, nystagmus, opisthotonus and convulsions in sheep and cattle but again salivation, bawling, anaesthesia and tenesmus do not occur. Listeriosis in cattle and sheep is usually manifested by localizing signs of circling and facial nerve paralysis. In sheep enterotoxaemia is usually confined to lambs on heavy carbohydrate diets, pregnancy toxaemia is entirely a disease of pregnant ewes and is readily differentiated by the presence of ketonuria, and louping ill is transmitted by insects, has a seasonal occurrence and a localized geographical distribution. Encephalopathy in pigs is a very wide field, and is discussed in some detail under Pseudorabies. In horses rabies is rare. Encephalopathy in this species may be caused by one of the encephalitides or by the other diseases described in the differential diagnosis of viral encephalomyelitis of horses.

Treatment

No treatment should be attempted after clinical signs are evident. Immediately after exposure irrigation of the wound with 20 per cent soft soap solution or a solution of Zephiran may prevent the establishment of the infection (5). Post-exposure vaccination is unlikely to be of value in animals, as death usually occurs before appreciable immunity has had time to develop. Euthanasia of suspect animals must be prevented, particularly if human exposure has occurred, since the development of the disease in the animals is necessary to establish a diagnosis. Antirabic serum may become available for animal treatment at some future date.

Control

It is not possible to give complete details of programmes for rabies control here. Such programmes include control of the disease in dogs, other domestic animals, wildlife and bats, and have been reviewed in detail (5, 16).

From the point of view of farm animals there are two useful control techniques: the prevention of exposure and vaccination. The former can be achieved to a degree by destruction of wild fauna, muzzling, restraint and vaccination of all cats and dogs, and keeping farm animals indoors. The need to protect feral animals and in many instances the impossibility or undesirability of completely eradicating them has led to the examination of the possibility of vaccinating wildlife. Foxes can be protected by vaccination with ERA vaccine and oral immunization is possible (17) and effective (18).

In some areas the most practical protection of farm animals is vaccination, repeated annually if rabies is enzootic in the area. This is particularly necessary where bats are the source of infection (5). High passage chick embryo attenuated vaccine is the only one suitable for large animals (23). It gives a strong immunity for at least 6 months after vaccination in adults, but vaccination of animals under 9 months of age may be less efficient. The Flury and ERA strains of the virus are in common use for the production of vaccines, but strains of higher antigenicity and lower pathogenicity are under constant review (19). The vaccine produced by attenuation on duck embryos is unlikely to be used in animals. Tissue culture vaccine produced from the ERA strain has given excellent results in the field (20). The field duration of immunity is 3 years in cattle and 2 years in horses and dogs (21). A vaccine produced from the Kelev strain has been safe and effective but requires 3 injections over a period of 6 months (22). Vaccinal antibodies are present in the colostrum of vaccinated cows and it is recommended that, where annual vaccination of all cattle is carried out, calves be vaccinated at 4 months of age and again when 10 months old. Post-vaccinal paralysis does not occur after its use. The value of post-exposure vaccination is unknown although in our own experience vaccination of a heifer with living, attenuated virus after exposure has been followed by death from rabies 30 days later. The vaccine must be administered intramuscularly and be kept in a viable state until used. Low passage virus intended for use in dogs has caused heavy mortality when used in cattle and the tendency has been to use high egg passage vaccine for all species. Occasional cases of anaphylaxis occur, presumably due to sensitivity to egg protein, but are preventable by the use of antihistamines.

The most effective method of preventing the entry of rabies into a country free of the disease is the imposition of a quarantine period of 4 to 6 months on all imported dogs. This system has successfully prevented the entry of the disease into island countries, but has obvious limitation in countries which have land borders. The occurrence of the disease in two dogs in the U.K. in 1969/70 in which the incubation period appeared to last 7 to 9 months suggests that the more usual period of 6 months may give incomplete protection and vaccination on two occasions with an inactivated vaccine while the animal is still in quarantine for 6 months is the current recommendation (1). To require a longer period of quarantine would encourage evasion of the law by smuggling.

REVIEW LITERATURE

Irvin, A. D. (1970). The epidemiology of wildlife rabies. *Vet. Rec.*, 87, 333.

REFERENCES

(1) Waterhouse, R. (1971). *Report of the Committee of Enquiry on Rabies, Final Report*, p. 129. London: HMSO.
(2) Toma, B. & Andral, L. (1970). *Cah. Méd. vét.*, 39, 98.
(3) Kauker, E. & Zettl, K. (1969). *Berl. Münch. tierärztl. Wschr.*, 82, 301.
(4) Hayles, L. B. & Dryden, I. M. (1970). *Canad. vet. J.*, 11, 131.
(5) Tierkel, E. S. (1959). *Advanc. vet. Sci.*, 5, 183.
(6) Andral, L. & Serie, C. (1965). *Ann. Inst. Pasteur*, 108, 442.
(7) Constantine, D. (1966). *Amer. J. vet. Res.*, 27, 13, 16, 20, 24; 29, 181.
(8) Correa-Giron, E. P. *et al.* (1970). *Amer. J. Epidem.*, 91, 203.
(9) Soave, O. A. (1966). *Amer. J. vet. Res.*, 27, 44.
(10) Baer, G. M. & Adams, D. B. (1970). *Publ. Hlth Rep. Wash.*, 85, 637.
(11) Schaaf, J. & Schaaf, E. (1968). *Dtsch. tierärztl. Wschr.*, 75, 315, 319.
(12) Henderson, J. A. (1942). *Vet. Med.*, 37, 88.

(13) Merriman, G. M. (1966). *J. Amer. vet. med. Ass.*, *148*, 809.

(14) Morehouse, L. G. *et al.* (1968). *J. Amer. vet. med. Ass.*, *153*, 57.

(15) Markson, L. M. *et al.* (1971). *Trop. Anim. Hlth Prod.*, *3*, 89.

(16) Fourth Report of the Expert Committee on Rabies (1960). *Wld Hlth Org. techn. Rep. Ser.*, 201.

(17) Black, J. G. & Lawson, K. F. (1970). *Canad. J. comp. Med.*, *34*, 309.

(18) Baer, G. M. *et al.* (1971). *Amer. J. Epidem.*, *93*, 487.

(19) Dreesen, D. W. *et al.* (1970). *J. Amer. vet. med. Ass.*, *157*, 826.

(20) Lawson, K. F. *et al.* (1967). *Vet. Med.*, *62*, 1073.

(21) Abelseth, M. K. (1967). *Canad. vet. J.*, *8*, 221.

(22) Kalmar, E. (1966). *Refuah vet.*, *23*, 151.

Pseudorabies

(*Aujesky's Disease*)

Pseudorabies is a viral disease affecting primarily pigs and rodents but occurring incidentally in most other species. In swine the disease is inapparent except in young pigs, in which it produces an acute fatal encephalitis. In the other species there is both encephalitis and marked local pruritus.

Incidence

Pseudorabies has a wide geographical distribution, including the U.S.A., and Britain, Europe, North Africa, Asia and South America. Cases in cattle occur only sporadically, but a number of animals may be affected when cattle and pigs are run together. The incidence in pigs may be quite high, but accurate figures are not available. In young, sucking pigs the morbidity and mortality rates approach 100 per cent, but in mature swine the disease may produce no clinical signs, and animals that are affected usually recover. Naturally occurring cases in other species are rare but the disease is usually fatal. In herds of pigs the highest morbidity occurs initially in unweaned piglets, but as the outbreak continues and piglets become passively immunized through the sow's colostrum, the major incidence may move to weaners (1).

Aetiology

The causative herpes virus can be passaged in rabbits and unweaned hamsters and can be grown in embryonated hen eggs and on tissue culture. More than one strain may exist. The virus can exist for 4 to 7 weeks or more in infected premises. The disease is known to occur naturally in pigs, cattle, sheep, dogs (2, 3) and cats (1), and it has been suspected in horses. It can be transmitted experimentally to horses, sheep, goats, foxes, dogs, cats and many small wild mammals and birds. Rare cases have been reported in man in which local pruritus occurs but the disease is not fatal.

In animals a strong natural immunity develops after an attack and artificial vaccination has been satisfactorily achieved. Unweaned pigs are most susceptible and weaning, even on to artificial diets at an early age, greatly reduces the susceptibility.

Transmission

Pigs and rodents appear to be the natural reservoir of the virus. The disease may spread from normal or clinically affected pigs to animals of other species, but does not usually spread between animals of the other species. For example, sheep and calves can be infected experimentally, but there is no evidence that they excrete the virus. Brown rats may be a minor source of infection but are unlikely to be an important reservoir. They are capable of spreading the disease to dogs.

The virus is present in the nasal discharge and in the mouth of affected pigs on the first day of illness and for up to 17 days after infection (5). The rarity of spread to other species is due to the scanty nasal discharge and the improbability of the discharge coming into contact with abraded skin or nasal mucosa of animals other than pigs.

The portal of entry is through abraded skin or via the intact nasal mucosa. Experimentally the disease can be transmitted by these routes and by intracerebral injection. Although the virus is detectable in the blood in the early stages of the disease, there is no evidence that biting insects act as vectors. Care should be exercised during necropsy examination, as infection of humans may occur through skin wounds.

Pathogenesis

The virus is pantropic and affects tissues derived from all embryonic layers. In the pig there is a short and ill-defined period of viraemia with localization of the virus in many viscera, but with multiplication occurring primarily in the respiratory tract. Spread to the brain is thought to occur by way of the olfactory, glossopharyngeal or trigeminal nerves. Virus disappears from the brain by the eighth day, coinciding with the appearance of neutralizing antibody in the blood (6). When the virus gains entry through a skin abrasion, it quickly invades the local peripheral nerves, passing along them centripetally and causing damage to nerve cells. It is this form of progression which causes local pruritus in the early stages of the disease and encephalomyelitis at a later stage when the virus has invaded the central nervous system. In pigs pruritus does not develop after intramuscular injection, but a local paralysis indicative of damage to lower motor neurones occurs prior to invasion of the central nervous system in some pigs.

When the virus is instilled into nasal cavities or inoculated into the brain, signs of encephalitis rather than local pruritus predominate. With intranasal inoculation there is an initial stage of viral proliferation in the nasal and tonsillar mucosa (7). Systemic invasion occurs and, as with intravenous injection, is followed by localization and invasion of the central nervous system along peripheral and autonomic nerve trunks and fibres (8).

Clinical Findings

The incubation period in natural outbreaks is about a week, whereas it may be as short as 2 days following experimental inoculation.

Pigs. Considerable difference in signs is apparent between adult and young pigs up to 3 months of age. Pruritus, as it occurs in cattle, does not occur in pigs of any age. In adult pigs complete anorexia may appear first, accompanied by dullness, agalactia and constipation. Temperatures are usually normal at 39·5°C (103°F). The skin may become dirty and there is a yellowish discoloration of the face and shoulders. Sows appear to be more susceptible about the time of farrowing, showing signs for a few days, but recovering promptly. A high incidence of mummified foetuses, late abortions, stillbirths and high neonatal mortality may occur in a group of infected sows. It is not uncommon for the signs to be so mild as to pass unnoticed in mature or half grown pigs.

Young pigs a few days to a month old show the greatest susceptibility. Very young sucklings develop an indistinct syndrome, but prominent nervous signs occur in older piglets. A febrile reaction, with temperatures up to 41·5°C (107°F), occurs prior to the onset of nervous signs. Incoordination of the hind limbs causing sideways progression is followed by recumbency, fine and coarse muscle tremors and paddling movements. Lateral deviation of the head, frothing at the mouth, nystagmus, slight ocular discharge and convulsive episodes appear in a few animals. A snoring respiration with marked abdominal movement occurs in many, and vomiting and diarrhoea in some affected pigs. Deaths occur about 12 hours after the first signs appear. In California a consistent sign has been blindness due to extensive retinal degeneration (9).

Cattle. There may be sudden death without obvious signs of illness. More commonly there is intense, local pruritus with violent licking, chewing and rubbing of the part. Itching may be localized to any part of the body surface, but is most common about the head, the flanks or the feet, the sites most likely to be contaminated by virus. There is intense excitement during this stage and convulsions and constant bellowing may occur. Maniacal behaviour, circling, spasm of the diaphragm and opisthotonus are often evident. A stage of paralysis follows in which salivation, respiratory distress and ataxia occur. The temperature is usually increased, sometimes to as high as 41 to 41·5°C (106 to 107°F). Final paralysis is followed by death in 6 to 48 hours after the first appearance of illness. The disease can occur in newborn calves.

The clinical picture in dogs and cats is similar to that in cattle, with death occurring in about 24 hours (10).

Clinical Pathology

Ante-mortem laboratory examinations are not ordinarily carried out, but specific virus neutralizing antibodies are detectable in the serum of recovered pigs and this test is in routine use for herd diagnosis and survey purposes. Injection of tissues from suspected animals into rats or mice is a highly regarded test (11).

Necropsy Findings

When pruritus has occurred there is considerable damage to local areas of skin and extensive subcutaneous oedema. The lungs show congestion, oedema and some haemorrhages. Haemorrhages may be present under the endocardium and excess fluid is often present in the pericardial sac. In pigs there are additional lesions of visceral involvement. Slight splenomegaly, meningitis and excess pericardial fluid are observed and there may be small necrotic foci in the spleen and liver. Histologically, in all species, there is severe and extensive neuronal damage in the spinal cord and brain. Perivascular cuffing and focal necrosis are present in the grey matter, particularly in the cerebellar cortex. Intranuclear inclusion bodies occur infrequently in the degenerating neurones particularly in cerebral cortex in the pig. These are of considerable importance in differential diagnosis.

The presence of the virus in frozen sections of brain is demonstrable by fluorescent antibody staining (12).

Material for transmission experiments in rabbits or unweaned hamsters should include local tissue at the site of infection, part of a local nerve trunk and its spinal segment and a piece of cerebellum.

Diagnosis

In cattle the diagnosis is usually suggested by the severe pruritus and short course. Confirmation can be obtained by transmission to the rabbit and a virus-neutralization test using known antipseudorabies serum. Subcutaneous transmission is preferred to intracerebral injection because of the characteristic local pruritus which occurs with the former method.

In pigs pseudorabies presents a similar clinical picture to viral encephalomyelitis (Teschen disease). The inclusion bodies of pseudorabies, serological tests and particularly the isolation of virus in tissue culture (13) are of help in diagnosis. Rabies is rare in pigs and is usually accompanied by pruritus at the site of the bite. Streptococcal meningitis is restricted in occurrence to sucking pigs of 2 to 3 weeks of age and the causative organism is readily cultured from the meninges. The response to treatment with penicillin is good and is of value as a diagnostic test. Hypoglycaemia of baby pigs has a very similar clinical picture.

In enzootic areas louping ill and Japanese B encephalitis may have to be considered as possible causes of encephalitis in pigs. Involvement of the nervous system with the development of encephalitis may occur in outbreaks of hog cholera and African swine fever, but there are other diagnostic features in these outbreaks. In a number of bacterial infections there may be similar involvement of the central nervous system. These include salmonellosis, Glasser's disease, *E. coli* septicaemia and erysipelas. Gut oedema and salt poisoning produce obvious nervous signs, but there is no fever and there are lesions at necropsy which aid in differentiation.

In cattle the local pruritus is distinctive but the disease may be confused with the nervous form of acetonaemia in which paraesthesia may lead to excitement. The rapid recovery which ordinarily occurs in this form of acetonaemia is an important diagnostic point. The furious form of rabies and acute lead poisoning cause signs of mania but pruritus does not occur.

Treatment

No treatment is likely to be of value.

Control

Destruction of rats and isolation of affected pigs is recommended. On affected premises separation of cattle and pigs should be instituted.

A strong immunity develops after natural infection in pigs and other species, and vaccination against the disease is widely practised in Europe. A killed, aluminium hydroxide saponin vaccine is usually used (14) and is credited with significantly reducing the prevalence of the disease (15). A live virus vaccine, with the virus attenuated by multiple passage through chick embryos or cell cultures, appears to produce satisfactory immunity in about 2 weeks. Two vaccinations several weeks apart are usually given (16, 17). Sucking pigs from vaccinated sows have a degree of passive immunity. Passive immunity can also be conferred by the use of globulin concentrates of hyperimmune serum.

REFERENCES

(1) Mackay, R. R. *et al.* (1962). *Vet. Rec.*, *74*, 669.
(2) Mullaney, R. & Murphy, E. C. (1962). *Irish vet. J.*, *16*, 161.
(3) Stepenko, M. F. (1962). *Veterinariya*, *39*, 61.
(4) McFerran, J. B. & Dow, C. (1970). *Brit. vet. J.*, *126*, 173.
(5) McFerran, J. B. & Dow, C. (1964). *Res. vet. Sci.*, *5*, 405.
(6) McFerran, J. B. & Dow, C. (1965). *Amer. J. vet. Res.*, *26*, 631.
(7) Sabo, A. *et al.* (1969). *Acta virol.*, *13*, 407.
(8) Blaskovic, D. *et al.* (1970). *Arch. exp. vet. Med.*, *24*, 9.
(9) Howarth, J. A. & dePaoli, A. (1968). *J. Amer. vet. med. Ass.*, *152*, 1114.
(10) Dow, C. & McFerran, J. B. (1963). *Vet. Rec.*, *75*, 1099.
(11) Fraser, G. & Ramachandran, S. P. (1960). *J. comp. Path.*, *79*, 435.
(12) Meyling, A. & Bitsch, V. (1967). *Acta vet. scand.*, *8*, 360.
(13) Pette, J. (1965). *Bull. Off. int. Épizoot.*, *63*, 1835.
(14) Berbinschi, C. *et al.* (1968). *Arch. vet.*, *5*, 99, 107.
(15) Skoda, R. *et al.* (1970). *Arch. exp. vet. Med.*, *24*, 167.
(16) Nochevnyi, V. T. & Osidze, D. F. (1970). *Veterinariya*, *6*, 44.
(17) Bran, L. *et al.* (1969). *Arch. vet.*, *6*, 15.

Viral Encephalomyelitis of Pigs

(*Teschen Disease, Talfan Disease, Poliomyelitis Suum*)

This encephalomyelitis occurs only in pigs. It is highly infectious, highly fatal and is characterized by hyperaesthesia, tremor, paresis and convulsions.

Incidence

Prior to the last war the incidence of known porcine viral encephalomyelitis was restricted to certain districts in Czechoslovakia. Since then reports of the disease have come from many countries and there is serological evidence that the disease occurs throughout the world (1). The most severe form of the disease—Teschen disease—appears to be limited to Europe, but the milder forms—Talfan disease, poliomyelitis suum and viral encephalomyelitis—are known to occur extensively in Europe, Scandinavia and North America. Losses due to the disease result primarily from deaths although there may be some crippling. The morbidity is usually about 50 per cent and the mortality rate 70 to 90 per cent in Teschen disease as it is described in eastern Europe. The disease in Denmark and the U.K. is much milder and the morbidity rate approximately only 6 per cent. Serological surveys in areas where the disease occurs indicate that a high proportion of the pig population is infected without showing clinical evidence of the disease.

Aetiology

A number of closely related but antigenically different enteroviruses, capable of growth in tissue culture, are known to be causes of encephalomyelitis in pigs (2) and additional, unidentified viruses are frequently isolated (3). The identified agents have been classified into two groups (4). Group 1, the Teschen viruses, includes three subgroups, Konratice, Talfan (Tyrol) and Reporyje. Group 2 contains the antigenically related viruses T80 and T52A. There is a great deal of variation in the severity of the disease in different countries and, although this is partly explainable in terms of the age at which infection occurs, baby pigs being much more susceptible, there is also a marked difference in pathogenicity between strains of the virus. The Konratice strain appears to be much more pathogenic than the others. Other enteroviruses, e.g. F.26, have been isolated from natural cases of polioencephalomyelitis in pigs (10).

The causative viruses will infect only pigs and are not related to any of the viruses which cause encephalomyelitis in other species. They are resistant to environmental conditions, including drying, and are present principally in the central nervous system and intestine of affected pigs.

Immunity after infection appears to develop since in some herds in enzootic areas the disease affects only newborn and introduced pigs. The results of vaccination experiments are conflicting but in some instances serviceable immunity has been produced. Pigs of all ages are susceptible, although pigs of 15 to 20 lb. weight are most readily infected experimentally. In field outbreaks a high incidence of the severe form of the disease is most common in baby pigs up to 2 weeks of age, and the mild transient form in pigs 1 to 6 months of age.

Transmission

Experimentally the disease is transmissible by ingestion, intranasal instillation and by intramuscular and intracerebral injection. It is presumed that in natural outbreaks the first two routes are of first importance. The source of the virus may be either clinically affected pigs or latent carriers which carry the virus on the tonsils or in the lower part of the alimentary tract. The ingestion of faeces from infected pigs is known to be a method of transmission, but not all infected pigs shed infective concentrations of virus in their droppings (5).

Pathogenesis

Available evidence suggests that the virus multiplies peripherally, probably in the intestine, and enters the brain via the blood stream. A viraemia occurs after infection, often 10 to 12 days before signs appear.

Clinical Findings

Acute viral encephalomyelitis (Teschen Disease). The experimental disease, which closely resembles the natural disease (6), commences with an incubation period of 10 to 12 days followed by several days of fever (40 to 41 °C or 104 to 106 °F). Signs of encephalitis follow, although these are more extensive and acute after intracerebral inoculation. They include stiffness of the extremities, and inability to stand, with falling to one side followed by tremor, nystagmus and violent clonic convulsions. Anorexia is usually complete and vomiting has been observed. There may be partial or complete loss of voice due to laryngeal paralysis. Facial paralysis may also occur. Stiffness and opisthotonus are often persistent between convulsions, which are easily stimulated by noise and often accompanied by loud squealing. The convulsive period lasts for 24 to 36 hours. A sharp temperature fall may be followed by coma and death on the 3rd to 4th day, but in cases of longer duration, the convulsive stage may be followed by flaccid paralysis affecting particularly the hind limbs. In milder cases early stiffness and weakness are followed by flaccid paralysis without the irritation phenomena of convulsions and tremor.

Subacute viral encephalomyelitis (Talfan Disease in the U.K., viral encephalomyelitis in North America, poliomyelitis suum in Denmark). The clinical findings in the subacute disease are much milder than in the acute disease and the morbidity and mortality rates are lower. The disease is most common and severe in pigs less than 2 weeks of age. Older sucking pigs are affected also but less severely and many recover completely. Sows suckling affected litters may be mildly and transiently ill. The morbidity rate in very young litters is often 100 per cent and nearly all the affected piglets die. In litters over 3 weeks old there may be only a small proportion of the pigs affected. The disease often strikes very suddenly—all litters in a piggery being affected within a few days—but disappears as suddenly, subsequent litters being unaffected. Clinically the syndrome includes anorexia, rapid loss of condition, constipation, frequent vomiting of minor degree and a normal or slightly elevated temperature. Nervous signs appear several days after the illness commences. Piglets up to 2 weeks of age show hyperaesthesia, muscle tremor, knuckling of the fetlocks, ataxia, walking backwards, a dog-sitting posture and terminally lateral recumbency, with paddling convulsions, nystagmus, blindness and dyspnoea. Older pigs (4 to 6 weeks of age) show transient anorexia and posterior paresis manifested by a swaying, drunken gait and usually recover completely and quickly.

Clinical Pathology

A virus-neutralization test in tissue culture and a complement-fixation test have been utilized in the diagnosis of the disease. The antibodies are detectable in the early stages and persist for a considerable time after recovery. Challenge of previously hyperimmunized pigs by the intracerebral injection of the suspect material is also a satisfactory diagnostic technique. Virus is present in the blood of affected pigs in the early stages of the disease and in the faeces in very small amounts in the incubation period before signs of illness appear, but brain tissue is usually used as a source of virus in transmission experiments.

Necropsy Findings

There is a diffuse non-suppurative encephalomyelitis of viral type with involvement of grey matter predominating. The brain stem and spinal cord show the most extensive lesions. Meningitis affecting particularly the meninges over the cerebellum is an early manifestation of the disease. Virus can be isolated from brain, from gastric mucosa and faeces in very small amounts, or from the blood during the incubation period. No inclusion bodies are present in neurones as there are in cases of pseudorabies.

Diagnosis

The diagnosis of diseases causing signs of acute cerebral involvement in pigs is extremely difficult and a confirmatory diagnosis usually depends on exhaustive laboratory work. In general, viral diseases, bacterial diseases and intoxications must be considered as possible groups of causes and careful selection of material for laboratory examination is essential. The differentiation of the possible causes of diseases resembling viral encephalomyelitis is described under pseudorabies and in general medicine under diseases of the nervous system.

Treatment

None is recommended.

Control

Immediate isolation of affected pigs is recommended because of the probable spread by direct contact. Vaccination is not generally accepted as a satisfactory method of control, but now that the virus has been grown in tissue culture, a suitable vaccine may become available. Vaccines prepared by formalin inactivation of infective spinal cord and adsorption on to aluminium hydroxide have been used extensively in Europe. Two or three injections are given at 10 to 14 day intervals and immunity persists for about 6 months (7). A modified live virus vaccine is also available (8).

In the event of its appearance in a previously free country eradication of the disease by slaughter and quarantine should be attempted if practicable. Austria recently reported eradication of the disease which had been present in that country for many years (9). A slaughter policy was supplemented by ring vaccination around infected premises.

REVIEW LITERATURE

Mills, J. H. L. & Nielsen, S. W. (1968). *Advanc. vet. Sci.*, 33.

REFERENCES

(1) Paterson, A. B. (1962). *Bull. Off. int. Épizoot.*, 57, 1569.
(2) Done, J. T. (1961). *Bull. Off. int. Épizoot.*, 56, 117.
(3) Girard, A. *et al.* (1964). *Res. vet. Sci.*, 5, 294.
(4) Darbyshire, J. H. & Dawson, P. S. (1963). *Res. vet. Sci.*, 4, 48.
(5) Alexander, T. J. L. (1962). *Amer. J. vet. Res.*, 23, 756.
(6) Dardiri, A. H. *et al.* (1966). *Canad. J. comp. Med.*, 30, 71.
(7) Lalonne, O. (1958). *Bull. Off. int. Épizoot.*, 50, 439.
(8) Korych, B. & Patocka, F. (1967). *Cslka Epidem. Mikrobiol. Imunol.*, 16, 257.
(9) Schaupp, W. (1968). *Wien. tierärztl. Wschr.*, 55, 346.
(10) Mason, R. W. (1970). *Brit. vet. J.*, 126, xix.

Sporadic Bovine Encephalomyelitis (SBE)

(Buss Disease, Transmissible Serositis)

Sporadic bovine encephalomyelitis is caused by a virus and characterized by inflammation of vascular endothelium and mesenchymal tissue. There is secondary involvement of the nervous system, with nervous signs, in some cases.

Incidence

The disease has been reported only from the United States, Japan and Israel but a provisional diagnosis has been made in Australia, where it is thought that the disease may have been present for some time, and in Canada, South Africa and Hungary. In the U.S.A. it occurs most commonly in the mid-western and western states. Sporadic cases or outbreaks occur in individual herds. Although the disease has not reached serious economic proportions in the enzootic areas, there is some serological evidence that widespread sub-clinical infections occur (1). As a rule only sporadic cases occur, but in some outbreaks there may be severe loss due to both deaths of animals and loss of condition (1). There is considerable variation in morbidity and mortality rates from herd to herd. Morbidity rates average 12·5 per cent (5 to 50 per cent), being highest in calves (25 per cent) and lowest in animals over a year old (5 per cent). Mortality rates average about 31 per cent and are higher in adults than in calves. In affected herds a stage of herd immunity is reached when only introduced animals and new-born calves are susceptible.

Aetiology

The disease is caused by a chlamydia (2). It resists freezing but is highly susceptible to sodium hydroxide, cresol and quaternary ammonium compounds in standard concentrations. The virus can be passaged in guinea pigs and hamsters and adapted to grow in the yolk sac of developing chick embryos. Only cattle are affected and calves less than 6 months of age are most susceptible. Other domestic and experimental species appear to be resistant. There is no seasonal incidence, cases appearing at any time of the year. A strong and apparently persistent immunity develops after an attack of the disease.

Transmission

Intracerebral inoculation of the virus in calves produces fever, anorexia, weight loss, inactivity, lacrimation and stiffness of gait, with histological but no clinical signs of encephalitis. Intraperitoneal inoculation results in peritonitis, perisplenitis and perihepatitis. The virus can be isolated from many organs, including liver, spleen and central nervous system and from the blood, faeces, urine, nasal discharges and milk in the early stages of the disease. There is some evidence that the virus is eliminated in the faeces for several weeks after infection.

The method of spread under natural conditions is not known. The pattern of incidence is variable. Spread from farm to farm does not occur readily. On some farms only sporadic cases may occur, but on others one or two cases occur every year. In still other herds the disease occurs in outbreak form, with a number of animals becoming affected within a period of about 4 weeks. The epizootiology of sporadic bovine encephalomyelitis resembles in many ways that of bovine malignant catarrh.

Pathogenesis

The virus is not specifically neurotropic and attacks principally the mesenchymal tissues and the endothelial lining of the vascular system, with particular involvement of the serous membranes. Encephalomyelitis occurs secondarily to the vascular damage.

Clinical Findings

In field cases the incubation period varies between 4 days and 4 weeks. Affected calves show depression and inactivity but the appetite may be unaffected for several days. Nasal discharge and salivation with drooling are frequently observed. Temperatures are raised (40·5 to 41·5°C or 105 to 107°F), and remain high for the course of the disease. About half of the animals have dyspnoea and cough and mild catarrhal nasal discharge and diarrhoea may occur. During the ensuing 2 weeks difficulty in walking and lack of desire to stand may appear. Stiffness with knuckling at the fetlocks is evident at first, followed by staggering, circling and falling. Opisthotonus may be present but there is no excitement or head-pressing. The course of the disease varies between 3 days and 3 weeks. Animals that recover show marked loss of condition and are slow to regain the lost weight.

Clinical Pathology

In experimental cases leucopenia occurs in the acute clinical stage. There is a relative lymphocytosis and depression of polymorphonuclear cells. Virus can be isolated from the blood in the early clinical phase and can be used for transmission experiments in calves and guinea pigs and for culture in eggs. Elementary bodies are present in the guinea-pig tissues and yolk-sac preparations. Serological methods, including a complement-fixation test, for the detection of circulating antibody are available although there is difficulty in differentiating antibodies to the virus from those to the typical psittacosis virus.

Necropsy Findings

A fibrinous peritonitis, pleurisy and pericarditis accompanied by congestion and petechiation are characteristic. In the early stages thin serous fluid is present in the cavities, but in the later stages this has progressed to a thin fibrinous net covering the affected organs or even to flattened plaques or irregularly shaped masses of fibrin lying free in the cavity. Histologically there is fibrinous serositis involving the serosa of the peritoneal, pleural and pericardial cavities. A diffuse encephalomyelitis involving particularly the medulla and cerebellum and a meningitis in the same area are also present. Minute elementary bodies are present in infected tissues and in very small numbers in exudate.

Diagnosis

The necropsy findings are diagnostic for sporadic bovine encephalomyelitis (SBE) and confirmation can be obtained by the complement-fixation test or virus-neutralization tests. Clinically the disease resembles other encephalitides of cattle. The epizootiology and pathogenesis resemble those of bovine malignant catarrh (BMC), but the mortality rate is much lower, there are no ocular or mucosal lesions and the serositis of SBE does not occur in BMC. A viral encephalomyelitis of calves (Kunjin virus) has been identified but has not been associated with clinical signs of disease of the nervous system (3). An encephalomyocarditis virus, a primary infection of rodents which also occurs in primates, and causes myocarditis in pigs (5) has been transmitted experimentally to calves but without causing significant signs of disease (4). Listeriosis is usually sporadic and is accompanied by more localizing signs, especially facial paralysis and circling. Rabies may present a very similar clinical picture, but the initial febrile reaction and the characteristic necropsy findings as well as the epizootiological history of SBE should enable a diagnosis to be made. Lead poisoning can be differentiated by the absence of fever, the more severe signs of motor irritation and the shorter course of the disease. Because of the respiratory tract involvement SBE may be easily confused with pneumonic pasteurellosis, especially if outbreaks occur, but in the latter disease nervous signs are unusual and the response to treatment is good.

Treatment

Broad spectrum antibiotics control the virus in vitro. Clinical results with chlortetracycline and oxytetracycline have been irregular (6), but they are likely to be effective if used in the early stages of the disease.

Control

Control measures are difficult to prescribe because of lack of knowledge of the method of transmission. It is advisable to isolate affected animals. No vaccine is available.

REFERENCES

(1) Harshfield, G. S. (1957). *Sporadic Bovine Encephalomyelitis, Tech. Bull. No. 8*, Agric. Exp. Sta., Sth. Dak. State Coll. Agric., Brookings, S.D., U.S.A.
(2) Harshfield, G. S. (1970). *J. Amer. vet. med. Ass.*, *156*, 466.
(3) Spradbrow, P. B. & Clark, L. (1966). *Aust. vet. J.*, *42*, 65.
(4) Spradbrow, P. B. *et al.* (1970). *Aust. vet. J.*, *46*, 373.
(5) Gainer, J. H. (1967). *J. Amer. vet. med. Ass.*, *151*, 421.

Ovine Encephalomyelitis

(*Louping Ill*)

Louping ill is an acute encephalomyelitis affecting chiefly sheep, but occurring occasionally in other animals and man. The causative virus is transmitted by the bite of an infective tick. Clinically the disease is characterized by fever, abnormality of gait, convulsions and paralysis.

Incidence

Louping ill is recorded only in Scotland, the border counties of England and Ireland, although a similar and probably identical disease, Russian spring-summer encephalitis, occurs in Russia and Central Europe. The distribution of these diseases is probably limited by the bionomics of the vector ticks. The morbidity rate of louping ill in Britain is low in areas where the disease is enzootic, only 1 to 4 per cent of adult sheep becoming infected. In lambs the morbidity rate may be as high as 60 per cent, although lambs born to immune ewes may resist infection for about 3 months. It would appear that in enzootic areas inapparent infection followed by immunity must be common, since the morbidity rate may be considerably higher in introduced mature sheep. The mortality rate is of the order of 10 to 15 per cent.

Aetiology

The causative arbovirus can be cultivated in all sites of the developing chick embryo and tissue culture and, after experimental injection, causes encephalitis in mice. It is not very resistant to environmental influences and is readily destroyed by disinfectants. Immunity after an attack persists for life. Sheep are the only animals commonly affected, but occasional cases occur in all other domestic species, various rodents and man. Rodents may act as reservoirs and amplifiers of the virus, especially in years of peak population (1). Red deer (*Cervus elaphus*) is an alternate host of the virus in Scotland (2) and the elk (*Alces a. alces*) may be in Sweden (3). The virus has also been isolated from birds (4, 5). Cases in man occur principally in laboratory workers, and the incidence in the human population does not vary with changes in the incidence in local sheep.

Transmission

Although the major method of spread is by the bites of infected ticks, spread by droplet infection may be of some importance. The vector ticks in the U.K. are *Ixodes ricinus* and *Rhipicephalus appendiculatus*, and in the U.S.S.R., *I. ricinus* and *I. persulcatus*. Only adult *I. ricinus* are infective; the virus persists in individual ticks for long periods, but whether it is transmitted through the egg is uncertain. Other ectoparasites, especially fleas, are suspected as vectors of the virus (4). The disease has a seasonal occurrence during spring and summer when the ticks are active.

Pathogenesis

After infection a viraemia occurs, concurrent with pyrexia. If entrance to nervous tissue is effected across the blood–brain barrier, a secondary febrile reaction occurs at the time of appearance of the nervous signs. In those animals in which invasion of nervous tissue does not occur recovery is rapid and uneventful and there is immunity to subsequent infection. The virus persists for some time in the blood of these animals, whereas it disappears immediately if the blood–brain barrier is passed. Because invasion of brain occurs in only a proportion of naturally or artificially infected animals, it has been suggested that a concurrent tick-borne fever infection may reduce the resistance of the blood–brain barrier to the louping ill virus. Recent work suggests that invasion of the central nervous system may occur in most if not all experimentally infected animals, although the lesions may be small and isolated (6). Haemagglutination inhibition antibodies are detectable 5 to 10 days after experimental infection provided the inoculation was not given intracerebrally (6).

Clinical Findings

After an incubation period of 6 to 18 days there is a sudden onset of high fever (up to 41·5°C or 107°F) followed by a return to normal, and then a second febrile phase starting about the 5th day during which nervous signs appear. Affected animals stand apart, often with the head held high. There is marked tremor of muscle groups and rigidity of the musculature, particularly in the neck and limbs. This is manifested by jerky, stiff movements and a bounding gait which gives rise to the name—louping ill. Inco-ordination is most marked in the hind limbs. The sheep walks into objects and may stand with the head pressed against them. Hypersensitivity to noise and touch may be apparent. The increased muscle tone is succeeded by paralysis and recumbency. In fatal cases death follows after a course of 7 to 10 days. The clinical picture in cattle is very similar to that observed in sheep although convulsions are more likely to occur in cattle, and in the occasional animals which recover from the encephalitis there is usually persistence of signs of impairment of the central nervous system. In man an influenza-like disease followed by meningo-encephalitis occurs after an incubation period of 6 to 18 days. Complete recovery is usual.

Clinical Pathology

The virus can be isolated from the blood of infected animals at the height of the initial viraemia, and for an indeterminate period afterwards in those which show no nervous signs. Intracerebral injection into mice produces a fatal encephalomyelitis. Neutralizing antibodies can be detected in the serum of recovered animals. Complement fixing antibodies are also detectable but are so transient that the test lacks dependability as a diagnostic tool (7). Mice immunized by the injection of serum are protected against experimental infection.

Necropsy Findings

No gross changes are observed. Histologically there are perivascular accumulations of cells in the meninges, brain and spinal cord with neuronal damage most evident in cerebellar Purkinje cells and to a less extent in the cerebral cortex. No pathognomonic inclusion bodies are present. For laboratory examination tissue fixed in formalin should be sent for histological examination and fresh tissue, unrefrigerated, in 30 per cent glycerol for virus isolation. The louping-ill virus can be consistently demonstrated in nervous tissue by the use of fluorescent antibody (8).

Diagnosis

The histological findings are not specific and transmission of the disease to mice, and serum-neutralization tests are required to confirm the diagnosis. Clinically the disease in sheep bears resemblance to some stages of scrapie, to inco-ordination due to plant poisons, to tetanus and to hypocalcaemia and pregnancy toxaemia. The short course and high fever differentiate it from scrapie and from plant poisonings. Tetanus is characterized by tetany of the limbs and occurs usually after skin wounds or minor surgery. Pregnancy toxaemia and hypocalcaemia are usually related to lambing and show no febrile reaction.

Treatment

An antiserum has been used and affords protection if given within 48 hours of exposure, but is of no value once the febrile reaction has begun.

Control

A formalinized tissue vaccine derived from brain, spinal cord and spleen provides excellent immunity and in enzootic areas vaccination of all animals over 4 months of age is recommended. The vaccine is not without risk for persons manufacturing it and it has been largely replaced by a new killed vaccine, prepared by growing the virus in tissue culture and mixing it with an adjuvant. This vaccine has been shown to give excellent results in field trials (9). Vaccination of ewes in late pregnancy is recommended to provide passive immunity to the lambs via the colostrum. Serial cultivation in hen eggs causes attenuation of the virus, but the potency of the avianized virus diminishes rapidly on storage. Control of ticks by frequent dipping helps to control tick-borne fever and lamb pyaemia as well as louping ill.

REFERENCES

(1) Gordon-Smith, C. E. *et al.* (1964). *Nature (Lond.)*, *203*, 992.
(2) Dunn, A. M. (1960). *Brit. vet. J.*, *116*, 284.
(3) Svedmyr, A. *et al.* (1965). *Acta path. microbiol. scand.*, *65*, 613.
(4) Varma, M. G. R. & Page, R. J. C. (1966). *J. med. Ent.*, *3*, 331.
(5) Timoney, P. J. (1972). *Brit. vet. J.*, *128*, 19.
(6) Reid, H. W. & Doherty, P. C. (1971). *J. comp. Path.*, *81*, 291, 331.
(7) Williams, H. E. (1968). *Amer. J. vet. Res.*, *29*, 1619.
(8) Doherty, P. C. & Reid, H. W. (1971). *J. comp. Path.*, *81*, 531.
(9) Brotherston, J. G. *et al.* (1971). *J. Hyg. Camb.*, *69*, 479.

Scrapie

Scrapie is a non-febrile, fatal, chronic disease of sheep characterized clinically by pruritus and abnormalities of gait, and by a very long incubation period.

Incidence

Scrapie occurs enzootically in the United Kingdom and Europe. Small outbreaks have been reported in Australia, New Zealand, Canada and the U.S.A., principally in sheep imported from enzootic areas. The flock morbidity ranges up to 20 per cent, and on occasions up to 40 per cent. A mortality rate of 100 per cent is usual although the possibility of recovery cannot be disregarded. The death loss is added to by the slaughter of infected and in-contact animals when eradication is undertaken. At the moment the disease is of major importance because of the embargoes maintained by several countries against sheep from enzootic areas. A similar disease to scrapie has been recorded in Iceland under the name of Rida, and there has been a positive identification of scrapie in a nondescript breed of mountain sheep in the foothills of the Himalayas (1). The disease is thought to have been introduced by Rambouillet rams imported into the flocks 20 years ago. A disease with marked similarity to scrapie has been described in mink (2).

Aetiology

Scrapie is caused by a particle which can be transmitted from one animal to another and which multiplies itself within these hosts. Although it is often referred to as virus-like, or a provirus, it has few of the characteristics of a virus. It is capable of withstanding the usual viricidal procedures and is destroyed neither by boiling for 30 minutes, by rapid freezing and thawing nor exposure to ether or 20 per cent formalin (3), although infectivity is greatly reduced by heating at 100°C for one hour (4). At present it is assumed that the scrapie transmitting agent is a small basic protein, or is associated with one, and may not contain nucleic acid (5). Experimentally, transmission of the disease to sheep is effected readily, and accidental transmission has been recorded in sheep vaccinated with louping ill vaccine prepared by formalinization of brain tissue infected with the scrapie agent. Under natural conditions scrapie occurs in sheep and occasionally in goats. Under experimental conditions scrapie has been observed to spread from sheep to goats by contact (6). Experimental transmission to goats is readily effected, the percentage of positive transmission being greater than in sheep (100 per cent as against 60 per cent). Only sheep over 18 months of age show clinical evidence of the disease in natural circumstances. Transmission of scrapie agent from sheep and goats to mice can be effected by intracerebral inoculation and force feeding and material from these mice can be used to produce scrapie in goats. Different strains of the agent may produce somewhat different pathological effects, e.g. a strain from a Dorset Down ram produced lesions in Cheviots in locations unusual for this breed (7). Also a mouse-adapted strain has been shown to undergo modification on passage through rats so that its reinoculation into mice produced different signs and lesions (6). The occurrence of scrapie in mice following the inoculation of biopsy material from a human patient with multiple sclerosis has been observed but not explained (8). All breeds of sheep are thought to be equally susceptible, but the disease does appear to occur more commonly in some breeds, and this has formed the basis for an hypothesis that the disease is inherited (9). In mice there appears to be a marked degree of genetic control over the length of the incubation period of the disease without any effect on absolute resistance being evident. Controversy over the importance of inheritance has been going on for some years, but it now seems indisputable that scrapie is caused by a biologically independent particle which is gene-determined. It is suggested that the disease is a genetic one, the physiological action of the gene being mediated by the specific particle, the provirus (10). The alternative explanation on the evidence is that there is vertical transmission of a slow virus from ewe to lamb. This does give a familial appearance to the occurrence of the disease and thus could suggest a genetic origin (10).

There is no evidence of the development of immunity in infected or apparently recovered animals.

Transmission

The agent is present in the brain, spinal cord, lymph nodes and spleen of infected sheep and has been extracted from sheep and goat brain. Experimental transmission can be effected by subcutaneous, intraocular and intracerebral injection with incubation periods of 20, 15 and 12 months respectively, and by oral dosing with scrapie brain suspension in sheep and goats. Vaccination against louping ill with vaccine contaminated by the agent of scrapie has in the one instance referred to above resulted in widespread dissemination of the disease.

Under natural conditions the method of spread is uncertain and there are unexplained regional differences in the ease with which it spreads. Scrapie appears to have been transmitted by mediate contagion of pasture (11) and is often restricted to particular farms and even to certain fields on these farms. In one instance it reappeared in a formerly infected area after the area had been clear of sheep for 3 years and the newly introduced sheep were from apparently uninfected flocks. Contact infection has also been observed in mice. Congenital infection deriving from either the ram or ewe is also thought to occur, even though neither parent may at any time show evidence of the disease.

The present views on the transmission of scrapie have been best summarized by Pattison (12) as follows: 'that field control of the disease and maintenance of animals under experiment should have regard to the considerable evidence that: (a) contact transfer of the agent from affected to healthy animals can occur in certain rare circumstances, that possibly involve ingestion of the agent: (b) hereditary or congenital transmission is important in sheep, but much less so, if at all, in goats.'

Pathogenesis

In mice, and probably in sheep, the virus shows a predilection first for lymphocytic tissues, where it replicates during the incubation period before invading other tissues, including the nervous system. The appearance of clinical signs is thought to be more closely related to the length of time the virus is present in the nervous system rather than to the amount of virus present (13). The essential lesion in scrapie is the vacuolation of neurones in the spinal cord, medulla, pons and midbrain and the consequential wallerian degeneration in dorsal, ventral and ventrolateral columns of the spinal cord and in nerve fibres in the cerebellar peduncles and in the optic nerves (14). In addition there is degeneration of the cerebellar and hypothalamo-neurohypophysial systems (15).

It has been suggested that there may be several forms of scrapie, e.g., the itching form and the muscle tremor form, and that these may be caused by different strains of the agent (16). There are some biological differences between the types but whether there are other differences is unknown (17). The distribution of the lesions in the brain are, within the limits imposed by lack of knowledge of the neuro-anatomy of the sheep and goat, easily reconciled with the clinical signs observed.

Clinical Findings

The incubation period varies from several months up to 3 years and a course of 4 years and 11 months has been recorded in a goat infected experimentally (18). The course is protracted, varying from 2 to 12 months, but lasting in most cases for about 6 months. The earliest signs are transient nervous phenomena occurring at intervals of several weeks or under conditions of stress. These episodes include sudden collapse and sudden changes of behaviour, with sheep charging at dogs or closed gates. Rubbing and biting at the fleece then begin but are often unobserved because of their infrequent occurrence. The apparent pruritus is manifested chiefly over the rump, thighs and tail base. The poll and dorsum of the neck may also be involved and, less commonly, the neck in front of the shoulder and the ribs behind the elbow. In all cases the affected areas are bilaterally symmetrical. In this early stage a stilted gait is often observed. A general loss of condition may also be observed as an early sign although the appetite may not be severely affected.

The stage of gross clinical signs is manifested by intense pruritus, muscle tremor and marked abnormalities of gait, and severe emaciation. Persistent rubbing causes loss of wool over the areas mentioned above. Scratching with the hind feet and biting at the extremities also occur. Haematoma of the ears and swelling of the face may result from rubbing. Light or deep pressure, pin pricking and application of heat or cold may elicit the characteristic 'nibbling' reaction, during which the animal elevates the head and makes nibbling movements of the lips and licking movements with the tongue. The sheep's expression suggests that the sensations evoked are pleasant ones. The reaction may not be observed consistently, often disappearing when the sheep is excited or in new surroundings.

Simultaneously with the development of pruritus there is serious impairment of locomotion. Hind limb abnormalities appear first. There is incomplete flexion of the hock, shortening of the step, weakness and lack of balance. The sense of spatial relationship appears to be lost and the sheep is slow to correct abnormal postures. Adduction occurs during extension and abduction during flexion. When the animal is attempting to evade capture, gross inco-ordination of head and leg movements is likely and the animal often falls. Convulsions, usually transient but occasionally fatal, may occur at this time. General hyperexcitability is evident. In the animal at rest an intermittent nodding and jerking of the head and fine tremor of superficial muscles may also be observed. In some cases nystagmus can be produced by rotating the head sideways. Other nervous signs include inability to swallow, although prehension is unaffected, vomiting, loss of bleat and blindness. A change of voice to a trembling note is often most noticeable. Anorexia is not evident until the last 4 to 5 weeks and results in rapid loss of body weight. Pregnancy toxaemia may occur as a complication in pregnant ewes during this stage of scrapie. Finally the sheep reaches a stage of extreme emaciation and inability to move without becoming readily fatigued. Sternal recumbency follows and lateral recumbency with hyperextension of the limbs is the final stage. Pyrexia is not evident at any time.

The experimentally produced disease in goats differs clinically from that of sheep in that pruritus is rare, the tail is always cocked up over the back and there is a characteristic posture of the hind legs.

Clinical Pathology

Ante-mortem laboratory examinations are not of positive value in diagnosis, but the examination of skin scrapings may help in the elimination of other diseases.

Necropsy Findings

Gross findings are restricted to traumatic lesions caused by rubbing and to emaciation and loss of wool. Histologically the characteristic lesions are in the grey matter of the brain and include vacuolation and degeneration of the neurones, particularly in the medulla, astrocytosis, and a spongy appearance in the neuroparenchyma. Although vacuolation of neurones does occur apart from cases of scrapie, the much higher incidence of vacuoles in the brains of animals affected with scrapie permits a positive diagnosis to be made on this basis. Some diagnostic use may be made of the development of clinical scrapie in white mice as early as the 96th day after intracerebral inoculation of brain emulsion from affected sheep. Although brain tissue is usually used as a source of virus in transmission experiments, almost every tissue, other than blood, is capable of causing the disease. The significance of the muscle lesions seen in some cases of scrapie is unknown, but it is probable that they are caused by a coincident disease.

Diagnosis

A final diagnosis can only be made on the basis of positive necropsy findings or transmission experiments. The characteristic signs of pruritus, inco-ordination and terminal paralysis occurring during a period of prolonged illness should suggest the possibility of this disease. The long incubation period, slow spread and high mortality rate should also be considered when making a diagnosis. Differentiation from louping ill, pseudorabies, photosensitization, pregnancy toxaemia and external parasitism is necessary. Louping ill occurs in sheep of all ages, has characteristic nervous signs and a short, acute course. Pseudorabies is very rare in sheep and is also characterized by an acute course. Photosensitive dermatitis may cause scratching but there are marked skin lesions which are distributed over the woolless part of the body. Pregnancy toxaemia has a seasonal incidence and a short course, there is ketonuria and pruritus is absent. External parasitism can usually be detected by simple examination of the skin. Visna has distinctive lesions.

Treatment

No treatment has proved capable of changing the course of the disease.

Control

Vaccines are not available. All clinical cases should be slaughtered. In herds and areas where the disease is not enzootic all in-contact animals should also be destroyed, and land on which the flock has run should be left unstocked for at least 2 months. Barns and shelter sheds should be cleaned and disinfected with a 2 per cent lye (caustic soda) solution.

In the United States and Canada the disease is under official control (19), and in those countries and the U.K. the disease has largely disappeared. In the U.S.A. the original eradication programme was as follows. Affected flocks were destroyed and animals transferred from them during the preceding 2 months traced, and they and their immediate progeny slaughtered. The recipient flock was placed under long-term surveillance. Currently a flock is destroyed if more than one family bears infected animals. Otherwise only the infected family is destroyed. The exposed unrelated sheep are quarantined and inspected.

REFERENCES

(1) Zlotnik, I. & Katiyar, A. D. (1961). *Vet. Rec.*, *73*, 542.
(2) Hartsough, G. R. & Burger, D. (1965). *J. infect. Dis.*, *115*, 387.
(3) Pattison, I. H. (1965). *J. comp. Path.*, *75*, 159.
(4) Hunter, G. D. & Millison, G. C. (1964). *J. gen. Microbiol.*, *37*, 251.
(5) Pattison, I. H. & Jones, K. M. (1967). *Vet. Rec.*, *80*, 2.
(6) Pattison, I. H. & Jones, K. M. (1968). *Res. vet. Sci.*, *9*, 408.
(7) Zlotnik, I. & Stamp, J. T. (1966). *Vet. Rec.*, *78*, 222.
(8) Field, E. J. (1966). *Brit. med. J.*, *2*, 564.
(9) Parry, H. B. (1962). *Heredity*, *17*, 75.
(10) Dickinson, A. G. *et al.* (1965). *Heredity*, *20*, 485.
(11) Gordon, W. S. (1964). *Vet. Rec.*, *58*, 516.
(12) Pattison, I. H. (1964). *Vet. Rec.*, *76*, 333.
(13) Eklund, C. M. *et al.* (1964). *Report of Scrapie Seminar, Washington D.C.*, pp. 288–91.

(14) Palmer, A. C. (1968). *Vet. Rec.*, *82*, 729.
(15) Beck, E. *et al.* (1964). *Brain*, *87*, 153.
(16) Brotherston, J. G. *et al.* (1968). *J. comp. Path.*, *78*, 9.
(17) Pattison, I. H. (1966). *Res. vet. Sci.*, *7*, 207.
(18) Pattison, I. H. (1965). *Vet. Rec.*, *77*, 1388.
(19) Hourrigan, J. L. (1963). *Proc. 17th World vet. Congr. Hanover*, *1*, pp. 619–24.

Visna

Visna is a disease of the central nervous system of sheep recorded only in Iceland (1). It can be transmitted by intracerebral injection of cell free filtrates of brain tissue and by intrapulmonary inoculation (2) but its mode of transmission in the field is unknown. The causative virus has been cultivated in tissue culture (3) and is closely related to the maedi virus. Progressive paralysis develops 1 to 2 years after inoculation in some animals. The characteristic histological lesion is an inflammation of the glial and ependymal cells, followed by demyelination, in the white matter of the cerebrum and cerebellum (4). There is an increased cell count in cerebrospinal fluid and neutralizing antibodies to the virus are present in the sera of affected sheep (5). The incubation period and the course of the disease are very long; clinical signs may not appear for 2 years after experimental inoculation and affected animals may show clinical signs for 1 to 2 years before final paralysis necessitates slaughter. During the course of the disease periods of relative normality may occur but the disease is usually fatal. Visna has been successfully eradicated from Iceland and is now thought to exist only as a laboratory model. However, lesions similar to those found in visna have been reported in Dutch sheep affected with zwoegerziekte (6).

REFERENCES

(1) Sigurdsson, B. & Palsson, P. A. (1958). *Brit. J. exp. Path.*, *39*, 519.
(2) Gudnadottir, M. & Palsson, P. A. (1965). *J. int. Dis.*, *115*, 217.
(3) Thormar, H. (1963). *Virology*, *19*, 273.
(4) Sigurdsson, B. *et al.* (1962). *Acta. neuropath.*, *1*, 343.
(5) Gudnadottir, M. & Palsson, P. A. (1965). *J. Immunol.*, *95*, 1116.
(6) Ressang, A. A. *et al.* (1966). *Path. Vet.*, *3*, 401.

'Hairy Shaker' Disease of Lambs

(Border Disease, Hairy Shakers, Hypomyelinogenesis Congenita)

This disease of newborn lambs of all breeds is recorded in the U.K. (5) and New Zealand (3). The cause is not known but all the evidence suggests an infectious agent, presumed to be transmissible horizontally from ewe to ewe, as well as by genital contact, and vertically from dam to offspring. Experimental transmission is effected by injection of lamb tissues into pregnant ewes during early pregnancy with the disease appearing in the next lambs (1). The causative agent appears to be more than usually viable and resists freezing and thawing. Abnormalities of lambs are only one of the disease's manifestations. There is also a lack of longevity and fertility (5).

Affected lambs are lighter than normal at birth. The trunk is thicker and the legs shorter than in normal lambs. The head is dome-shaped. Some kempy fibres are present in the fleece and the halo hairs persist and stick out over the normal level of fleece—hence 'hairy'. There are rhythmic tonic–clonic contractions of body muscles manifested as a coarse tremor, but only in some lambs. A high incidence of abortions occurs in experimentally infected ewes but has not been recorded in the natural disease (4). Ewes carrying affected lambs may suffer mild fever and lymphocytosis.

Diagnosis is largely on clinical grounds. The suspected virus has not yet been isolated. Experimental small animals are not susceptible and attempts at tissue culture and serological identification have been unsuccessful. At necropsy examination there is hypomyelinogenesis (3), a relative deficiency of myelin lipids and an excessive amount of esterified cholesterol in nervous tissue (2).

Affected lambs grow poorly and are weakly viable, most lambs dying soon after birth. Survivors have a poor life expectancy.

REFERENCES

(1) Barlow, R. M. et al. (1970). J. comp. Path., 80, 635.
(2) Patterson, D. S. P. et al. (1971). J. Neurochem., 18, 883.
(3) Manktelow, B. W. et al. (1969). N.Z. vet. J., 17, 245.
(4) Lewis, K. H. C. et al. (1970). Vet. Rec., 86, 537.
(5) Nott, J. A. & Shaw, I. G. (1967). Vet. Rec., 80, 534.

VIRAL AND CHLAMYDIAL DISEASES CHARACTERIZED BY SKIN LESIONS

Contagious Ecthyma

(*Contagious Pustular Dermatitis, Orf, Soremouth*)

Contagious ecthyma is a highly infectious viral disease of sheep and goats characterized by the development of pustular and scabby lesions on the muzzle and lips. The virus can also produce lesions on the teats of cattle.

Incidence

The disease occurs wherever sheep are raised and causes unthriftiness and some economic loss. The incidence within a flock may be as high as 90 per cent. The few deaths which occur are due to the extension of lesions into the respiratory tract, but the mortality rate may reach 15 per cent if lambs are badly cared for or if secondary infection and cutaneous myiasis are allowed to occur. In the rare outbreaks where systemic invasion occurs the mortality rate averages 25 per cent and may be as high as 75 per cent.

Aetiology

A dermatotropic ungulate pox virus, composed of at least six immunological strains, is the cause of the disease (1). The virus is immunologically distinct from vaccinia, but very similar to the causative agent of pseudocowpox. The virus withstands drying and is capable of surviving at room temperature for at least 15 years. Among farm animals, sheep, goats and cattle are affected naturally, and a few cases have occurred in humans working among sheep (2), and one in a dog (3). The disease has also been observed in chamois and wild thar goats. The virus can be passaged in rabbits if large doses are placed on scarified skin or injected intradermally. Mild lesions develop on the chorioallantois of the 9- to 12-day chick embryo. Guinea pigs and mice are not susceptible.

The disease is commonest in lambs 3 to 6 months of age although adult animals can be severely affected. Outbreaks occur at any time but they are most common in dry conditions when the sheep are at pasture. Recovered animals are solidly immune for 2 to 3 years, but no antibodies appear to be passed in the colostrum and newborn lambs of immune ewes are susceptible (1). In man typical lesions occur at the site of infection, usually an abrasion infected while handling diseased sheep or milking affected cows or by accidental means when vaccinating. The lesions are very itchy and respond poorly to local treatment.

Transmission

Spread in a flock is very rapid and occurs by contact with other affected animals or inanimate objects. The common occurrence in dry seasons suggests that abrasion of the skin by dry feed may provide a ready portal of entry for infection. The scabs remain highly infective for long periods.

Pathogenesis

Histologically the changes in the skin closely resemble those which occur in the pox diseases and the development of the diseases is very similar. That there is some relationship between the viruses of goat pox and contagious ecthyma is indicated by the finding that goat pox antiserum neutralizes the ecthyma virus, although the reverse does not hold.

Clinical Findings

Lesions develop initially as papules and then pustules, stages which are not usually observed, then as thick, tenacious scabs covering a raised area of ulceration, granulation and inflammation. The first lesions develop at the oral mucocutaneous junction, usually at the oral commissures. From here they spread on to the muzzle and nostrils, the surrounding haired skin and, to a lesser extent, on to the buccal mucosa. They may appear as discrete, thick scabs 0·5 cm. in diameter, or be packed close together as a continuous plaque. Fissuring occurs and the scabs are sore to the touch. They crumble easily but are difficult to remove from the underlying granulation. Affected lambs suffer a severe setback because of restricted suckling and grazing. Rarely systemic invasion occurs and lesions appear on the coronets and ears, around the anus and vulva or prepuce, and on the nasal and buccal mucosae. There is a severe systemic reaction and extension down the alimentary tract may lead to a severe gastroenteritis, and extension down the trachea may be followed by bronchopneumonia. In rams lesions on the scrotum may be accompanied by fluid accumulation in the scrotal sac. In benign cases the scabs dry and fall off, and recovery is complete in about 3 weeks. Affected lambs sucking ewes may cause spread of the disease to the udder. Secondary infection of the lesions by *Sphaerophorus necrophorus* occurs in some cases.

A related disease, pseudo-cowpox, occurs in dairy cattle as a mild erythema on the teats followed by extensive scabbing (4). In some acute cases the initial lesion observed is a vesicle or pustule. Healed lesions persist as small wartlike granulomas for several months. There is no evidence of direct transmission from sheep.

Clinical Pathology

Laboratory examination is not usually undertaken for diagnostic purposes but a definitive diagnosis requires transmission experiments to susceptible sheep or rabbits and the demonstration of resistance in previously immunized animals.

Recovered animals have a high level of neutralizing antibodies in their serum.

Necropsy Findings

In malignant cases there are typical ulcerative lesions in the nasal cavities and the upper respiratory tract, and in some cases erosion in the mucosae of the oesophagus, abomasum and small intestine.

Diagnosis

In most outbreaks of ecthyma the cases are sufficiently mild to cause no real concern about losses or about diagnosis. Violent outbreaks of a very severe form of the disease may occur, however, and are likely to be confused with bluetongue (5). Very severe cases are also commonly seen in housed experimental sheep especially colostrum free lambs.

Ulcerative dermatosis, and its causative agent, are sufficiently similar to cause confusion in diagnosis.

The lesions of proliferative dermatitis (strawberry footrot) are confined to the lower limbs. Bluetongue is always accompanied by a high mortality rate, a severe systemic reaction, and lesions occur on the muzzle and on the coronets and extensively on the buccal mucosa. It is more common in adults than sucking lambs. Because it is transmitted by insect vectors, the morbidity rate is usually much less than the 90 per cent commonly seen in contagious ecthyma. Sheep pox may present a rather similar clinical picture, but the scabs are typical hard crusts and there is a severe systemic reaction and heavy mortality rate.

Treatment

There is no specific treatment. Removal of the scabs and the application of ointments or astringent lotions are practised but delay healing in most cases. The provision of soft, palatable food is recommended.

Control

In the early stages of an outbreak, the affected animals should be isolated and the remainder vaccinated. Vaccination is of little value when a large number of animals are already affected. Persistence of the disease in a flock from year to year is common and in such circumstances the lambs should be vaccinated at 6 to 8 weeks of age. The vaccine is prepared from a suspension of scabs in glycerol saline and is painted on to a small area of scarified skin inside the thigh or by pricking the ear with an icepick dipped in the vaccine. Vaccination is completely effective for at least 2 years, but the lambs should be inspected 1 week after vaccination to ensure that local reactions have resulted. Absence of a local reaction signifies lack of viability of the vaccine or the existence of a prior immunity. The immunity is not solid until 3 weeks after vaccination. A small proportion of vaccinated lambs may develop mild lesions about the mouth because of nibbling at the vaccination site. The efficiency of this vaccine is approximately the same as that of one produced in the laboratory. The latter is produced by attenuation in tissue culture (6).

REFERENCES

(1) Hardy, W. T. (1964). *Proc. 67th ann. gen. Mtg U.S. Live Stock sanit. Ass.*, 293–9.
(2) Verdes, N. *et al.* (1970). *Rev. Path. comp. Med. exp.*, *70*, 71.
(3) Wilkinson, G. T. *et al.* (1970). *Vet. Rec.*, *87*, 766.
(4) Nagington, J. *et al.* (1965). *Nature (Lond.)*, *208*, 505.
(5) Gardiner, M. R. *et al.* (1967). *Aust. vet. J.*, *43*, 163.
(6) Kovalev, G. K. *et al.* (1971). *Veterinariya*, *3*, 46.

Papillomatosis

The common wart of cattle and horses is transmissible by intradermal injection and is caused by a virus with considerable host specificity.

Incidence

Warts are quite common in young cattle, especially when they are housed, but ordinarily they cause little harm and disappear spontaneously (1). In pure bred animals they may interfere with sales because of their unsightly appearance and in such groups the incidence may be as high as 25 per cent. Animals with extensive lesions may lose condition and secondary bacterial invasion of traumatized warts may cause concern. Warts on the teats of dairy cows often cause interference with milking. In horses the lesions are usually small and cause little inconvenience. They usually occur sporadically, although there is one report of 5 cases appearing within a 6-week period in a relatively small group, 4 of them occurring in a single inbred family (2). A similar condition has been described in goats, and in one outbreak, papillomatosis has been associated with a high incidence of carcinomas on the udder. The lesions were restricted to the white goats in the group (3). Papillomatosis in pigs commonly affects the genitalia (4).

Aetiology

A host-specific papavovirus is the cause of cutaneous warts in both cattle and horses. The bovine virus is the cause of the fibropapillomata of the bovine vulva and penis, although these are not true papillomata, consisting predominantly of connective rather than epithelial tissue. Transmission occurs at coitus and the lesions may interfere physically with copulation. The bovine virus, when injected intradermally in horses produces a lesion similar to sarcoid, the fibrosarcoma of moderate malignancy which occurs naturally on the legs and around the base of the ears in this species (5). Sarcoids do not metastasize, but commonly recur after excision. They have been successfully transmitted by application of infective material to skin scarifications (7) and horses resistant to infection with sarcoid material are susceptible to bovine papilloma virus (6).

The lack of susceptibility of adults to natural infection with warts is thought to be due to immunity acquired by apparent or inapparent infection when young. Immunity after an attack is solid and persists for at least 2 years.

Transmission

The method of spread is probably by direct contact with infected animals, infection gaining entry through cutaneous abrasions. Crops of warts sometimes occur around eartags or along scratches made by barbed wire and can be spread by tattooing implements. Warts can be spread experimentally by the intradermal injection of a suspension of wart tissue in both horses and cattle. The rare occurrence of congenital papillomatosis is difficult to explain other than by transmission of the infection across the placenta (8).

Clinical Findings

The incubation period after experimental inoculation in cattle is 3 to 8 weeks but is usually somewhat longer after natural exposure. Warts are solid outgrowths of epidermis and may be sessile or pedunculated. In young cattle and goats, they occur most commonly on the head, especially around the eyes, and on the neck and may spread to other parts of the body. They vary in size from 1·0 cm. upwards and their dry, horny, cauliflower-like appearance is characteristic. In adult cows the lesions are usually confined to the teats. In this location they are usually multiple, sessile, small (a millimetre or two in diameter) and elongated by milking machine action to tags up to 1 cm. long. They can usually be drawn out by the roots if sufficient traction is used. In horses warts are confined to the muzzle, nose and lips and are usually sessile and quite small, rarely exceeding 1 cm. in diameter. In both species spontaneous recovery is usual, but the warts may persist for 5 to 6 months and in some cases for as long as 18 months. In such cases there may be serious loss of condition.

Less common manifestations of the disease include the occurrence of papilloma in the oesophageal groove and reticulum, causing chronic ruminal tympany, and in the urinary bladder where they appear to cause no clinical signs (9).

Clinical Pathology

Biopsy of a lesion is rarely necessary to confirm a diagnosis, but it may be advisable when large growths are found on horses, particularly on the lower limbs, to determine whether or not they are sarcoids.

Diagnosis

Clinically there is little difficulty in making a diagnosis of papillomatosis. Differentiation from sarcoids in the horse may necessitate biopsy and histological examination. Carcinoma of the eye (cancer-eye) affects only eyelids or cornea.

Treatment

Commercial wart vaccines prepared from virus grown on eggs are available for the treatment of horses and cattle, but tissue vaccines, prepared from wart tissue of the affected animal, are preferable. The vaccine may be fully virulent or inactivated with formalin, and can be injected subcutaneously, but better results are claimed for intradermal injection. Two injections 1 to 2 weeks apart are recommended. Recovery in 3 to 6 weeks is recorded in 80 to 85 per cent of cases where the warts are on the body surface or penis of cattle, but in only 33 per cent when the warts are on the teats. The live vaccine remains fully viable at room temperature for at least 3 weeks. Other treatments include the injection of proprietary preparations containing antimony and bismuth and removal by traction or ligation, but results with these treatments have been very poor. In all cases the tendency for spontaneous recovery to occur makes assessment of the results of treatment very difficult. Surgical removal is sometimes necessary and removal of one or two warts may be followed by the rapid disappearance of the remainder. However, surgical intervention, and even vaccination, in the early stages of wart development may increase the size of residual warts and prolong the course of the disease. The causative virus is present in much greater concentration in the epithelial tissue of older warts than young ones, and this may have some effect on the efficiency of autogenous vaccines.

Control

Vaccination has been used to prevent the occurrence of the disease (10). Vaccines prepared from tissues produce satisfactory immunity but those prepared from egg-adapted virus are of dubious value. Tissue vaccines are capable of producing an immunity in epidermal tissues, but not in connective tissue, so that mild connective tissue outgrowths may occur after infection. Avoidance of close contact between infected and uninfected animals should be encouraged.

In horses surgical removal is recommended followed immediately by the administration of an autogenous vaccine, repeated with increasing dosage at 4-day intervals for about a month (11).

REFERENCES

(1) Huck, R. A. (1965). Vet. Bull., 35, 475.
(2) Ragland, W. L. et al. (1966). Nature (Lond.), 210, 1399.
(3) Moulton, J. E. (1954). N. Amer. Vet., 35, 29.
(4) Parish, W. E. (1962). J. Path. Bact., 83, 429.
(5) Ragland, W. L. et al. (1965). Lab. Invest., 14, 598.
(6) Ragland, W. L. et al. (1970). Equine vet. J., 2, 168.
(7) Voss, J. L. (1969). Amer. J. vet. Res., 30, 183.
(8) Njoku, C. O. & Burwash, W. A. (1972). Cornell Vet., 62, 54.
(9) Olson, C. et al. (1965). Cancer Res., 25, 840.
(10) Olson, C. et al. (1968). J. Amer. vet. med. Ass., 153, 1189.
(11) Page, E. H. et al. (1967). J. Amer. vet. med. Ass., 150, 177.

Lumpy Skin Disease
(Knopvelsiekte—S. Afr.)

Lumpy skin disease is a highly infectious skin disease of cattle caused by a virus. It is characterized by the sudden appearance of nodules on all parts of the skin.

Incidence

The disease is recorded only from South Africa (1, 5) and Kenya (6, 7), although sporadic cases of a similar disease (pseudo-lumpy skin disease) are reported from Britain (2). Although the mortality rate is low (less than 10 per cent), the economic loss caused is high due to loss of milk production, damage to hides and loss of bodily condition during the long course of the disease. In South Africa the morbidity in a group is high (5 to 50 per cent) and many animals may be affected at one time. Spread to neighbouring farms may be similarly rapid. In Kenya the disease is characterized by a much lower morbidity rate and the disease is much milder.

Aetiology

The herpes virus of lumpy skin disease occurs as at least three strains of which the 'Neethling' and

'Allerton' strains produce overt illness in cattle, the former causing typical lumpy skin disease, and the latter a mild form of it (3, 4). Although sheep pox virus confers immunity against at least one strain of the virus, there is doubt that the two viruses are the same because no cases of pox occur in sheep during outbreaks of LSD in cattle and vice versa (8). The 'Neethling' strain of LSD virus has similar cultural characteristics in tissue culture to sheep pox and other pox viruses (9), and resembles the virus of bovine ulcerative mammillitis.

All ages and types of cattle are susceptible to the causative virus except animals recently recovered from an attack, in which case there is a solid immunity lasting for about 3 months. The disease has been produced experimentally with Neethling virus in giraffe and impala, but wildebeeste were resistant (12).

Transmission

Although the method of spread under natural conditions is not known, the rapid spread of the disease and the ease with which it traverses long distances suggest an insect vector. Experimental transmission can be accomplished using ground-up nodular tissue and blood.

Pathogenesis

After an initial viraemia accompanied by a febrile reaction, localization in the skin occurs with development of inflammatory nodules.

Clinical Findings

An incubation period of 2 to 4 weeks is common in field outbreaks. In severe cases there is an initial rise of temperature sometimes accompanied by lacrimation, nasal discharge, salivation and lameness. Multiple nodules appear suddenly about a week later, the first ones usually appearing in the perineum. They are round and firm, varying from 1 to 4 cm. in diameter, and are flattened and the hair on them stands on end. They vary in number from a few to hundreds; they are intradermal and, in most cases, are confined to the skin area. In severe cases the lesions may also be present in the nostrils and on the turbinates causing respiratory obstruction and snoring. They may also be in the mouth. Oral and nasal lesions tend to be present as plaques, which later ulcerate. Nodules may develop on the conjunctiva causing severe lacrimation. Lesions on the prepuce or vulva may spread to nearby mucosal surfaces. In most cases the nodules disappear rapidly, but they may persist as hard lumps or become moist, necrotic and slough. Lymph nodes draining the affected area become enlarged and there may be local oedema. When sloughing of the yellow centre of nodules occurs there is often exposure of underlying tissues, e.g. testicles, tendons, especially if the nodules have coalesced. A convalescence of 4 to 12 weeks is usual. Pregnant cows may abort.

Necropsy Findings

Animals in which extension to the mucosae of the digestive and respiratory tracts occur often die. There is obstruction to respiration by the necrotic ulcers and surrounding inflammation in the nasal cavities. Similar lesions are present in the mouth, pharynx, trachea, bronchi, and stomachs and there may be accompanying pneumonia.

Diagnosis

The rapid spread of the disease and the sudden appearance of lumps in the skin after an initial fever make this disease quite unlike any other affliction of cattle. Diagnosis depends on recognition of inclusion bodies in sections of skin lesions, and in tissue cultures of the virus. Electron microscopy and fluorescent antibody tests would be applicable (13). An intradermal test has been described and may be of value in herd diagnosis (10).

Treatment

No specific treatment is available, but prevention of secondary infection is essential. The use of antibiotics or sulphonamides is recommended.

Control

A safe vaccine, produced by 60 passages of the virus through lamb kidney culture, is effective. It is administered to all animals over 6 months of age (11). An egg-adapted virus vaccine has also been tried, but caused the disease in inoculated animals. Vaccination of cattle with sheep pox virus, attenuated for cattle, and tissue culture produced, is effective in preventing infection with the 'Neethling' strain of lumpy skin disease virus—the only strain present in Kenya (8). A very small percentage of the vaccinates showed local reactions and there was no spread of sheep pox to sheep running with the cattle. The method has the obvious disadvantage that it can be used only in those countries where sheep pox exists.

REVIEW LITERATURE

Weiss, K. E. (1968). *Virol. Monogr.*, *3*, 111.

REFERENCES

(1) Thomas, A. D. & Mare, C. V. E. (1945). *J. S. Afr. vet. med. Ass.*, *16*, 36.

(2) Hyslop, N. St. G. & Hebeler, H. F. (1958). *Vet. Rec.*, *70*, 731.

(3) Haig, D. A. (1957). *Bull. epizoot. Dis. Afr.*, *5*, 421.

(4) Alexander, R. A. *et al.* (1957). *Bull. epizoot. Dis. Afr.*, *5*, 489.

(5) de Kock, G. (1948). *J. Amer. vet. med. Ass.*, *112*, 57.

(6) MacOwan, K. D. S. (1959). *Bull. epizoot. Dis. Afr.*, *7*, 7.

(7) Ayre-Smith, R. A. (1960). *Vet. Rec.*, *72*, 469.

(8) Capstick, P. B. & Coackley, W. (1961). *Res. vet. Sci.*, *2*, 362.

(9) Plowright, W. & Witcomb, M. A. (1959). *J. Path. Bact.*, *78*, 397.

(10) Capstick, P. B. & Coackley, W. (1962). *Res. vet. Sci.*, *3*, 287.

(11) Jansen, B. C. (1966). *Aust. vet. J.*, *42*, 471.

(12) Young, E. *et al.* (1970). *Onderspoort J. vet. Res.*, *37*, 79.

(13) Davies, F. G. *et al.* (1971). *Res. vet. Sci.*, *12*, 123.

Viral Papular Dermatitis

This disease of horses occurs in the U.S.A. (1), U.K. and Australia. It is characterized by cutaneous lesions in the form of firm papules 0·5 to 2 cm. in diameter. No vesicles or pustules are formed but after 7 to 10 days a dry crust is detached leaving small circumscribed areas of alopecia. The lesions are not itchy, there is no systemic disease and the distribution of the lesions, and the way in which they can develop simultaneously in large numbers in introduced horses, is suggestive of an insect borne disease. The course of the disease varies between 10 days and 6 weeks. A virus has been isolated from lesions and cultured on eggs. A febrile reaction, up to 40·5°C, precedes the appearance of skin lesions by about 24 hours. Recovery is usually complete and uncomplicated.

REFERENCE

(1) McIntyre, R. W. (1949). *Amer. J. vet. Res.*, *10*, 229.

Cowpox

Cowpox is a benign, contagious skin disease of cattle characterized by the appearance of typical pox lesions on the teats and udder.

Incidence

The clinical syndrome of cowpox occurs sporadically in most countries of the world but the incidence of true cowpox appears to have diminished considerably, most outbreaks being of the clinically similar pseudo-cowpox and bovine ulcerative mammillitis. In an affected herd most cows become infected unless there is immunity from previous attacks or suitable preventive measures are adopted. Losses result from inconvenience at milking time because of the soreness of the teats and from occasional cases of mastitis which develop when lesions involve teat sphincters. Milk from affected cows is suitable for human consumption.

Aetiology

The causative virus of true cowpox is closely related to the viruses of horsepox and smallpox. Probably the three are variants of the one virus produced by adaptation to the various animal species.

Transmission

Spread from cow to cow within a herd is effected by milkers' hands or teat cups. Spread from herd to herd is probably effected by the introduction of infected animals, by carriage on milkers' hands, and in the absence of either of the above methods, transport by biting insects is possible. In a herd in which the disease is enzootic only heifers and new introductions may develop lesions. The virus of horsepox can be transmitted to cattle and causes typical cowpox. Milkers recently vaccinated against smallpox may serve as a source of infection for cattle (1), although the smallpox vaccine virus, or vaccinia virus, is different from the cowpox virus (3).

Pathogenesis

In true cowpox, the five stages of a typical pox eruption can be observed. After an incubation period of 3 to 6 days, a roseolar erythema is followed by firm, raised papules light in colour but with a zone of hyperaemia around the base. Vesiculation follows, a yellow blister with a pitted centre being characteristic. The pustular stage, which develops soon afterwards, is followed by the development of a thick, red, tenacious scab.

In experimentally produced vaccinia virus mammillitis (produced by inoculation of smallpox vaccine) the lesions have three zones, a central brown crusty area of necrosis, surrounded by a grey-white zone of micro-vesicle formation, again surrounded by a red border due to congestion (3).

Clinical Findings

Typical lesions may be seen at any stage of development, but are mostly observed during the scab stage, the vesicle commonly having been ruptured during milking. True cowpox scabs are 1 to 2 cm. in diameter and are thick, tenacious and yellow-brown to red in colour. In cows being milked scab formation is uncommon, the scab being replaced by a deep ulceration.

Distribution of the lesions is usually confined to the teats and lower part of the udder. Soreness of the teats develops and milk let-down may be interfered with; the cow usually resents being milked. Secondary mastitis occurs in a few cases. Individual lesions heal quite quickly, within 2 weeks, but in some animals fresh crops of lesions may cause the disease to persist for a month or more. In severe cases lesions may spread to the insides of the thighs and rarely to the perineum, vulva and mouth. Sucking calves may develop lesions about the mouth. In bulls lesions usually appear on the scrotum.

Diagnosis

A number of skin diseases may be accompanied by lesions on the udder, but should not be confused with true cowpox. Cowpox is quite uncommon. Individual lesions are small and few, but severe. They are quite painful, but heal quickly in 2 to 3 weeks. Pseudo-cowpox lesions are larger, more numerous, less painful and more prolonged. Bovine ulcerative mammillitis is a much more severe disease and has characteristic plaques and ulceration of the skin of the teat. The differentiation of these diseases is not always easy on clinical grounds. Differentiation by use of the electron microscope has been described (1, 2). It is not infrequent that two or all three of the diseases are present in the one herd. Udder impetigo begins as thin-walled pustules and the lesions are variable in size and occur only on the udder, usually at the base of the teat. It spreads in a manner similar to cowpox and is often mistaken for this disease by farmers. Staphylococci can usually be isolated from unbroken lesions. A vesicular eruption may also occur on the udder in severe cases of foot-and-mouth disease, but always in conjunction with lesions on the buccal mucosa and coronet. Diffuse erythema and exfoliation with severe irritation may occur on the lateral aspects of the teats in photosensitized animals, but there are no discrete lesions. Mycotic dermatitis not infrequently affects the udder, although lesions are more usual on the dorsal aspect of the body. These are characteristic crusts usually with pus and a raw ulcerating surface beneath. The lesions in so-called 'black pox' are confined to the teats as crater shaped ulcers with raised edges and a black spot in the pitted centre. Most frequently the tip of the teat is involved and spread to the sphincter leads to the development of mastitis. Warts and chronic pseudo-cowpox have much in common, but lesions in various stages of development are usually present in the latter.

Treatment

Only palliative treatment is practicable. The application of a soft emollient cream before milking and an astringent lotion after milking facilitates recovery. Whitfield's ointment and 10 per cent sulphathiazole ointment are also used. A similar ointment (5 per cent sulphathiazole, 5 per cent salicylic acid) is recommended for 'black pox'.

Control

Prevention of spread is difficult, since the virus responsible for the disease is readily transmitted by direct or indirect contact. Udder cloths, milking machines and hands should be disinfected after contact with infected animals. Dipping of the teats in an alcoholic tincture of a suitable disinfectant, such as a quaternary ammonium compound, is usually satisfactory in preventing immediate spread. Control by vaccination has been attempted but is of dubious value (1, 2).

REFERENCES

(1) Gibbs, E. P. J. et al. (1970). Vet. Rec., 87, 602.
(2) Gibbs, E. P. J. & Johnson, R. H. (1970). J. comp. Path., 80, 455.
(3) Lauder, I. M. et al. (1971). Vet. Rec., 89, 571.

Pseudo-Cowpox

(Milkers' Nodule)

Pseudo-cowpox of cattle and 'milkers' nodule' of man are both caused by the same virus and are manifested by similar cutaneous lesions, on the teats in the former, on the hands in the latter.

Incidence

Pseudo-cowpox has been a common disease of cattle for many years and has been reported from most countries. It is a relatively benign disease, most losses occurring as a result of difficulty in milking and an increase in the incidence of mastitis. In an affected herd the rate of spread is relatively slow and this, together with the prolonged healing time in individual cows, may result in the disease being present in the herd for up to a year. The morbidity rate approximates 100 per cent, but at any given time varies between 5 and 10 per cent, and occasionally up to 50 per cent (1). The disease is transmissible to man, infection usually resulting in the development of 'milkers' nodule' on the hand.

Aetiology

The causative agent of pseudo-cowpox in cattle and 'milkers' nodule' in man is a pox virus of the 'orf' or paravaccinia (ungulate pox) group and has some similarity to the virus of infectious papular stomatitis and to that of contagious ecthyma (1, 2, 3, 4, 6). The virus can be propagated in tissue culture. Freshly calved and recently introduced cattle are most susceptible, but all adult cattle in a herd, including dry cows, are likely to be affected. The disease does not appear to occur in animals less than 2 years of age unless they have calved. However, the virus has been isolated from the mouth of a calf sucking an affected cow (5). It has also been isolated from the semen of two infertile bulls (8). There is no seasonal variation in incidence.

Transmission

The methods of spread of the disease have not been defined, but physical transport by means of contaminated milkers' hands, wash cloths and teat cups is considered to be the logical route.

Pathogenesis

The production of typical lesions by the introduction of the virus onto scarified areas of skin suggests that the lesions produced are the result of the local action of the virus.

Clinical Findings

Acute and chronic lesions occur and there may be up to 10 on one teat.

Acute lesions commence as erythema followed by the development of a vesicle or pustule which ruptures after about 48 hours resulting in the formation of a thick scab. Pain is moderate and present only in the pre-scab stage. The scab, varying in size from 0·5 to 2·5 cm. in diameter, becomes markedly elevated by developing granulating tissue beneath it. Seven to 10 days after lesions appear the scabs drop off, leaving a horseshoe-shaped ring of small scabs surrounding a small, wart-like granuloma which may persist for months. The disease tends to disappear from a herd after 18 to 21 days but may recur cyclically about one month later (9).

Chronic lesions also commence as erythema, but progress to a stage in which yellow-grey, soft, scurfy scabs develop. The scabs are readily rubbed off at milking leaving the skin corrugated and prone to chapping. There is no pain and the lesions may persist for months.

'Milkers' nodules' are clinically indistinguishable from human lesions caused by ecthyma virus.

The lesions vary from multiple vesicles to a single, indurated nodule.

Clinical Pathology and Necropsy Findings

Material for examination by tissue culture or electron microscopic examination, the latter being highly recommended as a diagnostic procedure (7), should include fluid from a vesicle.

Diagnosis

Differentiation of those diseases in which lesions of the teat are prominent is dealt with in the section on cowpox.

Treatment

Locally applied ointments of various kinds appear to have little effect on the lesions. The recommended treatment includes the removal of the scabs, which should be burned to avoid contaminating the environment, application of an astringent preparation, such as triple dye, after milking and an emollient ointment just before milking.

Control

Recommended measures such as treatment and isolation of affected cows, or milking them last, the use of disposable paper towels for udder washing and disinfection of teat cups appear to have little effect on the spread of the disease.

REFERENCES

(1) Nagington, J. et al. (1967). Vet. Rec., 81, 306.
(2) Lauder, I. M. et al. (1966). Vet. Rec., 78, 926.
(3) Friedman-Kein, A. E. et al. (1963). Science, 140, 1335.
(4) Liebermann, H. et al. (1967). Arch. exp. vet. Med., 21, 625.
(5) Moscovici, C. et al. (1963). Science, 141, 915.
(6) Huck, R. A. (1966). Vet. Rec., 78, 503.
(7) Gibbs, E. P. J. et al. (1970). Vet. Rec., 87, 602.
(8) Johnston, W. S. (1971). Vet. Rec., 89, 450.
(9) Cheville, N. F. & Shey, D. J. (1967). J. Amer. vet. med. Ass., 150, 855.

Bovine Ulcerative Mammillitis

Bovine ulcerative mammillitis is a viral disease manifested by severe ulceration of the skin of the teats and udder.

Incidence

Cowpox and pseudo-cowpox have been recognized diseases of cattle for many years. The description, for the first time, of bovine ulcerative mammillitis (1, 2, 3) may record the appearance of a new disease or the identification of one which has been present in the cattle population for some time. The morbidity rate varies between 18 and 96 per cent (average 50 per cent) and, although the mortality rate is negligible, losses due to the disease may be severe. Forms of loss include a much higher incidence of mastitis, reduction in milk yield in affected herds by up to 20 per cent, the culling of some cows because of severe mastitis and intractable ulcers, and a great deal of interference with normal milking procedure (2).

The disease is self-limiting, persisting in a herd for 6 to 15 weeks, the severity of the lesions decreases as the outbreak progresses. An incidence of 19 per cent of serologically positive cattle has been observed in U.K. (4).

Aetiology

A herpes virus, with a close resemblance to the Allerton virus of lumpy skin disease, has been identified as the causative agent, has been maintained in tissue culture and transmitted to rabbits and guinea pigs, and to day-old rats, mice and Chinese hamsters (4). Sheep and pigs show mild reactions and man, mice and rats appear to be refractory. The virus has no apparent relationship to other herpes viruses—infectious bovine rhinotracheitis or feline viral rhinotracheitis viruses. Only cows in milk appear to be affected, heifers more severely than adult cows. Whether appreciable immunity occurs after natural infection has not been determined, but the disease has recurred in herds 13 months after an initial attack. Herds infected for the first time have a high morbidity rate. Subsequently the incidence is low and is limited to fresh heifers (4). A high seasonal incidence in autumn and early winter has been noted.

Bovine ulcerative mammillitis is identical with the disease previously recorded as 'skin gangrene' (8, 9).

Transmission

Introduction of bovine ulcerative mammillitis into a herd may occur with the introduction of infected animals, but outbreaks have been observed in self-contained herds and because of the seasonal incidence in autumn, the possibility of insect transmission needs to be considered. Spread within a herd is thought to occur via teat cups, udder cloths and milkers' hands.

Pathogenesis

Typical clinical lesions and histopathological changes can be produced locally by introduction of the virus into scarifications of the skin of the teat and the oral mucosa and by intradermal and intravenous injection (5, 10).

Clinical Findings

In this disease there is an incubation period of 5 to 10 days. There is no systemic illness and lesions are confined to the teats and udder.

In cows calved for more than a few weeks the characteristic lesions are almost entirely confined to the skin of the teats; in recently calved cows they are restricted to the skin of the udder. The severity of the disease in recently calved cows appears to be directly proportional to the degree of post-parturient oedema which is present. Vesication occurs, commencing at the base of the teat and spreading over much of the udder surface, but rupture and confluence of the vesicles leads to weeping and extensive sloughing of the skin.

The severity of lesions on the teats in longer-calved cows varies, but in all cases the lesions are sufficiently painful to make milking difficult. In the most severe cases the entire teat is swollen and painful, the skin is bluish in colour, exudes serum and sloughs leaving a raw ulcer covering most of the teat. In less severe cases there are raised deep red to blue, circular plaques, 0·5 to 2 cm. in diameter, which develop shallow ulcers. In most cases scab formation follows but machine milking causes frequent disruption of them, resulting in frequent bleeding. The least severe lesions are in the form of lines of erythema, often in circles and enclosing dry skin or slightly elevated papules, which occasionally show ulceration. Mild lesions tend to heal in about 10 days but severe ulcers may persist for 2 or 3 months.

Vesicles occur but are not commonly seen. They are characteristically thin-walled, 1 to 2 cm. in diameter, variable in outline and easily ruptured during milking. Ulcers in the mouth of affected cows have been observed rarely and calves sucking affected cows develop lesions on their muzzles (11). During the recovery phase there is obvious scar formation and depigmentation. Lesions on the skin of the udder are similar to those on the teats but are usually less severe and heal more rapidly because of the absence of trauma.

Clinical Pathology and Necropsy Findings

Material for tissue culture or cutaneous transmission tests is best obtained by syringe from early vesicles. Swabs from early ulcers or oral lesions may also be used. Recovered animals show a high titre of antibodies which persist for at least two years (4). No necropsy reports of cases of bovine ulcerative mammillitis are available.

Diagnosis

Differentiation of other diseases of the skin of the teat and udder is dealt with in the section on cowpox.

Treatment

There is no specific treatment and the aim should be to develop scabs which can withstand machine milking. This is most easily effected by the application of a water-miscible antiseptic ointment just before putting the cups on, followed by an astringent lotion, such as triple dye, immediately after milking.

Control

Isolation of affected animals and strict hygiene in the milking parlour are practised but have little effect on the spread of the disease. An iodophor disinfectant is recommended for use in the dairy to prevent spread (7). Inoculation of the natural virus away from the teats produces a local lesion and good immunity, and the method has been tested as a control procedure (6).

REFERENCES

(1) Martin, W. B. *et al.* (1970). *Vet. Rec.*, *86*, 661.
(2) Deas, D. W. & Johnston, W. S. (1966). *Vet. Rec.*, *78*, 828.
(3) Pepper, T. A. *et al.* (1966). *Vet. Rec.*, *78*, 569.
(4) Rweyemamu, M. M. *et al.* (1969). *Brit. vet. J.*, *125*, 317.
(5) Rweyemamu, M. M. *et al.* (1968). *Brit. vet. J.*, *124*, 317.
(6) Rweyemamu, M. M. & Johnson, R. H. (1969). *J. comp. Path.*, *10*, 419.
(7) Martin, W. B. & Jaines, Z. H. (1969). *Vet. Rec.*, *85*, 100.
(8) Rweyemamu, M. M. *et al.* (1966). *Vet. Rec.*, *79*, 810; *85*, 698.
(9) White, J. B. *et al.* (1959). *Vet. Rec.*, *71*, 764.
(10) Martin, W. B. *et al.* (1969). *Amer. J. vet. Res.*, *30*, 2151.
(11) Gibbs, E. P. J. & Collings, D. F. (1972). *Vet. Rec.*, *90*, 66.

Sheep Pox and Goat Pox

In sheep pox typical pox lesions occur particularly under the tail. A malignant form with a general distribution of lesions occurs in lambs.

Incidence

Sheep pox is restricted in its distribution to the Middle East countries, south-eastern Europe and Scandinavia. It is the most serious of all the pox diseases in animals, often causing death in 50 per cent of affected animals. Major losses may occur in each new crop of lambs.

Aetiology

The causative ungulate pox virus affects only sheep, and animals of all ages are susceptible. A highly contagious pox occurs also in goats and is caused by a virus which is antigenically distinct from sheep pox virus (1), although it is sometimes transmissible experimentally to both goats and sheep. Goat pox in sheep is more severe than sheep pox, and lesions occur on the lips and oral mucosa, the teats and udder. The goat pox virus affords solid protection in sheep against both goat and sheep poxes but sheep pox vaccine does not protect goats against goat pox. The goat pox virus can be propagated in the developing hen's egg and egg-adapted virus can be used as a prophylactic (2). In areas where sheep pox is enzootic imported breeds may show greater susceptibility than the native stock. The virus has been cultivated on chick embryos and in tissue culture.

Transmission

Sheep pox is highly contagious and, although in most cases spread appears to occur by contact with infected animals and contaminated articles, spread by inhalation also occurs.

Pathogenesis

The development of typical pox lesions, as in vaccinia, is characteristic of the disease. Because of the close relationship between sheep pox and lumpy skin disease virus, a close study of the pathogenesis of sheep pox lesions has been made (3). The virus is present in greatest quantities between the 7th and 14th day after inoculation.

Clinical Findings

There is an incubation period of 2 to 14 days. In lambs, the malignant form is the more common type. There is marked depression and prostration, a high fever and discharges from the eyes and nose. Affected lambs may die during this stage before typical pox lesions develop. Skin lesions appear on unwoolled skin and on the buccal, respiratory, digestive and urogenital tract mucosae. The mortality rate in this type may reach 50 per cent. In the benign form, which is the common one in adults, only skin lesions occur, particularly under the tail, and there is no systemic reaction. The mortality rate is low, usually about 5 per cent. In ewes severe losses may occur if the udder is invaded because of the secondary occurrence of acute mastitis.

Necropsy Findings

In the malignant form pox lesions extend into the mouth, pharynx, larynx and vagina. Lesions may also appear in the trachea with an accompanying catarrhal pneumonia. Lesions occasionally reach the abomasum and are accompanied by a haemorrhagic enteritis.

Diagnosis

The disease occurs in enzootic areas and the lesions are characteristic of a pox disease. Confusion with bluetongue and contagious ecthyma may occur, but differentiation on the basis of clinical signs and lesions is ordinarily not difficult. An immunodiffusion technique for the identification of the sheep pox and goat pox viruses has been described (4). Attention has been drawn to the ease with which lesions of bovine skin can be diagnosed by electron microscopy (5).

Treatment

No specific treatment is advised, but palliative treatment may be necessary in severely affected animals.

Control

Control in free countries necessitates prohibition of importation from infected areas, and if the infection is introduced, the destruction of affected flocks and the quarantine of infected premises should be instituted. Vaccination with natural lymph is practised in affected areas but is capable of spreading the disease. Extensive use of a tissue vaccine adsorbed on aluminium hydroxide has been followed by no ill effects and by the establishment of immunity in 2 weeks which persists for 9 to 12 months. Also extensive field trials with a naturally occurring avirulent virus have given good results. A local reaction and a mild fever follow vaccination, but solid immunity persists for 14 months. A killed vaccine with adjuvant provides protection for five months (6, 7). Vaccination in the face of an outbreak is unlikely to prevent deaths during the subsequent 2 weeks.

REFERENCES

(1) Uppal, P. K. & Nilakantan, P. R. (1970). *J. Hyg. Camb.*, *68*, 349.
(2) Rafyi, A. & Ramyar, H. (1959). *J. comp. Path.*, *69*, 141.
(3) Plowright, W. *et al.* (1959). *J. comp. Path.*, *69*, 400.
(4) Bhambani, B. D. & Krishnamurty, D. (1963). *J. comp. Path.*, *73*, 349.
(5) Gibbs, E. P. J. *et al.* (1970). *J. comp. Path.*, *80*, 455.
(6) Sharma, S. N. & Dhanda, M. R. (1970). *Ind. J. Anim. Sci.*, *40*, 626.
(7) Uppal, P. K. *et al.* (1967). *Ind. vet. J.*, *44*, 815.

Swine Pox

Swine pox is usually a benign disease characterized by the appearance of typical pox lesions on the ventral abdomen.

Incidence

Swine pox occurs in most countries where swine are raised and, although the incidence in individual herds may be high, the disease is not usually widespread through an area. In some outbreaks the mortality rate in young sucking pigs may be heavy, but older animals seem to suffer little ill effect. An important feature of the disease is that its presence may increase the hazard of breaks occurring after hog cholera vaccination.

Aetiology

Two separate pox viruses, one of them closely related to the vaccinia virus, and one antigenically distinct, appear to be capable of causing the disease. Solid immunity appears to persist after infection with either virus. Swine pox virus has been cultured in tissue culture (2, 4).

Transmission

Outbreaks usually accompany infestation with the pig louse (*Haematopinus suis*) and transmission is usually effected by bites of this louse (1), although there is some evidence that flies and other insects may also act as transmitting agents. Young sucking pigs may have lesions on the face with similar lesions on the udder of the sow, and spread by direct contact may occur in these circumstances.

Pathogenesis

In field cases, the lesions do not proceed past the vesicle stage as a rule. Rupture of the vesicles and the formation of scabs which heal and drop off are the final stages.

Clinical Findings

Small, 1 cm. diameter papules develop first and may pass through the vesicular stage very quickly with the formation of red-brown, round scabs. In baby pigs the rupture of many vesicles at one time may cause wetting and scab formation over the cheeks, and conjunctivitis and keratitis are present in many affected animals (3). In most cases the lesions are restricted to the belly and inside the upper limbs, but may involve the back and sides and sometimes spread to the face. A slight febrile reaction may occur in the early stages in young animals and in sucking pigs some deaths are observed.

Diagnosis

The distribution of the pox-like lesions and the association of the disease with louse infestations suggest the diagnosis. Lesions caused by *Tyro-*

glyphid spp. mites are usually larger and occur anywhere on the body, and like those of sarcoptic mange, are usually accompanied by itching. The causative mites are detectable in skin scrapings. Ringworm and pityriasis rosea have characteristic lesions which do not itch and fungal spores are present in scrapings in the former disease.

Treatment

No specific treatment is available and lesions cause so little concern to the pig, and heal so rapidly, that none is attempted.

Control

Vaccination is not usually practised and control of the pig lice is the principal prophylactic measure attempted in most outbreaks (1).

REFERENCES

(1) Schang, P. J. (1952). *Rep. 14th int. vet. Congr.*, *2*, 421.
(2) Kasza, L. & Griesemer, R. A. (1962). *Amer. J. vet. Res.*, *23*, 443.
(3) Doman, I. (1962). *Magy. Állatorv. Lap.*, *17*, 121 & 365.
(4) Datt, N. S. (1964). *J. comp. Path.*, *74*, 62 & 70.

Horsepox

Horsepox is- a benign disease characterized by the development of typical pox lesions either on the limbs or on the lips and buccal mucosa.

Incidence

Horsepox occurs only in Europe and appears to be quite rare. In general it is a benign disease, but badly affected horses become debilitated and occasionally young animals may die.

Aetiology

The causative ungulate pox virus is identical antigenically with the virus of true cowpox and is transferable to cattle and to man. Immunity after an attack is solid.

Transmission

Horsepox may be spread by contact with infected grooming tools, harness and by handling.

Clinical Findings

Typical pox lesions develop either on the back of the pastern, the so-called 'leg form', or in the mouth, the 'buccal form'. In the leg form nodules, vesicles, pustules and scabs develop in that order on the back of the pastern and cause pain and lameness. There may be a slight systemic reaction with elevation of temperature. In the 'buccal' form similar lesions appear first on the insides of the lips and spread over the entire buccal mucosa, sometimes to the pharynx and larynx and occasionally into the nostrils. In very severe cases lesions may appear on the conjunctiva, the vulva and sometimes over the entire body. The buccal lesions cause a painful stomatitis with salivation and anorexia as prominent signs. Most cases recover with lesions healing in 2 to 4 weeks.

Diagnosis

The leg form may be confused with greasy heel, but no nodules, vesicles or pustules occur in the latter disease. Vesicular stomatitis occurs in horses but the lesions are much larger, rupture very readily and do not go through the typical stages of a pox lesion.

Treatment

Local astringent treatment, as in the other forms of pox, may facilitate healing.

Control

Because of the contagious nature of the disease rigid isolation and hygiene in the handling of infected horses is essential.

Ulcerative Dermatosis of Sheep

Ulcerative dermatosis of sheep is an infectious disease characterized by the destruction of epidermal and subcutaneous tissues, the development of raw, granulating ulcers on the skin of the lips, nares, feet, legs and external genital organs. The lesions on the lips occur between the lip and the nostril, those on the feet occur in the interdigital space and above the coronet, and the genital lesions occur on the glans and the external opening of the prepuce of rams and the vulva of ewes.

A virus, very similar but antigenically different to the ecthyma virus, is the cause of the disease (1, 2) which is likely to be confused with contagious ecthyma. However, the lesions are ulcerative and destructive rather than proliferative as in ecthyma. It is not highly infectious like bluetongue or sheep pox and the 'lip-and-leg' distribution of the lesions differentiates it from balanoposthitis of wethers, strawberry footrot, footrot and interdigital abscess. The presence of lesions on the glans penis and their absence from mucosae, the typical ulcerative form of the lesion, the absence of pus and the susceptibility of recovered animals to infection with ecthyma virus are diagnostic features of ulcerative dermatosis.

A morbidity rate of 15 to 20 per cent is usual, but up to 60 per cent of a flock may be affected. Mortality is low if the sheep are in good condition and the lesions are treated. Physical contact at breeding time seems to be the most probable method of spread.

REFERENCES

(1) Tunnicliffe, E. A. (1949). *Amer. J. vet. Res.*, *10*, 240.
(2) Trueblood, M. S. (1966). *Cornell Vet.*, *56*, 521.

VIRAL AND CHLAMYDIAL DISEASES CHARACTERIZED BY MUSCULO-SKELETAL LESIONS

Polyarthritis

A virulent chlamydia has been isolated from the joints of calves (1, 4) and sheep (2, 7) clinically affected by polyarthritis. The disease has also been produced experimentally and is characterized in calves by a chlamydaemia with subsequent localization in joints (6). In calves the disease has a high mortality; in lambs there is a high morbidity but deaths are few. The causative agent in calves is related to the chlamydia which causes sporadic bovine encephalomyelitis in that species.

In lambs it is one of the commonest, non-fatal diseases in feed-lots in the U.S.A., but also occurs in unweaned lambs at pasture (3). The morbidity rate in affected flocks ranges up to 80 per cent (8) but deaths are usually restricted to less than 1 per cent.

In lambs the clinical signs include stiffness, lameness, unwillingness to move, recumbency, depression, fever of 39 to 42°C and conjunctivitis. The clinical disease in calves is similar to that in lambs. The joints are often grossly swollen and the navel is unaffected. There may be clinical signs relating to lesions which occur in other tissues, e.g. pneumonia, encephalomyelitis and interstitial focal nephritis (4). Focal pneumonitis is a common lesion in lambs (5). Laboratory diagnosis is by complement fixation test and culture on chicken egg embryos. The disease is likely to be confused with polyarthritis caused by *Haemophilus* and *Mycoplasma* spp. Early treatment with tylosin and penicillin is recommended.

REFERENCES

(1) Storz, J. *et al.* (1966). *Amer. J. vet. Res.*, *27*, 633, 987.
(2) Mendlowski, B. & Segre, D. (1960). *Amer. J. vet. Res.*, *21*, 68, 74.
(3) Pierson, R. E. (1967). *J. Amer. vet. med. Ass.*, *150*, 1487.
(4) Kolbl, O. & Psota, A. (1968). *Wien. tierärztl. Mschr.*, *55*, 443.
(5) Page, L. A. & Cutlip, R. C. (1968). *Iowa Vet.*, *39*, 10, 14.
(6) Eugster, A. K. & Storz, J. (1971). *J. infect. Dis.*, *123*, 41.
(7) Tammemagi, L. & Simmons, G. C. (1968). *Aust. vet. J.*, *44*, 585.
(8) Cutlip, R. C. *et al.* (1972). *J. Amer. vet. med. Ass.*, *161*, 1213.

22

Diseases Caused by Rickettsia

Contagious Ophthalmia

CONTAGIOUS OPHTHALMIA is a disease of sheep and goats characterized by conjunctivitis and keratitis.

Incidence

The disease in sheep is widespread in most countries including Africa, Australia, the U.S.A., the U.K. and Europe. It causes only minor inconvenience by interfering with grazing for a few days in pastured animals. The disease occurs as widespread outbreaks in some years and in such circumstances may cause appreciable losses in weight gains. Outbreaks during the mating season can reduce the incidence of twinning. The morbidity rate varies widely depending on seasonal conditions. It is usually about 10 to 15 per cent but may be as high as 50 per cent.

Aetiology

Rickettsia (*Colesiota*) *conjunctivae* can be isolated from affected eyes and is capable of causing the disease in sheep and goats. The occurrence of rickettsial ophthalmitis in cattle is open to doubt, most cases of ophthalmia in this species being caused by *Moraxella bovis*. A rickettsia isolated from cases of keratoconjunctivitis in pigs less than two months of age is capable of causing the disease in piglets and can be passaged through chick embryos and mice.

In sheep a bacterium—*Neisseria catarrhalis* (*ovis*)—is commonly present in affected eyes but its aetiological significance is doubtful. It may be capable of causing disease when the resistance of the conjunctiva is lowered from other causes. All breeds of sheep are equally affected but the disease in lambs is less severe than in adults, and recently weaned animals are most severely affected. *Mycoplasma* spp. are frequently identified in the eyes of ewes with pinkeye and many are currently identified as aetiological agents of the disease (1, 2). *Mycoplasma* spp. have also been found in association with keratoconjunctivitis in goats (3). The disease is not transmissible experimentally to cattle, guinea pigs or rabbits. After a clinical attack recurrence of the disease is unusual before the following summer probably because of the persistence of the infection in the eye—a state of premunity. Resistance to infection seems to be reduced by concurrent diseases, poor nutrition and adverse weather.

Transmission

The disease is spread indirectly by flies, long grass and dust contaminated by the tears of infected sheep, or directly by means of exhaled droplets or immediate contact. The incidence is highest during the warm, summer months and when conditions are dry and dusty, and the fly population is heavy. Experimentally the disease can be transmitted by instillation of infected tears into the conjunctival sac but not by parenteral injection. Infection persists in the eye for periods up to 250 days and carrier animals are a source of reinfection in subsequent years (5). A degree of flock immunity appears to develop which may be sufficient to prevent the occurrence of acute outbreaks of the disease for 2 or 3 years.

Pathogenesis

Contagious ophthalmia commences as a conjunctivitis with frequent spread to the cornea.

Clinical Findings

Initially in sheep there is lacrimation and blepharospasm followed by keratitis with cloudiness of the cornea and some increase in vascularity. The watery discharge later becomes purulent but recovery commences in 3 to 4 days and is complete at about 10 days. In some animals the cloudiness of the cornea may persist for several weeks or even permanently. Local ulceration of the cornea may cause collapse of the eyeball. Both eyes are affected in many cases and spread through the flock is rapid. In goats the disease is milder with little apparent ophthalmia or keratitis. Conjunctivitis is followed by the development of granular lesions on the palpebral conjunctiva.

Clinical Pathology

Swabs or scrapings from the affected conjunctiva should be examined for the presence of rickettsiae in the epithelial cells.

Diagnosis

This is the only contagious ophthalmia known to occur in sheep. In goats *R. conjunctivae* causes only a mild conjunctivitis.

A more severe conjunctivitis and keratitis occurs in goats but its cause has not been established (8). All age groups are affected and although the morbidity is usually 10 to 20 per cent it may reach 50 per cent. Direct contact between animals appears to be necessary for spread of the infection, but the disease has not been transmitted experimentally. Conjunctivitis, opacity, vascularization and sometimes ulceration of the cornea are accompanied by an ocular discharge and blepharospasm. Recovery begins in 4 to 7 days but in severe cases healing may not be complete for 2 to 4 weeks.

In cattle *Mor. bovis* is the cause of most outbreaks of ophthalmia. Phenothiazine may also cause photosensitization of the cornea, but the resulting opacity is limited to the lateral half of the cornea.

Treatment

Local irrigation with astringent collyria, such as a 2·5 per cent solution of zinc sulphate, is usually used to allay the discomfort, but treated animals are more likely to relapse or become reinfected than the untreated. Chloramphenicol has appeared to have some beneficial effect in field studies but in controlled experiments aureomycin (0·5 per cent collyria) was much more effective, although relapses occurred quickly after the use of the latter. Ethidium bromide (0·5 per cent ointment or 0·5 to 1·0 per cent lotion once or twice daily for 3 to 4 days) and oxytetracycline (4) are also effective. Neither of these drugs appears to prevent the subsequent development of immunity after natural infection but do reduce the severity of the ocular lesion when they are applied. Clinically affected animals may require supplementary feeding if their sight is impaired.

Control

Complete eradication of the disease is not attempted but isolation of affected sheep, and removal to grassier, less dusty pasture may reduce the rate of spread. Confinement of affected sheep should also be avoided.

REFERENCES

(1) Surman, P. (1968). *Aust. J. biol. Sci.*, *21*, 447.
(2) Langford, E. V. (1971). *Canad. J. comp. Med.*, *35*, 8.
(3) McCauley, E. H. *et al.* (1971). *Amer. J. vet. Res.*, *32*, 861.
(4) Hofland, G. *et al.* (1969). *T. Diergeneesk.*, *94*, 353.
(5) Beveridge, W. I. B. (1942). *Aust. vet. J.*, *18*, 155.

Tick-Borne Fever

Tick-borne fever is a disease of cattle and sheep caused by rickettsiae, and characterized clinically by a mild fever and a short course.

Incidence

The disease, recorded in the United Kingdom, Scandinavia (1) and India (sheep only) is of minor importance because of its mild nature. It causes some loss of weight in lambs. It may recur each year on affected farms. One of the indirect effects of the disease is that it increases the susceptibility of lambs to staphylococcal pyaemia (2), staphylococcal pneumonia, and louping ill and possibly to other diseases. The mortality rate is negligible in cattle but may be higher in sheep.

Aetiology

The causative agents, *Rickettsia bovina* and *R. ovina* (also known as *Cytoecetes phagocytophila*) (3), resemble each other very closely and the disease produced experimentally in cattle by the ovine strain is almost identical with that produced by the bovine strain although slightly less severe. There is considerable cross-immunity between the two strains, the main difference between the two being the difficulty of establishing the bovine strain in sheep and vice versa. Attempts to grow the rickettsiae on hen eggs have not been successful. Cattle, goats and sheep are susceptible and calves and lambs are much less susceptible than adults. The rickettsia has been adapted to grow in mice and guinea pigs but is still infective for sheep after 90 serial passages. Information on immunity is scanty but under natural conditions the disease commonly recurs in the one animal in successive years. A state of low-grade premunity due to the presence of the rickettsia in the blood develops after infection and provides partial resistance to subsequent infections, the disease manifesting itself in a less severe form. Challenge of previously affected sheep did not produce any reaction during the next three months. Deep freezing of blood at −74°C preserves its infectivity for 8 months (4).

The necropsy lesions in cattle which die of tick-borne fever are very similar to those of bovine petechial fever (Ondiri disease) which occurs only in Kenya and is caused by a rickettsia closely related to that of tick-borne fever (5).

Transmission

The disease is transmitted by ticks, including *Ixodes ricinus* in Great Britain and *Rhipicephalus haemaphysaloides* in India and although the rickettsia persists in the tick through its stages of development, persistence to further tick generations has not been shown to occur. The rickettsiae persist in the blood stream of animals for a considerable period, up to 2 years in sheep, and this represents the major source of infection in an enzootic area.

Pathogenesis

The presence of the rickettsia in the leucocytes, and the emptied lymphoid deposits which are characteristic of the disease suggest that the disease is primarily leucolytic. The leucopenia combined with thrombocytopenia suggests myeloid inhibition and a similarity to other radiomimetic diseases such as bracken poisoning (6). This similarity is increased by the appearance in adult sheep of a haemorrhagic syndrome, with lesions particularly evident on the alimentary mucosa. It is not known whether the abortion which occurs in sheep, and less commonly in cattle, is due to the fever or to a specific effect of the rickettsia (5).

Clinical Findings

In cattle there is an incubation period of 6 to 7 days after experimental infection followed by a rise in temperature to about 40·5°C (105°F) which persists for 2 to 8 days. The temperature falls gradually and is followed by a secondary febrile period and, in some cases, further attacks of pyrexia occur. During each febrile period there is a marked fall in milk yield, lethargy and polypnoea and in experimentally produced cases, a mild cough (4). Cattle affected during the last two months of pregnancy commonly abort and occasionally animals die suddenly. The abortions occur shortly after the systemic disease.

In sheep the syndrome is similar to that observed in cattle except that respiratory distress is not observed. The reaction in young lambs is quite mild and manifested only by a moderate rise in temperature. Ewes exposed to the disease for the first time commonly experience outbreaks of abortion and affected rams are temporarily infertile. A haemorrhagic syndrome, affecting the intestinal mucosa, has been observed in experimentally infected adult sheep (6).

Clinical Pathology

Serological diagnosis is now possible with the development of an accurate specific complement fixation test (7).

The rickettsiae are present in the neutrophils and monocytes during each febrile period and for a few days afterwards in cattle and for several weeks in sheep, and can be detected in suitably stained blood smears. At the peak of the fever there is a marked leucopenia (4000 to 5000 per cmm.), due largely to a depression of the neutrophils. This is soon followed by a leucocytosis with a marked increase in immature neutrophils. At the commencement of the fever in the experimentally induced disease there is a severe but transient thrombocytopenia (6). Transmission of the disease may be effected by the intravenous injection of blood taken at the height of the fever.

Necropsy Findings

There are no gross changes other than splenomegaly in sheep, and histologically the only characteristic lesion is an apparent draining of lymphocytes from lymphoid tissue.

Diagnosis

The diagnosis is not difficult if the disease is suspected because of the ease with which the rickettsiae are found in leucocytes. The strict geographical restriction of the disease and its relation to tick infestation are diagnostic features. The disease in cattle has some similarity to bovine petechial fever (Ondiri disease) which occurs only in Kenya (8).

Treatment

Sulphadimidine is reported to be effective in sheep if treatment is continued for several days although the rickettsiae persist in treated animals which may subsequently suffer a relapse. Tetracyclines are effective against other rickettsiae and are recommended for trial in this disease.

Control

Control of tick-borne fever depends upon control of the tick population.

REFERENCES

(1) Bool, P. H. & Reinders, J. S. (1964). *Tijdschr. Diergeneesk.*, *89*, 1519.
(2) Foster, W. N. M. & Cameron, A. E. (1970). *J. comp. Path.*, *80*, 429.
(3) Foggie, A. *et al.* (1966). *J. comp. Path.*, *76*, 413.
(4) Ticomi, J. (1967). *Acta path. microb. scand.*, *70*, 429.
(5) Wilson, J. C. *et al.* (1964). *Vet. Rec.*, *76*, 1081.
(6) Foster, W. N. M. & Cameron, A. E. (1968). *J. comp. Path.*, *78*, 251, 255.
(7) Snodgrass, D. R. & Ramachandran, S. (1971). *Brit. vet. J.*, *127*, xliv.
(8) Danskin, D. & Bundin, M. L. (1963). *Vet. Rec.*, *75*, 391.

Erlichosis

Equine erlichosis has been recorded in the U.S.A. (1, 2). It is caused by a rickettsia and can be transmitted experimentally by the injection of blood collected from the donor at the peak of a febrile period. There are specific rickettsia for each species. Positive identification of the disease is made on the presence of inclusion bodies in neutrophil leucocytes. Clinically there is high fever 40 to 42°C (104 to 107°F) followed by mucosal pallor, anorexia, depression, increased respiratory movement, incoordination and reluctance to move, and after 3 or 4 days oedema and heat of the extremities. The oedema persists for 7 to 10 days. On laboratory examination there is a transient mild anaemia due to intravascular haemolysis. There is a marked, transient leucopenia. At necropsy there are petechia and oedema of the legs and at histological examination there is a vasculitis. The disease must be distinguished from equine anaemia.

REFERENCES

(1) Stannard, A. A. *et al.* (1969). *Vet. Rec.*, *84*, 149.
(2) Gribble, D. H. (1969). *J. Amer. vet. med. Ass.*, *155*, 462.

Diseases Caused by Fungi

SYSTEMIC AND MISCELLANEOUS MYCOSES

SYSTEMIC MYCOSES in animals are usually sporadic infections which occur by chance and cause non-specific syndromes because of variation in the organs in which they localize. An important development has been the observation that a proportion of bovine abortions, unrelated to other known infectious agents, are caused by infections with fungi and yeasts. Mycotic abortions have also been observed in ewes (4) and sows. The incidence of mycotic abortions is much greater in the winter months in housed cows than in any other group and the disease occurs rarely in cows running at pasture all the year round. The general impression is that cows confined to indoor housing are exposed to an environment which is likely to be heavily contaminated with spores from mouldy hay and ensilage. In these circumstances mycotic abortion may represent a high proportion (10 to 15 per cent) of all abortions that occur in the population. An incidence of 30 per cent has been observed in cattle housed in sheds all the year round (1). A strong positive correlation has been shown to exist between the incidence of mycotic abortion and the rainfall in the hay-making season prior to conception (3). Because of the common occurrence of fungal infections where antibiotics are used extensively, it has been suggested that the increasing incidence of mycotic placentitis may be related to the general use of antibiotic-treated semen in artificial insemination programmes. However, the incidence of the disease does not seem to be higher in artificially bred cows than in those mated naturally. It is more likely that infection occurs by inhalation or via abomasal ulcers (2) with subsequent localization in the pregnant uterus, and sometimes in other organs.

REVIEW LITERATURE

Smith, J. M. B. (1968). *N.Z. vet. J.*, *16*, 89–100.
Austwick, P. K. C. (1966). *Colston Pap.*, *18*, 321.
Kong, Y. C. M. & Levine, H. B. (1967). *Bact. Rev.*, *31*, 35–53.
Campbell, C. K. (1969). *Veterinary Annual*, pp. 129–39. Bristol: Wright.

REFERENCES

(1) Turner, P. D. (1965). *Vet. Rec.*, *77*, 273.
(2) Cordes, D. O. *et al.* (1964). *N.Z. vet. J.*, *12*, 95 & 101.
(3) Hugh-Jones, M. E. & Austwick, P. K. C. (1967). *Vet. Rec.*, *81*, 273.
(4) Gardner, D. E. (1967). *N.Z. vet. J.*, *15*, 85.

Coccidioidomycosis

Coccidioidomycosis is a comparatively benign disease of farm animals, usually causing no apparent illness. Sporadic causes are recorded in all species but are most common in dogs (1) and in cattle (2) and to a much less extent in pigs, sheep and horses (7). The disease is enzootic in south-western United States and up to 20 per cent of cattle fattened in feedlots in the area may be affected (7). The incidence of the disease in humans in the area provides a major problem in public health (8).

Coccidioides immitis is the cause of the disease in all species including man but the infection does not spread readily from animals to man, nor from animal to animal. Infection occurs by inhalation of spores of the fungus which grows in the soil, and possibly by ingestion and through cutaneous abrasions (5). The lesions produced in cattle and pigs (9) are granulomatous, contain a cream-coloured pus and are sometimes calcified. They are usually observed at necropsy or in abattoirs, and because of their appearance and location in the bronchial, mediastinal and rarely the mesenteric, pharyngeal and submaxillary lymph nodes and in the lungs, they may be mistaken for tuberculosis (3). Similar lesions in sheep bear some similarity to those of caseous lymphadenitis. Microscopic or cultural examination may be required to differentiate these diseases.

Two clinical cases have been recorded in horses (4, 6). In one there was severe emaciation, a fluctuating temperature, oedema of the legs, anaemia and a leucocytosis. Rupture of the liver caused death. In the other case intermittent colic also occurred and there were peritoneal adhesions at necropsy. Typical lesions were present in the lung, liver and spleen. The clinical disease has been recorded in sheep with fever and abscesses in peripheral lymph nodes. In diagnosis, an extract of the fungus, coccidioidin, has been used in an intradermal sensitivity test and a complement-fixation test. Isolation of the organism is preferred as evidence because of the non-specificity of coccidioidin (7). No effective treatment is available. Because infection occurs by the inhalation of soil-borne spores, control of dust in feedlots may help to prevent the spread of the disease. Dust control is a major factor in prevention of human coccidioidomycosis because there is no vaccine or effective therapeutic agent available and the eradication of *C. immitis* from the soil seems highly impracticable (8).

REFERENCES

(1) Maddy, K. T. (1958). *J. Amer. vet. med. Ass.*, *132*, 483.
(2) Prchal, C. J. (1948). *J. Amer. vet. med. Ass.*, *112*, 461.
(3) Maddy, K. T. (1954). *J. Amer. vet. med. Ass.*, *124*, 456.
(4) Zontine, W. J. (1958). *J. Amer. vet. med. Ass.*, *132*, 490.
(5) Stiles, G. W. & Davis, C. L. (1942). *J. Amer. med. Ass.*, *119*, 765.
(6) Rehkemper, J. A. (1959). *Cornell Vet.*, *49*, 198.
(7) Maddy, K. T. (1963). *Proc. 66th ann. gen. Mtg U.S. Livestock san. Ass.*, p. 396.
(8) Maddy, K. T. (1960). *Advances in Veterinary Science*, Vol. 6, pp. 251–286. New York: Academic Press.
(9) Prchal, C. J. & Crecelius, H. G. (1966). *J. Amer. vet. med. Ass.*, *148*, 1168.

Mucormycosis

Infections of animals with fungi of the family *Mucoraceae* include infections with the genera *Rhizopus*, *Absidia*, and *Mucor*. Fungal placentitis resulting in abortion has been recorded in cattle (1, 2). Abortions usually occur at 3 to 7 months. There is necrosis of the maternal cotyledons and the adherent necrotic material gives the placental cotyledon the appearance of a soft, yellow, cushion-like structure, and there are small yellow, raised leathery lesions on the intercotyledonary areas. Corresponding lesions occur on the endometrium and ringworm-like lesions occur on the foetal skin. Hyphae can be seen on examination of direct smears of cotyledons, foetal stomach and skin. If mycotic abortion is suspected the placental cotyledons offer the best source of material. Every effort should be made to obtain the entire placenta as the infection may be patchy and involve only a few cotyledons. The fungi can be cultured on suitable media. Preputial catarrh accompanied by slowness of service and masturbation has been associated with infection in bulls by an *Absidia* spp. fungus thought to be transmitted at coitus (3).

Granulomatous lesions, typical of those produced by fungal infections, may occur in the mesenteric lymph nodes and intestinal wall in pigs. Granulomatous lesions also occur in the mesenteric and mediastinal lymph nodes and other organs of cattle (4). The lesions closely resemble those of tuberculosis and require laboratory examination for accurate differentiation. They usually cause no apparent illness.

Mucormycosis of the alimentary tract occurs relatively commonly in pigs and also in young calves. It is often associated with prolonged antibiotic therapy. In pigs it may be manifested by gastroenteritis with vomiting and diarrhoea, or gastritis and gastric ulcer, again manifested by diarrhoea and oedema, haemorrhage and ulceration at necropsy (5). Oesophageal lesions are a common accompaniment (6). Similar outbreaks occur in calves (7, 8) and abomasal infection and ulceration are common lesions. Copper sulphate administered in the drinking water has been an effective agent in controlling the infection.

Primary rumenitis due to lactic acid fermentation after overloading of the rumen with concentrate is often complicated by invasion of the ruminal wall by the *Rhizopus* spp. fungi. The wall becomes much thickened, oedematous and black. The lesions may be diffuse or patchy and are usually located in the ventral sac of the rumen. There is necrosis of the cornified epithelium and an extensive peritonitis. Metastases may be present in the liver. Clinically the animal may respond to treatment for acute indigestion but relapses with the development of complete anorexia and ruminal atony and dies 3 to 4 days later.

Cutaneous candidiasis causing dermatitis has been recorded as a severe outbreak in pigs kept in moist conditions (9).

REFERENCES

(1) Austwick, P. K. C. & Venn, J. A. J. (1962). *Proc. 4th Int. Congr. Anim. Reprod., The Hague*, *3*, 562.
(2) Munday, B. L. (1967). *N.Z. vet. J.*, *15*, 149.
(3) Rollinson, D. H. L. & Haq, I. (1948). *Vet. Rec.*, *60*, 69.
(4) Cordes, D. O. *et al.* (1967). *N.Z. vet. J.*, *15*, 143.
(5) Gitter, M. & Austwick, P. K. C. (1959). *Vet. Rec.*, *71*, 6.
(6) Baker, E. D. & Cadman, L. P. (1963). *J. Amer. vet. med. Ass.*, *147*, 763.
(7) Mills, J. H. L. & Hirth, R. S. (1967). *J. Amer. vet. med. Ass.*, *150*, 862.
(8) Smith, J. M. B. (1967). *Sabouraudia*, *5*, 220.
(9) Reynolds, I. M. *et al.* (1968). *J. Amer. vet. med. Ass.*, *152*, 182.

Aspergillosis

Systemic aspergillosis is uncommon in large animals although *Aspergillus* spp. appears to be a relatively common cause of abortions in cattle

(1, 2) and has also been reported in mares (3) and sows (4). In cattle a placentitis, identical to that caused by infection with *Mucor* spp., is a characteristic feature and hyphae can be seen on examination of direct smears of the cotyledon or the foetal stomach, preferably the former. Most abortions occur during the sixth to eighth months of pregnancy. Material should be submitted for culture. A dermatomycosis occurs rarely in the aborted foetal calves, with discrete patches of alopecia, covered by a raised, greyish, felted covering occurring all over the body (5). Congenital infection may also occur, granulomatous lesions containing the fungus having been found in the lungs of a day old lamb (6).

Infection of the placenta is thought to originate from abomasal ulcers or from the respiratory tract which becomes infected by the inhalation of spores from mouldy hay or straw. Infection of the placenta and uterus can be established by intravenous injection during pregnancy (5) but not by intrauterine inoculation before fertilization.

Invasion of the alimentary tract occurs and is similar to candidiasis. In calves there is a severe fatal gastroenteritis. Areas of necrosis and ulceration occur in the oesophagus and stomach (7). Although pulmonary aspergillosis is uncommon in animals occasional cases have been recorded in all species, sometimes with generalization (8, 9). The pulmonary form of the disease appears as a chronic, subacute or acute pneumonia. The acute, fibrinous pneumonia is of very short duration and is accompanied by fever and dyspnoea. All forms are usually fatal (10). Occasional cutaneous granulomata, causing lesions similar to those of cutaneous tuberculosis, also occur in cattle. At necropsy the lungs have multiple discrete granulomas often with necrotic centres, giving a superficial resemblance to tuberculosis. In lambs the granulomas appear as very small nodules (1 to 3 mm. diameter) and resemble those caused by infestation with *Muellerius capillaris*. A persistent diarrhoea, which responded to treatment with nystatin, has been associated with *Aspergillus fumigatus* infection in foals (11).

REFERENCES

(1) Dijkstra, R. G. (1963). *T. Diergeneesk.*, *88*, 563.
(2) Austwick, P. K. C. & Venn, J. A. J. (1961). *Proc. 4th int. Congr. Anim. Reprod., The Hague*, *3*, 562.
(3) Mahaffey, L. W. & Adam, N. M. (1964). *J. Amer. vet. med. Ass.*, *144*, 24.
(4) Mason, R. W. (1971). *Aust. vet. J.*, *47*, 18.
(5) Hillman, R. B. & McEntee, K. (1969). *Cornell Vet.*, *59*, 269, 289.
(6) Nobel, T. A. & Shamir, A. (1956). *Refuah vet.*, *13*, 23.
(7) Barinov, V. N. (1968). *Veterinariya*, *2*, 57.
(8) Ainsworth, G. C. & Austwick, P. K. C. (1958). *Fungal Diseases of Animals*, Farnham Royal, Bucks, England: Commonwealth Agricultural Bureaux.
(9) Gracey, J. F. & Baxter, J. T. (1961). *Brit. vet. J.*, *117*, 11.
(10) Cordes, D. O. *et al.* (1964). *N.Z. vet. J.*, *12*, 101.
(11) Lundvall, R. L. & Romberg, P. F. (1960). *J. Amer. vet. med. Ass.*, *137*, 481.

Histoplasmosis

Histoplasmosis caused by infection with *Histoplasma capsulatum* is rare in farm animals compared to dogs and is unusual amongst fungal infections in that granulomatous lesions are not produced. Invasion of the cells of the reticuloendothelial system is characteristic of the disease and the lesions consist of groups of macrophages packed with fungal cells. Infection occurs by the inhalation of contaminated dust and primary invasion usually takes place in the lung. The disease may spread from animals to man. Attempts at experimental infection in cattle, sheep, horses and pigs have resulted in non-fatal infections, unless the agent is given intravenously, but the animals become positive to the histoplasmin test (1).

Cases have been recorded in horses, cattle and pigs (2). An affected cow showed chronic emaciation, dyspnoea, diarrhoea and anasarca. At necropsy there was ascites, enlargement of the liver, considerable oedematous thickening of the wall of the large intestine and moderate, pulmonary, interstitial emphysema. Histologically, typical eosinophilic round bodies were seen in endothelial cells in the portal triads. The incidence of hypersensitivity to the cutaneous histoplasmin test was high in other animals in the vicinity. The affected foal showed emaciation, dyspnoea and jaundice at 6 months of age. At death there was extensive consolidation of the lungs and gross enlargement of the bronchial lymph nodes.

As a diagnostic aid for herd or area use the histoplasmin skin test appears to be satisfactory and several surveys in animals have been reported (11).

The disease caused by infection with *H. farciminosum* is dealt with under the heading of epizootic lymphangitis.

REFERENCES

(1) Saslaw, S. *et al.* (1960). *Proc. Soc. exp. Biol.*, *105*, 76.
(2) Menges, R. W. *et al.* (1963). *Vet. Med.*, *58*, 331.

Rhinosporidiosis

Rhinosporidiosis is a chronic disease of the nasal mucosa in cattle and horses causing formation of large polyps in the posterior nares and interference with respiration. The causative fungus, *Rhino-*

sporidia seeberi, can be found in large sporangia in the polyps.

Nasal granuloma which are thought to be fungal in origin also cause obstruction to respiration in cattle. In these cases the lesions consist of small (0·5 to 2 cm. diameter) nodules, limited in distribution to the mucosa of the anterior third of the nasal cavity. Histologically there is a marked eosinophilic reaction and yeast-like bodies are present in cells or free in the tissue spaces. The fungi have not been positively identified but resemble *Rhinosporidia* spp. Clinically there is severe dyspnoea with a mucopurulent nasal discharge, sometimes blood-stained, from both nostrils. The lesions can be easily seen and palpated. The respiration is stertorous and can be heard from quite a distance. A high incidence of the disease may occur on some farms and in particular areas. Rhinosporidiosis of this type has been recorded in the U.S.A. (1), Australia (2), India and South America (3).

Clinically the disease resembles nasal obstruction caused by the blood fluke, *Schistosoma nasalis* (4, 5), and chronic allergic rhinitis seen in cattle and sheep.

REFERENCES

(1) Robinson, V. B. (1951). *Amer. J. vet. Res.*, *12*, 85.
(2) Albiston, H. E. & Gorrie, C. J. R. (1935). *Aust. vet. J.*, *11*, 72.
(3) Saunders, L. Z. (1948). *Cornell Vet.*, *38*, 213.
(4) Choudbury, B. (1955). *Indian vet. J.*, *31*, 403.
(5) Biswal, G. & Das, L. N. (1956). *Indian vet. J.*, *33*, 204.

Cryptococcosis

(European Blastomycosis, Torulosis)

Infection with the yeast *Cryptococcus neoformans* occurs in most species either as a generalized disease or as a granulomatous meningo-encephalitis (1). Two cases of meningitis have been recorded in horses which showed stiffness and hyperaesthesia or blindness and inco-ordination (2, 3). Myxomatous lesions of the nasal mucosa caused by *Crypt. neoformans* infection have been observed in horses and cattle, and pulmonary abscess in horses and goats (4, 5) and lymphadenitis in cattle have also been recorded. Mastitis caused by *Crypt. neoformans* is described elsewhere. Minute, focal lung lesions developing as metastases from cryptococcal mastitis have been observed in a cow (2).

REFERENCES

(1) Laws, L. & Simmons, G. C. (1966). *Aust. vet. J.*, *42*, 321.
(2) Barron, C. N. (1955). *J. Amer. vet. med. Ass.*, *127*, 125.
(3) Irwin, C. F. P. & Rac, R. (1957). *Aust. vet. J.*, *33*, 97.
(4) Sutmoller, P. & Poelma, F. G. (1957). *W. Ind. med. J.*, *6*, 225.
(5) Dickson, J. & Meyer, E. P. (1970). *Aust. vet. J.*, *46*, 558.

Moniliasis

(Candidiasis)

Moniliasis, caused by infection with the mycelial yeast *Candida albicans*, occurs in malnourished human infants as mycosis of the oral mucosa (thrush). Cases of a similar disease have been observed in baby pigs reared on an artificial diet (1, 3, 4). Frequent vomiting and emaciation develop at 2 weeks of age. A white pseudo-membrane covers the back of the tongue and extends down the oesophagus to the cardia of the stomach. The contents of the stomach and intestines are fluid. The fungus has been isolated from the bedding in pens in which the infection occurred, but it is thought that the fungus is not a primary pathogen, invasion of the mucosa occurring either in association with *E. coli* infection or because of the high sugar content of the artificial diet (5). Treatment of affected piglets with nystatin appears to effect little improvement.

A chronic pneumonia caused by *Cand. albicans* has been observed at a relatively high level of incidence in cattle in a feedlot (2). Clinical signs are those of pneumonia with a characteristically severe dyspnoea which may cause mouth-breathing but only a moderate febrile reaction. Profuse, stringy salivation and a mucopurulent, often brown streaked, nasal discharge appear. A profuse diarrhoea may occur and there may be crusting of the muzzle with dried exudate but there are no discrete ulcerative, erosive or vesicular lesions on the muzzle, nor in the nostrils or mouth. A profuse lacrimal discharge often mats the facial hair but there is no conjunctivitis. The disease is slowly progressive and the animal eventually dies or is slaughtered. At necropsy there is consolidation of the lungs, which may be extreme in advanced cases, and small caseated abscesses are present in the pneumonic tissue. Local lesions may also be present in the intestinal wall. The fungus can be seen in smears and sections and can be cultured on special media. *Cand. parapsilosis* has been implicated as the probable cause of abortion in a cow (6).

REFERENCES

(1) McCrea, M. R. & Osborne, A. D. (1957). *J. comp. Path.*, *67*, 342.
(2) McCarty, R. T. (1956). *Vet. Med.*, *51*, 562.
(3) Saunders, L. Z. (1948). *Cornell Vet.*, *38*, 213.
(4) Gitter, M. & Austwick, P. K. C. (1959). *Vet. Rec.*, *71*, 6.
(5) Osborne, A. D. *et al.* (1960). *Vet. Rec.*, *72*, 237.
(6) Bisping, W. *et al.* (1964). *Berl. Münch. tierärztl. Wschr.*, *77*, 260.

North American Blastomycosis

This disease appears to have been recorded only once in large animals (1). In the affected horse the appearance of a series of abscesses in the perineal region was followed by emaciation and death. In man and in dogs the disease usually takes the form of granulomatous lesions in the lung or on the skin. No effective treatment is available and the disease is an important zoonosis. The causative fungus is *Blastomyces dermatiditis*.

REFERENCE

(1) Benbrook, E. A. *et al.* (1948). *J. Amer. vet. med. Ass., 112,* 475.

DERMATOMYCOSES

Ringworm

Ringworm is caused by the invasion of the keratinized epithelial cells and hair fibres by dermatophytes.

Incidence

Ringworm occurs in animals in all countries but more commonly where animals are housed in close proximity to each other for long periods. Injury to affected animals is of a minor nature and little economic loss occurs. A high incidence of clinical cases in the winter and of spontaneous recovery in the spring is commonly reported. However, outbreaks often occur during the summer months and close confinement and possibly nutrition seem to be more important in the spread of the disease than other environmental factors such as temperature and sunlight.

Aetiology

The causative agents are fungi which grow on the hair or skin or both.

The common fungi which occur in each species are:

Horse: *Trichophyton equinum, Tr. quinckeanum, Tr. mentagrophytes, Microsporum equinum, Tr. verrucosum.*

Cattle: *Trichophyton verrucosum, Tr. mentagrophytes, Tr. megnini, Tr. verrucosum* var. *album, Tr. verrucosum* var. *discoides.*

Pig: *Tr. mentagrophytes, M. canis, Tr. verrucosum* var. *discoides, M. nanum, Tr. rubrum.*

Sheep: *Tr. verrucosum* var. *ochraceum, Tr. quinckeanum, Tr. mentagrophytes, Tr. gypseum, M. canis.*

Trichophyton spp. produce spores in long chains, *Microsporum* spp. produce a mosaic pattern of spores, and both are capable of growth on hair.

Transmission between species occurs readily and in rural areas 80 per cent of human ringworm may derive from animals (1). *Trichophyton* spp. infections are commonly contracted from horses and cattle and *M. canis* infections from dogs. Ringworm of animal origin affects adult humans as well as children and diagnosis and treatment are often very difficult.

Largely because of a developing interest in comparative mycology and the transmission of dermatomycoses from animals to man, an increasing number of previously unidentified fungi are being found in cutaneous lesions in animals. Three such fungi are *M. gypseum* in horses, *Keratinomyces allejoi* in horses and *Scopulariopsis brevicaulis* in cattle. Of particular interest is the observation of a widespread infection of pigs with *M. nanum* in which the lesions are often so mild as to go unnoticed by the farmer. The disease occurs chiefly in adult pigs.

It appears that deficiency of certain dietary factors contributes to the development of widespread and chronic lesions in cattle (2).

Transmission

Direct contact with infected animals is a common method of spread of ringworm but indirect contact with any inanimate objects, particularly bedding, harness, grooming kits and horse blankets is probably more important. Spores can exist on the skin without causing lesions, and 'carrier animals' of this type may act as important sources of infection. Premises may remain infective for long periods because fungal spores can remain viable for years provided they are kept dry.

M. gypseum, K. allejoi and *M. nanum* are soil saprophytes and the reasons for their assumption of pathogenicity are not understood.

Pathogenesis

Ringworm fungi attack chiefly keratinized tissues, particularly the stratum corneum and hair fibres resulting in autolysis of the fibre structure, breaking off of the hair and alopecia. Exudation from invaded epithelial layers, epithelial debris and fungal hyphae produce the dry crusts characteristic of the disease. The lesions progress if suitable environmental conditions for mycelial growth exist, including a warm humid atmosphere, and a slightly alkaline pH of the skin. Ringworm fungi are all strict aerobes and the fungi die out under the crust in the centre of most lesions leaving only the periphery active. It is this mode of growth which produces the centrifugal progression and the characteristic ring form of the lesions.

The significance of skin pH in the development of ringworm is widely known. The susceptibility of humans to ringworm infection is much greater before puberty than afterwards when the skin pH falls from about 6·5 to about 4·0. This change is largely due to excretion of fatty acids in the sebum and these fatty acids are often highly fungistatic. For this reason some treatments for human ringworm are based on ointments containing propionic and undecylenic acids. Calves are more commonly infected than adult cattle but whether this is due to increased susceptibility in calves or the development of immunity in adults has not been determined.

Secondary bacterial invasion of hair follicles is common. The period after experimental infection before distinct lesions appear is about 4 weeks in calves, but considerably less in horses. Spontaneous recovery occurs in calves in about 4 months, the duration and severity of the disease often depending upon the nutritional status of the host. A resistance to reinfection occurs after recovery from experimental infection even though a local mycotic dermatitis may occur at the reinfection site. The development of immunity and allergic dermatitis due to ringworm fungi has been reviewed (2).

Clinical Findings

In cattle the typical lesion is a heavy, grey-white crust raised perceptibly above the skin. The lesions are roughly circular and about 3 cm. in diameter. In the early stages the surface below the crust is moist, in older lesions the scab becomes detached and pityriasis and alopecia may be the only obvious abnormalities. Lesions are most commonly found on the neck, head and perineum but a general distribution over the entire body may occur, particularly in calves, and in severe cases the lesions may coalesce. Itching does not occur and secondary acne is unusual.

In horses the lesions may be superficial or deep. Superficial infections are more common and are manifested either by the development of thick crusts, or more generally a diffuse moth-eaten appearance with desquamation and alopecia. Less commonly deeper structures are infected through the hair follicles causing small foci of inflammation and suppuration. A small scab forms over the follicle and the hair is lost but extensive alopecia and crust formation do not occur. Some irritation and itching may be caused by this type. The distribution of lesions in the horse differs from that in

cows, lesions usually appearing first on the axillary/ girth area and spreading generally over the trunk and over the rump and may spread to the neck, head and limbs.

Ringworm lesions in pigs develop as a centrifugally progressing ring of inflammation surrounding a scabby, alopecic centre. The cutaneous lesion produced in pigs by *M. nanum* differs from the standard lesions of ringworm in this species. There is an absence of pruritus and alopecia and a minimal cutaneous reaction due to the superficial nature of the lesion. There is a characteristic centrifugal enlargement of each lesion which may reach an enormous size. Superficial, dry, brown crusts cover the affected area but are not obviously raised except at the edges in some cases. The crusts are formed of flakes or dust composed of epithelial debris. Most lesions occur on the back and sides. Spontaneous recovery does not occur in adult pigs. In sheep the lesions occur on the head and although they usually disappear in 4 to 5 weeks the disease may persist in the flock for some months. The disease is rare in pigs and very rare in sheep.

Clinical Pathology

Laboratory diagnosis depends upon the examination of skin scrapings for spores and mycelia by direct microscopic means and by culture. Skin scrapings should be made after defatting the skin with ether or alcohol if greasy dressings have been used. Scrapings are warmed gently in a 20 per cent solution of either potassium or sodium hydroxide. Spores are the diagnostic feature and appear as round or polyhedral, highly refractile bodies in chains (*Trichophyton* spp.) or mosaics (*Microsporum* spp.) in hair follicles, epithelial scales, and in or on the surface of hair fibres.

Examination of the skin of infected animals to detect the fluorescence caused by some fungal infections can also be a useful clinical aid. A source of possible error in this test is that many trichophyton fungi do not fluoresce, whereas petroleum jelly and other oily skin dressings may do so. The examination is made with a Wood's filter in front of a source of shortwave, ultra-violet light. A green fluorescence indicates hairs infected with ringworm fungi. Hairs which fluoresce should be selected for laboratory examination.

Specimens to be sent for laboratory examination should be packed in envelopes, as airtight jars and cans favour the growth of non-pathogenic fungi.

Diagnosis

The diagnosis of ringworm depends on evidence of infectivity, the appearance of characteristic lesions and the presence of fungal mycelia and spores. Clinically it may be confused with mycotic dermatitis in cattle, and in pigs with pityriasis rosea, exudative epidermitis and dermatitis caused by infestations with *Tyroglyphos* spp. mites. The two former diseases are common only in young pigs; *M. nanum* infection is rare in pigs of this age. Examination of skin scrapings may be necessary to differentiate ringworm from mange and miscellaneous cutaneous infections.

Treatment

Experimental work suggests that the treatments in current use have little effect on individual lesions and that most recorded cures are due to strategic treatment just prior to spontaneous recovery (15). However treatment is still widely practised and has the advantage that the contamination of the environment by infected animals is greatly reduced. Local or systemic treatments are used, the latter when lesions are widespread.

For local application the crusts should be removed by scraping or brushing with a soft wire brush and the medicament brushed or rubbed in vigorously. Care should be taken that the scrapings are removed and burnt. Suitable topical applications include a weak solution of iodine, Whitfield's ointment, 10 per cent ammoniated mercury ointment, and solutions of quaternary ammonium compounds (1 in 200 to 1 in 1000). Ointments containing propionic and undecylenic acids and their esters are effective, non-irritant and control secondary bacterial invasion. Rapid and effective cure of affected cattle, horses and pigs is claimed with 2 to 3 applications at 3- to 4-day intervals of 0·25 per cent hexadecamethylene-1:16-bis, isoquinolinium chloride (Tinevet). The preparation is best applied with a stiff brush and removal of thin scabs may not be necessary. Hexetidine (bis-1, 3 beta-ethyl-hexyl-5-methyl 5 aminohexa-hydropyrimidine), is reputed to be highly successful in young calves following one treatment. Borotannic complex is also an effective fungicide and has given good results in the treatment of equine ringworm. It has the particular advantage of being in a solvent—ethyl acetate and alcohol—which is a strong skin penetrant. Thiabendazole ointment, 2 applications of a 2 to 4 per cent ointment 3 to 5 days apart, gives excellent results. Local aqueous preparations and oral dosing with the anthelminthic are ineffectual (3). Other reports suggest that the preparation may be ineffective against new infections (4).

The above topical treatments are probably of greatest value in the early stages of an outbreak when the lesions are small and few in number. When infection in a group is widespread, washes or sprays which can be applied over the entire body surface of all animals are preferred. For example agricultural Bordeaux mixture has given good results in the control of ringworm in large groups of horses. Copper sulphate 4 lb. and unslaked lime 4 lb. should be dissolved in separate solutions and mixed in a wooden or earthenware container and made up to 40 gallons. Spraying with a handspray at weekly intervals gives good results. Copper naphthenate has given promising results in pigs (5) and Captan (N-trichloromethyl-mercapto-4- cyclohexene-1, 2-dicarboxamide) in a concentration of 1 in 300 to 1 in 400 has been used successfully in the control of ringworm in cattle when applied at the rate of 1 to 1½ gallons per animal on 2 occasions 2 weeks apart. Another preparation which has given good results when used as a spray for affected horses and their harness is N-trichloromethylthicotetrahydrophthalamide. Two ounces of a 45 per cent solution of this compound are mixed with 3 gallons of water and applied daily as a spray or wash to the horses and the harness scrubbed with it.

A systemic treatment in common use in farm animals is the intravenous injection of sodium iodide (1 g. per 30 lb. body weight) as a 10 per cent solution. More than one injection is often required and should be accompanied by topical application of fungistatic agents. Another systemic approach to the treatment of ringworm is the oral administration of griseofulvin. The original recommendation for calves of 0·5 g. per lb. body weight daily for 7 to 10 days was economically impracticable but a good response has subsequently been obtained from much smaller doses (125 mg. per 30 lb. body weight daily for 7 days). A dose rate of 1 g. per 100 kg. body weight has been recommended for pigs with a 30 to 40 day course of treatment (6). A fine particle preparation is used which can be given by drench or in the feed. It is highly effective and is now marketed as a premix of crude mycelia which is economically attractive. Human infection is reduced to a minimum and there is a prophylactic effect which lasts for 2 months (8). Another griseofulvin-like antibiotic, tricothecin, is on trial.

Spontaneous recovery is common in individual animals and careful appraisal of results in clinical trials is necessary. Carefully controlled trials suggest that the main virtue of topical applications with any fungicide to ringworm lesions in calves is 'to curtail the extension of recent lesions and limit the dissemination of infective material'. Many farmers overtreat their animals with irritant preparations administered daily for long periods. A crusty dermatitis, or even a neoplastic acanthosis (7) may result which is not unlike ringworm.

Control

Failure to control an outbreak of ringworm is usually due to the widespread contamination of the environment before treatment is attempted. Isolation and treatment of infected animals, the provision of separate grooming tools, horse blankets and feeding utensils, and disinfection of these items after use on affected animals are necessary if the disease is to be controlled. Cleaning and disinfection of stables with a commercial detergent or a strong solution (2·5 to 5 per cent) of phenolic disinfectant or sodium hypochlorite (0·25 per cent solution) is advisable where practicable. Good results are also claimed for the disinfection of buildings with a spray containing 2·0 per cent formaldehyde and 1·0 per cent caustic soda. In a control programme this is combined with spraying of all cattle in the herd, using a similar solution (0·4 per cent formaldehyde plus 0·5 per cent caustic soda), twice at intervals of a week.

There is an increasing interest in the possibility of vaccinating against ringworm (9). A formalized, aluminium hydroxide precipitated liquid culture of *Tr. gypseum* is reported to be an effective antigen (10). A live vaccine prepared from a highly immunogenic strain of *Tr. faviforme* is also favourably reported (11, 12). Only moderately good results are recorded with a killed vaccine (13).

Although ringworm occurs in well nourished as well as poorly fed animals, there does seem to be a tendency for the latter to become infected more readily and to develop more extensive lesions. Supplementation of the diet, particularly with vitamin A to young housed animals, should be encouraged as a preventive measure.

REFERENCES

(1) Medical Research Council (1956). *Vet. Rec.*, *68*, 357.
(2) Lepper, A. W. D. (1972). *Res. vet. Sci.*, *13*, 105.
(3) Neuman, M. & Platzner, N. (1968). *Refuah vet.*, *25*, 10.
(4) Hammerling, G. (1969). *Inaug. Diss. tierärztl. Hochschule, Hanover*, 73.
(5) Ginther, O. J. & Ajello, L. (1965). *J. Amer. vet. med. Ass.*, *146*, 361, 945; *148*, 1034, 1170.
(6) Kielstein, P. & Gottschalk, C. (1970). *Mh. Vet.-Med.*, *25*, 127, 130.
(7) Carter, G. R. & Glenn, M. W. (1966). *J. Amer. vet. med. Ass.*, *149*, 42.
(8) Edgson, F. A. (1970). *Vet. Rec.*, *86*, 58.
(9) Lepper, A. W. D. (1969). *Rev. med. vet. Mycol.*, *6*, 435.
(10) Sharapov, V. (1968). *Trudy vses. Inst. Vet. Sanit.*, *27*, 162.
(11) Podobedov, A. I. (1971). *Veterinariya*, *6*, 48.
(12) Sarkisov, A. K. *et al.* (1971). *Veterinariya*, *2*, 54.
(13) Kielstein, P. & Richter, W. (1970). *Mh. Vet.-Med.*, *25*, 334.

Epizootic Lymphangitis

(*Psuedoglanders*, *Equine*, *Blastomycosis*, *Equine Histoplasmosis*)

Epizootic lymphangitis is a chronic, contagious disease of horses characterized by suppurative lymphangitis, lymphadenitis and ulcers of the skin and by keratitis or pneumonia. The disease is of importance both in its own right and because of its similarity to glanders.

Incidence

The disease occurs chiefly in Asia, Africa and the Mediterranean littoral. It occurs in outbreaks rather than as an enzootic disease and although not highly fatal (the mortality rate is 10 to 15 per cent), the course is prolonged and loss of function of affected animals can cause serious economic loss. Most outbreaks occur when large numbers of horses are gathered together for military or other purposes.

Aetiology

A fungus *Histoplasma* (or *Zymonema*, *Cryptococcus*, *Saccharomyces*, *Blastomyces*) *farciminosum* is the cause of the disease. Horses and rarely cattle and man are the species affected, horses under 6 years of age being most susceptible. In enzootic areas most cases occur during the autumn and winter.

Transmission

Fungal spores are carried from infected animals by direct contact or on inanimate objects such as bedding, grooming utensils, horse blankets or harness, and gain entry through cutaneous abrasions. A saprophytic stage in the soil has been suggested to account for the difficulty experienced in eradicating the disease. Because of the frequent occurrence of abrasions on the lower limbs lesions are most commonly seen in this area. The organism has been isolated from the alimentary tract of biting flies and their possible role in the transmission of the diseases has been suggested (1).

Pathogenesis

There has always been a question about the pathogenesis of this disease. Is it a systemic disease or a disease of many forms, the cutaneous being one? The latter seems the more likely on the evidence and the disease might be best defined as 'being associated with *H. farciminosum* infection', and named equine histoplasmosis (2).

The fungus invades subcutaneous tissue, sets up a local granuloma or ulcer and spreads along the lymphatic vessels (3).

Clinical Findings

In the cutaneous form of the disease an indolent ulcer develops at the portal of entry, making its appearance several weeks to 3 months after infection occurs. Lymphatic vessels leaving the ulcer become thickened and enlarged and develop nodules along their course. These nodules rupture discharging a thick creamy pus. Local lymph nodes also enlarge and may rupture. Thickening of the skin in the area and general swelling of the whole limb are common. The lesions are quite painless.

In most cases the lesions develop on the limbs particularly about the hocks but may also be present on the back, sides, neck, vulva and scrotum. Occasionally lesions appear on the nasal mucosa, due usually to nibbling of lesions on the trunk and limbs, but are situated just inside the nostrils and do not involve the nasal septum. Ocular involvement, manifested by keratitis and conjunctivitis, and sinusitis and primary pneumonia occur in other forms of the disease.

The disease is chronic, persisting for 3 to 12 months, and affected animals lose much condition and cannot be worked. Spontaneous recovery occurs and immunity is solid after an attack but many animals are destroyed because of the chronic nature of the disease.

Clinical Pathology

Gram positive, yeast-like cells, with a characteristic double walled capsule are easily found in discharges but this is not a sure diagnostic method. The agent can be cultured on special media but the fungus dies quickly in specimens unless these are collected in antibiotic solutions, refrigerated and cultured promptly. The specimen should be collected into a solution containing 500 units penicillin per ml. The mallein test is negative but a sterile filtrate of a culture of *H. farciminosum* has been used in a cutaneous sensitivity test. A complement-fixation test, has been used but is positive in infected animals for only short periods and a fluorescent antibody technique is also available (4).

Necropsy Findings

Lesions are usually confined to the skin, subcutaneous tissues, and lymph vessels and nodes. In some cases granulomatous lesions may be found in the lungs, liver and spleen (5).

Diagnosis

Because of its characteristic clinical picture including cutaneous ulceration, lymphadenitis and lymphangitis, the disease may be confused with glanders. However, there is no systemic reaction, and rarely pulmonary involvement, lesions do not occur on the nasal septum and the pus is creamy. In ulcerative lymphangitis the pus is greenish, the lesions usually occur about the fetlocks and heal quickly. In sporotrichosis only small amounts of pus are discharged from the lesions and there is often no lymphatic involvement but differentiation should be made only on the basis of laboratory examinations.

Treatment

Many treatments have been tried largely without success. Early cases can be cured by extensive excision of affected parts followed by frequent local applications of silver nitrate or tincture of iodine. Parenteral iodides have been reported as effective in some cases (7).

Control

Strict hygienic precautions must be observed. Outbreaks in uninfected areas are probably best controlled by slaughter of affected animals. In enzootic areas severe cases should be destroyed and less severe cases kept in strict quarantine while undergoing treatment. All infected bedding, harness and utensils should be destroyed or vigorously disinfected. A formolized aluminium hydroxide adsorbed vaccine has been reported to give serviceable immunity (6).

REFERENCES

(1) Singh, T. *et al.* (1965). *Ind. J. vet. Sci.*, *35*, 102, 111.
(2) Singh, T. (1966). *Ind. J. vet. Sci.*, *36*, 45.
(3) Khater, A. R. *et al.* (1968). *J. Egypt. vet. med. Ass.*, *28*, 165.
(4) Fawi, M. T. (1969). *Brit. vet. J.*, *125*, 231.
(5) Fawi, M. T. (1971). *Sabouraudia*, *9*, 123.
(6) Noskov, A. I. (1960). *Trudÿ vses. Inst. Vet. Sanit.*, *16*, 368.
(7) Singh, S. (1956). *Indian vet. J.*, *32*, 260.

Sporotrichosis

Sporotrichosis is a contagious disease of horses characterized by the development of cutaneous nodules and ulcers on the limbs and may or may not be accompanied by lymphangitis.

Incidence

The disease is reported to occur in Europe, India and the U.S.A. Economic loss caused by sporotrichosis is not great because the disease spreads slowly, the mortality rate is low, and treatment is effective. Rare cases have been reported in man.

Aetiology

The cause of the disease, *Sporotrichum schencki* (*Sporothrix beurmannii, S. schencki, S. equi*), is a Gram positive fungus, which forms single walled spores. Horses are the only species commonly affected but cases have been recorded in man, dogs, cats, camels and cattle (1).

Transmission

The causative agent persists in organic matter and contamination of cutaneous wounds can occur either by direct contact with discharges from infected animals, or indirectly from contaminated surroundings. The disease spreads slowly and only sporadic cases occur in a group.

Pathogenesis

Local invasion through cutaneous wounds results in the development of abscesses and discharging ulcers.

Clinical Findings

Multiple, small, cutaneous nodules develop on the lower parts of the legs, usually about the fetlock. The nodules are painless, develop a scab on the summit, discharge a small amount of pus and heal in 3 to 4 weeks. Succeeding crops of lesions may cause the disease to persist in the animal for months. Lymphangitis, causing cording of the lymphatics, occurs in some outbreaks and not in others.

Clinical Pathology

Gram positive spores are present in the discharges but they may be few in number and difficult to find, and diagnosis by culture of pus is preferred. The hyphal stage is rare in tissues. Injection of pus into rats or hamsters produces a local lesion containing large numbers of the yeast-like cells. This may be of value when organisms are scarce in the pus from natural lesions.

Diagnosis

The disease occurs only sporadically in affected groups of animals and this helps to differentiate it from glanders, epizootic lymphangitis and ulcerative lymphangitis. In cases where there is lymphangitis identification of the yeast-like cells is necessary to complete the diagnosis. Maduromycotic mycetoma, in which small (0·5 to 1·0 cm. in diameter) nodules are present in the skin over most of the body has been reported in the horse (2). A few lesions discharge exudate; section of the nodules shows dark brown specks in pale pink tissue. The causative fungus has been identified as *Brachycladium spiciferum* Bainier.

Treatment

Systemic treatment with iodides (potassium iodide orally or sodium iodide intravenously) is the most effective treatment. Local application of tincture of iodine daily to ulcers may suffice in mild cases. A good response has been recorded in one case in a horse, which did not respond to iodine therapy, after the oral administration of griseofulvin (3).

Control

Prophylactic treatment of all cuts and abrasions, isolation and treatment of clinical cases, and disinfection of bedding, harness and gear will prevent spread of the disease in enzootic areas.

REFERENCES

(1) Saunders, L. Z. (1948). *Cornell Vet.*, *38*, 213.
(2) Bridges, C. H. & Beazley, J. N. (1960). *J. Amer. vet. med. Ass.*, *137*, 192.
(3) Davis, H. H. & Worthington, W. E. (1964). *J. Amer. vet. med. Ass.*, *145*, 692.

Swamp Cancer—Hyphomycosis Destruens

(*Florida Horse Leech, Bursattee*)

A common lesion of the skin and mucous membranes of horses in tropical climates is that referred to by one of the above names. The lesion occurs most commonly on the limbs, abdomen, neck, lips and alae nasi and consists of dense granulation tissue containing masses of yellow-grey necrotic tissue which are sometimes calcified, the masses often being present as cores in fistulae and being removable intact. Such masses are known as 'leeches' or 'kunkurs'. The granuloma ulcerates and extends peripherally and may reach a very large size in a short time. The aetiology of the disease has been in doubt for many years and has been thought to be either an infestation with the larvae of *Habronemia megastoma* or an infection with a fungus. It has recently been shown that infestation with *H. megastoma* larvae or infection with the fungus *Hyphomyces destruens* cause almost identical lesions and both qualify as causes of this disease (1). In a particular area one of these agents may be more common than the other.

Lesions caused by both agents spread rapidly, cause itching and have yellow necrotic foci in dense connective tissue. Both contain many eosinophiles and both appear to originate in wounds or areas of excoriation. The lesions of habronemiasis tend to regress in cold weather. Examination of a biopsy specimen is the only satisfactory way of determining which is the causative agent and care is necessary when taking the specimen to include a portion of necrotic tissue in which either the larvae or hyphae are most likely to be present. The treatment of the disease is outlined in the section on cutaneous habronemiasis.

Similar lesions in horses have been shown to be caused by the fungus *Entomophthora coronata* but the lesions have been restricted to the skin of the nostrils, the nasal mucosa and the lips. Surgical removal of the lesions is recommended in early cases (2).

REFERENCES

(1) Bridges, C. H. & Emmons, C. W. (1961). *J. Amer. vet. med. Ass., 138,* 579.
(2) Bridges, C. H. *et al.* (1962). *J. Amer. vet. med. Ass., 140,* 673.

24

Diseases Caused by Protozoa

Babesiasis

(Texas Fever, Redwater Fever, Cattle Tick Fever)

BABESIASIS includes those diseases caused by *Babesia* spp. in cattle, sheep, pigs and horses. They are all characterized by fever and intravascular haemolysis causing a syndrome of anaemia, haemoglobinaemia and haemoglobinuria, and are transmitted by blood-sucking ticks.

Incidence

The distribution of the causative protozoa is governed by the geographical distribution of the insect vectors that transmit them.

Bovine babesiasis caused by *Babesia bigemina* occurs in South America, the West Indies, Australia (northern part) and Africa; by *B. argentina* in Australia; by *B. bovis* in Europe, in Britain, South America and South Africa. Ovine babesiasis caused by *B. motasi* and by *B. ovis* occurs in south-eastern Europe, Africa and South America. Porcine babesiasis caused by *B. trautmanni* and *B. perroncitoi* occurs in south-eastern Europe and Africa. Equine babesiasis caused by *B. equi* occurs in south-eastern Europe, Africa and South America. Until 1961 babesiasis in horses caused by *B. caballi* was thought to occur only in south-eastern Europe, Africa, Asia, the Phillipines and South and Central America but at that time there was an unexpected occurrence of the disease in Florida, U.S.A. The disease was thought to have been introduced in horses imported from Cuba. One case of babesiasis due to *B. equi* has since been detected in Florida (1).

Bovine babesiasis is of the greatest economic importance both because of direct losses and because of restriction of movement by quarantine laws. Many animals die or undergo a long period of convalescence entailing loss of meat and milk production. Incidental costs of immunization and treatment add to the economic burden created by the disease.

In enzootic areas the animals most commonly affected are susceptible cattle introduced for breeding purposes, for slaughter, or in transit. Cattle indigenous to these areas are rarely affected because the natural resistance of the very young and passive immunity via colostrum from immune dams (42) is gradually replaced by a state of premunition. Severe clinical cases which occur in premunized cattle are usually caused by exposure to some stress such as parturition, starvation or intercurrent disease. Such breakdowns in premunity are most likely to occur if there is superimposed infection with a different parasite, especially *Anaplasma marginale*. Babesiasis is much more common in cattle of the European breeds than in Zebus, the difference probably being related to a difference in susceptibility to the vector tick.

Heaviest losses occur in marginal areas where the tick population is highly variable depending on the environmental conditions. In seasons when the tick population decreases, infection may die out and premunity be lost. Then in favourable seasons when ticks multiply, the disease spreads quickly amongst what has become a susceptible population. Comparable circumstances may be created artificially by an inefficient dipping programme which reduces the tick population to a low level and is subsequently unable to keep it under control. The morbidity rate in such circumstances is often 90 per cent and the mortality may be of the same order. There is also a seasonal variation in the prevalence of clinical babesiasis, the greatest incidence occurring soon after the peak of the tick population (2). With early, effective treatment the mortality rate can be reduced to 5 per cent. The morbidity and mortality rates and the losses caused by babesiasis in the other animal species are difficult to determine because they exist as enzootic diseases in areas where they occur. In the outbreak of equine babesiasis in Florida in 1961 the mortality rate was 10 per cent.

Aetiology

The protozoa vary in shape and size but all occur as intraerythrocytic parasites. Their classification has been uncertain but that suggested by Neitz (3) has been used here. The important species are listed in the section on incidence above. The diseases may have a seasonal incidence if the tick population varies with climate. For example in England babesiasis is largely a disease of spring, summer and autumn for this reason.

Strong premunity occurs after infestation with most babesia and persists for 1 to 2 years and indefinitely with repeated reinfection. Efficient treatment will destroy all the parasites and with them the premunity. There is no significant cross-immunity between the different species of babesia. Variation in susceptibility to babesiasis has been observed in the different races of cattle. All are equally susceptible to *B. bigemina* but Zebu and Afrikander cattle have a higher resistance to *B. argentina* than British and European breeds, Santa Gertrudis cattle occupying an intermediate position (5). Zebu-type cattle also enjoy a relative freedom from the disease because of their resistance to heavy infestations with ticks. Although the infection rate need not reflect the rate of occurrence of the clinical disease, there appears to be a variation in susceptibility to infection according to age in cattle. The greatest infection rate is in animals in the 6- to 12-months age group and infection is uncommon in animals over 5 years of age. Animals under one year of age are infected predominantly with *B. bigemina* and those over 2 years of age by *B. argentina* (4).

Specific antibodies to the parasites are produced and are used in serological diagnosis. The highest titres are obtained in the sera of cows which have had a series of infections and reinfections. The degree of immunity in the animal is not related to the complement fixing antibody titre. The antibodies can be passively transferred via serum (5) or colostrum (6).

Transmission

Ticks are the natural vectors of babesiasis and the causative parasites persist and pass through part of their life cycle in the invertebrate host (7). Both *B. argentina* and *B. bigemina* pass part of their life cycle in the tick *Boophilus microplus* and some mortality in ticks occurs when they ingest blood heavily infected with the former parasite (8). *Boophilus* (*Margaropus*) *annulatus*, *Boophilus microplus* and *Boophilus australis* are the major vectors of babesiasis but other *Boophilus* spp., *Rhipicephalus* spp. and *Haemaphysalis* spp. also act as vectors. *Ixodes ricinus* is the common carrier of *B. bovis* in England. *Rhipicephalus* spp. are the vectors in sheep; *Dermacentor* spp., *Rhipicephalus* spp., and *Hyalomma* spp. are the vectors in horses;

and *Rhipicephalus* spp. and *Boophilus* spp. are the vectors in pigs.

A knowledge of the life history of the tick is most important in applied control. Those ticks which parasitize only one host are easier to eradicate and cause less spread of the disease than those which parasitize two or three hosts. Control of ticks which are capable of surviving on both domestic and wild animals presents a major problem. The capacity of the protozoa to persist through several generations of ticks by passage through the egg is another important characteristic. *B. bigemina* and *B. caballi* (9) do persist in this manner, in *Boophilus microplus* and *Dermancentor nitens* (10), respectively, and transovarian transmission probably occurs in the other species of babesia also. *B. microplus* become infected in the adult stage when feeding on cattle undergoing a primary reaction to the infection, but transmission by the next generation of ticks does not occur until the ticks reach the nymphal or adult stages (11).

Pathogenesis

When an animal becomes infected, multiplication of the protozoa in the peripheral vessels (*B. bigemina*, *B. ovis*), or in the visceral vessels (*B. argentina*), reaches a peak with the development of clinically detectable haemolysis after an incubation period of 7 to 20 days. The haemolysis results in profound anaemia, jaundice and haemoglobinuria. Death is presumably due to anaemic anoxia. If the animal survives it becomes a carrier and is resistant to infection because of its premunized state. The duration of this carrier state in the absence of reinfection is usually about 1 year. Loss of virulence of blood from a carrier does not mean that the protozoa have died out, or that premunity has been lost. It may be due to periodic disappearance of infective forms from the peripheral blood.

A detailed study of the natural history in individual animals has been conducted in cattle run in a tick-free environment and after a single infective episode. With *B. argentina* recurrences of parasitaemia occurred for up to two years. With *B. bigemina* there were fewer, shorter recurrences. The ability of cattle to infect ticks was much longer (one year) with *B. argentina* than *B. bigemina* (4 to 7 weeks). Similarly the peak incidence was at a younger age and the reinfection rate was faster with *B. bigemina* (12).

When cows become infected during pregnancy there is no apparent infection of the calf in utero. But there is an apparent transfer of passive immunity via colostrum to the newborn calf. The resistance is specific to the strain of *B. argentina* which infects the cow (13).

Clinical Findings

Cattle. In field infections the incubation period is 2 to 3 weeks. Subclinical infections occur fairly commonly, especially in young cattle. *B. bigemina* and *B. argentina* produce syndromes which are clinically indistinguishable, and are characterized by an acute onset of high fever (41 °C or 106 °F), anorexia, depression, weakness, cessation of rumination and a fall in milk yield. Respiratory and heart rates are increased and the brick-red conjunctivae and mucous membranes soon change to the extreme pallor of severe anaemia. In the terminal stages there is severe jaundice, and the urine is dark red to brown in colour and produces a very stable froth. The febrile stage usually lasts for about a week and the total course about 3 weeks. Pregnant animals often abort. Animals that survive recover gradually from the severe emaciation and anaemia which are inevitable sequelae. A subacute syndrome also occurs, especially in young animals in which the fever is mild and haemoglobinuria is absent. Occasional animals infected with *B. bigemina* show cerebral babesiasis manifested by inco-ordination followed by posterior paralysis or by mania convulsions and coma. The mortality rate in these cases is high in spite of treatment (14).

The syndrome in infection with *B. bovis* is similar to the above, except that in addition there is spasm of the anal sphincter causing the passage of 'pipe stem' faeces. The faeces are evacuated with great force in a long, thin stream, even in the absence of diarrhoea.

Other species. In all other species the syndrome observed is clinically similar to the one seen in cattle except that haemoglobinuria is not always present in the horses and in this species subcutaneous oedema along the underline and in the supraorbital fossa, and petechial or ecchymotic haemorrhages on the conjunctival mucosa may occur. Colic also occurs relatively frequently. Afflicted horses may die within 24 to 48 hours of the first signs appearing. Chronic cases may survive for months and 'carriers' may persist for as long as four years (15).

Clinical Pathology

The detection of these diseases by laboratory methods presents some difficulties. Examination of smears of peripheral blood is the simplest diagnostic method, but although *B. bigemina* and *B. bovis* are numerous in peripheral capillaries *B. argentina* is much less readily found, but the difficulty can be largely overcome by the use of thick blood smears. A positive smear in all cases confirms the diagnosis but a negative smear does not eliminate it and for accurate diagnosis in these circumstances transmission tests are essential.

For a transmission test the animals to be inoculated must be susceptible and this can be ensured only by using animals from tick-free areas. To overcome the difficulty of subinfective numbers of the organism in donor blood it may be necessary to increase the susceptibility of the recipient by splenectomy. This technique is particularly necessary when infection with *B. argentina* is suspected. In transmission experiments 50 to 100 ml. of blood are injected into the recipient either subcutaneously or intravenously. In the latter case the incubation period will be shorter. The recipients are examined daily and the blood examined for protozoa at the peak of the febrile reaction.

A complement-fixation test is available but is of doubtful value as a diagnostic test in cattle because of the high incidence of false positives (16). An accurate, passive haemagglutination test for bovine babesiasis is also attracting attention (17), and an indirect fluorescent antibody test has been found to be efficient for the detection of *B. bigemina* (18) and *B. argentina* (19) antibodies. The complement-fixation test is useful in the diagnosis of babesiasis in horses (20). Other tests used for diagnosis of the disease in horses are a bentonite agglutination and a passive haemagglutination test (21), a fluorescent antibody inhibition test, and the rabbit antiserum precipitin test (15).

Severe anaemia with erythrocyte counts as low as 2 million per cmm. and haemoglobin levels down to 3 g. per cent is present in most clinical cases.

Necropsy Findings

In acute cases jaundice is marked, the spleen is enlarged, swollen and of a soft, pulpy consistency, the liver is grossly enlarged and dark brown in colour, and the gall-bladder is distended with thick, granular bile. The kidneys are enlarged and dark and the bladder contains red-brown urine. Ecchymotic haemorrhages are present under the epicardium and endocardium and the pericardial sac contains an increased quantity of blood-stained fluid. In cases of fairly long duration the carcase is emaciated but haemoglobinuria is absent and the other changes observed in acute cases are present but less pronounced. Smears for direct examination should be taken from peripheral blood, from kidney and heart muscle and, in the case of suspected *B. argentina* infection, from the brain (22).

Diagnosis

The presence of the insect vector must be verified before the diagnosis can be made unless the animal has left an enzootic area within the preceding month. Clinically, jaundice with haemoglobinuria and fever are suggestive but confirmation by examination of blood smears or by transmission experiments is essential. A necropsy which shows splenomegaly, jaundice, haemoglobinuria, swollen dark kidneys and liver, and myocardial ecchymoses, while highly suggestive, should also be confirmed by laboratory examination (23).

Differentiation from other diseases which are characterized by haemolytic anaemia may be difficult in cattle. Anaplasmosis is usually less acute, relapses are more common and haemoglobinuria is a rare occurrence. Eperythrozoonosis is less severe and the clinical findings are largely limited to those of anaemia. Theileriasis (*Theileria mutans*) is often an inapparent disease but severe clinical cases are occasionally observed (24). The protozoa are readily identifiable in a blood smear and primaquine is an effective treatment. Leptospirosis has a much shorter course and is more severe in young calves than in adults, the reverse of the picture in babesiasis and anaplasmosis. Equine babesiasis can be so similar to equine infectious anaemia that laboratory differentiation is usually necessary. Other causes of haemolytic anaemia in animals are discussed in detail elsewhere.

Treatment

Effective drugs are available for the treatment of these diseases in cattle but two important factors must always be kept in mind, especially when the drugs are being used to control a reaction produced artificially for purposes of premunization. The initial phase of the disease is acute and if treatment is delayed for too long the animal may succumb to the anaemia in spite of sterilization of the blood. Secondly, complete sterilization of the blood must be avoided if premunity is to be established.

Acaprin (a 5 per cent solution of akiron) is effective against *B. argentina* and *B. bigemina* but effective doses when given intravenously destroy all *B. bigemina*, especially if it is administered in the early stages of the disease. It can be given subcutaneously (1 ml. per 100 lb. body weight with a maximum dose of 6 ml.). Dose rates above 6 ml. are not recommended because of the danger of toxicity. After injection, salivation and anorexia may be observed, but only occasionally are the signs severe enough to require treatment with adrenaline (5 ml. 1 in 1000 subcutaneously). Repeated daily doses of Acaprin may be necessary if improvement is only temporary.

Ganaseg (P, P-diguanyl-diazoamino-benzene) at a minimum dose rate of 2 mg. per kg. body weight injected intramuscularly has given good control of clinical signs without complete elimination of the protozoa. Amicarbalide (3:3′—diamidino-carbanilide) given by deep intramuscular injection at the rate of 10 mg. per kg. body weight is also effective against *B. bigemina* infection but premunity is lost. At 7·5 mg. per kg. body weight, premunity is retained but some relapses occur. The more soluble di-isethionate salt of this compound appears to be equally effective at the same dose rate and premunity is retained (43). Homidium bromide (1 mg. per kg. body weight) and Berenil (diminazene aceturate) at a dose rate of 3·5 mg. per kg. body weight are also curative without loss of premunity (25). Imidocarb is an excellent treatment (26) and also protects cattle against artificial infection with *Babesia* spp. for 3 months (27, 28, 29).

An interesting new drug for the treatment of babesiasis is quinuronium (5,5′-methylene *bis* salicylate). It is not only effective but after administration its effect is maintained prophylactically for up to 35 days (30). Its disadvantage is renal toxicity at twice the therapeutic dose. Vaccination against *B. argentina* during the prophylactic period is effective (31).

Ancillary treatment in severely affected cases should include blood transfusions, and haematinics during convalescence.

Treatment of equine babesiasis is not well documented. Amicarbalide isethionate (Phenamidine) is effective against *B. caballi*, but not *B. equi* (32) when given intramuscularly at a dose rate of 9 mg. per kg. body weight on two consecutive days. The treatment also eliminates the carrier state but there may be some adverse side effects (20). Phenamidine isethionate and diminazene are effective against both infections but are rather toxic (32). Other drugs used in the horse are oxytetracycline (10 mg. per kg. body weight), Pirevan, Berenil and euflavine (15), and Phenamidine and Diampron (33).

Control

Eradication of bovine babesiasis from an area depends upon eradicating the vector tick—a problem in applied entomology. Eradication has been achieved in the U.S.A. by this technique.

In control not aimed at eradication, cattle introduced into enzootic areas and in marginal tick belts should be premunized. Although *B. bigemina* premunity may confer some degree of premunity against *B. argentina*, both protozoa are usually included in the injection if premunity against both is desired. To prepare donor animals as a source of blood for premunization purposes, susceptible animals from a babesiasis-free area are inoculated with either organism, or both simultaneously, and checked to ensure that they become infected. The preparation of donors which are infected by only one protozoan may be difficult. Pure infections with *B. bigemina* can be produced by serial passages in calves, blood being taken from each calf about 30 hours after inoculation when other protozoa have not yet appeared in the peripheral blood (11). Treatment to control severe infections is avoided whenever possible because of the danger of sterilization. If treatment is necessary, the dose rate should be reduced by about 50 per cent. Premunization against *A. marginale* by the injection of *A. centrale* may also be carried out at the same time. Cattle infected in this way can be regarded as adequate sources of infected blood for about 6 months. Donors which are kept for long periods at vaccination centres should be tested at frequent intervals by injection of their blood into susceptible (preferably splenectomized) animals. There can be a great deal of difference in infectivity of blood from different donors and of blood from the same donor at different times. Thus blood from a latently infected animal is much less infective than blood from an animal undergoing a reaction due to *B. argentina* at the time of the collection (34). Some of the difficulties of maintaining infected animals as permanent donors of vaccine are overcome by the technique of storing infective blood by deep freezing. Virulence of the blood is maintained for at least two years (35). The 'vaccine' used is stored at 1 to 5°C, contains 10^5 *B. argentina* organisms per dose as the minimum infecting dose (36) and 10^7 to 10^8 organisms is highly infectious (37). Reaction occurs 7 to 14 days after the vaccination. Treatment of cattle with excessive reactions, indicated by fever at greater than 40·5°C, with quinuronium sulphate at half the normal dose rate is effective.

The animals to be vaccinated are injected subcutaneously with 10 ml. of whole blood. If multiple premunization is desired, blood may be taken from a donor with a mixed infection or mixed bloods from donors with single infections may be used. Premunization of a large number of cattle is usually arranged by having a number of donors available, drawing blood as required and vaccinating on the spot. When vaccination is completed, the cattle should be housed or kept under close observation for a month in case excessive reactions occur.

Greater care is taken with pure-bred cattle pre-munized at centres en route to infected areas. It is most important that such animals be premunized before they are exposed to tick infestation. An excellent description of a premunization procedure is available (38). Blood from 'single infection donors' is used; *B. bigemina* premunization is given first, followed by *B. argentina*, when the reaction from the former has subsided. There does not seem to be much danger in simultaneous premunization with both protozoa but separate injections do permit a better assessment of the degree of reaction and the adequacy of each infection. This precaution is taken because of the rather common failure to transmit *B. argentina*. Temperatures are taken twice daily and blood smears from an ear vein once daily. Elevation of the temperature above 40°C (104°F) and the presence of protozoa in the smear indicate that the infection has been transmitted. The reaction begins at 10 to 14 days after vaccination and is at its peak at 15 to 20 days with *B. bigemina* infections and at 7 to 18 days with *B. argentina*. *B. bigemina* are detectable in very large numbers in blood smears but *B. argentina* are rare, even at the peak of the reaction, and in the latter the temperature reaction is used as the main guide to infection. If the reaction is too severe, treatment is indicated.

One of the major problems in premunization is the occasional apparent failure to transmit the protozoa. This may be due to the absence of the protozoa from the blood stream of the donor at the time that the blood is drawn, or to failure of individual animals in a group to become infected, due possibly to a low-grade natural immunity. In both instances a reaction does not occur after injection and the animals are still susceptible to natural infection. Revaccination is necessary in these circumstances, preferably with blood from a donor which is undergoing a severe reaction at the time. The duration of immunity in the absence of reinfection is less than one year with *B. bigemina* and more than 2 years with *B. bovis* (27). To provide effective immunity continuously vaccination should be carried out every 4 months.

Another problem has recently been described with the premunization of pregnant cows using whole blood, particularly when repeated premunizations are made. Antibodies to the donor red cells may be produced, absorbed from the colostrum, and produce iso-immune, haemolytic anaemia in the calves. As a safety precaution cows should not be premunized in the last 6 months of pregnancy (39).

Equine babesiasis is controlled similarly to the disease in cattle with attention focussed on eradicating the vector tick, selecting infected and carrier animals by the complement-fixation test and sterilizing the positive reactors by appropriate treatments (40).

A killed *B. argentina* vaccine has been developed for cattle (41). It is in incomplete Freund adjuvant and has not been field tested.

The prevention of introduction of the disease into an area depends on effective quarantine and other measures to prevent the introduction of the vector tick.

REVIEW LITERATURE

Riek, R. F. (1968). *Infectious Blood Diseases of Man and Animals*, pp. 219–68, New York: Academic Press.

REFERENCES

(1) Knowles, A. C. *et al.* (1966). *J. Amer. vet. med. Ass., 148,* 407.
(2) Johnston, L. A. Y. (1968). *Aust. vet. J., 44,* 265.
(3) Neitz, W. O. (1957). *Ann. N.Y. Acad. Sci., 64,* 56.
(4) Riek, R. F. (1965). *Aust. vet. J., 41,* 211.
(5) Mahoney, D. F. (1967). *Exp. Parasit., 20,* 119.
(6) Hall, W. T. K. (1963). *Aust. vet. J., 39,* 386.
(7) Riek, R. F. (1966). *Aust. J. agric. Res., 17,* 247.
(8) Riek, R. F. (1964). *Aust. J. agric. Res., 15,* 802.
(9) Roby, T. O. *et al.* (1964). *Amer. J. vet. Res., 25,* 494.
(10) Holbrook, A. (1970). *Proc. 2nd int. Conf. equine infect. Dis., Paris,* 1969, pp. 249–57.
(11) Callow, L. L. & Hoyte, H. M. D. (1961). *Aust. vet. J., 37,* 66, 381.
(12) Mahoney, D. F. (1969). *Ann. trop. Med. Parasit., 63,* 1.
(13) Hall, W. T. K. *et al.* (1968). *Aust. vet. J., 44,* 259.
(14) Callow, L. L. & McGavin, M. D. (1963). *Aust. vet. J., 39,* 15.
(15) Zavagli, Y. (1970). *Proc. 2nd int. Conf. equine infect. Dis., Paris,* 1969, pp. 244–48.
(16) Curnow, J. A. & Curnow, B. A. (1967). *Aust. vet. J., 43,* 286.
(17) Goodger, B. V. (1971). *Aust. vet. J., 47,* 251.
(18) Goldman, M. *et al.* (1972). *Res. vet. Sci., 13,* 77.
(19) Johnston, L. A. Y. & Tammemagi, L. (1969). *Aust. vet. J., 45,* 445.
(20) Frerichs, W. M. *et al.* (1969). *Amer. J. vet. Res., 30,* 697.
(21) Sibinovic, S. *et al.* (1969). *Amer. J. vet. Res., 30,* 691.
(22) Rogers, R. J. (1971). *Aust. vet. J., 47,* 242.
(23) Hoyte, H. M. D. (1971). *Aust. vet. J., 47,* 248.
(24) Rogers, R. J. & Callow, L. L. (1966). *Aust. vet. J., 42,* 42.
(25) Barnett, S. F. (1965). *Res. vet. Sci., 6,* 397.
(26) Brown, C. G. D. & Berger, J. (1970). *Trop. Anim. Hlth Prod., 2,* 196.
(27) Neitz, W. O. (1969). *J. S. Afr. vet. med. Ass., 40,* 419.
(28) Roy-Smith, F. (1971). *Aust. vet. J., 47,* 418.
(29) Callow, L. L. & McGregor, W. (1970). *Aust. vet. J., 46,* 195.
(30) Newton, L. G. & O'Sullivan, P. J. (1969). *Aust. vet. J., 45,* 404.
(31) Callow, L. L. & McGregor, W. (1969). *Aust. vet. J., 45,* 408.
(32) Kirkham, W. W. (1969). *J. Amer. vet. med. Ass., 155,* 457.
(33) Kirkham, W. W. (1966). *Ann. Rep. Univ. Fla agric. exp. St.,* 1965, p. 204.
(34) Callow, L. L. & Tammemagi, L. (1967). *Aust. vet. J., 43,* 286.
(35) Pipano, E. & Senft, Z. (1966). *J. Protozool., 13,* Suppl. 34.
(36) Callow, L. L. & Mellors, L. T. (1966). *Aust. vet. J., 42,* 464.
(37) Dalgliesh, R. J. (1968). *Aust. vet. J., 44,* 103.
(38) Ranatunga, P. & Wanduragala, L. (1972). *Brit. vet. J., 128,* 9.
(39) Langford, G. *et al.* (1971). *Aust. vet. J., 47,* 1.
(40) Bryant, J. E. *et al.* (1969). *J. Amer. vet. med. Ass., 154,* 1034.
(41) Mahoney, D. F. (1967). *Exp. Parasit., 20,* 125.
(42) Hall, W. T. K. (1963). *Aust. vet. J., 39,* 386.
(43) Riek, R. F. (1964). *Aust. vet. J., 40,* 261.

Anaplasmosis

Anaplasmosis of cattle, sheep and goats is caused by infection with *Anaplasma* spp. In cattle severe debility, emaciation, anaemia and jaundice are the major clinical signs. The disease is usually subclinical in sheep and goats.

Incidence

Anaplasmosis in cattle is common in South Africa, Australia, the U.S.S.R., South America and the U.S.A. Its spread is largely determined by the presence of suitable insect vectors and the incidence of the disease depends on the same factors, particularly the introduction of susceptible animals and sudden expansion of the vector population into previously free areas, which govern the incidence of babesiasis. Losses in enzootic areas may not be great because of widespread premunity. In general the disease has the same distribution as babesiasis but in both the U.S.A. and Australia it has spread beyond the boundaries of tick-infested areas. The disease is now present in 40 of the 50 states of the U.S.A. and is reputed to cost that country $35 million annually (1).

The morbidity rate is usually high in outbreaks but the mortality rate varies widely depending on susceptibility, and may be 50 per cent or more in introduced cattle. Recovered animals are emaciated and there is a prolonged convalescence.

Anaplasmosis of sheep and goats occurs in Africa, the Mediterranean countries, the U.S.S.R. and the U.S.A.

Aetiology

A. marginale is the causative agent in cattle and wild ruminants, and *A. ovis* in sheep and goats. Cross-infection and cross-immunity do not occur with *A. ovis* but subclinical infections with *A. marginale* can occur in sheep and goats. There may be a relationship between *A. marginale* and *Eperythrozoon wenyoni*, the latter interfering with the establishment of experimental anaplasmosis in splenectomized calves. Young animals are relatively resistant to the disease but susceptible to infection and remain permanently infected with a state of premunity. Animals over 3 years of age are usually affected by a peracute fatal form of the disease. The observed resistance to infection in very young calves is probably due to passive immunization as a result of the passage of antibodies from the dam to the calf in the colostrum. Inoculation of blood containing *A. marginale* into a bovine foetus in utero has resulted in infection and the development of complement fixing antibodies (2).

Zebu-type cattle are as susceptible as British breeds but under field conditions are not as commonly affected probably because of their relative resistance to heavy tick infestation. Deer can become infected and possibly act as reservoirs of infection for cattle. There is serological evidence of infection in elk and bighorn sheep but anaplasms have not been demonstrated in these animals. In Africa a large number of wild ruminants are considered to be susceptible to natural infection (3).

Exposure of infected, clinically normal animals to devitalizing environmental influences, particularly shortage of feed, and the presence of other diseases, may result in the development of acute anaplasmosis. For example cattle introduced into feedlots are highly susceptible and outbreaks among them are not uncommon 2 to 3 weeks after entry.

Transmission

The source of infection is always the blood of an infected animal. Once infected the animal remains a carrier for many years, probably for life, even though the parasite may not be always demonstrable in the blood. Spread from animal to animal occurs chiefly by insect vectors. In Australia the tick *Boophilus microplus* is the only vector but in the U.S.A. *Boophilus annulatus* and other ticks including *Dermacentor andersoni*, *Dermacentor variabilis*, *Argas persicus* and biting flies of *Tabanis* spp. also act as vectors (3) and many others are thought to do so. *Dermacentor occidentalis* (the Pacific Coast tick of the U.S.A.) parasitizes both deer and cattle and probably acts as a vector between the two species. The organism can survive for at least six months in *Dermacentor andersoni*. In sheep and goats a variety of ticks are known to spread the disease. Bovine anaplasmosis may also be spread mechanically by infected hyperdermic needles and castrating, spaying and dehorning instruments and by blood transfusions. The ease with which the infection is spread mechanically may vary with the virulence of the protozoan strain and this method of spread may be more important in some countries than others. Anaplasmosis may also be spread when cattle used

as donors of infected blood for premunization against babesiasis are infected with *A. marginale*, the reaction occurring some 3 weeks later than that due to the babesiae. There is a possibility that intrauterine infection may occur.

Pathogenesis

Anaplasmosis is primarily an anaemia, the degree of anaemia varying with the proportion of erythrocytes which are parasitized. The first appearance of the protozoa in the blood coincides with a fall in the haematocrit and erythrocyte levels, and the appearance of immature erythrocytes in blood smears and the development of fever. Acutely affected animals may die shortly after this phase is reached. If the animal recovers from the initial acute attack, periodic attacks of parasitic invasion of mature erythrocytes occur regularly, but with diminishing intensity. The degree of anaemia varies widely in young cattle up to 3 years of age but is always severe in adults and in splenectomized animals.

Clinical Findings

In cattle the incubation period varies with the amount of infected material injected but is usually recognized to be longer than in babesiasis, being about 3 to 4 weeks or more after tick-borne infection and 1 to 5 weeks after the inoculation of blood. In most cases the disease is subacute, especially in young animals. The temperature rises rather slowly and rarely to above 40·5 °C (105 °F). It may remain elevated or fluctuate with irregular periods of fever and normal temperature for from several days up to 2 weeks. Anorexia is seldom complete. The animal may die at this stage but many survive in an emaciated condition, and their fertility may be impaired. The mucous membranes are jaundiced and show marked pallor, particularly after the acute stage is passed, but haemoglobinuria is absent. Peracute cases, with a sudden onset of high fever, anaemia, icterus, severe dyspnoea and death often within 24 hours, are not uncommon in adult dairy cows. Affected animals are often hyperexcitable and tend to attack attendants just before death. Pregnant cows frequently abort. In convalescent bulls there may be depressed testicular function for several months.

In sheep and goats the disease is usually subclinical but in some cases, particularly in goats, a severe anaemia may occur and a clinical picture similar to that found in cattle may be seen. Severe reactions of this type in goats are most frequent when the animals are suffering from concurrent disease.

Clinical Pathology

Haemolysis may be so severe that the erythrocyte count is reduced to 1·5 million per cmm. Immature red cells are common at this stage and their presence is considered to be a favourable sign. The small dot-like protozoa are discernible at the periphery of up to 10 per cent of the red cells in subacute cases, but in peracute cases more than 50 per cent of the cells may be parasitized. *A. ovis* are usually situated at the periphery of erythrocytes but as many as 40 per cent of infested cells may show submarginal protozoa. Transmission experiments are best carried out on splenectomized animals and carriers can be detected by the same technique, severe relapses occurring after splenectomy. Calves often show anaemia without clinical signs after inoculation.

For the detection of carrier animals a highly accurate complement-fixation (CF) test has been developed in the U.S.A. The test is satisfactory for use in cattle, goats and sheep but the antibody titre is highest during the active phase of the disease and sufficiently low in carrier animals to give a proportion of false negative results (6). For unexplained reasons a small percentage of false positive reactions to the test also occur. A capillary tube agglutination test of comparable efficiency is available and is more economical and faster than the CF test (4, 5). A rapid card agglutination test, which tests serum or plasma for antibodies against *A. marginale*, is also available but little field testing is recorded (9).

Necropsy Findings

At necropsy the most obvious findings are emaciation, jaundice and pallor of the tissues, and thin, watery blood. The liver is enlarged and deep orange in colour, the kidneys congested, the spleen enlarged with soft pulp and there may be haemorrhages in the mycocardium.

Diagnosis

A positive diagnosis of anaplasmosis depends upon positive transmission and complement-fixation tests. The history of the outbreak, experience of the occurrence of the disease in the area and the presence of insect vectors or other means of spread of the disease may suggest the possible presence of anaplasmosis. Babesiasis is clinically much more acute, is accompanied by haemoglobinuria and can be distinguished on examination of smears of peripheral blood. The differential diagnosis of other causes of haemolytic anaemia has been discussed in detail elsewhere. The possible occurrence of more than one cause of haemolytic anaemia in the same group of animals should not be overlooked.

Treatment

In recent years interest in the treatment of anaplasmosis has centred around the use of broad spectrum antibiotics. In the control of clinical disease, 3 to 5 mg. of tetracycline per lb. body weight given in a single injection is effective, although it is more usual to give three such daily injections, but the parasite is not eliminated and immunity persists. Supportive treatment should include massive blood transfusions administered slowly to avoid cardiac embarrassment. Rough handling should be avoided at all cost. During treatment care must be taken to ensure sterilization of equipment between cases. A number of methods have been recommended for the treatment of carrier animals. Parenteral treatment with a tetracycline (5 to 15 mg. per lb. body weight daily for 10 to 16 days) has obvious disadvantages for large numbers of animals and oral administration of chlortetracycline (5 mg. per lb. body weight for 30 to 60 days) in the feed is preferred (6). Lower dosage for a longer period has also proved effective.

A carbazone (dithiosemicarbazone) has been found to be as effective in the treatment of anaplasmosis as tetracyclines (7) and a combination of a tetracycline and a carbasone is thought to be more effective as a treatment than either alone (8).

Control

The eradication of anaplasmosis is not in most countries a practicable procedure at the present time because of the wide range of insects which are capable of carrying the disease, the long period of infectivity of carrier animals, the inability to satisfactorily detect infected animals and, in some areas, the presence of carriers in the wild animal population (1). In enzootic areas some benefit is derived from the control or eradication of ticks, and the control of other vectors. Attention should also be given to preventing artificial transmission by instruments used for injections or surgical operations by disinfection after use on each animal. This is particularly important in feedlots where introduced groups are often subjected to multiple vaccinations and implantations at a time when their resistance is lowered by transport and change of feed. Some advantage can be gained when introducing animals into an enzootic area by limiting the introductions to animals of less than 2 years of age and by bringing them in when the insect population is least numerous.

Most control programmes in enzootic areas are

based on increasing the resistance of the population by premunization. Three forms of vaccination are used:

(i) Living *A. marginale* is used as a vaccine but its administration is limited to the relatively resistant age group below one year of age, to the winter months when vectors are sufficiently rare to avoid the chance of spread to other age groups, and to circumstances where animals which react severely can be restrained and treated adequately. The method has the serious disadvantage of creating a large population of carrier animals which may subsequently spread the disease.

(ii) Living *A. centrale*, which causes a mild, inapparent disease, does cause severe reactions in occasional animals. *A. centrale* is used extensively in Australia but not in the U.S.A. and there is some reluctance to introduce it into areas where it does not already occur. Premunization with *A. centrale* reduces the severity of the reaction when infection with *A. marginale* occurs, premunization with *A. marginale* eliminates the reaction (10).

(iii) Killed *A. marginale*, usually in an adjuvant vehicle, is receiving most attention as a vaccine at the present time. Its most serious disadvantage is that the immune response to one injection is poor and two vaccinations at least 6 weeks apart are required (11). The vaccine does not completely protect against infection but does significantly reduce the severity of the disease, thus permitting the development of a large population of carrier animals. It does have the advantage over the other vaccines of having a relatively short post-vaccination period (1 to 2 months) when animals remain positive to serological tests. The duration of the immunity is at least 5 months (24).

One of the problems with the living vaccines, the need to maintain a supply of living 'donor' animals at all times, may have been overcome by the observation that infective blood used as vaccine can be stored for up to $4\frac{1}{2}$ years by deep freezing (14). Whenever living vaccines are used vaccinated animals should be carefully observed to ensure that infection does in fact take place and that animals which suffer severe reactions are treated. An attenuated vaccine which gives excellent protection is also recorded as being free of serious defects (15). Another suggested method of reducing the severity of reactions which occur after premunization with *A. marginale* is that of injecting a minimum infective dose (0·01 ml. of infective blood) rather than the regular 5 ml. dose (16). An attenuated vaccine is under trial (17).

In any vaccination programme particular attention should be paid to the animals in high risk situations, particularly animals brought in from non-enzootic areas, those in surrounding similar areas to which infection may be spread by expansion of the vector population under the influence of suitable climatic conditions, and animals within the area which are likely to be exposed to climatic or nutritional stress.

The introduction of the disease into areas by carrier animals can be prevented by the use of the complement-fixation test or the capillary tube agglutination test. Vaccination with a killed vaccine in the area may be necessary when the risk of introduction by vector insects is high. If an outbreak does occur affected animals should be treated vigorously as described above and in-contact animals put onto a daily intake of 0·5 to 1 mg. oxytetracycline per lb. body weight for at least 10 days to prevent infection. Subsequently all exposed animals should be submitted to a suitable test and the reactors treated or preferably salvaged.

A killed vaccine with added adjuvant and containing *Anaplasma ovis* has produced resistance to challenge in sheep (12).

REVIEW LITERATURE

Ristic, M. (1968). In *Infectious Blood Diseases of Man and Animals*, pp. 473–542, New York: Academic Press.

REFERENCES

(1) Garlick, N. L. *et al.* (1965). *J. Amer. vet. med. Ass.*, *147*, 1565, 1567, 1570, 1573, 1576.
(2) Trueblood, M. S. *et al.* (1971). *Amer. J. vet. Res.*, *32*, 1089.
(3) Ristic, M. (1960). *Advanc. vet. Sci.*, *6*.
(4) Rogers, R. J. (1971). *Aust. vet. J.*, *47*, 364.
(5) Hibbs, C. M. (1966). *J. Amer. vet. med. Ass.*, *148*, 545.
(6) Roby, T. O. *et al.* (1971). *Proc. 74th ann. Mtg U.S. Anim. Hlth Ass.*, 1970, pp. 122–8.
(7) Kuttler, K. L. *et al.* (1970). *Res. vet. Sci.*, *11*, 334, 339.
(8) Kuttler, K. L. (1971). *Amer. J. vet. Res.*, *32*, 1349.
(9) Amerault, T. E. & Roby, T. O. (1968). *J. Amer. vet. med. Ass.*, *153*, 1828.
(10) Kuttler, K. L. (1967). *Res. vet. Sci.*, *8*, 467.
(11) Brock, W. E. *et al.* (1965). *J. Amer. vet. med. Ass.*, *147*, 948.
(12) Stepanova, N. I. & Kazakov, N. A. (1970). *Veterinariya*, *6*, 57.
(13) Wilson, J. S. & Trace, J. C. (1966). *Bull. Off. int. Épizoot.*, *66*, 897.
(14) Summers, W. A. & Matsuoka, T. (1970). *Amer. J. vet. Res.*, *31*, 1517.
(15) Lora, C. A. & Koechlin, A. (1969). *Amer. J. vet. Res.*, *30*, 1993.
(16) Franklin, T. E. & Huff, J. W. (1967). *Res. vet. Sci.*, *8*, 415.
(17) Welter, C. J. & Woods, R. D. (1968). *Vet. Med.*, *63*, 798.

Eperythrozoonosis

Although the causative agent of eperythrozoonosis—*Eperythrozoon* spp.—is a member of the Bartonella group and a rickettsia rather than a protozoa, the disease has been included here because of its close clinical resemblance to babesiasis and anaplasmosis. The disease occurs in swine, sheep and cattle, and is of particular importance in the former in which it is recorded in the mid-western and southern states of the U.S.A. (1). Latent eperythrozoonosis also occurs in mule deer and elk (2). The causative agent in swine is *Ep. suis*. Clinically the disease is characterized by weakness of the hind legs, mild fever (40°C or 104°F), increased pulse rate, pallor of the mucosae and emaciation. Jaundice is a frequent but inconstant feature of the disease. Haematological examination reveals extreme anaemia and the bartonellae are present in the erythrocytes. The infection causes a range of syndromes varying from mild anaemia to acute, fatal haemolytic anaemia with widespread haemorrhages but the mortality rate is usually low. Subclinical infections are also common.

A more acute form of the disease can be produced by the injection of infective blood into splenectomized pigs, death usually occurring on the 12th to 30th day after injection.

A complement-fixation test similar to that used in anaplasmosis can be used in diagnosis. Sera from affected animals give positive reactions on the third day of clinical illness, remain positive for 2 to 3 weeks, and then gradually revert to negative. Chronic carriers of the disease are usually negative reactors. A modified antiglobulin test is recommended now as a flock test for *Ep. ovis* infections (3) and a passive haemagglutination test is specific for *Ep. wenyoni* (4). A single intramuscular injection of tetracycline or oxytetracycline (1·5 mg. per lb. body weight, or more) is an effective treatment, with clinical improvement occurring in 24 hours. Neoarsphenamine given as a single intravenous injection (7 to 20 mg. per lb. body weight) has also been shown to be effective.

Eperythrozoonosis of cattle caused by *Ep. wenyoni* occurs in Africa and of sheep caused by *Ep. ovis* occurs in Africa, the U.S.A., France, Iran, Great Britain (5), Norway (6) and Australia. The disease in these species is similar to that described above for pigs, but in both species it is often subclinical (7, 8), and appears to require the presence of some other debilitating disease to manifest itself (9). In some areas it may be the principal cause of ill-thrift in lambs (10). Insects are thought to be the principal means of dissemination of the disease.

Treatment of affected lambs with neoarsphenamine (30 mg. per kg. body weight) or Antimosan (6 mg. antimony per kg. body weight) is effective but does not eliminate the carrier state.

REVIEW LITERATURE

Sutton, R. H. (1970). *N.Z. vet. J.*, *18*, 52, 55.

REFERENCES

(1) Biberstein, E. L. *et al.* (1956). *Cornell Vet.*, *46*, 288.
(2) Howe, D. L. & Hepworth, W. G. (1965). *Amer. J. vet. Res.*, *26*, 1114.
(3) Sheriff, D. & Geering, M. C. (1969). *Aust. vet. J.*, *45*, 505.
(4) Finerty, J. F. *et al.* (1969). *Amer. J. vet. Res.*, *30*, 43.
(5) Foggie, A. & Nisbet, D. I. (1964). *J. comp. Path.*, *74*, 45.
(6) Overas, J. (1969). *Acta vet. scand.*, Suppl. 28, 148.
(7) Harbutt, P. R. (1969). *Aust. vet. J.*, *45*, 493, 500.
(8) Campbell, R. W. *et al.* (1971). *Aust. vet. J.*, *47*, 538.
(9) Dodson, M. E. & Sheriff, D. (1965). *Aust. vet. J.*, *41*, 65, 68.
(10) Sheriff, D. *et al.* (1966). *Aust. vet. J.*, *42*, 169.

Coccidiosis

Coccidiosis is a contagious enteritis caused by infection with *Eimeria* spp. and occurs in all domestic animals. It is characterized by diarrhoea, dysentery, anaemia and emaciation.

Incidence

Coccidiosis occurs universally but is of most importance where animals are housed or confined in small areas. Most animals in a group become infected but only a minority show clinical signs. The disease is of minor economic importance because, although the mortality rate is relatively high (10 to 15 per cent) the morbidity rate is usually low. However, subclinical infection may cause retardation of growth and add greatly to the financial losses caused by the disease. The disease is of particular importance in young animals kept closely confined in overcrowded pens or paddocks or on irrigated pasture.

Aetiology

All domestic animals are susceptible but the coccidia are in general host-specific and infection does not pass readily from one animal species to another nor does cross-immunity between species of coccidia occur. In natural cases the infection is usually a mixed one and an immunity to a wide range of coccidia often develops. The immunity in coccidiosis is short-lived, of 3 to 4 months duration, and reinfection is common. Many coccidial species are virtually non-pathogenic. The species pathogenic to cattle include *Eimeria zurnii*, *Eim. bovis* (*smithii*), and *Eim. ellipsoidalis*; in sheep *Eim.*

arloingi, *Eim. ah-sa-ta* (1); in pigs *Eim. debliecki*, *Eim. scabra* and *Eim. perminuta*; in horses *Eim. leuckarti*. The pathogenic coccidia of goats have, in most instances, not been identified although *Eim. arloingi* and *Eim. faurei* are known to occur. Specific immunity to each coccidial species develops after infection so that young animals (2 to 12 weeks of age) exposed for the first time are more likely to develop a severe infection and clinical disease than older animals. However, acute attacks may occur in animals of any age when they are weakened by an intercurrent disease or exposure to inclement weather (2). In cattle, cases occur quite commonly in the 6- to 9-months age group and rare cases occur in adults. In sheep the pattern is the same with quite a high incidence in the 4- to 6-months age group. These outbreaks in older groups probably occur because of absence of exposure at an earlier age. Concurrent infestations with nematodes and coccidia occur commonly and the presence of the worms probably increases susceptibility to the coccidia.

Oocysts passed in the faeces required suitable environmental conditions if they are to become sporulated. Moist, temperate or cold conditions favour sporulation whereas high temperatures and dryness impede it. Dry conditions and high temperatures also destroy sporulated oocysts within a few weeks but the oocysts may survive for up to 2 years under favourable conditions.

Transmission

The source of infection is the faeces of clinically affected or carrier animals, and infection is acquired by ingestion of contaminated feed and water or by licking the hair coat contaminated with infected faeces. Ingestion of the sporulated, infected oocysts results in infection but very large numbers have to be taken in before clinical disease results. This level of ingestion usually comes about only by continual reinfection and building up of the degree of environmental contamination. This most commonly occurs when calves or lambs are crowded into small pens or confined in feedlots. However, overcrowding of pastured animals on irrigated pasture or around surface water holes in drought conditions may also cause heavy infestations. Animals brought into feedlots from sparse grazing may carry a few oocysts which build up into heavy infestations in the lots especially if conditions are moist. In such situations clinical signs of the disease usually appear about a month after the animals are confined.

On the other hand the disease in closely confined pigs is much less extensive if they are housed on concrete floors than if they are housed on dirt floors or pasture (3). Another factor which may be of importance in the development of very large coccidia populations is the fact that very young calves shed large numbers of oocysts for long periods (4).

Pathogenesis

The coccidia of domestic animals pass through all stages of their life cycles in the alimentary mucosa and do not invade other organs although schizonts have been found in the mesenteric lymph nodes of sheep and goats (5). The different species of coccidia manifest a tendency to localize in different parts of the intestine. *Eim. zurnii* and *Eim. bovis* occur chiefly in the caecum, colon and the last part of the ileum whereas *Eim. ellipsoidalis* and *Eim. arloingi* parasitize the small intestine.

The coccidial life history is self-limiting. Sporozoites released from ingested oocysts invade the intestinal epithelium and divide into asexual schizonts and then merozoites which in turn differentiate into male or female gametocytes. The fusion of the gametocytes produces the terminal oocyst which is discharged in the faeces. The merozoites and gametocytes are the pathogenic stages and cause rupture of the cells they invade with consequent exfoliation of the epithelial lining of the intestine. It is notable that the oocyst count is often low when the disease is at its peak as the oocysts have not yet formed. Exfoliation of the mucosa causes diarrhoea, and in severe cases haemorrhage into the intestinal lumen, and the resulting haemorrhagic anaemia may be fatal. If the animal survives this stage the life cycle of the coccidia terminates without further damage. The prepatent period varies with the species of coccidia but is usually within the range of 1 to 4 weeks. Under practical conditions, constant reinfection occurs and waves of pathogenic stages succeed each other.

The occurrence of villous atrophy in the intestinal mucosa of lambs affected by coccidiosis is probably related to the recurrence of diarrhoea and loss of body weight (6).

Clinical Findings

The incubation period after experimental dosing with oocysts varies. It is 16 to 30 days in cattle infected with *Eim. zurnii* and *Eim. bovis* (2), and about 14 days is usual in sheep. The clinical syndromes caused by the various coccidia are similar in all animal species. A mild fever may occur in the early stages but in most clinical cases the temperature is normal or subnormal. The first sign of illness is usually the sudden onset of severe diarrhoea with foul smelling, fluid faeces containing mucus and blood. The blood may appear as a dark, tarry staining of the faeces or as streaks or clots, or the evacuation may consist entirely of large clots of fresh, red blood. Severe straining is characteristic, often unaccompanied by the passage of faeces. Anaemia is variable depending on the amount of blood lost. It may be extreme with ash-white pallor of the mucosa, weakness, staggering and dyspnoea. Severe dehydration, emaciation and complete anorexia are usual. The course of the disease is usually 5 to 6 days. Survivors undergo a convalescent period of several weeks and regain condition slowly. In mild cases there is diarrhoea and poor growth but no dysentery, and subclinical cases show poor growth and anaemia only. Nervous signs, including convulsions, have been observed both in calves and older cattle during the course of an outbreak. In general, lambs and pigs show the same clinical signs but with much less dysentery than calves. In sheep a break in the wool may cause subsequent shedding of the fleece. Coccidiosis as a disease of horses has not been identified but the infection has been established experimentally (7).

Clinical Pathology

Affected animals subjected to a massive infestation may die of haemorrhagic anaemia some days before oocysts appear in the faeces, but oocysts can usually be recovered from the faeces in large numbers in the later stages of the disease. The period during which oocysts are discharged in significant numbers is quite short, 3 to 6 days, and this, together with the difficulty of finding oocysts in early cases, often makes it necessary to examine a number of animals in the group and rely upon a herd rather than an individual diagnosis.

A count of over 5000 oocysts per g. of faeces is considered to be significant. Although counts below 5000 per g. of faeces do not ordinarily suggest clinical infestation, they may indicate a potential source of severe infestation if environmental conditions for spread become favourable. Oocyst counts of over 100,000 per g. are common in severe outbreaks although similar counts may also be encountered in normal sheep (8). If oocysts are not found and the disease is suspected, merozoites can be looked for in direct smears; they do not float on the conventional concentrated sugar or salt solutions used for flotation of oocysts. The several species of coccidia can be differentiated up to a point on the characteristics of the oocysts. Haematological examination may reveal the presence of an anaemia due to blood loss, and dehydration.

Necropsy Findings

Congestion, catarrhal enteritis and thickening of the mucosa of the caecum, colon, rectum and ileum are the characteristic gross changes at necropsy. The thickening may be severe enough to produce ridges in the mucosa. Small white spots, formed by large schizonts, may be visible in the villi of the terminal ileum. Ulceration or sloughing of the mucosa may occur in severe cases. Whole blood or blood stained faeces may be present in the lumen of the large intestine and the carcase may show profound anaemia. Histologically there is denudation of the epithelium, and merozoites may be observed in some cells. Smears of the mucosa or intestinal contents should be examined for the various developmental stages. The necropsy findings in sheep are marked by more severe involvement of the small intestine than in cattle.

Diagnosis

Typical cases and outbreaks present a reasonably diagnostic syndrome and the detection of oocysts in large numbers is usually accepted as confirming the diagnosis. Diarrhoea with variable amounts of blood in the faeces also occurs in enteritis caused by *Escherichia coli*, *Salmonella* spp., and *Vibrio* sp. Differentiation can only be effected by faecal or necropsy examination. Scouring without dysentery, but associated with anaemia in young pigs, is usually due to iron deficiency, and in sheep and calves to infestation with gastric or intestinal nematodes. In adult cattle, sporadic cases of abomasal ulceration cause severe alimentary tract bleeding. Attention should also be given to the possible occurrence of coccidiosis in adult animals especially under the stress of another disease.

Treatment

Coccidiosis is a self-limiting disease and signs subside spontaneously in survivors when the multiplication stage of the parasite has passed and many treatments have been recommended without taking this into account. Sulphadimidine (sulphamezathine), sulphabromomezathine or phthalylsulphathiazole give excellent results when given orally at a dose rate of 1 g. per 15 lb. body weight daily for 3 to 4 days. Nitrofurazone is also recommended as a treatment and has the advantage that it can be given in the feed or drinking water and is particularly suitable when large numbers of pigs or lambs are to be treated. It is administered either mixed in the feed at a concentration of 0·04 per cent, or at a dose level of 5 mg. per lb. body weight daily for 7 days. Nitrofurazone in the drinking water (0·008 to 0·0133 per cent) for 7 days has also been shown to prevent mortality and reduce morbidity in affected lambs, but does not appear to be highly effective in calves even at dose rates as high as 5 mg. per lb. body weight (9). Dose levels of 15 mg. per lb. body weight were necessary for prophylaxis. Nicarbazin, an efficient coccidiostatic drug in chickens, cannot be used in calves because of its toxicity but amprolium (25 mg. per kg. daily) has been effective in experimentally-produced coccidiosis in calves (10) and lambs (11). In lambs treatment should be continued for at least 14 days. In calves treatment should be continued for 21 days and, as with other treatments, is most effective when given as a prophylactic to in-contact calves. A combination of amprolium (62·5 mg. per kg.) and ethopabate (3·2 mg. per kg.) has been shown to be highly effective in lambs. In naturally occurring cases in sheep, goats and calves a heavier dose rate of amprolium (50 to 100 mg. per kg.) for a shorter, more practicable period (4 days) has been recommended (12, 13). It should be remembered that amprolium is a thiamine metabolic antagonist and, theoretically at least, prolonged dosage could contribute to the development of polioencephalomalacia.

In an outbreak the clinically affected animals should be isolated and treated with one of the more efficient drugs. Individual treatment is preferred but may not be practicable when large numbers are involved. Clinically normal animals in the group may be protected by the prophylactic measures set out below.

In severe cases supportive treatment may be as important as the control of the coccidia. In acute bovine coccidiosis a high enema using a solution of electrolytes with one of the above drugs incorporated is commonly recommended. When anaemia is severe, blood transfusion and anticoagulants are suggested, and the rectal application of anaesthetic ointments or epidural anaesthesia may be indicated to control tenesmus.

Control

The control of coccidiosis depends largely upon hygiene and avoidance of overcrowding. As far as possible young animals should be separated from adults which provide the source or infection. Pens should be kept dry, cleaned out frequently and bedding disposed of so that oocysts do not have time to sporulate and become infective, and soiling of the coat, which may lead to infestation when calves lick themselves, is reduced. Feed and water troughs should be high enough to avoid faecal contamination. The ultimate in the control of the disease in calves is to rear in individual portable pens or on tether, with weekly movement to clean ground.

In groups of lambs at pasture, efficient control can be exercised by frequent rotation of fields. Special attention must be given to flocks where environmental conditions are conducive to spread, especially if the ewes have been exposed to the disease previously.

The elimination of carrier animals by treatment is impractical but when trouble is anticipated the prophylactic administration of drugs is a worthwhile procedure. Sulphaguanidine (2 g. per lamb daily or as 0·2 per cent of the ration) and elemental sulphur (0·5 to 1·5 per cent of the ration) have given good results in lambs in feedlots. Sulphaquinoxaline and sulphaguanidine (1 g. per 35 lb. body weight in the feed) are recommended in the prophylaxis of coccidiosis in calves and pigs. Amprolium at dose rates listed above is also a suitable prophylactic. Animals treated prophylactically become infected and develop immunity, showing as much resistance to subsequent infection as untreated animals (14). Care is required in the use of sulphaquinoxaline because of its toxicity for cattle but it is unlikely to cause toxic effects at the dose rates quoted above.

Nitrofurazone, at the dose rate recommended for treatment, should also be effective in control. In experimentally infected groups of lambs the addition of 0·0165 per cent of nitrofurazone to the feed for 21 days reduced the morbidity and improved gains in body weight and carcase quality compared with lambs fed less or no drug. Administration of the drug at this level did not prevent the development of infection, nor of clinical illness and no immunity to subsequent infection developed.

REVIEW LITERATURE

Niilo, L. (1970). *Canad. vet. J.*, *11*, 91.
Pout, D. D. (1969). *Vet. Bull.*, *39*, 609.

REFERENCES

(1) Mahrt, J. L. & Sherrick, G. W. (1965). *J. Amer. vet. med. Ass.*, *146*, 1415.
(2) Niilo, L. (1970). *Canad. J. comp. Med.*, *34*, 20.
(3) Vetterling, J. M. (1966). *Cornell Vet.*, *56*, 155.
(4) Niilo, L. (1969). *Canad. J. comp. Med.*, *33*, 287.
(5) Lotze, J. C. *et al.* (1964). *J. Parasit.*, *50*, 205.
(6) Pout, D. D. (1967). *Nature (Lond.)*, *213*, 306.
(7) Barker, I. K. & Remmler, O. (1970). *Vet. Rec.*, *86*, 448.
(8) Pout, D. D. *et al.* (1966). *Vet. Rec.*, *78*, 1455.
(9) Hammond, D. M. *et al.* (1965). *Amer. J. vet. Res.*, *26*, 83.
(10) Jolley, W. R. *et al.* (1971). *Proc. helminth. Soc. Wash.*, *38*, 117.
(11) Hammond, D. M. *et al.* (1967). *Cornell Vet.*, *57*, 611.
(12) Horak, I. G. *et al.* (1969). *J. S. Afr. vet. med. Ass.*, *40*, 293.
(13) Newman, A. J. *et al.* (1968). *Irish vet. J.*, *22*, 142.
(14) Baker, N. F. *et al.* (1972). *Amer. J. vet. Res.*, *33*, 83.

Globidiosis

(Besnoitiosis)

This disease is of limited importance outside of Africa. Alimentary globidiosis is an occasional cause of enteritis in animals. *Globidium gilruthi* has been observed as a cause of enteritis in sheep (1) and goats (2) in Australia and the United States with lesions occurring in the intestine and less commonly in the abomasum. A severe, fatal gastroenteritis in goats caused by *Globidium* spp. is recorded in Kenya (3). A profuse diarrhoea with dysentery, apparently caused by *G. fusiformis*, has been observed in cattle in India. Horses may develop enteritis as a result of infestations with *G. leuckarti*. Alimentary globidiosis is manifested by diarrhoea, dysentery and straining. There is no febrile reaction but dehydration, anaemia and much loss of condition occur. Clinically the disease is indistinguishable from coccidiosis and the two can only be differentiated by flotation examination of the faeces; the spores of *Globidium* spp. are banana-shaped in contrast to the oval oocysts of *Eimeria* spp. and are much smaller. Smears taken from the mucosa at necropsy will also contain the spores, and large cysts containing many spores can be seen in sections of the intestinal wall.

Cutaneous globidiosis is restricted in its distribution to south-western Europe and the African continent. *G. besnoiti* has been isolated from cutaneous lesions in cattle and horses. The method of transmission is incompletely known but transmission has been effected experimentally using *Glossina* sp., tabanids and *Stomoxys calcitrans* (4). In cattle in the early stages there is high fever, an increase in pulse and respiratory rates, and warm, painful swellings appear on the ventral aspects of the body, interfering with movement. The superficial lymph nodes are swollen, diarrhoea may occur and pregnant cows may abort. Affected bulls often become sterile for long periods. Lacrimation and an increased nasal discharge are evident and small, whitish, elevated macules may be observed on the conjunctiva and nasal mucosa. Cysts on the scleral conjunctiva are considered to be of particular diagnostic significance (5). The nasal discharge is serous initially but becomes mucopurulent later and may contain blood. Subsequently the skin becomes grossly thickened and the hair falls out. A severe dermatitis is present over most of the body surface. The mortality rate is about 10 per cent and the convalescence in survivors is protracted over a period of months. Horses are affected in much the same manner but the disease is less severe and the course less protracted. The disease also occurs in impala and blue wildebeeste in Africa (6) and caribou in Canada (7) but on the basis of cross-infection tests the individual isolates are distinct strains. Diagnosis depends upon detection of the cysts containing a number of spindle-shaped spores in scrapings or sections of skin. Many infected animals show no clinical signs of infection and laboratory diagnosis using a complement-fixation test has been attempted unsuccessfully (4). No specific treatment is available and affected animals should be treated symptomatically for enteritis or dermatitis.

REFERENCES

(1) Rac, R. & Wilson, R. L. (1959). *Aust. vet. J.*, *35*, 455.
(2) Soliman, K. N. (1960). *J. Parasit.*, *46*, 29.
(3) Mugera, G. M. & Bitakaramire, P. (1968). *Vet. Rec.*, *82*, 595.
(4) Bigalke, R. D. (1966). *Proc. 1st int. Congr. Parasit., Roma, 1964*, *1*, 288.
(5) Bigalke, R. D. & Nande, T. W. (1962). *J. S. Afr. vet. med. Ass.*, *33*, 21.
(6) Bigalke, R. D. *et al.* (1967). *Onderstepoort J. vet. Res.*, *34*, 7, 303.
(7) Choquette, L. P. E. *et al.* (1967). *Canad. vet. J.*, *8*, 282.

Toxoplasmosis

Toxoplasmosis is a contagious disease of all species, including man. Clinically it is manifested chiefly by abortion and stillbirths in ewes, and in all species by encephalitis, pneumonia and neonatal mortality.

Incidence

Toxoplasmosis is a true zoonosis occurring naturally in man, and in domesticated and wild animals and birds. It occurs in most parts of the world and surveys of its distribution indicate that a high incidence may occur in particular areas (1). In the United States, survey data based on serological findings include an incidence of 34 to 59 per cent in dogs, 34 per cent in cats, 47 per cent in cattle, 30 per cent in pigs and 48 per cent in goats.

Toxoplasmosis is one of the common causes of abortion in sheep and neonatal lamb deaths. Apart from this, animal losses, other than in dogs, appear to be small and the importance of the disease is in its potential threat to humans. In man and animals the proportion of latent cases is very high, especially in adults, and one of the major risks associated with the disease is its elevation to the clinical level when the host's resistance is reduced. The disease in man is likely to be occupational but may occur sporadically after the ingestion of infected milk and meat. The latter is unlikely as very light cooking kills the toxoplasma.

Extensive outbreaks in mink have been considered to result from the ingestion of carcases of animals dying of toxoplasmosis.

Ovine abortion and neonatal mortality have been observed in New Zealand, Australia, Canada and the United Kingdom. Perinatal mortality rates (including abortions and neonatal deaths) in affected flocks may be as high as 50 per cent.

Aetiology

The causative agent *Toxoplasma gondii* is of uncertain classification. It is provisionally described as a sporozoon but some exciting observations on its identity have been made in recent years. From natural cases of the disease in cats (2) and the experimental disease in that animal (3) it seems that *T. gondii* is a coccidian parasite closely related to genus *Isospora*.

It is also concluded that *Toxoplasma* is an intestinal coccidia in cats which has developed the ability to multiply in brain and muscle. Thus carnivorism is another means of transmission (4). This work is incomplete and its applicability to any species other than cat has not been examined but the probability is that the principles already elaborated will be applicable to toxoplasmosis generally. The organism is readily destroyed by heating, drying, and freezing and thawing, and dies quickly in the carcases of affected animals. The pseudocysts formed in the tissues of chronically sick animals are more resistant and may provide the most effective means of perpetuating the disease. Most species of animals and birds become infected and there is some variation in virulence of strains, these isolated from ovine abortions being of reduced pathogenicity. In sheep, a high rate of infection has been shown to be related to a high rainfall. Wild animals, especially water rats, and ravens may be infected (1).

Transmission

The method of transmission, apart from congenital infection from an inapparent carrier to the foetus, is uncertain (5). Mechanical transmission by insect vectors has been suggested but is unlikely to occur other than in exceptional circumstances. Ingestion is considered to be the most important route of infection, although pulmonary invasion after the inhalation of infected droplets may also occur.

Infected carcases, feed contaminated by saliva, nasal discharge or faeces, or infected milk are probable sources of infection. Rodents may be a reservoir of infection for man and house pets but are not known to be of much importance in farm animals. There are several specific instances in which transmission from wild rodents to ewes is thought to occur and other wild animals may serve as a reservoir of infection. Although clinically affected animals undoubtedly spread the disease it seems probable that inapparent carriers are the most significant source of continued infection.

Sheep are naturally rather resistant to toxoplasmosis and the occurrence of abortion as the most common clinical manifestation of the disease in this species suggests that the placenta and foetus are the most vulnerable tissues. Although transmission has been effected experimentally by the intravenous and subcutaneous injection of vegetative forms of the parasite (6) ingestion of cyst forms is thought to be the common mode of infection in sheep (7). It seems probable that only those sheep which become infected during pregnancy abort, those becoming infected at other times of the year developing sufficient immunity to prevent abortion. This probability is supported by the known higher incidence of abortion in young ewes. In pigs experimental infections can be set up by intramuscular injection or by inhalation. Piglets below the age of 12 weeks are much more susceptible than older animals (8).

Pathogenesis

T. gondii is an intracellular parasite which attacks most organs with predilection for the reticuloendothelial and central nervous systems. After invasion of a cell the parasite multiplies and eventually fills and destroys the cell. Liberated toxoplasms reach other organs via the blood stream after release from their development site. The clinical character of the disease varies with the organs attacked, which itself varies depending on whether the disease is congenital or acquired. In general the development of the disease in animals is the same as it is in man. The commonest syndromes are encephalitis when infection is congenital, and febrile exanthema with pneumonitis and enterocolitis when the disease is acquired postnatally. It is thought that a powerful exotoxin results in the granulomatous lesions which are characteristic of the disease. In pregnant animals the foetus is commonly invaded via an initial placentitis. The placentitis may result in foetal resorption or abortion and if the foetus is carried to term it is commonly born dead or affected with congenital toxoplasmosis (9). Maceration of foetuses is common and histological examination of foetuses may be necessary to demonstrate the presence of toxoplasma.

In the work in cats which demonstrates the relationship between *Isospora* spp. and *T. gondii* it is proposed that there are three developmental stages of the parasite: asexual development in reticulo-endothelial tissues, cyst development in skeletal muscle and central nervous system and sexual phases in intestinal epithelium (10).

Clinical Findings

The clinical syndrome and the course of toxoplasmosis vary a great deal between species and between age groups.

In cattle the disease usually runs an acute course with fever, dyspnoea, and nervous signs, including ataxia and hyperexcitability, in the early stages, followed by extreme lethargy. Stillborn or weak calves which die soon after birth may also be observed. Congenitally affected calves show fever, dyspnoea, coughing, sneezing, nasal discharge, clonic convulsions, grinding of the teeth and tremor of the head and neck. Death occurs after a course of 2 to 6 days.

In adult pigs there is debility, weakness, incoordination, cough, tremor and diarrhoea but no fever. Piglets may be premature or stillborn, or may become ill at 1 day to 3 weeks of age, with wasting and dyspnoea the major signs (11). Acutely ill piglets may have a high fever (40 to 42°C or 104 to 107°F).

In sheep although a syndrome of fever, dyspnoea, generalized tremor, abortions and stillbirths can occur the common finding is of abortion and neonatal deaths only. Abortion occurs during the last 3 to 4 weeks of pregnancy. Full term lambs from infected ewes may be born dead or alive but weak, with death occurring within 3 to 4 days of birth. Lambs affected after birth show fever and dyspnoea but a fatal outcome is uncommon (12). Foetal resorption can occur in ewes infected in early pregnancy but the significance of this is uncertain.

An association between high blood titres for toxoplasma and uveitis has been reported in horses (20).

Clinical Pathology

Serological tests are commonly used to determine the presence of toxoplasmosis but the results are apt to be equivocal. A complement-fixation test is adequate but a positive titre develops only late in the disease. The Sabin-Feldman dye test becomes positive at an earlier stage but is of limited value in the acute stages when titres are minimal. In these circumstances two tests are required, with the first one taken early to maximize any rise in titre (13). Titres of 1 in 256 or greater in the SF test are taken to indicate a recently acquired or activated

infection (14). An intradermal test using toxoplasmin or a similar antigen is usually considered to be of little value in animals but has shown efficiency in pigs provided they were not in the early stages of the disease (15). A positive reaction is an appreciable skin thickening 24 hours after injection.

In ovine abortion the complement-fixation test has been found to be of little value but reciprocal dye test titres have been uniformly high in natural and experimental cases (16). Immunofluorescence shows promise as a diagnostic aid (1, 17).

Necropsy Findings

Multiple, proliferative and necrotic granulomas are characteristic of toxoplasmosis and in cattle the lesions may undergo calcification. The lesions occur most commonly in the nervous system and lungs. When there is visceral involvement, pneumonitis, hydrothorax, ascites, lymphadenitis, intestinal ulceration and necrotic foci in the liver are common findings. Necrotic lesions may also be present in the spleen and kidneys. In sheep but not in the other species, there may be involvement of the uterine wall, the placenta and the foetus. The lesions in the foetal lambs are usually limited to focal necrotic lesions in brain, liver and lungs. Similar lesions are present in the foetal membranes (18).

On histological examination, granulomatous, necrotic lesions can be found in the viscera and in the brain. Toxoplasma can be found in the cells of most organs, particularly the lungs and brain. Material for transmission experiments should include brain and lung if there is evidence of visceral involvement. Intracerebral and intraperitoneal injection of aseptically collected material into mice is accepted as a suitable diagnostic procedure (1). Brain or diaphragm tissue is used as the donor material, with the highest recovery rate coming from the latter. A positive diagnosis depends upon the presence of toxoplasma cysts in the brains of the mice 8 weeks after the injection. Correlation between the Sabin-Feldman test and cultural examination in mice is good in the diagnosis of the disease in sheep.

Diagnosis

The reciprocal dye test and complement-fixation tests are the only satisfactory method of diagnosing toxoplasmosis in the living animal. Histological examination of tissues, particularly lung and brain, can also be used as a basis for diagnosis. Toxoplasmosis is clinically such a protean disease that it is likely to go unsuspected until detected by an observant pathologist. It should be considered particularly when there is a high incidence of un-identified abortions and stillbirths in sheep. The differential diagnosis of abortion in cattle is dealt with under brucellosis (p. 374), in sheep under brucellosis (p. 379), and in pigs under leptospirosis (p. 438). The causes of encephalitis in animals are listed under that heading (p. 212), and of pneumonitis under pneumonia (p. 168). Similar clinical syndromes of encephalopathy in newborn animals occur in vitamin A deficiency and as congenital defects after vaccination of pregnant dams with attenuated virus vaccines against hog cholera and bluetongue.

Treatment

Pyrimethamine (Daraprim) or sulphadiazine have limited value in treatment, curing less than 50 per cent of affected animals when used alone. Administration of both drugs together, however, is highly effective in mice and humans. Of the sulphonamides, the sulphapyrimidines (sulpha-dimidine, sulphamerazine and sulphadiazine) and sulphapyrazine are the most effective. Best results are obtained when they are combined with pyri-methamine. The drugs are effective against the proliferating parasites and not against the pseudo-cysts. SDDS (2-sulfamoyl-4,4'-diaminodiphenyl sulfon) has also been shown to completely prevent experimental infection in pigs. A dose rate of 5 mg. per kg. per day was necessary to achieve this (19).

Control

Because of lack of knowledge of the method of spread of toxoplasmosis, firm recommendations on methods for control cannot be made. Dams producing aborted or stillborn offspring should be considered as carriers and culled. Detection of in-fected animals by the complement-fixation or re-ciprocal dye tests may make it possible to lessen further the source of infection. Immediate contact appears to be necessary for spread of the disease and isolation of infected groups may also assist in controlling the disease. Because of the risk of trans-mission to humans, consideration should be given to the complete disposal of groups of animals in which the disease appears.

REVIEW LITERATURE

Siim, J. C. & Biering-Sorenson, U. (1963). *Advanc. vet. Sci.*, *8*, 335.

Anonymous (1969). *Wld Hlth Org. techn. Rep. Ser.*, No. 431, p. 31.

REFERENCES

(1) Munday, B. L. (1970). *The Epidemiology of Toxoplasmosis with Particular Reference to the Tasmanian Environment*, p. 95. Hobart, Tasmania, Australia: Department of Agriculture.

(2) Sheffield, H. G. & Melton, M. L. (1970). *Science, N.Y.*, *167*, 892.
(3) Hutchison, W. M. *et al.* (1971). *Trans. R. Soc. trop. Med. Hyg.*, *65*, 380.
(4) Frenkel, J. K. *et al.* (1970). *Science, N.Y.*, *167*, 893.
(5) Hartley, W. J. (1966). *N.Z. vet. J.*, *14*, 106.
(6) Wilson, S. G. *et al.* (1967). *Vet. Rec.*, *81*, 313.
(7) Jacobs, L. (1961). *N.Z. vet. J.*, *9*, 85.
(8) Folkers, C. (1964). *Vet. Rec.*, *76*, 747, 770.
(9) Work, K. *et al.* (1970). *Acta path. microbiol. scand.*, *78B*, 129.
(10) Werner, H. & Janischke, K. (1970). *Zbl. Bakt. ParasitKde*, *214*, 540.
(11) Harding, J. D. H. *et al.* (1961). *Vet. Rec.*, *73*, 3.
(12) Smith, I. D. (1962). *Aust. vet. J.*, *38*, 143.
(13) Cremers, F. X. M. M. (1969). *T. Diergeneesk.*, *94*, 695.
(14) Hartley, W. J. & Moyle, G. (1968). *Aust. vet. J.*, *44*, 105.
(15) Nobuto, K. *et al.* (1964). *Bull. Off. int. Épizoot.*, *61*, 437.
(16) Jacobs, L. *et al.* (1963). *Amer. J. vet. Res.*, *24*, 673.
(17) Archer, J. F. *et al.* (1971). *Vet. Rec.*, *88*, 206.
(18) Hartley, W. J. & Kater, J. C. (1963). *Res. vet. Sci.*, *4*, 326.
(19) Ohshima, S. *et al.* (1970). *Amer. J. trop. Med. Hyg.*, *19*, 422.

Dourine

Dourine is a contagious trypanosomiasis of horses transmitted by coitus and characterized clinically by inflammation of the external genitalia, cutaneous lesions and paralysis.

Incidence

Dourine is enzootic in Africa, Asia, south-eastern Europe, South America and a small area in the southern United States. It has been eradicated from Canada and the greater part of the U.S.A. and strict control measures have reduced the incidence to a low level in most parts of Europe. The mortality rate varies; in Europe it may be as high as 50 to 75 per cent but in other areas the milder form of the disease is much less fatal although many animals may have to be destroyed (1).

Aetiology

The causative protozoon, *Trypanosoma equiper-dum*, is incapable of surviving outside the host and dies quickly in cadavers. All equidae are susceptible but the disease is transmitted to ruminants only with great difficulty. At least one strain has been passaged in guinea pigs (3).

Transmission

Natural transmission occurs only by coitus but infection can be introduced artificially through other intact mucosae and the conjunctiva. The source of infection may be an infected male actively discharging trypanosomes from the urethra, or an uninfected male acting as a physical carrier after serving an infected mare. The trypanosomes in-habit the urethra and vagina but disappear periodically so that only a proportion of potentially infective matings result in infection. Invasion occurs through intact mucosa, no abrasion being necessary. Some animals may be clinically normal but act as carriers of the infection.

Pathogenesis

The trypanosomes multiply locally and produce an oedematous swelling. Subsequent systemic invasion occurs and localization in other tissues causes vascular injury and oedema, manifested clinically by subcutaneous oedema and paralysis.

Clinical Findings

The severity of the clinical syndrome varies depending either on the strain of the trypanosome or the general health of the horse population. The disease in Africa and North America is much more chronic than the disease in Europe (1, 2) and may persist for many years, often without clinical signs, although these may develop when the animals' resistance is lowered by other disease or malnutrition.

The incubation period varies between 1 and 4 weeks with much longer periods in occasional animals. In the stallion the initial signs are swelling and oedema of the penis, scrotum, prepuce and surrounding skin extending as far forward as the chest. Paraphimosis may occur and the inguinal lymph nodes are swollen. There is a moderate mucopurulent urethral discharge. In mares the oedema commences in the vulva and is accompanied by a profuse fluid discharge, hyperaemia and sometimes ulceration of the vaginal mucosa. The oedema spreads to the perineum, udder and abdominal floor.

Nervous signs appear at a variable time after genital involvement. Stiffness and weakness of the limbs are evident and inco-ordination develops. Marked atrophy of the hindquarters is common and in all animals there is loss of condition, in some to the point where extreme emaciation necessitates destruction.

In Europe the disease is more severe, genital tract involvement often being accompanied by sexual excitement and more severe swelling. Cutaneous urticaria-like plaques 2 to 5 cm. in diameter, develop on the body and neck and disappear within a few hours up to a few days. Succeeding crops of plaques may result in persistence of the cutaneous involvement for several weeks.

The course is variable. In Europe death occurs commonly and within a few weeks of the onset, but in the milder form of the disease the course may be as long as several years with recurrent mild attacks, or the disease may be subclinical, infected animals remaining spreaders of the disease for many years.

Clinical Pathology

The trypanosomes can be detected in oedema fluid and in the vaginal or urethral washings in the early stages of the disease. In the European disease the trypanosomes can also be found in the blood between the second and fifth weeks after infection. An efficient complement-fixation test is available and was the basis for a successful eradication programme in Canada (1).

Necropsy Findings

Emaciation, anaemia and subcutaneous oedema are always present and oedema of the genitalia may still be evident. There is softening of the spinal cord particularly in the lumbosacral area.

Diagnosis

The syndrome is diagnostic, no other disease having the clinical and epizootiological characteristics of dourine.

Treatment

Many trypanocidal drugs have been used in the treatment of dourine but results are variable, chronic cases in particular being unresponsive to treatment. Treatment should not be attempted if eradication is contemplated as many treated animals are likely to remain inapparent 'carriers' of the disease.

Control

In dourine-free countries an embargo should be placed on the importation of horses from countries where the disease is enzootic. In enzootic areas the disease can be eradicated on an area or herd basis by the application of the complement-fixation test. Positive reactors are disposed of and 2 negative tests not less than a month apart can be accepted as evidence that the disease is no longer present. The same measures can be applied when the disease occurs in a country for the first time.

REFERENCES

(1) Watson, E. A. (1920). *Dourine in Canada, 1904–1920. History, Research and Suppression*, Health of Animals Branch, the King's Printer, Ottawa.
(2) Parkin, B. S. (1948). *Onderstepoort J. vet. Sci., 23*, 41.
(3) Pavlov, P. & Christoforov, L. (1966). *Proc. 1st int. Congr. Parasit., Roma*, 1964, *1*, 323.

25

Diseases Caused by Helminth Parasites

INCIDENCE

IT is impossible to give an accurate estimate of the economic importance of parasitic disease because it varies so greatly between countries and between regions, depending both on climate and on the intensiveness of farming in the area. It is probably fair to say that the countries which have suffered most in the past have been those in which exploitative agriculture has been practised. In these countries periods of malnutrition are common and the effects of parasitic disease are exacerbated. The position seems to have changed, however, in the past 20 years in that the principal problem has moved to those areas of highly productive land on which large numbers of animals have been concentrated. As a result there has been a great increase in interest in the epizootiology of parasitic diseases, a rapidly expanding but relatively unexplored field of investigation, and in the control and treatment of parasitism.

AETIOLOGY

The incidence of parasitic diseases varies greatly between areas depending on the relative importance of many of the factors listed below. In most instances the importance of these individual factors is related to the level of agriculture in the area; nutritional deficiency, for example, achieves major importance in poorly developed countries where extensive grazing on native pastures is widely practised. Where agriculture is more intensive and land more productive pasture management tends to dominate other factors. Although a great deal of work has been, and is being, done on the bionomics of helminth larvae it is generally agreed that it is not yet possible to reliably predict the potential transmissibility of a particular parasite at a particular place and time. The micro- and macro-climate of the environment, the shade characters, volume and height of the pasture, the grazing habits and the immunological and nutritional status of the host, the presence of intermediate hosts and vectors and the numbers of infective larvae and eggs in the environment present a mesh-work of interacting variables which greatly confound even an understanding of epidemiological dynamics (1).

At our present state of knowledge of causes of parasitic disease it is difficult and even dangerous to lay down rigid rules for their control. For example, a programme for the control of haemonchosis in sheep in Australia may be ineffective in Scotland. For this reason a proper examination of the important predisposing factors in parasitic diseases should be carried out on a regional basis and recommended control measures should be similarly limited.

Nutrition

General nutritional status. It is a well established principle that poorly fed animals are more susceptible to the effects of internal parasites and are more inclined to carry heavy worm burdens because of their failure to throw off infestations quickly. However, optimum nutrition does not offer complete protection against overwhelming numbers of some kinds of worms. Thus in general terms trichostrongylosis achieves its greatest importance in sheep when nutrition is poor; on the other hand haemonchosis causes most losses when nutrition is excellent but environmental conditions are such that massive infestations occur. In calves both ostertagiosis and haemonchosis can be significant in either set of circumstances. Verminous pneumonia also is commonly thought of as a secondary disease which is likely to exacerbate the effects of poor nutrition and gastrointestinal helminthiasis, but it can be a major disease in its own right when fat calves on an excellent diet are exposed to large numbers of larvae. Although it has become fashionable, in terms of the above discussion, to categorize worms as primary or secondary, depending upon their ability to cause disease in the absence of nutritional or other stress, the concept is not a particularly valuable one because so many species can be primary or secondary depending on circumstances.

It has become evident that a number of factors, of which nutrition is only one, can have marked effects on the resistance of animals to helminths. Specific immunity, hypersensitivity (self-cure) which may or may not be accompanied by immunity, and age are some of these. It is often very difficult to separate the effects of these factors which may be acting in concert and it is particularly important to differentiate between resistance to the establishment of an infestation, such as occurs in an immune animal, and resistance to the effects of the established infestation, such as may occur in a well nourished animal (2).

Specific nutritional deficiencies. A dietary deficiency of a specific nutrient such as cobalt, copper, phosphorus or protein can lead to a reduction in the animal's resistance in much the same way as does general malnutrition. The anaemia, poor growth and condition associated with these deficiencies are generally accepted as predisposing to heavy worm burdens. There is an apparent contradiction to this in that *Haemonchus contortus* develops much better in sheep fed a cobalt supplement than in sheep on a cobalt-deficient diet. This and similar observations suggest that there may be some profit to be obtained from an examination of the dietary requirements of the helminths themselves.

Pasture Management

One of the important reasons for the increasing importance of parasitic diseases is the increase in productivity of pasture. By the introduction of new plants, new strains of existing plants, irrigation and improved fertilization, livestock are being maintained on smaller areas. As a result the faecal contamination of pasture is greater, the pasture is of greater length and bulk and provides more protection for eggs and larvae from sunlight and desiccation, and the manure of animals grazing the pasture is more fluid so that it spreads farther and the eggs or larvae are much more likely to develop than if they are imprisoned in a firm pat of manure. In most instances, the result is a greater rate of infestation in animals grazing improved pasture. However, in spite of these anticipated greater risks it is often found in practice that the helminthological status of animals actually improves on highly improved pastures. In these circumstances it is imperative to know the life cycles of the important worms in the area, the time intervals between infestation and egg laying, the ability of larvae to survive and their periods of survival, and all these under the pastoral conditions in question.

A heavy concentration of animals can also occur on extensive range, especially in bad seasons, when the only feed available is restricted to watercourses, around bores, wells and dugouts and in swampy areas. The opportunities for parasitic multiplication in such circumstances can be as great as on irrigated pasture and there is usually the added insult of malnutrition. Draining such areas, or fencing them to prevent access, may necessitate supplementary feeding but this may be more economic in the long run.

An important question in any pasture management programme is whether or not rotational grazing should be recommended, and if it is, what are the optimum periods for grazing and resting of the fields. From the standpoint of control of parasitic diseases it has been suggested that animals which are rotationally grazed may never assume a sufficiently large burden of worms to become immunized and may therefore be highly susceptible if the rotation programme breaks down and massive exposure occurs. It has also been suggested that if periods of grazing are very short, for example 7 days, livestock may be put back on to fields while they are still highly infective. In 'set-stocking' on the other hand animals may be overwhelmed by a rapid build-up of pastoral infestation especially if climatic conditions are favourable and the animals have gone on to the pasture with a moderately heavy worm burden. Although rotational grazing has been a very strong recommendation for parasite control in the past, sufficient information is now available to suggest that set-stocking may be a safer method in many circumstances (3). Because of the differences in profitability per acre which exist between these two systems, it is likely that a decision between them in a particular area may well be made on grounds other than purely parasitological ones. Two agronomic reasons for rotating pasture grazings are increased productivity of feed and preservation of some desirable plant species. If rotation is to be of much benefit the animals must be moved at intervals of no more than a week and moved to fields which have been rested for at least 3 and preferably 8 weeks. After such periods it is to be expected that the pastures will still be infective but at a reduced level. The bionomics of the parasites concerned and the managerial requirements in terms of how long pastures can be left ungrazed makes dependence on rotational grazing difficult as a control measure (4, 5). For complete elimination of infestation of pasture an interval of one year between grazings is necessary but is not usually practicable. Zero grazing with suitable hygiene provides the complete answer, especially if lambs are weaned early (16). Eventually it may be possible to create an artificial immunity by vaccination but this work is in its infancy and its applicability to all parasites is yet to be tested.

The problem of how animal droppings on pasture should be handled has some interesting aspects, especially in cattle and sheep (7). Dung pats, and presumably faecal balls, act as incubators by trapping heat but they also prevent migration of larvae unless their hard outer covering is softened by rain. Under relatively dry conditions and on short pasture where dung pats can act as reservoirs of larvae for up to 5 months in summer and 7 to 8 months in winter (8) it is probably advisable to break up dung pats frequently by the use of a chain harrow and expose the larvae to desiccation. When climatic conditions are warm and humid and skies overcast this procedure will probably facilitate contamination and infestation. Pasture harrowing to break up dung pats, or more importantly the introduction of appropriate dung beetles, can play an important role in worm control.

Some parasites of domestic animals are also able to survive in wild animals, and some may even be primary to them, so that when both groups have access to the one pasture cross-infestation can occur. The same applies to transfer of infestation from one domestic species to another. There is a great deal of confusion on this particular aspect of parasitic diseases and the degree of cross-infestation which actually occurs is uncertain. In many instances parasites of one species may be able to survive in another but not to the point of laying eggs or, if patency is achieved, the period of egg-laying is much reduced and the importance of the infestation, in terms of perpetuating itself in the environment is negligible. A great deal of work has been done on the zoological identification of parasitic species but little on the biological identification. The early phases of this work, such as has been carried out on *H. contortus* and *H. placei*, has been highly significant and further work in the same field will be watched with interest. It is probably time that the identification of helminths should be expanded to embrace physiological and biochemical behaviour as well as anatomical and immunological criteria. There are many examples of parasites which are classified in the same genus but which differ markedly in their metabolism.

Barn Management

Most parasitic diseases affect animals at pasture but animals kept indoors may be affected if management is inadequate. For example if faecal contami-nation of feed can occur when animals are fed on the floor or in very low troughs or are so over-crowded that defaecation into raised troughs occurs frequently, infestations can develop. If insufficient bedding is provided the entry of hookworm larvae through the skin is facilitated, and the coats of animals may be so contaminated with infective larvae of other worms that normal licking may result in infestation.

Inadequate nutrition is a constant hazard in animals housed for long periods. Young animals are most susceptible to parasitic infestation and if, when they are turned out to pasture, they are in poor condition because of poor feeding the stage is set for a serious outbreak. In the same way animals coming off pasture in good condition but carrying a heavy burden of worms may suddenly succumb to the effects of the worms when their diet is restricted during the stabling period. Some of these animals may have low faecal egg counts because their infestation, on entry into the barn, is restrained at the larval stage. Subsequently the larval population matures en masse for reasons which are not understood.

Because of the possibility of cross-infestation between animal species and the untoward results of infestation by a worm of an unnatural host, housing of different animal species in the one pen or sub-stitution of a different species without proper cleaning of the pen is not recommended. For example, cattle may suffer a massive pulmonary invasion by *Ascaris suum* if penned on pig litter containing infective eggs.

Climate

The most congenial surroundings for the great majority of helminth parasites are provided by warmth and wetness and larvae can survive in large numbers on pasture under suitable conditions for as long as 6 to 8 weeks. However, few species are able to withstand desiccation and high temperatures. On the other hand larvae appear to be relatively resistant to cold and many of them, particularly *Ostertagia* and *Nematodirus* spp. can survive in large numbers through a Canadian winter (9). However, in less extreme conditions the winter period may be an important factor in the maintenance of parasitic disease. Factors which are detrimental to larval survival may, if applied in lesser degree, prolong the rate of development. For example a mild winter instead of killing heavy infestations of larvae on pasture may so delay their development that when sheep are turned on to the pasture in the spring they are immediately exposed to a gross infestation (10). Another effect of climate is to vary the severity of infestations from year to year. Thus in areas with a severe winter and dry summer the parasite burden of the local livestock may be light in most years, but in those years when the winter is mild and the summer is wet the normally light burdens are rapidly multiplied so that severe outbreaks of parasitic diseases occur.

Insect vectors are important in some helminthic diseases, especially those caused by members of the order Filarioidea. The population of these vectors is dependent largely on climatic conditions and the incidence of the diseases is similarly subject to the vagaries of the climate. The same variations are implicit in those diseases in which snails, beetles and earthworms act as intermediate hosts.

Immunity

It is not easy to generalize on this aspect of parasitic diseases because immunity has been examined with reference to so few. In those species on which work has been carried out, particularly *Dictyocaulus viviparus*, *H. contortus* and *A. lumbricoides*, it is evident that immune antibodies are produced by the host against larval stages of the worm provided the larvae are alive and reach the histotrophic stages of development; in *H. contortus* the fourth- and fifth-stage larvae. Moreover the antibodies are effective particularly against these stages of larval development. Thus when infestation occurs the larvae are able to establish themselves and mature to the point where they are susceptible to the antibodies. They may of course cause some damage during this period.

The antigens responsible for the immune reaction are in the exsheathing fluid produced when the larvae moult. Immunity to nematodes appears to be specific, at least at the generic level. Thus sheep immune to *H. contortus* infestation are fully susceptible to *Trichostrongylus* spp. There are some serological cross reactions between nematodes but the antigens responsible for the production of these antibodies are apparently not the antigens which produce the preventive immune reactions.

Helminthic immunity is often less efficient and more transient than the immunity to unicellular organisms. In a highly immune animal infective larvae become established but are killed as they mature. In a partially immune animal the development of the larvae is inhibited but they are not killed so that, if the immunity wanes sufficiently, the larvae can resume their interrupted growth. It also seems likely that a degree of immunity is responsible for the maintenance of large numbers of larvae in an undeveloped stage in the presence of a developed worm population, and in the maturation of these inhibited larvae when the adults are removed. Another accepted feature of parasitic diseases is that the young are much more susceptible than adults but whether the increased resistance of older animals is due to age or to immunity because of prior infestation is seldom clear. At least in trichostrongylosis immunity due to prior exposure appears to be the effective factor. On the other hand resistance to infestation with *Nematodirus* spp. is specifically an age resistance, sheep over 6 months of age being resistant to the effects of the infestation whether they have been exposed previously or not.

Another important feature of the immune response is the occurrence of the post-parturient rise in egg production in sheep 6 to 8 weeks after lambing. It is probable that the increase in worm burden which occurs at this time is due to a temporary waning of the immunity in the ewe at the time of parturition. This phenomenon appears to be of very great importance in the epidemiology of parasitic gastroenteritis. It provides a very large number of worms in an environment inhabited by highly susceptible lactating ewes, which have temporarily lost their resistance, and highly susceptible young lambs who have not yet had time to develop theirs (11). A related phenomenon is the restriction by the immune response of the number of eggs laid by mature worms. Thus the faecal egg count in an immune animal may be a grossly inefficient measure of the actual worm burden.

Hypersensitivity to helminths also occurs, the two commonest manifestations being 'fog fever'—the allergic response of a sensitized animal to a massive pulmonary invasion by lungworm larvae—and the 'self-cure' phenomenon in parasitic gastroenteritis in sheep. In the latter there is a sudden evacuation of a heavy, adult, parasite load apparently because of a local hypersensitivity reaction in the stomach and intestine provoked by a second larval infestation. The larvae themselves are not necessarily affected and may reach maturity, sometimes in sufficient numbers to be fatal. Animals which evidence this phenomenon are not necessarily immune subsequently and the greatest practical importance of 'self-cure', other than a temporary remission, is in the misleading effect it may have on the assessment of control programmes.

The practical aspects of parasitic immunity are pertinent to the question of a planned immunity. The two obvious channels by which such immunity could be produced are by vaccination with antigenic material derived from helminths, or by animal husbandry manoeuvres by which the animals are exposed to planned larval infestations on pasture, the latter practice being fraught with obvious dangers. Vaccination, apart from vaccination against *D. viviparus*, is still not a practicable procedure and because of the many difficulties involved is unlikely to be so in the immediate future.

The question is often raised of the possibility of removing the stimulus to immunity, and hence the immunity, by over-zealous use of anthelminthics. At least with respect to *T. colubriformis* this seems unlikely unless the sheep are drenched at intervals of one week or less (12).

The development of immunity also has some relationship to the serological diagnosis of helminthiasis. Some serological techniques are in use, particularly in those diseases in which helminths invade tissues, but no reaction has been shown to detect protective antibody so that determination of a state of protective immunity is not presently possible. There is also a great deal of cross-reaction between many antigen–antibody systems, and serological reactions decline in titre quickly unless there is further stimulation (13).

THE HOST PARASITE ECOSYSTEM

Examination of worm populations in hosts with respect to numbers and maturation has been related to a study of immunity. But many aberrations were observed which were not accountable in terms of antibody levels. A number of factors have been identified. For example, a massive dose of larvae may not set up an infection whereas a smaller one may; comparable doses have different effects at different seasons; a change in abomasal pH will determine viability of a worm population (14, 15, 16). Also a population of *H. contortus* in the abomasum will significantly affect, via its effect on abomasal pH, the number and maturation of *Nematodirus* sp. in the intestine of sheep (17).

PRINCIPLES OF CONTROL OF PARASITIC DISEASES

'The fundamental ecological concepts of helminthic parasitism in general and especially of grazing animals are that every animal is infected and that contamination of the environment is continuous. The epizootiological factors which explain why outbreaks of helminthosis are not more numerous and more severe are the destruction of free-living stages and the development of resistance and immunity by the host' (18). This concept of helminthiasis includes two principles which are nowadays accepted as axioms; first there is sufficient potential

in most grazing animals to permit of the development of a major outbreak of helminthosis whenever the correct circumstances are provided; secondly, the appearance of clinical helminthosis indicates that proportionate losses due to subclinical levels of infestation are also occurring in the same group. Although the following principles of control are aimed at preventing both forms of loss it is necessary to remember that the objective of a parasite control programme must be the achievement of a maximum economic gain and this may not be synonymous with total control of infection. The objective may be different with different classes of stock. For example in fat lambs any restraint on speed and degree of growth is expensive and worm elimination is desirable. However, in lambs that are going to be flock replacements, mild infestations, sufficient to stimulate resistance, are desirable (19). Maintaining these infestations at moderate levels, below the point at which they adversely affect future productivity is one of the challenges of preventive veterinary medicine. The principles of a control programme are:

1. *The unit is the herd or flock and its environment.* The presence of one clinically affected animal suggests the presence of other developing clinical cases in the group. Treatment and control measures must be directed at the group together with its pasture or housing.

2. *Nutritional status.* In general a good nutritional status and freedom from specific nutritional deficiencies increase the resistance of livestock to the effects of helminth parasites but are insufficient protection against more than a moderate infestation.

3. *Pasture management and rotational grazing.* It is possible by careful study of the bionomics of specific helminths to plan pasture management so that animals are raised virtually free of worms but the results obtained and the recommendations made may be very specific to the area in which the information originates. To attempt to transfer the recommended management programme to other areas, particularly where the climate is different, may be dangerous and actually further the development of a parasitosis. The concentration of animals, their state of nutrition and the suitability of climate and herbage cover to the survival of larvae all influence the choice of which method of control is best in particular circumstances. Although set-stocking must be potentially more dangerous it cannot be generally recommended that rotational grazing is the superior method of management. If rotation is practised the animals

should be moved from a pasture after no more than a week and on to a pasture that has been rested for at least 4 weeks. Pasture which is short in length, besides being poor nutritionally, encourages infestation because larval concentration will be at a maximum—the distance they have to travel is so much less and some roots and soil are also taken. On the other hand, very short, dry pasture encourages desiccation and destruction of larvae because of the removal of leaf cover. Animals on range pasture should be denied access to marshes, wet areas around troughs and where surface water collects. In circumstances of very high risk, e.g. where flood-irrigated pastures are heavily stocked with ewes and lambs, satisfactory control may be possible only by the continuous feeding of an efficient anthelminthic, or in some cases by the use of zero-grazing—maintaining the animals in a dry lot and cutting and carrying the pasture to them.

4. *Barn management.* The important recommendations for housed animals are to avoid overcrowding, remove manure frequently, provide plenty of bedding, have feed and water troughs high enough off the floor to avoid faecal contamination and, probably most important of all, maintain the plane of nutrition. The provision of adequate feeding space so that all animals have access to feed at the same time is essential to avoid a 'tail' of poorly nourished individuals.

5. *The utilization of immunity to helminths.* Vaccines against *Dictyocaulus* spp. are available. Stimulation of immunity by controlling pastoral exposure to natural infestation is too hazardous to attempt on a practical scale with existing knowledge. It is dangerous to bring even adult animals from areas where a particular parasitic disease does not occur and expose them to heavy infestations in areas where it does.

6. *Avoidance of interspecies transmission.* Existing knowledge of the transmission of helminths from one animal species to another suggests that although the running of sheep and cattle together or successively on the one pasture can be a successful control procedure, neither method can be relied upon to reduce the degree of contamination of pasture. Incidentally, access to domestic pastures by wild fauna may lead to spread and multiplication of helminth parasites.

7. *Protection of young animals.* Control measures should be aimed primarily at protecting the most susceptible group—young animals up to 18 months of age which are exposed to infestation for the first time. Thus one of the major principles in the control of helminths is the regular treatment of breeding females, especially of ewes before or about the time of lambing to avoid the effect of the 'post-parturient rise' in worm egg production at 4 to 8 weeks after lambing. For the lamb the ewe is usually more important as a source of infection than is pasture contamination (20). Thus early weaning may be an important control measure in some circumstances, and lambing at different times of the year may reduce the importance of the ewe. For ewes the recommendation is to dose with an efficient anthelminthic 3 to 4 weeks after lambing and place them on a clean paddock. Returning ewes to their previous pasture is of no benefit. There is a known deficiency in this system. In many cases the 'post-parturient rise' is delayed rather than eliminated because the ewe remains in a susceptible state while lactating; she becomes reinfected quickly, and the net effect on the lambs can be negligible (21). Additional measures include frequent removal of manure from pens and the avoidance of running very young animals on fields previously grazed by yearlings particularly, but also by adults of any age group. On present knowledge such fields should not have been stocked for at least a year, an impractical requirement on many farms.

Although most work on the 'post-parturient rise' has been done on ewes, the phenomenon is not restricted to that species. It occurs in sows, at least with respect to *Oesophagostomum* spp. and *Hyostrongylus rubidus*. The rise begins 1 to 2 weeks before farrowing, peaks 6 weeks after that and ends abruptly when the pigs are weaned. The most satisfactory control measure to prevent infestation of the young pigs is confinement in concrete yards, and tri-weekly removal of dung (22).

8. *Control by protective treatments.* Protective dosing with anthelminthics has become an important part of most preventive programmes against clinical or subclinical parasitic disease. Two classes of treatment are usually programmed: strategic treatments carried out at the same time each year, or at the same stage in the management programme, with the specific purpose of eliminating known high risk periods; and tactical treatments which are added to the strategic programme, particularly in pastured animals, to abort outbreaks when abnormal climatic or nutritional conditions arise.

A good deal of controversy revolves around the question of how frequently and when strategic and tactical treatments need be applied. Much of the basis for the argument stems from the over-enthusiastic acceptance by farmers of the need for anthelmintics and the unnecessary expenditure which is often incurred. A moderate approach to the problem based upon a critical prediction of danger periods, usually results in an optimum use of preventive treatment programmes. Because there are such great differences between areas in the frequency and severity of danger periods, control programmes can also be expected to vary widely and still be optimum for the particular farm or area.

9. *Strategic treatments*. Strategic treatments are usually administered 2 to 4 times a year depending on the climate and management procedures. Because of the much greater susceptibility of young animals the most important strategic treatments are those planned to provide maximum protection until weaning and at weaning when the young animals suffer their greatest nutritional stress. The former can be accomplished in sheep by dosing of the ewes before lambing or preferably 3 to 4 weeks after lambing to eliminate the 'post-lambing rise'. In older animals the need for and the timing of strategic treatments depends upon the expected occurrence of periods of high pasture contamination by larvae or periods of nutritional stress (23). Treatments prior to the danger period are usually recommended and it may also be necessary to repeat them if the danger period is prolonged.

When animals are housed for part of the year, young animals are often exposed to a falling plane of nutrition when they leave the pasture and it is customary to provide a strategic treatment at this time.

10. *Tactical treatments*. Tactical treatments are provided on an ad hoc basis usually in periods of abnormally heavy rainfall and mild temperatures but also occasionally when nutrition is unusually poor or when animals from a worm-free environment, and thus lacking in acquired immunity, are introduced to a danger area. For proper use of tactical treatments the diagnosis of critical levels of infestation at which treatment is warranted becomes an important procedure. The emphasis has shifted in recent years from the need to prevent outbreaks to include the need to reduce losses caused by subclinical infestations. A number of methods have been used to monitor the parasite status of herds or areas (24); the principal ones are analysis of climate (25) and routine egg counts on faeces. If a bioclimatograph is available egg counts can be done when the graph indicates danger and if the counts are high prophylactic treatment can be carried out.

11. *The diagnosis of significant levels of infestation*. Many of the epidemiological studies of helminths have been directed to determining optimum conditions of climate and pasture for parasitic multiplication. Where suitable local data is available it is possible to predict the danger periods on climatic grounds and institute suitable treatment programmes. In the absence of this information there are other methods of assessing the helminth status of a group of animals. Visual appraisal of body weight and clinical evidence of parasitism is the time-honoured method but lacks sufficient definition for most situations. Assessment by faecal egg count has value if the counts are repeated a number of times and adequate numbers of animals are used as a sample, and if faecal cultures are used to determine the species of worms which are present. Egg counts have limitations as a measure of worm burden because they are so greatly influenced by the stage of maturity of the worms, the species present, the immune status and age of the host and the occurrence of the 'post-parturient rise,' but they do reflect significantly the contamination potential of the infestation (26). If prevention of loss is the aim the faecal egg count is the best indicator of the future worm status of the group, provided climatic and pastoral conditions are taken into account. The age of the group is important also. Yearling cattle are less susceptible than young calves. The older animals establish smaller worm burdens, stunting of worms occurs and there is a much lower worm egg output (27).

The total worm count, which has with modern methods become an accurate and simple field technique, is superior to a faecal egg count as a measure of the severity of an infestation but does not take into account whether or not the worms are in a highly contaminative phase. The method is often preempted by the unavailability of a sufficient number of guts for examination; there must be at least two. Because of the increasing availability of broad spectrum anthelminthics, there is an increasing tendency to avoid accurate diagnosis and to use the rate of body weight gain after dosing as a measure of the degree of parasitic infestation.

12. *Choice of treatments, dose rates and dose frequency*. Most naturally acquired helminth infestations are multiple, the incidence of individual species depending largely on the suitability of the climate and on the presence of suitable other primary and intermediate hosts. The emphasis on research into better anthelminthics has thus been directed towards the development of broad spectrum anthelminthics to avoid the use of mixtures.

Although recommendations on the choice of drugs for each helminth species are made in the sections which follow, it is not possible to lay down rigid rules on their order of preference. The range of parasites to be controlled may affect the selection, as may cost, the severity of the infestation and the physical status of the animals relative to possible toxic effects of the drug. In some circumstances, for example when large numbers of young, wild cattle are to be treated, the use of an injectable preparation may be essential.

To avoid injury to treated animals and to conserve costly drugs, the current tendency is to quote dose rates in terms of body weight and to adhere as strictly as possible to the recommendations. In an effort to standardize dose recommendations we have used the most favoured calibration of mg. per kg. body weight. The dose rates recommended in the text are based largely on published work but because of the large amount of high quality adaptive research carried out by the manufacturers their dose rates are more generally to be preferred.

Because a diagnosis of parasitic disease is a diagnosis of a herd or flock problem it is customary to treat all animals in the group to reduce environmental contamination to a minimum. An inescapable corollary to flock treatment is the immediate removal of the flock to pasture which has not been grazed for at least 4 and preferably 6 weeks. This action is further improved if the animals are kept in a holding yard or field overnight to avoid contamination of the new pasture by eggs which are already in transit through the alimentary tract.

It is necessary in many instances to repeat the treatment after several weeks to remove recently matured worms which were in an immature, and hence more resistant, stage at the time of the first treatment. The maturation which does occur need not be the result of reinfestation; it is known that the presence of an adult worm population can inhibit the development of a large number of larvae which mature rapidly when the mature worms are removed by treatment.

13. *Continuous or intermittent treatment.* In situations of very high risk, continuous or intermittent dosing at low levels calculated to inhibit egg production may be a suitable alternative to frequent repeated dosing at therapeutic levels. The method is used in the control of strongylosis in horses but has severe limitations for other species (see under haemonchosis, p. 642). In general it is satisfactory only for animals that are fed individually or at least in troughs in dry lots.

14. *Assessment of treatment response.* The efficiency of treatment used to be measured in terms of changes in egg counts or total worm burdens. It is becoming more common to accept mixed infections as the rule and assume a significant level of infection. It then becomes rational to assess the result of treatment in terms of liveweight gain improvement. Better still is the tendency to relate

the value of the weight gain to the cost of the treatment. The choice of anthelminthic is then related to the real objective (28).

15. *Causes of breakdown in control programmes.* Most of the principles laid down above, although they are implicit in any control programme, are applicable to the treatment of clinically affected animals. The need to treat such animals is usually an admission that the control programme has broken down. Breakdowns are usually due to (a) failure to move treated animals to an uncontaminated environment, (b) the use of an insufficient dose or incorrect anthelminthic, (c) failure to repeat treatment or repeating at overlong intervals in times of high risk, (d) failure to appreciate the relative resistance of the immature stages of most parasites, in some instances by virtue of their inaccessibility while migrating through tissue, (e) the introduction of non-immune sheep from a worm-free environment into a danger area, (f) failure to adequately protect young animals and (g) a very common inclination on the part of farmers to dose only that portion of the group which is not doing well or which is showing clinical signs of parasitic disease.

REVIEW LITERATURE

Gibson, T. E. (1969). Anthelminthics. *Veterinary Annual*, pp. 176–269. Bristol: Wright.
Michel, J. F. (1969). The epidemiology and control of some nematode infections of grazing animals. *Advanc. Parasit.*, 7, 211.

REFERENCES

(1) Levine, N. D. (1963). *Advanc. vet. Sci.*, 8, 215.
(2) Gordon, H. McL. (1960). *Proc. Aust. Soc. Anim. Prod.*, 3, 93.
(3) O'Sullivan, B. M. & Donald, A. D. (1970). *Parasitology*, 61, 301.
(4) Donald, A. D. (1968/69). *Vict. vet. Proc.*, 27, 34.
(5) Smeal, M. G. *et al.* (1969). *Aust. vet. J.*, 45, 554.
(6) Colglazier, M. L. *et al.* (1970). *Proc. helminth. Soc. Wash.*, 37, 230.
(7) Christie, M. G. (1963). *J. comp. Path.*, 73, 416.
(8) Durie, P. H. (1961). *Aust. J. agric. Res.*, 12, 1200.
(9) Smith, H. J. & Archibald, R. McG. (1965). *Canad. vet. J.*, 6, 257.
(10) Rose, J. H. (1965). *Vet. Rec.*, 77, 749.
(11) Heath, G. B. S. & Michel, J. F. (1969). *Vet. Rec.*, 85, 305.
(12) Gibson, T. E. *et al.* (1970). *Res. vet. Sci.*, 11, 138.
(13) Castelino, J. B. (1970). *Vet. Bull.*, 40, 751.
(14) Christie, M. G. (1970). *J. comp. Path.*, 80, 89.
(15) Anderson, N. *et al.* (1969). *Res. vet. Sci.*, 10, 18.
(16) Ross, J. G. *et al.* (1968). *Res. vet. Sci.*, 9, 314.
(17) Mapes, C. J. & Coop, R. L. (1970). *J. comp. Path.*, 80, 123.
(18) Gordon, H. McL. (1957). *Advanc. vet. Sci.*, 287.
(19) Southcott, W. H. (1971). *Aust. vet. J.*, 47, 170.
(20) Gibson, T. E. & Everett, G. (1971). *J. comp. Path.*, 81, 493.
(21) Arundel, J. H. & Ford, G. E. (1969). *Aust. vet. J.*, 45, 89.
(22) Connan, R. M. (1967). *Vet. Rec.*, 80, 424.
(23) Arundel, J. H. (1968/69). *Vict. vet. Proc.*, 27, 37.

(24) Ross, J. G. & Woodley, K. (1968). *Rec. agric. Res.*, Belfast, *17*, 23.
(25) Ollerenshaw, C. B. & Smith, L. P. (1969). *Adv. Parasit.*, *7*, 283.
(26) Michel, J. F. (1968). *Vet. Rec.*, *82*, 132.
(27) Smith, H. J. (1970). *Canad. J. comp. Med.*, *34*, 303.
(28) Cornwell, R. L. *et al.* (1971). *Vet. Rec.*, *89*, 659.

Hepatic Distomiasis

(*Hepatic Fascioliasis, Liver Rot, Fluke Disease*)

Hepatic distomiasis is caused by members of the genera *Fasciola, Fascioloides* and *Dicrocoelium*. With the first two genera acute or chronic hepatic insufficiency may result. Infectious necrotic hepatitis may develop as a result of infestation by any of the three genera and this is considered to represent the only pathogenic effect of flukes of the genus *Dicrocoelium*. The term hepatic fascioliasis is reserved for infestation with *Fasciola hepatica*.

Incidence

Hepatic fascioliasis is an important disease of ruminants in all countries where climatic conditions suitable for the proliferation of host snails prevail. Although many animals are infested without showing clinical signs the disease causes many deaths and much loss of condition. Control of host snails and prophylactic and therapeutic dosing of cattle and sheep are expensive undertakings and are themselves not without danger. Affected livers are rejected at meat inspection and add to the financial loss. Preliminary data on economic loss caused by fascioliasis in cattle indicates that productive efficiency is reduced by 8 per cent in mild infections and to over 20 per cent in severe ones (1). In sheep wool production can be reduced by 20 to 39 per cent by similar subfatal infections (2).

Morbidity and mortality rates vary widely but an infection rate of 90 per cent, as indicated by rejection of livers at meat inspection, is not unusual in areas where *F. hepatica* is endemic. Mortality rates depend very much on the efficiency of treatment and control measures but are generally low. Dramatic death losses occur with massive invasion of the liver, and with infectious necrotic hepatitis. Although the acute form of fascioliasis is restricted largely to sheep, it can occur in cattle. Human cases of hepatic fascioliasis occur not infrequently after the ingestion of marsh plants such as watercress.

Aetiology

F. hepatica is the most common and important liver fluke and has a cosmopolitan distribution. Although it may infest all domestic species, it is of economic importance only in sheep and cattle. A high incidence has also been reported in donkeys in the U.K. (3). The other animal species may provide a source of reinfection for domestic ruminants.

Ruminants of all ages are subject to hepatic fascioliasis but young sheep are most commonly affected with the acute form of the disease usually during the summer months, although the most serious losses are from the chronic form of the disease which usually appears in the late summer and early winter. However, in countries where winters are relatively mild the major outbreaks of acute fascioliasis and black disease of sheep may not appear until the winter months especially when animals congregate on small marshy areas to obtain green feed. Clinical fascioliasis does occur in cattle and losses may result but cattle are much less susceptible to the effects of the parasite and are used in preference to sheep to graze a known snail habitat (4).

Although hepatic fascioliasis is most commonly associated with low lying, swampy areas, land which carries many small streams or which has large areas of shallow surface water must also be considered dangerous. Areas subjected to frequent flood irrigation are also highly suitable for the development of fascioliasis and acute outbreaks may occur soon after irrigation is carried out. Infested snails tend to lie dormant in intervening dry periods but release large numbers of cercariae after each irrigation. No solid immunity appears to develop and individual flukes may live for years in the one host. Apparent recovery may occur but is usually due to improvement in nutrition and not to 'self-cure'.

F. gigantica is more common in Africa, India, where it occurs commonly in goats and buffalo, and southern U.S.A. and *Fascioloides magna* in North America and Europe. In Canada *F. magna* is widely distributed in elk, deer and moose and has caused isolated outbreaks of fascioliasis in cattle and sheep. Sheep and goats are particularly susceptible to infestation with *F. magna* especially when they share pasture with deer. The incidence of infestation in cattle may be very high but only in rare cases are these animals affected clinically. The position in the U.S.A. is obscure but it seems that *Fasciola hepatica*, *F. gigantica* and a hybrid of these and *F. magna* may all occur. *Dicrocoelium dendriticum* has a restricted distribution in North America but is widespread in Europe and Asia and in those countries is causally related to infectious necrotic hepatitis.

The spread of hepatic fascioliasis to new areas depends upon the spread of the host snail or of infested ruminants. The snails themselves may be infested and spread the disease without any movement of the host. Important host snails for *Fasciola hepatica* are *Lymnaea tomentosa* in Australia, *L. truncatula* in Great Britain and Europe, and *Galba bulimoides*, *G. b. techella* and others in the U.S.A. For *Fascioloides magna* they are *G. b. techella* and at least five other lymnaeid snails. Intermediate hosts for *D. dendriticum* in the U.S.A. are the land snail *Cionella lubrica* and the ant *Formica fusca*.

Life Cycle

All of the above parasites, with the exception of *Fascioloides magna* in cattle and in sheep, mature in the bile ducts of the host and their eggs pass down the bile ducts and are excreted with the faeces. The eggs may hatch miracidia which actively invade the host snails (*Fasciola* and *Fascioloides* spp.) or be eaten by the snails and hatch in their gut (*D. dendriticum*). In either instance sporocysts develop in the tissues of the snail. Suitable climatic and environmental conditions are required for the persistence and hatching of the eggs, viability of the miracidia and persistence of the snails. In general terms the life cycle is assisted at this point by warm, moist conditions and the presence of free surface water. The interaction between temperature and moisture makes possible all degrees of severity of infestation. For example metacercariae do not survive long on pasture in Australia and infections are usually due to recent contamination (5). This is in contrast to conditions in U.K. and Europe where massive levels of metacercariae can build up (4).

Similar conditions are necessary for the development of the next stage of the parasite, the free-swimming cercaria, which leaves the host snail, attaches itself to herbage, becomes encysted and may be ingested by the final host. Under severe winter conditions the cercariae do not survive. Housed animals are protected against the disease unless hay infested with cercariae is sufficiently moist to enable the cercariae to survive. Cercariae may survive in hay for as long as 17 months but are killed by ensiling the material for 3 months. In general terms and under average conditions, and provided suitable host snails are present, pasture becomes infective about 2 months after infested animals carrying mature flukes are grazed on it and such pasture can remain infective for up to 12 months after animals are removed from it. Those cercariae which reach the alimentary tract of a ruminant escape from their cysts, invade the intestinal wall and, in the case of *Fasciola* and *Fascioloides* spp., migrate through the peritoneal cavity to the liver. The migration is often misdirected and many ectopic flukes can be found in the lungs. *D.*

dendriticum migrates to the liver via the bile ducts. After invasion of the liver, the young fluke follows a definite pattern of free migration in the parenchyma before following a more localized migratory pattern prior to entering the bile duct (6). Young *Fasciola hepatica* migrate through the hepatic parenchyma for about 4 days before they reach the bile ducts. Here they remain fixed and commence laying eggs about 55 days after infestation. Adult sheep and cattle may remain as carriers of *F. hepatica* for many years because of the longevity of the individual mature flukes in bile ducts.

A special exception to this general life history is the passage of *D. dendriticum* through a snail and then through an ant before it is infective for sheep. *Fascioloides magna* also differs from this pattern in that it is essentially a parasite of elk and deer. In cattle these flukes encyst in the liver and do not reach the bile ducts to release eggs to the exterior, but they may cause serious impairment of hepatic function if the infestation is heavy and may migrate as far as the lungs. It is doubtful if this fluke ever matures in sheep but because it does not encyst but continues to migrate, it causes severe and often fatal damage to the liver.

Pathogenesis

Acute and chronic hepatic fascioliasis are caused by different stages of *Fasciola hepatica* in the liver. Acute hepatic fascioliasis is caused by the sudden invasion of the liver by masses of young flukes, sufficient parenchyma may be destroyed to cause acute hepatic insufficiency and to this may be added the effects of haemorrhage into the peritoneal cavity (7, 8, 9). Flukes are tissue feeders and besides devouring hepatic parenchyma also incidentally ingest large quantities of blood. Chronic hepatic fascioliasis develops slowly and is the result of the activities of mature flukes in the bile duct. It is a combination of cholangitis, biliary obstruction, destruction of hepatic tissue with resultant fibrosis and liberation of a haemolytic toxin by the fluke. *Fascioloides magna* infestations in cattle cause a syndrome similar to chronic hepatic fascioliasis, *F. gigantica* in cattle can cause severe anaemia and acute liver damage (10), and *F. magna* and *F. gigantica* in sheep (11) cause a syndrome similar to acute hepatic fascioliasis. *D. dendriticum* is of low pathogenicity.

As might be expected the number of metacercariae ingested governs to a large extent the way in which fascioliasis is manifested. For example, the prepatency period is much shorter with smaller numbers, with larger numbers hepatic fibrosis and damage retards migration (9). The number of meta-cercariae ingested at any one time is probably not the only factor which determines whether acute or chronic fascioliasis occurs, or whether the pathogenesis is related chiefly to hepatic parenchymal damage or to biliary tract obstruction. Previous exposure to infection appears to reduce bile duct populations and to inhibit migration (12). Cattle are more resistant to infection than sheep. This is partly innate, many first infection cercariae not persisting in the bovine liver, but also resistance after previous infection has been demonstrated in cattle (13).

Migration of the young *Fasciola hepatica*, and in some areas *D. dendriticum*, through hepatic tissue containing quiescent spores of *Clostridium novyi* may cause the development of infectious necrotic hepatitis in sheep and cattle. This migration has also been thought to stimulate the development of occasional cases of bacillary haemoglobinuria in cattle.

Clinical Findings

Acute fascioliasis in sheep is often a syndrome of death without other apparent clinical abnormality (14). If the disease is observed clinically in sheep it is manifested by dullness, weakness, lack of appetite, pallor and oedema of mucosae and conjunctivae, and pain when pressure is exerted over the area of the liver. Death occurs quickly, often in less than 48 hours, and may be accompanied by the passage of blood-stained discharges from the nostrils and anus. Outbreaks are most common and severe in young sheep and are of relatively short duration, most deaths occurring within a period of 2 to 3 weeks.

A subacute fascioliasis is also described in sheep (14, 15). The same clinical findings occur as in the acute disease but the course is longer, one to two weeks. Additional signs are loss of body weight and resentment on palpation of the anterior abdomen.

Chronic fascioliasis is much more prolonged and 'fluky' sheep lose weight, develop submandibular oedema (bottle-jaw) and pallor of the mucosae over a period of weeks. Diarrhoea and shedding of the wool are common occurrences. The course of the disease is often as long as 2 to 3 months in those which die; many survive but are emaciated for longer periods. Cattle also lose weight, especially when there is the added drain of lactation, milk production falls and anaemia and chronic diarrhoea develop. The latter sign is usually associated with concurrent nematodiasis.

The clinical findings in black disease (necrotic

hepatitis) and bacillary haemoglobinuria are described under those headings (pp. 332 and 334).

Clinical Pathology

In acute fascioliasis there is marked macrocytic anaemia, and eosinophilia, there are high SGOT levels and severe hypoalbuminaemia. There are no fluke eggs in the faeces. In the subacute disease the findings are the same but there are fluke eggs in the faeces. The bromsulfalein liver function test is significantly prolonged (8).

A diagnosis of chronic hepatic fascioliasis can be confirmed by the detection of large numbers of characteristic, operculated fluke eggs in the faeces. The eggs are thin-walled and stained yellow-brown by biliary pigments but are not suspended satisfactorily by all flotation solutions. Special sedimentation tests appear to be more accurate and counts of over about 2000 epg seem to be associated with probable mortalities. The presence of any eggs suggests that treatment may cause improvement (16). It is important to collect faecal samples in the middle of the day because there is a peak in egg production at that time. Operculated fluke eggs are also characteristic of paramphistomiasis but in this latter disease the eggs are somewhat larger, are not stained yellow, have a transparent shell, a much more distinct operculum and well defined embryonic cells. Anaemia is characteristic of fascioliasis and persists for many months in affected animals. Characteristically there is a rise in blood eosinophils and serum albumin and a slight fall in serum calcium and magnesium levels (17). Hyperimmunoglobulinaemia occurs but total proteins are normal. Liver function tests are not significantly affected (18). Intradermal sensitivity tests and laboratory tests using serum agglutination techniques are used in Europe in the diagnosis of the disease (19) but their efficiency is open to some doubt (20).

Necropsy Findings

Acute hepatic fascioliasis is characterized by a badly damaged, swollen liver. The capsule shows many small perforations and subcapsular haemorrhages and the parenchyma shows tracts of damaged tissue and is much more friable than normal. The immature flukes are often so small that they are not readily discernible. They are most easily demonstrated by slicing a piece of liver thinly and shaking in water permitting the flukes to settle to the bottom. The peritoneal cavity may contain an excess of blood stained serum (14).

Chronic hepatic fascioliasis is characterized by the presence of large, leaf-like flukes in grossly enlarged and thickened bile ducts which protrude above the surface of the liver. Calcification of the bile duct walls is a common finding in cattle but not in sheep. The hepatic parenchyma is extensively fibrosed and the hepatic lymph nodes are dark brown in colour. Anaemia, oedema and emaciation are attendant abnormalities.

One of the important facets of a necropsy examination is to estimate the duration of the infection from the length of the flukes. This may help locate the habitat of the snail and be an important factor in a control programme (21). In infestations with *D. dendriticum* the lesions are much less marked and comprise fibrosis of the parenchyma and thickening of the smaller bile ducts. The flukes are smaller and lanceolate in shape. In *Fascioloides magna* infestations in sheep the lesions are large, black tracts and in cattle the liver shows dark, black cysts up to 4 cm. in diameter and elevated slightly above the surface, and tracts of necrotic hepatic tissue in the parenchyma.

Diagnosis

In an area where liver flukes occur every case of chronic ill-health in sheep must be considered as a possible case of fascioliasis. To support the diagnosis there should be fluke eggs in the faeces and hepatic lesions characteristic of the disease in the liver at necropsy. However, the infestation may be incidental to or even secondary to another debilitating disease such as a nutritional deficiency of cobalt or copper, other internal parasitisms or such chronic infections as Johne's disease and it is relatively easy to mistake the diagnosis. In a flock where fluke is present probably every adult sheep will show the characteristic necropsy lesions and it is necessary to estimate the severity of the lesions to determine whether or not they could be the sole or main contributing factor to the ill-health or death of the animal. In cattle the common presence of fascioliasis and ostertagiasis has caused diagnostic problems, resolved in a general sense by the preponderance of anaemia in the former and diarrhoea in the latter (22).

Acute fascioliasis of sheep is most difficult to differentiate from infectious necrotic hepatitis because of the small lesions which may, in the latter disease, require histological examination for identification. In general, acute fluke disease occurs only in young animals whereas black disease is usually confined to animals in the 2- to 4-year age group. If vaccination against black disease has been carried out the disease can be rejected as a possible cause of mortality. The friable, badly damaged liver of acute fascioliasis and the presence of immature parasites are usually sufficient to differentiate the disease from other causes of acute, heavy mortality, especially haemonchosis, anthrax and enterotoxaemia. There are also characteristic necropsy findings which help to identify these latter diseases.

Treatment

Little work has been done on the treatment of hepatic distomiasis other than on that caused by *Fasciola hepatica* and the bulk of the following information refers specifically to that disease. The optimum treatment of hepatic fascioliasis must destroy the migrating immature flukes as well as the adult flukes fixed in the bile ducts. Relative lack of toxicity is also essential because of the already impaired efficiency of hepatic detoxicating mechanisms. There is no available drug which satisfies all criteria and there are at present insufficient data on which to base a strong recommendation for any particular treatment or method of administration.

Oral treatments. Carbon tetrachloride and hexachloroethane have been in use for many years but some new oral drugs show promise.

Carbon tetrachloride is used chiefly in sheep because of its cheapness but should not be used in cattle because of its toxicity. It is not effective against *D. dendriticum* and is generally ineffective against immature *Fasciola hepatica*. The recommended oral dose rate in sheep used to be 1 ml. per 18 kg. body weight diluted in mineral oil and repeated 4 weeks later. However, because of the inefficiency of this dose rate against immature flukes, it is now customary to use 1 ml. per 9 kg. body weight. No prior starvation or purgation is necessary. Carbon tetrachloride is not highly poisonous and mortalities are rare but a common recommendation is to dose a small portion of the flock 48 to 72 hours prior to completing drenching to avoid major losses such as sometimes occur with this drug. The difficulty with carbon tetrachloride is that outbreaks of poisoning are unpredictable except in instances where the drug is given to sheep with acute fascioliasis or black disease, and its toxicity is influenced by a number of nutritional and other factors.

Hexachloroethane given orally has been a longstanding treatment in cattle and is usually purchased as a prepared suspension. It is not as efficient in sheep as carbon tetrachloride. It is reputed to be effective against immature *F. hepatica* and against *D. dendriticum*. The dose rate is 220 mg. per kg. body weight but should be reduced or divided for emaciated animals. In spite of the relative efficiency of the drug against immature flukes repeated drenchings are probably advisable where fascioliasis is a problem. The milk of treated animals may be tainted for several days and although the drug is less toxic than carbon tetrachloride signs of poisoning do occur in animals fed heavily on concentrates or in animals with severe liver damage. Some deaths can be expected in debilitated animals.

Hilomid (a mixture of two brominated salicylanilids) at a dose rate of 30 mg. per kg. body weight (23), and Zanil or oxyclozanide (24) have low toxicity and high efficiency against mature flukes but the double dose rates required against immature flukes are lacking in safety. Oxyclozanide is usually administered at a dose rate of 10 mg. per kg. for bile duct infestations. For heavy cattle over 350 kg. a standard dose rate of 3·4 g. is recommended (25). Hexachlorophene is an efficient treatment for cattle and sheep but some difficulty exists with the preparation of a suitable formulation for oral dosing. Hetol, bithional, freon 112, rafóxanide also are effective fasciolicides in sheep (26, 16, 27, 28). Bithional is also effective against *F. gigantica* (29). Rafoxanide is an efficient treatment for cattle (30). Clioxonide is an effective treatment but its efficiency at 40 mg. per kg. by oral dosing depends on whether it goes into the rumen or into the abomasum (31). If it passes directly to the abomasum it is very inefficient against young flukes (32). Menichlopholan (33) has the same deficiency (34). Both drugs need to be given at double the usual rate if acute infestations with immature flukes are the problem.

Treatments administered by injection. Carbon tetrachloride given by intramuscular injection has proved to be 90 per cent effective in cattle (26). The recommended dose rate is 1 ml. per 9 kg. body weight with a maximum of 30 ml. and a maximum injection of 15 ml. at any one site. Subcutaneous injections produce too severe a reaction to be satisfactory and intramuscular injections, even though there is little clinical evidence of injury, produce extensive muscle necrosis. The injection should consist of carbon tetrachloride alone and should be given into the cervical muscles. Treated animals should not be sold for meat within 3 months of the injection (35). In milking cows very small quantities of the drug are excreted in the milk which may have an abnormal flavour and odour for several days. The method has the advantage that large numbers of wild cattle can be treated much more quickly than by drenching. Excellent results have also been recorded in lambs after the injection intramuscularly of 4 ml. of a 50 per cent

carbon tetrachloride–liquid paraffin mixture (36) and in pigs after the injection of 1 to 6 ml. of a 3:1 mixture of carbon tetrachloride and liquid paraffin (37). Subcutaneous injections of carbon tetrachloride and oil mixtures are not recommended for horses because of the severe necrosis they cause. Hexachlorophene is effective against mature flukes in cattle when given by subcutaneous injection but has had no extensive field trial. Severe local reactions are common after the injections. Dose rates are the same as for oral use. Nitroxynil, 10 mg. per kg. injected subcutaneously, is an effective and safe treatment for cattle (38) and sheep (39). When combined with hexachlorophene, a fasciolicide normally given by mouth, in an injection a significant additive effect is obtained (40).

One of the most active research fields in veterinary chemotherapy is the search for the perfect treatment for liver fluke. The important criteria are efficiency against immature fluke and low toxicity. All of the drugs currently used can deal with immature flukes but at dose rates which are too toxic and too expensive. This is especially so because the serious infestations with young fluke that require treatment are cases of acute fluke disease with serious hepatic damage. In prophylactic situations where the objective is to remove as many flukes as possible with minimum number of drenches the matter of toxicity is not quite so serious.

For subacute infections with treatment aimed at mature flukes, over 12 weeks of age, there is very little to choose between almost all of the drugs listed above. Although carbon tetrachloride is occasionally toxic it seems to be as safe as any drug available. For acute infections, and at some risk, the drugs recommended are hexachlorophene and Bayer 9015A (27). Carbon tetrachloride is specifically contraindicated.

Infections with *F. gigantica* in sheep and cattle are susceptible to treatment with carbon tetrachloride, hexachloroethane, hexachlorophene, oxyclozanide, nitroxynil, bilevon and Hilomid. The same limitations of efficiency apply as they do with the treatment of immature *F. hepatica* (42, 43, 44, 45).

Control

In general adult and well nourished animals are less susceptible to the effects of the disease and maintenance of a good plane of nutrition may help to reduce its severity. Disruption of the life cycle of the liver fluke, with the eventual aim of control or eradication, can be effected by a combined attack on the egg-laying adult flukes in the sheep and on the host snails in the pasture. However, because of the extreme 'efficiency' of this parasite and the way in which it takes advantage of environmental conditions to multiply enormously, careful study of its ecology is necessary to predict periods of danger and initiate strategic attacks on both snails and flukes. The most dangerous times are when wet seasons, which allow snail multiplication, are followed immediately by dry seasons which force sheep to graze on small, heavily infested areas. In temperate winter rainfall climates the period of maximum infestation is in spring but in summer rainfall areas the infestation period of pasture may occur during the winter months, thus necessitating a variation in the times at which control measures are carried out.

Forecasting liver fluke disease. Although there are general patterns of development of outbreaks of fascioliasis it has become increasingly evident that because the costs of fluke control and snail control are so great and because strategic operations may be completely swamped in a bad season, great emphasis must be placed on tactical manoeuvres. Work in the U.K. by Ollerenshaw (46) and Ross (47) has directed attention at forecasting the development of dangerous escalations of metacercarial infestations of pasture by analysis of weather records. This makes it possible to apply a molluscicide to the pasture at an appropriate time without actually checking the snail population (48). Only careful preparation of the predictive bioclimatographs can avoid errors in forecasting and obviate the need for the use of a molluscicide and a fasciolicide in the same situation (49). These matters should be taken into consideration when planning the general programmes set out below.

Fluke control. Because of the gross multiplication of the fluke population during the life cycle from egg to egg it is vital that all living flukes in the sheep or cattle be destroyed. For general use, carbon tetrachloride or hexachloroethane should be used as recommended above. In winter rainfall areas three treatments are given annually, one in midwinter and one in spring to prevent contamination of pasture and one in late autumn to reduce the clinical effects of the flukes already parasitizing the animal. Complete eradication is seldom achieved but the fluke population is kept to a minimum. Tactical dosing may also be necessary especially when seasonal conditions favour rapid snail multiplication or outbreaks of acute fascioliasis occur. Maximum doses of carbon tetrachloride (5 ml. for adults) are usually recommended in the latter instance, because of the greater efficiency of large doses against immature flukes, and immediate

vaccination against black disease should be considered in areas where the disease occurs. Repeated treatments at monthly intervals are advisable to kill immature flukes. A much heavier programme of drenching may be necessary in badly infested areas and has been recommended in Great Britain. In breeding flocks repeated heavy dosing could have deleterious effects on reproductive efficiency. The nil effect of nitroxynil observed in this matter (5) could be repeated with other drugs. Other possible hosts which frequent the same pasture should be treated or removed. Rabbits especially should be destroyed.

Snail control. Eradication of the host snails from the environment has been a major facet of fluke control for many years but this eradication may be extremely difficult, sometimes impossible, in lowlying, wet areas with a temperate climate. Multiplication of the snails is extremely rapid and incomplete eradication achieves only a temporary reduction in their population. Snail numbers increase mostly during the summer months and this contributes to the high incidence of fascioliasis in the autumn and early winter. Light outbreaks may occur during spring and early summer because of over-wintering of encysted cercariae and such outbreaks are not prevented by snail control.

Because of the poor practicability of snail control and its high cost the emphasis on it has decreased in recent years and its implementation is probably best restricted to farms which have a small localized area suitable for snail growth. These small areas are best neutralized in a permanent manner by drainage or being fenced off.

In larger areas where control of the snails is necessary it is usual to apply a molluscicide. The time of application of the molluscicide is governed by a number of factors. It is most effective during hot, wet weather when the snails are active but their numbers are small and, if copper sulphate is used, before the snail-breeding season because this compound does not kill snail eggs. Thus spring and early summer are best and the administration should be repeated 2 to 3 months later. Copper pentachlorphenate is effective against snail eggs and the restriction to the pre-breeding period does not apply.

Copper sulphate is an effective killing agent for snails but must be applied intensively. On marshy land where a large area is to be treated 9 kg. of finely ground copper sulphate (usually mixed with sand to facilitate distribution) are applied per acre. Similar amounts may be applied by spray, and sprays containing 0·5 per cent. copper sulphate applied at the rate of 137 gallons per acre have been recommended. Stagnant water may be effectively cleared by the addition of copper sulphate to make a solution of 1 in 100,000. However, suspended organic matter in such captive bodies of water renders the copper sulphate ineffective as a molluscicide. The concentration should be increased to 1 in 50,000 in these circumstances. Running water can be effectively treated but only after careful computation of the rate of flow. Edible fish in the treated water die and in some areas this may upset the natural balance of insects or interfere with the supply of human food. The application of copper salts to large areas of land is not without danger especially where chronic copper poisoning or hepatitis due to plant poisoning occur.

Copper pentachlorphenate has been found to be much more effective as a molluscicide than copper sulphate (51) when applied at the rate of 4·5 kg. per acre in a high volume spray (400 gallons per acre). It has the advantage of not being inactivated by organic matter. The nitrogenous fertilizer calcium cyanamide has been given a preliminary trial as a molluscicide and has significantly reduced the new infection rate (52). N-Tritylmorpholene (Frescon) is a very effective molluscicide which has been shown to reduce the new infection rate of sheep with fluke, after administration to the pasture (41). It is most effective in small, low density snail habitats. When it is used on large high snail density areas the infestation rate of lambs can be dangerously high (53). The application of any molluscicide is made more efficient if the area to be treated is surveyed and marked beforehand and a dye marker included in the material applied. Where irrigation is the principal hazard it may be possible to add the molluscicide to the water by means of a mechanical metering device such as is used in streams.

Because of the habits of snails in sheltering under foliage beside water a control measure of great importance is the cleaning of the banks of streams and water reservoirs. Herbage cleared from these areas should not be available to animals as it may be heavily infested with cercariae. Cattle are more inclined to graze in marshy areas than sheep and may serve as a means of carrying infection to sheep on the same pasture. Separation of cattle from sheep, especially during warm periods when infestation of snails is more likely, is particularly desirable. Many livestock owners do not appreciate that cattle can carry the parasite.

The implementation of control measures against D. dendriticum are complicated by the existence of two intermediate hosts, a land snail and an ant.

Infestation with *Fascioloides magna* can be avoided by keeping wild ruminants, particularly elk, and to a lesser extent deer, off the pasture.

REVIEW LITERATURE
Brunsdon, R. V. (1967). *N.Z. vet. J.*, *15*, 9.
Boray, J. C. (1969). Experimental fascioliasis in Australia. *Advanc. Parasit.*, *7*, 95.

REFERENCES
(1) Ross, J. G. (1970). *Brit. vet. J.*, *126*, xiii.
(2) Roseby, F. B. (1970). *Aust. vet. J.*, *46*, 361.
(3) Pankhurst, J. W. (1963). *Vet. Rec.*, *75*, 434.
(4) Ross, J. G. & Todd, J. R. (1968). *Vet. Rec.*, *82*, 695.
(5) Boray, J. C. (1969). *Aust. vet. J.*, *45*, 549.
(6) Dow, C. *et al.* (1968). *Parasitology*, *58*, 129.
(7) Ross, J. G. *et al.* (1966). *J. comp. Path.*, *76*, 67.
(8) Roberts, H. E. (1968). *Brit. vet. J.*, *124*, 433.
(9) Boray, J. C. (1967). *Ann. trop. Med. Parasit.*, *61*, 439.
(10) Bitakaramire, P. K. & Bwangamoi, O. (1970). *Bull. epizoot. Dis. Afr.*, *18*, 149.
(11) Alibasoglu, M. & Guralp, N. (1969). *Vet. Fak. Derg. Ankara Üniv.*, *16*, 110.
(12) Ross, J. G. (1967). *J. Helminth.*, *41*, 217, 223.
(13) Doyle, J. J. (1971). *Res. vet. Sci.*, *12*, 527.
(14) Ross, J. G. *et al.* (1967). *Vet. Rec.*, *80*, 543.
(15) Reid, J. F. S. *et al.* (1970). *Vet. Rec.*, *86*, 242.
(16) Happich, F. A. & Boray, J. C. (1969). *Aust. vet. J.*, *45*, 326, 329.
(17) Ross, J. G. (1967). *Vet. Rec.*, *80*, 214.
(18) Simesen, M. *et al.* (1968). *Nord. Vet.-Med.*, *20*, 638, 651.
(19) Babenskas, M. (1967). *Proc. 18th World vet. Congr.*, Paris, *1*, 131.
(20) Blancou, J. *et al.* (1971). *Rev. Élev. Méd. vét. Pays trop.*, *24*, 373.
(21) Ross, J. G. (1968). *Irish vet. J.*, *22*, 62.
(22) Reid, J. F. S. *et al.* (1967). *Vet. Rec.*, *80*, 371.
(23) Boray, J. C. *et al.* (1965). *Vet. Rec.*, *77*, 175; *79*, 358.
(24) Froyd, G. (1968). *Brit. vet. J.*, *124*, 116.
(25) Froyd, G. (1969). *Vet. Rec.*, *85*, 705.
(26) Horak, I. C. (1965). *J. S. Afr. vet. med. Ass.*, *36*, 561.
(27) Boray, J. C. *et al.* (1967). *Vet. Rec.*, *80*, 218.
(28) Campbell, N. J. & Hotson, I. K. (1971). *Aust. vet. J.*, *47*, 5.
(29) Guralp, N. & Ozcan, C. (1966). *Brit. vet. J.*, *122*, 450.
(30) Knapp, S. E. & Presidente, P. J. A. (1971). *Amer. J. vet. Res.*, *32*, 1289.
(31) Pearson, I. G. *et al.* (1970). *Aust. vet. J.*, *46*, 480.
(32) Boray, J. C. & Roseby, F. B. (1969). *Aust. vet. J.*, *45*, 363.
(33) Lane, P. J. & Stewart, J. M. (1967). *Vet. Rec.*, *80*, 702.
(34) Boray, J. C. *et al.* (1969). *Aust. vet. J.*, *45*, 94.
(35) Boray, J. C. (1965). *Aust. vet. J.*, *41*, 291, 295.
(36) Downey, N. E. (1962). *Vet. Rec.*, *74*, 453.
(37) Winterhalter, M. & Delak, M. (1956). *Vet. Arh.*, *26*, 225.
(38) Colegrave, A. J. (1968). *Vet. Rec.*, *82*, 343, 373.
(39) Reid, J. S. F. *et al.* (1970). *Vet. Rec.*, *86*, 41.
(40) Kendall, S. B. & Parfitt, J. W. (1971). *Brit. vet. J.*, *127*, 149.
(41) Crossland, N. O. *et al.* (1969). *Vet. Rec.*, *84*, 182.
(42) Mathur, P. B. & Dutt, S. C. (1970). *Ind. J. Sci. Ind. B (Anim. Sci.)*, *4*, 1, 11.
(43) Berger, J. (1971). *Bull. epizoot. Dis. Afr.*, *19*, 37.
(44) Hildebrandt, J. (1968). *Vet. Rec.*, *82*, 699.
(45) Roy, R. M. & Reddy, N. R. (1969). *Vet. Rec.*, *85*, 85.
(46) Ollerenshaw, C. B. & Smith, L. P. (1969). *Advanc. Parasit.*, *7*, 283.
(47) Ross, J. G. (1970). *Vet. Rec.*, *87*, 278, 370.
(48) Ross, J. G. (1970). *Brit. vet. J.*, *126*, 401.

(49) Urquhart, G. M. *et al.* (1970). *Vet. Rec.*, *86*, 338.
(50) Lucas, J. M. S. (1970). *Brit. vet. J.*, *126*, 487.
(51) Gordon, H. McL. *et al.* (1959). *Aust. vet. J.*, *35*, 465.
(52) Ross, J. G. (1970). *Vet. Rec.*, *87*, 373.
(53) Ross, J. G. *et al.* (1970). *Brit. vet. J.*, *126*, 283.

Paramphistomiasis

(*Stomach Fluke Disease, Intestinal Amphistomiasis*)

The intestinal phase of amphistomiasis is a common parasitic disease of cattle, and to a lesser extent sheep, caused by paramphistome flukes and characterized by a severe enteritis.

Incidence

As a serious disease intestinal amphistomiasis has been recorded in cattle in the U.S.A., Australia and India, in sheep in the U.S.A., South Africa, New Zealand and India and in goats in India. Cattle are most commonly affected and the mortality rate in groups of heavily infested animals may be as high as 96 per cent (1). The mortality rate in sheep has been as high as 90 per cent. Acute mortalities appear to be the only manifestation of the disease.

Aetiology

Paramphistomum cervi, *P. microbothrioides*, *P. liorchis*, *P. ichikawai*, *Calicophoron calicophorum*, *Ceylonocotyle streptocoelium*, *Calicophoron ijimai*, and *Cotylophoron cotylophorum* are the commonly recorded species in sheep and cattle. Most outbreaks occur during the late summer, autumn and early winter when pastures have become heavily contaminated with encysted cercariae.

All ages of cattle, sheep, goats and wild ruminants may be affected but young cattle in the yearling class are the usual subjects. It is probable that some degree of immunity develops; this is suggested by the uncommon occurrence of the disease in adults.

Life Cycle

All of these flukes have as intermediate hosts aquatic planorbid snails which require deep water for proliferation. They are thus quite different in their distribution to the lymnaeid snails with corresponding differences in the incidence of hepatic and stomach flukes. The immature flukes settle in the duodenum and as they mature migrate through the abomasum to the rumen and reticulum. The period required for maturation varies from 6 weeks to 4 months and the factors which cause this variation have not been determined (2, 7).

Pathogenesis

Clinical illness is produced only when there are enormous numbers of the immature flukes in the duodenum and abomasum, the migrating flukes setting up an acute enteritis. Mature flukes in the forestomachs appear to cause little harm.

Clinical Findings

With an infestation by immature fluke a persistent foetid diarrhoea is characteristic and is accompanied by weakness, depression, dehydration and anorexia. There may also be submaxillary oedema and obvious pallor of the mucosae. Death usually occurs 15 to 20 days after the first signs appear.

A syndrome has also been ascribed to heavy infestations with adult flukes (8). The disease is chronic and signs include loss of weight, anaemia, rough dry coat and a drop in production.

Clinical Pathology

The characteristic fluke eggs which identify the presence of the flukes in the alimentary tract are usually not detectable in the faeces of clinically affected animals although they may be detectable in older animals in the same herd. A sedimentation method is preferred to detect the presence of eggs and it may be advisable to use a sedimentation and decanting technique to find immature flukes which have been passed. The latter is in fact a more common basis for diagnosis than identification of the eggs. The larvae are characterized by their round shape and the presence of anterior and posterior suckers. The eggs have a distinct operculum, the shell is thin and colourless and the embryonic cells are clearly outlined. There is a knob at the posterior pole. There is a marked drop in total plasma protein, due largely to a fall in plasma albumin (6).

Necropsy Findings

There is muscular atrophy, subcutaneous oedema and accumulations of fluid in the body cavities, and the fat depots are gelatinous. In the upper part of the duodenum the mucosa is thickened, covered with blood-stained mucus and there are patches of haemorrhage under the serosa. Large numbers of small, flesh-coloured flukes (3 to 4 mm. long and 1 to 2 mm. wide) are present in this area but decrease in number towards the ileum. There may be none in the abomasum and forestomachs. There may be a few in the peritoneal cavity and on histological examination the young flukes are present not only on the mucosal surface but are also embedded in the mucosa and deeper layers (6).

Diagnosis

Intestinal amphistomiasis may be easily missed because, although intestinal parasitism is often suspected in animals of this age group, immature flukes, which usually cause clinical illness, will not be laying eggs and even at necropsy the small parasites may be missed. The occurrence in yearling cattle of a severe enteritis, unaccompanied by fever, in environmental conditions suitable for the propagation of flukes and where host snails can be found should arouse suspicion of the disease. A nutritional deficiency of copper and infestation with liver flukes or intestinal round worms are the diseases with which it is most likely to be confused. The infectious enteritides, including the viral and bacterial infections, are usually accompanied by fever and other diagnostic signs. Johne's disease in adult animals is a much more chronic disease. Poisonings, including many weeds, inorganic arsenic and lead, can only be differentiated by their detection in the environment and in tissues at necropsy.

Treatment

Carbon tetrachloride and hexachloroethane, as used in the treatment of hepatic fascioliasis, appear to give good results against adult flukes in the forestomachs but variable, and generally poor, results against immature flukes in the duodenum. Freon is ineffective and hexachlorophene and methyridine (Promintic) are only moderately effective after a single dose but multiple doses give almost complete elimination. Bayer 2353 (Yomesan or Lintex) at 50 mg. per kg. body weight is highly effective against paramphistomes in the abomasum and intestine of sheep but ineffective against these parasites in the forestomachs and in cattle (3). Bithionol is highly effective in sheep at dose rates of 25 to 100 mg. per kg. body weight but is not recommended for cattle because it causes ataxia and abdominal pain at therapeutic levels (4). Niclosamide (90 mg. per kg.) and menichlopholan are also effective with the former preferred. Treatment with intestinal sedatives to control the enteritis and parenteral fluids to repair the dehydration are recommended. During an outbreak it is essential that affected animals be immediately removed from the pasture.

Control

Control measures are generally the same as those for hepatic fascioliasis and include periodic treatment against adult flukes with hexachloroethane and destruction of host snails by the use of molluscicides and drainage of low-lying areas. Small scale

experiments have shown that vaccination with irradiated larvae of *P. microbothrium* is an efficient procedure in sheep, goats and cattle (5).

REVIEW LITERATURE

Dinnik, J. A. (1964). *Bull. epizoot. Dis. Afr.*, *12*, 439.
Horak, I. G. (1971). *Advanc. Parasit.*, *9*, 33.

REFERENCES

(1) Butler, R. W. & Yeoman, G. H. (1962). *Vet. Rec.*, *74*, 227.
(2) Dinnik, J. A. & Dinnik, N. N. (1962). *Bull. epizoot. Dis. Afr.*, *10*, 27.
(3) Horak, I. G. (1964). *J. S. Afr. vet. med. Ass.*, *35*, 161.
(4) Horak, I. G. (1965). *J. S. Afr. vet. med. Ass.*, *36*, 361, 561.
(5) Horak, I. G. (1966). *J. S. Afr. vet. med. Ass.*, *37*, 428.
(6) Boray, J. C. et al. (1969). *Aust. vet. J.*, *45*, 133.
(7) Durie, P. H. (1953). *Aust. J. zool.*, *1*, 192.
(8) McFadden, G. M. (1968/69). *Vict. vet. Proc.*, *27*, 69.

Tapeworm Infestation

Tapeworm infestations have little apparent effect on the health of farm livestock but heavy infestations in young animals may cause failure to thrive. Disease caused by infestation with the intermediate stages of tapeworms is not dealt with because of its lack of applicability to clinical disease. Coenurosis is dealt with under diseases of the nervous system (p. 217).

Incidence

The common tapeworms have a cosmopolitan distribution and the incidence of the less common is indicated below. Occasional outbreaks in calves cause poor growth and some deaths and the disease has been produced experimentally in lambs.

Aetiology

Those tapeworms which have been recorded as occurring commonly in farm livestock are:

Ruminants—*Moniezia expansa*, *M. benedini* and *Thyanosoma actinioides* (*Taenia fimbriata*). Of lesser importance are infestations with *Avitellina* sp. (Mediterranean countries and India), *Stilesia globipunctata* (Europe and India) and *S. hepatica* (Africa), and *Thysaniezia* (*Helictometra*) *giardi* (Europe, Africa and America).

Horses—*Anaplocephala magna*, *A. perfoliata* and *Paranoplocephala mamillana*.

Although tapeworms may infest animals of any age they appear to have little if any deleterious effects on adults and heavy infestations are necessary to cause clinical illness in the young. The relationship between heavy tapeworm burdens and enterotoxaemia in lambs is described under the heading of that disease.

Life Cycle

The eggs of mature tapeworms pass in the faeces of the host to the exterior, either singly or protected by the tapeworm segment or in egg capsules or parauterine organs. At this time the eggs contain developed embryos. All of the above tapeworms require an intermediate host which ingests the eggs and in which the intermediate state is produced. Mature tapeworms develop only when the primary host ingests the intermediate stage either by eating the intermediate host or its infested organ. As far as is known the intermediate hosts of the worms under consideration are orobatid mites.

Pathogenesis

Tapeworms, according to their species, are either confined to the small intestine or invade its associated organs, the biliary and pancreatic ducts (*Thyanosoma actinioides* and *Stilesia hepatica*). In the former instance the mechanisms by which the worms affect the host are by competing for nutrients, by the excretion of toxic materials and, because of their length, by interfering with the motility of the gut. Blockage of pancreatic and biliary ducts appears to cause little harm and the most serious effect is the rejection of damaged livers at meat inspection. Some interference with the flow of digestive juices and with digestion is to be expected and very heavy infestations with *M. expansa* in lambs have been associated with outbreaks of enterotoxaemia (1). In horses *Anaplocephala perfoliata* causes inflammation and ulceration at its point of attachment to the mucosa. The faeces may be covered with blood-stained mucus and rupture of the caecum has been known to occur.

In general the gastrointestinal signs commonly attributed to tapeworm infestation occur in very young animals when the diet is inadequate and the infestation is gross (2).

Clinical Findings

The hallmarks of tapeworm infestation in ruminants are unthriftiness, poor coat, vague digestive disturbances including constipation, mild diarrhoea and dysentery and sometimes anaemia. These signs are restricted chiefly to animals less than 6 months of age, which may also show stunting and become pot bellied. In infestations with *Thyanosoma actinioides* signs may be delayed to a later age. Infested animals may be more susceptible to the effects of other internal parasites and to other diseases or adverse environmental conditions. In horses diarrhoea, emaciation and anaemia may be seen in heavily infested animals.

Clinical Pathology

Segments of the tapeworms may be visible macroscopically in the faeces. On microscopic examination of flotation specimens the thick walled, embryonated eggs may be present singly or in egg capsules.

Necropsy Findings

Most commonly tapeworms are present in the small intestine. The site of attachment may be indicated by the presence of an ulcer. Secondary, non-specific lesions include emaciation and anaemia. In the case of infestations with *Thyanosoma actinioides* and *Stilesia hepatica* the immature worms may be present in the biliary and pancreatic ducts and be accompanied by fibrosis and thickening of the duct walls.

Diagnosis

A diagnosis of tapeworm infestation as a cause of illness is made rarely except on necropsy because of the general view that the worms are of low pathogenicity. Young lambs up to 6 months of age and young horses are the only groups in which the diagnosis needs to be seriously entertained. Other causes of stunting and emaciation in these groups include many diseases but the two common ones are heavy infestations with nematodes and malnutrition. A positive diagnosis depends upon finding large numbers of eggs or proglottides in the faeces or large numbers of worms in the intestine at necropsy.

Treatment

In ruminants lead arsenate (0·5 g. for lambs, 1·0 g. for adult sheep, 0·5 to 1·5 g. for young cattle) is effective against all tapeworms and is often administered combined with phenothiazine to control other parasites. The toxic dose of lead arsenate for adult sheep is about 4 g. although debilitated animals may be more susceptible. A new lead compound, dibutyl lead diacetate, shows promise although it is toxic to unweaned lambs (7). A mixture of 40 per cent nicotine sulphate and copper sulphate as recommended for infestations with *Haemonchus contortus* is fairly effective, and dichlorophen (diphenthane, Dicestal) at a dose rate of 500 mg. per kg. body weight is highly efficient. Tin arsenate (200 mg. per animal) has also been used extensively in ruminants in recent years but care is needed to avoid serious toxic effects. Another effective taenicide is niclosamide (Yomesan, Lintex) which has proved to be highly effective against *Moniezia*, *Thysaniezia* and *Avitellina* spp., in lambs and calves

(3, 4). The recommended dose rate is 75 mg. per kg. body weight except for very young lambs which require 1 g. irrespective of their weight. Bithionol (200 mg. per kg. body weight) is effective against *T. actinioides* (5) in sheep but some diarrhoea and weight loss occur after its use. Bunamidine hydroxynaphthoate is highly effective against *M. expansa* in sheep at a dose rate of 25 mg. per kg. (6). There are no drugs effective against young tapeworms which have migrated to the biliary or pancreatic ducts. There is no highly effective treatment in horses; Bithionol acetate or dichlorophen should be effective.

Control

Control of the mites which act as intermediate hosts is impractical and in areas where infestation is sufficiently heavy to retard the growth of lambs periodic dosing, particularly during the summer and autumn, with one of the above taenicides may be necessary.

REVIEW LITERATURE

Euzeby, J. (1967). *Veterinary Medical Review* (Farben-fabriken Bayer A. G.), *2/3*, 169.

REFERENCES

(1) Thomas, P. L. *et al.* (1956). *N.Z. vet. J.*, *4*, 161.
(2) Rees, G. (1967). *Helminth. Abstr.*, *36*, 1.
(3) Hall, C. A. (1966). *Vet. med. Rev.*, Leverkusen, *1*, 59–66.
(4) Allen, R. W. *et al.* (1967). *Proc. helminth. Soc. Wash.*, *34*, 195.
(5) Allen, R. W. *et al.* (1962). *Amer. J. vet. Res.*, *23*, 236.
(6) Czipri, D. *et al.* (1968). *Vet. Rec.*, *82*, 505.
(7) Graber, M. & Gras, G. (1969). *Rev. Elev. Méd. vét. Pays trop.*, *22*, 85.

Ascariasis

Heavy infestations of the intestine with adult ascarid worms can cause digestive disturbances and poor growth in young animals and this is the major source of economic loss caused by the worm, but in individual animals more acute signs are caused by migration of the immature worms through the liver and lungs and occasionally other organs.

Incidence

Ascarids occur generally throughout the world but the occurrence of ascariasis is limited largely to farms on which the concentration of horses or pigs is high, where the animals run at pasture and on the same pasture year after year. The incidence may also be high in penned pigs when they are fed on the floor in pens which are seldom or never cleaned.

Aetiology

Each animal species has its specific ascarid, *Ascaris suum* in pigs, *Parascaris equorum* in horses and *Neoascaris vitulorum* in cattle. *Ascaris* spp. do not occur in sheep. *A. suum* of the pig has only minor anatomical differences from *A. lumbricoides* of man but each is host-specific and although cross-infestations occur the infestations do not mature. Infections of an atypical host can be produced experimentally (1) but there is no evidence that such cross-infections occur naturally in large animals other than with *A. suum*.

Life Cycle

The life cycles of all *Ascaris* spp. are very similar, with the possible exception of *N. vitulorum* in which infestation may occur in utero. The following details relate only to *A. suum* in pigs but it is probable that the same data apply generally to other ascarid species. The adult worms live in the small intestine and lay very large numbers of eggs. The larvae develop inside the eggs and no free-living larvae occur, the only mode of infestation being the ingestion of eggs containing these larvae. Because the eggs have very thick walls the infective stage is very resistant to deleterious environmental influences. They can be killed by phenolic disinfectants but this is obviously impractical on pastures. The eggs are very resistant to cold and survive most readily in cool, moist surroundings. Periods of survival of up to 5 years have been recorded. When the egg is passed it is not infective but under suitable environmental conditions, particularly high humidity (2), the ovum develops into a first and then a second stage larva which, after a period of several weeks, is infective. These infective eggs hatch quickly in the intestine of the new host and the larvae migrate through the intestinal wall, reach the portal vein and are transported to the liver, sometimes within 24 hours of being swallowed. They again enter blood vessels and pass to the lungs and some may pass through the lungs to other parts of the body although prenatal infestation does not appear to occur. Those which remain in the lung are passed up the bronchi and trachea to the pharynx, are swallowed and come to rest again in the intestine where they mature. Those which reach other organs may cause damage but do not re-enter the intestine. The total period required for re-entry into the intestine after infestation is 3 to 4 weeks and the worms are mature and commence laying eggs about 5 weeks later, or 8 to 9 weeks after infestation.

Details of the life cycle of *P. equorum* are sparse but eggs do not usually appear in the faeces until the foal is 12 to 13 weeks of age. In occasional foals eggs are present from as early as the 22nd day of life but these are thought to be due to the ingestion of uninfective eggs by the foal rather than to prenatal infestation. The peak of egg production is reached very quickly (about 16 to 18 weeks) and then declines gradually so that most foals cease to pass eggs after 6 months of age, due presumably to the development of immunity.

The adult worms are long (20 to 50 cm.), cylindrical, pointed at both ends and have a thick, glistening, yellow-white cuticle.

Pathogenesis

In the intestine the second stage larvae cause irritation to the mucosa, and mature worms, in addition, compete with the intestinal wall for metabolites. Migration of worms into the biliary ducts may cause biliary obstruction, cholangitis and jaundice in some cases. Occasionally the intestine may be completely obstructed by large masses of worms. During their migration through the liver the larvae cause necrotic and haemorrhagic tracts which heal by fibrosis, appearing as white spots under the capsule, or as diffuse fibrosis if the infestation is massive. In the lungs they provoke alveolar injury with oedema and consolidation; there is obstructive bronchiolitis in heavy infestations. Sensitization to antigens prepared from ascarids can be produced experimentally in pigs and a second administration 11 to 20 days after the first can cause fatal anaphylaxis. Immunity to migrating larvae is acquired and can be transferred through colostrum or immune serum (3).

In infestations by *A. suum* in animals other than pigs larval migration and development occur but adult worms are not recovered. During larval migration severe clinical signs of pulmonary involvement may appear. The disease has been produced experimentally in lambs (4) and calves (1, 5) and has also been observed as a field occurrence in yearling cattle (6, 7).

Clinical Findings

In all animal species only the young are seriously affected. In pigs up to 4 to 5 months old, the important clinical signs are poor growth and lowered resistance to other diseases. Enzootic pneumonia of pigs and swine influenza are reported to be much more serious diseases when accompanied by ascariasis and breaks in hog cholera vaccination with live virus are often attributed to this cause. There may be cough but this is not marked and there is seldom sufficient damage to the lungs to cause a noticeable increase in respiratory rate or

depth. In rare cases the infestation may be so severe that pigs manifest severe dyspnoea or die of acute hepatic insufficiency. Adult worms may be vomited up and occasional cases of obstructive jaundice and intestinal obstruction or rupture occur.

The effects in calves due to infestation with *N. vitulorum* and foals up to about 8 months of age with *P. equorum* are similar to those observed in young pigs and include poor coat, diarrhoea and occasionally colic. In addition, in foals, convulsions, intestinal obstruction and perforation may occur. In calves reduced weight gains, anaemia and steatorrhea are additional signs (8).

In older animals no clinical signs are observed but infested animals, particularly adult sows and yearling horses, continue to contaminate the surroundings and are an important link in the chain of infection. With infestation by *A. lumbricoides* (*suum*) in other species fever, dyspnoea and anorexia occur about the 8th day after infestation (4).

Clinical Pathology

Ascarid eggs are thick walled, the walls having a radially striated appearance and a pitted surface. The eggs are usually present in very large numbers in the faeces of clinically affected animals. A marked eosinophilia often accompanies the early stages of infestation in pigs and in other species, and in experimentally infested pigs there is an appreciable rise in serum transaminase levels, the peak being reached about the 2nd to 3rd day after infestation, presumably due to damage to the liver during larval migration. Egg counts in excess of 1000 epg are considered to be indicative of significant infections. Some attention has been given to serological examination for antibodies as a diagnostic tool but no practical techniques have transpired (9).

Necropsy Findings

Necropsy findings vary with the stage of development of the disease. In the early stages of a massive infestation the liver is enlarged and congested and there may be haemorrhages under the capsule. Microscopically, necrotic tracts and sections of larvae are observed. There are subpleural haemorrhages, and oedema and cyanosis of the lungs. The larvae are too small to be observed by the naked eye and should be looked for by microscopic examination of scrapings of bronchial mucus. The pleural cavity may contain blood-stained fluid.

In chronic cases the capsule of the liver is marked with white spots of small diameter which may, in severe cases, be confluent and constitute a network of connective tissue. Histologically the necrotic tracts have been replaced by fibrous tissue. The carcase is usually in poor condition and may be jaundiced. Large numbers of mature worms may almost fill the lumen of the small intestine. In species other than the pig infestation with *A. suum* is accompanied by congestion and haemorrhage in the lungs and necrotic tracts in the liver.

Diagnosis

In young pigs chronic cough and increased rate and depth of respiration are caused much more commonly by enzootic pneumonia and there are many other causes of debilitation including malnutrition and chronic enteritis due to infections with *Salmonella* spp. and *Vibro coli*. In young foals the chronic form of corynebacterial pneumonia may be mistaken for ascariasis but auscultation of the lungs reveals gross abnormality of the lung sounds. Ascariasis of calves must be differentiated from the many other causes of enteritis.

Treatment

A number of satisfactory treatments are available for horses and the choice depends upon cost, palatability to permit dosing via the feed, and the spectrum of susceptible parasites. A common aim is the provision of a single preparation which will be effective against ascarids, strongyles and botfly larvae.

Piperazine is the drug of choice against ascarids (10) in horses and is commonly combined with thiabendazole as a treatment for strongyles and ascarids (11) and with an organophosphate to combat botfly larvae.

Thiabendazole at the standard dose rate (44 mg. per kg. body weight) is highly efficient against strongyles but needs to be given at double the dose rate (80 to 100 mg. per kg. body weight) to be uniformly effective against ascarids. It is not efficient as a botfly larvacide but can be safely combined with carbon disulphide if this is desired. Pyrantel (12·5 mg. per kg.) is effective either by stomach tube or mixed in the feed (19).

All of the above treatments are effective against ascarids residing in the gut; there is no treatment which is effective against ascarid larvae migrating through tissues.

In pigs the piperazine salts (at 200 mg. per kg. body weight) are effective and economical. Sodium fluoride administered in the feed has several disadvantages but is cheap and efficient and is still used in many areas. Dichlorvos (12) and haloxon (13) are effective in pigs, as is parbendazole at a dose rate of 20 mg. per kg. mixed in the feed (14), and pyrantel tartrate at 22 mg. per kg. (15). Cambenda-

zole (at 0·01 and 0·03 per cent in the feed) gives complete protection against infection (16) and tetramisole at 15 mg. per kg. has the advantages of being well accepted in feed and having high efficiency against *Ascaris*, *Hyostrongylus*, *Metastrongylus* and *Oesophagostomum* spp. as well as *Ascaris suum* (17).

Control

The important features of the ascarid life cycle which must be taken into account when devising a control programme are that the worms are prolific egg-layers, the infective eggs are very long lived and resistant to damaging influences and young animals are most susceptible. Emphasis must be placed on avoiding exposure of young pigs and foals to infested adults and soil contaminated by them and by periodic treatment of the young animals. In pigs these principles are laid down in more detail in the 'McLean County System' of control of ascariasis. In this system the sow is washed with warm soap and water and placed in a farrowing pen which has been thoroughly cleaned with boiling lye solution (4 g. per 30 gallons water) 3 to 4 days before her due date. It is not imperative that the sow be treated with an ascaricide at this time but such a treatment should still further lessen the chances of infection of the piglets. If the litter and sow are turned out to pasture they must not walk over infested ground but be drawn in an enclosed vehicle and the pasture should preferably be one on which pigs have not previously been grazed or has been rested for at least 2 years. This exacting control of the young pigs must be maintained until they are at least 4 months old.

If the pigs are kept in houses and allowed access to small earthen yards, these must be kept well drained and the manure moved frequently to an area to which neither pigs nor cattle have access. The eggs do not become infective until about 4 weeks after deposition and deep burial of contaminated soil should prevent their maturation. With modern pig-raising methods of keeping pigs confined at all times in concrete pens the risk of ascarid infestation is very greatly reduced if normal hygienic precautions are maintained.

If the above methods are impracticable periodic dosing of young pigs with sodium fluoride or piperazine compounds is recommended. Piperazine salts are more effective against immature worms, cause no toxic effects and can be purchased already mixed in feed. The dose rate is approximately 200 mg. per kg. body weight. Ascarid infestations in pigs are kept to a low level if large quantities of skim or whey are fed. Continuous low-level feeding with cambendazole (16) or thiabendazole (18) of pigs from 3 weeks of age until marketing is an effective way of reducing worm burdens in fattening pigs.

Young foals present more of a problem especially as concurrent infestations with ascarids, strongyles and botfly larvae are not uncommon. The foals run with the mares which occasionally may act as a source of infestation, and they almost always run at pasture on which foals have run the previous year and which can become very heavily contaminated with eggs. Because of their curiosity the foals often nibble at foreign material, including faeces. Recommendations for control include thorough cleaning and disinfection of the maternity stall after each foaling, the use of small paddocks for exercise which have been rested from occupation by horses for a year if possible, and weekly removal of manure from the pasture. The foals should be routinely treated at about 10 to 12 weeks of age when the worms are first becoming mature and the treatment repeated bi-monthly. In this way heavy egg contamination of the pasture can be avoided. Carbon bisulphide (2·5 ml. per 100 lb. body weight) by nasal tube or in a capsule by mouth is effective but piperazine is more easily administered and is more effective against immature worms.

REFERENCES

(1) Kennedy, P. C. (1954). *Cornell Vet.*, *44*, 531.
(2) Enyenihi, U. K. (1969). *J. Helminth.*, *43*, 3.
(3) Kelley, G. W. & Nayak, D. P. (1965). *Cornell Vet.*, *55*, 607.
(4) Fitzgerald, P. R. (1962). *Amer. J. vet. Res.*, *23*, 731.
(5) Greenway, J. A. & McCraw, B. M. (1970). *Canad. J. comp. Med.*, *34*, 227, 247.
(6) Morrow, D. A. (1968). *J. Amer. vet. med. Ass.*, *153*, 184.
(7) McCraw, B. M. & Lautenslager, J. P. (1971). *Canad. vet. J.*, *12*, 87.
(8) Enyenihi, U. K. (1969). *Bull. epizoot. Dis. Afr.*, *17*, 171.
(9) Castelino, J. B. (1970). *Vet. Bull.*, *40*, 751.
(10) Round, M. C. (1968). *Brit. vet. J.*, *124*, 248.
(11) Taffs, L. F. (1968). *Vet. Rec.*, *83*, 219.
(12) Isenstein, R. S. & Todd, A. C. (1965). *J. Parasit.*, *51*, Suppl. 33.
(13) Czipri, D. A. (1970). *Vet. Rec.*, *86*, 306.
(14) Chang, J. (1969). *Amer. J. vet. Res.*, *30*, 77.
(15) Arakaua, A. *et al.* (1971). *Vet. Med.*, *66*, 108.
(16) Egerton, J. R. *et al.* (1970). *Res. vet. Sci.*, *11*, 590.
(17) Walley, J. K. (1967). *Vet. Rec.*, *81*, 617.
(18) Taffs, L. F. & Davidson, J. B. (1967). *Vet. Rec.*, *81*, 421.
(19) Cornwell, R. L. & Jones, R. M. (1968). *Vet. Rec.*, *82*, 586; *85*, 196.

Oxyuriasis

Infestation of the horse by the worm *Oxyuris equi* is not a serious disease, but its major manifestation, that of intense irritation of the perianal region, is annoying and may cause disfigurement of valuable animals. Affected horses rub and bite their tails, causing loss of hair at the base and sometimes physical damage to the tissues of the area. The mature worms are grey in colour and inhabit the caecum and colon. The male worm is about 1·2 cm. long, but the female is much longer, up to 15 cm., and has a long thread-like tail.

The life cycle is simple. Mature females migrate down the gut and crawl onto the perianal area where they lay their eggs in yellow patches of egg clusters. An embryo develops in the egg in about 3 days under favourable conditions and is then infective. Infestation occurs by ingestion of these eggs either by biting at the area or by feeding on contaminated material. The eggs resist desiccation, may be airborne in dust and remain viable in stables for long periods. Diagnosis is by detection of the operculated eggs, which may be flattened on one side, in scrapings from around the anus, or by the presence of worms in the faeces.

Treatment comprises the application of a mild disinfectant ointment to the perianal region and the administration of a piperazine compound (200 mg. per kg. body weight up to a maximum of 80 g.) or thiabendazole (44 mg. per kg. body weight), the latter being more effective. This treatment should be repeated in 3 weeks. Hygromycin B, as described under ascariasis, has high efficiency against whipworms.

Strongyloidosis

Infestations of farm animals with *Strongyloides* spp. are recorded from most countries and although their overall economic importance does not appear to be very great, individual outbreaks of severe intestinal strongyloidosis in sheep and calves are encountered. The effects in terms of profitability have been estimated in young cattle. When evaluated in living animals the loss was 15 per cent. At slaughter the loss was 25 per cent (1). The following species have been observed: *Sheep and cattle—Strongyloides papillosus*; *horse—S. westeri*; *pig—S. westeri, S. suis, S. ransomi*. All are parasites of the small intestine and the mature females lay thin-shelled, flat-sided eggs which contain embryos. The eggs may hatch in the intestine and free-living larvae be passed, but most eggs hatch externally. However, trans-colostral infection has been observed in pigs and pigs kept separate from their infected dams do not become affected (2). The larvae may be parasitic or non-parasitic and the latter forms may reproduce themselves several times before a parasitic generation is produced. It is the ability of the worm to live and reproduce free from the host which makes the disease so difficult to control. Parasitic larvae enter the body via the skin and entering capillaries are carried to the lungs where they migrate into the air passages, up the trachea and down the oesophagus to the intestine. They may also be ingested on infested feed. The minimum prepatent period in lambs and calves is 9 days (3). Some larvae are carried to unusual sites, particularly muscles, and prenatal infections may result (4). During their migration through the skin heavy infestations may cause dermatitis or balanoposthitis in the bull.

In young animals diarrhoea is the most common sign of heavy infestation. Experimental infestations in calves cause pallor and coughing (5) and in lambs dermatitis, pulmonary haemorrhage and enteritis occur (3). Pigs may show abdominal pain, vomiting, restlessness, anorexia and weight loss, but in many cases signs are restricted to unthriftiness (4). Sheep may also develop lameness or be more susceptible to footrot when subjected to heavy infestations. Methyridine, thiabendazole and tetramisole are effective in the treatment of this parasite in lambs. These preparations and Neguvon are also recommended for treatment of the disease in calves (4). For pigs trichlorophon injected subcutaneously is moderately effective (6) but thiabendazole in the feed is preferred. Some difficulty is experienced with pigs which have alternative food supplies and a failure of weight gain has occurred in these circumstances (7). Cambendazole is also effective in pigs (8). Thiabendazole is highly effective in foals. Control depends upon repeated treatment and elimination of the source of infestation. The larvae survive most readily in warm, moist surroundings and suitable pasture rotation, and keeping pens dry and clear of debris, may reduce the rate of infestation.

REFERENCES

(1) Restani, R. *et al.* (1971). *Vet. ital.*, *22*, 342.
(2) Supperer, R. & Pfeiffer, H. (1967). *Wien. tierärztl. Mschr.*, *54*, 101.
(3) Turner, J. H. *et al.* (1960). *Amer. J. vet. Res.*, *21*, 536.
(4) Stewart, T. B. *et al.* (1968). *Vet. Med.*, *63*, 1145.
(5) Eckert, J. & Abdel, A. F. (1963). *J. Parasit.*, *49*, 5, Sec. 2, 45.
(6) Leland, S. E. & Neal, F. C. (1966). *Amer. J. vet. Res.*, *27*, 280.
(7) Leland, S. E. *et al.* (1968). *Amer. J. vet. Res.*, *29*, 1235.
(8) Egerton, J. R. *et al.* (1970). *Res. vet. Sci.*, *11*, 590.
(9) Hiepe, T. *et al.* (1971). *Angew. Parasit.*, *12*, 65.

Rhabditis Dermatitis

Dermatitis caused by the larvae of the nematode *Rhabditis strongyloides* is rare and is recorded most commonly in the dog. Several outbreaks in cattle have been observed (1, 2). Alopecia is marked, particularly on the neck and flanks. In moderate cases the skin on affected areas is thickened, wrinkled and scurfy and some pustules are present on the ventral abdomen and udder. The pustules are up to 1 cm. in diameter and contain thick yellow caseous material, and larvae or mature worms. In severe cases affected areas are swollen, raw and exude serum, and there is marked irritation. Infestation is encouraged by housing animals on warm, wet bedding conducive to multiplication of the worm, and under highly favourable conditions the disease may spread rapidly (2). In these circumstances the lesions occur most commonly where the skin contacts the bedding.

Granulomatous lesions involving the maxillae, nasal bones and lymph nodes of a horse have been described (3).

The worm is a facultative parasite; that is, it can lead a free-living or parasitic existence, and usually lives free in the soil or in decaying organic matter. Only infrequently do the larvae invade the skin of an animal host. The nematodes are easily detected in skin scrapings or biopsy specimens, and in samples of the bedding, preferably taken from the top few inches in the pen.

Recommended control measures include frequent removal of manure from the sides of the body, frequent additions of bedding to avoid over heating and keeping the bedding dry. Spontaneous recovery usually occurs if these precautions are taken but local application of a parasiticide should be effective.

REFERENCES

(1) Levine, N. D. *et al.* (1950). *J. Amer. vet. med. Ass.*, *116*, 294.
(2) Rhode, E. A. *et al.* (1953). *N. Amer. Vet.*, *34*, 634.
(3) v.d. Linde-Sipman, J. S. & Gruys, E. (1970). *T. Diergeneesk.*, *95*, 242.

Trichuriasis

(*Whipworm Infestation*)

Trichuris spp. infestations in farm livestock are usually considered to be innocuous. They all inhabit the caecum of the host and if they are present in large numbers may cause sufficient irritation to result in diarrhoea, sometimes accompanied by the passage of mucus and blood. Experimentally produced trichuriasis in pigs causes much weight loss and the formation of nodules in the caecal wall. Naturally occurring cases in pigs and lambs are recorded (1, 2), the clinical signs including diarrhoea, anorexia, and weight loss. The mortality rate can be high in recently weaned pigs (3). A fatal case has been recorded in a heifer (4). The common species are: *Ruminants—Trichuris ovis*, *Tr. discolor*; *sheep—Tr. globulosa*; *pig—Tr. suis*, *Tr. trichiura*.

The life cycle is direct and eggs, which become embryonated, are very resistant to external environmental conditions and can survive for up to 6 years in pigs in old pigsties. Hatching occurs only after ingestion, infective eggs producing mature adults in about 7 weeks after ingestion in pigs and 12 to 20 weeks in lambs and goats. Diagnosis depends on detection in the faeces of the yellow oval eggs, which have a transparent plug at each end, and possibly adult worms which are 2 to 5 cm. long and shaped characteristically like a whip, the anterior third being much thinner than the handle-like posterior end. Egg counts in excess of 6000 epg are considered to be indicative of significant worm burdens.

In ruminants methyridine, organophosphates including trichlorphon, coumaphos, haloxon, laevamisole and parbendazole are effective but thiabendazole is reported to have a low efficiency (1).

In pigs effective treatments are parbendazole, 20 mg. per kg. in the feed (5) and organophosphates but a low efficiency is recorded for thiabendazole, tetramisole, pyrantel and piperazine (1). Dichlorvos has been shown to be an effective treatment in this species (6). If a control programme is necessary the one recommended for the control of ascariasis should be effective because of the similar difficulty encountered in destroying the infective eggs.

REFERENCES

(1) Beer, R. J. (1971). *Vet. Bull.*, *41*, 343.
(2) Farleigh, E. A. (1966). *Aust. vet. J.*, *12*, 462.
(3) Schoneweis, D. A. & Rapp, W. R. (1970). *Vet. Med.*, *65*, 63.
(4) Georgi, J. R. *et al.* (1972). *Cornell Vet.*, *62*, 58.
(5) Chang, J. & Westcott, R. B. (1969). *Amer. J. vet. Res.*, *30*, 77.
(6) Beer, R. J. *et al.* (1971). *Vet. Rec.*, *88*, 436.

Strongylosis of Horses

(Redworm Infestation)

Infestation with nematodes of the genera *Strongylus*, *Triodontophorus* and *Trichonema* commonly cause debility and anaemia in horses. Other less common lesions produced by *Strongylus vulgaris* include verminous aneurysm, rupture of the aorta and iliac thrombosis.

Incidence

Strongylosis appears to be common in horses all over the world and causes deaths when control measures are neglected. However, the greatest losses caused are probably the failure of young horses to grow properly and the inefficiency of working horses which are moderately parasitized.

It is only in relatively recent years that attention has been drawn to the association between performance in racehorses and their haemoglobin levels. There are a number of factors which may cause anaemia and although the importance of strongylosis compared to that of dietary deficiency and frequent racing for long periods has not been determined, it is generally accepted that strongylosis is probably the most important of these causes.

Aetiology

The common nematodes found in the large intestine of the horse are *Strongylus equinus*, *S. edentatus*, *S. vulgaris*, *Trichonema* spp. and *Triodontophorus tenuicollis*. The *Strongylus* spp. are larger (2 to 5 cm.) and are referred to generally as large strongyles. They are blood suckers and their grey colour is usually over-shadowed by the redness caused by blood in their alimentary tracts. *Trichonema* and *Triodontophorus* spp. are smaller (0·5 to 2·5 cm.), hence the general name small strongyles. They are less easily seen and because of their habit of feeding on intestinal contents rather than sucking blood they are normally white in colour. There are numbers of other small strongyles of limited importance including *Craterostomum*, *Oesophagodontus*, *Poteriostomum* and *Gyalocephalus* spp. In natural infections most strongylid genera are present in the one animal and the clinical picture presented here represents the net effect of such a mixed infestation.

Life Cycle

The life cycle is direct. Eggs are passed in the faeces of the host and, in a suitable environment, hatch to produce two non-parasitic larval stages, followed by an infective third stage in 5 to 7 days. As in other gastro intestinal helminthiasis the important factors governing hatching of the eggs and longevity of the larvae are shade, moisture and temperature. The larvae are relatively resistant, except to desiccation, and usually live for about 3 months but under optimum conditions may survive for over a year. Neither eggs nor larvae appear to be killed by freezing but their development ceases. Optimum chances for infestation of the host are in the early morning and evening and in warm, wet weather, conditions which encourage migration of the larvae onto forage plants.

The further development of the larvae of the different species and genera varies and may cause differences in the clinical signs observed. Infestation occurs only by the ingestion of the third stage larvae. The larvae of *S. equinus* migrate through the wall of the caecum and colon and produce nodules around themselves in the subserous tissues. Here they mature to fourth-stage larvae and migrate through the peritoneal cavity to the liver, then to the pancreas and back again to the caecum and colon as young adult worms. This migration and maturation stage takes about 5 months. There is some dissension about the route followed by *S. edentatus* but it appears to be similar to that of *S. equinus* except that the larvae reach the liver by the portal vessels and there develop into fourth-stage larvae.

The larvae of *Trichonema* spp. also enter the intestinal wall to form subserous nodules but migration across the peritoneal cavity to the liver does not occur. In about 3 months the larvae return to the lumen of the gut and mature there.

A number of differing routes have been described for the migration of *Strongylus vulgaris* larvae (1, 2). Although the question is still to an extent undecided it appears probable that *S. vulgaris* larvae migrate via the arterial wall rather than being transported in arterial blood to reach the aorta and intestinal arteries. Whichever route is followed adult *S. vulgaris* are not present in the large intestine until foals are about 6 months old.

Although young horses appear to be most susceptible, adults may carry very heavy loads of strongylid worms. They are often unaffected clinically but suffer a degree of anaemia sufficient to interfere with their racing performance, and neglected brood mares running at pasture may die of gross infestation. Infested adults provide the major source of infestation for young horses running with them. The average age of foals at which patent infections are present and eggs commence to appear in the faeces are as follows: *Trichonema* spp., 12 to 14 weeks; *Triodontophorus* spp., 16 to 26 weeks; *S. vulgaris*, 26 weeks; *S. edentatus*, 50 to 55 weeks.

Pathogenesis

The clinical signs caused by strongylosis are in two groups, those caused by the migrating larvae and those caused by the presence of adults in the intestine. The larvae of *Trichonema* spp., *S. equinus* and *Triodontophorus tenuicollis* may cause nodules and ulcers in the wall of the caecum and colon. The ulcers are usually of most significance when a blood vessel is eroded causing serious haemorrhage. The larvae of *S. edentatus* cause quite large haemorrhagic nodules under the peritoneum which may cause signs of colic and anaemia. *S. vulgaris* larvae cause more serious damage because of their localization in arteries, particularly the cranial mesenteric and its branches and to a lesser extent the

trunk of the aorta (3) and the iliac arteries; arteritis of the iliac arteries has long been considered to be due to strongylosis but there is some doubt that this is so. It is possible that portions of thrombi protruding into the abdominal aorta may break off and lodge in one or both iliac arteries. Less common sites for verminous arteritis are the renal, splenic, hepatic, cerebral and coronary arteries. Involvement of these vessels results in the development of aneurysms, occlusion, obstruction by thrombi and emboli and in some cases rupture of the vessel. In the cranial mesenteric site restriction of blood flow to the intestine and pressure on the nearby mesenteric plexus may cause recurrent colic; complete occlusion by thrombus and emboli may result in mesenteric vessel thrombosis and acute intestinal haemorrhage or in gangrene of a segment of intestine. Clinical descriptions of these disorders are included in the chapter on diseases of the alimentary tract.

The adults of the large strongylid worms are all heavy blood suckers and may cause bleeding ulcers, both factors contributing to anaemia. The tendency to ulceration is even more marked in infestations of *Tridontophorus tenuicollis* and such ulcers when they occur in the colon may lead to the development of splenic abscess. Heavy infestations with adult small strongyles are sometimes associated with profuse watery diarrhoea.

Clinical Findings

In foals weakness, poor coat and loss of condition parallel the development of anaemia. In severe cases scouring and subcutaneous oedema of the ventral abdominal wall may also occur. Acute haemorrhagic anaemia without apparent cause in adult horses may occur occasionally due to bleeding from an intestinal ulcer. In most cases the blood loss is so rapid that the animal dies before evidence of haemorrhage is present in the manure.

Adult mares in the last few weeks of pregnancy and carrying very heavy infestations may become very weak even to the point of recumbency. On clinical examination the mucosae are pale, the heart rapid and loud and respiration moderately increased. Intestinal sounds are increased to the point where enteritis may be suspected although the faeces are usually normal. Abortion may occur and a fatal outcome is to be expected.

The clinical syndromes caused by aneurysms of the mesenteric artery, aorta and iliac artery are described in detail elsewhere.

Clinical Pathology

Examination of the faeces for strongylid eggs does not permit accurate differentiation between the different strongylid genera, nor from *Trichostrongylus axei*. Larval cultures are essential for this purpose. An estimation of the degree of infestation can be made, however, by faecal examination because *T. axei* is a comparatively poor egg-layer and for practical purposes differentiation of the strongylid genera is not necessary. The levels of eggs per gramme (epg) of faeces which can be considered to be significant have not been accurately established although the usual classification in adult horses is: up to 500 epg probably not significant, 500 to 1000 epg moderate infestation, more than 1000 epg severe infestation. Horses with more than 1000 epg usually show improved performance after treatment. However, normal horses with normal blood counts may carry 2000 epg. It should be remembered also, that egg production is higher in the summer than in the winter.

Care must be taken in interpreting egg counts on the faeces of foals. Adult worms even of *Trichonema* spp., do not become established and commence egg laying until they are about 12 weeks old. Eggs present before this age have probably been swallowed by the foal when it has eaten its dam's droppings. These eggs are not infective and have no significance.

Estimations of haemoglobin levels, erythrocyte counts and packed cell volumes of the blood are often taken as an indication of the degree of infestation with strongyles but a number of other factors including dosing with phenothiazine, excitement, dietary deficiency, continued racing over long periods, toxic depression of bone marrow by infectious processes and a number of infectious diseases may also cause depression of these values. Appreciable differences have been noted by various authors between normal horses in different countries and between different breeds (e.g. Thoroughbreds and Standardbreds) but it can be assumed that any horse with a haemoglobin level of less than 12·0 g. per cent, an erythrocyte count of less than 8 million per cmm. or a packed cell volume of less than 35 per cent will profit by treatment for anaemia, which may include treatment for strongylosis (4).

Indirect tests are important in strongylosis when one is concerned with attempting to assess the burden of worms which have invaded tissue, rather than those present in the gut. The only estimation with significance in this respect is the measurement of serum proteins, a marked rise in beta-globulins and a marked fall in albumins being associated with heavy infestations (5). This measurement also provides a safer diagnostic tool than an egg count on faeces or a haemoglobin estimation in the early cases of infestation causing severe weight loss in previously unexposed horses. In these animals serious damage can be done before the worms are patent and accurate diagnosis is essential (6).

Necropsy Findings

Because most cases of strongylosis are caused by mixed infestations with all genera, necropsy findings usually include most of the lesions characteristic of each worm.

In cases dying of anaemia and enteritis, the basic disease in strongylosis, very large numbers of adult worms will be found in the caecum and colon: there may be so many that they appear to form a living cover to the contents of these organs. *Triodontophorus tenuicollis* are often found in large numbers in the right dorsal colon in association with small circular haemorrhages, and they are sometimes attached in groups to the base of deep mucosal ulcers.

There may be larvae in many subserous sites, especially in nodules in the intestinal wall, and the body cavities may contain an excess of blood-stained fluid. Verminous aneurysms of varying size are common at the root of the cranial mesenteric artery and occasionally in the iliac artery. The affected arterial wall is greatly thickened and contains loculi on its internal surface, many of which contain living larvae. Lamellated thrombi are also common at this site and these are sometimes infected. The thickening of the arterial wall often extends along the caecal and colic arteries and complete occlusion of these may be followed by gangrene of a segment of intestine. Similar lesions of arteritis may be present at the base of the aorta. Spontaneous rupture of the vessel may occur (7).

Diagnosis

Ascariasis is another common cause of poor growth and debility in foals but anaemia is not a prominent sign. A satisfactory differentiation can be made by examination of the droppings for eggs. A gross nutritional deficiency, or agalactia in the mare, may have the same effect but these causes are usually evident. Specific nutritional deficiencies in foals and adults are not commonly recorded as causes of anaemia and are unlikely in horses running at pasture but horses fed stored feeds in stables may require dietary supplementation with a mineral containing iron and copper. Of the infectious causes of anaemia, babesiasis and equine infectious anaemia are usually accompanied by other clinical signs of diagnostic significance.

Treatment

Thiabendazole (50 mg. per kg.) is highly efficient against both large and small strongyles and is the drug of choice for the treatment of strongylosis but not for ascariasis (8). Yearlings and older horses should be dosed with thiabendazole every 4 to 8 weeks. Foals from the 8th to 28th week after birth should be treated every 4 weeks with a mixture of thiabendazole and piperazine. The only disadvantage of the drug is its cost. If it is too expensive the second choice for treatment is a mixture of piperazine, phenothiazine and Neguvon. Piperazine or phenothiazine alone have too many limitations in efficiency to be popular as general equine anthelminthics and Neguvon alone is too toxic at recommended dose levels. Of the modern anthelminthics pyrantel tartrate (12·5 mg. per kg.) is effective in strongylosis, and also in ascariasis (9). Tetramisole (12·5 to 20 mg. per kg.) is highly effective against ascarids and *S. vulgaris* but less effective against *S. edentatus* and *Oxyuris equi* (10). Dichlorvos is a successful broad-spectrum anthelminthic for horses and is extensively used in the feed in the form of PVC granules.

A major clinical problem is the treatment of animals with verminous aneurism or parasitic arteritis, in which larvae are still likely to be migrating. Thiabendazole at 440 mg. per kg. by mouth on two successive days appears most effective (7, 11) compared with diethylcarbamazine, parbendazole, pyrantel and tetramisole.

Control

As in most parasitic infestations adequate control measures depend upon an accurate knowledge of the life cycle of the worms. Because of the heavy egg-laying capacity of adult strongyles, the heavy worm burdens carried by older animals, especially yearlings, and the longevity of the larvae on pasture, the control of strongylosis by management alone is impossible. Foals are the group which are most seriously affected and because of the universal practice of running them at pasture with their dams they are easily exposed to gross infestation.

Because of the impracticability of maintaining pastures used for horses free from strongyle larvae much attention has been given to reducing the strongyle population in horses on breeding farms by the daily administration of very small doses (1 to 2 g.) of phenothiazine. Although adult strongyles may persist in the gut in spite of such a regimen their egg-laying activities are markedly reduced and the eggs laid are of reduced fertility. A heavy infestation of strongyles may take several months to bring under control by this method and an initial treatment as above followed by low level administration continuously is preferred (12). No toxic effects appear even when horses are fed phenothiazine at this low level for years. There are no reports of the emergence of phenothiazine-resistant worms and the programme has been widely adopted. Phenothiazine-resistant strongyles have been encountered (13) but only on farms where phenothiazine was administered in full therapeutic doses and treatment with phenothiazine and piperazine was still effective. Best results are obtained by feeding the phenothiazine, preferably mixed with bone meal or a mineral supplement, intermittently for the first three weeks in every month. On breeding farms the mares are subjected to this regimen at all times and the foals from weaning onwards. The method appears to be effective against large and small strongyles but not against *T. axei*, *Habronema muscae* or *Oxyuris equi*.

The alternative is to treat all the horses (alternating thiabendazole with the phenothiazine, piperazine and Neguvon mixture) at strategic intervals. As a general rule three treatments a year are administered; in the spring, the autumn and winter although more intensive programmes of dosing 6 times a year at 2 monthly intervals are highly recommended (14). Mares are treated 6 to 8 weeks before foaling. The foals enter the routine dosing programme when they are 4 to 6 months old and are treated until that time for ascarids only.

REFERENCES

(1) Poynter, D. (1969). *Proc. 2nd int. Conf. equine infect. Dis.*, *Paris*, 1969, pp. 269–89.
(2) Enigk, K. (1969). *Proc. 2nd int. Conf. equine infect. Dis.*, *Paris*, 1969, pp. 259–68.
(3) Farrelly, B. T. (1954). *Vet. Rec.*, *66*, 53.
(4) Steel, J. D. & Whitlock, L. E. (1960). *Aust. vet. J.*, *36*, 136.
(5) Round, M. C. (1968). *Vet. Rec.*, *82*, 39.
(6) Round, M. C. (1971). *Equine vet.*, *3*, 31.
(7) Coffman, J. R. & Carlson, K. L. (1971). *J. Amer. vet. med. Ass.*, *158*, 1358.
(8) Round, M. C. (1968). *Brit. vet. J.*, *124*, 248.
(9) Cornwell, R. L. & Jones, R. M. (1968). *Vet. Rec.*, *82*, 586.
(10) Lyons, E. T. & Drudge, J. H. (1970). *Amer. J. vet. Res.*, *31*, 1477.
(11) Drudge, J. H. & Lyons, E. T. (1969). *Proc. 2nd int. Conf. equine infect. Dis.*, *Paris*, 1969, pp. 310–22.
(12) Todd, A. C. (1952). *Bull. Ky agric. Exp. Sta.*, No. 582.
(13) Drudge, J. H. *et al.* (1961). *J. Parasit.*, *47*, 4, Sec. 2, 38–9.
(14) Drudge, J. H. & Lyons, E. T. (1966). *J. Amer. vet. med. Ass.*, *148*, 378.

Lungworm Infestation in Cattle

(*Verminous Pneumonia*, *Verminous Bronchitis*)

Invasion of the lungs of cattle by *Dictyocaulus viviparus* results in the development of any one of several disease states including verminous pneumonia, acute atypical pneumonia and secondary bacterial pneumonia. All are serious diseases which must be differentiated from pneumonia caused by infectious agents because they do not respond satisfactorily to treatment and control measures used for pneumonias caused by bacteria or viruses. Lungworm infestations in pigs, sheep and horses are dealt with in a separate section (p. 626).

Incidence

Infestation of cattle with lungworm has a very wide distribution through temperate and cold areas and, depending on climatic conditions and season, can cause serious losses. Great Britain appears to be the country in which the disease reaches its greatest importance. The disease is often restricted to particular areas and to particular farms where it is likely to recur each autumn.

Aetiology

D. viviparus is the only lungworm of cattle. All lungworm species are host-specific and cross-infections to other hosts do not occur. For all practical purposes only animals grazing on pasture are exposed to the disease and although calves 4 to 10 months of age are most commonly affected, all ages are susceptible. For example under conditions of heavy exposure outbreaks in adults are not uncommon.

The most important factor governing the incidence of lungworm disease is climate, the highest incidence occurring in warm, wet summers. At these times distribution of faeces, pasture management and grazing behaviour also assume major importance; practices which in normal years are without danger may lead to rapid and serious spread of the infestation. Immunity to reinfestation with D. viviparus occurs after an initial infestation but is variable in degree and duration. In most animals a serviceable immunity persists for about 7 months. A highly effective vaccination procedure against this parasite is based on the known immunological data.

Life Cycle

The mature lungworms live in the bronchi and air passages and their eggs are coughed up and swallowed by the host. The eggs hatch in the air passages or alimentary canal and only larvae are passed in the faeces. The first-stage larvae of D. viviparus develop in the internal environment into second- and then third-stage infective larvae, provided conditions are suitable. The worm is a heavy egg producer and it has been estimated that a single

infested calf may contaminate a pasture with 33 million larvae. Moisture is essential for the survival and development of the larvae and a moderate temperature of 18 to 21 °C (65 to 70 °F) permits their full development to the infective state in 3 to 7 days. Under optimum conditions the larvae may survive in the pasture for over a year. They are quite resistant to cold although it greatly delays their maturation. They can withstand temperatures of 4·5 °C (40 °F) for a year. Observations in Canada indicate that they can overwinter on pasture in Ontario and Quebec although the principal source of infection in spring is carrier animals (1). For example in some parts of Great Britain a small percentage of larvae do survive the winter, but in Canada persistence of the parasite depends upon survival of some adult worms in carrier animals and possibly some larvae in barnyard manure. The ability of the larvae to survive best in cool damp surroundings, especially when the environment is stabilized by the presence of long herbage or free water is the reason for the build-up of lungworm infestation in the autumn months and the appearance of the clinical disease in late autumn and early winter.

The infective larvae are quite inactive and the mortality rate amongst them is high for this reason. Factors which encourage their spread on pasture, and thus their infectivity include soft fluid faeces, mechanical spreading and concentration of animals. Toadstools (Pilobolus spp.) have been shown to have a striking influence on larval distribution (2). The explosive discharge of the sporangia of these fungi can propel D. viviparus larvae inhabiting the same dung pat for distances up to 10 feet. Reticence is often desirable and it is probably good advice to keep one's mouth shut when examining dung pats.

The third-stage larvae must be ingested to infest the primary host. On entering the intestine they migrate through its wall and reach the mesenteric lymph nodes where they become fourth-stage larvae. From here they enter the lymphatics and pass eventually to the venous blood stream, through the heart and reach the lungs where they escape into the alveoli. Three to 6 weeks after infestation they have migrated up to the bronchi and are mature and laying eggs. Adult worms survive in the bronchi for about 7 weeks at which time immunity has developed and the 'self-cure' process causes death and discharge of a high proportion of the worms. The approximate timing of these phases in D. viviparus infestations in calves is: penetration phase (ingestion to arrival of larvae in lung), day 1 to day 7; prepatent phase (larvae in lung), day 7 to day 25; patent phase (mature worm in lung), day 25 to day 55; post-patent phase (lungworm disappearing from lung), day 55 to day 70 (3).

Pathogenesis

The migrating larvae cause little damage until they reach the lungs and all of the effects of the worms, except possibly for minor irritation of the intestinal mucosa during migration, are centred there. However, the response of the lung varies widely depending largely on the number of larvae which are ingested but also on the nutritional status and age of the host and whether or not it is being exposed for the first time. Studies on the ecology of *D. viviparus* have shown that those larvae which are picked up by a calf in the first 9 days of exposure have most effect on the course of the disease in the animal. Thus the infectivity of the pasture (the concentration of larvae that it carries) during this period largely determines whether disease develops and at what degree of severity. This is in contradistinction to the more general situation of gradual accumulation of worm load.

Although the severity of the clinical disease is not directly proportional to the number of larvae ingested it is generally accepted that there is an acute and a subacute syndrome depending on the degree of infestation. A massive invasion of the lungs of calves with a very large number of larvae causes an acute, general involvement of the parenchyma. Moderate infestations usually lead to the subacute form of the disease and with light infestations no clinical signs may be apparent.

In the acute form of the disease the reaction of pulmonary tissue to a massive invasion of larvae is initially one of areas of collapse throughout all lobes, oedema of the septa, interstitial emphysema and the accumulation of eosinophiles. This is followed by alveolar epithelialization, oedema and hyaline membrane formation. The lesions are widespread and irreversible and cause severe dyspnoea, cough and usually a fatal outcome. Frothy fluid containing many larvae is present in the air passages terminally but death usually occurs before adult worms are present.

In the chronic form of the disease the areas of collapse are widespread but initially are much fewer than in the acute disease. There is a more marked bronchiolar reaction and the bronchi are soon filled with mucus, pus and larvae. The collapsed portion of the lung becomes much more extensive, particularly in the diaphragmatic lobes, and although many adult worms may be present in the bronchi, the lesions persist for long periods after the worms

have died. Secondary bacterial bronchopneumonia is a common sequel.

It is evident that the presence of adult worms and exudate in the air passages contribute little to the severity of the acute form of the disease. Collapse of the alveoli, and in acute cases oedema, hyaline membrane formation and emphysema, are the major causes of the anoxic dyspnoea and death of the animals. It is notable that alveolar epithelialization, a major cause of collapse and consolidation in this disease, is most marked in the later stages and often reaches its greatest magnitude when no larvae or adult worms are present. It is also worthy of mention that treatments which kill the worms, especially adults, will not affect the lesions already present. If, as has been suggested, the epithelialization is a reaction to lungworm tissues this may explain the continued development of the lesion after the worms are dead (4).

Although it is common to find a combined infestation of lungworms and gastrointestinal helminths in which the latter appear to play the more important role, and although poorly nourished animals appear less able to throw off an infestation of lungworms, it is not unusual, provided the right environmental conditions exist, for severe lungworm infestations to be fatal to well fed calves. This refers not only to the hypersensitivity reaction in the lungs of cattle sensitized to lungworm tissues by previous infestation but also to primary infestations with large numbers of larvae as described above. That a hypersensitivity reaction, particularly in yearlings, can occur and cause acute atypical pneumonia seems highly probable. However, very many cases of atypical pneumonia can occur without lungworms being present and it must be considered to be a hypersensitivity caused by one of a number of sensitizing agents. Animals recovered from a natural infestation are partially immune for about 7 months but are also in a sensitized state which may result in atypical pneumonia as described above (5, 6). Larvae may invade the tissues of immune animals but appear to be destroyed in lymph vessels and mesenteric lymph nodes. This information on immunity to *D. viviparus* in calves has been utilized dramatically in the production of vaccines against parasites.

Clinical Findings

The disease in cattle is almost entirely confined to those running at pasture and occurs most frequently in young animals, particularly those in the 4- to 6-months age group but severe outbreaks of the acute form are occurring more commonly in adults. All degrees of severity are observed in calves but individual cases can usually be classified as acute or subacute.

Acute verminous pneumonia. The first sign in experimentally produced cases (7) is diarrhoea preceding the onset of respiratory signs but this is often not noticed in natural cases. There is a sudden onset of rapid shallow breathing which is largely abdominal in type and often reaches a rate of 100 per minute. There is a frequent bronchial cough, a slight nasal discharge and a high temperature of 40 to 41 °C (104 to 105 °F) The heart rate is increased to 100 to 120 per minute. On auscultation all parts of the lungs are involved approximately equally, the abnormalities including a markedly increased vesicular murmur and bronchial tones. The animal is bright and active and will attempt to eat although the severe respiratory distress often prevents this. Progress of the disease is rapid and within 24 hours dyspnoea may become very severe and be accompanied by mouth breathing, a violent respiratory heave and grunt, cyanosis and recumbency. Changes in the sounds heard on auscultation are also evident. Consolidation, evidenced by loud bronchial tones and absence of vesicular murmur, becomes more apparent, moist râles are heard over the bronchial tree and the crackling of interstitial emphysema commences over the dorsal two-thirds of the lung but is never as evident as in subacute cases. Fever persists until just before death, which usually occurs in 3 to 14 days and is greatly hastened by exercise or excitement. The mortality rate in this form of the disease is high, probably of the order of 75 to 80 per cent. As a rule a number of animals are affected at one time and the calves have often been moved onto the pasture 7 to 12 days previously.

Subacute verminous pneumonia. This is more common in calves than the acute form. The onset is usually sudden, there is evidence of recent scouring, the temperature is normal or slightly elevated and there is an increase in the rate (60 to 70 per minute) and depth of respiration. An expiratory grunt is heard in severe cases and expiration may be relatively prolonged. There are frequent paroxysms of coughing. The course of the disease is quite long, 3 to 4 weeks, and auscultation findings vary widely with the duration of the illness and the area of lung involved. In general, there is consolidation and bronchitis ventrally, and marked emphysema dorsally. Affected animals lose weight very quickly and although the mortality rate is much less than in the acute form, many of the surviving calves have badly affected lungs and may have laboured breathing for several months, are very

susceptible to secondary bacterial bronchopneumonia and remain stunted for long periods. A proportion of the surviving calves may show a sudden exacerbation of the dyspnoea during the 7th and 8th weeks and many of these animals die, the important lesion appearing to be the development of a proliferative pneumonia which is probably allergic in origin.

Clinical Pathology

The important observation to be made in *D. viviparus* infestation is the presence of larvae in the faeces. These may not be present in the early stages of clinical illness because the worms in the bronchi are not yet mature. In general larvae can be found about 12 days after signs appear, that is to say 24 days after infestation occurs. They may be few in number at first but may be as numerous as 500 to 1500 per g. of faeces 3 to 4 weeks after the illness commences. A common but not diagnostic finding is that of eosinophilia which is apparent in subacute cases from the first day of illness but is most marked about 3 weeks later (7). A detectable level of complement-fixing antibodies against *D. viviparus* antigen occurs in calves on the 30th to 35th day after infestation with this worm and rises to a peak about the 75th day but this is unlikely to be used as a diagnostic procedure. An intradermal sensitivity test is being investigated.

If the disease is suspected but the lungworms are still in the prepatent stage, and confirmation of the diagnosis by necropsy is impracticable, examination of pasture clippings for larvae may be necessary. This is a laborious procedure because large amounts of herbage must be used and the yield of larvae is low. Counts of less than 1 larva per 500 g. indicate a non-fatal level of infestation, a count of 1 to 3 larvae per 500 g. indicates a lethal level and counts of over 3 larvae per 500 g. are associated with the acute syndrome and heavy mortalities. Attention must also be given to the fact that the number of larvae on pasture will vary from day to day and at different times during the day depending on the humidity and temperature in the pasture.

Necropsy Findings

The wide variation in necropsy findings in this disease necessitates caution during the examination (4). In subacute cases the total number of adult worms in the bronchi may be as high as 3000 and counts of 10,000 to 20,000 are not uncommon. However, if the case is of sufficient duration and self-cure has been completed, no worms may be visible and careful microscopic examination of bronchial mucus is necessary to find the causative larvae.

The morphological changes in the lung in acute cases include enlargement of the lungs due to oedema and emphysema, widespread areas of collapsed tissue of a dark pink colour, haemorrhagic bronchitis with much fluid filling all the air passages and enlargement of the regional lymph nodes. Histologically the characteristic lesions are oedema, eosinophilic infiltration, dilatation of lymphatics, filling of the alveoli and bronchi with inflammatory debris and larvae in the bronchioles and alveoli.

In subacute cases interstitial emphysema is usually gross, areas of dark pink consolidation are present in all lobes but particularly in the diaphragmatic lobe and occupy about two-thirds of the lung volume and tend to be gathered around the bronchi. There is froth in the bronchi and the lymph nodes are enlarged. Histologically eggs and larvae can be seen in the air passages, the bronchial epithelium is much thickened, the bronchioles are obstructed with exudate and the alveoli show epithelialization and foreign-body giant-cell reaction.

Diagnosis

Verminous pneumonia in calves can be easily confused clinically with bacterial bronchopneumonia, with acute and chronic atypical pneumonia and with viral pneumonia. Ante mortem the important factors which suggest lungworm infestation are a history of exposure to pasture previously grazed by animals of the same species, and of the presence of the disease in the area, failure to respond to standard treatments for bacterial or viral pneumonia and the occurrence of the disease in outbreak form in autumn. The presence of fever, cough and auscultation findings suggesting a consolidation of the lungs and interstitial emphysema are common to all of these diseases, and, although absence of bronchial involvement characterizes early cases of viral and atypical pneumonia, secondary bacterial bronchopneumonia occurs sufficiently commonly to make this an undependable criterion. One clinical feature which may be of some value in differentiation is the relative softness and paroxysmal nature of the cough in parasitic pneumonia as compared to viral pneumonia. The cough in the latter is harsher and drier. The presence of larvae in the faeces supports the diagnosis but it must be remembered that there is a prepatent period of 3 weeks and affected animals may be ill for as long as 2 weeks before larvae appear and may still show obvious clinical signs for some weeks after larvae disappear from the faeces. Faecal samples should be collected from all of the animals in the group and for a complete examination samples of pasture, preferably selected from wet, low-lying areas, should also be checked for larvae. Deaths are sufficiently frequent to make necropsy diagnosis a common practice.

In adult cattle the major problem in diagnosis is to differentiate the acute form of the disease from acute atypical pneumonia due to other causes. Clinically the diseases are indistinguishable, and a history of movement onto a new pasture 1 to 2 weeks before the onset of the disease is common to both. Careful examination of the pasture for larvae and of the faeces of the young cattle for evidence of infestation and of necropsy material should make definition possible. That all cases of atypical pneumonia are not due to lungworm infestation is shown by the persistence of the disease on farms on which lungworm disease is controlled by vaccination (8). Heavy infestations with ascarid larvae in young and adult cattle occur rarely but should be suspected when cattle and infested pigs run together.

Treatment

At least two effective treatments are available. Tetramisole (laevamisole) is highly effective by oral dosing or injection at the standard dose rate of 15 mg. per kg. (9). Diethylcarbamazine (10) is effective at 40 mg. per kg. but lacks the wide spectrum of the former drug and for a broad cover treatment to include parasitic gastroenteritis needs to be combined with another anthelminthic such as pyrantel.

For the veterinarian in the field the effects of treatment are often unpredictable. If the infestation is massive and much damage has been done by larvae, treatment will effect no clinical improvement. If, however, treatment is administered in the early patent stages, when much of the damage is being caused by adults in the bronchi, clinical improvement is often dramatic. The difficulty for the veterinarian is to predict which of these will occur.

Because the disease in calves depends for its severity on the number of larvae which invade the lungs, treatment of early clinical cases is recommended in a control programme to reduce pasture contamination.

In most cases of acute verminous pneumonia the temperature is high and pus is evident in the bronchi at necropsy but this is seldom due to the development of a secondary bacterial pneumonia. However, most veterinarians find it advisable to administer broad spectrum antibiotics or sulphonamides to guard against such infection. In many cases the antibiotic has little or no effect on the temperature. Antihistamines are almost always administered in an attempt to reduce the severity of the reaction to the larvae. Because acute verminous pneumonia is so highly fatal a combined and expensive treatment with an anthelmintic, an antihistamine and a broad spectrum antibiotic is justifiable.

Control

The sources of larvae must be reduced and attention should be directed to the following points. Young, susceptible animals should not be grazed on pasture contaminated by older animals especially in wet summers, on permanent pastures containing low-lying or swampy, shaded areas and where pasture is long and succulent. A recommended method is to raise calves by grazing, and bucket feeding once daily in large paddocks which they graze rotationally ahead of the cows. Deer, although they appear to be unaffected clinically, may carry heavy infestations and provide a source of lungworm for cattle grazing the same pasture. Contamination is much more widespread when the faeces of carrier animals are loose due to lush grazing or other causes. On problem farms periodic dosing with a recommended drug is a routine practice. Where animals are housed during the winter, treatment of yearlings, who are the chief carriers, should be carried out just before they go to pasture in the spring and the calves should be treated at monthly intervals until winter. Animals should not have access to manure piles, to fields over which barn effluent runs or to fields which are dressed with barnyard manure. As has been pointed out previously the factor which governs the severity of the disease produced is the concentration of larvae on the pasture for the first 9 days after the calves are turned onto the field. Any control procedure which can reduce the concentration of larvae at this time will reduce the severity of the disease. Exposure to a few larvae will not result in clinical disease but will result in the development of some immunity.

Because of the solidity of the immunity which occurs after natural infestation a great deal of attention has been given to preventing infestation by the use of vaccines prepared from irradiated third-stage larvae (3, 4, 11, 12). An effective method of preventing *D. viviparus* infestation in calves has been shown to be two oral vaccinations with 1000 irradiated larvae on two occasions 6 weeks apart. Infective larvae attenuated by exposure to triethylene melamine have also been used to make a

vaccine which is as effective as the irradiated larvae (13). It is recommended that calves be confined indoors until at least 2 weeks after the second vaccination. Although vaccinated calves can act as carriers and cause clinical verminous pneumonia in non-vaccinated calves running with them (14), the vaccination is claimed to be 98 per cent effective in preventing clinical lungworm disease in average conditions (8). There are some limitations. For example it is recommended that vaccinated calves should not be exposed to grossly infested pastures nor be mixed with heavily infested calves and that on problem farms they be allowed only gradual access to pasture. In both naturally and artificially immunized animals, subsequent infestations of larvae migrate to the lungs where their further development is suppressed, but not before the occasional appearance of mild signs of the disease and death in some cases (15).

The vaccine has a relatively short shelf life and is rather expensive. The requirement to house cattle during vaccination is most inconvenient and it is possible, by avoiding periods when massive pasture contamination is likely, to vaccinate at pasture (16). Provided satisfactory control procedures are maintained during production of the vaccine this vaccination procedure offers the most efficient method of controlling verminous pneumonia in calves. Although natural immunity can achieve the same effect it can never be accurately measured nor predetermined but artificial immunization provides a known and calibrated weapon. The development of a satisfactory immunity as a result of natural exposure probably occurs in a significant number of beef calves sucking cows, especially if their condition is well maintained. Other methods of vaccination which have been investigated include the parenteral injection of living fourth-stage *D. viviparus* larvae (17) and oral dosing with *D. filaria* larvae (18).

In areas where enzootic pneumonia of calves and verminous pneumonia both occur a difficult decision may have to be made—whether to have the calves out on pasture to avoid spread of enzootic pneumonia or to keep them housed to avoid lungworm infestation. In such a situation it is preferable to run them at pasture and treat periodically as suggested above or confine them in outdoor pens without access to infested pasture.

REFERENCES

(1) Gupta, R. P. & Gibbs, H. C. (1970). *Canad. vet. J.*, *11*, 149.
(2) Robinson, J. (1962). *Nature* (*Lond.*), *193*, 353.
(3) Jarrett, W. F. H. *et al.* (1961). *Amer. J. vet. Res.*, *22*, 492.
(4) Jarrett, W. F. H. *et al.* (1959). *Amer. J. vet. Res.*, *20*, 522.
(5) Michel, J. F. (1958). *Vet. Rec.*, *70*, 554.

(6) Weisman, J. (1970). Proefschrift Fac. Diergeneeskunde Rijksuniv. Utrecht, p. 123.
(7) Djafar, M. I. *et al.* (1960). *J. Amer. vet. med. Ass.*, *136*, 200.
(8) Poynter, D. *et al.* (1970). *Vet. Rec.*, *86*, 148.
(9) Ross, D. B. (1968). *Vet. Rec.*, *83*, 69.
(10) Walley, J. K. (1957). *Vet. Rec.*, *69*, 819, 850.
(11) Jarrett, W. F. H. *et al.* (1962). *Amer. J. vet. Res.*, *23*, 1183.
(12) Edds, G. T. *et al.* (1963). *Amer. J. vet. Res.*, *24*, 139.
(13) Cornwell, R. L. & Jones, R. M. (1970). *Res. vet. Sci.*, *11*, 533.
(14) Cornwell, R. L. (1962). *Vet. Rec.*, *74*, 622.
(15) Downey, N. E. (1965). *Vet. Rec.*, *77*, 890.
(16) Downey, N. E. (1968). *Vet. Rec.*, *82*, 338.
(17) Cornwell, R. L. (1962). *J. comp. Path.*, *77*, 181.
(18) Lucker, J. T. *et al.* (1964). *Proc. helminth. Soc. Wash.*, *31*, 153.

Lungworm Infestation in Other Species

Sheep and Goats

Infestations with *Dictyocaulus filaria*, *Muellerius capillaris* and *Protostrongylus rufescens* are all encountered. Lambs 4 to 6 months of age are most severely affected but sheep of all ages are susceptible. Lungworm infestation in sheep needs to be differentiated from maedi and jaagsiekte. Infestations with *Cystocaulus ocreatus* and *Neostrongylus linearis*, the latter similar in most of its characters to *M. capillaris*, have also been observed in sheep in Great Britain (1) but their economic significance has not been defined.

D. filaria infestations in sheep appear to follow the same pattern as those of *D. viviparus* in calves; the life cycle is direct and the third-stage larvae are long-lived in damp, cool surroundings. However, acute cases, caused by massive infestations with larvae, do not appear to occur. Adult worms live in the bronchi and cause alveolar and bronchiolar damage. The resulting blockage of bronchioles by exudate leads to the collapse of portions of lung. The area of lung damaged is usually not sufficiently extensive to cause severe dyspnoea. Clinically the emphasis is on bronchial irritation and its resulting cough, on moderate dyspnoea and loss of condition. There may be added fever and evidence of toxaemia if secondary bacterial infection occurs. Laboratory diagnosis depends upon the detection of first-stage larvae in the faeces of infested animals. Although *D. filaria* is primarily a lungworm of sheep it can infest and grow to maturity in cattle and can, after experimental infestation, cause the death of calves (2). It is highly pathogenic to young goats.

At necropsy the lesions are similar to those of the subacute disease in calves with exudate in the bronchioles and scattered patches of consolidation.

Cyanacethydrazide and diethylcarbamazine are effective treatments but tetramisole is efficient not only against *D. filaria* but also against gastro-intestinal helminths (3, 4) and appears to be the superior treatment available at present. It can be administered orally or by subcutaneous injection. Control by vaccination with irradiated *D. filaria* larvae is undergoing examination (5). Immunity after natural exposure is strong and durable (at least 46 months) in sheep but less so in goats (13).

Infestation with *Muellerius capillaris* in sheep has been recorded from most parts of the world and although the worm appears to be relatively innocuous it may constitute a limiting factor in the production of choice market lambs and it has been suggested as a causative factor in outbreaks of enterotoxaemia in sheep. Massive invasion with larvae is improbable because the intermediate host snails and slugs are usually not ingested in large numbers nor are they grossly infested with larvae. Those larvae which reach the lungs of sheep remain in the parenchyma and become encysted in fibrous nodules and because such nodules may not contain adults of both sexes, fertile eggs may not be deposited in the air passages. For this reason the number of larvae in the faeces is often no indication of the degree of infestation. Also, in many animals the infestation is carried over from one year to the next. Massive infestations with this worm do not develop acutely and heavy infestations, when they occur, appear to develop over a long period of time (6).

At necropsy the worms are found in small fibrous nodules up to 5 mm. in diameter. Most of the nodules are in the parenchyma of the lung immediately under the pleura. Many of them are calcified and they often contain only one live or dead worm. None of the drugs used in the treatment of other lungworms has been found to be of any value against *M. capillaris*, but emetin hydrochloride (7) appears to be effective against this worm and against *Cystocaulus ocreatus* and *Protostrongylus rufescens*.

P. rufescens infestations in sheep and goats cause clinical signs similar to those of *D. filaria*. The adult worms live in the bronchi, causing verminous bronchitis and pneumonia. Only lambs and kids show serious clinical involvement. Because the life cycle is indirect, requiring a land snail for completion of the second stage larval development, massive infestations are unlikely to occur. Cyanacethydrazide is reported to be effective as treatment but clinical improvement in field outbreaks may not be great. Tetramisole is considered to be highly effective against this worm.

Pigs

The lungworms which infest pigs are *Metastrongylus apri* (*M. elongatus*), *M. salmi* and *M. pudendodectus*. *M. apri* is the most common species but mixed infestations are not uncommon (8). They have an indirect life history, passing their intermediate stages in earthworms. Eggs laid by adult worms in the lungs are coughed up and swallowed and, passing out with the manure in an embryonated stage do not hatch till they reach the exterior. The eggs first appear in the faeces 3 to 4 weeks after infestation and at their peak reach levels of 25 to 50 epg. The embryonated eggs or first-stage larvae are either eaten by the earthworms or the larvae migrate actively into the worms. Here they develop successively into second- and third-stage larvae in about 2 weeks. Details of the ability of the first-stage larvae to survive before they infest the intermediate host are lacking but they appear to be fairly resistant. The larvae of *M. apri* may survive for as long as a year after hatching. The primary host must ingest an intermediate host to become infested and this is an important factor influencing the spread of the disease. Once ingested the infective larvae migrate to the lungs in much the same manner as do *D. viviparus* larvae.

In natural cases bronchitis accompanied by sporadic bouts of a barking cough which is easily stimulated by exercise, pneumonia in severe cases, poor growth and debility are the obvious signs but minimal clinical signs are apparent after experimental production of the disease (9). These worms are suggested as vectors in the transmission of swine influenza virus, and possibly hog cholera virus, from pig to pig.

At necropsy the lesions in early cases comprise small areas of consolidation due to verminous pneumonia. More chronic cases have bronchitis, emphysema, peribronchial lymphoid hyperplasia and bronchiolar muscular hypertrophy. The lesions are small and discrete, appearing as greyish nodules up to 1 cm. in diameter and are present particularly at the ventral border of the diaphragmatic lobes (9). In more severe experimental cases acute and chronic lesions are more widely disseminated and often involve the anterior lobes.

Cyanacethydrazide and diethylcarbamazine have good reputations as treatments but tetramisole is highly efficient and has the advantage of a wide spectrum dealing efficiently with *Ascaris*, *Oesophagostomum* and *Hyostrongylus* spp. (12).

Horses

Infestations with *D. arnfieldi* are recorded more commonly in donkeys than in horses and the former are considered to be the more normal host. Heavy infestations in donkeys do not cause clinical illness but young horse foals may be affected with a disease similar to that which occurs in calves. Adult horses appear to have an age immunity. *D. arnfieldi* infestations appear to have been recorded only once in North America (10). Cyanacethydrazide has been tested as a treatment in donkeys (11) and although it reduced the number of larvae in the faeces by half it did not completely remove worms from the lungs. Dose rates used were the same as those prescribed for cattle.

Control of Miscellaneous Lungworm Infestations

Those worms which have direct life cycles, *D. filaria* and *D. arnfieldi*, can be controlled by the methods set out at the beginning of this chapter. All lungworms are host-specific and thus sheep can be used to graze a pasture heavily contaminated with cattle lungworm larvae without risk of infestation. Combined infestations of lungworms and intestinal trichostrongylids are common and because of the similarity of their life cycles control of the two groups is effected by the same programme. The major difference is that the lungworm larvae live longer than most of the intestinal nematodes. Insufficient work has been carried out to determine the exact environmental conditions required by the larvae and it is therefore impossible to lay down strict management rules, nor does the efficiency of the new drugs, cyanacethydrazide, diethylcarbamazine and tetramisole in control programmes appear to have been determined.

In those worm species which have indirect life cycles, *Muellerius capillaris*, *Protostrongylus rufescens* and *Metastrongylus* spp. the control measures must include avoidance of the intermediate hosts. Snails and slugs are most active in wet weather and in the early morning or evening. Pasturing of animals on wet, undrained areas at those times of the day should be avoided where possible. Little can be done to control earthworm populations, and pigs which run in dirt yards or at pasture should be moved at short intervals to prevent ingestion of infested worms. Rooting by pigs can be discouraged by providing adequate feed and by the insertion of nose rings. Pastures which are known to be contaminated should be left for at least 6 months before restocking, although infested earthworms may persist in hog lots for up to 4 years.

REVIEW LITERATURE

Poynter, D. & Selway, S. (1966). *Vet. Bull.*, **36**, 539.

REFERENCES

(1) Rose, J. H. (1965). *Res. vet. Sci.*, **6**, 189.

(2) Parfitt, J. W. (1963). *Vet. Rec.*, *75*, 124.
(3) Gibson, T. E. & Parfitt, J. W. (1968). *Vet. Rec.*, *82*, 238.
(4) Skerman, K. D. *et al.* (1968). *Vet. Rec.*, *82*, 736.
(5) Sokolic, A. *et al.* (1965). *Brit. vet. J.*, *121*, 212.
(6) Rose, J. H. (1959). *J. comp. Path.*, *69*, 414.
(7) Durbin, C. G. (1954). *Vet. Ext. Q. Univ. Pa*, *133*, 49.
(8) Ewing, S. A. & Todd, A. C. (1961). *Amer. J. vet. Res.*, *22*, 606, 1077.
(9) McKenzie, A. (1959). *Vet. Rec.*, *71*, 209.
(10) Baker, D. & Guralp, N. (1957). *Cornell Vet.*, *47*, 456.
(11) Thomas, R. E. & Jones, L. P. (1960). *Vet. Med.*, *55*, 38.
(12) Walley, J. K. (1967). *Vet. Rec.*, *81*, 617.
(13) Wilson, G. I. (1970). *Res. vet. Sci.*, *11*, 7.

Oesophagostomiasis

(*Oesophagostomosis, Nodular Worm Disease, Pimply Gut*)

Infestations with worms of *Oesophagostomum* spp. occur in all farm animals except horses. The disease produced is characterized clinically by emaciation and the passage of soft droppings containing more than normal amounts of mucus and in most species at necropsy by the presence of necrotic nodules in the wall of the intestine.

Incidence

Infestations with *Oesophagostomum* spp. occur most commonly in temperate and subtropical climates with summer rainfall and cause economic loss in sheep and cattle. Although deaths may occur the major losses are caused by failure to thrive. The damage done to intestines renders them unsuitable for use as sausage casings and results in much financial loss.

Aetiology

All of the species of the genus *Oesophagostomum* are thick, white roundworms (0·5 to 2·5 cm. long) which inhabit the large intestine. The important species are:

Sheep and goats—*Oesophagostomum columbianum*; *Oe. venulosum*; *Oe. asperium* (goat only).
Cattle—*Oe.* (*Bosicola*) *radiatum*; *Oe. venulosum*.
Pig—*Oe. dentatum*; *Oe. quadrispinulatum*.

Oe. dentatum is rather smaller than the others being only 0·5 to 1·5 cm. long. All ages and classes of livestock are affected. In some areas lambs and calves suffer from a more acute form of the disease. Adults probably develop some immunity, expressed by nodule formation but losses may be heavy in adult cattle and ewes particularly if their resistance is lowered by poor nutrition. Although there is obvious species specificity some cross infection occurs. Thus *Oe. columbianum* can develop in cattle to the point of penetrating the mucosa and producing lesions similar to those in lambs, but without any apparent effect on health (1). The infection does not confer any resistance against infection with *Oe. radiatum*.

Life Cycle

The life cycle is direct. Eggs passed in the faeces hatch and, after undergoing two moults, become infective third-stage larvae; under optimum conditions this takes 6 to 7 days. The requirements of the free-living larvae are quite strict, both eggs and larvae of *Oe. columbianum* being susceptible to cold and dryness. Thus in young animals exposed to infestation for the first time, an acute form of the disease is most common in the summer months especially when the temperature is high. In older animals which have some immunity the clinical disease is more likely to appear in the winter after such summers, presumably when the immunity fades. In spite of the predilection of the worm for warm, moist conditions the more chronic form of the disease is quite common in eastern Canada and the New England states of the U.S.A.

Infestation occurs only by ingestion. The larvae of all species, except those of perhaps *Oe. venulosum*, invade the intestinal wall at any level. In young sheep exposed to infestation for the first time the larvae of *Oe. columbianum* stay in the intestinal wall for about 5 days and the adults commence egg-laying about 6 weeks after infestation occurs. Persistence of the larvae in the intestinal wall for long periods is usually taken to indicate immunity on the part of the host and is followed by nodule formation. Thus in older sheep nodules develop in the intestinal wall at any level and occasional nodules may also be present in nearby organs. In these animals the larvae remain in the nodules for periods up to a year. When the resistance of the animal is lowered, due for example to poor nutrition, the larvae leave the nodules, re-enter the intestinal lumen and pass down to the colon, where they complete their development and become adults. The adults attach themselves to the colonic mucosa and commence egg laying. This is the probable explanation for the three common findings at necropsy; young sheep with many adult worms and no nodules, adult sheep with many nodules and no adult worms, and adults with both.

The life cycle of *Oe. radiatum* is not so accurately defined in young animals exposed for the first time, larvae leave the intestinal wall about the 10th day and egg laying commences at about 6 weeks.

Pathogenesis

There are many aspects of the pathogenesis of oesophagostomiasis which are poorly understood. The adult worms exert quite serious effects although they are not blood suckers nor do they cause much trauma. The effects of infestations with *Oe. radiatum* in calves include changes other than the physical ones usually described (2). These include lack of appetite, reduction in the efficiency of food utilization, a normocytic, normochromic anaemia due apparently to malnutrition rather than blood loss, and hypoproteinaemia. The hypoproteinaemia has been shown to be due to loss of albumin into the caecum and colon during the period of severe swelling and oedema of that organ (3). The lack of appetite in itself exerts a marked effect on the decline of the affected calves. Emergence of the larvae from the intestinal wall appears to cause irritation resulting in the development of a catarrhal colitis and diarrhoea. Experimentally produced oesophagostomiasis in lambs is marked by anorexia, loss of body weight, diarrhoea and a fall in packed cell volume, haemoglobin, plasma protein, plasma albumin, and albumin–globulin ratio, and an increase in plasma globulin (4, 5). The degree of nodule development varies, depending apparently on whether the animal has any immunity to the infestation, and has been discussed under life cycle. The persistence of the larvae in the intestinal wall gives rise to local necrosis, fibrous tissue formation, calcification and nodule formation. If the nodules become infected varying degrees of local peritonitis and adhesion formation interfere with intestinal movement and may terminate in intussusception or stenosis. The nodules caused by *Oe. radiatum* in cattle and *Oe. dentatum* in pigs are much fewer in number but have similar significance; those caused by *Oe. quadrispinulatum* are rather larger and develop into ulcers.

The lesions produced experimentally in pigs have been well defined (6). With *Oe. dentatum* the prepatent period is 35 days, the histotrophic stage is between 2 and 10 days after infection. Oedema and marked thickening of the wall of the caecum and colon develop. With heavy infestations outbreaks of necrotic enteritis may be activated in pigs carrying resident *Salmonella* spp. populations (7).

A marked 'post-parturient rise' in egg count occurs at least in some sows, and can be a critical factor in increasing the effects of the disease on the sow and the spread of the infection to the young pig. It commences about a week before farrowing, peaks 6 weeks after farrowing, and terminates abruptly when lactation ends (8). There is also a seasonal variation in egg count which is independent of parturition status, the egg count being highest in spring (9).

Clinical Findings

In heavy infestations in young sheep there may be severe persistent diarrhoea but in the more common syndrome observed in older sheep in the winter months there is an intermittent passage of semi-soft droppings containing more than normal amounts of mucus, and occasionally blood. There is rapid loss of condition, hollowing of the back, stiffness of gait and elevation of the tail. Nodules may be palpated on rectal examination. Anaemia is not characteristic and is never marked. Severe outbreaks of intussusception sometimes occur in young sheep and oesophagostomiasis is often implicated as a primary cause.

In cattle losses due to *Oe. radiatum* are not common but calves and occasionally adults are affected. The clinical signs are similar to those observed in sheep and include anaemia, persistent mucoid-type diarrhoea, straining at defaecation, loss of condition and stiffness of gait. In pigs, although loss of condition and diarrhoea have been attributed to this disease, clinical signs are rarely observed even with massive infestations (10).

Clinical Pathology

The severity of the disease may bear no relation to the number of eggs in the faeces, counts varying widely with the season of the year and the stage of development of the disease. In the early stages of a massive infestation signs may be evident but there may be no eggs in the droppings. After the prepatent period in young sheep eggs are usually present in large numbers and may be accompanied by living adult worms. However, in chronic cases there may be very few eggs in the droppings. The eggs cannot be readily distinguished from those of other strongylid worms.

Necropsy Findings

In early acute cases there is a mild catarrhal enteritis and larvae may be detectable in scrapings of intestinal mucosa. In the later, more chronic stage there are adult worms in the colon. The adult worms are usually lying in thick mucus overlying a chronic catarrhal colitis. Nodules, when they are present, may be found at all levels of the intestine. They are up to 6 mm. in diameter and, depending on their age, contain a green, pasty material or yellow-brown, crumbly, partly calcified material. There may be a great deal of thickening of the intestinal wall and local peritonitis.

The number of worms in the lumen of the colon

is usually quite small and 200 *Oe. columbianum* adult females is considered to be a heavy infestation.

Diagnosis

A definite diagnosis of oesophagostomiasis can only be made by necropsy examination or identification of larvae from a faecal culture. The diseases with which it is most likely to be confused are trichostrongylosis, which is also at its peak during the winter but in which diarrhoea is more evident, and malnutrition, especially when sheep are housed and poorly fed. The disease has a relatively restricted geographical distribution and this should be taken into account.

Oesophagostomum dentatum and, to a less extent, *Hyostrongylus rubidus* infections are commonly thought to be significant factors in causing the 'thin sow syndrome'. The sows lose condition in late pregnancy and this continues for up to 6 months. In many herds the majority of sows are affected with disastrous effects on the economy. The sows are emaciated but eat well and behave normally, usually rearing their litters satisfactorily. The skin is usually dry and obviously scaly. Other suggested causes are a too low protein content of the diet, bullying of timid sows and discomfort in stalls. There are probably a number of causes and, at least in some, control of internal parasites has a salutory effect.

Treatment

Thiabendazole (50 mg. per kg. body weight) or tetramizole (15 mg. per kg. body weight) are the drugs of choice because of their efficiency against these and other gastrointestinal helminths. For greatest efficiency against larvae of *Oe. columbianum* a dose rate of thiabendazole of 125 mg. per kg. body weight is recommended (11).

Piperazine is also an effective single treatment but the drug is of no value against the common causes of parasitic gastroenteritis of ruminants and, because infestations are usually mixed, other anthelmintics are usually preferred.

Phenothiazine is effective against adults living in the colon but not against larvae in nodules and is not used extensively. Although organic phosphate compounds are ineffective in the large bowel of sheep they are of value in cattle. For example, Neguvon is effective orally and by injection but the dose rate necessary to affect larvae is toxic to the calf.

In pigs thiabendazole (100 mg. per kg.) and haloxon (45 mg. per kg.) (12), parbendazole 20 mg. per kg. in the feed (13) and pyrantel tartrate at 22 mg. per kg. (14) all give good results. Tetramisole at 15 mg. per kg. is well taken in food and is highly efficient, with a broad spectrum including *Ascaris* spp. and lungworms (15). Dichlorvos is similarly effective against ascarids and hyostrongylids as well as *Oesophagostomum dentatum* and is well taken in feed (16).

Control

The rather narrow range of climatic conditions in which the non-parasitic larval stages of *Oe. columbianum* can survive reduces the ability of the genus to persist from year to year. However, this is compensated by the ability of parasitic larvae to survive for up to a year in nodules in the intestinal wall.

To keep infestation at a minimum level in sheep flocks and at pasture all the year round three strategic dosings with an efficient anthelmintic in early spring, midsummer and late autumn are recommended. The flock should be moved to a clean pasture after each drenching. The aim should be to treat the flock immediately after a period when climatic conditions, particularly a dry summer or a cold winter, are likely to have destroyed the majority of larvae on the pasture. Sheep which are housed in the winter months and suffer greatest damage at this time are usually dosed only once a year, preferably 1 to 2 months before lambing. The observation that grazing sheep on a field of green oats is highly effective in removing *Oe. columbianum* from the colon may have some significance as a control measure. The use of a vaccine using irradiated larvae has shown limited promise (19).

In pigs the control programme must take the 'post-parturient rise' into account. Dosing of the sow before farrowing is recommended. Housing is not a protection unless there is an absence of litter and manure is removed frequently (8). For fattening pigs continuous low-level feeding is useful. Thiabendazole at 0·05 per cent in feed for 5 weeks from 3 to 8 weeks of age and then at 0·01 per cent until just before marketing significantly reduces populations of *Oesophagostomum* spp., *H. rubidus*, *Metastrongylus* spp., *Trichuris* spp., and *Ascaris suum* (17). To increase the efficiency of thiabendazole against *Ascaris suum* it is sometimes given with piperazine carbodithoic acid (18).

REFERENCES

(1) Herlich, H. (1970). *Amer. J. vet. Res.*, *31*, 263.
(2) Bremner, K. C. (1961). *Aust. J. agric. Res.*, *12*, 498.
(3) Bremner, K. C. (1969). *Exp. Parasit.*, *24*, 364.
(4) Horak, I. G. & Clark, R. (1966). *Onderstepoort J. vet. Res.*, *33*, 139.
(5) Dobson, C. (1967). *Aust. vet. J.*, *43*, 291.
(6) McCracken, R. M. & Ross, J. G. (1970). *J. comp. Path.*, *80*, 619.

(7) Stockdale, P. H. G. (1970). *Brit. vet. J.*, *126*, 526.
(8) Connan, R. M. (1967). *Vet. Rec.*, *80*, 424.
(9) Jacobs, D. E. & Dunn, A. M. (1968). *Nord. Vet.-Med.*, *20*, 258.
(10) Nickel, E. A. & Haupt, W. (1964). *Berlin Münch. tierärzt. Wschr.*, *77*, 193.
(11) Smith, H. J. & Archibald, R. McG. (1964). *Canad. vet. J.*, *5*, 331.
(12) Czipri, D. A. (1970). *Vet. Rec.*, *86*, 306.
(13) Chang, J. & Wescott, R. B. (1969). *Amer. J. vet. Res.*, *30*, 77.
(14) Arakaua, A. *et al.* (1971). *Vet. Med.*, *66*, 108.
(15) Walley, J. K. (1967). *Vet. Rec.*, *81*, 617.
(16) Jacobs, D. E. *et al.* (1971). *Res. vet. Sci.*, *12*, 189.
(17) Taffs, L. F. & Davidson, J. B. (1967). *Vet. Rec.*, *81*, 426.
(18) Taffs, L. F. (1968). *Vet. Rec.*, *83*, 219.
(19) Dhar, D. N. & Singh, K. S. (1970). *J. Helminth.*, *44*, 11.

Chabertiasis

Chabertiasis of sheep, goats and cattle is caused by *Chabertia ovina*, a worm 1 to 2 cm. in length, which inhabits the colon and causes a clinical syndrome similar to that of oesophagostomiasis. The life cycle is direct and resembles that of other strongylid worms. After hatching two non-parasitic larval stages are followed by a third infective stage which, when ingested, sets up the infestation in the colon. The non-parasitic larvae are relatively resistant to cold and heavy infestations may occur in mild winters. No migration through body tissues occurs but the fourth-stage larvae, which develop within a few hours of ingestion, attach to the colonic mucosa or enter the intestinal wall causing marked petechiation but without causing nodule formation (1). Eggs begin to appear in the droppings of infested lambs 7 to 8 weeks after infestation.

Clinical signs are caused by both larvae and adult worms. The adults attach to the mucosa of the colon and cause thickening of the bowel wall, excessive production of mucus and petechiation. Less commonly there is ulceration and haemorrhage, leading to the development of anaemia. In either case the predominant sign is the passage of semi-soft faeces, sometimes containing blood and mucus. Infestations may be sufficiently heavy in young lambs to cause severe diarrhoea and some deaths. In these lambs there is often an unexplained inability to rise without apparent loss of muscular power. The clinical illness may commence a month after infestation when the worms are still immature so that although examination of the faeces for eggs, and faecal cultures for larvae are standard diagnostic procedures these may be negative or indicative of only a light worm burden. In experimental infestations diarrhoea, dysentery and anaemia are the significant clinical signs and these can be caused by the immature worms (4).

Changes seen at necropsy are thickening, oedema and petechiation of the wall of the colon, with blood sometimes present in the intestinal contents. The number of worms present is often surprisingly small and severe morphological changes may be evident with only 5 to 10 worms. More than 100 worms is considered to be a heavy infestation (2).

Chabertiasis is similar in many ways to oesophagostomiasis and the control measures described there apply here also, with the exception that heavy infestations are more common in late winter and early spring and tactical treatments may be necessary. Most of the newer anthelminthics including methyridine, thiabendazole and tetramisole are highly effective against *Ch. ovina* and 1:8 dihydroxy-anthraquinone (2 g. per sheep) is also recommended. Piperazine and the organic phosphate compounds are not effective (3).

REFERENCES

(1) Threlkeld, W. L. (1947). *J. Parasit.*, *33*, Dec. Supp., p. 12.
(2) Seddon, H. R. (1950). *Cwlth Aust.*, *Div. Vet. Hyg.*, Serv. Pub. No. 5.
(3) Gordon, H. McL. (1957). *Aust. vet. J.*, *33*, 1.
(4) Ross, J. G. *et al.* (1969). *Brit. vet. J.*, *125*, 136.

Stephanuriasis

(*Kidney Worm Disease*)

Stephanuriasis is a disease of swine caused by the migration of larvae and young adults of *Stephanurus dentatus* through the body. Poor growth and feed utilization is characteristic in mildly affected animals whereas badly affected animals become emaciated and develop ascites and muscle stiffness.

Incidence

Kidney worms occur commonly in most tropical and subtropical countries such as Africa, the East and West Indies, Brazil, Hawaii, Philippines, southern U.S.A. and Australia where the climate is sufficiently mild to permit the survival of eggs and larvae. The mortality rate is not high, the important causes of loss being poor growth and condemnation of parts or all of the infested carcase.

Aetiology

St. dentatus are large (2 to 5 cm.) thick roundworms which inhabit the perirenal tissues, and less commonly the other abdominal organs and spinal canal of the pig. They have been observed rarely in cattle. Experimentally dosed calves develop severe hepatic injury similar to that which occurs in pigs but the life cycle is not completed and no perirenal lesions develop.

Life Cycle

Adult worms inhabit cysts around the renal pelvis and the wall of the ureter. The cysts communicate with the urinary passages and the eggs are passed out into the urine of the host. They are very heavy egg layers and an infective adult sow may void as many as a million eggs in a day. Under suitable environmental conditions the eggs hatch and, after undergoing two moults, the non-infective larvae develop into the infective third stage in about 4 days. The eggs and larvae are very sensitive to cold and desiccation, eggs in a dry situation dying within an hour. Exposure to temperatures below 10°C (50°F) are damaging and 4°C (40°F) is lethal. Most larvae in optimum conditions of moisture, warmth and shelter from sunlight survive for about 3 months, some for as long as 5 months. There is some suggestion that larvae may survive for long periods as facultative parasites in earthworms and this may enable the larvae to survive even though the micro-climate of the soil is adverse (1, 2).

The host is invaded actively via the skin or through the stomach wall if the larvae are ingested. After undergoing a moult in the stomach wall or skin the larvae reach the liver. From the stomach the route of migration is the portal vessels, migration taking about 3 days; from the skin the larvae reach the systemic circulation and pass to the liver via the lungs in 1 to 6 weeks. In the liver the larvae migrate from the blood vessels through the parenchyma and eventually, about 3 months after infestation, having undergone a fourth moult, penetrate the capsule of the liver and reach the perirenal tissues to establish themselves as adults. Egg laying usually commences about 6 months after infestation but the pre-patent period may be very much longer, i.e. 2 to 3 years, and individual worms appear to live as long as 2 years (4).

During their migration the larvae, as in *Strongylus vulgaris* infestations, often follow an erratic path and cause the development of atypical lesions and clinical signs. These larvae often reach maturity in these aberrant sites and prenatal infection can occur in this way (3).

Pathogenesis

The principal effects of these worms is the damage caused by the migrating larvae and young adults. The migrating worms cause a great deal of necrosis, fibrosis and occasional abscess formation along the path of their migration and this is most marked in the perirenal tissues and the liver. Many apparently unrelated clinical signs are produced by aberrant larvae which may invade the spinal cord causing paralysis, or blood vessels, particularly portal veins, hepatic artery and posterior vena cava, causing thrombus formation, and psoas muscles, causing the local pain and stiffness so marked in some badly affected pigs. Passage through the peritoneum and pleura causes the formation of adhesions and many larvae become encysted in the lung.

Clinical Findings

Poor growth in spite of a good appetite may be the only sign in mild cases. Severely affected pigs are emaciated and may have ascites. Stiffness and lameness of the hind legs followed by weakness and eventually paralysis occur in a number of pigs. In the early stages nodules in the skin of the belly wall and enlargement and soreness of the peripheral lymph nodes may be evident (4).

Clinical Pathology

The large, thin-walled, embryonated eggs are present in the urine when adult worms are present in the ureteral wall. A marked eosinophilia (33 to 34 per cent) occurs in the 2nd to 4th weeks after infestation but this is of little diagnostic significance.

Necropsy Findings

The common findings include fibrosis and abscess formation in perirenal tissues with large adult worms present here and occasionally in the pelvis of the kidney and ureter, infarcts and scars in the kidney and enlargement and scarring of the liver, sometimes accompanied by ascites. The hepatic lesions include irregular whitish tracts in the parenchyma, extensive fibrosis, haemorrhage and eosinophilic abscess formation (8). Larvae may also be present in peripheral lymph nodes and cutaneous nodules, in small abscesses in the lung and pancreas and in thrombi of blood vessels, particularly in the liver and lungs. Pleurisy and peritonitis if they are present are usually manifested by adhesions.

Diagnosis

Poor growth and emaciation in pigs is commonly associated with poor nutrition and sporadically with a number of chronic bacterial diseases. Most of the latter, including necrotic enteritis and vibrionic dysentery, affect the alimentary tract and are accompanied by intermittent diarrhoea. Other parasitic diseases such as ascariasis and hyostrongylosis may cause similar clinical syndromes. Posterior weakness in pigs may be caused by stephanuriasis but is more commonly caused by vitamin

A deficiency, osteodystrophia, sometimes by fracture of a lumbar vertebra, brucellosis, erysipelas when intervertebral joints are involved, or by spinal cord abscess or lymphoma. Experimental visceral larval migrans, caused by infestations of pigs with larvae of *Toxocara canis*, can also cause a syndrome of ataxia and posterior paralysis (5) but the natural occurrence of this disease does not seem to have been observed.

A definite diagnosis of stephanuriasis may be made by finding eggs in the urine but necropsy examination is preferred. Young pigs with a heavy infestation of larvae may present a problem in diagnosis because adult worms and characteristic renal lesions may not yet be present.

Treatment

No treatment is effective.

Control

In the absence of a suitable treatment control depends upon hygienic measures to prevent the spread of infestation. The age group most heavily infested and the most potent source of infestation are sows 6 to 7 years old and it is particularly important to prevent infestation of baby pigs by the sow. The important points in the programme are those suggested for the control of ascariasis. Pigs running at pasture and in dirt yards are most likely to be infested, and sleeping shelters should be placed on high dry ground, preferably bare of vegetation, so that the infectivity of the urine is reduced. Because pigs in yards commonly urinate against the fences it is recommended that a 6- to 10-foot strip of earth inside the fence be kept free of pasture and preferably packed hard. Muddy spots and water holes must be filled in and drainage provided. Water and feed troughs should be on a concrete apron. Young animals should be segregated from adults and fields rested for 3 to 6 months after the adults are removed. Results are excellent if the programme is carried out diligently and intelligently but the extra work involved has militated against the general acceptance of the programme (6). A control programme based on the long pre-patent period of about 10 months has been devised. Infected sows are replaced by first litter gilts which are in turn replaced by their own first progeny. The method works satisfactorily and has the advantage that the piggery can be kept fully stocked (7).

Indoor pens should be constructed with a good slope to the floor to avoid dampness. A recommended control measure is weekly spraying of the pens with 10 per cent copper sulphate solution or a 5 per cent solution of Kerol. These sprays are also recommended for the spraying of dirt yards, the latter being particularly effective when applied at the rate of 1 gallon per 10 sq. yards, maintaining the toxicity of mud for larvae for a period of at least 66 days. Neither spray is toxic for pigs kept in the treated yards. Because of the importance of mature animals as sources of infestation, early replacement of breeding stock is recommended in problem herds.

REFERENCES

(1) Seddon, H. R. (1950). *Div. vet. Hyg. Cwlth Aust. Dept. Hlth Service Pub.*, No. 5.
(2) Batte, E. G. *et al.* (1960). *J. Amer. vet. med. Ass.*, *136*, 622.
(3) Batte, E. G. *et al.* (1966). *J. Amer. vet. med. Ass.*, *149*, 758.
(4) Ross, I. C. & Kauzal, G. P. (1932). *Counc. sci. ind. Res.*, *Cwlth Aust. Bull.*, No. 58.
(5) Done, J. T. *et al.* (1960). *Res. vet. Sci.*, *1*, 133.
(6) Spindler, L. A. & Andrews, J. S. (1955). *Proc. 58th ann. gen. Mtg U.S. Live Stock sanit. Ass.*, 296.
(7) Stewart, T. B. *et al.* (1964). *Amer. J. vet. Res.*, *25*, 1141.
(8) Peneyra, R. S. & Naui, V. C. (1967). *Philipp. J. vet. Med.*, *4*, 129.

Bunostomiasis

(*Hookworm Disease*)

Infestations with hookworms (*Bunostomum* spp.) cause poor growth and blood loss manifested by anaemia and anasarca.

Incidence

Hookworm infestations are most common and cause greatest losses in subtropical and temperate countries including southern United States, Africa, Australia and Europe where climatic conditions are most suited for completion of the worms' life cycles. However, the disease is encountered in such countries as Scotland and Canada, especially when animals are housed during the winter in dirty surroundings with insufficient bedding.

Aetiology

Hookworms are small (1 to 2·5 cm.), reddish roundworms which inhabit the small intestine of their hosts. The important species are:

Cattle—*Bunostomum phlebotomum* is the important hookworm in this species. *Agriostomum vryburgi* may occur in cattle in India and Sumatra.

Sheep—*Bunostomum trigonocephalum* and in India and Africa *Gaigeria pachyscelis*.

Pigs—Infestations with some species of hookworms occur but are rarely important.

Immunity to *B. phlebotomum* in cattle appears to develop with age (1) and calves affected one year appear to be completely immune the next.

Calves 4 to 12 months of age are most commonly affected and the degree of infestation is always greatest in the winter months.

Life Cycle

The life cycle of all the hookworms is direct. The eggs hatch and a parasitic larva is produced in about a week. As in most strongylids there are two free-living, non-parasitic larval stages which are very susceptible to desiccation, and an infective larva which is, in all hookworms, capable of entering the body of the host through the skin. Larvae of *G. pachyscelis* enter only in this way; *Bunostomum* spp. larvae enter by this route and via the mouth. Percutaneous entry greatly enhances the chances of infestation when the surroundings are wet, and this, together with the susceptibility of the larvae to desiccation, leads to the higher incidence of the disease in humid subtropical countries.

The larvae, after cutaneous penetration, enter the blood stream, are carried to the heart and lungs, enter the alveoli where the fourth-stage larvae develop, pass up the air passages to the pharynx, are swallowed and reach the small intestine. Ingested larvae penetrate the intestinal wall and return to its lumen without further migration. In *B. trigonocephalum* infestations the fourth-stage larvae reach the intestine in about 11 days and egg-laying adults are present about 10 weeks after infestation. The prepatent period in *B. phlebotomum* infestations is about 8 weeks and in *G. pachyscelis* 10 weeks.

Pathogenesis

Hookworms are active blood suckers, especially the immature forms, and cause severe anaemia in all animal species. Total worm numbers as low as 100 may cause clinical illness and 2000 may cause death in young cattle. There is a loss of whole blood and hypoproteinaemic oedema may result. Some irritation to the intestinal mucosa is inevitable and mild or intermittent diarrhoea follows. Penetration of the skin by larvae may cause signs of irritation and lead to the introduction of pathogenic bacteria.

In the experimental disease in lambs and kids (2) most deaths occurred 8 to 18 days after percutaneous infection with the principal lesion an acute congestion of the lungs and pneumonia.

Clinical Findings

In mild infestations in stabled cattle fidgeting, stamping and licking of the feet may be observed. Constipation, accompanied by mild abdominal pain, is seen in the early stages and is followed by bouts of diarrhoea. The cattle are unthrifty and anaemic. In severe infestations there is obvious pallor of mucosae, weakness, anasarca under the jaw and along the belly, prostration and death in 2 or 3 days. Signs in sheep are similar to those in cattle. The convalescent period, even after treatment, is prolonged unless the diet is supplemented to stimulate erythrocyte production.

Clinical Pathology

The blunt ends and deeply pigmented embryonic cells of hookworm eggs enable them to be differentiated fairly accurately from the eggs of other strongylid worms. Egg counts of 400 to 500 epg are usually associated with fatal infestations. The adult worms are heavy egg-layers and both they and the immature worms are strong blood suckers. Clinical signs are often evident in the prepatent period before eggs appear in the faeces (3). The presence of severe anaemia and occult blood in the faeces are only contributory evidence but can be used as a measure of the severity of the infestation.

Necropsy Findings

The number of worms present may be quite small. In calves total worm counts of 100 or more suggest a significant level of infestation, counts of over 2000 worms indicate a degree of infestation likely to be fatal. In sheep and goats 24 adult *G. pachyscelis* represent a fatal load. Most of the worms are found in the first few feet of the small intestine and the intestinal contents nearby are often deeply blood stained. Some of the worms may have been washed down into the colon and are likely to be mistaken for *Oesophagostomum* spp.

Diagnosis

Hookworm infestations in young animals may be confused with many diseases in which anaemia, diarrhoea and anasarca occur. Haemonchosis is probably the most similar disease and mixed infestations of these two worms are not uncommon in some countries. Hepatic fascioliasis may also be manifested by a similar clinical picture and the anaemia and diarrhoea of coccidiosis and the anaemia caused by heavy louse infestation may also cause difficulty in diagnosis. A dietary deficiency of cobalt or copper, and chronic molybdenosis should also be considered in the differential diagnosis of bunostomiasis in lambs and calves.

Treatment

Tetramisole (15 mg. per kg. body weight orally) is highly efficient against hookworms in calves.

Neguvon (110 mg. per kg. body weight orally) is also effective against adult and immature *B. phlebotomum* but is not without toxic effects in calves at this dose rate. It is also effective by subcutaneous injection at 60 mg. per kg. body weight (4). Supportive treatment is essential in this disease because of the severe anaemia which occurs. The provision of a mineral mixture containing iron, copper and cobalt is recommended and a general improvement in the quality of the diet, particularly in respect of protein, may shorten the convalescent period.

Control

Wet surroundings, in pastures, in yards and in barns, should be avoided to reduce the chances of percutaneous infestation and reduce the viability of the free-living larvae. Pens should be cleaned frequently and ample bedding provided. Heavy stocking of sheep or calves in small pens should be avoided. Under conditions of heavy risk periodic treatment should be administered. *B. trigonocephalum* is known to occur in Scottish red deer and these animals may provide a source of infestation for sheep grazing the same pasture. The hookworms of cattle and sheep are not host-transferable, and it is often suggested that rotation of the two animal species on a pasture may tend to clear up the infestation.

REFERENCES

(1) Roberts, F. H. S. (1951). *Aust. vet. J.*, 27, 274.
(2) Srivastava, V. K. *et al.* (1969). *Ind. J. Anim. Sci.*, 39, 219, 315, 317.
(3) Soulsby, E. J. L. *et al.* (1955). *Vet. Rec.*, 67, 1124.
(4) Little, R. K. (1964). *Aust. vet. J.*, 40, 402.

Trichostrongylosis, Ostertagiasis, Cooperiasis, Nematodiriasis

(*Scour Worms, Hair Worms*)

Although infestations with these worms *Trichostrongylus* spp., *Ostertagia* spp., *Cooperia* spp., and *Nematodirus* spp. are specific diseases they commonly occur together and, being closely related and inhabiting the abomasum and small intestine, have very similar effects. The disease they cause is characterized by persistent diarrhoea and wasting.

Incidence

These infestations have their major effects in lambs and calves and cause heavy losses, in both deaths and in poor growth, in most countries in temperate regions. Although these worms are probably the most important single cause of losses in lambs and calves in most countries where young ruminants are at pasture all the year, the diagnosis is frequently missed, partly because the disease occurs commonly in association with malnutrition and partly because the worms are not easily seen. It is this association with so-called 'weaner illthrift' in sheep that has attracted so much attention to the economic effects of parasitism and the need to economically assess every treatment programme. As a result emphasis is tending to move away from the effects of treatment on egg and total worm counts and towards the effects of drenching on body weight gains and wool production (1, 2). When experiments of this sort are done the results can be staggering. Gains of 300 per cent total liveweight production and 1000 per cent return on investment are recorded in the treatment of ostertagiasis in calves (3).

The disease in all species is one of pastured animals but there are exceptions to this rule. Nematodiriasis, for example, occurs quite commonly in stabled calves which have never been outside and ostertagiasis has been observed in yearling cattle up to 5 months after they have been removed from the pasture to the barn. A carryover of infestation in indoor pens is quite possible, especially with *Nematodirus* spp., and if calves are fed on the floor severe infestations can occur.

Aetiology

All of these helminths with the exception of *Nematodirus* spp. (1 to 2·5 cm.) are difficult to see in a necropsy specimen. Their anatomical predilection sites are indicated in the table facing.

In most natural infestations a mixture of genera and species is found but in sheep trichostrongylosis is the most important disease; in calves ostertagiasis and, to a less extent, nematodiriasis are more important. Although the same species may occur in both sheep and cattle there appears to be some degree of host specificity and ovine strains of, for example, *T. colubriformis* do not persist in calves. However, *T. axei* of equine origin do develop in lambs and calves and *C. oncophora* and *C. punctata* of cattle develop in sheep.

These worms are predominantly parasites of young animals. In sheep the two age groups most commonly affected are weaner lambs and yearlings. Sheep over 18 months of age are less commonly affected because of immunity resulting from previous infestation and also possibly because of an age effect. Malnutrition and conditions suitable to the development of overwhelming infestations, particularly overcrowding and wet weather in the cooler months of the year, are important predisposing causes.

Anatomical Distribution of Trichostrongylid Worms in Ruminants*

Parasite	Cattle		Sheep and Goats	
	Abomasum	Small Intestine	Abomasum	Small Intestine
Trichostrongylus spp.				
T. axei	×		×	
T. colubriformis, T. longispicularis		×		×
T. falculatus, T. vitrinus, T. capricola, T. rugatus, T. probolurus				×
Ostertagia spp.				
O. ostertagi	×		×	
O. circumcincta,			×	
O. trifurcata			×	
Cooperia spp.				
C. punctata, C. oncophora		×		×
C. pectinata		×		
C. curticei		-		×
Nematodirus spp.				
N. spathiger, N. battus, N. filicollis		×		×
N. helvetianus		×		

* *Trichostrongylus axei* occurs in the stomach of horses.

In all species the disease is of most importance when the plane of nutrition is low but massive infestations can overwhelm well fed animals. Moderate infestations can be borne by animals on good feed while poorly nourished animals may succumb. In weaner lambs it is the reduction of food intake because of weaning which increases the susceptibility while in yearlings in the winter months it is the general reduction in available feed combined with optimum conditions for worm multiplication. In cattle the disease is most common in calves 3 to 6 months of age although it can cause significant illness in animals up to 2 years of age and occasionally in adults.

Climatically trichostrongylosis is favoured by cool, wet weather so that in Australia and South Africa this is a disease of the winter months in those areas where the rainfall occurs chiefly at this time of the year. This state of affairs is subject to variation. If the conditions for worm multiplication are good the effects of the worms may be offset because of a general improvement in nutrition occasioned by the climate. In such circumstances the effects of the worm burden may not be felt until nutrition declines. Thus the clinical disease may not be manifested until the next summer. However, the important fact that does emerge is that strategic dosing to control the worm population must be concentrated in the winter months when the infestation is heaviest. In arid areas the disease is of little significance except in years of unusually heavy precipitation. Although the eggs and larvae of *Trichostrongylus* spp. are resistant to cold they

are not resistant to freezing and in cold climates trichostrongylosis may be more common in the late summer and autumn when rainfall is heavy and temperatures generally cool. However, the disease under these conditions is rarely as severe as in winters in temperate climates. Thus it is much less important in Canada than in Australia. The eggs and larvae of *Ostertagia* and *Nematodirus* spp. are much more resistant to cold and can survive the coldest winter. The larvae of *Cooperia* spp. are less affected by high temperatures and the disease occurs in all seasons in temperate climates.

Life Cycle

The life cycle in all of these genera is direct. The eggs of most species are passed in the faeces and under suitable environmental conditions hatch producing two successive non-parasitic larval stages. A parasitic larva is then produced which, when ingested by the host, sheds its sheath, enters the mucosa, undergoes a third moult and returns to the surface in the abomasum or small intestine where it matures. The eggs of *Nematodirus* spp. do not hatch until the third-stage infective larvae are produced.

The eggs and free-living larvae of most of these species can survive and develop at much lower temperatures than *Haemonchus* and *Oesophagostomum* spp. Upper temperature limits for survival are, however, lower. Although the eggs and larvae of all the worms under discussion can survive through a moderate winter, the bulk of the infective larvae of *Trichostrongylus* spp. disappear even in favourable weather in about a month and the perpetuation of infestation is due largely to carrier animals. This is not so with *Nematodirus* spp., the eggs of which may survive in large numbers on the pasture from one spring to the next.

The behaviour of infective strongyle larvae in pats of cattle manure can have an appreciable effect on persistence of the disease. Pats present in the summer time may remain as a source of larvae for 5 months and in winter for as long as 7 to 8 months. Migration of larvae from pats occurs only when they are moist on the surface and may therefore occur continuously or in waves.

Minimum prepatent periods are quite short; in *Trichostrongylus* spp. infestations in sheep 2 to 3 weeks with maximum egg production 4 weeks later; *T. axei* in the horse 25 days; *O. ostertagi* in calves 3 to 4 weeks; *C. punctata* in calves 12 to 15 days; and *C. oncophora* in this species 17 to 22 days; *Nematodirus spathiger* in sheep 3 to 4 weeks; and *N. helvetianus* in 21 days. However, these periods may be very much longer (4) probably because the host has a degree of immunity from a prior infestation. In this circumstance the development of the larvae is retarded until the animal's resistance is lowered for example by intercurrent disease or nutritional stress (5). One of the most interesting recent developments in the study of parasitic diseases is the proposal that the inhibition of larvae in tissue may be due to factors other than an immune response in the host, and that the 'inhibition' may in fact be due to an innate susceptibility of larvae to such factors as season of the year (6). In fact, the ingestion of a large number of larvae in the autumn appears to be a prerequisite for the development of type 2 ostertagiasis in cattle (7).

There is a good deal of evidence to suggest that 'self-cure' and increased resistance to infestation with these worms occurs in the field. Immune reactions to *T. colubriformis* have been shown to occur in sheep (8) and to *O. ostertagi* in cattle (5) and the level of titratable antibodies influences the number of eggs laid by female worms in subsequent infestations and future contamination of pasture may be reduced by the immune reaction. Although immunity does cause an increased resistance in cattle to infection with *O. ostertagi* the degree of resistance is much less than it is with *Dictyocaulus viviparus* and the chances of producing an effective commercial vaccine are remote (6). There is an increasing resistance in lambs to *N. battus* and *N. spathiger* infestation due solely to increasing age (9). The demonstration that in sheep resistance to this group of worms can be inherited (10) is a major development but determination of its practical significance awaits investigation.

One of the most important considerations in the epidemiology of intestinal parasites in sheep is the post-parturient rise in helminth eggs which occurs in ewes 6 to 8 weeks after lambing (11). Lambs running with these ewes are exposed to heavy infestation when they are in a most susceptible state. If lambing occurs in the spring months, the opportunity for a rapid, massive build-up of helminthiasis is provided.

There are many factors which affect the degree of infection of animals at pasture. Two significant ones of relatively recent recognition are the relationship of speed of new infection (infection rate) and the degree of infection; the same number of larvae ingested in a short period producing a much more severe infection than when they are taken in slowly. There is also a marked 'overcrowding' effect, as the degree of infestation increases the total egg output is reduced (12).

Pathogenesis

Parasitic gastroenteritis of ruminants is currently undergoing intensive study, especially as regards its pathogenesis and clinical pathology. In general terms the effects of the infestation will vary depending on the identity of the parasites and the number and site of their establishment in the host. In cattle these will in turn determine the severity of the damage to the abomasal mucosa. In these animals the principal effects of parasitic gastroenteritis are lack of appetite, a fall in the abomasal acidity and pepsin content (16), and serum albumin levels and rises in plasma pepsinogen levels and, in chronic cases, serum globulin (13). Other characteristics include weight loss, intermittent or continuous diarrhoea and haemoconcentration.

T. axei larvae cause irritation of the abomasal mucosa and other species, especially *Nematodirus* sp., cause damage to the duodenal mucosa. It is presumed that interference with digestion and absorption occurs as a result of damage to abomasal and duodenal mucosae and leads to the loss of condition and eventually scouring which develops only at a relatively late stage in the disease. But it is not only the shorter alimentary tract sojourn which is important in pathogenesis. In chronic infections with *T. colubriformis* in sheep the significant pathogenetic changes which accompany the characteristic decline in food intake and body weight are an initial fall in serum protein due to a decline in serum albumin, although elevation of gamma globulin later restores the serum protein level, anaemia and hypophosphataemia. In acute trichostrongylosis the effects are the same but more severe so that death follows in two to three weeks (14).

The depression of serum protein levels to 4 to 5 g. per 100 ml. is not due to blood loss or liver damage. There is little doubt that the main factor causing this, at least in ostertagiasis, is a continuous loss of protein through the damaged abomasal and intestinal mucosa (15).

Modes of pathogenesis in ostertagiasis. Clinical ostertagiasis manifests itself in several forms depending on which mode of pathogenesis is important in a particular situation. The larvae of *Ostertagia* spp. penetrate the abomasal mucosa and develop in microscopically apparent nodules which are gastric glands. There is severe irritation as a result and oedema follows. This oedema of the submucosa is often so severe that it remains after the larvae have moved on. Emergence of the larvae produces another insult to the mucosa, manifested as mucosal sloughing (46).

The development of two clinical forms of ostertagiasis depends on the behaviour of the invading larvae. If they are uninhibited and pass in, then out of the mucosa and quickly come to lie in the lumen of the gut, the effects are largely those caused by the mature parasites lying in the lumen. This is the type 1 of contemporary literature. However, if the larvae are inhibited and reside semi-permanently in the submucosa the more severe type 2 occurs (6). In type 2 faecal egg counts are variable and usually low and the response to anthelminthics is very poor. The damage to the mucosa which is more severe and of much longer duration in type 2 causes destruction of acid producing glands, with a rise of abomasal pH (6 to 7 as against 2·5 to 4·5) and of pepsin producing cells, so that abomasal pepsin levels fall and plasma/serum pepsinogen levels rise (17). In type 1 ostertagiasis there is an added insult, the blood-sucking capacity of the mature worms which causes a significant but not gross anaemia.

The pathogenesis of trichostrongylosis in calves and lambs is similar especially with respect to the loss of abomasal acidity and its loss of digestive function, the protein loss and the haemoconcentration (18). *T. axei* infestations in horses cause hyperaemia, catarrhal inflammation, necrosis, erosion and chronic proliferative irritation of the mucosa of stomach and duodenum (19). Although the larvae of *Cooperia* and *Nematodirus* spp. have similar behaviour patterns there is only circumstantial evidence that the anaemia, lack of appetite, weight loss and diarrhoea have the same pathogenesis as described above.

Clinical Findings

In all species the onset is insidious and the young animals start to lose weight and fail to grow. They are unthrifty and lack vitality and bloom. If they are observed sufficiently closely their food intake can be seen to be markedly reduced. This may be the full clinical picture in many flocks which are considered to have 'weaner ill-thrift' (16). More severely affected sheep pass dark green, almost black, soft faeces which foul the wool of the breech. Lamb and yearling flocks are most seriously affected and a constant mortality begins, a few animals dying each day. The losses are not acute but may eventually exceed 35 per cent. A rather more dramatic picture may occur with heavy infestations of *Nematodirus* spp. in young lambs, especially those in the 6- to 12-weeks age group. Clinical signs are similar to those described above but deaths may start within 2 days of the first observed illness.

Calves show the same clinical signs as lambs but being kept under closer observation more details of signs are available. The calves lose weight, pass soft manure which eventually becomes very thin and dark green to yellow in colour, develop a long, dry haircoat and become dehydrated with sinking of the eyes in the terminal stages. Until the last they continue to eat although the amount of food taken is much below normal. Gross anaemia is not evident but the mucosae are pale and dry. Submandibular oedema is common, especially in the type 2 disease. The temperature may be elevated (39·5°C or 103°F) and the heart rate increased (120 per minute) in calves showing dehydration. In the terminal stages the calves become so weak and emaciated that they are unable to stand but they may persist in this recumbent state for several weeks if they are provided with a good diet. A characteristic of the disease is that scouring often continues in badly affected calves even though most of the adult worms are removed by treatment. Standard treatments for diarrhoea are also unsuccessful. Although the effects of these worms can be exerted when the burden is heavy and nutrition poor the commonest occurrence is in calves running on very good pasture when nutritional deficiency can hardly be a factor. In the latter circumstances the worm burden itself appears to be the sole aetiological factor, contributed to by overcrowding and optimum conditions for parasite development. Clinical differentiation between types 1 and 2 ostertagiasis in calves is not easy, although the signs generally are more severe in the latter and the prognosis is a great deal poorer. The absence of eggs from the faeces and the poor response to treatment are the diagnostic features of type 2. Although parasitism generally, and ostertagiasis in particular, is a disease principally affecting the young, it can be encountered, especially the type 2 disease, in adults and is relatively common in cattle of 2 to 3 years of age.

In horses *Trichostrongylus* may be present in the stomach in very large numbers, often associated with localized thickening and irritation of the mucosa, but it is impossible to define the signs caused by this infestation because it always occurs concurrently with infestations of other, more pathogenic, strongylid worms.

Clinical Pathology

It has become apparent in recent years that too much dependence has been placed on faecal egg counts as a measure of the severity of an animal's worm burden. Because of the high pathogenicity of larvae which may be inhibited in their development there is often so little relation between egg counts and the bodily condition and worm burden of the host that a critical diagnosis should not be made on egg counts alone (12). A post mortem examination and a total worm count is a more favoured diagnostic test, preferably with a peptic digest of mucosa.

The eggs of *Trichostrongylus, Cooperia* and *Ostertagia*, cannot be readily differentiated by examination of faecal smears or flotation specimens. The eggs of *Nematodirus* spp. are larger than the others and can be detected by even an inexperienced observer. Therefore, it is usual to classify these species as a group and egg counts of individual species cannot be estimated unless faecal cultures are used to determine which worm predominates. Counts of over 1000 epg are usually associated with heavy infestations and obvious clinical illness. *Nematodirus* spp. are the exception in that they are poor egg-layers and severe clinical signs in calves have been associated with egg counts as low as 10 to 40 epg. In lambs counts of 1000 epg of *Nematodirus* spp. are usually associated with fatal infestations (20).

Because of the prevalence of type 2 ostertagiasis it is now routine in diagnostic laboratories to carry out plasma pepsinogen estimations to identify those animals with large populations of inhibited larvae. Levels of plasma pepsinogen in excess of 3000 I.U. are usually considered to be positive results (6, 21, 12). We have come to rely heavily on this test but some doubt has been cast on its accuracy (22). The results of plasma pepsinogen estimations in horses infected with *T. axei* are suggestive but not conclusive (23). Plasma and serum pepsinogen levels in other species, and with other nematodes, are being examined.

Haemoglobin levels are usually in the vicinity of 6 to 8 g. per cent and serum protein levels 4 to 5 g. per cent with a marked reduction in serum albumin levels. Anaemia is more evident in *Cooperia* and *Ostertagia* spp. infestations whereas in trichostrongylosis there may be polycythaemia.

Necropsy Findings

The adult worms are found in the abomasum or small intestine depending on the predilection site of the individual species. A total worm count is the critical measure of the degree of infestation. Counts of less than 500 are considered to be light infestations, counts of over 5000 are heavy but massive counts of over 400,000 in calves and 50,000 in lambs are not uncommon.

Most of these worms are sufficiently small to evade detection by the naked eye. Milking out a loop of intestine and examination of the material in saline in a petrie dish over a black surface makes it possible to see them. A more satisfactory method of demonstrating the worms is to roll a loop of duodenum inside out on a test tube or piece of glass rod and immerse this in aqueous iodine solution (iodine 30 g., potassium iodide 4 g., water 100 ml.) for several minutes and then into a 5 per cent solution of sodium thiosulphate for a few seconds. The mucosa is decolourized but the brown-stained worms retain their colour and are easily seen. This method has been satisfactorily adapted as an efficient, rapid field technique for performing a total worm count.

Gross pathological findings are often not apparent, that is apart from the non-specific lesions of emaciation, dehydration, moderate anaemia and evidence of scouring. The mucosa of the abomasum and upper duodenum may be hyperaemic and swollen in severe cases, and on histological examination, there is a fibrino-catarrhal gastritis. In chronic cases of type 2 ostertagiasis there are diagnostic lesions including a morocco-leather-like appearance of the mucosa with some umbilicated nodules present, epithelial cytolysis and a putrid smell resulting from the growth of bacteria in the lowered acid medium. Estimation of the pH is a worthwhile procedure. Ringworm-like lesions of hyperplastic gastritis have been described in chronic cases of trichostrongylosis in lambs, calves and horses.

Diagnosis

In most outbreaks of gastrointestinal helminthiasis in sheep, and to a less extent in calves, the two factors of malnutrition and parasitism are probably of equal importance and to place undue emphasis on one may lead to neglect of the other when treatment and control programmes are outlined. It is not uncommon to neglect completely the presence of the parasites. However, it is important not to fall into the opposite error, that of diagnosing parasitic gastroenteritis solely on the basis of a faecal egg count. The clinical signs, the age of the animals and the season of the year must be taken into account when assessing the importance of a known level of infestation and the critical test is the degree of response obtained by treatment with the relevant anthelmintic. Other common causes of emaciation and diarrhoea in groups of young animals include secondary copper deficiency in calves and coccidiosis. In adults Johne's disease, secondary copper deficiency again and chronic fascioliasis are the common causes of a similar syndrome.

It is not usual in routine diagnostic work to attempt differentiation between trichostrongylosis, ostertagiasis and cooperiasis, nor is it necessary because treatment and control measures are approximately the same.

Treatment

Thiabendazole has such efficiency in the treatment of this disease that the performance of all drugs is usually measured in terms of comparison with thiabendazole. A large number of drugs are currently available. The earliest and as yet most significant contender for popularity with thiabendazole is laevamisole, which replaced tetramisole and thus avoided the mild toxicity of that compound. Laevamisole has two outstanding virtues: it can be administered parenterally and it is highly effective against intestinal nematodes and lungworms. Apart from these superiorities, and they are significant ones, there is very little to choose between the following compounds. They have approximately the same efficiency through the length of the alimentary tract (24, 25, 26). Dose rates and other pharmacological data are available from the manufacturers and are not duplicated here.

The range of effective drugs includes methyridine (27), the benzimidazoles, thiabenzole (20, 28), parbendazole (29, 30, 31), laevamisole (32, 33, 44) and cambendazole (34, 35); to provide a wider spectrum of activity thiabendazole is also used as a combination with oxyclozanide which has high efficiency over gastrointestinal worms, lungworms and liver fluke (36). The pyrimidine group of anthelminthics includes morantrel (37, 38) and

pyrantrel (39, 40) both of which are efficient; morantrel is marketed as a combination with diethylcarbamazine to provide a mixture effective against intestinal worms and lungworms (41). The organophosphates such as coumaphos and naphthalophos are in general too narrow in their spectrum, with comparative inefficiencies against *Nematodirus* and lower bowel inhabitants, to be recommended.

The choice of which drug to use will depend on price, safety, ease of administration and spectrum of activity. The comparison of the relative efficiencies of the drugs in improving rate of gain over controls is becoming a more commonly used criterion of efficiency than the effect on egg counts or worm populations (42). Because of modern intensification of cattle raising and the need to cut down labour costs, anthelminthics for cattle which can be given by injection or in the feed are more popular than preparations for drenching by mouth. Pellets medicated with laevamisole have been shown to be highly effective (49) and many other similar preparations are available. In this respect it is perhaps wise to give some consideration to the possibility of resistance to an anthelminthic developing when it is used frequently. Resistance of *Tr. colubriformis* to the benzimidazoles is recorded (43) but there are few other reports in the literature.

In ostertagiasis in calves it is important to remember that a single treatment in cases of type 2 ostertagiasis will have very little effect and multiple treatments will be necessary to catch the emerging larvae as they mature (44).

Irrespective of the treatment used it is imperative that the importance of removing the animals from the infested pasture be realized. It may be necessary to use a barn or drylot when suitable fields are not available. The use of such confined areas has an additional advantage; a good balanced ration can be fed in suitable amounts without the need for exercise by the sick animals. The feeding of dried brewer's yeast has been recommended as a means of stimulating the appetite, a major problem in these parasitoses. A mineral supplement containing iron, copper and cobalt should also be provided preferably combined with bonemeal or other source of calcium and phosphorus. Rumen transplants and blood transfusions may hasten recovery and are justifiable in valuable animals. These measures are more likely to be implemented in cattle than in sheep and are particularly important in severe cases of ostertagiasis in calves, in which total removal of the worm burden by an anthelminthic may not effect clinical improvement. They are also of value in building up the strength of the patient before it is treated with a full dose of the anthelminthic. This is probably most important when phenothiazine is to be used: severely parasitized animals succumb rather readily to full doses of this drug.

Control

The general principles of the control of helminthoses have been dealt with in the introductory part of this chapter. Specific recommendations for the control of trichostrongylosis, cooperiasis, ostertagiasis and nematodiriasis are difficult to make because of the wide variety of conditions in which the different diseases occur.

The first and most important step is to improve the nutritional status. This is particularly important in trichostrongylosis in sheep. Calves are more likely to be afflicted with ostertagiasis on an overcrowded, lush pasture but infestation with all of these worms can occur in the late autumn months when the feed supply is failing badly and in these circumstances bringing the animals indoors and providing a balanced diet is recommended. The provision of a diet sufficiently high in protein, minerals and vitamins is essential and specific deficiencies particularly cobalt, copper and phosphorus should be made good.

The second important step is to provide worm-free pasture. Although infested pastures may retain viable *Trichostrongylus* spp. larvae for periods of up to a year, the numbers are probably not highly significant after a month in average weather and the chances for reinfestation are small. This is not so in *Nematodirus* spp. infestations in which the carry-over from spring to spring may be very heavy. It is necessary when dealing with this worm to avoid putting lambs onto pasture in the spring which was grazed by lambs during the previous spring. Inter-species transmission of these worms occurs with some worms and not with others and because of the incompleteness of the information available, it is probably safest not to depend on alternating cattle and sheep on pastures to clean up the infestation unless adult animals are used. Rotational grazing has been recommended as a control measure but the desirability of the procedure in many circumstances is open to doubt. Light infestations in animals on good feed do no harm and probably enhance immunity so that set-stocking has its advantages. However, if the animals are overcrowded and climatic conditions favour rapid multiplication of the worms, animals running on the one field continuously can be overcome by sheer weight of numbers of worms. Rotational grazing after treatment may reduce the immune status

of the animals but at least will avoid an unsuspected sudden outbreak of severe parasitism.

Step 3 in a control programme is the strategic dosing with a suitable anthelminthic. In areas where the disease is a problem sheep up to 1 year old running at pasture during winter should be drenched at intervals of 4 to 6 weeks, depending on weather conditions, from autumn till spring. Some economy can be effected when multiple drenchings are necessary by using the expensive, highly efficient drugs, such as thiabendazole, for the important treatments and the less expensive drugs, such as Rametin-H or phenothiazine, for the others. In less dangerous situations it is possible to do with less treatments. The two danger periods are those of the 'post-parturient rise' in egg production and the period immediately after weaning. Drenching of the ewes four weeks after the commencement of lambing is adequate to control the former (11) and drenching on the day of weaning is recommended for the latter (45). Sheep that are housed in the winter should be drenched when they go into the barn and again 3 weeks later. After drenching sheep should be put onto a rested field. Thiabendazole has an advantage in this respect in that it is markedly ovicidal and droppings passed eight hours after drenching will not infest pasture (20). Because of the special longevity of the larvae of *Nematodirus* spp. control of this worm depends largely on reducing the degree of contamination of the pasture. For lambs three treatments at 3-weekly intervals are recommended for this purpose (46). The importance of a massive hatching of over-wintered *N. battus* larvae in the spring is so great that techniques have been devised to predict danger periods of infestation depending on soil temperatures (47).

A suitable strategic programme for calves and ostertagiasis is less well defined. If clean pasture is available the task is relatively simple; weaned calves can be treated once in early summer and be put immediately onto the sterile pasture. The average dairy farmer's procedure of running calves at pasture in small fields increases the chances of infestation greatly and while they are on such fields they should probably be treated at 3 months of age and then at intervals which may be as short as one month until they are turned out onto clean country or are housed. One of the advantages of a mixed sheep/cattle economy is that fields grazed by sheep are effectively clean as far as cattle are concerned.

Calves running at pasture in areas where the disease is common would probably profit by periodic treatments during the danger season. Nematodiriasis in housed calves can be reduced by raising troughs well off the floor to avoid contamination of feed and water and keeping the pens well bedded. Continuous low-level administration of phenothiazine as a control measure is discussed under haemonchosis (p. 645).

REFERENCES

(1) Banks, A. W. et al. (1966). Aust. vet. J., 42, 116.
(2) Brunsdon, R. V. (1966). N.Z. vet. J., 14, 77.
(3) Brunsdon, R. V. (1968). N.Z. vet. J., 16, 176.
(4) Anderson, N. et al. (1965). Vet. Rec., 77, 1196.
(5) Ross, J. G. (1965). Vet. Rec., 77, 16.
(6) Armour, J. (1970). Vet. Rec., 86, 184.
(7) Jennings, F. W. et al. (1967). Parasitology, 57, 20P.
(8) Stewart, D. F. & Gordon, M. McL. (1958). Nature (Lond.), 181, 921.
(9) Gibson, T. E. & Everett, G. (1963). Brit. vet. J., 119, 214.
(10) Scrivner, L. H. (1964). J. Amer. vet. med. Ass., 144, 1024.
(11) Brunsdon, R. V. (1966). N.Z. vet. J., 14, 118.
(12) Brunsdon, R. V. (1969). N.Z. vet. J., 17, 161.
(13) Ross, J. G. et al. (1969). Res. vet. Sci., 10, 133, 142.
(14) Horak, I. G. et al. (1968). Onderstepoort J. vet. Res., 35, 195.
(15) Neilsen, K. (1966). Gastrointestinal Protein Loss in Cattle, p. 148. Copenhagen: Carl Fr. Mortensen.
(16) Ritchie, J. D. S. et al. (1966). Amer. J. vet. Res., 27, 659.
(17) Murray, M. et al. (1970). Res. vet. Sci., 11, 417.
(18) Ross, J. G. et al. (1970). Brit. vet. J., 126, 149, 159.
(19) Leland, S. E. et al. (1961). Amer. J. vet. Res., 22, 128.
(20) Gordon, H. McL. (1964). Aust. vet. J., 40, 9.
(21) Allen, W. M. et al. (1970). J. comp. Path., 80, 441.
(22) Mylrea, P. J. & Hotson, I. K. (1969). Brit. vet. J., 125, 379.
(23) Waddell, A. H. & McCosker, P. J. (1969). Aust. vet. J., 45, 360.
(24) Kates, K. C. (1971). J. Parasit., 57, 356.
(25) Arundel, J. H. (1967). Aust. vet. J., 43, 455.
(26) Colglazier, M. L. et al. (1971). Proc. helminth. Soc. Wash., 38, 203.
(27) Walley, J. K. (1962). Vet. Rec., 74, 927.
(28) Armour, J. et al. (1967). Vet. Rec., 80, 510.
(29) Ross, D. B. (1970). Vet. Rec., 86, 60.
(30) Rubin, R. (1969). J. Amer. vet. med. Ass., 154, 177.
(31) Johns, D. R. & Mendel, G. J. (1969). Aust. vet. J., 45, 460.
(32) Forsyth, B. A. (1968). Aust. vet. J., 44, 185.
(33) Lyons, E. T. et al. (1972). Amer. J. vet. Res., 33, 65.
(34) Benz, G. W. (1971). Amer. J. vet. Res., 32, 399.
(35) Baker, N. F. & Walters, G. T. (1971). Amer. J. vet. Res., 32, 29.
(36) Walley, J. K. (1970). Vet. Rec., 86, 222.
(37) Cornwell, R. L. & Jones, R. M. (1970). Brit. vet. J., 126, 134, 142.
(38) Cornwell, R. L. & Jones, R. M. (1970). Vet. Rec., 86, 430, 465.
(39) Cornwell, R. L. (1966). Vet. Rec., 79, 590, 626, 723; 80, 434, 676.
(40) Gibson, T. E. et al. (1969). Res. vet. Sci., 10, 307.
(41) Cornwell, R. L. et al. (1972). Vet. Rec., 90, 123.
(42) Cornwell, R. L. et al. (1971). Vet. Rec., 89, 352.
(43) Hotson, I. K. et al. (1970). Aust. vet. J., 46, 356.
(44) Reid, J. F. S. et al. (1968). Vet. Rec., 83, 14.
(45) Gibson, T. E. & Everett, G. (1968). J. comp. Path., 78, 427.
(46) Gibson, T. E. (1964). Vet. Rec., 76, 295.
(47) Smith, L. P. & Thomas, R. J. (1972). Vet. Rec., 90, 388.
(48) Brunsdon, R. V. (1966). Proc. N.Z. Soc. Anim. Prod., 26, 165.
(49) Presidente, P. J. A. et al. (1971). Amer. J. vet. Res., 32, 1359.

Haemonchosis

(Barber's Pole Worm)

Haemonchosis is a serious parasitosis in sheep, cattle and goats during the summer months in most countries. It is characterized clinically by severe anaemia and anasarca.

Incidence

Haemonchosis is an important disease of sheep and cattle wherever they are kept but the disease exerts its greatest economic effect in sheep in temperate and tropical countries especially where there is a good summer rainfall. It is not uncommon for serious outbreaks to occur in colder climates such as those of Canada and the United States when humidity is high in summer. The disease is uncommon in semi-arid regions. Haemonchosis causes heavy death losses and poor growth and production. In sheep, losses occur mostly in lambs, especially those recently weaned, but yearlings and mature sheep may also be affected. Poor growth in lambs results when their ewes' milk production is restricted by a heavy infestation. Dairy calves are the most commonly affected group amongst cattle but steers and other young cattle up to 3 years of age may also be affected.

Aetiology

Sheep, cattle and goats are affected by haemonchosis in that order of frequency. *Haemonchus contortus* is the species most commonly found in sheep and goats. It inhabits the abomasum and is easily seen, being 1 to 2·5 cm. long and relatively thick. Adult males are homogeneously red, the females are a spiral red and white. *H. placei* also develops well in sheep and causes clinical haemonchosis but of less severity than that caused by *H. contortus*. *H. placei* is the usual *Haemonchus* spp. in cattle, and also inhabits the abomasum. *H. contortus* may also be present but usually only when the cattle are grazing the same pasture as sheep or goats. The infestations are usually not as heavy and are eliminated sooner than *H. placei* infestations. Infestations with *Mecistocirrus digitatus* occur in the Orient and in Central America. Adults of this species inhabit the abomasum of sheep, cattle and buffalo and cause a disease very similar to haemonchosis.

Haemonchosis is for the most part a primary parasitosis, predisposing causes for infestation including overcrowding, lush pasture and hot, humid climatic conditions. However, development of clinical illness is favoured by a fall in the plane of nutrition particularly in calves. This infestation can occur in several ways. Lambs in excellent condition and running on the very best pasture may be suddenly overcome by a massive infestation. In sheep this is by far the most important occurrence of the disease but sheep in poor condition may become clinically affected by a worm burden which would not bother a fat sheep. Under excellent nutritional conditions cattle may develop a subclinical infestation but when the pasture subsequently fails the disease appears.

The importance of diet as a predisposing cause has been debated but there is good evidence that a ration very low (less than 3 per cent) in protein makes sheep and calves much more susceptible to heavy infestation than a normal diet; the worms become established more readily and persist for longer periods. Diets as low as this in protein are commonly encountered in range sheep and cattle. Sudden depression of the protein content of the diet can cause a serious fall of resistance in an animal and permit progression of a latent infestation. This may be why the epizootiology in calves differs somewhat from that in sheep, heavy infestations occurring in summer but clinical signs not appearing until winter when the plane of nutrition declines. The cobalt status of sheep is also important in haemonchosis, animals on a cobalt-deficient diet being much less susceptible to the effects of infestation with *H. contortus* (1). Hay-free rations have been shown to inhibit fertile egg production, the inhibition being overcome by the addition of 5 per cent alfalfa (2).

A great deal of effort has been devoted to determining the conditions in which haemonchosis occurs in sheep so that outbreaks can be predicted and preventive measures taken. The production of climatographs for geographical areas has been undertaken and makes such predictions possible. Months which have mean temperatures of over 18°C (64°F) and rainfall of over 5·25 cm. are months in which the disease is likely to occur. Thus in wet summers the disease may continue unchecked whereas in drier years there may be a peak of incidence in early summer and another in autumn.

Development of a strong sensitivity reaction to *H. contortus* has been demonstrated in sheep and 'self-cure' occurs under natural conditions. Circulating antibodies are detectable by a complement-fixation test in recovered sheep. The antigenic substances appear to be derived from the third- or fourth- and fifth-stage larvae and it is the latter group which is most susceptible to the immune reaction (3). Titrable antibodies do not appear to develop in the serum of calves infested with *H. placei* nor does complete 'self-cure' occur but after an initial infestation there is a rapid decline in egg-laying power, and the development of resistance to the worm is indicated by rapid expulsion of adults and retardation of development of larvae. How significant immunity to *H. contortus* is in limiting infections under natural conditions is not known but it has been shown that prolonged, uninterrupted infection is followed by strong resistance (4, 5).

Life Cycle

As in other trichostrongylid worms the life cycle is direct, infestation of the host occurring by the ingestion of food contaminated by infective larvae. Adult *H. contortus* are prolific egg-layers, individual females laying up to 10,000 eggs per day for several months and under optimum climatic conditions gross contamination of the pasture can occur in a very short time. Eggs passed in the faeces hatch under optimum conditions and pass through two non-infective larval stages before developing into the third-stage infective larva about 4 days after hatching. In a less suitable environment the period required for development through these stages may be prolonged and this may affect control procedures generally recommended. For example, in Scotland the shortest period required for development from egg to third-stage larva is 2 weeks and may be a great deal longer. Preinfective larvae are susceptible to desiccation but not to freezing and the infective larvae are resistant to both. After ingestion the larvae grow to maturity in the abomasum and commence egg-laying in about 18 days but egg production is not heavy until the 25th to 30th day. The ingested third-stage larvae migrate into the abomasal mucosa and develop into fourth-stage larvae. Adult *Haemonchus* spp. attach themselves to the abomasal mucosa. The life cycle of *H. placei* is similar except that in cattle the first eggs do not appear in the faeces until the 26th day after infestation, rising to a peak at 6 to 7 weeks and declining rapidly to low levels by the 11th to 14th week (6).

Pathogenesis

Both fourth-stage larvae and adults are vigorous blood suckers and by passing large amounts of the host's blood through their alimentary tracts cause loss of all blood components including erythrocytes and plasma protein. Anaemia and hypoproteinaemia result. There is no evidence that any factor other than simple blood loss causes the anaemia, although intravascular haemolysis and depression of bone marrow activity have both been suggested as accessory causes. The migration of the larvae into the pits of the gastric glands in the abomasal wall and the physical injury caused to the mucosa by the attachment of adults cause abomasitis. The presence of *H. contortus* in the abomasum appears to interfere with the digestibility and absorption of protein, calcium and phosphorus but whether this is due to the damage to the mucosa and its digestive function by the worms or to the effects of toxic principles elaborated by the worms has not been determined. There is a significant rise of abomasal pH soon after infection due to loss of gastric acidity and plasma pepsinogen levels rise at the same time (7).

Clinical Findings

Lambs and young sheep are commonly affected by the acute form of the disease in which animals are found dead without premonitory signs having been observed. The mucosae and conjunctivae of such sheep are always extremely pale. More chronic cases show lethargy and muscular weakness, pallor of the mucosae and conjunctivae, and anasarca, particularly under the lower jaw and to a less extent along the ventral abdomen. Affected sheep are often noticed for the first time when the flock are being driven; they lag behind, breathe faster, have a staggery gait and often go down; some may die as a result of exercise but most can rise and walk a little further after rest. Grazing animals lie down a good deal of the time, often around the water troughs, the energy needed to walk and eat appears to be lacking. Most cases show constipation rather than diarrhoea. There is a loss of body weight but this may not be noticeable. Sheep not fatally affected develop a break in the wool and the fleece may be lost at a later date. Calves show a similar syndrome.

Clinical Pathology

Eggs of *Haemonchus* spp. cannot be easily differentiated from those of *Oesophagostomum* spp., *Trichostrongylus* spp., *Ostertagia* spp., and *Cooperia* spp., and identification and quantification depends on counting larvae in faecal cultures, a procedure not readily applicable in routine diagnosis. Although egg counts of the above worms in the range of 500 epg in cattle and 5000 epg in sheep are considered to be pathogenic, it must be remembered that low counts of eggs may be encountered in gross haemonchosis when the bulk of the pathogenic worms are in the larval stage.

Severe infestations, usually mixed, are accompanied by egg counts of about 10,000 epg.

Necropsy Findings

Gross necropsy findings include severe anaemia, gelatinization of fat depots, general anasarca and the presence of large numbers of readily visible *H. contortus* or *H. placei* in the abomasum. If the cadaver is fresh the worms may still be attached or swimming actively in the ingesta but a careful search may be necessary if the animal has been dead for some time. Total counts of up to 500 worms may cause no illness in fat sheep but 1000 mature worms are considered to be a heavy infestation. Counts of 3000 in lambs and 9000 in adult sheep are usually associated with heavy mortalities. The abomasal wall is hyperaemic and blood clots may be present in the mucosa where larvae have migrated. Small ulcerations may be present where adult worms have been attached. The abomasal contents usually have a distinct brownish colour due to the presence of free blood.

Diagnosis

In sheep other causes of sudden death, such as lightning stroke, snake-bite, anthrax or enterotoxaemia are often suggested by the farmer and can only be differentiated by necropsy. The other common causes of acute anaemia in sheep include coccidiosis, in which diarrhoea and dysentery are usually present, and acute hepatic fascioliasis in which hepatic damage is characteristic. Less acute cases have to be differentiated from nutritional deficiencies of copper and cobalt and chronic hepatic fascioliasis in which anasarca is more evident than anaemia. Other parasitic infestations, particularly trichostrongylosis, are characterized by diarrhoea rather than anaemia but infestations with *Haemonchus* spp. and *Oesophagostomum* spp. commonly coexist and the soft manure caused by the latter infestation may be confusing.

In calves, coccidiosis, heavy infestations with *Bunostomum* spp., and sucking lice, haemolytic anaemia caused by drinking large quantities of cold water, the ingestion of rape, kale and chou moellier, bacillary haemoglobinuria, leptospirosis, babesiasis and anaplasmosis are characterized by acute anaemia.

Treatment

Many drugs are effective in sheep including phenothiazine, carbon tetrachloride, the organic phosphates, thiabendazole, laevamisole (8, 9) and parbendazole (10, 11), and a final selection will probably depend on criteria such as cost and the presence of other parasites, e.g. liver fluke, to be included in the objectives of the drenching programme. Copper sulphate-nicotine sulphate mixtures are relatively efficient and are still sometimes used for routine treatments. Copper sulphate–arsenic–nicotine sulphate mixtures are similarly used for their broad-spectrum efficiency but their safety margin is too narrow for general use (12). Methyridine and the bephenium compounds are erratic and are not recommended. Several organic phosphates are being used at a single dose level for all body weights, older sheep getting proportionately less but still sufficient to control haemonchosis and lighter sheep getting a high dose rate per kg. body weight which controls a wider range of parasites. The relative inefficiency of the organophosphates against parasites resident in the large bowel limits their use (13) but if *H. contortus* is the only target the relative cheapness of these compounds is in their favour. Clioxanide and rafoxanide are efficient fasciolicides and are also effective as oral treatments for haemonchosis (14, 15) but have limited efficiency against *Trichostrongylus* spp. (9). Clioxanide has a further limitation; it is much less effective against *H. contortus*, as it is against *F. hepatica*, when it enters the abomasum directly, instead of entering the rumen (16). To overcome the inefficiency of haloxon against *Oesophagostomum columbianum* when it occurs together with *H. contortus*, the compound has been effectively mixed with piperazine (12).

Because of the practical difficulty of treating large numbers of beef calves by drenching an injectable anthelmintic is sought. Neguvon, 15 mg. per kg. body weight, is effective against *H. placei* by subcutaneous injection (17). Laevamisole is similarly effective and has a much wider spectrum of efficiency. Methyridine is too erratic against *Haemonchus* spp.

Some strains of *H. contortus* now show a degree of resistance to thiabendazole and parbendazole but not to the point that it seriously interferes with their use (18).

Control

Apart from the general recommendations for control of parasitic gastroenteritis as set out in the first part of this chapter, especially as they apply to the epizootiology of this disease, the important control measure in haemonchosis is strategic dosing to keep the worm population at a minimum combined with rotation of pastures.

In sheep flocks strategic dosings are carried out in the spring and autumn with a varying number of treatments in the summer. For these treatments

phenothiazine in standard therapeutic doses is effective but copper sulphate-nicotine sulphate, copper sulphate-arsenic and, where *Oe. columbianum* is a problem, copper sulphate-piperazine mixtures are commonly used in sheep because of their reduced cost. Organic phosphates at low dose rates are also used for the same reason. Alternation of treatments is recommended, the most common method being to dose with phenothiazine for the spring and autumn treatments and the cheaper remedies for the remainder. The number and frequency of summer treatments varies with the climate. In areas of moderate infestation two treatments are often satisfactory but in bad areas treatment every 3 to 4 weeks is commonly practised. In very bad years this may be increased to treating every 10 days. If phenothiazine is used the intervals can be longer because of its greater efficiency against immature worms. As a general guide it can be assumed that drenching will be necessary about 3 weeks after every summer rainfall of 1·25 cm. especially if the weather is overcast and humid. Repeat treatments can be relaxed in dry weather and when cold weather begins. After each treatment the animals should be turned onto pasture which has been rested for at least 6 weeks.

Although a number of investigations have been conducted on the efficiency of vaccination against *H. contortus* with X-irradiated larvae, the method has not achieved any practical utilization.

REFERENCES

(1) Downey, N. E. (1965). *Brit. vet. J.*, *121*, 362.
(2) Theuer, R. C. *et al.* (1965). *Amer. J. vet. Res.*, *26*, 123.
(3) Ross, J. G. (1963). *J. Helminth.*, *37*, 359.
(4) Silverman, P. H. *et al.* (1970). *Amer. J. vet. Res.*, *31*, 841.
(5) Donald, A. D. *et al.* (1969). *Parasitology*, *59*, 497.
(6) Roberts, F. H. S. (1957). *Aust. J. agric. Res.*, *8*, 740.
(7) Coop, R. L. (1971). *J. comp. Path.*, *81*, 213.
(8) Lyons, E. T. *et al.* (1972). *Amer. J. vet. Res.*, *33*, 65.
(9) Colglazier, M. L. *et al.* (1971). *Proc. helminth. Soc. Wash.*, *38*, 203.
(10) Bennett, D. G. (1968). *Amer. J. vet. Res.*, *29*, 2325.
(11) Gibson, T. E. & Parfitt, J. W. (1968). *Brit. vet. J.*, *124*, 69.
(12) Kingsbury, P. A. & Heffer, B. (1967). *Aust. vet. J.*, *43*, 171.
(13) Kingsbury, P. A. & Curr, C. (1967). *Aust. vet. J.*, *43*, 166.
(14) Pearson, I. G. *et al.* (1970). *Aust. vet. J.*, *46*, 480.
(15) Campbell, N. J. & Hotson, I. K. (1971). *Aust. vet. J.*, *47*, 5.
(16) Symons, L. E. A. & Roseby, F. B. (1969). *Aust. vet. J.*, *45*, 385.
(17) Keith, R. K. (1963). *Aust. vet. J.*, *39*, 264.
(18) Theodorides, V. J. *et al.* (1970). *Amer. J. vet. Res.*, *31*, 859.

Parasitic Gastritis of Pigs

Parasitic gastritis of pigs is recorded commonly but clinical illness appears to be the exception rather than the rule. Sporadic death losses occur and poor growth and anaemia have been observed occasionally.

Incidence

Most countries of the world report the occurrence of the causative nematodes but in only rare instances are death losses or poor growth recorded.

Aetiology

Hyostrongylus rubidus occurs in most countries where pigs are kept; *Ollulanus tricuspis* is seldom recorded; *Ascarops strongylina, A. dentata*, and *Physocephalus sexalatus*, occur in pigs in the United States, the Malayan peninsula, the East Indies and Australia; *Simondsia paradoxa* occurs in Europe and India. *Hyostrongylus rubidus* is a small (0·5 to 1·25 cm.) thin, red worm, and *Ascarops*, *Physocephalus* and *Simondsia* spp. are thick white worms 1 to 2·5 cm. long. Young pigs are most susceptible but adult sows especially when lactating may also be affected. Although among farm animals pigs are the only common host for these worms, *H. rubidus* has been propagated in a calf and the larvae of this worm have been found in the intestinal wall of the kid and rabbit and of domestic birds. Encapsulated larvae of *P. sexalatus* have been found in the intestinal wall of fowls, ducks and geese. In some birds they were present in very large numbers. It is possible that such larvae could complete their life cycles in pigs fed on the intestines of infected birds.

Life Cycles

H. rubidus has a direct life cycle similar to that of most strongylid worms, infective larvae, which are quite susceptible to desiccation and cooling, developing 7 days after hatching. Infestation occurs by ingestion of the infective larvae, and the first eggs appear 20 to 25 days later. *Ascarops* spp. and *Physocephalus* spp. have indirect life cycles; eggs passed in the faeces of the pig are eaten by dung beetles in which hatching and development to infective larvae occur. Infestation of the final host occurs when they eat infested beetles.

A post-parturient rise in egg count, similar to the one encountered in sheep, has been suggested in pigs (1) but is not always evident (2).

Pathogenesis

All of these worms burrow into the gastric mucosa and cause some irritation but there is little evidence of clinical illness unless the resistance of the animal is reduced by poor nutrition or other diseases. Even then infestations, with the exception of *H. rubidus*, are usually quite light. *H. rubidus*, having a direct life cycle, may be present in very large numbers and, besides burrowing into the gastric mucosa and causing ulceration and nodules, may suck large amounts of blood. Its effect on young pigs may not be clinically apparent and the contribution the parasite makes to the 'thin-sow syndrome' still needs to be clarified. Perhaps in combination with *Oesophagostomum quadrispiculatum* it may have such an effect (3). Massive infestations produced experimentally in young pigs have caused fever, listlessness, lack of appetite, diarrhoea, and a reduced weight gain (5) but smaller infestations are without apparent effect (6).

Clinical Findings

Young pigs infested with *H. rubidus* may show anaemia, unthriftiness, poor growth and diarrhoea (4). The appetite is poor but there is marked thirst. In adult sows there is emaciation, pallor due to anaemia and often a depraved appetite. Poor reproductive performance often results and if the disease is not controlled, unnecessary heavy culling may result (7). Adult sows may carry heavy infestations without clinical illness but sudden death due to haemorrhage from gastric ulcers or to peritonitis by ulcerative perforation has been observed (4, 8).

As discussed under pathogenesis there are doubts about the practical importance of *H. rubidus* infections and the clinical pictures described above may subsequently need to be modified.

Clinical Pathology

The eggs of *H. rubidus* are typical strongylid eggs and in the pig are indistinguishable from those of *Oesophagostomum* spp.; those of *Physocephalus* and *Ascarops* spp. are small and thick shelled, and contain larvae when laid. Examination of larvae which develop in faecal cultures may enable an ante-mortem diagnosis of hyostrongylosis to be made. The differentiation is important as the two worms commonly occur together in nature but have different egg-laying capacities and susceptibilities to anthelminthics. Faecal counts of 300 to 1200 epg are recorded in *H. rubidus* infestations in adults and counts greater than 500 epg must be considered significant.

In spite of the pallor observed clinically in adult infested sows, there is no evidence of anaemia in experimentally infected young pigs (6).

Necropsy Findings

Adult *Physocephalus, Ascarops* and *Simondsia* spp. are readily visible but careful examination of a mucosal scraping mixed with water and held against a black background may be necessary to find *H. rubidus*. There may be several thousand of the latter worms present in the one pig. In moderate cases there is hyperaemia of the mucosa which is covered with an excess of thick mucus beneath which the worms lie. In severe cases the mucosa may be thickened and oedematous and covered with a diphtheritic pseudomembrane. Deep, extensive ulcers may also be present.

Diagnosis

The clinical picture of unthriftiness, weakness, emaciation and anaemia of young pigs may also be the result of vibrionic dysentery, necrotic enteritis caused by *Salmonella* spp., coccidiosis, infestation with *Oe. dentatum* and malnutrition. A satisfactory definitive diagnosis can only be made on a necropsy specimen.

Treatment

Thiabendazole is recommended at a dose rate of 50 mg. per kg. (2, 7); haloxon is considered to be moderately effective (9); and laevamisole (15 mg. per kg.) includes *H. rubidus* in its broad spectrum of efficiency (10). Dichlorvos in the feed is effective (11).

Control

Standard hygienic precautions including frequent removal of manure, the provision of drainage in outside pens and rotation of pastures will reduce environmental contamination. Control of dung beetles, the intermediate hosts of *Physocephalus* and *Ascarops* spp. is impracticable.

To avoid the effects of the post-parturient rise on young and old the pigs should be housed on concrete with an absence of deep litter and the frequent removal of manure (1, 7).

The sows should be treated just before farrowing and if the post-parturient rise is likely to be high, again one or two weeks afterwards. In the young pigs effective control is reported by the feeding of thiabendazole continuously and at a low level of 0·05 per cent from 3 to 8 weeks of age and then 0·01 per cent from 8 weeks until sale (12).

REFERENCES

(1) Connan, R. M. (1967). *Vet. Rec.*, *80*, 424.
(2) Thomas, R. J. & Smith, W. C. (1968). *Vet. Rec.*, *83*, 489.
(3) Baskerville, A. & Ross, J. G. (1970). *Brit. vet. J.*, *126*, 538.
(4) Dodd, D. C. (1960). *N.Z. vet. J.*, *8*, 100.
(5) Castelino, J. B. *et al.* (1970). *Brit. vet. J.*, *126*, 579.
(6) Lean, I. J. *et al.* (1972). *Brit. vet. J.*, *128*, 138, 147.
(7) Davidson, J. B. *et al.* (1968). *Vet. Rec.*, *83*, 582.
(8) Mouwen, J. M. V. M. *et al.* (1968). *T. Diergeneesk.*, *93*, 211.
(9) Czipri, D. A. (1970). *Vet. Rec.*, *86*, 306.
(10) Walley, J. K. (1967). *Vet. Rec.*, *81*, 617.
(11) Jacobs, D. E. (1968). *Vet. Rec.*, *83*, 160.
(12) Taffs, L. F. & Davidson, J. B. (1967). *Vet. Rec.*, *81*, 426.

Habronemiasis

(*Summer Sores, Swamp Cancer, Bursattee*)

Infestation of skin wounds of horses by larvae of *Habronema* spp. causes the formation of extensive granulation tissue. Infestation of the gastric mucosa causes gastritis and the development of suppurative granulomas in the stomach. Invasion of the conjunctiva may lead to the development of a granular conjunctivitis.

Incidence

These worms have a world wide distribution but are of importance only in warmer climates and especially in wetter areas where the intermediate hosts are common.

Gastric habronemiasis is relatively common and although it may cause sporadic deaths most affected horses show no signs of illness. Cutaneous and conjunctival habronemiasis are rarely fatal but may cause considerable inconvenience.

Aetiology

There are three genera, *Habronema muscae*, *H. microstoma* and *H. (Draschia) megastoma*, all of which infest the stomach of horses. Adults of the first two genera are larger (1 to 2·5 cm.); those of *H. megastoma* rarely exceed 1·25 cm. in length. Gastric granulomas and most cutaneous lesions appear to be caused by *H. megastoma* although typical cutaneous lesions do occur naturally and have been produced experimentally in horses by the cutaneous implantation of *H. muscae* or *H. microstoma* larvae (1). Horses of all ages are susceptible but the disease is most common in adults.

Life Cycle

The life cycle is indirect, all three genera passing their intermediate stages in flies. *H. muscae* and *H. megastoma* in the house fly (*Musca domestica*) and numerous bush and blowflies, and *H. microstoma* in the stable fly (*Stomoxys calcitrans*). The larvae are passed in the manure, there to invade the larval maggots of the respective host which breeds in horse manure. In the maggot they develop and reach the infective stage in the pupal stage of the fly. The larvae may be ingested if dead flies are present in water or feed, or may pass from the fly through its proboscis when it feeds on the lips or on wounds of the horse. Larvae that are swallowed reach maturity in the stomach, those deposited in wounds cause cutaneous habronemiasis. Although occasional stray larvae are known to migrate widely in the animal body there are several records of massive invasion of, for example, lungs (2).

Pathogenesis

Gastric habronemiasis. The larvae of *H. megastoma* invade the gastric mucosa and cause the development of large granulomatous masses. These large cauliflower-shaped 'tumours' are perforated by sinuses which open into the gastric lumen and contain adult worms. In many horses the lesions cause only a mild, chronic gastritis. In rare cases ulceration is followed by perforation with the development of local peritonitis which may involve the intestine causing constriction, or the spleen causing splenic abscess. *H. microstoma* and *H. muscae* do not produce 'tumours'. Although they do not invade the gastric wall but lie on the mucosal surface they cause irritation, leading to clinical gastritis, and in rare cases ulceration (1).

Cutaneous habronemiasis. *Habronema* spp., larvae deposited in wounds cause local inflammation and the development of extensive granulation tissue. There is some doubt that the lesions of so-called 'swamp cancer' are caused solely by these worms.

Conjunctival habronemiasis. Small subconjunctival lesions similar histologically to those of the cutaneous form develop.

Clinical Findings

Gastric habronemiasis is manifested by a poor condition and coat and a variable appetite which is often depraved. Large tumours may cause pyloric obstruction and gastric distension. When perforation occurs there is depression, a fever of $39 \cdot 5$ to $40 \cdot 5 °C$ (103 to 105°F) and pain and heat on the left side just behind the costal arch. Mild to moderate colic may be evidenced when intestinal stenosis is present. If the spleen is involved there is marked anaemia and a gross increase in the total leucocyte count with a shift to the left.

Cutaneous habronemiasis (Swamp Cancer, Summer Sores, Bursattee). This is manifested by the appearance of lesions on those parts of the body where skin wounds or excoriations are most likely to occur and where the horse cannot remove the vector flies. Thus they are most common on the face below the medial canthus of the eye and on the midline of the abdomen, extending in males onto the prepuce and penis. Less commonly lesions may be found on the legs and withers but those occurring in the region of the fetlocks and coronary band are especially serious. The cutaneous lesions commence as small papules with eroded, scab-covered centres. Development is rapid and individual lesions may increase to 30 cm. diameter in a few

months. The centre is depressed and composed of coarse, red granulation tissue covered with a greyish necrotic membrane and the edges are raised and thickened. Although the lesions do not usually heal spontaneously, they may regress in colder weather and recur the following summer. There is little discharge. The sores are unsightly and inconvenient and appear to cause some irritation.

Conjunctival habronemiasis. Lesions on the nictitating membrane may be as large as 5 mm. diameter. The conjunctivitis is manifested by small, yellow, necrotic masses about 1 mm. diameter under the conjunctiva. It is accompanied by soreness and lacrimation and does not respond to standard treatments for bacterial conjunctivitis. In conditions conducive to the development of flies extensive outbreaks with acute, severe signs may occur.

Clinical Pathology

Diagnosis is difficult in the gastric form of the disease because the larvae are not easy to find in the faeces. Biopsy of a cutaneous lesion reveals connective tissue containing small, yellow caseous areas up to 5 mm. in diameter. In early lesions a larva may be found in the centre but in old lesions larval debris is all that is apparent. This is a marked local eosinophilia.

Necropsy Findings

Granulomatous lesions may be found in all the sites mentioned in the description of clinical signs, and although varying in size are of essentially the same composition as described under biopsy above. Horses which have had the cutaneous form of the disease may have small nodules in the parenchyma of the lung. These are hard, yellowish and contain inspissated pus and larvae.

Diagnosis

Infestations with *Habronema* spp. are strongly associated with infestations of *Strongylus* spp., and *Gasterophilus* spp. and it is difficult to differentiate the gastric form of the disease from these infestations. The cutaneous lesions are characteristic and are not likely to be confused with other diseases. There is no other communicable conjunctivitis of horses.

Treatment

For gastric habronemiasis treatment in the past has comprised gastric lavage with 1 to 2 gallons of 2 per cent sodium bicarbonate solution to remove excess mucus followed by carbon bisulphide (2·5 ml. per 45 kg. body weight). *H. muscae* and *H. megastoma* are effectively removed but *H. microstoma* residing in 'tumours'are not affected. Thiabendazole (50 mg. per kg. body weight) is effective but double this dose rate is required to remove immature *H. microstoma* (3).

Cutaneous habronemiasis does not respond well to standard wound treatments and local applications of camphor and phenol in mineral oil, or arsenic, either as arsenic trioxide dusted on the raw surface or as an organic arsenical injected into the mass have been used extensively. Daily applications of a mixture of 2 per cent formalin and 5 per cent glycerine in water are also recommended (1). Results are only moderately good but a reduction in size may make surgical excision more practicable. Small lesions should be excised or cauterized. Ronnel (an organo-phosphatic compound) has been given orally to a large number of cases of cutaneous habronemiasis with excellent results (4). The recommended dose is 90 mg. per kg. body weight by nasal tube and repeated at 2-week intervals. Improvement is usually seen in 1 to 2 weeks and complete recovery in several more weeks is to be expected. Surgical and local treatment is still recommended to hasten recovery. Treatment with organo-phosphates should be effective against gastric and conjunctival habronemiasis.

Control

Interruption of the life cycle by careful disposal of horse manure and control of the fly population are obvious measures. In enzootic areas all skin wounds and excoriations should be treated to promote healing and protect them against flies.

REFERENCES

(1) Jesus, Z. de (1963). *Philipp. J. vet. Med.*, 2, 133.
(2) Bain, A. M. *et al.* (1969). *Aust. vet. J.*, 45, 101.
(3) Noda, R. *et al.* (1964). *J. Japan vet. med. Ass.*, 17, 565.
(4) Wheat, J. D. (1961). *Vet. Med.*, 56, 477.

Neurofilariasis

This is a disease of sheep caused by infestation of the brain and spinal cord with the filarid worm *Pneumostrongylus tenuis* (*Elaphostrongylus tenuis*, *Neurofilaria cornellensis*). The life cycle of the worm has not been accurately defined but the worm is primarily a parasite of white-tailed deer in which it migrates and passes through the central nervous system without causing apparent clinical signs (1). When infestation occurs in an atypical species migration occurs via the central nervous system and the clinical disease occurs. In lambs (2) the thread-like female migrates through nervous tissue causing limping and incoordination followed by almost complete paralysis of the hind limbs or of the neck, body and all four legs. There are no signs of cerebral involvement and affected lambs are alert and continue to eat and, if given supportive treatment, can survive for at least a month. This worm also occurs commonly in deer and moose in the U.S.A. and Canada and is the cause of nervous signs in 'moose sickness' of these species (3). The disease has been produced experimentally in moose and caribou calves with worms obtained from deer (4). A similar disease in reindeer appears to be caused by *E. rangiferi* (5). The clinical disease in moose includes weakness, unsteadiness, incoordination, circling, impaired vision, blindness, abnormal carriage of the head, paralysis, lack of fear of man and occasionally aggressiveness (3).

The experimental disease in goats may be characterized by colitis and peritonitis in the early stages, with nervous signs occurring only in those animals which survive this first form of illness (6). In other wild cervidae, e.g. wapiti, there is always damage to the central nervous system but the severity of the clinical illness varies widely from species to species (2).

REFERENCES

(1) Anderson, R. C. & Strelive, U. R. (1967). *Canad. J. Zool.*, 45, 285.
(2) Anderson, R. C. *et al.* (1966). *Canad. J. Zool.*, 44, 851, 889.
(3) Smith, H. J. & Archibald, R. McG. (1967). *Canad. vet. J.*, 8, 173.
(4) Anderson, R. C. (1964). *Path. vet.*, 1, 289.
(5) Roneus, D. & Nordkreist, M. (1962). *Acta vet. scand.*, 3, 201.
(6) Anderson, R. C. & Strelive, U. R. (1969). *Canad. J. comp. Med.*, 33, 280.

Epidemic Cerebrospinal Nematodiasis

(*Lumbar Paralysis, Kumri*)

Filarid worms of the genus *Setaria* are commonly found in the peritoneal cavity of most domestic animals but *Setaria digitata* of cattle are reputed to invade the central nervous system and eye of other animal species and to cause paralysis and blindness. *Setaria equina, S. cervi* (*labiatopapillosa*) and *S. congolense* occur in the peritoneal cavity of horses, cattle and pigs respectively and are thought to have little pathogenic significance. A high incidence of *S. equina* infestation has been observed in horses in Europe and although no clinical illness was observed there was evidence of recent peritonitis at slaughter (1). A new nomenclature for the genus *Setaria* was introduced in 1959 in which two genera, *Setaria* and *Artionema*, were identified (2). For clarity the older names are retained in this description.

Incidence

Although infestations of cattle with *Setaria* spp. are recorded from many countries the occurrence of cerebrospinal nematodiasis is recorded only from Israel, Japan, Korea, India and Ceylon. Ocular filariasis appears to have been observed only in Japan. No details of the incidence of the two diseases are available but they appear to be quite common, the cerebrospinal form sometimes occurring in epidemic proportions, causing death losses in horses, sheep and goats.

Aetiology

S. digitata, a long (5 to 10 cm.), threadlike worm, occurs commonly only in the peritoneal cavity of cattle, its natural host. However, it can infest unnatural hosts, especially horses, sheep, goats and man in which it migrates in an abnormal manner, causing epizootic cerebrospinal nematodiasis (3). when it invades the brain and spinal cord. The disease has been produced experimentally in goats, foals and lambs (4). Similar behaviour of another setaria (*S. marshalli*) of cattle has also been observed in sheep (5).

Life Cycle

Microfilariae are taken up from the peripheral blood of the infected animal by blood-sucking mosquitoes which transmit the disease to others. The number of microfilariae in capillary blood varies: in horses *S. equina* microfilariae are present in greatest numbers in capillary blood between 8 and 12 p.m., at lower temperatures and at higher barometric pressures. All of these factors would probably increase the chances of spread by insect vectors and infective larvae have been shown to develop in *Aedes vittatus* and *Armigeres obturans*, but not *Culex fatigans* or *Stomoxys calcitrans* (6). In cattle *S. digitata* and *S. marshalli* migrate only to the abdominal cavity where they reach maturity in 8 to 10 months. An occurrence of congenital infection in a goat has been recorded (10). Cerebrospinal nematodiasis and ocular filariasis are diseases of the summer and autumn when the vectors are most prevalent.

Pathogenesis

In horses, sheep and goats invasion of the eye may cause endophthalmitis (7) and of the nervous system an acute focal encephalomyelomalacia (8). The clinical picture which develops depends on the site and severity of the lesions.

Clinical Findings

In cerebrospinal nematodiasis there is acute or subacute paresis with weakness and inco-ordination or paralysis involving the hind legs most commonly, but sometimes all four legs. The onset may be sudden with affected animals dying within a few days but many animals partially recover or persist in a state of impaired nervous function. There are no systemic signs and the animals may continue to eat.

Clinical Pathology

Ante-mortem diagnosis has been accomplished by detection of microfilariae in the blood stream but the procedure is laborious and the results inconclusive.

Necropsy Findings

There are no macroscopic changes and sections taken from many levels of the spinal cord should be submitted to careful histological examination. The tracts of migrating worms are indicated by necrosis of nervous tissue. Occasionally the whole or part of a worm may be found in a case where nervous signs have been present for only a few days.

Diagnosis

There are many diseases which are capable of producing a similar clinical syndrome. A feature of cerebrospinal nematodiasis is its occurrence in the late summer and autumn when insect vectors are most common. In horses enzootic equine ataxia (wobbles) is clinically almost identical, in sheep and goats paralytic rabies must be considered. In all species traumatic injury, spinal cord abscess and migration of other parasites, e.g. warble fly in cattle, may cause similar clinical signs.

Treatment

There is no treatment which could be reasonably expected to have any effect on the lesion but systemic anthelmintics may prevent further damage. Diethylcarbamazine (Caricide) has given encouraging results in early experimental work in sheep and goats, horses and cattle (9).

Control

Control of the vector mosquitoes is usually impracticable in those countries where the disease is common. Diethylcarbamazine (10 mg. per kg. body weight daily for 10 days by mouth) effectively kills *Setaria* spp. in cattle and a control programme to prevent cerebrospinal nematodiasis in sheep and goats by eliminating the worm from cattle in the area by the use of this drug has been recommended.

REFERENCES

(1) Jirina, K. (1959). *Dtsch. tierärztl. Wschr.*, *66*, 439.
(2) Yea, L. S. (1959). *J. Helminth.*, *33*, 1.
(3) Saunders, L. Z. (1959). *Vet. Rec.*, *71*, 631.
(4) Shoho, C. & Nair, V. K. (1960). *Ceylon vet. J.*, *8*, 2.
(5) Kadenatsii, A. N. (1955). *Helminth. Abstr.*, *24*, 316.
(6) Varma, A. K. *et al.* (1971). *Z. ParasitKde*, *36*, 62.
(7) Ahmed, S. A. & Gupta, B. N. (1965). *Indian vet. J.*, *42*, 140.
(8) Innes, J. R. M. & Pillai, C. P. (1952). *Brit. vet. J.*, *108*, 71.
(9) Katiyar, R. D. (1960). *Indian vet. J.*, *37*, 167.
(10) Patnaik, B. (1966). *Ind. J. Anim. Hlth*, *5*, 1.

Thorn-headed Worm of Pigs

(*Macracanthorhyncus hirudinaceus*)

Infestations in pigs with these thick-bodied (0·5 to 1·25 cm.), long (up to 38 cm.) transversely wrinkled worms are not usually heavy and cause relatively little loss. They inhabit the small intestine and eggs passed in the pig's faeces are very resistant to environmental stress, surviving for up to 2 years in average conditions. The life cycle is indirect, the intermediate hosts being 'June-bug' or 'Christmas' beetles. The beetle larvae become infested by eating the worm eggs and a new infestation is set up in a pig when it eats an infested grub or adult beetle. Periodic increases in the degree of infestation by this worm has been related to the 3-year life cycle of these beetles (1). The adult female commences egg-laying in 2 to 3 months, is a very heavy egg-layer and lives in the host for about a year.

Heavy infestations cause slow growth and loss of body weight and occasional deaths may occur due to perforation of the intestinal wall. Damage to the intestinal wall may reduce its suitability as sausage casing.

There is no highly efficient treatment but sodium fluoride as used for the treatment of ascariasis removes some worms (2) and carbon tetrachloride is also used. Phenothiazine is not effective. Suitable disposal of pig manure and avoidance of contact with the beetles which are intermediate hosts are recommended as control measures.

REFERENCES

(1) Swales, W. E. & Gwatkin, R. (1948). *Canad. J. comp. Med.*, *12*, 297.
(2) Seddon, H. R. (1950). Cwlth of Aust., Dept. of Hlth, Div. Vet. Hygiene. Service Pub. No. 5.

Thelaziasis

Thelazia spp. worms occur in the conjunctival sacs of mammals and although they may cause or contribute to the development of conjunctivitis, keratitis, ophthalmia and abscess formation on the eyelids (1, 2, 3), their pathogenic importance is uncertain. In those species in which they have been studied the life cycles are indirect, the intermediate hosts being flies (*Musca* spp.) which deposit larvae of the worms in the conjunctival sac when feeding around the eyes. Most clinical cases occur in the summer and autumn when flies are plentiful. Diagnosis is made by finding adult worms in the conjunctival sac or by microscopic examination of rinsings from the lacrimal duct (5). Treatment in the past has comprised local irrigation with 1 in 2000 aqueous iodine solution or 0·5 per cent aqueous lysol solution. The former is often administered by a catheter inserted in the nasolacrimal duct. Systemic treatment with diethylcarbamazine or methyridine, local irrigation with a 3 per cent aqueous solution of piperazine adipate or manual removal of worms are all used in treatment (2). Tetramisole by mouth (15 mg. per kg.) is also highly effective in cattle (4). The application of insect repellents around the eyes may help to reduce the incidence.

REFERENCES

(1) Fitzsimmons, W. M. (1963). *Vet. Rec.*, *75*, 1024.
(2) Vohradsky, F. (1970). *Bull. epizoot. Dis. Afr.*, *18*, 159.
(3) Franzos, G. (1964). *Refuah vet.*, *21*, 33.
(4) Corba, L. *et al.* (1969). *Trop. Anim. Hlth Prod.*, *1*, 19.
(5) Sander, W. (1971). *Mh. Vet.-Med.*, *26*, 648.

Onchocerciasis

(*Worm Nodule Disease*)

Infestations by the filarid worms of *Onchocerca* spp. cause rejection of meat for human consumption and are thought to cause fistulous withers and poll evil in horses.

Incidence

Onchocerciasis of cattle, Indian buffaloes and horses occurs in a number of tropical and subtropical countries including South Africa, the Malay peninsula, India and Australia. A high incidence of infestation has also been recorded in cattle in Great Britain. Losses caused by *Onchocerca* spp. are slight although *O. cervicalis* is thought to be of importance in the production of fistulous withers and poll evil (nuchal disease) in horses and *Onchocerca* spp. in cattle cause rejection of beef carcases from the high-class meat trade and unsightly trimming is necessary at the abattoir. Hide damage may also be important (1).

Aetiology

In cattle *Onchocerca gibsoni* infests the subcutaneous tissues, especially the brisket, *O. ochengi* causes a dermatitis resembling demodectic mange and pox (1), and *O. gutturosa* (*O. bovis*, *O. lienalis*) infests the ligamentum nuchae. *O. armillata* is recorded as causing aortitis in cattle, Indian buffalo and goats in India (2). In horses *O. cervicalis* (*O. reticulata*) infests the ligamentum nuchae and the connective tissue around the flexor tendons. *O. cervicalis* larvae have also been found in the cornea of large numbers of horses and occasionally in cases of dermatitis. The worms are thin and thread-like and vary in length, those of the horse being 15 to 18 cm. long, but cattle species may be as long as 75 cm.

Life Cycle

As with most filarid worms the microfilariae in the cutaneous blood vessels are picked up by blood-sucking insects, in this case midges, sandflies or black-flies (*Culicoides* spp., *Simulium* spp.), and deposited in the skin of other animals. Development of the microfilariae to an infective stage in the intermediate host appears to take some time, e.g. *O. gutturosa* up to 3 weeks in *Simulium ornatum* (3). In the final host the microfilariae are deposited where and when the vector feeds, in the case of *Simulium ornatum* around the umbilicus (4), from where they migrate in connective tissue and become fixed in a predilection site and, in *O. gibsoni*, from a fibrous nodule. Microfilariae produced by adult female worms appear to migrate to nearby blood and lymph vessels, particularly the latter. Some filariae migrate to the eyes of horses and have been linked with periodic ophthalmia but most authors agree that there is no causal relationship. Similar ocular lesions have been described in cattle with heavy infestations of *O. armillata*. In horses *O. cervicalis* produces a great variety of ocular lesions (5). Onchocerciasis is a major cause of human blindness in West Africa.

Pathogenesis

The characteristic nodules of *O. gibsoni* consist of fibrous tissue canalized by the long body of the worms. Other species of *Onchocerca* cause the formation of fibrous tissue without producing nodules.

Clinical Findings

In cattle there are no specific clinical signs other than the presence of nodules about 3 cm. in diameter in the subcutaneous tissue. They are usually freely movable but may be attached to the skin. The brisket is the most common site but nodules are also often found around the stifle and on the lateral surface of the thigh. In infestations with *O.*

ochengi, the cutaneous lesions are most common on the scrotum and udder.

In horses fistulous withers and poll evil and swelling and nodule formation around the fetlock, especially of the foreleg (6), may be associated with the infestation. There may be an acute inflammatory reaction in the eye similar to periodic ophthalmia (5).

Clinical Pathology

Microfilariae are not detectable in the blood stream but excision of a subcutaneous nodule will show the presence of an adult worm or debris, and microfilariae may be found in surrounding lymph spaces. Large adult worms may be found in the connective tissue around the ligamentum nuchae during surgical operations.

Diagnosis

In cattle 'skin tuberculosis' and demodectic mange cause lesions which may be confused with those of onchocerciasis.

Control

No completely satisfactory treatment is known but diethylcarbamazine (4 mg. per kg. mixed in the food daily for 4 days and repeated in one week) has been recommended (7). The drug is contraindicated during the ocular inflammatory phase (5). Control of the insect vector is virtually impossible but valuable horses can be partially protected by housing at night, by the use of insect repellents and by avoidance of areas where the insects are likely to be present in large numbers. In cattle herds animals showing large numbers of nodules should be disposed of.

REFERENCES

(1) Bwangamoi, O. (1969). *Bull. epizoot. Dis. Afr.*, *17*, 435.
(2) Sristavasta, S. C. & Pande, B. P. (1964). *Indian J. vet. Sci.*, *34*, 222.
(3) Steward, J. S. (1937). *Parasitology*, *29*, 212.
(4) Eichler, D. A. & Nelson, G. S. (1971). *J. Helminth.*, *45*, 245, 259.
(5) Cello, R. M. (1971). *Equ. vet. J.*, *3*, 148.
(6) Marolt, J. *et al.* (1960). *Schweiz. Arch. Tierheilk.*, *102*, 571.
(7) McMullan, W. C. (1972). *SWest. Vet.*, *25*, 179.

Elaeophoriasis
(*Filarial Dermatitis of Sheep*)

Elaeophoriasis is a chronic disease of sheep characterized chiefly by a dermatitis and caused by the nematode *Elaeophora schneideri*.

Incidence

The disease has been recorded in sheep in North America (1) and Italy (2). Deer may be infested with the causative nematode but lesions have not been recorded. In most cases affected sheep have been grazed at high altitudes during the summer months. The incidence in affected sheep flocks is usually about 1 per cent and sheep over 2 years old are most commonly affected. Losses result from the inconvenience of the disease and the scarred nodules which affect the market value of hides.

Aetiology

Microfilarial forms of the blood worm *E. schneideri* produce the lesions. The adult worms are present in large blood vessels.

Life Cycle

The common occurrence of the disease after high summer pasturing and the occurrence of the worm in deer suggest that these animals may act as a reservoir of infection and that transmission occurs by insect vectors when deer and sheep are in close contact.

Pathogenesis

Although adult worms can be recovered from the arteries supplying affected parts of the body and from the heart, the lesions are almost completely confined to the skin, conjuctiva and the oral and nasal mucosae. This suggests either a positive heliotropism or requirement of a surface membrane for viability (3). The remissions and exacerbations of the itching associated with the disease are thought to be due to the periodic arrival at the surface of new generations of microfilarids. Signs do not usually appear until the year after exposure suggesting a protracted period of maturation of the worms.

Clinical Findings

Lesions are found most commonly on the head, particularly the poll, but extending over the face to involve the lips and in some cases the oral and nasal mucosae. Abnormalities of the eye are common including cataract, iridocyclitis and corneal opacity. Sight usually remains adequate in sheep although it is often lost in deer (4). The feet and ventral abdomen are other common sites. Initially the lesions are small, circumscribed areas of dermatitis but the irritation produced by them is so intense that scratching causes the development of extensive areas of bleeding, granular surface containing numerous small abscesses. On the feet the lesions extend from the coronary band to above the fetlock and cause much local swelling. Recurrent periods of quiescence occur and scabs form over the lesions, but 2 to 3 days later scratching recommen-

ces and the lesions are spread further. The course is long, often 7 months and up to 3 years, but recovery may eventually occur. Residual lesions include deformity of the hooves and bare, thickened patches of skin.

Clinical Pathology

Microfilarids may be detected by a skin biopsy and maceration of the specimen to release the worms, or by histological examination. Skin scrapings are not usually satisfactory.

Necropsy Findings

A search for adult worms in arteries supplying affected parts can be supplemented by cutting the sheep's throat and allowing the blood to pass through a wire gauge to trap any free worms. The adult worms are not usually attached and cause no vascular lesions. Lesions, especially those in the oral and nasal mucosae, are often unilateral.

Diagnosis

Other forms of dermatitis particularly photosensitization, contagious ecthyma, mycotic dermatitis and strawberry footrot, are likely to be confused with elaeophoriasis. The latter two conditions do not have the same distribution on the body, mycotic dermatitis occurring chiefly along the back and strawberry footrot only on the lower legs. No irritation occurs in either of these diseases. Contagious ecthyma lesions are restricted to the lips in most cases and have a characteristic granulomatous structure with a thick scab. Photosensitization lesions may have a very similar distribution and appearance to those caused by the elaeophorid filaria but there is usually marked oedema and swelling and a history of access to photosensitizing or hepatotoxic plants.

Treatment

Systemic treatment with arsenic, antimony and bismuth preparations is effective. Most satisfactory results are obtained by the intramuscular injection of 35 ml. of Fuadin or Anthiomaline (150 mg. antimony per gramme) on two occasions 10 days apart (1).

Control

Avoidance of grazing sheep in close proximity to deer seems a logical control procedure.

REFERENCES

(1) Kemper, H. E. (1957). *J. Amer. vet. med. Ass.*, *130*, 220.
(2) Micozzi, G. (1956). *Zooprofilassi*, *11*, 441.
(3) Jensen, R. & Seghetti, L. (1955). *J. Amer. vet. med. Ass.*, *127*, 499.

(4) Abdelbaki, Y. Z. & Davis, R. W. (1972). *Vet. Med. small Anim. Pract.*, 67, 69.

Miscellaneous Filarial Dermatidites

(*Cutaneous Stephanofilarosis*)

A number of filarid worms, other than *Elaeophora schneideri* and *Onchocerca* spp., which are dealt with elsewhere, cause intramuscular subcutaneous and cutaneous lesions in domestic animals.

Parafilaria multipapillosa occurs in eastern countries and Europe (1), and in horses causes the development of subcutaneous nodules which ulcerate, bleed, heal and disappear spontaneously. The lesions are evident only in summer time and flies which feed on the bleeding nodules have been suggested as vectors. *P. bovicola* causes similar lesions in cattle in Eastern Europe, India and the Philippines and again the lesions are most common in summer. This parasite has been imported into Canada in cattle imported from France (2). *Suifilaria suis* causes similar lesions in the pig in South Africa.

Stephanofilaria spp. also cause connective and subcutaneous tissue lesions. *Stephanofilaria dedoesi* occurs in the East Indies in cattle, causing a dermatitis called 'cascado'; *S. kaeli* and *S. assamensis* cause dermatitis in cattle in Malaya and India known as 'humpsore'; *S. assamensis* has also been recovered from dermatitis in buffalo and goat (3). *S. assamensis* is viviparous and the disease can be produced experimentally only by deposition of the microfilariae in abraded skin (4). The common site for lesions caused by this worm is on the hump which is frequently damaged when the cattle rub against rough objects. Lesions are also produced around the base of the dewclaws, each lesion having a superficial resemblance to a papilloma (5). The insect vector for *S. assamensis* is the biting fly *Musca conducens* (6). *S. zaheeri* causes a dermatitis around the ears of buffalo, referred to as 'earsore' or contagious otorrhoea. *S. stilesi* causes a dermatitis, mostly on the ventral abdomen of cattle in the U.S.A. Unidentified *Stephanofilaria* spp. filarids cause dermatitis in cattle in Germany and a pruritic dermatitis of the muzzle in cattle in Japan (9).

The lesions in cutaneous stephanofilarosis vary from 3 to 15 cm. in diameter. Initially there are small papules which later coalesce to form lesions up to 25 cm. diameter. The lesions are itchy and a good deal of irritation and rubbing are evident (7). Part but not all of the hair is lost and dried exudate forms a thick, crumbly scab which may crack with the appearance of bloodstained moisture in the crack. If healing occurs the scab disappears and a scar is left. Most lesions are seen along the midline of the abdomen. Worms or parts of them can be found in dry skin scrapings made after scabs are removed.

Treatment of stephanofilarial dermatitis by three subcutaneous injections at weekly intervals of stibophen (12 mg. per kg. body weight) has given moderately good results in cattle. Neguvon given as a single oral dose (60 mg. per kg. body weight) repeated if necessary a month later has shown comparable efficiency. Local application is also recommended, a 40 per cent chlorophos (trichlorphon) ointment being very effective (8). The disease is probably spread by insects, *Lyperosia* spp. are common vectors, and projected control measures should take this into account.

REFERENCES

(1) Gibson, T. E. *et al.* (1964). *Vet. Rec.*, 76, 764.
(2) Niilo, L. (1968). *Canad. vet. J.*, 9, 132.
(3) Patnaik, B. & Roy, S. P. (1968). *Ind. J. vet. Sci.*, 38, 455.
(4) Srivastava, H. D. & Dutt, S. C. (1963). *Ind. J. vet. Sci.*, 33, 173.
(5) Pal, A. K. & Sinha, P. K. (1971). *Indian vet. J.*, 48, 190.
(6) Shamsul, A. V. M. (1971). *Veterinariya*, 3, 112.
(7) Dewan, M. L. (1971). *Veterinariya*, 3, 113.
(8) Ivashkin, V. M. *et al.* (1971). *Veterinariya*, 3, 66.
(9) Kono, I. (1965). *Japan. J. vet. Sci.*, 27, 33.

26

Diseases Caused by Arthropod Parasites

Gasterophilus spp. Infestation

(*Botfly*)

INFESTATIONS with larvae of *Gasterophilus* spp. may cause chronic gastritis and occasionally perforation of the stomach in horses.

Incidence

Botflies appear to have a general distribution and parasitize horses wherever they are kept. They rarely cause deaths but loss of condition and reduced performance is often attributed to them.

Aetiology

There are five species of flies, *Gasterophilus nasalis*, *G. intestinalis*, *G. haemorrhoidalis*, *G. pecorum* and *G. inermis* and their larvae are the parasitic 'bots' of horses. *G. intestinalis* is the most important species. The larvae inhabit the stomach and are thick, fat, transversely striated and about 5 to 12 mm. long. They are creamy pink in colour. The adult, fly stage is brown and hairy, about the size of a bee and has only two wings.

Life Cycle

The adult fly does not feed and lives from a few days to 2 weeks solely for the purpose of laying eggs. It is most prevalent in the summer months, the different species often appearing at different times. The eggs are laid on the horse's coat. *G. pecorum* may lay its eggs on inanimate objects in the horse's environment. The eggs of *G. pecorum* and *G. haemorrhoidalis* are dark brown, the eggs of the others are yellow and are readily visible glued to the hairs, usually one to a hair. The eggs of *G. intestinalis*, the most common fly, are laid on the front legs, particularly the lower parts; those of *G. nasalis* in the intermandibular area; the others on the cheeks and lips.

The eggs hatch in about 10 days and the larvae enter the mouth either by biting or licking or by migration through the cheeks. The eggs of *G. intestinalis* require licking to hatch. The larvae are not swallowed directly into the stomach but after penetration of the buccal mucosa migrate in the direction of the stomach, entering the lumen of the alimentary tract again at various points beyond the pharynx about a month after infestation. Occasional larvae migrate to abnormal sites including the brain, the cranial sinuses, the heart and lungs.

G. intestinalis larvae are found in the tongue and subsequently the cardiac area of the stomach, where they become attached to the mucosa usually in bunches. *G. nasalis* larvae are found in the pyloric region of the stomach and the duodenum. *G. pecorum* larvae may be found in the cheeks, the pharynx and upper part of the oesophagus and in the fundus of the stomach. *G. haemorrhoidalis* larvae are found in the tongue, the pharynx and the gastric fundus.

In the host two moults are made and the larvae pass out in the droppings 10 to 12 months after infestation, usually in the spring and early summer. Some larvae may attach temporarily to the rectal mucosa on their way through. The larvae migrate into the ground, pupate and adult flies emerge after 3 to 5 weeks to recommence the late summer attacks on horses.

Pathogenesis

There is some doubt as to the importance of the lesions caused by the larvae. At the sites where they adhere there is an area of thickening and inflammation and in rare cases gastric perforation occurs. It is probable that there is some chronic gastritis and interference with digestion in most infestations. The larvae do not suck sufficient blood to cause anaemia, feeding mostly on tissue exudate. In very heavy infestations with *G. pecorum* the presence of large numbers of larvae (100 to 500) on the soft palate and base of the tongue can cause stomatitis and some deaths.

Clinical Findings

A non-specific syndrome of unthriftiness, poor coat, occasional mild colic and lack of appetite, plus bad temper and unwillingness to work is usually ascribed to 'bot' infestations. Adult flies frighten horses by their hovering, darting flight, especially around the head of the horse, and may be a cause of shying and balking.

Clinical Pathology

The eggs on the hairs can be seen by direct inspection but the presence of larvae in the stomach and intestines can only be detected after treatment with a suitable boticide.

Necropsy Findings

A few larvae are present in the stomach of most horses at necropsy but clinical illness is usually associated with very large numbers. The areas of attachment of the larvae are pitted and the gastric wall thickened and there may be an adhesive peritonitis and attachment and abscessation of the spleen over such areas.

Diagnosis

The syndrome produced is not sufficiently characteristic to make ante-mortem diagnosis possible and 'bot' infestations are commonly associated with helminth infestations which may produce most of the signs observed.

Treatment

Dosing with carbon bisulphide as described for gastric habronemiasis has been recommended for many years and is effective. Transitory abdominal pain occurs in some horses shortly after dosing but the treatment is generally without risk. Some of the organophosphatic insecticides including Butonate or Ruelene (100 mg. per kg. body weight by stomach tube, 50 mg. per kg. body weight in feed), Metriphonate (75 mg. per kg. body weight by stomach tube, 25 to 100 mg. per kg. body weight in feed) and Bayer 37341 (50 mg. per kg. body weight by nasal tube or in the feed) (1, 2) are effective and are commonly combined with anthelmintics as described under strongylosis. A recent USDA recommendation is a single administration of 40 mg. per kg. body weight metriphonate in feed. Dichlorvos (10 mg. per kg.) in a paste smeared on the tongue is effective against both bots and ascarids (3).

Control

On most horse farms treatment is administered routinely at times when the larvae can be expected to be present in the stomach. Two doses are usually given, one in late autumn and one in spring.

The use of repellents or agents to kill the larvae in manure has not been successful and the main aim is to kill the eggs deposited on the hairs. This is most effectively done by frequent vigorous bathing of the infested parts with hot water (over 38°C or 100°F). This stimulates mass hatching and rapid death of the larvae. Singeing or the application of cresolic disinfectants can be used for the same purpose but must also be repeated frequently and energetically. The use of fringes, veils and tassels on the head harness helps protect horses against the fly but are of little use in preventing bot infestation.

REFERENCES

(1) Smith, J. P. & Bell, R. R. (1968). *SWest. Vet.*, *21*, 293.
(2) Drummond, R. O. (1965). *Vet. Rec.*, *77*, 1418.
(3) Bennett, D. G. & Bickford, A. A. (1971). *Vet. Med. small Anim. Clin.*, *66*, 441.

Oestrus ovis Infestation

(*Sheep Nasal Botfly, Nasal Bots*)

The adult fly is about the size of a bee and is dark grey to brown in colour. It is active only in the summer time, except in very warm climates, and deposits its larvae around the nostrils of sheep. The larvae migrate into the nasal cavities where they develop for several weeks, then pass into the frontal sinuses from which they emerge within several more weeks and are then snorted out or crawl out and enter the ground to pupate. The adult fly may emerge in 3 to 6 weeks. All stages of development are much longer during the winter. The larvae are thick yellow-white grubs about 2·5 cm. long with dark transverse bands. Sheep are the only domestic animals affected but the larvae have been observed in deer.

Adult flies attempting to lay eggs annoy the sheep and cause them to seek shelter. Stamping of the feet and shaking of the head are common. In bad seasons the sheep may lose a good deal of grazing time. The spiny surface of the larvae causes irritation of the nasal mucosa resulting in catarrhal rhinitis with sneezing, a mucopurulent nasal discharge, and difficult, snoring respiration. Secondary bacterial infections are uncommon but may cause occasional deaths. The infestations are not usually severe enough to necessitate treatment but it is often attempted. The organophosphates are in general effective as treatment but vary in their efficiency against the more mature larval stages. Oral dosing with Bayer 37341 or dimethoate (both 40 mg. per kg. body weight), Bayer 37342 or Dowco 109 (both 50 mg. per kg. body weight), Famophos or Fenchlorphos (both 100 mg. per kg. body weight), Fenthion (30 mg. per kg.) and Ruelene (125 mg. per kg. body weight) or intramuscular injection of Bayer 37342 or dimethoate (both 25 mg. per kg. body weight) is effective (1, 2). Nasal sprays of 3 per cent dichlorvos are less effective. Annual treatments have been shown to greatly reduce the incidence of infestation in isolated sheep flocks (3) but eradication is impracticable because of the probability of reinfestation.

REFERENCES

(1) Knapp, F. W. & Drudge, J. H. (1964). *Amer. J. vet. Res.*, *25*, 1686.
(2) Drummond, R. O. (1965). *Vet. Rec.*, *77*, 1418.
(3) Meleney, W. P. *et al.* (1969). *J. Amer. vet. med. Ass.*, *155*, 136.
(4) Peadt, R. E. (1967). *J. econ. Ent.*, *60*, 1420.

Hypoderma spp. Infestation

(*Warble Flies, Warbles*)

Infestations of cattle with the larvae of *Hypoderma* spp. cause serious damage to hides, occasional deaths due to anaphylactic shock or toxaemia and damage to the central nervous system or oesophagus.

Incidence

Warble flies are common parasites of cattle in most countries in the northern hemisphere. They do not occur in Australia in spite of having been introduced to that country on several occasions. The migrating larvae cause severe damage to the most valuable portion of the hide and heavy infestations may make it completely valueless. The average infestation costs a depreciation in hide value of about $2 and in carcass value of $7 due to excessive trimming.

Aetiology

There are two species which parasitize cattle, *Hypoderma bovis*, and *H. lineata*. The two flies have slightly different geographical distributions. *H. lineata* favours a warmer climate and is the only warble fly present in the southern states of the United States. In the northern states and Canada both flies occur. The adult flies are heavy-set and hairy, about the size of a bee (12 to 18 mm. long), are yellow-orange in colour and have two wings. They are not easily seen because of the rapidity of their flight. Young animals are usually more seriously affected than adults. Occasional cases of warble fly infestation are seen in horses.

H. aeratum and *H. crossi* are similar to the above and parasitize sheep and goats in Cyprus and India respectively. Although the larvae of these two flies migrate through tissues they do not do so as extensively as cattle warbles, the eggs being laid on the sides of the animals and the larvae emerging at almost the same site. *H. silenus* has been reported to cause losses in goats in Russia (1).

The larvae of *Dermatobium hominis*, a small (12 mm. long) related fly, parasitize man in a manner similar to the way in which warbles parasitize cattle. Infestations may also occur in most other animals. The habitat of the fly is Central and South America where it causes heavy losses in cattle. Larvae have been found on at least two occasions in imported animals in U.S.A. but the fly does not seem to have become established. The larva is about 2·5 cm. long and causes a painful cutaneous swelling. The life cycle is similar in many ways to that of *Hypoderma* spp. except that the eggs are transported by mosquitoes and migration through tissues does not occur. Some strains of cattle in Colombia are completely resistant to *D. hominis* which points to the possibility of control by breeding. Treatment and control measures are the same as for *H. bovis*.

Life Cycle

Adult flies are active in the hottest part of the summer and lay their eggs attached to hairs on the legs and occasionally on the body. Hatching occurs in about 4 days and the emerging larvae penetrate the skin and migrate through the tissues towards the dorsal surface of the body. This migration takes most of the autumn and winter and in early spring the larvae come to rest under the skin of the back where they develop a breathing pore to the exterior, enlarge further and in about a month perforate the skin, wriggle out and fall to the ground where they pupate for about 5 weeks. The fully developed larvae are thick (8 mm.), transversely ridged and about 3 cm. long.

During their migration the larvae of *H. bovis* may enter the epidural space and the larvae of *H. lineata* commonly enter the submucosal tissue of the oesophagus. The larvae can be anticipated to be present in these sites about 4 months after oviposition. *H. lineata* is rarely found in the epidural space and *H. bovis* seldom in the oesophageal wall. This variation between the species probably depends on the site of deposition of the eggs. *H. bovis* lays its eggs on the rump, loins and upper parts of the hind legs. By migrating in interfascial planes they generally reach the back but many pass through the epidural space. *H. lineata* lays its eggs on the dewlap and on the forelegs particularly at the heels. Migration in fascial planes to the thoracic inlet leads to passage along the oesophagus to the diaphragm and thence up to the back. Thus the larvae occur commonly in the oesophageal wall and in many of the thoracic organs.

The timing of the life cycle, that is the period when grubs are present under the skin of the back and the time at which the flies are present in large numbers, varies with the climate and is of importance in a control programme. *H. lineata* generally is 1 to 2 months ahead of *H. bovis* and where the two flies are present both 'grub' and 'fly' seasons may be very long. In the southern United States the 'fly season' is February and March, in Canada June to August. The period when grubs are present in the back is December in the south and February to May in Canada.

Pathogenesis

Larvae maturing under the skin of the back cause local discrete swellings and later perforations of the skin. 'Anaphylactic' attacks are often ascribed to the death of migrating larvae but these are most often associated with unsuccessful attempts to remove the larvae mechanically. These reactions are more common in adult animals. Inflammation of the oesophageal wall may result in stenosis and obstructive bloat.

Clinical Findings

If the fly population is heavy, cattle at pasture may be worried by their attacks and be prevented from feeding properly. Heavy infestations with larvae are commonly associated with poor growth, condition and production but such heavy infestations are often complicated by other forms of mismanagement including malnutrition and parasitic gastroenteritis.

The presence of the larvae causes obvious swelling with pain on touch. The swellings are usually soft and fluctuating and about 3 cm. in diameter. There may be as many as 200 to 300 such lesions on the back of one animal.

With involvement of the spinal cord there is a sudden onset of posterior paralysis without fever and without other systemic signs. The suddenness of onset and the failure of the disease to progress usually suggest traumatic injury. A similar disease can occur in horses and is reputed to be more common in horses than in cattle (4).

Clinical Pathology

The presence of warble fly larvae cannot be detected in the living animal. Eggs on the hair coat in late summer suggest that larvae will appear in the spring.

Necropsy Findings

The larvae are usually found in an area of tissue surrounded by a zone of red or green discoloration. Mature larvae lie in a cyst-like structure surrounded by a yellow, cloudy fluid.

Diagnosis

No other disease causes the characteristic swellings on the back. The differential diagnosis of posterior paralysis and anaphylaxis are discussed in detail under the respective headings of disease of the spinal cord and anaphylaxis.

Treatment

Systemic insecticides, particularly the organophosphates, are the only means of destroying migrating warble larvae. These preparations can be applied by spray or a 'pour-on' technique, by individual oral dosing or by mixing in the feed. They are highly effective but unless used in strict accordance with the recommendations of the manufacturer toxic effects may occur.

There has been so much activity in this field during the past few years that it is impossible to make specific recommendations on the drugs to be used, the most efficient dose rates and the most suitable methods and times of application. Drugs currently in use include coumaphos, fenchlorphos, Ruelene and metriphonate (Neguvon) all of which can be administered percutaneously or as feed additives (2). Other drugs which show promise are Fenthion, Tamaphos and Imidan (3).

The time of administration varies with climate. The emphasis on timing is to provide treatment early in the autumn after all eggs have hatched and larvae are in subcutaneous sites. Later dosing means that the third-stage larvae, which are less susceptible to these drugs, may not be controlled and larvae killed in some sites, especially spinal cord and oesophagus may cause serious illness.

All routes of treatment appear to be effective, including feeding in grain for 7 days. Administration in the feed has the advantage that individual dosing, often a problem in young beef cattle, is unnecessary but the method requires at least twice the amount of drug and individual animals may refuse to eat the treated feed, or in free-choice feeding be prevented from eating it, and have very heavy infestations of grubs.

Application in the form of a spray should ensure that the skin is wetted by using a pressure spray (300–400 lb. per sq. in.) and spraying the flat body surfaces such as the neck, back, shoulders, sides and thighs. Use of a low pressure spray or wash should be followed by vigorous use of a curry comb or brush. Pour-on applications should be made carefully along the mid-line in a thin stream which penetrates the hair coat (5).

Although these compounds disappear very quickly from tissues, recommendations are that they should not be administered to milking animals, and beef animals should not be slaughtered for at least 60 days after dosing.

Toxic effects of organo-phosphates have been described elsewhere. The pitfalls in their use in warble control are related chiefly to the time of administration. If they are administered when the larvae are well grown, severe systemic reactions may occur and the dead larvae may cause severe local tissue necrosis. Either of two well recognized sequelae may follow but the actual relationship between the treatment and the lesion is strongly contested (6). One manifestation is perforation of the oesophageal mucosa when larvae in this site are killed. An extensive cellulitis develops under the mucosa causing failure to eat and persistent bloat. If the lesion is in the cervical oesophagus the thickening of the oesophagus can be palpated but lesions in the thoracic oesophagus may only be assumed. There is great difficulty in passing a stomach tube and attempts to do this may cause laceration of the necrotic tissue. If the larvae are in the spinal canal posterior paralysis may result.

Dosing late in the season may also be accompanied by other signs of toxicity including staggering, mild bloat and salivation. In northern climates this is thought to be due to reduced water intake in cold weather. Severe signs and heavy mortalities, such as occur after accidental administration of large quantities of these compounds, seldom occur if the manufacturers' recommendations are followed accurately. The antidote is atropine sulphate administered subcutaneously, $\frac{1}{2}$ grain per 300 lb. body weight. The frequency of reactions to organo-phosphatic treatment is about 1 in every 10,000 treated.

When small numbers of cattle are affected with relatively few warble grubs manual removal of the larvae is practised. Incomplete removal or breaking the larvae during removal may cause a severe systemic reaction. This reaction and the one which sometimes occurs after systemic treatment of cattle infected with warble fly has been ascribed to anaphylaxis. However, there is evidence that it is due directly to toxins liberated from dead warble maggots (7). The clinical signs include dullness, salivation, lacrimation, dyspnoea, wrinkling of skin on the side of the neck and oedema under the jaw (8).

Control

Control of this parasite depends on preventing the larvae from reaching the ground to pupate. This can be done quite effectively and cheaply by applying a contact insecticide (usually derris powder containing about 5 per cent rotenone) to the animal's back and sides at the time that the larvae are present in the subcutaneous tissues.

The method is cheap but is ineffective unless it is carried out over a large area. In North America co-operation between local agricultural authorities and groups of farmers has been outstandingly successful in reducing warble fly losses over large areas by annual spraying with derris. In recent years control by the use of systemic insecticides (principally organo-phosphates as described in treatment above) has attracted much attention because damage to the hides of the treated cattle is also prevented. This method has a further big advantage in that warble damage can be prevented each year on an individual farm irrespective of the control programme on nearby farms. It is also preferred over rotenone for young beef cattle because of the ease of administration. A sample recommended programme is the application of one coumaphos spray in the autumn or three sprays, at 3-week intervals, in the summer. It is possible to eradicate the pest temporarily by this sort of programme being applied over a large area (8). Although administration of the systemic parasiticide in the autumn has some disadvantages it is recommended in ordinary circumstances and has the distinct advantage that it restricts the build-up of louse infestations for the winter.

Rotenone applications. To be effective these must be applied at the time when the grubs are in the subcutaneous tissue of the back. If the grub season is an extended one the application may have to be repeated at 3- to 4-week intervals. Normally two applications are necessary and three are recommended. A power spray is needed (400 to 600 lb. pressure) and the spray nozzle must be held close enough for the spray to penetrate the breathing pores of the grubs: simple wetting of the skin is not sufficient. Great care is needed to ensure that all grub sites are sprayed and that cattle are not sprayed in the eyes; a painful kerato-conjunctivitis may result. A suitable spray solution contains 0·045 per cent rotenone. Breakdowns in control are usually due to treatment too early and to inefficient application of the spray.

When small numbers of cattle are to be treated and a community sprayer is not available a wash

(2 kg. derris powder per 25 litre water) or dust (0·5 kg. derris powder per 2 kg. talc) can be applied but again the preparation must be brushed or rubbed vigorously into the back to ensure that it penetrates the breathing pore and comes into contact with the larva. Derris powder is difficult to wet and should be mixed to a paste first, preferably with a detergent 8 g. per 10 litres water for spray or wash) or soft soap (0·5 kg. per 25 litres for wash).

REFERENCES

(1) Kamarli, A. P. & Filatov, I. P. (1960). *Veterinariya* (*Moscow*), *37*, 65.
(2) Beesley, W. N. (1965). *Vet. Bull.*, *35*, 1.
(3) Drummond, R. O. & Graham, O. H. (1965). *Vet. Rec.*, *77*, 1418.
(4) Olander, H. J. (1967). *Path. Vet.*, *4*, 477.
(5) Khan, M. A. (1964). *Canad. vet. J.*, *5*, 20.
(6) Khan, M. A. (1969). *Res. vet. Sci.*, *10*, 355.
(7) Anderson, P. H. & Kirkwood, A. C. (1968). *Brit. vet. J.*, *124*, 569.
(8) Khan, M. A. (1968). *Vet. Rec.*, *83*, 97, 345.

Screw-worm Infestation

Myiasis caused by screw-worms has been a cause of great financial loss in livestock in the Western Hemisphere, Africa and Asia.

Incidence

The disease is of importance in tropical and subtropical areas of Africa, Asia, North and South America, especially Central America, the Caribbean islands, Mexico and American states bordering on Mexico. Death losses may be heavy in groups of livestock which are at range and are seen only infrequently. The prevalence of the fly in enzootic areas places severe restriction on the times when prophylactic surgical operations can be carried out.

Screw-worm infestation has been an important disease in the southern states of the U.S.A. and although it is still potentially a major disease, losses have been greatly reduced by rigid control measures.

Aetiology

Larvae of the flies *Callitroga americana* (*Cochliomya hominivorax*) and *Chrysomyia bezziana* cause 'screw-worm disease) of animals. The flies are typical blow-flies, *Ch. americana* being blue-green with an orange head; *Ch. bezziana* is of similar colouring. *C. americana* occurs in the Americas, *Ch. bezziana* in Africa and Asia. The occurrence of *Ch. bezziana* in Papua, New Guinea provides a constant threat to livestock on the Australian mainland (1).

A similar fly is *Callitroga* (*Cochliomyia*) *macellaria* which is not a true 'screw-fly' in that it infests only cadavers or badly necrotic sores. True 'screwflies' are obligatory parasites of all domestic and wild, warm-blooded animals and birds, laying their eggs only in fresh wounds. The navel of a newborn animal is the most favoured site but fresh accidental or surgical wounds, especially those produced by castration, docking and dehorning are readily infested. Wounds which have already been infested are markedly attractive to the flies because of their odour. In bad seasons the flies will lay eggs on minor wounds such as areas of excoriation, tick bites, running eyes, peeling brands and on the perineum soiled by vaginal and uterine discharges in animals which have recently given birth.

The development of the fly is favoured by hot, humid weather. The disease can be spread either by migration of flies or by shipment of infested cattle or other livestock. In the new environment the flies may die out if the climate is unsuitable or persist to set up a new enzootic area. Persistence of the fly in an area may depend upon persistence in wild life or in neglected domestic animals, although the latter do not usually survive unattended for more than about 2 weeks. In many enzootic areas it is common for the fly to persist in neighbouring warmer areas during winter, returning to its normal summer habitat as the temperature rises. This pattern is exemplified by the introduction of screw-worms into the southeastern United States in 1933 where they had not previously occurred. The flies died out in most areas in winter but persisted in southern Florida. In succeeding summers migrations of flies northwards caused outbreaks. The disease has since been eradicated from the area.

Life Cycle

The adult female fly lays 150 to 500 white eggs in shingle-like clusters at the edges of fresh wounds. Larvae hatch in about 12 hours and penetrate the tissues surrounding the wound. They mature in 5 to 7 days reaching a length of about 2 cm., and then leave the wound, falling to the ground. The larvae feed as a group and at their time of maturation will have created a cavity 10 to 12 cm. in diameter. The period of pupation in the ground varies widely depending on climatic conditions. It may be as short as 3 days or as long as 2 months. Emerging flies commence egg-laying in about 1 week, having completed the life cycle, under optimum environmental conditions, in less than 3 weeks.

The susceptible point in the life cycle is the

pupal stage which is unable to survive freezing for more than short periods and soil temperatures below 15°C (60°F) inhibit development. Temperatures below this point for more than 2 months cause death of the pupa. Thus the occurrence of the disease is limited to warm climates.

Pathogenesis

Secondary bacterial infection, toxaemia and fluid loss contribute to the death of the animal. Surviving calves frequently develop infectious polyarthritis.

Clinical Findings

The young larvae invade the surrounding tissues vigorously and, unlike other maggots, burrow deeply rather than feed on necrotic superficial tissue. A profuse brownish exudate pours from the wound and an objectionable odour is apparent. This is highly attractive to other flies and multiple infestations of a single wound may occur within a few days. The resulting tissue damage may be so extensive that the animal is virtually eaten alive.

Affected animals do not feed but wander about restlessly, seeking shade and shelter.

Clinical Pathology

It is imperative to differentiate screw-worm infestation from infestation with other fly larvae. The appearance and smell of the wound are significant but careful examination of the larvae is necessary to confirm the diagnosis. Mature larvae are 1 to 2 cm. long and pink in colour; they are pointed anteriorly and blunt posteriorly; two dark lines are visible reaching from the blunt posterior to the middle of the body and are diagnostic for screw-worm larvae. Specimens forwarded to a laboratory for identification should be preserved in alcohol.

Necropsy Findings

Superficial examination of infested wounds is usually sufficient to indicate the cause of death.

Diagnosis

The presence of maggots in the wound is usually apparent. It is important to differentiate them from blowfly larvae as described above.

Treatment

Affected wounds should be treated with a dressing containing an efficient larvicide and preferably an antiseptic. The larvicide should be capable of persisting in the wound for some time to prevent reinfestation. A number of proprietary prepara-

tions containing 5 per cent lindane or an organophosphate are available. An ointment or gel base is preferred so that as much of the medicament as possible is left in the site. It should be liberally and vigorously applied with a paint brush to ensure that larvae in the depths of the wound are destroyed. To avoid reinfestation in extensive lesions or in bad seasons the treatment should be repeated twice weekly.

When large numbers of animals are affected and individual treatment is impractical spraying with a 0·25 per cent solution of Co-Ral (Bayer 21/199), coumaphos, Chlorfenvinphos or Dow ET-57 (Ronnel, Korlan), using a power sprayer is recommended (2). The spray is directed forcibly into wounds and except for young calves, applied generally over the body to provide protection for about 2 weeks. Young calves may show signs of toxicity if sprayed too liberally and application should be restricted to the belly. These sprays can be used to protect animals which are not infested but are exposed to considerable risk or are to be shipped to free areas. In the latter situation dusts are also available if spraying is undesirable in cold weather. A pyrophyllite dust containing 5 per cent Co-Ral and 2 per cent mineral oil is effective as a protectant if applied at the rate of 60 to 180 g. per animal. Residual protection lasts for 3 to 7 days.

Control

In an enzootic area the incidence of the disease can be kept at a low level by the general institution of measures designed to break the life cycle of the fly. Surgical procedures should be postponed where possible until cold weather. In the warm months all wounds including shearing cuts must be immediately dressed with one of the preparations described under treatment. All range animals should be inspected twice weekly and affected animals treated promptly. Infestation of fresh navels is common and newborn animals should be treated prophylactically. If possible the breeding programme should be arranged so that parturition occurs in the cool months.

In the United States an eradication programme has been successfully carried out in the southeastern states, where the screw-worm fly population was independent of that in the Texas area, and on the island of Curacao. Cultured pupae were exposed to the sterilizing effects of cobalt 60 and the emerging flies liberated to compete with natural males for available females which mate only once. Because of the high proportion of sterile matings the incidence of infestation fell markedly and in two years infestations ceased altogether (3). This programme was subsequently extended to cover parts of Texas and northern Mexico (4).

REFERENCES

(1) Norris, K. R. & Murray, M. D. (1964). *Aust. vet. J.*, *40*, 148.
(2) Drummond, R. O. *et al.* (1966). *J. econ. Ent.*, *59*, 395.
(3) Bushland, R. C. (1960). *Advanc. vet. Sci.*, *6*, 1.
(4) Baumhover, A. H. (1966). *J. Amer. med. Ass.*, *196*, 240.

Calliphorine Myiasis

(*Blowfly or Fleece-fly Strike*)

Cutaneous infestation by blowfly maggots causes serious loss of sheep and wool in many countries. The disease is called calliphorine myiasis to differentiate it from myiasis caused by screw-worms.

Incidence

Calliphorine myiasis can be a highly important cause of losses in sheep in most countries where large numbers are kept. In bad years many sheep may die (up to 30 per cent of a flock) and the expense of controlling the flies and failure of wool to grow after recovery may be a serious strain on the local sheep economy. Merino sheep, especially those with heavy skin wrinkles, are by far the most susceptible breed and accordingly Australia, South Africa and Great Britain are the greatest sufferers from this disease. The problem is a mild one in New Zealand, India and the United States. In the latter country screw-worm infestations are much more important.

Aetiology

There are a large number of species capable of causing the disease and they are grouped geographically below:

North America—*Phormia regina, P. terrae-novae.*
Britain—*Calliphora erythrocephala, C. vomitoria, P. terrae-novae, Lucillia (Phoenicia) cuprina, L. (Phoenicia) sericata.*
New Zealand—*L. sericata, Calliphora stygia.*
Australia—*L. cuprina, L. sericata, C. stygia, C. australis, C. nociva, C. augur, C. fallax Microcalliphora varipes, Sarcophaga spp., Chrysomia rufifacies, C. micropogon.*

Cutaneous myiasis is principally a disease of sheep although it may occur sporadically in any species. In sheep the incidence varies widely depending largely on the climate, warm humid weather being most conducive to a high incidence. Outbreaks are therefore most common when there is abnormally heavy rain in summer and autumn

and when the climate is humid and sunshine intermittent. Two factors operate to encourage the development of the disease, a large fly population and the presence of susceptible sheep.

The fly population. The number of flies present in the environment depends on suitable climatic conditions and the presence of rotting organic matter to provide a source of food. In countries where sheep raising is carried on extensively there is usually no dearth of the latter, the cadavers of sheep, cattle and wild animals being left to decompose on the range. The climate determines the rate of decomposition of the carcass which in turn governs the numbers and proportions of primary, secondary and tertiary flies. Primary flies attack cadavers only in the early stages of decomposition, secondary flies when liquefaction is taking place and tertiary flies during the mummification stage. Tertiary flies do not ordinarily attack living animals although they may infest wool matted with dried exudate. They are of no economic importance. Primary and secondary flies succeed each other on the living as they do in the dead. In countries where a large number of fly species are present successive waves of infestation occur. Some flies, especially the important *Lucillia cuprina*, prefer live sheep to cadavers.

Important primary flies are: *Lucillia cuprina, L. sericata, Calliphora stygia, C. augur, C. australis, C. novica, C. fallax.*

Important secondary flies are: *Chrysomyia rufifacies, C. albiceps, C. micropogon, Microcalliphora varipes, Sarcophaga* spp.

Susceptibility of sheep. Wounds, especially castration incisions, docking wounds and head wounds on rams caused by fighting, are likely to provide good sites for blowfly strike. However, by far the most common site is the breech and infestation occurs here because of soiling and excoriation by soft faeces and the urine of ewes. Lush pasture and parasitic gastroenteritis are predisposing factors but individual sheep are predisposed because of the conformation of this part of their anatomy. Excessive wrinkling of the skin on the back of the thighs and the perineum, a narrow perineum and crutch and an excessively long or short tail favour continuous soiling of the area and encourage 'crutch or breech strike' or 'tail strike'. Less common sites for infestation are around the prepuce ('pizzle strike'), on the dorsum of the head when there is excessive folding of the skin ('poll strike') and along the dorsum of the body ('body strike') in very wet seasons when fleece rot is common. Sheep grazing on tall, dense pasture are commonly affected by body strike because of the way in which the wet plants keep the fleece on the lower part of the body wet (1). Young sheep are in general more susceptible to both diseases because of the openness of the fleece and its greater liability to wetting. Ewes which have lambed recently may be struck on the back of the udder where it is soiled with uterine discharge. In bad fly years the total number of sheep affected at these less common sites may reach alarming proportions.

Life Cycle

Adult flies are attracted by the smell of decomposing organic matter, particularly animal tissues. When fly numbers are small they largely restrict their activities to cadavers but in wet seasons when the fly population is high they attack infected wounds and wet wool, especially when it is contaminated by urine or faeces. Large numbers of eggs are laid near or on these sites and larvae hatch in 12 to 72 hours. The larvae feed on the decomposing organic matter and become fully grown in 2 days to 3 weeks depending on the suitability of the environment. When fully grown they are 6 to 12 mm. long, thick, yellow-white in colour and move actively. Some are smooth, others (*Chrysomyia rufifacies*, *C. albiceps* and *Microcalliphora varipes*) are hairy. When mature they fall to the ground and pupate, adult flies emerging in as short a period as 3 days, although this period may be very much longer in winter. Thus the life cycle can be completed in a period as short as 7 days but hibernation of larvae or pupae can carry a generation through from autumn until the next spring.

Pathogenesis

Moisture and warmth are essential for the hatching of eggs and the development of the larvae. The larvae shun light and burrow into the fleece surrounding the struck area. They also prefer an alkaline medium and prosper in decomposing fleece and tissues. From here the larvae burrow into normal skin and often undermine it, thus spreading the original lesion. They may also migrate from the original area of strike, along the surface of skin to set up another focus of damage —a secondary strike. The effects of strike include toxaemia due to absorption of toxic products of tissue decomposition, loss of skin and subsequent fluid loss, and secondary bacterial invasion.

Clinical Findings

Individual sheep may be 'struck' at any time from spring to autumn provided they are in a sus-

ceptible condition. Massive outbreaks tend to be confined to periods of humid, warm weather and are therefore usually limited in length to relatively short periods of 2 to 3 weeks.

The clinical effects of 'blowfly' strike vary with the site affected but all struck sheep have a basic pattern of behaviour caused by the irritation of the larvae. The sheep are restless, sometimes markedly so, will not feed, and move about from place to place with their heads held close to the ground. They tend to bite or kick at the 'struck' area and continually wriggle their tails. If the area is large there is an obvious odour and the wool can be seen to be slightly lifted above normal surrounding wool. The affected wool is moist and usually brown in colour although in wet seasons when fleece rot is prevalent other colours may be evident. In very early cases the maggots may still be in pockets in the wool and not yet in contact with the skin. When they have reached the skin it is inflamed and then ulcerated and the maggots commence to burrow into the subcutaneous tissue. Tracts of discoloured wool may lead to other affected areas of skin. As the struck area extends a scab forms over the centre, the wool falls out and the maggots are active only at the periphery.

Blowfly strike in sheep is commonly classified according to the site involved. This has more than casual significance because the site of strike is usually closely related to predisposing conditions which can, in some instances, be corrected.

Clinical Pathology and Necropsy Findings

A clinical examination is all that is necessary to make the diagnosis but identification of the flies responsible may be important if epizootiology is being considered. Some information can be obtained by examination of the larvae but the trapping of flies makes identification easier. The deficiency of trapping is that not all species of flies are equally attracted by the commonly used baits. *Lucillia cuprina* particularly does not occur in trap samples in the proportion in which it occurs on sheep.

Diagnosis

Predisposing diseases such as footrot, wound infections and diarrhoea due to parasitic gastroenteritis are usually easily detected and fleece rot is indicated by matting of the wool and discoloration.

Treatment

A local dressing containing a larvicide and an antiseptic is applied. The prevention of reinfestations is also an important aim and as repellents have been largely unsatisfactory, it has become apparent that the larvicide in a suitable dressing must be one with maximum retention in the treated area. Efficient older type dressings are BTB (boric acid, tar oil, bentonite mixture) and BKB (boric acid, kerosene, bentonite mixture). When these older type dressings are used affected areas should be clipped as closely as possible, ensuring that all tracts are followed and pockets of maggots and secondary strike areas are exposed. Because of the general prohibition on the use of chlorinated hydrocarbons, these compounds have been largely superseded in fly dressings by the organophosphates which are listed under control measures. They give a complete kill of maggots within about 12 hours and have the advantage of not having to be applied directly to the skin so that the wool need not be clipped. Powder and liquid dressings containing diazinon are most generally favoured.

Control

Control of cutaneous myiasis in small sheep flocks depends mainly on the prevention of unnecessary injury and of infection of wounds when they occur. Under conditions of extensive sheep raising, such as occur in Australia and South Africa and where climatic conditions are conducive to the development of the disease, the control of blowfly strike is a major undertaking and an extensive bibliography on the subject is available (2). Only a summary can be presented here.

The subject can be divided into three phases: reduction in fly numbers, prediction of fly waves followed by prophylactic crutching and application of larvicides, and reduction in susceptibility of sheep. Eradication by the use of sexually sterilized males has not proved to be a practicable procedure (3).

(a) *Reduction of fly numbers.* Although the activities listed below are of limited value in bad years they should not be neglected. If the primary fly responsible for initiating strikes can be controlled the importance of secondary flies is greatly reduced. The measures used include trapping, early treatment of clinical cases and the disposal of carcasses and wool waste. Biological control by the use of insects parasitizing blowflies has been generally unsuccessful. Trapping, provided the traps are carefully looked after and satisfactory baits are used, can reduce the number of blowflies in a small area but they are not efficient in reducing the primary fly population. For example, *L. cuprina* is

almost impervious to trapping. Destruction of carcasses must be prompt. Burying is adequate provided the carcasses are either poisoned with a larvicide or buried at least 60 cm. below the surface. Burning is more effective and is preferred if there is no fire hazard. In either instance disposal must take place within 72 hours or many primary larvae will have left the carcass. Clippings (crutchings) from infested sheep must be disposed of similarly. Clinically affected sheep must be detected before larvae have had time to mature. When affected areas are clipped, the clippings should be disposed of and larvae on the sheep destroyed with a suitable dressing.

(b) *Prediction of fly waves.* Sporadic cases of cutaneous myiasis may occur in sheep at any time and cannot reasonably be prevented, but if the environmental circumstances conducive to high fly populations and high susceptibility of sheep are recognized fly 'waves' can be predicted and short term prophylactic measures taken. The two most important predisposing factors are high environmental temperature and humidity which favour sheep susceptibility and fly reproduction rates. Lush pastures are also important but these are an inseparable corollary to the type of climate mentioned. Ideal weather for fly-strike is warm, showery weather extending over several weeks. Heavy rainfalls for a day or two are less important especially when temperatures are low or drying winds are experienced. Sheep with long fleeces are more susceptible and the time at which shearing is carried out may exert an influence on the frequency and severity of outbreaks.

If an outbreak is predicted or has begun 'crutching' and the prophylactic application of larvicides will reduce the severity of the infestation.

'Crutching' refers to clipping of the wool around the breech or crutch of the sheep to avoid it becoming wet with urine and faeces and providing a focus of attraction for flies. It is carried out routinely before lambing and immediately prior to a strike wave but provides protection for no more than 6 weeks. All the wool from above the tail, to the posterior aspect of the thighs and down to the hocks must be removed. Because of the labour and loss of wool involved most sheep farmers depend on prophylactic dressing with a larvicide.

Prophylactic dressing with a larvicide has been a major part of blowfly control for many years but the preparations used and the methods of their administration have undergone many important changes. Arsenical preparations are effective provided they are applied by a strong jet spray in such a way that they reach the skin, but they may cause arsenical poisoning if applied to a struck sheep and their protective effect is short lived. They have been almost completely superseded by more potent insecticides. They were replaced by the chlorinated hydrocarbons, DDT and benzene hexachloride, which have in turn given way to dieldrin and aldrin, which in field use have been much superior. The latter two give comparable results under average conditions with dieldrin giving better results in bad seasons and providing a rather longer period of protection. The period of protection is about 10 weeks for body strike and 4 to 6 weeks for crutch strike. Concentrations recommended are 0·1 per cent for aldrin and 0·05 per cent for dieldrin.

The chlorinated hydrocarbons are still widely used in some countries but the search for other effective compounds has been greatly stimulated by the discovery of highly resistant strains of flies and larvae in the areas where dieldrin and aldrin have been extensively used and by prohibition of the use of chlorinated hydrocarbons in some countries. Of the organophosphates, which are now the favoured compounds, Diazinon is probably the most popular. Dow ET-57 (Korlan), Chlorfenvinphos (0·05 to 0·1 per cent) (4, 5), coumaphos (0·25 per cent) (6), fenchlorphos (0·25 per cent) (7) and Bromophos (0·05 per cent) (8) have all given good results in extensive field trials. Most organophosphates appear to be effective but they vary in the duration of the protection they provide. The protection period also varies widely with the season of application (9). Lucijet (S 1751 or Lujet) and Bromophos have superior characteristics of longevity and low toxicity respectively (10) and may become the favoured preparations.

The methods of application used include dipping, when small numbers of sheep are involved, low power spraying sufficient to wet only the tip of the fleece (tip-spraying) and high power jetting in which the spray is forced through the wool to reach the skin. 'Tip-spraying' methods are based on the unusual capacity of dieldrin to diffuse down the wool fibres and are favoured by many because of the ease and speed of application. However, a much larger weight of insecticide must be used to achieve protection comparable with that of jetting and the method cannot be used with organophosphates. For crutch-strike jetting is still recommended even though it means a special chute and spray equipment and individual spraying for each sheep. Dipping has the usual disadvantages of high equipment and labour costs and unless a dis-

infectant is included in the solution laminitis caused by *Erysipelothrix rhusiopathiae* may occur.

(*c*) *Reduction in susceptibility of sheep*. Because of the prevalence of myiasis in Merino sheep with a heavily wrinkled skin most attempts have been directed towards removing the wrinkles. A breeding programme aimed at the selection of plain-bodied animals suggests itself as a suitable control measure but because wrinkliness is not inherited in a simple manner, a genetic approach to the problem has not been well accepted. The easiest method of reducing wrinkliness is by the 'Mules' operation (2). Originally the important folds of skin in the breech area were removed with sharp sheep-shears after shearing or crutching. The method has been modified and is applied to all sheep in the flock. Rather than removing the wrinkles the aim is to increase the width of the woolless area in the crutch or breech region by removing a crescentic strip of skin on both sides starting just above and to the side of the butt of the tail, continuing down the back of the thigh to just above and inside the beginning of the gastrocnemius tendon. Only woolled skin is removed, the strip terminating at a point at either end and being widest (5 to 6 cm.) opposite the vulva. Young sheep (5 to 10 months old) are easier to handle and are preferred for this operation. The technique has been developed extensively in Australia and is not described in detail here. It appears to be relatively painless and in the hands of an experienced technician the time required to improve the perineal topography need be no longer than 1 to 2 minutes. The improvement is permanent and does away to a large extent with the need for prophylactic medication and crutching.

The Mules operation is often supplemented by including a tail-strip operation in which a thin strip of woolled skin is removed from each side of the tail to above its butt. This results in a reduction of the amount of wool on the tail and less chance of faecal and urinary contamination. This operation is usually carried out at docking, the major operation being left until later. Tail stripping is important when tails are left at the longer recommended length, that is to the tip of the vulva. Docking so that the tail is of the correct length and so that a flap of ventral woolless skin is left to seal over the stump is important. The latter can be effected by pushing the skin back with the back of the docking knife before severing the tail.

Although removal of wool and skin wrinkles from the breech of sheep by surgical means or by selective breeding reduces the susceptibility of sheep, it is not anticipated that these measures alone will prevent calliphorine myiasis, nor will crutching or ringing (shearing of the breech and pizzle areas respectively). These are recommended control procedures but the protection provided will be efficient only when the blowfly population is relatively low. When flies are present in great numbers only the periodic application of an insecticide will prevent blowfly strike.

REFERENCES

(1) Axelsen, A. & Willoughby, W. M. (1968). *Aust. vet. J.*, *44*, 15.
(2) Deen, R. B. & Connelly, F. B. (1965). *Aust. J. exp. Agric. Anim. Husb.*, *5*, 6.
(3) Yeoman, G. H. & Warren, B. C. (1965). *Vet. Rec.*, *77*, 922.
(4) Thompson, G. E. (1965). *J. S. Afr. vet. med. Ass.*, *36*, 245.
(5) Wood, J. C. *et al.* (1965). *Vet. Rec.*, *77*, 896.
(6) Beesley, W. N. (1963). *Ann. appl. Biol.*, *52*, 295.
(7) Brown, F. G. & Rose, G. J. (1965). *Agric. vet. Chem.*, *6*, 131.
(8) Harrison, I. R. (1965). *Vet. Rec.*, *77*, 1145.
(9) Greenwood, E. S. (1964). *N.Z. J. agric. Res.*, *1*, 375.
(10) Fiedler, O. G. H. (1965). *J. S. Afr. vet. med. Ass.*, *36*, 233.

Ked and Louse Infestations

Although infestations with these insects are important diseases of domestic animals it is possible to deal with them only briefly here.

SHEEP KED (*Melophagus ovinus*)

This flat brown insect, which measures about 6 mm. in length, occurs on sheep in most parts of the world. It is a blood sucker and although the degrees of infestation usually encountered cause only irritation with resulting scratching, biting and damage to the fleece, very heavy infestations may cause severe anaemia. There is good evidence that keds transmit Q fever in sheep (1). Staining of the wool by the faeces of the ked also causes depreciation in its value. Heavy infestations cause skin blemishes which are costly to the leather industry. Sheep in poor condition suffer most from infestations. Goats may also be infested.

Keds live their entire life cycle on the host and spread for the most part is by direct contact between hosts. Single larvae are deposited directly on the wool and soon pupate, a complete life cycle taking 5 to 6 weeks in optimum warm conditions but very much longer in cold weather. Heavy infestations are usually encountered in the winter months and in cool climates but spread appears to occur most commonly during periods of bright sunlight. Resistance is acquired in time, related in part to the nutritional status of the animal (2).

Because the ked does not leave the host, control of the parasite must include power-spraying or dipping in an insecticidal solution. The chlorinated hydrocarbons, where applicable, and organophosphates are effective and have the advantage over rotenone and arsenical preparations that they persist in the fleece sufficiently long to destroy keds emerging from pupae subsequent to dipping. One treatment is usually sufficient. Dusting with a powder containing dieldrin, Ronnel or Diazinon is also highly effective and avoids wetting the sheep. It is most effective if carried out after shearing; later treatments may require three times as much insecticide (3, 4). Persistence of the infestation is usually due to prolongation of the pupal stage during cold weather. Failure to dip all sheep, improper use and mixing of medicaments are other causes of persistence. A control programme usually consists of one dipping or dusting a year, preferably carried out soon after shearing. When it is necessary to treat young lambs only derris or rotenone should be used because of the toxicity of the other compounds for this age group.

LOUSE INFESTATIONS (PEDICULOSIS)

All species of lice can cause sufficient irritation of the skin to stimulate scratching, rubbing and licking leading to restlessness, damage to fleece and hides and loss of weight gain or milk production. The coat of affected animals is rough and shaggy and there is usually marked pityriasis. Cattle heavily infested with sucking lice may develop serious and even fatal anaemia (5). The pig louse spreads swine pox. Foot lice of sheep may cause lameness, and hairballs may be common in heavily infested calves because of continued licking. In searching for lice special attention should be paid to the back, the sides of the neck, escutcheon and tail switch. The feet of sheep should be searched carefully for foot lice. Animals in poor condition, improperly fed and exposed to cold and debilitating disease carry heaviest infestations (10), especially if they are housed in overcrowded conditions. Lice of cattle and sheep are small and pale coloured and are not readily visible unless seen in a strong light, although the eggs can usually be detected fixed to dark coloured hairs.

Life cycles of all lice are similar and are normally passed entirely on the host although some species can survive for up to 2 weeks away from the host. The eggs are laid attached to coat fibres and there are three nymphal stages before mature lice appear. The life cycle of most species varies from 2 to 4 weeks under optimum conditions. Most louse populations show a seasonal periodicity with greatest numbers in winter and virtual disappearance in summer and under very wet conditions (6, 11). Transmission is effected by direct contact but inert objects such as blankets, grooming tools and harness may remain infective for several days and the foot-louse of sheep may remain infective on pasture for 3 days.

The important species are:

Cattle—*Linognathus vituli* (long-nosed sucking louse), *Solenoptes capillatus* (small blue sucking louse), *Haematopinus eurysternus* (short-nosed sucking louse), *Damalinia* (*Bovicola*) *bovis* (biting louse), *H. quadripertusus* (tail louse).

Sheep—*Haematopinus quadripertusus* (tail louse), *H. tuberculatus* (buffalo louse), *Linognathus ovillus* (sucking face louse), *L. africanus*, *L. stenopsis* (sucking goat louse), *L. pedalis* (sucking foot louse), *Damalinia* (*Bovicola*) *ovis* (biting louse).

Goats—*Linognathus stenopsis* (sucking blue louse), *Damalinia* (*Bovicola*) *caprae* (biting red louse), *Bovicola painei*, *Damalinia* (*Bovicola*) *limbata*, *Damalinia* (*Bovicola*) *crassipes*.

Pig—*Haematopinus suis* (sucking louse).

Horse—*Haematopinus asini* (sucking louse), *Damalinia* (*Bovicola*) *equi* (biting louse).

Affected animals can be effectively treated with sodium arsenite in a dip or with sprays, dips or dusts containing rotenone or synergized pyrethrins, chlorinated hydrocarbon insecticides (e.g. lindane, toxaphene, methoxychlor, dieldrin) or organo-phosphatic insecticides (7, 8). The manufacturer's recommendations should be accurately followed especially with the latter group and when using dusts or surface sprays (4). Lice develop resistance to insecticides quite rapidly and strains of *D. ovis* which are resistant to the chlorinated hydrocarbon insecticides are common in the U.K. Control programmes include treatment of all animals and spraying of housing in early winter and further treatments as required in winter and early spring. Eradication is a practicable procedure but should not be undertaken unless reinfestation can be prevented (9).

REFERENCES

(1) Pavilanis, V. (1959). *Canad. J. publ. Hlth*, *50*, 31.
(2) Nelson, W. A. & Hironaka, R. (1966). *Exp. Parasit.*, *18*, 274.
(3) Pfadt, R. E. & Lavigne, R. J. (1965). *J. econ. Ent.*, *58*, 37.
(4) Sinclair, A. N. (1963). *Aust. vet. J.*, *39*, 81.
(5) Collins, R. C. & Dewhirst, L. W. (1965). *J. Amer. vet. med. Ass.*, *146*, 129.
(6) Murray, M. D. (1963). *Aust. J. Zool.*, *11*, 153, 157, 173 & 183.
(7) Khan, M. R. (1964). *Canad. vet. J.*, *5*, 20.
(8) Greenwood, E. S. (1964). *N.Z. J. agric. Res.*, *7*, 382.
(9) Anthony, D. W. *et al.* (1963). *J. Amer. vet. med. Ass.*, *142*, 130.
(10) Utech, K. B. W. *et al.* (1969). *Aust. vet. J.*, *45*, 414.
(11) Murray, M. D. & Gordon, G. (1969). *Aust. J. Zool.*, *17*, 179.

Tick Infestations

Tick infestations are of great importance in the production of diseases of animals. Apart from their role as vectors and potential reservoirs of infectious diseases, as outlined below, heavy infestations can cause direct losses. Many are active blood suckers (e.g. *Ixodes ricinus*, *Argas* spp.) and may cause death from anaemia. Some species cause tick paralysis and it is possible that other ticks may elaborate toxins other than those causing paralysis (1). As with louse infestations heavy tick burdens cause sufficient worry to interfere with feeding which may lead to loss of production and weight gain (2).

The life cycles of the ticks vary widely. Some species pass their entire life on the one host, others pass different stages of the cycle on successive hosts, and others are parasitic only at certain stages. The eggs are laid in the soil and larvae attach themselves to a passing host on which they may develop through one or more nymphal stages (instars) before becoming adults. Adult females engorge on blood or lymph and drop to the ground to lay their eggs. Single host ticks are more easily controlled than those which pass part of their life cycles away from the host. A list of the single and multiple host ticks is provided below.

SINGLE-HOST TICKS

Boophilus spp.
Margaropus winthemi
Otobius megnini

TWO-HOST TICKS

Rhipicephalus evertsi
R. bursa
Hyalomma spp. (most have two or three hosts)

THREE-HOST TICKS

Ixodes spp.
Rhipicephalus spp. (except *R. evertsi* and *R. bursa*)
Haemaphysalis spp.
Amblyomma spp.
Hyalomma spp. (most have two or three hosts)
Ornithodorus spp.—many hosts
Dermacentor spp.
Argas persicus—many hosts

Although many ticks favour a particular host they are usually not completely host-specific and may parasitize a wide variety of animals. In the limited space available here the species are listed according to whether they cause worry only or transmit infectious diseases of large domestic animals.

For more detailed information on transmission of infectious diseases and the biology and distribution of ticks the papers by Neitz (3) and Theiler (4) from which much of the following information has been drawn should be consulted.

TICKS CAUSING PARALYSIS

Paralysis is not uncommon in young domestic animals which are heavily infested with the ticks listed in the next column. Details of the clinical syndrome are provided in Chapter 31. Recovery is usual in early mild cases if the ticks are removed.

Ticks Reported to Cause Paralysis

Animal Affected	Tick	Country
Sheep, calves, goats	*Dermacentor andersoni*	U.S.A.
	D. occidentalis (5)	U.S.A.
Calves, lambs	*Ixodes holocyclus*	Australia
Sheep, goats, calves	*I. pilosus*	South Africa
Sheep, goats, calves, antelope	*I. rubicundus*	South Africa
Lambs	*Rhipicephalus evertsi*	South Africa
Calves, sheep, goats	*Haemaphysalis punctata*	South Africa, Europe, Japan
Sheep	*Ornithodorus lahorensis*	Central Asia
Sheep	*Hyalomma aegyptium*	Yugoslavia
Sheep, goats	*Ixodes ricinus*	Crete

TICKS WHICH TRANSMIT PROTOZOAN DISEASES

Ticks are the most important vectors of many protozoan diseases, the protozoa in most instances surviving from generation to generation of ticks by infecting their eggs. Where control of these diseases is to be undertaken it is necessary to know which ticks are vectors, how many hosts the tick parasitizes during a life cycle and which animals can act as hosts. Much of the information on these points is fragmentary and only a summary is presented in the table on p. 669.

BACTERIAL, VIRAL AND RICKETTSIAL DISEASES TRANSMITTED BY TICKS

The transmission of diseases caused by these agents may be effected by means other than insect vectors and by insect vectors other than ticks. A list is provided in the table on p. 670.

TICKS WHICH CAUSE WORRY

Most ticks cause a great deal of worry to farm animals when they are present in large numbers. A list of ticks which have this effect but are not known to cause paralysis or transmit infectious diseases in farm animals is given below.

Ticks which Cause Worry Only

Otobius megnini, the 'spinose ear tick' of the U.S.A. and Canada
Amblyomma americanum, the 'Lone Star Tick' of the U.S.A.
A. maculatum, the 'Gulf Coast Tick' of the U.S.A.
Margaropus winthemi of South America and Africa
Ixodes canisuga, the English dog tick
Ornithodorus moubata of Africa and South-east Asia
O. savignyi of Africa and South-east Asia.

Treatment and Control of Tick Infestations

Choice of insecticide. Individual animals can be effectively treated by the application of any one of a number of insecticides applied either as a spray or by dipping. The choice of insecticides depends largely on three factors: the persistence of the compound on the skin and hair coat, the likelihood of residues of insecticide toxic to man appearing in the milk or meat, and whether or not the ticks in the area have developed resistance to the particular insecticide. The more modern insecticides have the advantage over arsenical preparations, which have served so well for so long, of ease of administration and persistence on the skin but resistance to chlorinated hydrocarbons, organophosphates (6) and carbamates (7) appears to develop quite rapidly. Resistance to arsenic also occurs and although it develops much more slowly than, for example, resistance to benzene hexachloride it may make its use unwarranted over large areas. The problem of resistance of ticks to insecticide is increasing rapidly to the point where a selection of new drugs, even some with toxicity problems, must be kept on hand (9).

The same criteria apply in control as in treatment except that cost becomes a limiting factor when large numbers of animals require frequent treatments and it is obvious in some circumstances that the effect of tick infestation on Brahman-cross steers is insufficiently great to warrant treating them (10). It is impossible to make specific recommendations on methods of application and the most efficient insecticide to use because these vary widely between species of ticks. In general, arsenic preparations are most satisfactory for the control of multiple-host ticks, the more modern ixodicides for one-host ticks. The insecticides which are safe to use in all classes of cattle are arsenic, rotenone

Ticks Reported to Transmit Protozoan Diseases (2, 5)

Disease	Protozoan	Vector Tick	Country
Bovine Babesiasis	*Babesia bigemina*	*Boophilus annulatus* *B. australis (microplus)* *B. (annulatus) calcaratus, B. decoloratus, Rhipicephalus appendiculatus, R. bursa, R. evertsi, Ixodes ricinus* *Haemaphysalis punctata*	N. America Australia and S. America Africa Europe
	Babesia bovis	*Ixodes persulcatus* *I. ricinus* *Boophilus annulatus*	Russia Europe Iran
	Babesia argentina	*B. australis (microplus)*	Australia
	Babesia berbera	*B. annulatus (calcaratus), Rhipicephalus bursa*	Africa
Ovine and Caprine Babesiasis	*Babesia motasi*	*Dermacentor silvarum, Rhipicephalus bursa, Haemaphysalis punctata, Ixodes ricinus*	Europe
	Babesia ovis	*Rhipicephalus bursa* *Haemaphysalis bispinosa*	Russia India
Equine Babesiasis	*Babesia caballi*	*Hyalomma dromedarii* *Dermacentor (reticulata) marginatus, D. pictus, D. silvarum, Hyalomma (excavatum) anatolicum, H. marginatum, H. volgense, Rhipicephalus bursa, R. sanguineus*	Africa Russia and the Balkans S. America and Florida U.S.A.
	Babesia equi	*Hyalomma dromedarii, Rhipicephalus evertsi, R. sanguineus, Dermacentor marginatus, D. pictus, Hyalomma anatolicum, H. marginatum, H. uralense, Rhipicephalus bursa, R. sanguineus*	Africa the Balkans S. America
Porcine Babesiasis	*Babesia trautmanni*	*R. sanguineus (turanicus)*	Russia
Bovine Anaplasmosis	*Anaplasma marginale*	*Boophilus annulatus, Argas persicus, Dermacentor albipictus, D. andersoni, D. occidentalis, D. variabilis, Ixodes scapularis, Rhipicephalus sanguineus* *Boophilus australis (microplus)* *B. decoloratus, Hyalomma excavatum, Rhipicephalus bursa, R. simus* *Haemaphysalis punctata, Ixodes ricinus* *Boophilus (annulatus) calcaratus*	North America Australia and S. America Africa Europe Russia
Ovine and Caprine Anaplasmosis	*Anaplasma ovis*	*Dermacentor silvarum, Rhipicephalus bursa, Ornithodorus lahorensis*	Russia

(derris) and pyrethrum. They can all be used on milking cows with little danger provided they are carefully mixed.

Arsenic is usually used as a dip containing 0·1 to 0·2 per cent arsenic trioxide. The proportion of arsenic used is varied depending on the frequency of dipping. Arsenic preparations are used only as dips because of the danger of contaminating surroundings with sprays. As in all dips the concentration of insecticide is likely to be gradually reduced by repeated use and this 'stripping' must be repaired by periodic replenishment of the dip.

Rotenone (2 to 4 oz. of 5 per cent derris dust per gallon of water) and pyrethrum (pyrethrins 0·1 per cent plus piperonyl butoxide 1·0 per cent—synergized pyrethrins) are used as sprays or dips.

For beef cattle and all other species lindane and toxaphene may be used as dips at concentrations of 0·025 per cent and 0·25 per cent respectively or as sprays at similar concentrations. Carbamate

Diseases Caused by Bacteria, Viruses and Rickettsia Reported to be Transmitted by Ticks (5)

Disease	Causative Agent	Vector Tick	Country
Tick Pyaemia (lambs)	*Staphylococcus aureus*	*Ixodes ricinus*	Great Britain
Tularaemia (sheep)	*Pasteurella tularense*	*Haemaphysalis leporispalustris, H. otophila, Dermacentor andersoni, D. variabilis D. pictus, D. marginatus, Ixodes luguri*	U.S.A. Norway, Europe, Russia
Brucellosis	*Brucella abortus* and *Br. melitensis*	Many ticks may be infected but infection of host appears to occur only if ticks or their faeces are eaten (8)	Russia
Encephalomyelitis of Horses	Western type Virus	*Dermacentor andersoni* *Ixodes ricinus, Dermacentor* spp. (lab. only)	U.S.A. Russia
Louping Ill	Virus	*Rhipicephalus appendiculatus* (lab. only) *Ixodes ricinus*	Africa England
Tick-borne Fever	*Rickettsia* spp.	*I. ricinus* *Rhipicephalus haemaphysaloides*	Great Britain, Norway India
Caseous Lymphadenitis of Sheep	*Cor. pseudo-tuberculosis*	*Dermacentor albipictus*	North America

compounds, including carbaryl and RD 12308, have been successful as acaricide dips and sprays. The organophosphates as a group are also highly effective. Drugs in current use include Co-Ral, Ronnel, coumaphos, Diazinon, Delnav, ethion, ciodrin, carbophenothion, dioxathion (7) and Chlorfenvinphos (8). Recommended strengths for dips and sprays are 0·05 per cent for weekly application and 0·075 per cent to 0·15 per cent for applications at intervals of 3 to 4 weeks. A mixture of toxaphene and Delnav gives good control of mange, hornfly (*Lyperosia irritans*) and *Dermatobia hominis*. Ticks in the ears of horses present a problem because of the difficulty of applying topical preparations. Metriphonate (20 mg. per kg. body weight daily for 10 days) in the feed is an effective remedy (11). In other species it is more common to use a topical preparation squirted into the ears with a syringe. These preparations vary in the duration of the protection they afford and local conditions of rainfall and tick population must be taken into account when determining the time intervals between sprayings or dippings. Chlorphenamidine gives 80–90 per cent kill of *B. microplus* when used in a spray at a concentration of 0·012 per cent but because of its toxicity it is more valuable as an additive to a preparation containing organophosphates (9).

A special case is that of young lambs which are exposed to tick pyaemia. Sprays, dips and ointments are too toxic and the most effective procedure is the application of a liquid emulsion cream containing the insecticide to the woolless parts of the body.

Control and Eradication

In most countries all that is attempted is reduction of the tick population by periodic dipping or spraying. Complete eradication is extremely difficult because of the persistence of ticks, especially multi-host ticks, on wild fauna, and the ability of adult ticks to live for very long periods apart from a host. On the other hand, continuous treatment to restrain the tick population is highly conducive to the development of resistance, a problem which has become apparent in many tick areas. *Boophilus annulatus* was eradicated from the south-eastern U.S.A. by a programme of continuous dipping at short intervals of all livestock in the area. *B. microplus* was also eradicated from Florida by a similar procedure but 20,000 head of deer, the important alternate host in the area, had to be slaughtered (12). Attempts to eradicate other single-host ticks in other countries have not been generally successful. Although both dipping and spraying are recommended for the control of ticks, complete wetting of the animal, which can only be effected by dipping, is essential if eradication is to be undertaken. This adds another impediment to eradication plans because of the cost of constructing proper dips and yards. When one considers that dipping may have to be carried out every 14 days for 15 months, that every animal in the eradication area must be dipped and that a strict quarantine of the area must be maintained, it is obvious that eradication cannot be undertaken lightly.

Measures other than the application of insecticides used in the control of tick infestation include burning of pasture, removal of native fauna, ploughing of fields, and rotational grazing. So little is known of the bionomics of specific ticks in specific areas that these measures have been largely unsuccessful and it is impossible to provide details for their proper implementation (4). Pasture spelling and rotational grazing have been shown to be capable of greatly reducing the tick population on farms in some areas. The practicability of the procedure depends upon a full-scale financial assessment of the increased weight gains relative to the costs of management. Duration of the spelling period varies between 4 and 18 weeks. Aerial spraying of pasture with DDT (20 lb. per ton of superphosphate) has been used in an attempt to control *Haemaphysalis bispinosa* infestation in New Zealand (13). All livestock must be removed from the area during dusting and allowed to return only when rain has fallen. Other insecticides have also been similarly used but this procedure is still in the experimental stage.

It is possible to reduce the ravages of ticks and tickborne diseases by the introduction of genetically resistant strains (14) or breeds of cattle. Brahman cattle are notably more resistant than British breeds and crossbreds of the two races retain this characteristic (15, 10). In Australia the possibility that *B. microplus* might escape from its control area because of increased resistance to acaricides has been realized. For this reason a great deal of attention is being paid to the possibility of selecting cattle for tick resistance (9, 15, 16). With successive infestations cattle differ in their response to *B. microplus*. Thus there is increased irritation and more licking (16) and a decrease in the number of ticks carried. There are some prospects that an artificially created immunity to the tick could have practical application (1).

Other special cases include *Otobius megnini*, the nymphs of which drop off to moult and lay eggs in protected spots, necessitating the spraying of buildings, fence posts, feed troughs and tree trunks in feedlots where heavy infestations are most common. *Ornithodorus* spp. ticks are difficult to control because the nymphs and adults attach to feed for brief periods only. Where ticks which cause paralysis are common it may be necessary to apply an insecticide as a dust and dip at short intervals.

REVIEW LITERATURE
Wharton, R. H. & Roulston, W. J. (1970). Resistance of ticks to chemicals. *Ann. Rev. Entom.*, *15*, 381.

REFERENCES
(1) Riek, R. F. (1965). *Aust. vet. J.*, *41*, 211.
(2) Little, D. A. (1963). *Aust. vet. J.*, *39*, 6.
(3) Neitz, W. D. (1956). *Onderstepoort J. vet. Res.*, *27*, 115.
(4) Theiler, G. (1959). *J. S. Afr. vet. med. Ass.*, *30*, 195.
(5) Loomis, E. C. & Bushnell, R. B. (1968). *Amer. J. vet. Res.*, *29*, 1089.
(6) Shaw, R. D. & Malcolm, H. A. (1964). *Vet. Rec.*, *76*, 211.
(7) Roulston, W. J. & Wilson, J. T. (1965). *Bull. ent. Res.*, *55*, 617.
(8) Drummond, R. O. *et al.* (1966). *J. econ. Ent.*, *59*, 395.
(9) Roulston, W. J. *et al.* (1971). *Aust. vet. J.*, *47*, 521.
(10) Gee, R. W. *et al.* (1971). *Aust. vet. J.*, *47*, 257.
(11) Drummond, R. O. & Graham, O. H. (1965). *Vet. Rec.*, *77*, 1418.
(12) Anonymous (1959). *Proc. 67th ann. gen. Mtg U.S. Live Stock sanit. Ass.*, 1958, pp. 187–91.
(13) Smythe, E. B. (1959). *N.Z. vet. J.*, *7*, 66.
(14) Wharton, R. H. (1970). *Aust. J. agric. Res.*, *21*, 163.
(15) Watts, R. M. (1969). *Aust. vet. J.*, *45*, 437.
(16) Hewetson, R. W. (1972). *Aust. vet. J.*, *48*, 299.

Miscellaneous Flies, Midges and Mosquitoes

Although these insects differ quite markedly they are dealt with together because they exert similar deleterious effects, particularly the worry they cause livestock and the capacity they have for transmitting infectious diseases.

STABLE FLIES

The stable fly, *Stomoxys calcitrans*, occurs in most countries. Other species, including *S. nigra*, occur in South Africa. *S. calcitrans* is about the size of a housefly, is grey in colour and sits head upwards. It is a blood sucker attacking particularly horses and cattle and to a lesser extent pigs. Bites from the fly are quite painful and often bleed freely when fresh. The eggs are laid in rotting hay and straw, especially when it is contaminated with urine, and in horse manure, A complete life cycle may be completed in 30 to 60 days, the larval and pupal stages taking place in the organic matter. Warm, moist conditions favour multiplication of the flies and in bad seasons the large numbers of flies may cause anaemia, worry, loss of grazing time and reduction of growth and yield. With very heavy infestations some deaths may occur. Among the important infectious diseases transmitted by

S. calcitrans are anthrax, infectious equine anaemia and surra. The fly is not a true intermediate host but acts only as a mechanical vector. The fly also acts as the intermediate host for *Habronema microstoma* and is reputed to be a cause of allergic dermatitis in horses in Japan.

Control of the fly necessitates removal or close covering of rotting organic matter from the environment. Silage stacks and compost heaps are favoured breeding spots. Destruction of flies is difficult because they feed for only short periods. Spraying of cattle with repellents such as one litre of an emulsion of pyrethrins 0·05 per cent and piperonyl butoxide 0·5 per cent per head or the proprietary preparations Tabutrex or R. 326 (1) is recommended and the spraying of fixtures, barns, stables and foliage where flies alight with a suitable barn spray containing pyrethrins, methoxychlor, lindane, chlordane or an organophosphate should also reduce fly numbers (2).

HORSE FLIES, MARCH FLIES OR BREEZE FLIES (*Tabanus* spp.)
DEER FLIES
(*Chrysops* spp., *Haematopota* and *Pangonia* spp.)

These large brown robust flies are widespread in many countries and like *S. calcitrans* worry large animals, particularly horses and cattle and being blood suckers can cause anaemia. They can also act as mechanical vectors of such diseases as infectious equine anaemia, surra and anthrax. *Haematopota* spp. are commonly suspected of acting as vectors for corynebacterial mastitis (summer mastitis) of cattle. The life cycle differs from that of *S. calcitrans* in that the eggs are laid on the leaves of plants growing in or near water. The larval and pupal stages are passed in water or mud and the life cycle takes 4 to 5 months to complete. The flies are active in summer and attack animals principally on the legs and ventral abdomen. Control is difficult unless wet areas can be drained or livestock kept away from these areas where the flies are most active. Repellents have been used and are reasonably effective in horses subject to fly-worry. Dimethyl phthalate and Huon pine oil (3) and the pyrethrin–piperonyl butoxide emulsion listed above are recommended but afford protection for only a few days. A number of commercial products are available which can be applied automatically to the udders of milking cows (4)

BUFFALO FLIES (*Lyperosia* (*Haematobia*, *Siphona*) *exigua*),
HORN FLIES (*L. irritans* and *L. minuta*)
. These small (6 mm.) greyish flies have fairly limited geographical distributions, *L. exigua* in

Australia and South-East Asia, *L. irritans* in the continental U.S.A. and Hawaii and *L. minuta* in Africa. They have similar life cycles and habits. Although they are primarily parasites of cattle and water buffalo and are unable to survive apart from these animals, they can be a nuisance to horses and man in bad seasons. They are blood suckers but are not known to transmit diseases, their chief importance being to worry animals and interfere with their grazing. Very heavy infestations (over 1000 flies) can cause serious loss of condition and deaths in cattle. The flies congregate chiefly on the withers, shoulders and flanks and around the eyes. Zebu cattle are less affected by the flies than British breeds. Horses may develop sores around the eyes and under the belly which provide sites for infestation of larvae of *Habronema megastoma*. The flies are easily recognized by the way in which the wings are held at rest, slightly divergent and angled upwards away from the body. Adult flies stay on the host most of the time, leaving it only to lay eggs in fresh cattle manure. The eggs and larvae have narrow environmental limits in which they can survive; they are very susceptible to drying, requiring 60 to 80 per cent free moisture; the optimum temperature for development is 26 to 30°C (80 to 85°F), higher or lower temperatures arresting development. Thus the flies can only persist in warm moist climates, requiring an annual rainfall of at least 50 cm. and a mean temperature of 22°C (72°F). The larvae live in the fresh manure and pupate in the soil, a complete life cycle ending in 8 days to 3 weeks under optimal environmental conditions. Adult flies are active only in warm weather and particularly in the vicinity of water and shade. They may be carried long distances by prevailing strong winds but the main method of spread is by the movement of cattle.

Control of these flies is difficult on a large scale because of their large numbers and the lack of control of cattle in the areas where they are common. Trapping and periodic spraying can be used to reduce the fly numbers greatly where cattle are in sufficiently small groups to be handled easily. Pour-on preparations of coumaphos, Co-Ral or Ruelene (all 0·5 per cent) or Neguvon (1 per cent), sprays of Diazinon (0·1 per cent) and dimethoate (1·0 per cent) and dusts of Diazinon powder (2 to 25 per cent) or Guthion (10 per cent) all give excellent protection for 14 days (5). Strategically placed 'back-oilers' containing 5 per cent toxaphene, 5 per cent DDT in fuel oil, Co-Ral 0·25 per cent, Ronnel 1 per cent in oil also provide effective control in beef cattle herds (6) as do self-treatment dust bags containing 1 per cent coumaphos (15).

Milking cows can be effectively protected by daily spraying from an automatic spraying device and effective control is recorded in beef cattle at pasture with similar devices. A suitable spray mixture contains fenchlorphos (0·25 per cent), pyrethrins (0·05 per cent), piperonyl butoxide (0·25 per cent) in petroleum distillate (99·45 per cent). Aerial spraying with trichlorfon has been tried with some success (7). Self-applied and hand-applied dusts containing organophosphates are effective if application is frequent (8).

Observations on *L. irritans* showed that flies which inhabit the lower legs of cattle are predominantly male. A spraying programme, using an organophosphate, has eliminated whole horn-fly populations (9).

HORSE LOUSE-FLIES

(Hippobosca equina, H. rufipes and H. maculata)

Hippobosca equina is the common fly and is a parasite of horses and cattle in most countries with a warm climate. It is a flat, glossy, reddish brown fly, slightly bigger than a housefly. It is a blood sucker and lives most of the time on the host, particularly on the perineum and between the hind legs. Female flies deposit individual puparia in dry humus in which they mature to adult flies. The flies appear to cause little annoyance in horses which are accustomed to them but horses experiencing them for the first time manifest fright and fly-worry. Being blood suckers they may act as mechanical vectors for infectious diseases. Topical spraying of susceptible areas of the body with chlorinated hydrocarbons appears to keep these parasites in check.

BITING MIDGES

These tiny flies are members of the family Ceratopogonidae, the important genera being *Culicoides* spp. They are 1 to 3 mm. long, suck blood and, apart from causing annoyance and worry, can transmit infectious diseases such as bluetongue in sheep, horse sickness, ephemeral fever in cattle and act as intermediate hosts for *Onchocerca* spp. filarid worms. Hypersensitivity to the bites of *Culicoides* spp. is the cause of allergic dermatitis (Queensland Itch) in horses in Australia. The flies are plentiful in the warmer months and are most active at dusk and in the early morning. Because of their small size they are capable of being carried long distances by wind. Control of the flies is virtually impossible and most measures to reduce their importance are based on preventing access of the flies to the animals. Repellents, especially dimethyl phthallate, are effective on a short-term basis but mosquito screens are insufficient protection. Keeping horses away from areas where the flies are present in large numbers is advisable.

BLACK FLIES, BUFFALO GNATS, SANDFLIES

These small grey to black flies (5 mm.) are members of the family Simuliidae and include a number of species and genera. In North America the important flies appear to be *Cnephia pecuarum* common in the southern states of the U.S.A., *Simulium arcticum* in northern Canada, *Austrosimulium pestilens* and *A. bancrofti* in Australia, and *Simulium ornatum* in Great Britain. These very small flies occur in most parts of the world and with the exception of *S. arcticum* are troublesome only in warm climates. They are particularly active in the summer months, especially at dusk and in the early morning, and frequent areas where fresh, surface water and shade-trees are plentiful. Very large numbers of flies are often present after periods of flooding or in areas with many streams. The flies congregate in swarms and attack all animals, causing much worry and annoyance. They tend to bite animals around the legs, on the belly and around the head, causing weals and papules. The annoyance may be so intense that animals stampede or mill about and young animals may be injured or even trampled to death and are frequently separated from their dams. Cattle may spend much of their time wallowing in mud or kicking up dust to keep the flies away. Sudden deaths in cattle have also been recorded after attacks by very large numbers of flies. The cause of death is unknown although swelling of the throat causing suffocation, anaphylaxis or direct toxicity are suspected. (10). Filarid worms of *Onchocerca* spp. are also transmitted by these flies.

Because the larval stages of these worms are passed in flowing streams, large-scale control measures must be directed at killing the larvae at this stage. Aerial distribution of DDT has been effective when added to streams and water supplies (11). For less ambitious control programmes, efforts should be directed towards keeping flies away from animals by the application of repellents or the use of smudge fires.

MOSQUITOES

A number of mosquitoes including *Psorophora* spp., *Aedes* spp., *Mansonia* spp. and *Culex* spp. are important parasites of domestic animals. When present in large numbers they cause annoyance and worry to animals and have been known to kill young pigs and puppies by the severe anaemia they produce. Although such occurrences are rarely recorded this is surprising in the light of the blood loss that can occur in severe infestations (12). This is apparently sufficient to cause a brake on productivity even in mature large animals. Their most important role is as vectors of disease. *Culex tarsalis*, *Aedes dorsalis*, and *A. nigromaculis* transmit equine encephalomyelitis, *Culex tritaeniorhyncus* is the principal vector of Japanese B encephalitis in Japan (6), *Psorophora confinnis* is instrumental in spreading the eggs of *Dermatobia hominis*, the tropical warble fly, and *Mansonia* spp. transmits Rift Valley fever. The filarid worm *Setaria digitata* is also spread by mosquitoes.

Control over a large area must include drainage of collections of still surface water or destruction of the larvae by the addition of any one of a number of insecticides, particularly DDT. For small groups of animals protection from the attacks of mosquitoes can only be satisfactorily effected by mosquito-proof screens. Temporary protection by repellents such as dimethyl phthalate is partial only.

HOUSE-FLY (*Musca domestica*)

The common house-fly has a world wide distribution and achieves veterinary importance because it is capable of transmitting, in a mechanical manner, the causative bacteria of many infectious diseases. It is often cited as a means whereby anthrax, erysipelas and brucellosis are spread but its importance in this regard is largely unproven. It acts as an intermediate host for the larvae of *Habronema muscae* and *H. megastoma*. The eggs are laid in decaying organic matter of any kind but fresh horse manure is preferred. A life cycle may be completed in 12 to 14 days in warm weather so that in wet summers the fly population may increase very rapidly causing annoyance to livestock and farm workers.

To reduce the fly population it is necessary to remove all manure and organic matter or spray it in situ. In dry weather the manure can be spread thinly on fields but a more dependable method is to place it in a special fly trap, e.g. Baber's fly traps, from which larvae and adult flies cannot escape. Measures to control fly emergence from manure include spraying with diazinon (100 mg. per sq. foot).

To reduce the fly population in buildings is an important procedure in public health work and many measures are recommended. It is not possible to give details of them here because so many factors have to be taken into consideration, including toxicity of the products used for man and animals, development of resistance to the insecticides and contamination of food products such as milk by the insecticides.

BUSH FLIES
(*Musca vetustissima*, *M. fergusoni*, *M. terraeregina*, *M. hilli*)

These flies occur commonly in Australia in drier areas and are a cause of much worry to livestock in the summer months. *Musca vetustissima* in particular occur in very large numbers and during the day congregate around the eyes, on the lips, on any visible mucous membrane and on wounds. They are thought to carry contagious ophthalmia of sheep, infectious kerato-conjunctivitis of cattle and contagious ecthyma of sheep, to delay the healing of wounds, to contribute to the lesions produced by buffalo flies (*Lyperosia exigua*) and to act as intermediate hosts for the larvae of *Habronema* spp. Control of the fly population is virtually impossible in the areas where it occurs but individual animals may be protected by repellents such as dimethyl phthalate or the pyrethrum-piperonyl butoxide emulsion described under stable flies.

FACE-FLY (*Musca autumnalis*)

This small fly, indigenous to Europe and Asia, first appeared in North America in 1952 and is now present over large areas of eastern Canada and north-eastern and north-central U.S.A. The flies resemble the house-fly but are slightly larger. They congregate on the face of cattle, feeding on nasal and lacrimal secretions and saliva. Very large numbers cause a certain amount of fly-worry and they are thought to be instrumental in transmitting infectious kerato-conjunctivitis (pink-eye) of cattle. Fly numbers are greatest in summer and cattle are worried particularly when outdoors. Repellents have been extensively used but are not highly successful. Syrup baits containing organophosphatic insecticides and applied 3 times weekly to the forehead of cows may help to eliminate these flies (13). Self-applied or hand-applied dusts containing organophosphatic insecticides are more extensively used (8). Faeces of cattle fed low levels of organophosphates inhibit the development of face-fly larvae but the usefulness of this procedure in the field is limited by the migration of flies from surrounding infested areas (14).

Several other species of Muscidae, *Musca larvipara*, *M. convexifrons* and *M. amica* act as intermediate hosts for *Thelazia* spp. worms which infest the conjunctival sacs and lacrymal ducts of domestic animals.

REFERENCES

(1) Bruce, W. N. & Decker, G. C. (1957). *J. econ. Ent.*, *50*, 709.
(2) Parr, H. C. M. (1959). *Nature* (*Lond.*), *184*, Suppl. 11, 829.
(3) McCulloch, R. N. & Waterhouse, D. F. (1947). *Cwlth Aust. Counc. sci. ind. Res. Bull.*, 213.
(4) Cheng Tien-Hsi *et al.* (1959). *J. econ. Ent.*, *52*, 866.
(5) Dorsey, C. K. (1962). *J. econ. Ent.*, *55*, 425.
(6) Hoffman, R. A. & Roberts, R. H. (1963). *J. econ. Ent.*, *56*, 258.
(7) Knapp, F. W. (1966). *J. econ. Ent.*, *59*, 468.
(8) Poindexter, C. E. & Adkins, T. R., Jun. (1970). *J. econ. Ent.*, *63*, 946.
(9) Witherspoon, B. & Burns, E. C. (1967). *J. econ. Ent.*, *60*, 1280.
(10) Lukyanov, N. I. & Ivanenko, N. M. (1965). *Veterinariya*, *42*, 89.
(11) Fredeen, F. J. H. (1963). *Nature* (*Lond.*), *200*, 1024.
(12) Standfast, H. A. & Dyce, A. L. (1968). *Aust. vet. J.*, *44*, 585.
(13) Hansens, E. J. & Granett, P. (1963). *J. econ. Ent.*, *56*, 24.
(14) Treece, R. E. (1964). *J. econ. Ent.*, *57*, 881, 962.
(15) Janes, M. J. *et al.* (1968). *J. econ. Ent.*, *61*, 1176.

Infestation with Trombidiform Mites

Infestations with trombidiform mites cause dermatitis in horses, pigs and sheep. Except for *Psorergates ovis* in sheep and *P. bos* in cattle, they are all harvest or grain mites, primarily attacking harvested grain and infesting animals only secondarily and usually transiently. *P. bos* has no significant pathogenicity (1).

PSORERGATES OVIS OR 'ITCH-MITE' OF SHEEP

The 'itch-mite' has been recorded as a parasite of sheep in Australia, New Zealand, South Africa, and the United States. The life cycle, comprising egg, larvae, three nymphal stages and adults, takes 4 to 5 weeks and appears to be completed entirely on the sheep. Adult mites are extremely small and can be seen only with a microscope. Only the adults are mobile and they effect spread of the disease by direct contact between recently shorn sheep. All stages occur in the superficial layers of the skin and cause irritation leading to rubbing and biting of the affected parts (principally the sides, flanks and thighs) and raggedness, sometimes shedding, of the fleece. Wool over these areas becomes thready and tufted and contains dry scales. The skin shows no gross abnormality but carries more scales than normal and histologically there is hyperkeratosis and desquamation. In the individual sheep and in flocks the disease spreads slowly so that it may be several years before clinical cases are observed and an appreciable number are visibly affected. The incidence of clinical cases in a neglected flock may be as high as 15 per cent. Amongst sheep, Merinos are most commonly affected and the highest incidence is observed in this breed, particularly in areas where the winter is cold and wet. Clinically, the disease resembles louse infestation. Diagnosis depends on detecting the mites in skin scrapings taken over an extensive area which has been closely clipped and smeared with oil. A search can be made of the scraping mounted in oil or after digestion. Best results are obtained if the scrapings are taken over the shoulders or high ribs and in the winter or spring (2, 4).

The mites are about half the size of a mange mite, are fragile and care must be taken not to digest the scrapings too vigorously. Dipping in lime sulphur dip (containing 1 per cent polysulphide sulphur and a wetting agent) is most effective but arsenical dip (containing 0·2 per cent arsenic trioxide), although slightly less efficient against 'itch-mite' also has activity against lice and keds. Rotenone dips (0·01 per cent in miscible oil) are also highly effective but benzene hexachloride and organophosphates are not (3). Commercial dips are available containing diazinon, rotenone and piperonyl butoxide and should be effective in the control of sheep ked, lice and itch mite.

HARVEST MITE INFESTATIONS

Chigger Mites

The larvae of *Pediculoides ventriculosus*, *Trombicula autumnalis*, *Leptus ryleyi*, *Trombicula alfreddugesi*, *T. splendens*, *T. batatasis* are parasitic on man and most animals causing dermatitis and, in man, transmitting important diseases. The natural hosts are small rodents. Engorged larvae drop off and develop into non-parasitic nymphs and larvae which live in grain and hay. The larvae are most active in the autumn at harvest time and may cause dermatitis in animals grazing at pasture or those confined in barns and being fed newly harvested grain.

Horses and cattle are usually affected on the face and lips, which, in white-faced horses, may suggest a diagnosis of photosensitization, and about the feet and lower limbs, especially in the flexures. Affected areas are itchy and scaly but, with rubbing, small fragile scabs and absence of hair may become apparent. The infestation is self-limiting and treatment is not usually necessary but the local application of an efficient parasiticide should hasten recovery.

Infestation with *Tyroglyphus* spp. in pigs appears to be manifested by itchiness and the development of fragile scabs about 3 cm. in diameter scattered over the body. Unlike the thick scabs of sarcoptic mange, the skin beneath appears normal. The infestations occur in pigs eating dry ground grain from automatic feeders, lesions appearing several weeks after the dry feeding is begun and disappearing spontaneously about 3 weeks later. No treatment is necessary although spraying with lindane is usually recommended. Affected pigs show no ill effects but the lesions may be mistaken for those of swine pox or sarcoptic mange. The ingestion of large numbers of mites appears to have no ill effects.

REFERENCES

(1) Roberts, I. H. & Meleney, W. P. (1965). *J. Amer. vet. med. Ass.*, *146*, 17.
(2) Sutherland, A. K. (1964/65). *Vict. vet. Proc.*, pp. 53–57.
(3) Downing, W. & Mort, P. (1962). *Aust. vet. J.*, *38*, 269.
(4) Sinclair, A. N. & Gibson, A. J. F. (1970). *Aust. vet. J.*, *46*, 311.

Demodectic Mange

(*Follicular Mange*)

Mites of *Demodex* spp. infest hair follicles of all species of domestic animals. The disease causes little concern except in cattle in which there may be significant damage to the hide.

Incidence

Demodectic mange occurs in all species. Cattle in some areas or herds may be affected at a high level of incidence and in these circumstances the disease may cause significant losses from rejection of hides, and rarely deaths due to gross secondary bacterial invasion may occur (1). The disease can also be severe in goats (2, 3).

Aetiology

Mites infesting the different host species are considered to be specific and are designated as *Demodex bovis* for cattle, *D. ovis* for sheep, *D. caprae* for goats, *D. equi* for horses and *D. phylloides* for pigs. The alternate nomenclature is *D. folliculorum* var. *bovis*, etc. Demodicidosis may occur in animals of any age, especially those in poor nutritional condition, but most cases in cattle occur in adult dairy animals, particularly in the late winter and spring.

Life Cycle

The life cycle appears to be completed on the host although adult mites can survive for several days away from the host. The mites differ from other mange mites in that they invade hair follicles and sebaceous glands. The disease does not spread rapidly on individual animals nor in a group and sometimes seems to disappear spontaneously especially in the summer. However, lesions are likely to recur in such animals during the succeeding winter.

In cattle transmission is probably direct although the common occurrence of lesions around the brisket and shoulders suggests that spread may occur by the contamination of inert objects such as feed troughs and stanchions. In horses grooming tools and rugs are probably instrumental in spreading the mites.

Pathogenesis

Invasion of hair follicles and sebaceous glands leads to chronic inflammation (3), loss of the hair fibre and in many instances the development of secondary staphylococcal pustules or small abscesses. It is these foci of infection which cause the small pinholes in the hide which interfere with its industrial processing and limit its use. In goats the commonest site is the finely-haired area behind the elbows and from here to the mid-line. A squamous form of the disease in which superficial scaling and alopecia occur is common in the dog and although uncommon in large animals may occur in association with the follicular form. An internal phase of this disease, such as occurs in dogs, does not appear to occur in cattle (1).

Clinical Findings

Because of its deep situation demodectic mange does not cause itching. The important sign is the appearance of small (3 mm. diameter) nodules and pustules which may develop into larger abscesses, especially in pigs. The small lesions can be seen quite readily in short-coated animals and on palpation feel like particles of bird-shot in the hide. In severe cases there may be a general hair-loss and thickening of the skin in the area. The contents of the pustules are usually white in colour and cheesy in consistency. In large abscesses the pus is more fluid. In cattle and goats the lesions occur most commonly on the brisket, lower neck, forearm and shoulder. Larger lesions are easily visible but very small lesions may only be detected by rolling a fold of skin through the fingers. In horses the face and around the eyes are predilection areas. Demodicidosis in pigs usually commences on the face and spreads down the ventral surface of the neck and chest to the belly. There is little irritation and the disease is observed mainly when the skin is scraped at slaughter (5). The disease may be especially severe in goats, spreading extensively before it is suspected and in some instances causing deaths. Severe cases in goats are commonly affected with several skin diseases such as mycotic dermatitis, ringworm, besnoitiosis and myiasis (3). Demodicidosis is rare in sheep. In this species pustules and scabs appear on the coronets, nose, tips of the ears and around the eyes (4).

Clinical Pathology

The characteristically elongated mites are usually easy to find in large numbers in the waxy material which can be expressed from the pustular lesions. They are much more difficult to isolate from squamous lesions. Lesions in hides can be detected as dark spots when a fresh hide is viewed against a strong light source (1).

Diagnosis

The commonest error is to diagnose the disease as a non-specific staphylococcal infection. In cattle and goats the disease often passes unnoticed unless the nodules are palpated. Deep-seated ringworm in horses has much in common with demodicidosis. A satisfactory diagnosis can only be made by demonstration of the mite.

Treatment and Control

Repeated dipping or spraying with the acaricides recommended for other manges is usually carried out but is more likely to prevent spread than cure existing lesions.

REFERENCES

(1) Smith, H. J. (1961). *Canad. J. comp. Med.*, *25*, 165, 201, 243 & 307.
(2) Baker, D. W. & Fisher, W. F. (1966). *Proc. 70th ann. Mtg U.S. Live Stock sanit. Ass.*, *Buffalo*, 1966, pp. 409–16.
(3) Bwangamoi, O. (1971). *Brit. vet. J.*, *127*, 30.
(4) Murray, M. D. (1959). *Aust. vet. J.*, *35*, 93.
(5) Harland, E. C. *et al.* (1971). *J. Amer. vet. med. Ass.*, *159*, 1752.

Sarcoptic Mange

(*Barn Itch, Red Mange*)

Sarcoptic mange occurs in all species causing a severe itching dermatitis.

Incidence

Amongst domestic species pigs are most commonly affected and sheep least commonly and the disease is a common and important one in camels (3). It is a notifiable disease in most countries and is important because of its severity and the difficulty experienced in treating it. Affected animals are constantly itchy and lose much grazing time. Loss of condition, production and vitality may be severe and the appearance of affected animals is aesthetically displeasing.

Aetiology

The causative mite, *Sarcoptes scabiei*, is usually considered to have a number of subspecies each specific to a particular host and designated *S. scabiei* var. *bovis*, *S. scabiei* var. *suis* etc., but this host-specificity is not complete and transference from one host species to another can occur, a point of some importance when attempting to control the disease. Animals in poor condition appear to be most susceptible but conditions, especially overcrowding, in which sarcoptic mange occur often go hand in hand with poor feeding and general mismanagement. The disease is most active in cold, wet weather and spreads slowly during the summer months.

Life Cycle

The eggs are laid in tunnels in the skin made by the adults, the larvae either remaining in the tunnels or migrating to the skin surface to continue their development as nymphs. The nymphs burrow superficially in the skin and the adult stage is reached about 17 days after the eggs are laid.

The infestation is spread chiefly by direct contact between hosts, all three stages being capable of migration, but inert materials such as bedding, blankets, grooming tools and clothing may act as carriers. Adult mites do not usually survive for more than a few days away from the host but in moist, protected sites they may persist for as long as 3 weeks. In pigs adult sows are often the source of infestation for young pigs even though they show no signs of the disease. Large numbers of mites can often be found in the ears of normal sows and it is presumed that the mites are in a latent stage.

Pathogenesis

Although all stages feed on cutaneous debris the adult females, by burrowing deeply, cause inflammation and severe itching.

Clinical Findings

Early lesions are characterized by the presence of small red papules and general erythema of the skin. The affected area is intensely itchy and frequently excoriated by scratching and biting, Loss of hair, thick brown scabs overlying a raw surface, and thickening and wrinkling of surrounding skin soon follow. In pigs the lesions commence on the trunk, in sheep and goats on the face, in cattle on the inner surface of the thighs, the underside of the neck and brisket and around the root of the tail, and in horses on the neck. Except in sheep where the lesions do not spread to the woolled skin, lesions become widespread if neglected and such animals may show systemic effects including emaciation, anorexia and weakness and in neglected cases death may occur.

The course of sarcoptic mange is rather more acute than in the other forms of mange and may involve the entire body surface of cattle in a period as short as 6 weeks.

Clinical Pathology

Necropsy examinations are not usually undertaken. Examination of deep scrapings after digestion in warm 10 per cent potassium hydroxide solution usually reveals mites, often in relatively small numbers.

Diagnosis

Sarcoptic mange is the only mange which occurs in pigs. It can be confused with infestation with *Tyroglyphus* spp. mites or lice, or with swine pox, parakeratosis, infectious dermatitis, pityriasis rosea and ringworm. In most of these diseases there are clinical features which are characteristic and final diagnosis can be made on the presence or absence of the mite. The same comments apply to the differentiation in cattle of sarcoptic mange from chorioptic and psoroptic mange and from chlorinated naphthalene poisoning and ringworm. Horses may be affected by psoroptic or chorioptic mange but the lesions are most common at the base of the mane and tail and at the back of the pastern respectively. Infestation with the trombidiform mites and photosensitization may resemble sarcoptic mange. The disease is uncommon in sheep.

Treatment and Control

Treatment must be thorough so that all parts of the skin, especially under the tail, in the ears and between the legs are wetted by the acaricide. Although buildings, bedding, and other inert materials do not support the mite for more than a few days they should also be treated unless they can be left in a dry state for 3 weeks.

None of the treatments used can penetrate the burrows in the skin and repeated treatments are necessary. The older treatments, sulphur dioxide fumigation and spraying or dipping in lime-sulphur dip, were effective but difficult to apply and they have been largely superseded by more modern insecticides. Rotenone and derris are effective but the standard treatment is lindane (0·06 per cent) as a spray or dip repeated in 10 to 12 days. Other chlorinated hydrocarbons, including chlordane, toxaphene and dieldrin are also effective. Where the use of these compounds on animals is prohibited the organophosphatic insecticides, e.g. malathion (a single application of a 0·5 per cent spray), on badly infested pigs are also recommended. If the number of animals to be treated is small, vigorous application of the dipping fluid to affected parts with a brush before dipping will hasten recovery. A suspension of Diazinon (25 g. per 150 litres water) poured onto the skin twice at intervals of about a month is reported as an effective treatment in cattle (1, 2).

A suitable control programme can be based on quarantine of infested herds and frequent treatments until the disease is eradicated. All animals on the farm should be treated.

REFERENCES

(1) Lodha, K. R. (1966). *Vet. Rec.*, 79, 41.
(2) Bouvier, G. (1965). *Schweiz. Arch. Tierheilk.*, *107*, 163.

Psoroptic Mange

(*Sheep Scab, Common Scab of Cattle*)

Psoroptic mange is of greatest importance in sheep in which it causes 'sheep-scab'.

Incidence

Psoroptic mange occurs in all species but, as 'sheep-scab' it is a disease of major importance where large numbers of sheep are raised for wool-growing purposes. In most progressive countries the incidence has been so greatly reduced that it can be considered to be virtually eradicated. The disease was widespread in cattle in the United States but has been largely brought under control. Because of the ease with which it spreads it can cause serious losses in cattle if neglected. This is exemplified by the serious losses which can occur in feedlots.

Aetiology

Psoroptes communis is more selective in its host specificity than *Sarcoptes scabiei* and on biological grounds the varieties are considered to be species. Hence *Psoroptes communis ovis* is specific to sheep, *P. communis caprae* to goats, *P. communis equi* to horses and *P. communis bovis* and *P. natalensis* to cattle. *P. hippotis* is also recorded in horses (1). *P. cuniculi* is recorded as a cause of ear mange in goats (2).

Life Cycle

In sheep the eggs of *P. communis ovis* are laid on the skin at the edge of a lesion, the larval and nymphal stages last 2 to 4 days each and a life cycle is completed in 8 to 9 days. All stages are capable of survival away from the host for up to 10 days and under optimum conditions adult females may survive for 3 weeks. Optimum conditions for development include moistness and cool temperatures. Thus the disease is most active in autumn and winter months. This is due not only to increased activity of the mites but also to the more rapid development in housed animals and to the tendency for the disease to be most severe in animals in poor condition. Although individual mites survive for only 4 to 6 weeks the disease is continuous, and even when conditions are adverse a few mites are likely to survive in protected spots, in the ear canals, skin folds around the horns and the breech and the prepuce. The life cycles of the other species are thought to be similar.

Pathogenesis

Unlike *Sarcoptes scabiei* this mite migrates to all parts of the skin and prefers areas covered with hair or wool. The adults puncture the epidermis to feed on lymph and cause local inflammation resulting in itchiness and the exudation of serum which accumulates to form a crust. The mites are most active at the edges of the crust and the lesion spreads peripherally.

Clinical Findings

Sheep. Cutaneous lesions may occur on any part of the body but characteristically in badly affected sheep they are most obvious on the sides. Very early lesions are small (6 mm. diameter) papules which ooze serum. Attention may be attracted to the area by raggedness of the wool caused by biting and scratching. In older lesions thin yellow crusts are present and the wool commences to shed. The wool may contain large masses of scab material which bind the fibres together in a mat.

In a typical outbreak of 'sheep-scab' many animals are affected and show itchiness and shedding of the fleece. Some become markedly emaciated and weak and deaths may occur. However, it is possible to have the disease in a flock at a very low level of incidence and with minimal lesions. This usually occurs when the sheep are highly resistant because of good nutrition, or climatic conditions are adverse for mite development, or treatment has been carried out but has been incomplete. In such cases there may be little or no clinical evidence of the disease and a careful search for latent cases may be necessary. This is facilitated by packing the animals into a confined space, so that the mites become active, and watching for signs of itchiness. Sheep which bite or scratch should be carefully examined by palpating the surface of the skin in search of papules and scabs. Special attention should be paid to the ears, the base of the horns, the infra-orbital fossa and the perineal and scrotal areas in rams.

Goats are usually described as having ear mange, and typical scabs are common inside the ears and on the outside extending over the poll, but they may also be present on the lower parts of the limbs in severe cases (2).

Horses. Large, thick crusts are found on those parts of the body carrying long hair, the base of the mane and the root of the tail, and hairless areas such as the udder, prepuce and axilla. Affected parts are itchy, the hair is lost and with constant rubbing the surrounding skin becomes thickened. *P. hippotis* infestations in horses cause severe irritation in the ear accompanied by discharge, shaking of the head, rubbing of the head and tenderness of the poll (1).

Cattle. Typical lesions appear first on the withers, neck and around the root of the tail. In severe cases they may spread to the rest of the body. The lesions are intensely itchy. They commence as papules but soon are covered with a scab which enlarges peripherally and coalesces with other lesions so that very large areas of skin may become involved. The hair is lost, the skin becomes thickened, wrinkled and covered with scabs. Badly affected animals become weak and emaciated and may die.

Clinical Pathology

The mites can be easily demonstrated in scrapings taken from the edges of the lesions. Examination is facilitated by prior digestion of the scraping in warm, 10 per cent potassium hydroxide solution.

Diagnosis

Severe cases of psoroptic mange in sheep are similar to fleece rot except that there is no itching in the latter. Diseases causing itchiness such as scrapie, ked and louse infestations and infestations with *Psorergates ovis* and harvest mites do not have typical cutaneous lesions and the latter group can usually be detected by examination for the causative parasites.

Treatment and Control

Psoroptic mange in sheep is a notifiable disease in most countries and local legislation may determine the agents to be used and the method and frequency of its application. Factors which influence the treatment are as follows. Although the mite is easily killed by most acaricides it is important to wet the skin thoroughly and pay special attention to severe cases where mites are likely to be present in inaccessible sites on the body. Thus a plunge dip is almost essential and the sheep must be kept immersed in the dipping fluid for 2 minutes. Prior shearing may be advisable but may lead to further spread of the infestation. Care must be taken to ensure that the concentration of the acaricide in the dip is maintained, especially when large numbers of sheep are being treated. Badly affected animals should be set aside and inaccessible sites including ears, horn bases and perineum treated manually with the dipping fluid. Dipped sheep should not be returned to their pastures, nor to the barn unless the latter has been thoroughly cleaned and sprayed with the dipping fluid.

Lime-sulphur dip (containing not less than 1·5 per cent polysulphide sulphur) is highly efficient but has little residual effect and dipping must be repeated in 10 days, and after a further 10 days in severely affected sheep flocks. Lindane (0·06 per cent), or toxaphene (0·5 per cent) are preferred in sheep (3). The other chlorinated hydrocarbons, benzene hexachloride (0·013 per cent gamma isomer), dieldrin and chlordane (0·25 to 0·4 per cent) are effective and single dippings are sufficient because of the persistence of these compounds in wool. Dipping or spraying of affected cattle on 2 occasions 10 to 14 days apart with a benzene hexachloride solution is also effective but some signs of toxicity may be expected in emaciated young animals. Gammexane has also been used successfully in goats (2). The organophosphates have given equivocal results in the treatment of psoroptic mange in sheep, but provided they were in a liquid formulation diazinon (0·06 per cent) and crotoxyphos (0·3 per cent) were effective in preventing infection (4).

Eradication of 'sheep-scab' on an area basis is usually undertaken by quarantine and compulsory dipping of all susceptible animals in the area at the same time. The necessity to dip all animals in the area during a short period presents difficulties and the cost of construction of dips and lack of desire to dip in cold climates are other obstructing factors. Where it is desired to keep the disease at a low level short of eradication, the disease is made notifiable and infested farms are quarantined and the sheep dipped until clean.

REFERENCES

(1) Johnston, L. A. Y. (1963). *Aust. vet. J.,* 39, 208.
(2) Littlejohn, I. (1968). *Vet. Rec.,* 82, 148.
(3) Meleney, W. P. & Roberts, I. H. (1967). *J. Amer. vet. med. Ass.,* 151, 725.
(4) Roberts, I. H. & Meleney, W. P. (1971). *J. Amer. vet. med. Ass.,* 158, 372.

Chorioptic Mange

(*Tail Mange of Cattle, Leg Mange of Horses*)

Chorioptic mange is the commonest form of mange in cattle and horses. In the latter it causes leg-mange, a source of annoyance and inefficiency at work.

Incidence

Although the disease is common in cattle it appears to cause little other than aesthetic damage. The disease is widespread in horses as leg mange. In sheep it has been suggested as contributing to testicular hypoplasia or atrophy when it occurs on the scrotum (1).

Aetiology

The mites *Chorioptes equi* occur on the horse, *C. bovis* on cattle, *C. caprae* on goats and *C. ovis* on sheep. In cattle the mites are much more active in the latter part of the winter and tend to disappear in cattle at pasture. This diminution in activity is not noted in cattle kept housed in the summer time.

Life Cycle

Details of the life cycle are not available but it appears to be similar to that of *Psoroptes* spp. Transmission is probably effected by direct contact in most instances although in animals housed in barns, grooming tools may be an additional method of spreading the disease. Infestation of bedding is not a common method of transmission.

In horses the parasites occur almost entirely in the long hair on the lower parts of the legs and are rarely found on other parts of the body. In cattle the disease is most evident in the winter time, lesions occurring most commonly on the perineum, and back of the udder, extending in severe cases to the backs of the legs and over the rump. In the summer months the mites migrate to the area above the hooves, particularly the pasterns of the hind leg, and around the muzzle. In sheep, lesions are confined to the woolless areas, chiefly the lower parts of the hind legs.

Pathogenesis

In horses the mites cause severe irritation and itchiness. The initial lesion in cattle is a small nodule which exudes serum causing matting of the hair. In severe cases these coalesce to form heavy scabs and cause thickening and wrinkling of the skin. Mites can be isolated from many animals which show no clinical evidence of the disease. *C. bovis* is known to be a common parasite of sheep in the U.S.A. but appears to be without pathogenicity in this species (2).

Clinical Findings

The first sign in horses is usually violent stamping of the feet and rubbing of the back of the hind pasterns on wire, rails or stumps. This is most evident during periods of rest and at night. Examination of the area is difficult because of the long hair present and the horses may resent manipulation. In cases of long duration the skin is seen to be swollen, scabby, cracked and usually greasy.

Cattle show little evidence of cutaneous irritation but the small crusty scabs (3 mm. diameter) on the escutcheon, udder and thighs are unsightly. Although the mites appear to cause little trouble in the summer time, occasional animals are seen which have thick, crusty scabs on the skin, just above the coronets and around the muzzle.

Clinical Pathology

Scrapings from the affected areas usually contain large numbers of mites.

Diagnosis

Greasy heel in horses resembles chorioptic mange except that pain is more evident in the former and itchiness in the latter. It has been suggested that the two diseases are aetiologically related. The lesions in cattle may go unnoticed but are not likely to be mistaken for those of any other disease with the possible exception of other manges. The presence of chorioptic mites in footrot and mucosal disease lesions may be purely coincidental, but cases of chorioptic mange which have lesions around the coronet and muzzle may be mistaken for one of the erosive diseases. Sheep with itchy, scabby legs may be infested with other forms of mange or have contagious ecthyma or strawberry footrot.

Treatment and Control

Although control of the mites appears to be effected easily complete eradication from an animal or herd is not, and apparent eradication in a herd is often followed by a reappearance of the disease the following winter, even if multiple treatments are undertaken.

Effective treatments include lime-sulphur and lindane sprays and dips as used in other manges. An advantage of lindane is its persistence on the hair coat for 9 to 10 days. Lindane (0·06 per cent solution) applied as a spray has been used extensively but is disappointing in sheep and cattle unless care is taken to spray inaccessible spots such as between the udder and thighs. Several sprayings with lindane at 10-day intervals are usually required. Ciodrin (0·25 per cent solution) applied as a spray is highly effective, is claimed to leave no residue in meat or milk (3) and is recommended as the superior treatment for cattle and sheep (4). Diazinon is also recommended. Local treatment may be necessary for feet and scrotum. Many compounds and formulations and methods of administration are now in use for bulk application to animals to control external parasites especially mange mites and lice. The selection of the most appropriate treatment is fast becoming a task for a specialist entomologist (5). Lime-sulphur needs to be applied on six occasions 6 to 10 days apart and is no longer popular. Frequent local applications of these preparations to horses' legs, after prior clipping, is usually effective.

REFERENCES

(1) Crawford, R. *et al.* (1970). *N.Z. vet. J.*, *18*, 209.
(2) Roberts, I. H. *et al.* (1964). *Amer. J. vet. Res.*, *25*, 478.
(3) Smith, H. J. (1967). *Canad. vet. J.*, *8*, 88.
(4) Sutherland, A. K. (1967–68). *Vict. vet. Proc.*, pp. 58.
(5) Matthysse, J. G. *et al.* (1967). *J. econ. Ent.*, *60*, 1615, 1645.

27

Metabolic Diseases

AMONGST domestic farm animals the metabolic diseases achieve their greatest importance in dairy cows and pregnant ewes. In the other species these diseases occur only sporadically. The high-producing dairy cow always verges on abnormality and the breeding and feeding of dairy cattle for high milk yields is aetiologically related to the diseases of metabolism so common in these animals. In dairy cows, the incidence of metabolic diseases is highest in the period commencing at calving and extending until the peak of lactation is reached, and their susceptibility appears to be related to the extremely high turnover of fluids, salts and soluble organic materials during the early part of lactation. With this rapid rate of exchange of water, sodium, calcium, magnesium, chlorides and phosphates, a sudden variation in their excretion or secretion in the milk or by other routes, or a sudden variation in their intake because of changes in ingestion, digestion or absorption, may cause abrupt, damaging changes in the internal environment of the animal. It is the volume of the changes in intake and secretion and the rapidity with which they can occur that reduce the metabolic stability of the cow. When one considers that the continued nutritional strain of a pregnancy is often exacerbated by an inadequate diet in the dry period this point becomes obvious. The effect of pregnancy is particularly important in ewes, especially those carrying more than one lamb.

In the next phase of the production cycle parturition is followed by the sudden onset of a profuse lactation which, if the nutrient reserves have already been seriously depleted, may further reduce them to below critical levels and clinical metabolic disease then occurs. The essential metabolite which is reduced below the critical level determines the clinical syndrome which will occur. Most attention has been paid to variations in balances of calcium and inorganic phosphates relative to parturient paresis, of magnesium relative to lactation tetany, of blood sugar and ketones and hepatic glycogen relative to ketosis, and of potassium relative to hyperkalaemia on cereal grazing, but it is probable that other imbalances are important in the production of as yet unidentified syndromes.

During the succeeding period of lactation, particularly in cows on test schedules and under the strain of producing large quantities of milk, there is often a variable food intake, especially when pasture is the sole source of food, and instability of the internal environment inevitably follows. The period of early lactation is an unstable one in all species. Hormonal stimulation at this stage is so strong that nutritional deficiency often does not limit milk production and a serious drain on reserves of metabolites may occur.

The fact that some dams are affected much more by these variations than others is probably explainable on the basis of variations in internal metabolism and degree of milk production between species and between individuals. Between groups of cows variations in susceptibility appear to depend on either genetic or management factors. Certainly Jersey cows are more susceptible to parturient paresis than cows of other breeds, and Guernseys, in our experience, seem to be more susceptible to ketosis. Even within breeds considerable variation is evident in susceptibility between families. Under these circumstances it seems necessary to invoke genetic factors, at least as predisposing causes.

Management practices of most importance are housing and nutrition. In those sections of North America where cattle are housed during the winter, and in poor pasture areas, ketosis is prevalent. In the Channel Islands local cattle are unaffected by lactation tetany whereas the disease is prevalent in Great Britain. In New Zealand metabolic diseases are complex and the incidence is high, both probably related to the practice of having the cows calve in late winter when feed is poor, to the practice of depending entirely on pasture for food, and to the high proportion of Jerseys in the cattle population.

A knowledge of these various factors is essential before any reasonable scheme of prevention can be undertaken. It should also indicate that although the commoner disease entities are set out in this chapter there is high probability that a disturbance of more than one of the metabolites mentioned may occur simultaneously in the one animal and give rise to complex syndromes which are not described here. The disease entities dealt with must be considered as arbitrary points in a long scale of metabolic disturbances.

Finally, only a knowledge of the aetiological factors involved will help in understanding the incidence of the various syndromes. Largely because of variations in climate the occurrence of metabolic disease varies from season to season and from year to year. In the same manner variations in the types of disease occur. For example in some seasons most cases of parturient paresis will be tetanic; in others most cases of ketosis will be complicated by hypocalcaemia. Further, the incidence of metabolic disease and the incidence of the different syndromes will vary from region to region. Ketosis may be common in low rainfall areas and on poor pasture. Lactation tetany may be common in colder areas and where natural shelter is poor. Recognition of these factors can make it possible to devise means whereby the incidence of the diseases can be reduced.

The metabolic diseases, because of high prevalence and high mortality rate, are of major importance in some countries, so much so that predictive systems are being set up. Rapid analysis of soil, pasture and stored feed is being used in Europe (1) and the use of biochemical profiles has grown rapidly in the U.K.

REFERENCE

(1) Mudd, A. J. (1969). *Vet. Rec.*, *84*, 627.

Parturient Paresis

(*Milk Fever*)

Parturient paresis is a metabolic disease occurring most commonly about the time of parturition in adult females and is characterized by hypocalcaemia, general muscular weakness, circulatory collapse and depression of consciousness. A similar disease has been dealt with separately as lactation tetany of mares because of its more frequent occurrence during lactation and after transport.

Incidence

In cattle the disease is essentially one of domestication and occurs in high-producing cows in all countries. Few figures are available on the incidence of the disease although an annual morbidity rate of 3·54 per cent has been quoted for Great Britain (1). Generally the disease is sporadic but on individual farms the incidence may rarely reach

25 to 30 per cent. With standard treatment relatively few deaths occur in uncomplicated cases but incidental losses due to aspiration pneumonia, mastitis and limb injuries are often quite high. The occurrence of parturient paresis causes some loss by significantly increasing the inter-calving period in affected cows (2). Several surveys suggest that 75 to 85 per cent of those cases clinically diagnosed as parturient paresis are uncomplicated and respond to calcium therapy alone. A proportion of these animals require more than one treatment, either because complete recovery is delayed, or because relapse occurs. The remaining 15 to 25 per cent are either complicated by other conditions or are incorrectly diagnosed. The economic importance of the disease has been minor since the introduction of calcium borogluconate as treatment and depends almost entirely on the cost of veterinary treatment and losses due to intercurrent disease. However, during late years the position appears to have changed considerably in most countries. Simple cases of parturient paresis which respond to treatment with calcium borogluconate seem to have decreased and there has been an increase in cases which are apparently complicated by metabolic factors other than hypocalcaemia.

Parturient paresis is rare in sows but does occur in outbreak form in groups of sheep in which 25 per cent of a flock may be affected at one time. Besides the disease in lactating ewes the disease also occurs in young sheep up to about a year old, especially when they are grazed on green oats, but also when pasture is short in winter and spring in south-east Australia. The disease is manifested by paresis but in the rest of the flock poor growth, lameness and bone fragility can be detected.

Aetiology

It is generally conceded that a depression of the levels of ionized calcium in tissue fluids is the basic biochemical defect in parturient paresis. There is a fall in serum-calcium levels in all cows at calving and a significantly greater fall occurs in cows which develop the disease. The importance of the calcium ion in maintaining muscle tone is well known and affected cows respond rapidly to the parenteral administration of calcium solutions. Although total serum-calcium levels are used to express the animals' status with regard to calcium, it is possible that differences between the ionized and non-ionized compartments of total calcium may be more important than the total level. Little is known of intrinsic factors, such as levels of serum protein and acid–base balances, which influence the proportion of total serum calcium which is ionized, but those observations which have been made on cows with parturient paresis indicate that both total and ionized serum calcium levels fall proportionately (3).

Serum-calcium levels fall in all adult cows at calving due to the onset of lactation. This has been satisfactorily demonstrated by comparing the effects of parturition on serum-calcium levels in normal and mastectomized cows. The important fact is that the serum-calcium levels fall more in some cows than in others and it is this difference which results in the varying susceptibility of animals to parturient paresis. There are 3 factors which affect calcium homeostasis and variations in one or more of them may be instrumental in causing the disease in any individual. Firstly, it may simply be the excessive loss of calcium in the colostrum beyond the capacity of absorption from the intestines and mobilization from the bones to replace. Variations in susceptibility between cows could be due to variations in the concentration of calcium in the milk and the volume of milk secreted. Secondly, there may be an impairment of absorption of calcium from the intestine at parturition and there is evidence suggesting that this does occur (1). The third and probably most important possibility is that mobilization of calcium from storage in the skeleton may not be sufficiently rapid to maintain normal serum levels. Certainly the calcium mobilization rate and the immediately available calcium reserves are sufficiently reduced in cows in later pregnancy to render them incapable of withstanding the expected loss of calcium in the milk (4). This deficiency in mobilization and reserves is not a permanent characteristic of cows prone to parturient paresis; in fact their rate of mobilization appears to be better than that of non-susceptible animals except at parturition (5). Failure to mobilize skeletal calcium could arise because of parathyroid insufficiency, as first suggested by Dryerre and Greig who postulated that the gland was relatively quiescent due to the decreased calcium and phosphorus metabolism of the dry period. There is conflicting evidence on this point and although susceptibility to parturient paresis may be associated with parathyroid dysfunction, it is unlikely that the relationship is a simple one (4, 6, 7). However, parturient paresis can be prevented by the feeding of a ration high in phosphorus and low in calcium during late pregnancy. Such a ration would stimulate parathyroid activity during the dry period and condition the gland for the increased activity required at parturition. Conversely the observation that feeding a diet high in calcium at this time increases the incidence of the disease, probably by depressing the activity of the gland, lends additional support to the hypothesis. The possibility exists that rather than a deficiency of parathormone the presence of excess calcitonin, or thyrocalcitonin, the serum-calcium depressing hormone of the thyroid gland, may be an important factor (8), but the normal function of this hormone tends to be limited to the fine adjustment of calcium homeostasis rather than causing major adjustments like those we are concerned with in parturient paresis (9). This is in spite of the observation that the intravenous injection of the hormone causes severe hypocalcaemia and signs of parturient paresis, reversible by treatment with calcium injections (10).

In summary it is assumed that in dairy cows parturient paresis is a hypocalcaemia caused by a failure to mobilize calcium reserves, and by a depletion of these reserves caused by the development of a negative calcium balance in late pregnancy. Prevention of the disease therefore seems to depend largely upon the preservation of a positive balance in susceptible cows.

There is no convincing evidence that adrenal hypofunction is the cause of the disease and the administration of adrenal corticosteroids appears to have no prophylactic effect.

In goats a depression in serum levels of calcium and phosphorus occurs similar to that in cows but in ewes no such depression occurs at lambing (11) and the intervention of a precipitating factor appears to be necessary to further reduce the serum-calcium level below a critical point. For example in sheep sudden deprivation of feed or forced exercise can cause marked depression of the serum-calcium levels. However, ewes are in a susceptible state in early lactation because they are in negative calcium balance. In late lactation a state of positive balance appears due largely to a low rate of bone resorption (12).

Occurrence

Amongst cattle mature cows are most commonly affected, usually in the 5- to 10-year age group, although rare cases have been observed at the first and second calvings. This age relationship also appears in serum-calcium levels, a hypocalcaemia occurring at calving in most cows with their 3rd to 7th calves but infrequently in first-calf heifers. There is considerable difference in susceptibility between the breeds. Jerseys are most susceptible, an incidence of 33 per cent having been observed in a sample compared with 9·6 per cent incidence in other breeds (13). Although there is no definite evidence on the point, the consensus of opinion is that cows are more susceptible if they are heavily fed before and after calving especially if the protein level of the diet is high. There is no specific seasonal occurrence or relationship to weather conditions.

Individual cows, and to some extent families of cows, are more susceptible than others, the disease tending to recur at successive parturitions. Complete milking in the first 48 hours after calving, as opposed to normal sucking by a calf, appears to be a precipitating factor and is probably related to the high incidence of the disease in domesticated cattle.

Parturient paresis in cattle occurs at three main stages in the lactation cycle. Most prepartum cases occur in the last few days of pregnancy and during parturition but rare cases occur several weeks before calving. The great majority of cases occur within the first 48 hours after calving and the danger period extends up to about the 10th day post-partum. Occasional cases occur 6 to 8 weeks after the commencement of lactation. Such cases are most often recurrences of the disease in highly susceptible cows which were affected at calving. Undue fatigue and excitement may precipitate such attacks and there is a special susceptibility at oestrus. In the latter case the depression of appetite by the elevation of blood oestrogen levels may be a significant factor (4). Starvation for 48 hours also causes severe depression of serum-calcium levels and this may be of importance in the production of hypocalcaemic paresis in this species at times other than in the post-parturient period (4, 5). As another explanation of the heightened susceptibility of cows at oestrus a possible depression of the degree of ionization of calcium under the influence of increased serum oestrogens is suggested (14).

In sheep, goats and pigs only sporadic cases occur except under special circumstances. Forced exercise, long distance transport, sudden deprivation of food, and grazing on oxalate-containing plants or green cereal crops commonly precipitate outbreaks of hypocalcaemic paresis in sheep, mature ewes being most susceptible, particularly in the period from 6 weeks before to 10 weeks after lambing. Under the local name of 'moss-ill' the disease occurs endemically in the north of England (15).

Pathogenesis

The bulk of evidence points to hypocalcaemia as the cause of the signs of classical 'milk fever' with hypophosphataemia and variations in levels of serum-magnesium playing subsidiary roles. Serum-calcium and serum-phosphate levels are significantly lower in clinical cases than in normal, comparable cows and there is some relationship between the severity of the signs and the degree of biochemical change. The complete response to the parenteral administration of calcium salts in most cases, and the occurrence of tetany coincident with hypocalcaemia after the intravenous administration of disodium ethylenediamine tetraacetate (16) is further proof. In addition some signs reminiscent of parathyroprivic tetany in other species are observed in the initial stages of parturient paresis. Early excitement, muscle twitching, tetany, particularly of the hind limbs, hypersensitiveness and convulsive movements of the head and limbs fall within this category. The demonstration of failure of neuromuscular transmission of stimuli in cows with parturient paresis is in accord with the clinical signs of the disease (17). The high incidence of prolapse of the uterus in cows or of the vagina in ewes (18) is often ascribed to depression of muscle tone due to hypocalcaemia, but often without other clinical signs especially in the latter.

When hypomagnesaemia coexists these signs continue but where serum-magnesium levels are normal or high, relaxation, muscle weakness, depression and coma supervene. It is likely that the hypocalcaemic tetany is overcome by the relative hypermagnesaemia (the ratio of Ca:Mg may change from 6:1 to 2:1) approximating the ratio at which magnesium narcosis develops. There is normally a rise in serum-magnesium levels at calving but in those cases of parturient paresis in which tetany is a feature serum-magnesium levels are low. These low levels are in many cases expressions of a seasonal hypomagnesaemia.

Low serum-phosphorus levels have been observed in clinical cases of parturient paresis and have been credited with an influence on the signs which occur. It has been observed that some cases do not respond to calcium injections even though serum-calcium levels return to normal, but do recover when the udder is inflated and serum-phosphorus levels rise. In addition there are unpublished reports on the efficacy of orally or intravenously administered sodium acid-phosphate in some cases of parturient paresis. The high content of phosphorus in colostrum and milk suggests that the onset of lactation might be the cause of low serum-phosphorus levels (4). There is difficulty in reconciling the biochemical and clinical findings because in other circumstances long periods of profound hypophosphataemia can occur without neuromuscular signs.

Clinical Findings

Cattle. Three arbitrary stages of the disease have been described. The first stage is a brief one of excitement and tetany with hypersensitiveness and muscle tremor of the head and limbs. The animal is disinclined to move and does not eat. There may be shaking of the head, protrusion of the tongue and grinding of the teeth. The rectal temperature is usually normal to slightly above normal. Stiffness of the hind legs is apparent and the animal is ataxic and falls easily and, on going down, the hind legs are stuck out stiffly.

The second stage is one of sternal recumbency. Consciousness is usually depressed, the cow having a very drowsy appearance and sitting up, usually with a lateral kink in the neck or the head turned into the flank. Tetany of the limbs has disappeared and the cow is unable to rise. The muzzle is dry, the skin and extremities cold, and the rectal temperature subnormal (36 to 38°C or 97 to 101°F). The pupils are dilated and the eyes are dry and staring. There is relaxation of the anus and loss of the anal reflex. Circulatory signs are prominent including a marked decrease in the intensity of the heart sounds and an increase in rate (about 80 per minute). Also the pulse is weak, the pressures and amplitude being considerably reduced. Venous pressure is also low and difficulty may be experienced in raising the vein. Ruminal stasis and constipation are characteristic. Respiration is not markedly affected although a forced expiratory grunt may be heard. The pupillary light reflex is incomplete or absent and the diameter of the pupil varies from normal to maximum dilatation.

The third stage is that of lateral recumbency. The cow is almost comatose and although the limbs may be stuck out there is complete flaccidity on passive movement and the cow cannot sit up. In general, the depression of temperature and the circulatory signs are more marked. The pulse is, in most cases, impalpable, the heart sounds almost inaudible and increased in rate up to 120 per minute, and it may be impossible to raise the jugular vein. Bloat is usual because of the posture.

Without treatment very rare cases recover spontaneously, a few remain unchanged for several days and most deteriorate rapidly during a period of 12 to 24 hours, the animal dying imperceptibly from cessation of respiration, or during a convulsion.

A concurrent hypomagnesaemia has a modifying effect on the classical syndrome. Tetany and hyperaesthesia persist beyond the first stage. There is considerable excitement and fibrillary twitching of the eyelids, and tetanic convulsions are readily precipitated by sound or touch. Trismus may be present. The cardiac and respiratory rates are greatly increased and the heart sounds are much increased in intensity. Without treatment death occurs during a convulsion. The clinical picture when there is a concurrent hypophosphataemia is one of classical parturient paresis which responds to calcium therapy in all respects except that the cow is unable to rise.

Sheep. The syndrome is very similar to that in cattle. Early signs include a stilty, proppy gait and tremor, particularly of the shoulder muscles. Recumbency follows, sometimes with tetany of the limbs. The characteristic posture is sternal recumbency, with the legs under the body or stretched out behind. Ruminal movements are absent, the head is rested on the ground, there may be an accumulation of mucous exudate in the nostrils and the respiratory rate is increased. The venous blood pressure is low and the pulse impalpable. Mental depression is evidenced by a drowsy appearance and depression of the corneal reflex. Constipation is usual. Response to parenteral treatment with calcium salts is rapid, the ewe being normal 30 minutes after a subcutaneous injection. Death often occurs within 6 to 12 hours if treatment is not administered. The syndrome is usually more severe in pregnant than in lactating ewes.

Swine. As in cattle signs develop within a few hours of farrowing. There is restlessness, a normal temperature, and anorexia followed by inability to rise and later lateral recumbency and coma. Milk flow is decreased.

Clinical Pathology

No completely satisfactory field test is available. The Sulkowitch test, based on the detection of calcium in the urine, is not an accurate guide to the calcium status of the animal. A rapid semi-quantitative test, based upon the amount of sodium ethylene diamine tetraacetate (EDTA, Sequestrene) required to prevent clotting of a sample of blood and hence the approximate calcium concentration, seems worthy of a trial as a field test for calcium concentrations in serum (20). Total serum-calcium levels are reduced to below 8 mg. usually to below 5 mg. and sometimes to as low as 2 mg. per cent. The reduction is usually, but not always, proportional to the severity of the clinical syndrome. Serum levels of magnesium are usually moderately elevated to 4 to 5 mg. per cent but in some areas low levels may be encountered especially in cows at pasture. Serum inorganic-phosphorus levels are usually depressed to 1·5 to 3·0 mg. per cent. Blood sugar levels are usually normal although they may be depressed if ketosis occurs concurrently.

Changes in the leucocyte count include an eosinopenia, a neutrophilia and a lymphopenia suggestive of adrenal cortical hyperactivity but similar changes occur at calving in cows which do not develop parturient paresis. Clinico-pathological findings in the other species are not described in detail except for depression of total serum-calcium levels.

Necropsy Findings

There are no gross or histological changes unless concurrent disease is present.

Diagnosis

A diagnosis of parturient paresis is usually based on the occurrence of paresis and depression of consciousness in animals that have recently given birth to young. The diagnosis is confirmed by a favourable response to treatment with parenteral injections of calcium solutions, and by biochemical examination of the blood. In ewes the history usually contains some reference to recent physical stress and the disease is quite common in the period preceding lambing.

In the immediate post-partum period there are many conditions which cause recumbency in cows. Hypomagnesaemia may accompany the hypocalcaemia so that the case presented is one of parturient paresis complicated by lactation tetany. Hyperaesthesia and tetany are present instead of the classical signs of coma and flaccidity. A complicating hypophosphataemia is suggested as a cause of continued recumbency in cows after partial response to calcium therapy (21). Ketosis may complicate parturient paresis, in which case the animal responds to calcium therapy by rising but continues to manifest the clinical signs of ketosis, including in some cases the nervous signs of licking, circling and abnormal voice.

Toxaemia during the immediate post-parturient period is likely to occur in coliform mastitis, aspiration pneumonia, acute diffuse peritonitis resulting from traumatic perforation of the reticulum or uterus, and acute septic metritis. The depression in these instances may be profound and the animal be unable to rise, but careful clinical examination reveals a much more rapid heart rate than is usual in a corresponding stage of parturient paresis, and some localizing signs of abnormality of the milk and udder, of the lungs or of the uterus. Aspiration pneumonia should be suspected if the animal has been lying on its side, especially if there is evidence of regurgitation of ruminal contents from the nostrils, no matter how small the amount, or if there is a history of the animal having been drenched. Abnormal auscultatory findings may not be detectable until the second day. Early diagnosis is imperative if the animal is to be saved and the mortality rate is always high (22).

Although some elevation of the temperature may be observed in these severe toxaemic states it is more usual to find a subnormal temperature. The response to calcium therapy is usually a marked increase in heart rate, and death during the injection is common. Every case of recumbency must be carefully examined as these conditions may occur either independently or as complications of parturient paresis. In our experience about 25 per cent of cases of post-parturient recumbency in cows are due primarily to toxaemia or injury rather than to hypocalcaemia.

Injuries to the hindquarters are common at the time of parturition because of the marked relaxation of the ligaments of the pelvic girdle. Fenwick (23) records seven types of leg abnormality in this group at an incidence level of 8·5 per cent in 400 consecutive cases of parturient paresis. The abnormalities included radial paralysis, dislocation of the hips and rupture of gastrocnemius muscle. In most instances the affected animals are down and unable to rise but they eat, drink, urinate and defaecate normally, show no rise in temperature or pulse rate and make strong efforts to rise particularly with the forelimbs. Maternal obstetric paralysis is the most common injury. Although this occurs most frequently in heifers after a difficult parturition it may also occur in adult animals following an easy birth, and occasionally before parturition especially in cows in poor condition. The mildest form is evidenced by a frequent kicking movement of a hind leg as though something was stuck between the claws. All degrees of severity from this, through knuckling and weakness of one or both hind legs to complete inability to rise may occur, but sensation in the affected limb is usually normal. The cause of the condition is thought to be trauma to peripheral nerves during passage of the calf, or in pregnant animals to compression of the sciatic nerve by a calf crammed into the pelvic canal. In many cases of maternal obstetric paralysis there are gross haemorrhages, both deep and superficial, and histopathological degeneration of the sciatic nerves (24). Individual animals may show involvement of the obturator nerve with defective adduction of the thighs. The position of the hind limbs is often normal but in severe cases, especially those with extensive haematoma along the sciatic nerve trunk, the leg may be held extended with the toe reaching the elbow as in dislocation of the hip, but in the latter case there is exaggerated lateral mobility of the limb. Additional injuries causing recumbency near parturition include those associated with degenerative myopathy, dislocation of the hip and ventral hernia.

Degenerative myopathy (ischaemic muscle necrosis), affecting chiefly the heavy muscles of the thighs, occurs commonly in cattle which are recumbent for more than 48 hours (43). At necropsy large masses of pale muscle can be found surrounded by muscle of normal colour. Clinically the condition is indistinguishable from sciatic nerve paralysis. Markedly increased serum levels of glutamic-oxaloacetic transaminase have been observed in some cows recumbent for long periods after an initial attack of parturient paresis. Such increased SGOT activity may be related to muscle damage of this sort but it is apparent that a dietary deficiency of selenium is not associated with the muscular lesion (25). Other conditions which may have their origin in lesser degrees of this myopathy include rupture of the gastrocnemius muscle or separation of its tendon either from the muscle or the tuber calcis. Most of these injuries occur rather commonly in cattle but rarely in other species. Shock at parturition may occur with prolapse or rupture of the uterus but the cause is usually obvious.

One of the major problems in dairy cattle practice is the so-called 'Downer Cow' syndrome in which the animal goes down during the period of susceptibility to parturient paresis but fails to respond to treatment. Clinically the animal may be normal except for recumbency, or show nervous signs varying from lateral recumbency with opisthotonous to constant clonic convulsions.

Paresis with mental depression and associated with low total serum-calcium levels can occur in cows at times other than at parturition. The cause is largely unexplained but the syndrome occurs rarely in animals other than ruminants. Hypocalcaemia may occur after gorging on grain and may be a significant factor in particular cases. Sudden rumen stasis due to traumatic reticulitis may rarely cause hypocalcaemic paresis. Diarrhoea, particularly when cattle or sheep are placed on new lush pasture, may also precipitate an attack. Access to plants rich in oxalates may have a similar effect particularly if the animals are unaccustomed to the plants. Affected animals respond well to calcium therapy but relapse is likely unless the primary cause is corrected.

Hypocalcaemic paresis in sheep must be differentiated from pregnancy toxaemia in which the course is much longer, the signs indicate cerebral involvement and the disease is restricted to pregnant ewes. There is no response to calcium therapy and a positive test for ketonuria is almost diagnostic of the disease. In horses transit tetany is virtually identical clinically but occurs in both sexes and is always associated with transport. In sows the absence of fever may help to differentiate the disease from metritis and mastitis, but in hot weather a temperature of 40 to 41°C (104 to 105°F) is not unusual in sows with parturient paresis. At parturition goats are susceptible to enterotoxaemia and hypoglycaemia, both of which present clinical signs reminiscent of parturient paresis (26).

Treatment

The treatment of parturient paresis by the parenteral injection of calcium salts is standard practice. Calcium borogluconate is the preparation of choice. For cattle 100 to 200 g. of the compound as a 20 to 30 per cent solution is the usual dose (i.e. 400 to 800 ml. of a 25 per cent solution). Calcium laevulinate in 60 to 120 g. doses is also used (27). Calciumcarboxymethyl dextran (Cadexil) has been used experimentally but some deaths due to cardiac failure during the injection have been reported. There is a tendency among veterinarians to underdose with calcium salts largely because of toxic effects which tend to occur when all of the calcium is given intravenously. As an initial dose a heavy cow (1200 to 1300 lb.) requires 800 to 1000 ml. of a 25 per cent solution and a small cow (700 to 800 lb.) 400 to 500 ml. Underdosing increases the chances of incomplete response, with inability of the cow to rise, or of relapse.

For a quick response the solution is given by intravenous injection although subcutaneous injection is satisfactory for cows which are still standing. As a general rule half the dose should be given by each route to combine the rapid action and prolonged effect of the two methods. This also tends to avoid deaths due to over dosage and too rapid intravenous injection. Subcutaneous or intraperitoneal administration is preferred in cows with severe toxaemia due to aspiration pneumonia, metritis and mastitis. Toxaemic cows are very susceptible to voluminous intravenous injections and death may occur due to overloading of the circulation. In such cases the heart rate increases markedly (up to 180 per minute), there is respiratory distress, trembling and collapse and the cow dies within a few minutes. Sows should receive 100 to 150 ml. of a 15 per cent solution intraperitoneally and ewes 50 to 100 ml. of a similar solution intravenously or subcutaneously.

Cows suffering from hypocalcaemic paresis show a definite pattern of response to specific therapy. The classical response includes belching, muscle tremor, particularly of the flanks and often extending to the whole body, slowing, and improvement in the amplitude and pressures of the pulse, increase in the intensity of the heart sounds, sweating of the muzzle and defaecation. The faeces are characteristically in the form of a firm stool with a hard crust and covered with mucus containing a few flecks of blood. Urination usually does not follow until the cow rises. Tetany may also be observed to return transitorily in the limbs.

Unusual reactions include a marked increase in heart rate in cows suffering from toxaemia and acute heart block in apparently normal animals especially with overdosage, too rapid injection and cases in which treatment has been unduly prolonged. In the latter the maximum tolerated dose of calcium borogluconate by intravenous injection is likely to be of the order of 250 ml. of 25 per cent solution (28). Overdosage may occur when farmers treat cases unsuccessfully by multiple subcutaneous injections and these are followed by an intravenous injection. When the peripheral circulation is very poor it is probable that the calcium administered subcutaneously is not absorbed until the circulation improves following the intravenous injection and the massive doses of calcium then absorbed cause acute toxicity. In all cases of intravenous injection close watch should be kept on the circulation. Some degree of irregularity occurs in most cases but if there is gross irregularity or sudden increase in heart rate the injection should be stopped temporarily or continued with great caution. In normal circumstances at least ten minutes should be taken to introduce the standard dose. The acute toxic effect of calcium salts seems to be exerted specifically on heart muscle, a bradycardia being followed by a terminal tachycardia and magnesium sulphate (300 ml. 10 per cent solution) injected intravenously is the specific antidote. Sudden death may also occur after calcium injections if the cow is excited or frightened. It has been suggested that these deaths are caused by undue sensitivity to adrenaline. When affected cows are exposed to the sun or a hot, humid atmosphere, heatstroke may be a complicating factor. In such cases an attempt should be made to bring the temperature to below 39·5 °C (103 °F) before administering calcium.

Chronic toxicity may also occur. In rabbits and rats severe uraemia due to extensive calcium deposits in the kidney occur after the subcutaneous injection of calcium chloride and borogluconate and similar deposits are often seen at necropsy in cows dying after multiple injections of calcium salts administered at short intervals.

Failure to respond to treatment may be due to incorrect or incomplete diagnosis, or inadequate treatment. An inadequate response also includes relapse after a temporary improvement. The same factors which cause poor response apply but relapses are much the most common in middle-aged Jersey cows who may have as many as 5 or 6 attacks around one calving. In all cases the incidence of relapses is much higher in cases which occur just before calving than in those which occur afterwards (29). The needs of individual animals for calcium replacement vary widely, depending on their body weight and the degree of hypocalcaemia. In cattle, cows that have very recently calved, and older cows, are likely to show an incomplete response. In the latter instance the poor response is probably an indication of diminished skeletal reserves of calcium and inability of the normal mechanisms to maintain serum-calcium levels in the face of excessive drain in the milk. The duration of the illness and the posture of the cow are also important in relation to response. Thus, in an extensive study, there were no downer cows or deaths in cows still standing at treatment, 13 per cent downers and 2 per cent deaths in cows in sternal recumbency and 37 per cent downers and 12 per cent deaths in cows in lateral recumbency at treatment (30). The longer the period from onset of illness to treatment the longer the period of post-treatment recumbency and the more cows lost by destruction or sale for slaughter. After routine treatment 37 per cent of cases rose unassisted within 10 minutes and 23 required some assistance, 26 per cent recovered after longer periods of recumbency and 14 per cent died, or were destroyed or sold for slaughter. Another interesting relationship is the observation that a low body temperature due probably to exposure to low environmental temperature and increased wind velocities is positively correlated with a high proportion of deaths and poor responses (28). The best procedure to follow if response does not occur is to revisit the animal at 12-hourly intervals and check the diagnosis. If no other cause of the recumbency can be determined the initial treatment should be repeated on a maximum of 3 occasions. Beyond this point further calcium therapy is seldom effective. At the second visit alternative treatments, including inflation of the udder, and the injection of solutions containing either phosphorus, magnesium or dextrose, may also be administered, depending upon the clinical signs presented and the results of available biochemical tests. Glucose is usually administered as 500 ml. of a 40 per cent solution, sodium acid-phosphate as 200 ml. of a 15 per cent solution, and magnesium sulphate as 200 to 400 ml. of a 15 per cent solution.

Udder inflation has been largely superseded because of the possibility of damage to the udder but it is still a valuable alternative treatment, particularly in cows which do not respond completely to the injections described above. It is recommended as the routine treatment for cows which are likely to relapse. Serum calcium and phosphorus levels are raised but hypercalcaemia, such as occurs after injected calcium solutions, is avoided and the depression of homeostatic mechanisms is also avoided (19). The response is good and often prompt, but may not be apparent for up to 12 hours. Serum-magnesium levels are not affected by udder inflation and in view of the high levels of calcium and phosphorus and low level of magnesium in colostrum, it seems probable that udder inflation acts by preventing the further secretion of milk and slowing down the excretion of calcium and phosphorus (31). Inflation is best carried out with a special hand pump carrying an air filter and teat siphon. The udder is pumped up to a uniform, moderate firmness and the teats taped with broad tape which must be removed, the teats massaged and the tape replaced, at half-hourly intervals. Scrupulous cleanliness is necessary to prevent the introduction of infection into the quarters.

A further aid to parenteral therapy with solutions of calcium salts, especially for the purpose of increasing recovery rates and preventing relapses, is the oral administration of gels containing calcium chloride (32) described under prevention.

General nursing procedures are important. The calf should be removed and for the first 48 hours only sufficient milk drawn for its maintenance. A gradual return to full milking can then be permitted. If the cow is down for any length of time she must be kept propped up, since to leave her lying flat is to invite regurgitation and aspiration pneumonia. She should be moved from side to side 3 or 4 times a day and the legs and bony prominences massaged. Erection of a shelter over the cow is advisable if she cannot be moved to permanent shelter. If a cow is recumbent for more than 48 hours she should be raised in a hip sling several times daily. However, drastic measures to get cows up should be avoided. Gentle nudging in the ribs or the use of an electric prod are the maximum stimulants advised. The best assistance that can be given to a cow attempting to rise is a good heave at the base of the tail when she is half way up. In many cases of parturient paresis which fail to rise after treatment it seems that there is no physical reason for the recumbency and that 'tonic immobility' is the cause. The common ways of testing this possibility are to bring on a dog, remove or stimulate the calf, open the door of the pen or cause fright in some way.

Control

Although no completely satisfactory method of prevention is available much attention has been directed to this aspect of the disease. The feeding of additional calcium is contraindicated and may in fact increase the incidence especially if the diet is alkaline, so much so that the feeding of an acid-type diet has been suggested as a preventive measure (33). On the other hand the maintenance of appetite and the avoidance of alimentary tract stasis in late pregnancy appear to be important preventive measures which are likely to ensure an adequate calcium absorption (4). Testosterone derivatives with anabolic actions are undergoing trials to assess their efficiency as stimulators of appetite in cows near parturition. To improve mobilization the efficiency of prepartum milking and high-phosphate feeding have been examined. If the sudden onset of profuse lactation precipitates the hypocalcaemia it might be expected that milking before calving would prevent the sudden drop in serum-calcium levels which occurs in all cows. However, prepartum milking does not reduce the incidence of parturient paresis, nor significantly affect the changes in serum which normally occur in cows at parturition.

The administration of large quantities of phosphate in the ration should result in increased phosphate, and concurrently calcium, excretion in the urine. If the ration is also low in calcium the resulting negative balance of calcium can be expected to stimulate activity of the parathyroid gland. Boda and Cole have made use of this physiological mechanism by feeding a high phosphorus-low calcium ration to cows during the last month of pregnancy. With a Ca:P ratio of 6:1 30 per cent of cows developed parturient paresis, at a Ca:P ratio of 1:1 15 per cent developed the disease and at a ratio 1:3·3 no cases occurred. Although there is no apparent effect on the subsequent lactation there is the possibility, if the negative balance of calcium is prolonged or repeated frequently, that such a ration may contribute to the development of osteoporosis. The inclusion of 5 per cent of monosodium phosphate in a concentrate ration is also recommended as a preventive. The phosphate-treated diet is fed continuously (34).

A ration high in protein, designed to stimulate maximum milk production at calving is thought to increase the incidence of parturient paresis although the opposite view is also held. From our own observations, herds which are 'steamed up' before calving do, as a rule, have a higher incidence of the disease.

The most recent addition to the list of preventive measures is the provision by mouth of supplementary calcium in the form of a calcium gel (35, 36). This is given by drench or in the feed at a level to provide 100 g. of calcium daily. Excellent results are claimed provided the dose is raised to 150 g. and 3 doses are given 24 hours before, 1 to 2 hours before and 10 to 14 hours after calving.

In an attempt to reverse the negative calcium balance of susceptible cows the administration of vitamin D is now commonly used as a preventive measure. Oral dosing with vitamin D_2, the intravenous administration of vitamin D_3 and the intramuscular injection of dihydrotachysterol all have their proponents. Oral dosing with 20 million units of vitamin D_2 per day for 5 days to cows immediately prior to calving greatly reduces the expected incidence of parturient paresis. The exact date of calving is often difficult to determine and if the administration is discontinued for up to 4 days before calving an unusually high incidence of the disease may follow, probably because of the depression of parathyroid activity which follows the administration (44). The danger of causing metastatic calcification also exists as this has been produced with smaller doses (10 to 20 million units daily for 10 days). Pregnant cows are more susceptible to calcification than non-pregnant animals. Treatment with larger doses or for longer periods than those recommended above should be avoided because of the danger of toxic effects. Smaller doses reduce the risk of calcification but also reduce the degree of calcium retention (37). The optimal dose as a single injection is probably of the order of 10 million units (250 mg.) repeated as necessary at 8-day intervals (38). Clinically symptomless calcification may occur in vessel walls but this is unlikely if dietary phosphorus and magnesium intake is adequate. Single doses of 40 million units can be lethal. The injection can be intravenous or intramuscular and is repeated every 8 days until the cow calves. Variable results have been recorded (39, 36). One of the disadvantages of the method is the likelihood that cows which do not calve at the anticipated time can be more seriously affected than if they receive no treatment. Occasional cases of shock occur after the intravenous injection, especially if more than one injection is given, and the intramuscular route is preferred (40). The injection of vitamin D is preferred to feeding it and a protection rate of up to 80 per cent can be anticipated. It is estimated that 95 per cent of Jersey cattle are protected (41).

Dihydrotachysterol has a much stronger calcaemic effect than vitamin D and good results are claimed for the intramuscular injection of 10 mg. as a prophylactic measure. Used simultaneously with calcium therapy at first treatment it may also reduce the incidence of relapses. Hypercalcaemia results after 24 hours and persists for 72 hours. Up to 50 mg. has been injected without ill effect. Most observers find little benefit from the use of dihydrotachysterol as a prophylactic against either initial attacks or relapses and the drug appears to have no effect on calcium retention (37). In spite of its limitations it may still have value as an ancillary treatment. To be effective against initial attacks it must be given immediately the cow calves, and must thus be left to the farmer to give: if an attack of parturient paresis does occur within 24 hours—as it commonly does—it will probably be less severe than if no treatment had been given. The same comment applies to relapses with the additional finding that cows suffering many attacks during a short time can usually have the sequence terminated by an injection of dihydrotachysterol. One important corollary to therapy with this drug is that it will not prevent relapses which are the result of insufficient calcium therapy in the first place.

Miscellaneous prophylactic measures include injections of parathyroid extract which have no apparent effect, incomplete milking after calving which is similarly disappointing, and the prophylactic injection of calcium solutions as soon after calving as possible, which may be effective but is largely impractical. Years ago the administration of ammonium chloride by mouth to produce acidosis and enhance calcium mobilization and ionization was recommended to prevent milk fever. There is some support for its use on the same basis now (42). The ammonium chloride is fed with grain over the last few weeks of pregnancy, commencing with 25 g. and increasing to 100 g. per day at calving.

In species other than cattle the disease is commonly caused by errors in management, and prevention depends on their avoidance. Pregnant and lactating ewes and cows should not be subjected to unnecessary exercise or excitement. It is good practice to improve the plane of nutrition during late pregnancy in ewes to avoid pregnancy toxaemia but changes, particularly to lush pasture, should be made gradually, and sheep moved from wooded pasture to open fields with little natural shelter should be provided with some protection from the weather.

REFERENCES

(1) Moodie, E. W. (1965). *Brit. vet. J.*, *121*, 338.
(2) Belonje, P. C. & Van der Walt, K. (1971). *J. S. Afr. vet. med. Ass.*, *42*, 135.
(3) Carlstrom, G. (1970). *Acta vet. scand.*, *11*, 89.
(4) Payne, J. M. (1964). *Vet. Rec.*, *76*, 77, 1275.
(5) Payne, J. M. *et al.* (1963). *Vet. Rec.*, *75*, 588.
(6) Mayer, G. P. *et al.* (1969). *Amer. J. vet. Res.*, *30*, 1587.
(7) Capen, C. C. & Young, D. M. (1967). *Lab. Invest.*, *17*, 717.
(8) Ochs, B. O. *et al.* (1964). *J. Dairy Sci.*, *47*, 542.
(9) Care, A. D. *et al.* (1967). *J. Endocrin.*, *37*, 155.
(10) Barlet, J. P. (1968). *C. R. Acad. Sci. (Paris)*, *267D*, 2010.
(11) Barlet, J. P. *et al.* (1971). *Ann. Biol. anim. Biochim.*, *11*, 415.
(12) Braithwaite, G. D. *et al.* (1969). *Brit. J. Nutr.*, *23*, 827.
(13) Hibbs, J. W. *et al.* (1964). *J. Dairy Sci.*, *29*, 617.
(14) Bach, J. S. & Messervy, A. (1969). *Vet. Rec.*, *84*, 210.
(15) Littlejohn, A. I. (1969). *Vet. Rec.*, *84*, 130.
(16) Mayer, G. P. *et al.* (1966). *J. Amer. vet. med. Ass.*, *149*, 402.
(17) Bowen, J. M. *et al.* (1970). *Amer. J. vet. Res.*, *31*, 831.
(18) Stubbings, D. P. (1971). *Vet. Rec.*, *89*, 296'
(19) Mayer, G. P. *et al.* (1967). *J. Amer. vet. med. Ass.*, *151*, 1673.
(20) Mayer, G. P. *et al.* (1965). *J. Amer. vet. med. Ass.*, *146*, 839.
(21) Hoffman, W. & El Amrousi, S. (1971). *Dtsch. tierärztl. Wschr.*, *78*, 156.
(22) Fenwick, D. C. (1969). *Aust. vet. J.*, *45*, 450.
(23) Fenwick, D. C. (1969). *Aust. vet. J.*, *45*, 118.
(24) Galabinov, G. (1966). *Mh. Vet.-Med.*, *21*, 601.
(25) Jonsson, G. *et al.* (1969). *Acta vet. scand.*, *10*, 104.
(26) Linzell, J. L. (1965). *Vet. Rec.*, *77*, 767.
(27) Blood, D. C. *et al.* (1965). *Aust. vet. J.*, *31*, 245.
(28) Fenwick, D. C. (1969). *Aust. vet. J.*, *45*, 114, 123.
(29) Roine, K. (1970). *Nord. Vet.-Med.*, *22*, 567.
(30) Fenwick, D. C. (1969). *Aust. vet. J.*, *45*, 111, 454.
(31) Payne, J. M. & Vagg, M. J. (1966). *Brit. vet. J.*, *122*, 163.
(32) Jonsgard, K. *et al.* (1971). *Nord. Vet.-Med.*, *23*, 606.
(33) Ender, F. (1964). *3rd int. Mtg Dis. Cattle, Copenhagen, Reports*, *2*, 408.
(34) Stott, G. H. (1965). *J. Dairy Sci.*, *48*, 1485.
(35) Simesen, M. G. & Hyldgaard-Jensen, C. (1971). *Nord. Vet.-Med.*, *23*, 35.
(36) Jonsson, G. & Pehrson, B. (1970). *Vet. Rec.*, *87*, 575, 583.
(37) Manston, R. & Payne, J. M. (1964). *Brit. vet. J.*, *120*, 167.
(38) Payne, J. M. & Manston, R. (1967). *Vet. Rec.*, *81*, 214.
(39) Gustafsson, B. *et al.* (1971). *Nord. Vet.-Med.*, *23*, 44.
(40) Seekles, L. *et al.* (1964). *Vet. Rec.*, *76*, 486.
(41) Gregorovic, V. *et al.* (1967). *Vet. Rec.*, *81*, 161.
(42) Vagg, M. J. & Payne, J. M. (1970). *Brit. vet. J.*, *126*, 531.
(43) Flagstad, T. *et al.* (1970). *Medlemsbl. danske Dyrlægerforen*, *53*, 363.
(44) Capen, C. C. (1966). *Amer. J. vet. Res.*, *27*, 1177.
(45) Littledike, E. T. (1969). *J. Amer. vet. med. Ass.*, *155*, 1955.

The 'Downer Cow' Syndrome

A number of metabolic disturbances, serious infections, and injuries to the musculoskeletal system occur at the time of parturition in dairy cows. Many entities can be detected by clinical, clinico-pathological and necropsy examinations but, when these have all been identified, one is still left with a residuum of animals which show paresis of unknown origin. There may be more than one entity but, for lack of a better classification, these cases are described under the heading the 'downer cow' syndrome.

Incidence

The incidence of illness classified as 'downer cow' syndrome is distressingly high, particularly because so many of the affected animals are heavy producers and of great value. It is impossible to give accurate figures on incidence because of variations in nomenclature and in the accuracy of diagnoses. Cases included in this classification by some veterinarians are classified by others as maternal obstetric paralysis, as obturator paralysis or as hypophosphataemia. Because it is a syndrome lacking in definition, and comprising the residual cases which cannot be otherwise classified, it varies in size depending largely upon the clinical acuity of the individual veterinarian, and probably also on varying environmental factors in different areas. Nevertheless the incidence seems to be increasing, particularly in intensive farming areas, although this impression could arise from the increased necessity to effect a cure in valuable animals.

Aetiology

The aetiology is unknown and a number of factors may operate. Clinical, clinico-pathological and necropsy findings suggest that a severe circulatory crisis occurs near parturition in affected animals but the exact nature of the crisis and whether it is primary or secondary has not been determined. Hypoproteinaemia due to inadequate protein feeding during a period of increased protein requirement and an unspecified digestive disturbance (1) have been suggested as causes. Hypopotassaemia has also been suspected as an important part of the pathogenesis, particularly in the so-called 'creeper' cows which are alert and crawl and struggle but are unable to rise. Treatment by injection with solutions containing 5 to 20 g. potassium per infusion is used with apparent success (2, 3). However, the toxicity of potassium, either orally or parenterally, for cows limits its use as a treatment (4).

Occurrence

The disease occurs most commonly in the first 2 or 3 days after calving in heavy milk producers, and in many cases occurs concurrently with parturient paresis.

Pathogenesis

Because of its similarity to parturient paresis, one forms the impression that this is a functional or metabolic disease affecting particularly the circulatory and neuromuscular systems. Albuminuria is a common accompaniment and probably results from damage to renal glomerular epithelium either primarily or as a result of the circulatory failure. There may be an associated hypocalcaemia in the early stages. The alternative proposition that downer cows are always a sequel to hypocalcaemia and due largely to ischaemic muscle necrosis (5) is a worthy one. At least early detection and treatment of cases of parturient paresis and careful nursing of them reduces the prevalence of downer cows (6, 7).

Clinical Findings

Affected cows usually show no signs of illness until they go down, either at calving or usually within the succeeding 48 hours. They are bright and alert and, although the appetite is reduced, the cow eats and drinks moderately well. The temperature is normal or slightly elevated, the heart rate is increased to 80 to 100 per minute, and the pulse is small and weak, but the respiration is unaffected. Defaecation and urination are normal. Initially affected cows may make frequent attempts to rise but are unable to completely extend their hind legs.

This is the clinical picture in the typical case but, in others, the signs may be more marked and include particularly a tendency to lie in lateral recumbency with the head drawn back. When lifted and supported, these cows appear quite normal but, when they are left alone, they always revert to the position of lateral recumbency within a short time. Still more severe cases show hyperaesthesia and some tetany of limbs but only when lying in lateral recumbency. These more severe cases do not usually eat or drink.

The 'downer cow' syndrome may occur independently, or follow apparent recovery after treatment for parturient paresis, except for the continued recumbency which, in effect, constitutes the disease. The course of the disease varies from 1 to 2 weeks in subacute cases, after which slaughter is often necessary, or death may occur within 48 to 72 hours in the more acute cases.

Clinical Pathology

The calcium, phosphorus, magnesium and glucose levels of the blood are within the normal range and the results of haematological examinations are usually consistent with those found in normal cows which have recently calved. There may be moderate ketonuria and, in many cases, there is marked albuminuria with some hyaline and granular casts also present in the urine (8). Low arterial blood pressures and abnormal electrocardiograms have been observed in some animals (8).

Necropsy Findings

There are no characteristic gross findings. The heart is dilated, flabby and thin-walled, the liver shows moderate fatty degeneration and the adrenal glands are enlarged. Histologically there are degenerative changes in the glomerular and tubular epithelium of the kidneys.

Diagnosis

Differentiation from parturient paresis is based on failure to respond to treatment with calcium salts and an absence of narcosis, hypothermia and paralysis of plain muscle. Great care should be taken not to overdose with calcium while arriving at a diagnosis. The other common causes of persistent recumbency in cattle during the immediate post-parturient period are described under the diagnosis of parturient paresis (p, 687). Lymphomatosis involving the spinal cord is not restricted to cows which have recently calved and recumbency is usually preceded by a period during which there is paresis evidenced by knuckling at the fetlocks and difficulty in getting up. Acute impaction of the rumen also occurs in animals other than those recently calved and is accompanied by complete ruminal atony and severe depression.

Treatment

Many treatments, including the injection of magnesium salts, phosphates, isotonic saline solutions, cortisone and ACTH, stimulant tonics and cholinergic drugs, have been tried without consistent success. Attempts at slinging are usually unsuccessful because the cows will not take weight on the hind legs. The most satisfactory treatment programme consists of maintaining the comfort and the nutritional status of the animal in the hope that spontaneous recovery will occur. Suggested measures include slinging to prevent damage to the thigh muscles, frequent turning from side to side, and the provision of ample bedding, food and water. Parenteral injections of fluids, dextrose and electrolytes and, where possible, protein hydrolysates or amino-acids may be prescribed depending on clinical and biochemical findings.

Control

Insufficient is known of the aetiology for suitable control measures to be recommended.

REFERENCES

(1) Jacobsson, S. O. & Knudson, O. (1962). *Cornell Vet.*, *52*, 173.
(2) Johnson, B. L. (1963). *Vet. Med.*, *53*, 217.
(3) Johnson, B. L. (1967). *J. Amer. vet. med. Ass.*, *151*, 1681.
(4) Ward, G. M. (1966). *J. Amer. vet. med. Ass.*, *148*, 543.
(5) Bjorsell, K. A. *et al.* (1969). *Acta vet. scand.*, *10*, 36.
(6) Fenwick, D. C. (1969). *Aust. vet. J.*, *45*, 184.
(7) Curtis, R. A. *et al.* (1970). *Mod. vet. Pract.*, *51*, 7, 25.
(8) Sellers, A. F. *et al.* (1956). *Proc. 92nd ann. gen. Mtg Amer. vet. med. Ass.*, 1955, pp. 35–7.

Transit Tetany of Ruminants

Transit tetany is a disease which occurs after prolonged transport, usually in cows and ewes in late pregnancy. It is characterized by recumbency, alimentary-tract stasis and coma and is highly fatal. It has a wide distribution and can be expected to occur in most countries. Most affected animals die and heavy losses are encountered when cows and ewes in late pregnancy are moved long distances by rail or on foot.

Although cows of any age in late pregnancy are most commonly affected the disease has also been recorded in cows recently calved, in bullocks, steers and dry cows (1). Precipitating causes include heavy feeding before shipment, deprivation of food and water for more than 24 hours during transit and unrestricted access to water and exercise immediately after unloading. There is an increased incidence during hot weather. The cause is unknown although physical stress is an obvious factor and the observation that prolonged intravenous infusion of norepinephrine induces hypocalcaemia in sheep (4) is suggestive in this connection.

Clinical signs may occur while the cattle are still on the train or up to 48 hours after unloading. In the early stages there may be excitement and restlessness, trismus and grinding of the teeth. A staggering gait with paddling of the hind legs and recumbency occur, and are accompanied by stasis of the alimentary tract and complete anorexia. Animals that do not recover gradually become comatose and die in 3 to 4 days. There may be a moderate hypocalcaemia and hypophosphataemia (3) but there are no lesions at necropsy. The relationship of the disease to transport or forced exercise is diagnostic.

Some cases respond to treatment with combined calcium, magnesium and glucose injections. Udder inflation, induced abortion and general stimulants, such as strychnine are of no apparent value. Repeated parenteral injections of large volumes of electrolyte solutions are recommended.

If prolonged transport of cows or ewes in advanced pregnancy is unavoidable, they should be fed on a moderately restricted diet for several days beforehand and provided with adequate food, water and rest periods during the trip. The administration of an ataractic before loading is highly recommended especially for nervous animals (2). On unloading they should be allowed only limited access to water for 24 hours and should be allowed a minimum of exercise for 2 or 3 days.

REFERENCES

(1) McBarron, E. J. (1952). *Aust. vet. J.*, *28*, 36.
(2) Walt, K. van der (1961). *J. S. Afr. vet. med. Ass.*, *32*, 283.
(3) Tunger, G. (1966). *Inang. Diss.*, Freie Univ., Berlin, p. 48.
(4) Luthman, J. (1970). *Acta vet. scand.*, *11*, 327.

Lactation Tetany of Mares

(*Eclampsia, Transit Tetany*)

Lactation tetany of mares appears to have been a common occurrence when draught horse breeding was widely practised but is observed rarely nowadays. The mortality rate is high in untreated animals.

Hypocalcaemia occurs constantly, with serum levels in the range of 4 to 6 mg. per cent, and response to treatment with injections of calcium salts is excellent. Hypomagnesaemia (with serum-magnesium levels of 0·9 mg. per cent) has been observed in some cases (1) but only in association with recent transport. Hypermagnesaemia has been reported in other cases (2).

A number of factors appear to predispose to the disease. Most cases occur in lactating mares, either at about the tenth day after foaling or 1 to 2 days after weaning (4).

Mares which are grazing on lush pasture and have an exceptionally heavy flow of milk appear to be most susceptible and in many instances hard physical work (5), the housing of wild ponies (6), or prolonged transport (2) appears to precipitate an attack. The latter has been a particularly important factor in the aetiology of the disease in Britain and has been credited with precipitating it even in stallions and dry mares (6). Occasional cases occur without there being any apparent cause (3).

Many mild cases which recover spontaneously occur after transport but the mortality rate in some shipments may be greater than 60 per cent. Mares affected at the foal heat or at weaning are usually more seriously affected and the mortality rate appears to be higher still.

Severely affected animals sweat profusely and have difficulty in moving because of tetany of the limbs and inco-ordination. Rapid, violent respirations and wide dilatation of the nostrils are accompanied by a distinct thumping sound from the chest, thought to be due to spasmodic contraction of the diaphragm. Muscular fibrillation, particularly of the masseter and shoulder region, and trismus are evident but there is no prolapse of the membrana nictitans. Affected animals are not hypersensitive to sound but handling may precipitate increased tetany. The temperature is normal or slightly elevated, and, although the pulse is normal in the early stages, it later becomes rapid and irregular. The mare may make many attempts to eat and drink but appears to be unable to swallow and passage of a stomach tube may be impossible. Urination and defaecation are in abeyance, and peristalsis is reduced.

Within about 24 hours the animal goes down, tetanic convulsions develop and become more or less continuous, the mare dying about 48 hours after the onset of illness. The tetany and excitement in the early stages may suggest tetanus but there is no prolapse of the third eyelid and there is the usual relationship to recent foaling or weaning and physical exertion. The anxiety and muscle tremor of laminitis may also be confused with those of lactation tetany, especially as it may occur in mares which have foaled and retained the placenta. Pain in the feet is the diagnostic feature of this latter disease. Treatment by the intravenous injection of calcium solutions as recommended in the treatment of parturient paresis causes rapid, complete recovery. One of the earliest signs of recovery is the voiding of a large volume of urine. Occasional cases which persist for some days are recorded (7).

REFERENCES

(1) Green, H. H. *et al.* (1935). *J. comp. Path.*, *48*, 74.
(2) De Gier, C. J. (1935). *T. Diergeneesk.*, *62*, 1186.
(3) Baird, J. D. (1971). *Aust. vet. J.*, *47*, 402.
(4) Forsyth, H. & Hodgkinson, E. J. (1945). *Vet. Rec.*, *57*, 503.
(5) Kjos-Hanssen, J. (1943). *Norsk vet. Tidsskr.*, *55*, 116.
(6) Montgomerie, R. F. *et al.* (1929). *Vet. Rec.*, *9*, 319.
(7) Rach, D. J. *et al.* (1972). *Canad. vet. J.*, *13*, 78.

THE HYPOMAGNESAEMIC TETANIES

Tetany associated with depression of serum-magnesium levels is a common occurrence in ruminants, but probably in no other disease of domestic animals is there as much confusion in relation to aetiology and pathogenesis as there is in this group of diseases. The position is made even more confusing by the variety of circumstances in which they occur, and by their common association with other metabolic and nutritional deficiency diseases.

The syndrome associated with hypomagnesae-mia is relatively constant, irrespective of the cause, but the group of diseases in which it occurs has been divided into hypomagnesaemic tetany of calves, which appears to be due specifically to a deficiency of magnesium in the diet, and lactation tetany, in which there may be a partial dietary deficiency of magnesium but in which nutritional or metabolic factors reduce the availability, or increase the body's loss, of the element so that serum-magnesium levels fall below a critical point. Lactation tetany is a misnomer because, although this disease occurs more commonly in lactating cows, it also occurs at other times and even occasionally in males. In general the occurrence is related to three sets of circumstances. Most common is the occurrence in lactating cows turned out on to lush, grass-dominant pasture in the spring after wintering in closed housing—the classical lactation or grass tetany of Holland. Wheat pasture poisoning may occur when any type of cattle or sheep is grazed on young, green cereal crops. The third occurrence is in beef or dry dairy cattle running at pasture in the winter time, usually when nutrition is inadequate and where no shelter is provided in changeable weather, rather than in severe, prolonged cold. Hypomagnesaemia of sheep, although it is less common, occurs in the same general groups of circumstances as the disease in cattle.

It may be less confusing to consider these three occurrences of lactation tetany as separate diseases because the aetiology in each instance is probably different but they have so much in common with respect to clinical findings, clinical pathology, necropsy findings and methods of treatment and control that they are dealt with as one.

Lactation Tetany

(Hypomagnesaemic Tetany, Grass Tetany, Grass Staggers, Wheat Pasture Poisoning)

Lactation tetany is a highly fatal disease of all classes of ruminants but reaches its highest incidence in lactating cows. It is characterized by hypomagnesaemia, and usually hypocalcaemia, and clinically by tonic and clonic muscular spasms and convulsions, and death due to respiratory failure.

Incidence

Lactation tetany of dairy cows turned out to graze on lush, grass-dominant pasture after winter housing is most common in northern Europe and the U.K. and a similar condition occurs in Australia and New Zealand, where the cows are not housed but have access to a phenomenal flush of pasture growth in the spring. In cases where an autumn flush of pasture occurs a high incidence of hypomagnesaemic tetany may occur in the autumn or early winter. Wheat pasture poisoning has been recorded in many countries but is most prevalent where young cereal crops are utilized for winter grazing. The south-western United States has experienced heavy losses of cattle caused by this disease. Hypomagnesaemic tetany in cattle wintered in the open causes some losses in Britain, New Zealand, Southern Australia and the east-central states of the U.S.A. Although the disease is preeminently one of animals at pasture, it can occur in housed cattle if the total energy intake is low.

In all of these forms of the disease the morbidity rate is highly variable, reaching as high as 12 per cent in individual herds, and up to 2 per cent in particular areas. The incidence varies from year to year depending largely on climatic conditions and management practices, and the disease is often limited in its occurrence to particular farms and even to individual fields.

Hypomagnesaemia has been recognized as a disease of sheep in Australia and Great Britain and although the incidence is not great it appears to be increasing and can cause heavy losses in individual flocks.

Aetiology

It is conventional to speak in terms of 'seasonal hypomagnesaemia', in which no clinical signs occur and lactation tetany which is the clinical syndrome. The following account deals with factors which cause lactation tetany but *inter alia*, many of them are causes of the purely biochemical disturbance.

The most constant and significant biochemical disturbance reported in lactation tetany in both cattle and sheep is hypomagnesaemia. Hypocalcaemia is often present concurrently and, although it is of less severe degree than in parturient paresis, there is increasing evidence that the actual onset of clinical tetany may be associated with a rapid fall in serum-calcium levels superimposed on a pre-existing seasonal hypomagnesaemia (1, 2). Most investigations into the causes of lactation tetany are directed at determining the causes of the hypomagnesaemia and little information exists on the causes of the hypocalcaemia. It is known that a short period of starvation (24 to 48 hours) in lactating cows and ewes is capable of causing a significant sudden depression of calcium and magnesium levels (3) and this may be the important factor in many instances. It is of interest to note that the hypocalcaemia may not occur for some hours after the fast ceases. When the disease occurs in associa-

tion with transport (4) a similar mechanism may be involved.

Some attention has been given to the high serum levels of potassium which occur in ruminants on lush grass pasture and green cereal crops, and the relationship of this hyperkalaemia to the development of tetany. It seems probable that the mechanism is one of competition with magnesium for absorption, a secondary hypomagnesaemia then being the cause of tetany (5). For example it has been shown that pasture heavily top-dressed with potash is low in calcium and phosphorus and the availability of the calcium is low. Because the dry matter content of the feed is low cows on this pasture are in negative balance for calcium, and for magnesium because of the high magnesium content in the urine. The mechanisms which maintain magnesium homeostasis in ruminants are still very much under review (5) with a general consensus at present that there is no significant, effective mechanism for this purpose in ruminants. These species appear especially vulnerable with regard to magnesium because there is no readily mobilizable large store of magnesium in the body and the delicate balance of serum- (or more properly extracellular fluid) magnesium levels depends largely on the daily intake of magnesium in the diet. In lactating animals the daily loss of magnesium in the milk, urine and digestive secretions is high and a marked reduction in intake or availability of ingested magnesium can cause hypomagnesaemia (6). Although there is no large, mobilizable store of magnesium in the body, some reserves do exist in soft tissues and bones and can be of importance in delicate situations.

Until relatively recent years the hypomagnesaemia, which is characteristic of lactation tetany, was thought to arise because of defects in internal metabolism. This view derived partly as a heritage from the work on hypocalcaemia and partly because of the absence of any apparent deficiency of magnesium in the diet. The fact that the disease could be produced experimentally in cattle and sheep on artificial diets was interpreted as an indication that a dietary deficiency could be a cause but was unlikely to be so under natural conditions. This view has been re-examined in the light of work which shows that young, green grass has a lower content of available magnesium than mature grass, that lush grass pasture has a lower content of total magnesium than mature pasture (7), that grasses have a lower magnesium content than clovers and other dicotyledonous plants, and that heavy applications of potassium- and nitrogen-rich fertilizers reduce the availability of soil magnesium (8). As a result it is now generally accepted that cattle and sheep, particularly those in heavy lactation, may be receiving a diet deficient in magnesium when they graze many grass-dominant, lush, heavily fertilized pastures. In view of the estimation that milking cows need to ingest about 20 g. and to absorb about 4 g. of magnesium daily the observation that cows fed on winter rations usually receive 32 to 34 g. per day and cows on dangerous pasture receive only 10 to 22 g. daily is a significant one (9). The critical figure for concentration of magnesium in pasture is 0·20 per cent of the dry matter. Pasture with a magnesium content below this level is likely to cause hypomagnesaemia.

Apart from the question of the concentration of magnesium in the diet there is the question of the amount of food ingested. A reduction in dry matter intake must reduce the magnesium intake and, in situations where hypomagnesaemia is already present, a further depression of serum-magnesium levels can be anticipated when complete or partial starvation occurs. Whether hypomagnesaemia pre-exists or not, a period of starvation in lactating cows and ewes is sufficient to produce a marked hypomagnesaemia and the fall may be sufficiently great to cause clinical tetany (3). A period of bad weather, yarding, transport or movement to new pastures or the production of unpalatable pastures by heavy top dressing with nitrogenous fertilizers may provide such a period of partial starvation.

A number of factors are thought to reduce the availability of the magnesium which is ingested. Experimental intoxication with ammonia produces a clinical syndrome not unlike that of lactation tetany and it has been suggested that the production of large quantities of ammonia in the rumen when the diet is very rich in protein may, by a process akin to chelation, reduce the availability of magnesium (10). *Trans*-aconitate has also come under suspicion as a plant constituent which could reduce the biological efficiency of magnesium by forming non-ionizable complexes with it (11). The suspicion currently appears to have been exorcised (12, 13). The failure of the disease to develop on legume-dominant pasture suggests that protein intake per se is not the critical factor, although this has to be viewed in the light of the higher magnesium content of clovers. The rise in serum-magnesium which follows the feeding of cottonseed meal to ewes grazing tetany-prone pasture is further evidence that protein intake is not critical (14). The presence of chelating agents, e.g. alpha keto-butyric acid, in plants or in the ruminal contents is not unlikely and these would of course be inimical to magnesium absorption (5). Diarrhoea is commonly associated with lactation tetany on spring pasture and by decreasing the alimentary sojourn may also reduce magnesium absorption.

In areas where the disease is common, grass pastures top dressed with nitrogenous fertilizers are dangerous and their toxicity may be increased by the application of potash. Potash is known to compete with sodium for absorption by plants and thus interfere with magnesium absorption by them (7). Experimentally the administration of potassium to sheep diets decreases the apparent absorption of magnesium (35) and seriously increases the hypomagnesaemic effect of a low magnesium intake (15). The reduction of magnesium intake of high-producing dairy cows from 25 to 5 g. per day produced hypomagnesaemia and some clinical cases but the administration, in addition, of di-sodium hydrogen phosphate or sodium sulphate precipitated acute attacks of the disease (16).

A close association between climatic conditions and serum-magnesium levels has also been observed. Reduced levels occur in adult cattle and sheep exposed to cold, wet windy weather with little sunshine and with no access to shelter or to supplementary feed. Supplementary feeding appears to reduce the effect of inclement weather on serum-magnesium levels and it is possible that failure to eat during bad weather may be the basic cause of hypomagnesaemia.

Alternatively attention has been drawn to the possible role of hyperthyroidism in the production of seasonal hypomagnesaemia. Depression of serum-magnesium levels and clinical 'grass staggers' have been produced in recently calved cows by reducing the dietary intake or by feeding thyroprotein. This has led to the rather wider concept of a negative energy balance as a possible cause of hypomagnesaemia, with increased activity of the thyroid gland as the hormonal mediator. It is likely that hypomagnesaemia and hyperthyroidism occur concurrently without there being any cause–effect relationship between them.

In summary it appears that a number of factors are capable of causing hypomagnesaemia in ruminants and that under particular circumstances one or other of them may be of major importance. In lactation tetany of cows and ewes turned on to lush pasture in the spring, a primary dietary deficiency of magnesium or the presence of some factor in the diet which reduces the absorption or internal metabolism of magnesium and calcium appears probable. In wheat pasture poisoning the ingestion of abnormally large amounts of potassium in the diet probably leads to a relative or absolute hypomagnesaemia as serum-postassium levels rise. Hypomagnesaemic tetany occurring in cattle wintered at pasture (1) and exposed to inclement weather may be related to inadequate caloric intake and possibly to the resultant hyperactivity of the thyroid gland. Although the above suggestions as to the most important aetiological factors in each set of circumstances in which lactation tetany occurs may be valid, undoubtedly combinations of these and other factors have aetiological significance in individual outbreaks of the disease. One other important factor which must be borne in mind is the variation between individual animals in their susceptibility to hypomagnesaemia and to the clinical disease. These variations are quite marked in cattle (17) and in intensively managed, high-producing herds it is probably worth while to identify susceptible animals and give them special treatment.

Occurrence

The major occurrence of lactation tetany is in cattle and sheep turned out to lush, grass-dominant pasture in the early spring after wintering indoors, and in late autumn. Most cases occur during the first 2 weeks after the animals leave the barn. Pasture which has been heavily top dressed with fertilizers rich in nitrogen and potash are potentially most dangerous. The disease may also occur on this type of pasture even when the cattle have wintered outdoors.

The high incidence on cereal crops has given rise to the name of wheat pasture poisoning although the disease occurs on all types of cereal, including oats and barley. The pasture is usually dangerous for only a few weeks but heavy losses may occur in all classes of sheep and cattle, particularly when the pasture is in the early stages of growth.

Exposure to bad weather is exacerbated by absence of trees or other shelter in fields and by failure to supply supplementary feed, circumstances particularly likely to arise in stubble fields, or when dry dairy cattle, beef cattle or sheep are not housed in the winter time in moderately cold climates. The disease does not seem to occur in cattle kept outside in prolonged winters where environmental temperature is consistently very low. Although the disease is not specifically related to parturition it is most common in the first 2 months after calving, hence the name 'lactation tetany'. The disease is most common in lactating dairy cattle, may reach a moderate level of incidence in beef cattle and calves and has occurred in dry cows and bulls. Cattle in the 4- to 7-year age group are most susceptible but adult sheep and calves and

lambs may be affected. Ewes which have lambed during the preceding month are by far the most susceptible group. As in cattle the greatest incidence is on cereal grazing and lush grass pasture, losses usually ceasing when the flock is moved onto rough, unimproved pasture. Cases also occur in sheep which are exposed to inclement weather when on a low nutritive intake.

Pathogenesis

Most evidence points to hypomagnesaemia as the cause of the tetanic signs observed but the concurrent hypocalcaemia may have a contributory effect and in many instances may even be the dominant factor (1). Most clinical cases of the disease have serum-magnesium levels below 1·0 mg. per cent compared with the normal levels in cattle of 1·7 to 3·0 mg. per cent and there is a striking relationship between the incidence of the clinical disease and the occurrence of a seasonal hypomagnesaemia. The reduction in serum levels of magnesium is concurrent with a marked fall in the excretion of magnesium in the urine. Unfortunately field outbreaks do not always follow the classical picture. In affected herds many clinically normal cows have low serum-magnesium levels and in these circumstances a concurrent hypocalcaemia may be the precipitating cause.

In sheep the experimentally induced disease is characterized by hypocalcaemia (4·5 to 6·9 mg. per 100 ml.) and hypomagnesaemia (0·5 to 0·7 mg. per 100 ml.) and hypophosphataemia (0·9 to 1·2 mg. per 100 ml.). The clinical disease did not occur in ewes with hypophosphataemia and hypomagnesaemia if normal calcium levels existed (18).

There has been little investigation of the mechanism by which the tetany and convulsions are produced. In parallel to work in other species it has been shown in calves that the increased, excessive muscular contractions of hypomagnesaemic tetany are due to facilitation of transmission of impulses through the neuromuscular system (19).

Clinical Findings

For convenience lactation tetany can be described in acute, subacute and chronic forms.

Acute lactation tetany. The animal may be grazing at the time and suddenly cease to graze, adopt a posture of unusual alertness and appear uncomfortable, and twitching of the muscles and ears is evident. There is severe hyperaesthesia and slight disturbances precipitate attacks of continuous bellowing and frenzied galloping. The gait becomes staggering and the animal falls with obvious tetany of the limbs which is rapidly followed by clonic convulsions lasting for about a minute. During these convulsive episodes there is opisthotonus, nystagmus, champing of the jaws, frothing at the mouth, pricking of the ears and retraction of the eyelids. Between episodes the animal lies quietly but a sudden noise or touch may precipitate another attack. The temperature rises to 40 to 40·5 °C (104 to 105 °F) after severe muscle exertion; the pulse and respiratory rates are also high. The absolute intensity of the heart sounds is increased so that they can be heard some distance away from the cow. Death usually occurs within a half to one hour and the mortality rate is high because many die before treatment can be provided. The response to treatment is generally good.

Subacute lactation tetany. In this form of the disease the onset is more gradual. Over a period of 3 to 4 days there is slight inappetence, wildness of the facial expression and exaggerated limb movements. The cow often resists being driven and throws her head about as though expecting a blow. Spasmodic urination and frequent defaecation are characteristic. The appetite and milk yield are diminished and ruminal movements decrease. Muscle tremor and mild tetany of the hind legs and tail with an unsteady, straddling gait may be accompanied by retraction of the head and trismus. Sudden movement, noise, the application of restraint or insertion of a needle may precipitate a violent convulsion. Animals with this form of the disease may recover spontaneously within a few days or progress to a stage of recumbency with a similar but rather milder syndrome than in the acute form. Treatment is usually effective but there is a marked tendency to relapse.

Chronic lactation tetany. Many animals in affected herds have low serum-magnesium levels but do not show clinical signs. A few animals do evidence a rather vague syndrome including dullness, unthriftiness and indifferent appetite and may subsequently develop one of the more obvious syndromes. The chronic type may also occur in animals which recover from the subacute form of the disease.

Parturient paresis with hypomagnesaemia. This syndrome is described under parturient paresis (p. 668) and consists of paresis and circulatory collapse in an adult cow which has calved within the preceding 48 hours but in which dullness and flaccidity are replaced by hyperaesthesia and tetany.

Clinical Pathology

Diagnostic clinical pathology depends upon estimation of total calcium and magnesium levels in serum. The majority of healthy animals will have a serum-magnesium concentration of 1·7 to 3·0 mg. per 100 ml. (5). These levels in cattle are often reduced in seasonal subclinical hypomagnesaemia to between 1 and 2 mg. per cent but tetany is not usually evident until the level falls to below 1·2 mg. per cent. However, levels may fall as low as 0·4 mg. per cent without clinical illness. These discrepancies may be explainable in terms of variations between animals in the degree of ionization of the total magnesium. It is also possible that a transitory elevation of the level occurs after violent muscular exercise. Total serum-calcium levels are often reduced to 5 to 8 mg. per cent and this may have an important bearing on the development of clinical signs. Serum-inorganic-phosphate levels may or may not be low. Similar changes occur in lactation tetany in sheep. In wheat pasture poisoning of cattle there is hypocalcaemia, hypomagnesaemia and hyperkalaemia. The occurrence of low urine magnesium levels is good presumptive evidence of hypomagnesaemia and a field test is available (20).

Necropsy Findings

Extravasations of blood may be observed in subcutaneous tissues and under the pericardium, endocardium, pleura, peritoneum and intestinal mucosa. Agonal emphysema may also be present. A low magnesium content of heart muscle has attracted attention as providing evidence of hypomagnesaemia at necropsy examination (21). The procedure is time-consuming and expensive and is insufficiently accurate to justify its use (22).

Diagnosis

Inco-ordination, hyperaesthesia and tetany are the major clinical abnormalities which should arouse suspicion of hypomagnesaemic tetany especially if they occur in ruminants exposed to bad weather or grazing green cereal crops or lush grass-dominant pasture. Lactating animals are likely to be affected first. There are many other diseases which present a similar clinical picture. Acute lead poisoning is usually accompanied by blindness and mania, sometimes with an attack complex and there is usually a history of access to lead. Rabies may also resemble hypomagnesaemic tetany but is characterized by straining, ascending paralysis, anaesthesia and an absence of tetany. The nervous form of ketosis is not usually accompanied by convulsions or tetany and there is marked ketonuria. Poisoning caused by *Claviceps paspali* occurs only if there is access to the ergots and the syndrome is typically one of cerebellar ataxia.

In sheep it is almost impossible to differentiate between an uncomplicated hypocalcaemia and one which is complicated by hypomagnesaemia. The latter is to be expected in recently lambed ewes on lush spring pasture. Failing estimation of serum levels of magnesium and calcium the response to treatment may be the best indication of the disease state present.

Treatment

Most authors have recorded satisfactory results with solutions containing both calcium and magnesium salts or even calcium salts alone. The former is recommended for general use in all forms of lactation tetany and details are provided under the treatment of parturient paresis. However, solutions containing only magnesium salts are also used and the final choice must depend upon the results of biochemical tests and the response obtained. The efficiency of the various treatments appears to vary from area to area, and even within areas under different conditions of management and climate. The safest general recommendation is to use a combined calcium-magnesium preparation (e.g. 500 ml. of a solution containing 25 per cent calcium borogluconate and 5 per cent magnesium hypophosphite for cattle, 50 ml. for sheep) intravenously followed by a subcutaneous injection of a concentrated solution of a magnesium salt. When magnesium solutions are used 200 to 300 ml. of a 20 per cent solution of magnesium sulphate may be injected intravenously: this is followed by a rapid rise in serum-magnesium levels which return to pre-injection levels within 3 to 6 hours. A much slower rise and fall occurs after subcutaneous injection. For optimum results the subcutaneous injection of 4 oz. (200 ml. of a 50 per cent solution) of magnesium sulphate has been recommended. A rise in serum-magnesium of 0·5 mg. per cent occurs within a few minutes and subsequent levels do not go above 5·0 mg. per cent. In cases where serum-magnesium levels are low because of a seasonal hypomagnesaemia, the injection of magnesium salts is followed by a rise and then a return to the subnormal pre-injection levels.

The intravenous injection of magnesium salts is not without danger. There may be cardiac embarrassment or medullary depression may be severe enough to cause respiratory failure. If signs of respiratory distress or excessive slowing or increase in heart rate are noticed the injection should be stopped immediately and, if necessary, a calcium solution injected.

The substitution of magnesium lactate for magnesium sulphate has been recommended to provide a more prolonged elevation of serum-magnesium levels. A dilute solution (3·3 per cent) causes no tissue injury and can be administered intravenously or subcutaneously. Magnesium gluconate has also been used as a 15 per cent solution and good results were obtained with dose rates of 200 to 400 ml. High serum magnesium levels are obtained more slowly and are maintained longer than with magnesium sulphate (23). The feeding of magnesium-rich supplements, as described under *Control*, is recommended after parenteral treatment. Because of the tendency for acute cases to have convulsions during treatment, it is a common practice to give a large intramuscular dose of an ataractic drug before commencing specific treatment and to continue this until recovery is apparent.

Control

Feeding of magnesium supplements. The preventive measure which is now universally adopted is the feeding of magnesium salts to cows during the danger period. The feeding of magnesite (containing not less than 87 per cent magnesium oxide) prevents the seasonal fall in serum-magnesium levels and daily administration by drenching or in the feed of at least 60 g. of magnesium oxide per day is recommended to prevent the disease. This is not always completely effective and in some circumstances larger doses may be necessary. Daily feeding of 120 g. is safe and effective but 180 g. daily may cause scouring. The dose for sheep is 7 g. daily or 14 g. every second day (24). The protection afforded develops within several days of commencing administration and terminates abruptly after administration ceases. Difficulty may be experienced in getting the stock to eat the required amount of magnesite, especially when it is in the powder form. It is not unpalatable but the powdery consistency is unattractive. This can be countered by mixing it with molasses, in equal parts and allowing free access to the mixture. The problem with any sort of feed supplement that the cattle are not forced to eat to get subsistence is to ensure that animals take any of it and that all animals take enough because this disease is sufficiently dangerous that in many circumstances an unprotected animal is a dead one. In field circumstances the provision of magnesium in tasty mixtures for cattle has been disappointing and is not recommended (25). Magnesium acetate–molasses mixtures in ball feeders are satisfactory but are expensive (26). The more common practice is to mix the magnesite with molasses and dilute with water which is then sprayed on to the hay in the windrows when it is being made, injected into the bales before feeding or sprayed on to the hay at feeding. The preparation may also be used in a granular form, or in a cake or pellets or by mixing in damp feed.

The use of heavy 'bullets' of magnesium to prevent hypomagnesaemia has shown early promise in laboratory trials but in field trials the results have varied. The objective is to place a heavy 'bullet' of magnesium in the reticulum from which site it constantly liberates small amounts of magnesium, about 1 g. daily. This objective is achieved and the occurrence of the clinical disease is usually greatly reduced (27, 28) but serum magnesium levels are often little altered and it is felt that the animals are still very susceptible (29). In dangerous situations it is customary to administer up to 4 'bullets' at a time. As with all 'bullets' there is a proportion lost by regurgitation and by passage on through the gut. A special sheep-sized 'bullet' is used in ewes with similar results (30).

Top dressing of pasture with magnesium-rich fertilizers raises the level of magnesium in the pasture and decreases the susceptibility of cattle to hypomagnesaemia. For top dressing calcined magnesite ($\frac{1}{2}$ ton per acre) or magnesic limestone ($2\frac{1}{2}$ tons per acre) are satisfactory, the former causing the greater increase in pasture magnesium. The duration of the improved magnesium status is unknown, but the degree varies with the type of soil, being greatest on light sandy loams on which a dressing of $\frac{1}{4}$ ton of calcined magnesite per acre can provide protection for 3 years. On heavy soils protection for only one year is to be expected (32). To avoid unnecessary expense it may be possible to top dress one field with the magnesium fertilizer and keep this field in reserve for spring grazing.

The magnesium content of pastures can be raised much more quickly by spraying with a 2 per cent solution of magnesium sulphate at fortnightly intervals (7) or by application of very finely ground magnesium oxide to the pasture (28 lb. per acre or 30 kg. per hectare) before grazing commences (31). The technique is referred to as 'foliar dusting or spraying' and has the advantage over feed supplementation that the intake is standard. It is very effective in cattle in maintaining serum magnesium levels and preventing the occurrence of the clinical disease (33).

In some high risk situations it may be advisable to provide magnesium in several forms to ensure adequate intake.

Management of pasture fields. The economics of dairy farming make it necessary to produce maximum pasture growth, and the development of tetany prone pastures is unavoidable in many circumstances. It may be possible to reduce the danger of such pastures by encouraging the development of legumes, by restricting the amount of potash added especially in the early spring and by ensuring that ample salt is available during the danger period to counteract the high intake of potassium. The addition of magnesite to the fertilizer, as described above, is strongly recommended.

Whenever magnesium supplements are used in the diet of cattle, attention must be given to the phosphorus intake of the herd. It is strongly suspected that a high magnesium intake reduces the availability of phosphorus (34) and the possibility of provoking clinical hypophosphataemia seems to be a real one.

Provision of shelter. In areas where winter pasturing is practised the observation that serum-magnesium levels fall during the winter and in association with inclement weather suggests that cattle and sheep should be provided with shelter at such times. If complete housing is impractical it may be advisable to erect open access shelters in those fields that have no tree cover or protection from prevailing winds. Fields in which lactating cows are kept should receive special attention in this regard. Unfortunately the disease is most common on highly improved farms where most natural shelter has been removed and it is desired to keep the cows on the highly improved pasture to maintain milk production or fatten calves rapidly.

Time of calving. In areas where the incidence of the disease is high it may be advisable to avoid having the cows calve during the cold winter months when seasonal hypomagnesaemia is most likely to develop. Unfortunately it is often important to have cows calve in late winter to take advantage of the flush of spring growth when the cows are at the peak of their lactation.

Feeding on hay and unimproved pasture. Because of the probable importance of lush, improved, grass pasture in producing the disease, the provision of some grain, hay or rough grazing may reduce the incidence. It is most important that the periods of fasting, such as occur when cattle or sheep are yarded, or moved or during bad weather, should be avoided especially in lactating animals and when seasonal hypomagnesaemia is likely to be present.

REVIEW LITERATURE

Burns, K. M. & Allcroft, R. (1967). *Brit. vet. J.*, *123*, 340, 383.

REFERENCES

(1) Hemingway, R. G. & Ritchie, N. S. (1965). *Proc. Nutr. Soc.*, *24*, 54.

(2) Seekles, L. (1964). *Proc. 3rd int. Mtg Dis. Cattle, Copenhagen*, *1*, 120.

(3) Herd, R. P. (1966). *Aust. vet. J.*, *42*, 269.

(4) Hjerpe, C. A. & Brownell, J. R. (1966). *Vet. Rec.*, *79*, 396.

(5) Wilson, A. A. (1964). *Vet. Rec.*, *76*, 1382.

(6) Rook, J. A. F. et al. (1964). *J. agric. Sci.*, *62*, 273.

(7) Bould, C. (1964). *Vet. Rec.*, *76*, 1377.

(8) Moodie, E. W. (1965). *Brit. vet. J.*, *121*, 338.

(9) Kemp, A. et al. (1960). *Brit. vet. Ass. Conf. Hypomagnesaemia*, *23*, 13.

(10) Ashton, W. M. & Sinclair, K. B. (1965). *J. Brit. Grassld Soc.*, *20*, 118.

(11) Bohman, V. R. et al. (1969). *J. Anim. Sci.*, *29*, 99.

(12) Kennedy, G. S. (1968). *Aust. J. Biol. Sci.*, *21*, 529.

(13) Wright, D. E. & Wolff, J. E. (1969). *N.Z. J. agric. Res.*, *12*, 287.

(14) Barrentine, B. F. (1966). *J. Anim. Sci.*, *25*, 249.

(15) Suttle, N. F. & Field, A. C. (1969). *Brit. J. Nutr.*, *23*, 81.

(16) Dishington, I. W. & Tollersrud, S. (1967). *Acta vet. scand.*, *8*, 14.

(17) Halse, K. (1970). *Acta vet. scand.*, *11*, 394.

(18) Schuster, N. H. et al. (1969). *Aust. vet. J.*, *45*, 508.

(19) Todd, J. R. & Horvath, D. J. (1970). *Brit. vet. J.*, *126*, 333.

(20) Mershon, M. M. (1964). *Proc. 101st ann. gen. Mtg Amer. vet. med. Ass.*, Chicago, 47.

(21) Kershaw, G. F. & Wilson, A. A. (1969). *Vet. Rec.*, *84*, 525.

(22) Field, A. C. (1969). *Vet. Rec.*, *23*, 591.

(23) Fischer, W. (1968). *Dtsch. tierärztl. Wschr.*, *75*, 8.

(24) Herd, R. P. (1966). *Aust. vet. J.*, *42*, 160, 369.

(25) Horvath, D. J. et al. (1967). *J. Anim. Sci.*, *26*, 875.

(26) Ross, E. J. & Gibson, W. W. C. (1969). *Vet. Rec.*, *84*, 520.

(27) Davey, L. A. & Gilbert, G. A. (1969). *Vet. Rec.*, *85*, 194.

(28) Foot, A. S. et al. (1969). *Vet. Rec.*, *84*, 467.

(29) Kemp, A. & Todd, J. R. (1970). *Vet. Rec.*, *86*, 463.

(30) Smyth, P. J. & Egan, D. A. (1971). *Irish vet. J.*, *25*, 4.

(31) Todd, J. R. & Morrison, N. E. (1964). *J. Brit. Grassld Soc.*, *19*, 179.

(32) Todd, J. R. (1965). *Brit. vet. J.*, *121*, 371.

(33) Rogers, P. A. M. & Poole, D. B. R. (1971). *Irish vet. J.*, *25*, 197.

(34) Mudd, A. (1970). *J. agric. Sci. (Cambridge)*, *74*, 11.

(35) Newton, G. L. et al. (1972). *J. Anim. Sci.*, *35*, 440.

Hypomagnesaemic Tetany of Calves

(*Whole-Milk Tetany*)

Hypomagnesaemic tetany of calves is a disease with a close clinical similarity to lactation tetany.

Incidence

The disease is common in some areas, particularly where animals are housed during the winter and are inadequately fed. Cases may occur sporadically or a number of deaths may occur on the one farm within a short period of time.

Aetiology

Hypomagnesaemia is a common finding and is accompanied in many cases by hypocalcaemia. A condition closely resembling the field syndrome has been produced experimentally by feeding an artificial diet with a very low content of magnesium and the evidence points to the disease being caused by a dietary deficiency of magnesium (1) exacerbated by a high intake of calcium which causes depletion of magnesium stores and lower serum and bone levels of magnesium (2). Milk, in spite of its low magnesium content, is an adequate source of the element for very young calves because their absorptive capacity is good. However, the efficiency of magnesium absorption decreases markedly up to about 3 months of age when maximum susceptibility to the disease occurs (3). The efficiency of absorption is also decreased by a reduction in transit time in the intestine and this may be related to the occurrence of the disease in scouring calves. A significant loss of magnesium in the faeces also occurs in calves allowed to chew fibrous material such as bedding, the chewing stimulating profuse salivation and creating greater loss of endogenous magnesium. Peat and wood shavings are bedding materials known to have this effect (4).

Hypomagnesaemic tetany in calves is often complicated in field cases by the coexistence of other diseases, especially enzootic muscular dystrophy. The situation is further confused by the apparent occurrence of hypocalcaemic tetany in calves kept indoors and fed a heavy grain diet without added calcium or vitamin D.

Occurrence

Hypomagnesaemic tetany occurs in calves 2 to 4 months of age or older which are fed solely on a diet of whole milk and calves receiving the greatest quantity of milk and growing most rapidly are more likely to be affected because of their greater need for magnesium for incorporation into developing soft tissues. It is most likely to occur in calves being fattened for veal. Cases have also been reported in calves fed milk replacer diets or milk, concentrates and hay, and in calves running at pasture with their dams (5). Those cases which occur on milk replacer appear to be related to chronic scours and low magnesium content of the replacer.

Pathogenesis

On affected farms calves are born with normal serum-magnesium levels of 2 to 2·5 mg. per cent but the levels fall gradually in the succeeding 2 to 3 months, often to below 0·8 mg. per cent. Tetany does not occur until the serum-magnesium falls below this point and is most severe at levels below 0·6 mg. per cent, although calves may have levels even lower than this and show few clinical signs. It seems probable that depression of the serum-calcium level precipitates tetany in animals rendered tetany prone by low serum-magnesium levels. It is also apparent that tetanic convulsions can occur in hypocalcaemic calves in the absence of hypomagnesaemia (6). The disease is not related in any way to enzootic muscular dystrophy although the diseases may occur concurrently. The depletion of body stores of magnesium in the bones by a continued nutritional deficiency of magnesium places calves in a vulnerable position if further deprivation occurs—in such circumstances the serum-magnesium in the bones, and the estimation of the Ca:Mg ratio in bones can be used in the diagnosis of the disease.

Clinical Findings

The first sign in the experimental disease is constant movement of the ears. The temperature is normal and the pulse rate accelerated. Hyperaesthesia to touch, and grossly exaggerated tendon reflexes with clonus are present. Shaking of the head, opisthotonus, ataxia without circling, and a droopy, backward carriage of the ears are constant. There is difficulty in drinking due to inability to get to the bucket. The calves are apprehensive, show agitation and retraction of the eyelids when approached, and are hypersensitive to all external stimuli but show no tetany. Later, fine muscle tremors appear followed by kicking at the belly, frothing at the mouth and spasticity of the limbs. Convulsions follow, beginning with stamping of the feet, head retraction, champing of the jaws and falling. During the convulsions the jaws are clenched, respiratory movements cease and there are tonic and clonic movements of the limbs, and involuntary passage of urine and faeces, and cycles of protrusion and retraction of the eyeballs. The pulse rate rises to 200 to 250 per minute and the convulsions disappear terminally. The pulse becomes impalpable and cyanosis appears before death. In field cases the signs are almost identical but are rarely observed until the terminal tetanic stage. Older calves usually die within 20 to 30 minutes of the onset of convulsions but young calves may recover temporarily only to succumb to subsequent attacks. Cases which occur in young calves with scours, usually at about 2 weeks of age, show convulsions as the earliest sign. The convulsion is usually continuous and the calves die in a half to one hour.

Clinical Pathology

Serum-magnesium levels below 0·8 mg. per cent indicate severe hypomagnesaemia and clinical signs occur with levels of 0·3 to 0·7 mg. per cent. Normal values are 2·2 to 2·7 mg. per cent (3). Serum-calcium levels tend to fall when serum-magnesium levels become very low and are below normal in most clinical cases. The estimation of the magnesium in bone (particularly ribs and vertebrae) is a reliable confirmatory test at necropsy. Values below a ratio of 70:1 for Ca:Mg may be regarded as normal and above 90:1 are indicative of severe magnesium depletion. Absolute bone-calcium values are not decreased and are often slightly elevated. An incidental change is the marked increase in serum creatinine phosphokinase levels observed in calves after an acute attack of hypomagnesaemic tetany. SGOT levels are marginally elevated (7).

Necropsy Findings

There is a marked difference between the necropsy lesions of some natural and the experimental cases. In some field cases there is calcification of the spleen and diaphragm, and calcified plaques are present in the aorta and endocardium, together with hyaline degeneration of musculature. In other cases necropsy lesions similar to those in enzootic muscular dystrophy occur. In experimentally produced cases these lesions are not evident but there is extensive congestion in all organs, and haemorrhages in unsupported organs, including the gall-bladder, ventricular epicardium, pericardial fat, aorta, mesentery and intestinal wall. The lesions are obviously terminal and are associated with a terminal venous necrosis. Some field cases present a picture identical with this and doubtless some factor other than hypomagnesaemia is responsible for the calcification of tissues described above.

Diagnosis

Clonic convulsions in calves may occur as a result of acute lead poisoning, tetanus, strychnine poisoning, polioencephalomalacia, enterotoxaemia caused by Clostridium perfringens type D and avitaminosis A. It may be virtually impossible to distinguish between these diseases clinically and a careful examination of the history with particular reference to feeding, water supply, and possible access to poisons may be the only basis on which a tentative diagnosis can be made. Tetanus has a longer course and is usually accompanied by bloat and prolapse of the third eyelid. Tetany is persistent between convulsions which do not occur until the late stages of the disease. Poisoning by organic arsenical or mercurial compounds is less common but the syndrome is essentially the same as that of hypomagnesaemic tetany. Viral encephalitides including rabies and sporadic bovine encephalomyelitis are not restricted to calves and have other signs of diagnostic value, and the signs do not fluctuate as much as in hypomagnesaemic tetany; in rabies there is anaesthesia and ascending paralysis; and in SBE a high fever and serositis. Bacterial meningitis and encephalitis are usually accompanied by fever.

Treatment

Response to magnesium injections (100 ml. of a 10 per cent solution of magnesium sulphate) is only transitory because of the severe depletion of bone reserves of magnesium. This dose provides only a single day's requirements. Follow-up supplementation of the diet with magnesium oxide or carbonate as described below is advisable. Chloral narcosis or tranquillization with an ataractic drug may be essential to avoid death due to respiratory paralysis.

Control

The provision of hay in the diet helps to prevent the disease. Supplementary feeding of magnesium, if begun during the first 10 days of life, will prevent excessive falls of serum-magnesium but if begun after the calf is 7 weeks old may not prevent further depression of the levels. Supplementation should continue until at least 10 weeks of age. Daily feeding of the magnesium compound is necessary and fairly accurate dosing is necessary to avoid scouring or inefficient protection. Detailed dose schedules are available but for calves of average growth rate appropriate dose rates are 1 g. daily for calves to 5 weeks, 2 g. for calves 5 to 10 weeks and 3 g. for 10 to 15 week calves of magnesium oxide or twice this dose of carbonate (3). Supplementation of the diet with magnesium restores serum-calcium levels to normal as well as correcting the hypomagnesaemia, but hypomagnesaemia occurs when administration is stopped (5). Magnesium alloy bullets, two of the sheep size per calf, have shown high efficiency in preventing the clinical disease and also the hypomagnesaemia which precedes it (8). Calves kept indoors and fed largely on milk should get adequate mineral supplement and vitamin D (70,000 I.U. vitamin D3 per day). Magnesium utilization will not be affected but calcium absorption, which is often sufficiently reduced to cause a concurrent hypocalcaemia, will be improved.

REFERENCES

(1) Larvor, P. et al. (1964). Ann. Biol. anim. Biochem. Biophys., 4, 345 & 371.
(2) Ivins, L. N. & Allcroft, R. (1969). Brit. vet. J., 125, 548.
(3) Smith, R. H. (1964). Proc. 3rd int. Mtg Dis. Cattle, Copenhagen, 1, 143.
(4) Ivins, L. N. & Allcroft, R. (1970). Brit. vet. J., 126, 505.
(5) Allcroft, R. (1960). Brit. vet. Ass. Conf. on Hypomagnesaemia, 102–19.
(6) Holtenius, P. et al. (1970). Nord. Vet.-Med., 22, 463.
(7) Todd, J. R. et al. (1969). Vet. Rec., 84, 176.
(8) Hemingway, R. G. & Ritchie, N. S. (1969). Vet. Rec., 84, 465.

Ketosis of Ruminants

(Acetonaemia of Cattle, Pregnancy Toxaemia of Sheep)

Ketosis in ruminants is a disease caused by impaired metabolism of carbohydrate and volatile fatty acids. Biochemically it is characterized by ketonaemia, ketonuria, hypoglycaemia and low levels of hepatic glycogen. Clinically, the diseases in cattle (acetonaemia) and in ewes (pregnancy toxaemia) are rather different entities and occur in different parts of the pregnancy–lactation cycle, but the biochemical disturbance is essentially the same and they occur under similar conditions of management.

Incidence

Ketosis of dairy cattle is prevalent in most countries where intensive farming is practised. It occurs mainly in animals housed during the winter months although it is seen occasionally in animals at pasture. The wastage due to the disease is difficult to assess accurately; its high incidence and known effects suggest that it is one of the major causes of loss to the dairy farmer. In rare instances the disease appears to be irreversible and the affected animal dies but the bulk of the economic loss is due to the loss of production while the disease is present and failure to return to full production after recovery. Subclinical ketosis is also common and although it has received little attention it may rank with the clinical disease in its economic effects.

Ketosis of pregnant ewes is highly fatal, and in individual flocks can reach a level of incidence sufficient to be classed as an outbreak. The disease in cattle may also occur in outbreak form with virtually every cow being affected but this is unusual and most herds suffer only sporadic cases. Ketosis in recently farrowed sows is rare.

Aetiology

Bovine ketosis. The major biochemical manifestation of ketosis in cattle is hypoglycaemia, and treatment of affected cattle which returns the blood-glucose level to normal is followed by at least a transient recovery. There are as many theories on the cause of ketosis as there are potential causes of hypoglycaemia and without doubt the disease must be considered as one in which there are many signi-

Schematic Representation of Carbohydrate Metabolism in Ruminants (1)

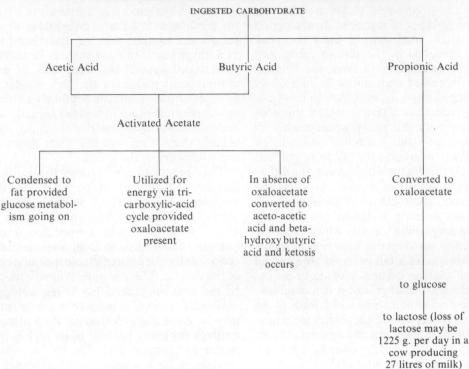

INGESTED CARBOHYDRATE

Acetic Acid   Butyric Acid   Propionic Acid

Activated Acetate

| Condensed to fat provided glucose metabolism going on | Utilized for energy via tri-carboxylic-acid cycle provided oxaloacetate present | In absence of oxaloacetate converted to aceto-acetic acid and beta-hydroxy butyric acid and ketosis occurs | Converted to oxaloacetate |

to glucose

to lactose (loss of lactose may be 1225 g. per day in a cow producing 27 litres of milk)

ficant predisposing causes. This hypothesis is supported by the variety of circumstances in which the disease can occur. As a general statement it is safe to say that clinical ketosis occurs in ruminants at times when they are subjected to heavier demands on their resources of glucose and glycogen than can be met by their digestive and metabolic activity. Most argument on the causation of the disease centres around the exact manner in which this failure to provide available glucose arises. This failure could be purely relative if the requirement is greater than the maximum carbohydrate intake could physically provide. It would be absolute if an adequate supply of carbohydrate is not provided by the ration. Again it could be a defect of digestion or metabolism in converting what is an adequate dietary supply of carbohydrate into available glucose. Bovine, and to a less extent ovine, ketosis occur in the field when the failure of supply of available glucose to tissues results from any of the above causes. A direct result of this deficiency is an increase in gluconeogenesis in the liver with a parallel rise in ketone body formation. If the latter rise is beyond the limit of physiological needs clinical ketosis ensues (1).

In more detail, the salient points of the aetiology of ketosis can be set out as follows. All carbo-

hydrate ingested is converted in the rumen to acetic and butyric acids which are potentially ketogenic, and to propionic acid which is glycogenic. These two groups of acids are produced under normal conditions in the ratio of about 4 to 1. The production of propionic acid and its conversion to glucose in the liver must continue at a normal level if glucose supplies to tissues are to be maintained. If this system is inefficient the alternative pathway of providing glucose by synthesis from amino-acids and glycerol increases in volume. The stimulation of this type of energy producing reaction results in a much increased demand for oxalo-acetate which is used preferentially for this purpose. As a result the utilization of ketone bodies by tissues, which also requires oxaloacetate, is impeded. The ketone bodies then accumulate to the point where ketosis occurs (see table above).

Ruminants are in a particularly vulnerable position compared to other species with regard to their carbohydrate metabolism because, although very little carbohydrate is absorbed as such, a direct supply of glucose is essential for tissue metabolism, particularly the formation of lactose, and in addition the utilization of volatile fatty acids for energy purposes is also dependent upon a supply of available glucose. This vulnerability is further exacerbated, particularly in the cow, by the tremendous rate of turnover of glucose and the relatively poor reserves of glycogen. In the period from immediately after calving until the peak of lactation is reached in the case of cattle, and the last third of pregnancy in ewes, the demand for glucose is increased and cannot be completely restrained. Even though the milk flow in cows can be reduced by reduction of energy intake, this does not follow automatically nor proportionately in early lactation because hormonal stimuli for mammary activity overcome the effects of reduced food intake. It is this factor which makes the difference between the ketosis of simple starvation and the more severe spontaneous ketosis of high-producing cows in early lactation (2). In ovine ketosis it is the developing foetuses which cause the unremitting drain on available maternal nutrients although in this species a fall in blood glucose and an elevation of plasma ketones also occur on exposure to inclement weather and it is a combination of undernutrition and stress which leads to the development of most cases of pregnancy toxaemia. A combination of cold stress and undernutrition, each alone readily tolerated by ewes in late pregnancy, may together prove fatal (3).

Most of the investigational work of recent years has been directed towards elucidating the pathogenesis of ketosis in cows that are fed heavily on rations which at first glance appear to contain adequate carbohydrate. However, such a diet need be deficient only in precursors of propionic acid to be ketogenic.

In the search for causative factors in high-producing animals a number of endocrinal and metabolic mechanisms have been investigated. The claim that dysfunction of the adrenal gland is the primary cause of bovine ketosis has not been substantiated. The stress of parturition and lactation in cattle, and of late pregnancy in ewes, must lead to increased adrenocortical activity, and this may be further stimulated by the additional stress of malnutrition. In such circumstances some diminution of the hormonal reserves of the gland may follow, leading to a state of relative adrenocortical insufficiency which exacerbates the metabolic defect inaugurated by the stress factors mentioned. That there is only a relative insufficiency is evidenced by the ability of affected animals to respond to adrenocorticotrophins. It is probable therefore that the endocrinal changes observed are secondary only.

A relative hypothyroidism has also been suggested as a cause on the basis of low protein-bound iodine levels in the serum of affected cows, because iodine and thyroprotein are preventative and curative in some instances, and because of the tendency for the disease to occur in ewes and cows which get insufficient exercise. On the other hand injections of L-thyroxine into cows early in lactation has led to induced ketosis (4). That lack of exercise is entirely responsible for the high incidence of the disease in housed animals is unlikely although clinical cases rarely occur in well fed animals at pasture, and plasma-ketone levels of lactating dairy cows usually show a marked fall when they are turned out to pasture in the spring.

The composition of rations fed to dairy cattle has been examined in an effort to determine whether it has any effect on their glucose-ketone status. Ensilage and hay are the common feeds likely to vary widely in composition from year to year and from farm to farm and therefore be responsible for the unpredictable sporadic occurrence of the disease. There is some evidence that this may be the case. In general hay is less ketogenic than ensilage, and ensilage made from succulent material may be more highly ketogenic than other types of ensilage probably because of its higher content of preformed butyric acid. The factors which make ensilage more ketogenic than hay, other than the higher content of butyric acid in some samples, have not been determined.

The composition and metabolic activities of the ruminal flora are likely to change under differing dietary conditions and variations in diet may change the end products of digestion and their relative concentrations. This may be the basis for differences in ketogenicity between feeds. For example, grass and corn ensilage may have this effect apart from their butyric acid content. High protein diets lead to greater butyric acid production in the rumen. They also reduce the digestibility of rations and probably contribute to ketosis by providing additional ketone precursors in the form of ketogenic amino acids (5). Whatever the mechanism high protein diets have been shown to increase susceptibility to ketosis induced by L-thyroxine injections. Starvation leads to a relative lowering of the propionic acid concentration in the rumen and this probably adds to the effects of starvation on internal metabolism, particularly the excessive utilization of fat, in producing ketosis. From quantitative and qualitative estimations on the ketone bodies present in ruminal liquor and body fluids, it appears that abnormal ruminal conditions may play an important part in the production of clinical ketosis.

From time to time factors other than those mentioned above have come under consideration.

Hepatic insufficiency has been shown to occur in bovine and ovine ketosis but whether it occurs in all cases and whether it is primary or a result of ketosis is unknown. As one of the reactions to hypoglycaemia is mobilization of fat reserves and deposition of fat in the liver, some degree of hepatic insufficiency is to be expected as a secondary development of the disease.

Ovine ketosis. Although hypoglycaemia and hyperketonaemia are the primary metabolic disturbances in ovine ketosis as they are in the bovine disease, and although the precipitating causes are similarly a dietary deficiency of nett energy exacerbated by the increased demand for energy in the latter part of pregnancy, there are some biochemical differences between the two diseases, e.g. an elevation of plasma cortisol levels in pregnancy toxaemia, and in the terminal stages their pathogenesis appears to be quite dissimilar. The most important aetiological factor in pregnancy toxaemia is a decline in the plane of nutrition during the last 2 months of pregnancy, particularly in ewes that are carrying twins and which have been well fed beforehand (6). There is a great deal of variation between sheep in the ease with which the disease can be produced experimentally, and the incidence of the naturally occurring disease in conditions which appear to be conducive to its development. It seems likely that the difference between sheep depends upon the metabolic efficiency of the liver. Ewes which, because of impaired hepatic function, are predisposed to the disease may react to the continued, preferential demands for glucose by well grown twin foetuses by being unable to effectively carry on gluconeogenesis, leading to hypoglycaemia and the accumulation of ketone bodies and cortisol. Exposure to inclement weather or a heavy worm infestation, e.g. with *Haemonchus contortus* (7), would add a similar drain on glucose metabolism and increase the chances of development of the disease.

The elevation of plasma cortisol levels which is commonly encountered in ewes with pregnancy toxaemia has attracted attention because of its possible indication of adrenocortical involvement in causing the disease. It seems more likely that the observed increase is in response to environmental and nutritional stresses (8), and possibly to failure by the liver to metabolize the cortisol.

Occurrence

Cattle. Bovine ketosis occurs under the following conditions:

(*a*) In high-producing, heavily fed dairy cows housed in barns.

(*b*) In cattle at pasture, and less frequently when housed and fed on rations of inadequate caloric content.

(*c*) Under conditions of specific nutritional deficiency.

(*d*) As a complication of another primary disease.

Ketosis of heavily fed, high-producing cows— so-called 'estate acetonaemia'— is the most important occurrence of the disease. Genetic susceptibility may be a factor but adequate proof on this point is lacking. The tendency for the disease to recur in individual animals is probably a reflection of variation between cows in digestive capacity or metabolic efficiency but these characters may or may not be inherited. It is more probable that the rations fed cause abnormal internal metabolism or ruminal function and lead to the development of ketosis in these circumstances. Other factors which are known to influence the development of the disease are excessive feeding of ensilage, particularly when it has a high content of butyric acid, inadequate exercise, over fatness at calving time and inadequate energy intake during early lactation.

Specific dietary deficiencies of cobalt and possibly phosphorus may also lead to a high incidence of ketosis. This may be due in part to a reduction in the intake of TDN, but in cobalt deficiency the essential defect is a failure to metabolize propionic acid (9). It may be necessary to re-evaluate the role of cobalt in view of the observation that blood and liver levels of vitamin B_{12} are significantly reduced during the early stages of lactation in apparently normal cows and may sometimes fall below the critical level necessary for adequate gluconeogenesis from propionic acid (10).

A secondary ketosis may also develop, due usually to a reduction in appetite as a result of abomasal displacement, traumatic reticulitis, metritis, mastitis or other diseases common to the postparturient period. A high incidence of ketosis has also been observed in herds affected with fluorosis. The proportion of cases of acetonaemia which are secondary, and their diagnosis as such, are both matters of great interest which are generally neglected in veterinary literature. In one sample of 120 cases 42 per cent of the affected animals had an accompanying disease (11).

Regardless of the specific aetiology bovine ketosis occurs most commonly during the first month of lactation, less commonly in the second month, and only occasionally in late pregnancy. Cows of any age may be affected and the disease is not uncommon in heifers calving for the first time.

Sheep. Ovine ketosis occurs only in ewes in late pregnancy, usually during the last month in ewes carrying more than one lamb, although ewes bearing a single, large lamb may be affected. It is primarily a disease of intensive farming systems and is relatively rare in extensive grazing units. Most commonly the precipitating cause is a prolonged and gradual fall in the plane of nutrition followed by sudden, short periods of starvation of up to 48 hours caused by management changes. In ewes on a good plane of nutrition such changes lead more commonly to the development of hypocalcaemia. The level of nutrition at which the disease occurs may appear to be good but in such instances the plane of nutrition will usually be found to have fallen recently. This may be an explanation for the common occurrence of the disease in over fat ewes. In some outbreaks the ewes have been moved on to better pasture during late pregnancy to prevent the occurrence of ketosis but it occurs because the ewes are unaccustomed to the type of feed and do not eat well, or because they are more exposed to bad weather and seek shelter rather than graze. Cold, inclement weather and an absence of shelter also appear to markedly increase the incidence (6). Another common occurrence is when ewes are bred too early and the pasture is not sufficiently advanced to provide a rising plane of nutrition in late pregnancy. The disease occurs in goats during late pregnancy and is identical with ovine ketosis.

Pathogenesis

The principal metabolic disturbances observed, hypoglycaemia with a low level of hepatic glycogen, and ketonaemia may both exert an effect on the clinical syndrome. In many cases the severity of the clinical syndrome is proportional to the degree of hypoglycaemia and this, together with the rapid response to parenterally-administered glucose, suggests hypoglycaemia as the predominant factor. This hypothesis is supported by the development of prolonged hypoglycaemia and a similar clinical syndrome to that of ketosis, after the experimental, intravenous or subcutaneous injection of insulin (2 units per kg. body weight). Moreover in the experimentally induced disease in ewes, pregnancy toxaemia, the onset of clinical signs was always preceded by hypoglycaemia and hyperketonaemia although the onset of signs was not related to minimum glucose or maximum ketone levels (30).

The evidence that the irreversible stage of ovine ketosis is a hypoglycaemic encephalopathy is further support for hypoglycaemia as the important factor, although it has been suggested alternatively that the effects of the hypoglycaemia are added to by inhibition of glucose utilization and a resulting depression of cerebral metabolism. This may provide the reason for the irreversible cerebral lesion. In affected ewes there is an abnormally high level of cortisol in plasma—an expected reaction to continued environmental stress and hypoglycaemia, especially if hepatic metabolism of cortisol is reduced. Renal dysfunction is also apparent in the terminal stages of ovine ketosis, and may also contribute to the development of clinical signs and the fatal outcome. Azotaemia and proteinuria should be especially looked for in ewes showing no neurological signs. At histopathological examination the lesions are similar to human pre-eclampsia (12). Those ewes which are carrying only one lamb and have been well fed prior to a short period of undernutrition may develop a subacute syndrome both clinically and biochemically.

However, in most field cases the severity of the clinical syndrome is also roughly proportional to the degree of ketonaemia. This is an understandable relationship as ketone bodies are produced in larger quantities as the deficiency of glucose increases. However, the ketone bodies may exert an additional influence on the signs observed. Aceto-acetic acid is known to be toxic and probably contributes to the terminal coma in diabetes mellitus in man. The nervous signs which occur in some cases of bovine ketosis are thought to be caused by the production of isopropyl alcohol, a breakdown product of acetoacetic acid in the rumen, although the requirement of nervous tissue for glucose to maintain normal function may also be a factor in these cases.

Spontaneous ketosis in cattle is usually readily reversible by treatment; incomplete or temporary response is usually due to the existence of a primary disease with ketosis present only as a secondary development, although fatty degeneration of the liver in protracted cases may prolong the recovery period. Changes in ruminal flora after a long period of anorexia may also cause continued impairment of digestion.

Clinical Findings

In many herds and flocks in which clinical cases occur, biochemical examination of the urine and blood of clinically normal animals may show degrees of hypoglycaemia and ketonaemia suggestive of early ketosis. It is probable that there is some reduction in milk yield of cattle in this subclinical stage.

Bovine ketosis. Two major forms of the disease are described, the wasting and the nervous forms, but these are the two extremes of a range of syndromes in which wasting and nervous signs are present in varying degrees of prominence.

The purely wasting type is the commoner of the two and is manifested by a well-known syndrome which has recently been assessed in one of the very few statistical appraisals of symptomatology in veterinary literature (11). The syndrome is based primarily on the gradual but moderate decrease in appetite and milk yield over 2 to 4 days. On the statistical assessment these were present in 85 per cent and 87 per cent respectively of the cases seen. The pattern of appetite loss is often unusual in that the cow first refuses to eat grain, then ensilage but may continue to eat hay. The appetite may also be depraved. Body weight is lost rapidly, usually at a greater rate than one would expect from the decrease in appetite. Farmers usually describe affected cows as having a 'woody' appearance due to the apparent wasting and loss of cutaneous elasticity due presumably to disappearance of subcutaneous fat. The faeces are firm and dry but serious constipation does not occur. The cow is moderately depressed and the hang-dog appearance and disinclination to move and to eat may suggest the presence of mild abdominal pain.

The temperature and the pulse and respiratory rates are normal and although the ruminal movements may be decreased in amplitude and number they are within the normal range unless the course is of long duration when they may virtually disappear. A characteristic odour of ketones is detectable on the breath and often in the milk. Very few affected animals die but without treatment the milk yield falls and although spontaneous recovery usually occurs over about a month, as equilibrium between the drain of lactation and food intake is established, the milk yield is never fully regained. In the wasting form nervous signs may occur in a few cases but rarely comprise more than transient bouts of staggering and partial blindness.

In typical cases of the nervous form the signs are usually bizarre and begin quite suddenly. The syndrome is suggestive of delirium rather than of frenzy and the characteristic signs include walking in circles, straddling or crossing of the legs, head-pushing or leaning into the stanchion, apparent blindness, aimless movements and wandering, vigorous licking of the skin and inanimate objects, depraved appetite and chewing movements with salivation. Hyperaesthesia may be evident, the animal bellowing on being pinched or stroked. Moderate tremor and tetany may be present and the gait is usually staggery. The nervous signs usually occur in short episodes which last for 1 or 2 hours and may recur at intervals of about 8 to 12 hours. Affected cows may injure themselves during the nervous episodes.

Ovine ketosis. In ewes the syndrome is similar to that of the nervous form of ketosis in cows. The earliest sign is separation from the flock and apparent blindness which is manifested by an alert bearing but a disinclination to move. The ewe will stand still when approached by men or dogs and will turn and face them but make no attempt to escape. If it is forced to move it blunders into objects and when an obstacle is encountered, presses against it with the head. Many stand in water troughs all day and lap the water. Constipation is usual, the faeces are dry and scanty and there is grinding of the teeth. In later stages marked drowsiness develops and episodes of more severe nervous signs occur but they may be infrequent and are easily missed. In these episodes tremors of the muscles of the head cause twitching of the lips, champing of the jaws and salivation, and these are accompanied by a cog-wheel type of clonic contraction of the cervical muscles causing dorsiflexion or lateral deviation of the head, followed by circling. The muscle tremor usually spreads to involve the whole body, the sheep goes down and has a tonic-clonic convulsion. The ewe lies quietly after each convulsion and rises normally afterwards but is still blind. In the periods between convulsions there is marked drowsiness which may be accompanied by head-pressing, the assumption of abnormal postures including unusual positions of the limbs and elevation of the chin—the 'star-gazing' posture —and inco-ordination and falling when attempting to walk. A smell of ketones may be detectable on the breath.

Affected ewes usually become recumbent in 3 to 4 days and remain in a state of profound depression or coma for a further 3 to 4 days. Foetal death occurs commonly and is followed by transient recovery of the ewe, but the toxaemia caused by the decomposing foetus soon causes a relapse. Affected ewes commonly have difficulty in lambing. Recovery may ensue if the ewe lambs or the lambs are removed by Caesarian section in the early stages of the disease. In an affected flock the disease usually takes the form of a prolonged outbreak, a few ewes becoming affected each day over a period of several weeks.

Clinical Pathology

Hypoglycaemia, ketonaemia and ketonuria are characteristic of the disease and there is an increase in plasma-free fatty acids in some cases (13) due probably to accelerated gluconeogenesis from tissues. Blood-glucose levels are reduced from the normal of 50 mg. per cent to 20 to 40 mg. per cent in cattle and sheep. In cattle, ketosis secondary to other diseases is usually accompanied by blood-sugar levels above 40 mg. per cent and often above normal. Blood-ketone levels in bovine ketosis are elevated from a normal of up to 10 mg. per cent to 10 to 100 mg. per cent. The levels are high also in secondary ketosis but are rarely above 50 mg. per cent. Quantitative estimation of urinary ketones may be unsatisfactory because of the wide variations that occur depending upon the concentration of the urine. In clinically normal cattle urinary ketones may be as high as 70 mg. per cent although usually they are lower than 10 mg. per cent. Levels of 80 to 1300 mg. per cent indicate the presence of ketosis which may be primary or secondary. Ketone levels in milk are rather less variable, ranging from a normal of 3 up to an average level of 40 mg. per cent in cows with ketosis. Liver-glycogen levels are low and the glucose tolerance curve is normal. Volatile fatty acid levels in blood and rumen are much higher in ketotic than in normal cows and the ruminal levels of butyric acid are markedly increased relative to acetic and propionic acids (27). However, the severity and rate of onset of clinical signs are more closely related to blood sugar levels than to plasma acetone-plus-aceto-acetate or free fatty acid levels (11).

There is a small but significant fall in serum-calcium levels (down to about 9 mg. per cent) due probably to increased loss of base in the urine to compensate for the acidosis. Changes in the leuco-cyte count include eosinophilia, lymphocytosis and neutropenia. The neutrophil count may be as low as 10 per cent, the lymphocytes may be as high as 60 to 80 per cent and the eosinophils 15 to 40 per cent. Severe cases show an increase in serum glutamic-oxaloacetic transaminase but the reason for this increase in serum enzyme activity is unexplained.

Field tests to detect ketosis are in general use and may be carried out on urine or milk. They are subject to several minor sources of error. The concentration of ketone bodies in these fluids will depend not only on the ketone level of the bood but also on the amount of urine excreted or on the milk yield. Milk is less variable and suitable laboratory procedures are available but field reagents in general use are only sufficiently sensitive to detect severe cases. The other disadvantage of these tests is that they measure only the aceto-acetic acid content of the urine, beta-hydroxybutyric acid giving no reaction and acetone very little. This is not of major importance as the ketone bodies are usually present in approximately the same proportions.

Tests on urine are based on Rothera's reaction and many commercial reagents are now available. A reagent should be used in conjunction with a colour chart to give an approximate estimate of the amount of ketones present in the specimen. In most cases the test must be read at a specified time, usually 30 seconds, for accurate appraisal. There is some difference of opinion as to whether primary and secondary ketosis can be differentiated on the basis of the degree of colour change in the reagent, but primary cases always give a strong reaction whereas a moderate reaction is more common in secondary cases. Rough quantitative estimations of blood ketones can also be quickly made with some commercial reagents.

In sheep a terminal uraemia, indicated by a rise in plasma non-protein nitrogen levels, may occur but may be due to the death and decomposition of the foetuses. Now that estimations of steroid hormones are becoming diagnostically common-place, the elevation of plasma cortisol which occurs in pregnancy toxaemia in ewes has been used as a diagnostic feature; pregnancy toxaemia and clinical hypocalcaemia can both cause sufficient stress to promote such an elevation (14).

Necropsy Findings

The disease is not usually fatal in cattle but fatty degeneration of the liver and secondary changes in the anterior pituitary gland and adrenal cortex may be present. In ewes there are usually twin lambs, a fatty friable liver and evidence of constipation. The lambs may be dead and in varying stages of decomposition. Hepatic glycogen levels are usually very low in both sheep and cattle.

Diagnosis

The clinical picture is usually too indefinite, especially in cattle, to enable a diagnosis to be made solely on clinical grounds. General consideration of the history, with particular reference to the time of calving, the duration of pregnancy in ewes and the feeding programme, and biochemical examination to detect the presence of hypoglycaemia, keto-naemia and ketonuria are necessary to establish a diagnosis.

Cattle. Traumatic reticulitis, bovine pyelon-phritis, indigestion and abomasal displacement may be confused with the wasting form of ketosis, and a secondary ketosis, due to these diseases and to metritis and mastitis, often presents a problem in diagnosis. Careful clinical examination of these cases usually reveals a mild fever, an increased heart rate, only a moderate ketonuria and some localizing signs of the primary disease. Traumatic reticulitis does not necessarily have the same relationship to recent calving, the onset of anorexia and fall in milk production is much more acute and severe, and pain can usually be elicited on percussion over the hypogastrium. In the early stages ruminal movements are completely absent. A leucocyte count and blood glucose examination are useful aids in difficult cases. Vagus indigestion may also lead to a secondary ketosis but is usually accompanied by marked stasis of the alimentary tract, abdominal distension and moderate bloat. A diagnosis of indigestion usually depends on a history of improper diet, the presence of ruminal stasis and an absence of other clinical signs. Abomasal displacement occurs usually right at calving, anorexia develops suddenly and persists intermittently, there is a reduction in abdominal size, the faeces are pasty and passed in small amounts, and abomasal sounds may be audible over the lower left abdomen. There is incomplete and temporary response to treatment for ketosis. Rare cases of diabetes mellitus have been recorded in cattle (15) and its diagnosis must depend on the detection of a high blood-sugar level and reduced glucose tolerance. The response to insulin is good.

The nervous form of bovine ketosis is usually distinguished by the marked signs of delirium and the ketonuria. The episodes are transient, unlike those of listeriosis, and there is no fever. Rabies is characterized by mania, ascending paralysis and anaesthesia and is always fatal. Convulsions such as occur in lactation tetany, acute lead poisoning and poisoning with *Claviceps paspali* are not observed. The nervous form of bovine ketosis is never fatal and responds quickly to treatment.

Some difficulty may be encountered in cows which have ketosis and parturient paresis concurrently. Cows which show a partial response to treatment for parturient paresis but fail to eat well should be examined for evidence of ketosis. The nervous form of bovine ketosis combined with early parturient paresis is manifested by a reeling, staggery gait and signs of nervous involvement including narcosis and drunken behaviour. Later these animals go down and may show hyperaesthesia and clonic convulsions.

Sheep. Ovine ketosis is usually suspected in heavily pregnant ewes which show nervous signs and die within 6 or 7 days. Parturient paresis occurs in pregnant and lactating ewes, is manifested by paralysis, has a much shorter course of 12 to 24 hours, usually affects a considerable proportion of the flock at one time, and is accompanied by a history of exertion or sudden deprivation of food. Affected animals respond well to treatment with solutions of calcium salts. Listeriosis and rabies are differentiated as in cattle. Local lesions caused by *Coenurus cerebralis* larvae, and cerebral abscess, and otitis media usually affect only one or two sheep, and have a long course and localizing signs. Louping ill occurs only when the vector ticks are present, is accompanied by fever and has a characteristic histopathology.

Treatment

In cattle a number of effective treatments are available but in some affected animals the response is only transient and in rare cases the disease may persist and cause death or necessitate slaughter of the animals. Most of these cases are secondary and failure to respond satisfactorily to treatment is due to the primary disease.

Although the pathogenesis of the disease in ewes is similar in some ways to that in cows, the response to the same treatments as are used in cattle is variable and in general much less satisfactory. This is probably due to the added biochemical lesions of decreased glucose utilization, hypoglycaemic encephalopathy and increased plasma cortisol levels which occur in severe cases. Neither replacement therapy nor hormonal treatments are likely to have any effect in these cases, and the variability of response to treatment in ewes probably depends on the severity of the cases and the duration of the disease. When clinical cases are obvious the rest of the flock should be examined daily for any evidence of ketosis and affected animals treated with propylene glycol or glycerol immediately. Supplementary feeding of the flock should be commenced immediately, particular attention being given to an increase in carbohydrate intake. With clinical cases an immediate Caesarean section to remove the lambs is favoured by many but results are not good. If expense is not a great object parenteral treatment with glucocorticoids plus glucose or glycerol is recommended (16, 8).

The only rational treatment in ketosis is to relieve the need for glucose formation from tissues and allow ketone body utilization to continue normally. Theoretically the simplest means of doing this is by the administration of glucose replacement therapy.

Replacement therapy. The intravenous injection of 500 ml. of a 50 per cent solution of glucose (dextrose) effects marked improvement in most cows but relapses occur commonly unless repeated treatments are used. This is probably due to the transience of the hyperglycaemia, or insufficient dosing, the dose required varying directly with the amount of lactose being lost in the milk. Subcutaneous injections prolong the response but are not recommended as they cause discomfort, and large unsightly swellings, which often become infected, may result. Intraperitoneal injections of 20 per cent solution of dextrose may be used alternatively. Other sugars, especially fructose, have been used in an effort to prolong the response but idiosyncrasy to some preparations, in the form of polypnoea, muscle tremor, weakness and collapse, occur rather commonly while the injection is being given. To overcome the necessity for repeated injections propylene glycol or glycerine (8 oz. twice daily for 2 days followed by 4 oz. daily for 2 days to cattle) can be administered as a drench or in the feed and give excellent results; administration in feed is preferred because the dangers of aspiration with drenching are avoided. It is recommended that for best results dosing with these preparations be preceded by an intravenous injection of glucose. Parenteral infusions of glucose solutions and the feeding of glycerol depress the fat content of milk, and the nett saving in energy may favourably influence response to these drugs. Glycerol and propylene glycol are not as efficient as glucose because this conversion to glucose does utilize oxaloacetate (1), but they are probably least damaging in this respect of all glucose precursors and for practical reasons their use is justified.

The results of replacement therapy in sheep vary widely. Propylene glycol or glycerine (4 oz. daily by mouth) have given excellent results for some workers but poor results for others. Parenteral treatment with glucose solutions is not recommended because relapses occur commonly unless the injections are repeated.

Because of its glucogenic effect sodium propionate is theoretically a suitable treatment but when administered in 4 to 8 oz. doses daily the response in cattle is often very slow. Lactates are also highly glucogenic but both calcium or sodium lactate (2 lb. initially followed by 1 lb. daily for 7 days) and sodium acetate ($\frac{1}{4}$ to 1 lb. daily) have given less satisfactory results than those obtained with sodium propionate. Ammonium lactate (200 g. daily for 5 days) has, however, been used extensively with reported good results. Sodium ethyloxaloacetate given intravenously is effective in natural and experimental cases in ewes but is unlikely to be a practicable form of treatment because of cost.

Hormonal therapy. The efficiency of adrenocortical hormones in the treatment of bovine ketosis has been amply demonstrated in both experimental and field cases. Their chief attractions are their ease of administration and the fact that glucose or its precursors need not be administered concurrently. Many preparations are available and have been used successfully, the newer preparations being more potent, requiring less dosage, and having fewer side effects. Gluconeogenesis is stimulated for about 48 hours after a single injection of a suitable preparation (17). It is not proposed to review the literature on this subject as the number of preparations is too extensive but in general the recommendations of the manufacturer with regard to dosage should be followed. In sheep the results are generally poor. The major disadvantage of treatment with adrenocortical preparations is that gluconeogenesis is stimulated at the expense of other body tissues and possibly at the expense of oxaloacetate utilization in removing excess ketone bodies. It is also noted that successful treatment with glucocorticoids is often accompanied by a significant depression in milk yield, which may contribute to the recovery rate (18, 19).

Insulin has been used from time to time in conjunction with glucose or glucocorticoids but does not appear to confer marked therapeutic advantage (17).

Miscellaneous treatments. Chloral hydrate has long been used in the treatment of both forms of bovine ketosis. An initial oral dose of 30 g. can be followed by 7 g. doses twice daily for several days. The larger dose is usually given in a capsule and subsequent doses as drenches in molasses and water. The method of action of chloral hydrate appears to be its capacity to increase the breakdown of starch in the rumen and stimulate the production and absorption of glucose (20). It is also thought to selectively influence rumen fermentation in the direction of increased production of propionate (28). Potassium chlorate is widely used and highly regarded but there is no apparent explanation for its reputed anti-ketogenic activity. It is also inclined to cause severe diarrhoea (21). Vitamin B_{12} and cobalt are sometimes administered either as a sole treatment or in conjunction with more standard therapy. Because of the suspected deficiency of coenzyme A in ketosis of cattle, cysteamine (a biological precursor of coenzyme A) and also sodium fumarate have been used to treat cases of the disease (22). Results reported initially were good but the method has not been generally adopted. The recommended dose rate of cysteamine is 750 mg. intravenously for 3 doses at 1- to 3-day intervals. Affected animals should be provided with adequate food and water, and in hot weather sheep at pasture should be driven into the shade to avoid heat stroke.

Control

In is difficult to make general recommendations for the control of the disease because of the many conditions under which it occurs and its probable multiple aetiology. A list of the recommended procedures is set out below.

Cattle. (*a*) Cows should neither have been starved nor be overfat at calving. An adequate caloric intake should be ensured in the early part of lactation and especially after treatment. In heavy producing, heavily fed herds the big problem is to provide enough food to avoid a deficient caloric intake relative to utilization, but at the same time to avoid imbalance, to avoid ruminal acidosis on a too-high carbohydrate diet and to avoid acetonaemia on a diet too high in protein. Careful estimation of diets by reference to food value tables is recommended but as a rough guide the following procedure is suggested (23): 3 lb. hay per 100 lb. bodyweight, 3 lb. ensilage per 1 lb. hay, 1 lb. grain per 3 lb. of 4 per cent milk produced. (*b*) Cows that are housed should get some exercise each day and in herds where the disease is a particular problem during the stabling period, the cattle should be turned out to pasture as soon as possible in the spring. (*c*) Ensure that the ration contains adequate cobalt, phosphorus and iodine. (*d*) If there is a high incidence in a herd receiving large quantities of ensilage, reduction of the amount fed for a trial period is indicated. (*e*) The prophylactic feeding of sodium propionate may be considered in problem herds: 110 g. daily for 6 weeks, commencing at calving, has given good results in reducing the incidence of clinical bovine ketosis and improving production. Propylene glycol (350 ml. daily for 10 days after calving) has been similarly used with moderately good results (24).

Experimental observations have tended to reduce the importance of heavy feeding of grass ensilage, failure to provide an adequate mineral mixture and failure to provide grain to stall-fed cows in late pregnancy but, in view of the known multiple-factor aetiology of this disease, these experiments do not prove that under particular sets of circumstances one or other of these factors may not be the precipitating cause. In fact in many field outbreaks adoption of the recommendations made above appears to markedly reduce the incidence of the disease.

Sheep. The same general recommendations apply in the prevention of ovine ketosis as in the prevention of ketosis in cattle. Ensure that the plane of nutrition is rising in the second half of pregnancy even if it means restricting the diet in the early stages. The last 2 months are particularly important. During this period the provision of a concentrate containing 10 per cent protein at the rate of $\frac{1}{2}$ lb. per day, increasing to 2 lb. per day in the last 2 weeks, has provided good protection. Sudden changes in type of feed should be avoided and extra feed provided during bad weather. Shelter sheds should be available, and in purely pastoral areas lambing should not occur before the pasture is well grown.

A high incidence is often encountered in small, well fed flocks where the ewes get insufficient exercise. In such circumstances the ewes should be driven about for half-an-hour twice daily and, if pasture is available, only concentrate should be fed so that they will be encouraged to forage for themselves.

It has been suggested that the control of ketosis may be achieved by manipulation of the ration so that the production of propionate in the rumen is increased relative to that of acetate (25). Not only is propionate antiketogenic, but its increased production, and a corresponding decrease in acetate production in the rumen is associated with a reduction in the percentage of fat in the milk and, as a result, a reduction in energy loss. Under experimental conditions the proportion of propionate produced in the rumen has been increased both by feeding a ration of finely ground roughage and cooked grain, and by the feeding of cod liver oil and certain unsaturated fatty acids. If these experimental results can be duplicated under conditions of practical dairy cattle feeding a satisfactory method of controlling ketosis by dietary means may be within reach.

With the current emphasis on monitoring to provide early warning of the probable occurrence of a largely subclinical disease it has been suggested that blood glucose estimations be carried out on a sample of cows in their 2nd to 6th weeks of lactation (26). Blood glucose levels of below 35 mg. per 100 ml. should raise the alarm. Regular tests for ketones in milk might be equally useful (29).

REVIEW LITERATURE

Bergman, E. N. *et al.* (1971). Symposium: ketosis in dairy cows. *J. Dairy Sci.*, *54*, 936.

Pehrson, B. (1966). Studies on ketosis in dairy cows. *Acta vet. scand.*, suppl. *15*, 59.

Reid, R. L. (1968). The physiopathology of undernourishment

in pregnant sheep, with particular reference to pregnancy toxaemia. *Advanc. vet. Sci.*, *12*, 163.

REFERENCES

(1) Krebs, H. A. (1966). *Vet. Rec.*, *78*, 187.
(2) Thin, C. & Robertson, A. (1953). *J. comp. Path.*, *63*, 184.
(3) Panaretto, B. (1968). *Aust. J. agric. Res.*, *19*, 273.
(4) Hibbitt, K. G. & Baird, G. D. (1967). *Vet. Rec.*, *81*, 511.
(5) Hibbitt, K. G. *et al.* (1969). *Res. vet. Sci.*, *10*, 245.
(6) Fookes, T. J. & Singleton, A. G. (1964). *Brit. vet. J.*, *120*, 56.
(7) Bennett, D. G. *et al.* (1968). *Amer. J. vet. Res.*, *29*, 2315.
(8) Saba, N. *et al.* (1966). *J. agric. sci. Camb.*, *67*, 129.
(9) Marston, H. R. *et al.* (1961). *Nature (Lond.)*, *190*, 1085.
(10) Elliot, J. M. (1966). *Proc. 1966 Cornell Nutr. Conf.*, 73.
(11) Cote, J. F. *et al.* (1969). *Canad. vet. J.*, *10*, 179.
(12) Ferris, T. F. *et al.* (1969). *J. clin. Invest.*, *48*, 1643.
(13) Kronfeld, D. S. (1965). *Vet. Rec.*, *77*, 30.
(14) Saba, N. & Cunningham, N. F. (1971). *Res. vet. Sci.*, *12*, 483.
(15) Phillips, R. W. *et al.* (1971). *Cornell Vet.*, *61*, 114.
(16) Hazzard, T. C. & Russell, A. M. (1968). *Vet. Rec.*, *82*, 359.
(17) Cote, J. F. (1971). *Canad. vet. J.*, *12*, 19.
(18) Braun, R. K. *et al.* (1970). *J. Amer. vet. med. Ass.*, *157*, 941.
(19) Baird, G. D. & Heitzman, R. J. (1969). *Brit. vet. J.*, *125*, xiii.
(20) Quaghebeur, D. & Oyaert, W. (1971). *Zbl. vet. Med.*, *18A*, 55, 64.
(21) Burns, K. N. (1963). *Vet. Rec.*, *75*, 763.
(22) Bach, S. J. & Hibbitt, K. G. (1962). *Vet. Rec.*, *74*, 965.
(23) Kronfeld, D. S. (1969). *Mod. vet. Pract.*, *50*, No. 4, 45.
(24) Emery, R. S. *et al.* (1964). *J. Dairy Sci.*, *47*, 1074.
(25) Shaw, J. C. (1959). *Feedstuffs*, *31*, 18.
(26) Schafer, M. & Schwarzer, E. (1971). *Mh. Vet.-Med.*, *26*, 582.
(27) Simeonov, S. (1969). *Vet. Med. Nauki, Sofia*, *6*, 25.
(28) Prins, R. A. & Seekles, L. (1968). *J. Dairy Sci.*, *51*, 882.
(29) Emery, R. *et al.* (1968). *J. Dairy Sci.*, *51*, 867.
(30) Procos, J. & Gilchrist, F. M. C. (1966). *Onderstepoort J. vet. Res.*, *33*, 161.

Neonatal Hypoglycaemia

(*Baby Pig Disease*)

Neonatal hypoglycaemia is a metabolic disease of piglets caused by restriction of food intake.

Incidence

The disease has been recorded mainly from the United States and Britain. Most affected pigs die if left untreated and the morbidity is usually 30 to 70 per cent and may be as high as 100 per cent in individual litters. Apart from deaths due to hypoglycaemia many piglets are too weak to avoid the sow and are killed by overlaying.

Aetiology

An inadequate intake of milk is always the primary cause of hypoglycaemia of piglets. This may be due to failure of the sow's milk supply or to failure of the piglets to nurse. Failure to nurse may be due to such diseases as coliform septicaemia,

transmissible gastroenteritis, streptococcal infections, myoclonia congenita and haemolytic disease of the newborn (1). Piglets under 4 days of age rapidly develop hypoglycaemia under fasting conditions; older pigs do not (8).

In many instances failure to nurse occurs for no apparent reason, although an anaphylactic reaction to colostral antibodies has been suggested as a cause (2). An unusual probable occurrence of hypoglycaemia is reported in baby pigs produced in a newly constructed SPF piggery. The disease occurred apparently because of failure of piglets to become populated with lactobacilli necessary for milk digestion. Inoculation with an appropriate lactobacillus corrects the condition (7).

Occurrence

Only pigs during the first week of life are affected and sows of any age or condition may have affected litters. Other than the occurrence of primary diseases there are no special circumstances in which the disease occurs and the general nutritional status of the sow appears to have no effect on the incidence of the disease. Although there is no record of hypoglycaemia as a disease of young lambs and calves it does occur in these species. In lambs it is usually caused by mismothering and complete absence of the mother in lambs only a few days old. The lambs are in lateral recumbency, make slow uncontrolled athetoid movements, have subnormal temperatures and respond well to parenteral treatment with glucose. In calves hypoglycaemia is also recorded as a concurrent disease in calves with scours. It seems probable that the hypoglycaemia is secondary to the interference with absorption and digestion caused by the diarrhoea. The signs are characteristic but the disease does not respond to glucose therapy (6).

Pathogenesis

The piglet is born with good hepatic stores of glycogen (10 to 14 mg. per cent) and a blood-glucose level at 24 hours after birth of 80 to 90 mg. per cent although there may be considerable variation between litters or even between litter-mates (3). Satisfactory gluconeogenesis does not develop in piglets until the 7th day after birth, and during this period glycogen stores are likely to be rapidly exhausted if the intake of milk is restricted. The blood-glucose level is then extremely unstable and dependent entirely upon dietary sources. The first week of life is thus the danger period (1). Deprivation of food after this produces only loss of weight and has no effect on blood-glucose levels. This particular susceptibility to hypoglycaemia in the early postnatal period seems to be characteristic of the pig and may play a major role in causing losses in piglets by contributing to the effects of various infectious and non-infectious agents.

Signs appear first when blood-glucose levels fall to about 50 mg. per cent, although further depression to levels as low as 7 mg. per cent has been observed. Even in such extreme cases complete recovery is possible after the administration of glucose (1). Experimental hypoglycaemia produced by the injection of insulin causes a clinical syndrome similar to that of the naturally occurring disease.

Clinical Findings

Only piglets less than a week old are affected. Uncertainty in gait is apparent first and the piglet has progressive difficulty in maintaining balance until recumbency becomes permanent. There is shivering, dullness and anorexia, and often a typical weak squeal. A characteristic feature is the subnormal rectal temperature and the cold, clammy skin which also evidences marked pallor and ruffling of the hair. The pallor is related to the failing circulation. The heart rate becomes increasingly feeble and slow and may fall as low as 80 per minute. In many cases there are few additional signs but convulsions are recorded as a common occurrence by some observers (1). These vary from aimless movements of the head and fore limbs to severe tetanic convulsions. In the latter there are violent galloping movements, particularly with the hind legs, opisthotonus and champing of the jaws. Tortuous movements and rigidity of the neck and trunk also occur. Terminally coma develops and death follows 24 to 36 hours after the onset of signs.

Clinical Pathology

Blood-glucose levels of less than 50 mg. per cent can be considered as pathognomonic. Significant rises in blood non-protein-nitrogen and urea nitrogen are often observed but appear to be related to increased metabolism rather than to renal dysfunction (4).

Necropsy Findings

There are no visible lesions. Absence of curd in the stomach is good contributory evidence but in many cases it will be obvious that some food has been taken. Hepatic glycogen levels are usually negligible.

Diagnosis

Unless blood-glucose levels are estimated the predominantly nervous signs may lead to an error in diagnosis. However, hypoglycaemia and a good response to treatment with glucose may occur when the hypoglycaemia is secondary to another disease. A definite diagnosis of neonatal hypoglycaemia must depend on elimination of other diseases as primary causes. Viral encephalomyelitis and pseudo-rabies cause an almost identical clinical picture but are not restricted in occurrence to pigs less than a week old. Bacterial meningo-encephalitis including streptococcal septicaemia and listeriosis may also affect pigs of this age. Necropsy examination should make definition of viral and bacterial infections a relatively easy task.

Treatment

Intraperitoneal injections of glucose (15 ml. of 5 per cent solution), repeated at intervals of 4 to 6 hours, should be given until the piglet will suck a foster-mother or eat an artificial diet. Cortisone is ineffective as treatment (5). Protection from cold is most important and an environmental temperature of 80 to 90°F (27 to 32°C) will prolong the life of affected pigs (4).

Control

Avoidance of the causative factors listed above constitutes prevention. Piglets should be carefully observed during the first week for early signs of any disease and treatment instituted promptly. Maintenance of a stable environmental temperature at 32°C (90°F) may delay the onset of the disease, or in marginal circumstances prevent its occurrence.

REFERENCES

(1) Goodwin, R. F. W. (1955). *Brit. vet. J.*, *111*, 361.
(2) Young, D. A. & Underdahl, N. R. (1947). *Cornell Vet.*, *37*, 175.
(3) Schoop, G. *et al.* (1963). *Dtsch. tierärztl. Wschr.*, *70*, 345.
(4) Morrill, C. C. (1952). *Amer. J. vet. Res.*, *13*, 164, 171, 322, 325, 327.
(5) Goodwin, R. F. W. (1957). *Vet. Rec.*, *69*, 1290.
(6) Tennant, B. *et al.* (1968). *Cornell Vet.*, *58*, 136.
(7) Henry, D. C. (1967). *Aust. vet. J.*, *43*, 175.
(8) Swiatek, K. R. *et al.* (1968). *Amer. J. Physiol.*, *214*, 400.

Post-parturient Haemoglobinuria

Post-parturient haemoglobinuria is a disease of high-producing dairy cows occurring soon after calving and characterized by intravascular haemolysis, haemoglobinuria and anaemia.

Incidence

Although this disease has been observed in many countries its relatively low incidence makes it one of minor importance. The mortality rate may be as high as 50 per cent but only one or two animals in a herd are affected at a time.

Aetiology

Rations low in phosphorus and a diet of cruciferous plants are usually associated with the development of the disease. Experimental production of the disease in one cow has been reported after feeding a low-phosphorus ration for three pregnancies (1). In this instance other signs of phosphorus deficiency occurred 18 months before haemoglobinuria developed, and the case responded well to supplementary feeding with bone meal. The disease may be associated with heavy feeding on plants which normally have a low content of phosphorus. At least hypophosphataemia is a predisposing cause of the disease and feeding on cruciferous plants may be a precipitating factor (2, 3). For example, in a group of animals in which the disease occurs it is sometimes found that dry cows and yearlings have normal serum-inorganic-phosphorus levels, milking cows are in the low–normal range, and cows that calved within the preceding 2 months have low levels.

Occurrence

Only adult cows develop the typical haemolytic syndrome, usually in the period from 2 to 4 weeks after calving. Heavy producing cows in their 3rd to 6th lactations are most commonly affected. The disease does not occur commonly in beef cattle. Phosphorus-deficient soils and drought conditions are thought to be predisposing and the disease is often a problem on particular farms. Cases occur more commonly when the cows graze rape, turnips or other cruciferous plants (2) or when large quantities of beet pulp are fed. In areas of severe phosphorus deficiency the disease may occur at pasture, but in Europe and North America it is more common during prolonged periods of housing. The ingestion of cold water or exposure to extremely cold weather may precipitate attacks of the disease (4). A similar condition accompanied by hypophosphataemia, has been observed in late pregnancy in Egyptian buffaloes (5) and in the post-parturient period in Indian buffaloes (6).

Pathogenesis

There is a constant association with hypophosphataemia and a low dietary intake of phosphorus, and it is presumed that the drain of lactation causes further depletion of phosphorus reserves.

The reason for the sudden development of intravascular haemolysis is unknown. Erythrocyte fragility is not increased and haemolysis does not always occur in cases of hypophosphataemia. The signs observed are those of acute haemolytic anaemia and in fatal cases death is due to anaemic anoxia.

Clinical Findings

Haemoglobinuria, inappetence and weakness develop suddenly and there is a severe depression of the milk yield although, in some less acute cases, the cow continues to eat and milk normally for 24 hours after discolouration of the urine is evident. Dehydration develops quickly, the mucous membranes are pallid, and the cardiac impulse and jugular pulse are much augmented. A moderate temperature rise (to 40 °C or 103·5 °F) often occurs. The faeces are usually dry and firm. Shortness of breath and tachycardia are evident and jaundice may be apparent in the late stages. Pica may be observed in the other animals in the group. The disease runs an acute course for 3 to 5 days, the cow becoming weak and staggery and finally recumbent. Gangrene and sloughing of the tip of the tail or the digits has been observed occasionally. Death follows within a few hours. In non-fatal cases convalescence requires about 3 weeks and recovering animals often show pica. Ketosis commonly occurs coincidentally.

In a herd where the disease occurs there may be additional signs of phosphorus deficiency although when the deficiency is marginal the general condition of the herd may be excellent. A similar acute syndrome to that described above, and less severe cases of anaemia, may occur sporadically in animals on lush spring pasture.

Clinical Pathology

In marginal phosphorus-deficient areas normal non-lactating animals in an affected herd may have serum-inorganic-phosphorus levels in the normal range. Lactating cows in an affected herd may have moderately low levels of 2 to 3 mg. per cent and affected animals extremely low levels of 0·4 to 1·5 mg. per cent. Erythrocyte counts and haemoglobin levels are also greatly reduced. Heinz bodies may be present in erythrocytes (7). The urine is dark red-brown to black in colour and usually moderately turbid. No red cells are present.

Necropsy Findings

The blood is thin and the carcase jaundiced. The liver is swollen, and fatty infiltration and degeneration are evident. Discoloured urine is present in the bladder.

Diagnosis

Post-parturient haemoglobinuria is characterized by an acute haemolytic anaemia in cows calved within the preceding 4 weeks. Other causes of acute haemolytic anaemia are not confined to the post-calving period. Laboratory examination is usually necessary to confirm the diagnosis and to eliminate haematuria as a cause of the discolouration of the urine.

Treatment

The transfusion of large quantities of whole blood may be the only treatment capable of saving the life of a severely affected animal. The treatment must be given quickly. A delay of 12 hours often seems to lead to an irreversible state. A minimum of one gallon is recommended. The administration of phosphorus to acutely ill animals should include the intravenous injection of 60 g. of sodium acid-phosphate in 300 ml. of distilled water and a similar dose subcutaneously, followed by further subcutaneous injections at 12-hour intervals on three occasions and similar daily doses by mouth. Oral dosing with bone meal (4 oz. twice daily) or including it in the ration is a suitable alternative. Haematinics during convalescence are recommended and a phosphorus supplement, bone meal if it is available, should be fed. Ketosis is a not uncommon accompaniment and additional treatment for it may be required.

Control

An adequate dietary intake of phosphorus (1 oz. of acid sodium phosphate or 3 oz. of bone meal daily) should be ensured particularly in early lactation if the diet contains large quantities of beet pulp or cruciferous plants.

REFERENCES

(1) Madsen, D. E. & Nielsen, H. M. (1944). *J. Amer. vet. med. Ass.*, *105*, 22.
(2) Tarr, A. (1947). *J. S. Afr. vet. med. Ass.*, *188*, 167.
(3) Parkinson, B. & Sutherland, A. K. (1954). *Aust. vet. J.*, *30*, 232.
(4) Penny, R. H. C. (1956). *Vet. Rec.*, *68*, 238.
(5) Awad, F. I. & El-Latif, K. A. (1963). *Vet. Rec.*, *75*, 11, 298.
(6) Nagpol, M. *et al.* (1968). *Indian vet. J.*, *45*, 1048.
(7) Martinovich, D. & Woodhouse, D. A. (1971). *N.Z. vet. J.*, *19*, 259.

Paralytic Myoglobinuria

(*Azoturia*)

Paralytic myoglobinuria is a disease of horses, occurring during exercise after a period of inactivity on full rations. It is characterized by myoglobinuria and muscular degeneration.

Incidence

The disease was once of great economic importance in draught horses but is now reduced to sporadic cases occurring particularly in racehorses fed heavily on grain.

Aetiology

The commonly accepted theory is that large stores of glycogen are laid down in muscles during a period of idleness and when exercise is taken the glycogen is rapidly metabolized to lactic acid. If the rate at which lactic acid is produced exceeds the rate at which it can be removed in the blood stream, accumulation occurs and causes coagulation of the muscles and liberation of myoglobin which escapes in the urine. The possible role of a dietary deficiency of vitamin E in this disease has been suggested.

Occurrence

In most instances there is a history of a period of complete inactivity for 2 or more days immediately preceding the onset of the disease. An attack is unusual if the period of rest is as brief as 1 day or as long as 2 weeks. Horses taken off track work because of minor injuries or illness, are often maintained on full working rations and become affected when taken back to work. Attacks are not uncommon after general anaesthesia. Sporadic cases have also been recorded in horses running at pasture (1). A severe outbreak in horses maintained at pasture during the week but ridden at the weekend has been reported (2). A clinically similar disease has been recorded in single cases in cattle 2 to 8 days after their release onto pasture from winter housing (3).

Pathogenesis

Coagulation necrosis of muscle fibres causes hard, painful swelling of the large muscle masses. The gluteal muscles are most commonly involved and this is thought to be due to their high content of glycogen. The primary myopathic lesion may cause pressure on the sciatic and other crural nerves and result in a secondary neuropathic degeneration of the rectus femoris and vastus muscles. These latter muscles are said to be the only ones which subsequently atrophy in surviving animals (4). The liberation of myoglobin from the necrotic muscle fibres is followed by the passage of dark red-brown urine. Death is usually due to decubital septicaemia or myohaemoglobinuric nephrosis and uraemia, depending upon the extent of muscle damage. Degeneration of myocardium is sometimes observed and may in some instances be the cause of death.

Clinical Findings

Signs develop 15 minutes to 1 hour after the beginning of exercise which need not be vigorous. There is profuse sweating, stiffness of the gait and reluctance to move. The signs may disappear in a few hours if the horse is given complete rest immediately but the condition usually progresses to recumbency, the horse first assuming a dog-sitting position followed by lateral recumbency.

Severe pain and distress are accompanied by restlessness, struggling and repeated attempts to rise. The respirations are rapid, the pulse small and hard and the temperature may rise to 40·5°C (105°F) in the late stages in severe cases. One limb or all four may be affected but the common finding is involvement of both hind legs. The quadriceps femoris and gluteal muscles are hard and board-like. The urine is of deep red-brown colour and urination may be inhibited. Appetite and water intake are often normal.

Many subacute cases in which signs are mild and myoglobinuria is absent occur in circumstances in which azoturia might be expected to occur. There is lameness, soreness over the rump, crouching, and great restriction of movement of the hind limbs. If exercise is stopped as soon as lameness occurs the horse may recover in 2 to 4 days. The prognosis is good if the animal remains standing, recovery occurring in 2 to 4 days, but recumbency is usually followed by fatal uraemia or decubital septicaemia.

Clinical Pathology

The urine contains myoglobin which can only be differentiated from haemoglobin by spectroscopic examination. There is no discolouration of the serum because the renal threshold for myoglobin is very low. Protein and casts are present in the urine which has a high specific gravity. There is a marked polycythaemia.

In horses the creatinine phosphokinase levels are highest in skeletal and cardiac muscles. SGOT is high in these muscles and liver. Because of its specificity to muscle SCPK levels are the preferred indicator of degree of muscle necrosis (5).

Necropsy Findings

Gross and microscopic changes are present, mainly in the large gluteal and quadriceps groups of thigh muscles, and in the iliopsoas and vastus muscles. There is extensive, pale discolouration with a waxy, cooked appearance of the cut surface. Similar degenerative lesions have also been observed in myocardium and muscles of the larynx and diaphragm in some cases (6) but this has not been a general finding. Dark brown urine is present in the bladder and the renal medulla shows dark brown streaks.

Diagnosis

Severe cases present no major difficulty in diagnosis. Similar lameness may occur in laminitis but the history is different, there is no discolouration of urine and pain is evident at the coronet. Reddish discolouration of the urine is more commonly due to the presence of haemoglobin, and diseases in which haemoglobinuria occurs are not usually accompanied by lameness or local pain. A local maxillary myositis and a generalized polymyositis have also been recorded in horses (7). The former develops slowly and affects only the muscles of the jaw, and the latter is a muscular dystrophy comparable to that caused by vitamin E deficiency. Iliac thrombosis can be detected on rectal palpation. 'Tying-up', which occurs primarily in light horses, includes a number of conditions, one of which may be mild paralytic haemoglobinuria.

Treatment

Further exercise should be avoided and the animal either cared for where it is or taken home by low-level trailer and kept in a box-stall. Every effort should be made to keep the horse standing, and slinging may be advisable in some cases. Narcosis with chloral hydrate or ataractic drugs may be necessary if pain is severe or the horse makes repeated efforts to rise. Corticosteroids, administered intravenously, are recommended. Thiamine hydrochloride is claimed to give favourable results. Intramuscular injections of 0·5 g. are usually repeated daily (8, 9). The administration of antihistamines and vitamin E is probably warranted, especially in the early stages of the disease. Ancillary treatment includes the intravenous or oral administration of large quantities of electrolyte solutions to maintain a high rate of urine flow and avoid tubular blockage, catheterization if urination is difficult and the maintenance of soft faeces. The urine should be kept alkaline to avoid precipitation of myoglobin in renal tubules. Hot applications to the affected parts may ease the discomfort.

Control

The disease can be avoided by reducing the grain ration to half when the horse is getting no exercise. If there is a chance that the disease may develop exercise should be kept very light initially and increased only gradually.

REFERENCES

(1) Pope, D. C. & Heslop, C. H. (1960). *Canad. vet. J.*, *1*, 171.
(2) Tritschler, L. A. & Miles, D. (1966). *Vet. Med.*, *61*, 649.
(3) Christl, H. (1971). *Dtsch. tierärztl. Wschr.*, *78*, 204.
(4) Merillat, L. A. (1944). *J. Amer. vet. med. Ass.*, *104*, 223.
(5) Gerber, H. (1969). *Equine vet. J.*, *1*, 129.
(6) Goto, M. *et al.* (1953). *Jap. J. vet. Sci.*, *15*, 227.
(7) Alstrom, I. (1948). *Skand. vet. Tidskr.*, *38*, 593.
(8) Bauch, R. E. (1945). *Vet. Med.*, *40*, 169.
(9) Stroup, N. L. (1945). *Vet. Med.*, *40*, 170.

28

Diseases Caused by Nutritional Deficiencies

INTRODUCTION

THE following criteria are suggested for the assessment of the importance of nutrition in the aetiology of a disease state in a single animal or in a group of animals:

(i) Is there evidence from an examination of the diet that a deficiency of a specific nutrient or nutrients may be occurring?
(ii) Is there evidence from an examination of the animals that a deficiency of the suspected essential nutrient or nutrients could cause the observed disease?
(iii) Does supplementation of the diet with the essential nutrient or nutrients prevent or cure the condition?

The difficulties encountered in satisfying these criteria and making an unequivocal diagnosis of a nutritional deficiency have increased as investigations have progressed into the area of trace elements and vitamins. The amounts of such substances as selenium present in feedstuffs and body tissues are exceedingly small and their estimation difficult and expensive. Because of these difficulties it is becoming more acceptable to describe individual syndromes as 'responsive diseases', i.e. which satisfy only the third of the above criteria. The practice leaves much to be desired but has the advantage that applicable control measures are more readily available.

(i) *Evidence of existence of deficiency*. General evidence will include either evidence of deficiency in the diet or abnormal absorption, utilization or requirement of the nutrient under consideration. Special evidence may be obtained by chemical or biological examination of the feed.

(a) *Diet*. The diet for a considerable period prior to the occurrence of the disease must be considered because body stores of most dietary factors may delay the appearance of clinical signs. Specific deficiencies are likely to be associated with particular soil types and in many instances soil and geological maps may predict the probable occur-

rence of a nutritional disease (1). Diseases of plants may also indicate specific soil deficiencies, e.g. 'reclamation disease' of oats indicates a copper deficiency in the soil. Domination of the pasture by particular plant species may also be important, e.g. subterranean clover selectively absorbs copper, legumes selectively absorb molybdenum and *Astragalus* spp. are selector plants for selenium.

Farming practices may have a marked bearing on the presence or absence of specific nutrients in livestock feed. For example heavy applications of nitrogen fertilizer can reduce the copper, cobalt, molybdenum and manganese content of the pasture. On the other hand, many applications of lime reduce plant copper, cobalt, zinc and manganese levels but increase the molybdenum content (2). Effects such as these are sufficiently severe to suggest that animals grazing the pasture might suffer trace element deficiency (3). Modern hay-making methods, with their emphasis on the artificial drying of immature forage, tend to conserve vitamin A but may result in a gross deficiency of vitamin D. Soil and pasture improvement by exaggeration of the depletion of nutrients, particularly trace elements, from marginally deficient soil may give rise to overt deficiency disease. Thus local knowledge of farming and feeding practices in a particular area is of primary importance in the diagnosis of nutritional deficiency states.

(b) *Abnormal absorption*. Even though a diet may contain adequate amounts of a particular nutrient some other factor, by decreasing the absorption of the nutrient, may reduce the value of the dietary supply. For instance excess phosphate reduces calcium absorption, excess calcium reduces the absorption of iodine, and absence of bile salts prevents proper absorption of the fat-soluble vitamins. Chronic enteritis reduces the absorption of most dietary essentials.

(c) *Abnormal utilization* of ingested nutrients may also have an effect on the development of conditioned deficiency diseases. For example molybdenum and sulphate reduce copper storage, vitamin E has a sparing effect on vitamin A and thiamine reduces the dietary requirement of essential fatty acids.

(*d*) *Abnormal requirement.* Stimulation of the growth rate of animals by improved nutrition or other practices may increase their requirement of specific nutrients to the point where deficiency disease occurs. There seems to be little doubt that there is a genetic variation in mineral metabolism and it has even been suggested that it may be possible to breed sheep to 'fit' actual deficiency conditions, but the significance of the inherited component of an animal's nutritional requirement is unknown and probably small (2). It should not be overlooked, however, when policies of upgrading livestock in deficient areas are initiated.

(ii) *Evidence of a deficiency as the cause of the disease.* Evidence is usually available from experimental work to indicate the clinical signs and necropsy findings one can expect to be produced by each deficiency. Several modifying factors may confuse the issue. Deficiencies under natural circumstances are unlikely to be single and the clinical and necropsy findings will be complicated by those caused by deficiencies of other factors or by intercurrent infections. In addition most of the syndromes are both variable and insidious in onset and the minimal nature of the necropsy lesions in many nutritional deficiency diseases adds further difficulty to the making of a diagnosis.

Special clinical and laboratory examinations of the animals are valuable aids to diagnosis in many instances. Impaired night vision is a good indication of vitamin A deficiency. Roentgenological examination of joints in rickets, and electrocardiographic examination in thiamine and vitamin E deficiency are examples of the special aids that can be used. The levels of most nutrients in the blood, urine and liver can be assayed in the living animal or at necropsy, and metabolic defects caused by nutritional deficiencies may also be detected.

(iii) *Evidence based on cure or prevention by correction of the deficiency.* The best test of the diagnosis in suspected nutritional deficiency is to observe the effects of specific additions to the ration. Confounding factors are frequently encountered. Spontaneous recoveries may occur and adequate controls are essential. Curative responses may be poor because of an inadequate dose rate or because of advanced tissue damage or the abnormality may have been only a predisposing factor or secondary to a complicating factor which is still present. Another common cause of confusion in therapeutic trials is the impurity of the preparations used, particularly when trace elements are involved. Finally the preparations used may have intrinsic pharmacological activity and produce some amelioration of the disease without a deficiency having been present.

REVIEW LITERATURE

McDonald, I. W. (1968). The nutrition of grazing ruminants. *Nutr. Abst. Rev.*, *38*, 381.

REFERENCES

(1) Thornton, I. *et al.* (1972). *Vet. Rec.*, *90*, 11.
(2) Pope, A. L. (1971). *J. Anim. Sci.*, *33*, 332.
(3) Mudd, A. J. (1970). *Brit. vet. J.*, *126*, 38.

DEFICIENCIES OF MINERAL NUTRIENTS

Cobalt Deficiency

The disease caused by a deficiency of cobalt in the diet is characterized by anorexia and wasting.

Incidence

Cobalt deficiency is known to be of major importance in Australia, New Zealand, the United Kingdom and North America and probably occurs in many other parts of the world. Where the deficiency is extreme large tracts of land have been found to be unsuitable for the raising of ruminants and in marginal areas suboptimal growth and production may be limiting factors in the husbandry of sheep and cattle.

Aetiology

The disease is caused by a primary deficiency of cobalt in the diet. Cattle and sheep are similarly affected and the signs are identical in both species. Cattle are slightly less susceptible than sheep, and lambs and calves are more seriously affected than adults. Frank deficiency is unlikely to occur in pigs, or in other omnivores or carnivores because Vitamin B_{12} is present in meat and other animal tissues, but there are some reports of improved weight gains following supplementation of the ration with cobalt. Horses appear to be unaffected.

Occurrence

Primary cobalt deficiency occurs only on soils which are deficient in cobalt. Such soils do not appear to have any geological similarity, varying from wind-blown shell sands to soils derived from pumice and granite. Although soils containing less than 2 ppm cobalt are likely to produce pastures containing insufficient cobalt, the relationship between levels of cobalt in soil and pasture is not always constant. The factors governing the relationship have not been determined although heavy liming is known to reduce the availability of cobalt in the soil. Manganese appears to have a similar action but the agricultural significance of the relationship is unknown (1).

Pastures containing less than 0·07 and 0·04 ppm DM lead to the development of clinical signs in sheep and cattle respectively. The daily requirement for sheep at pasture is 0·08 mg. of cobalt per day; for growing lambs the need is somewhat greater (2). Variations in the cobalt content of pasture occur with seasonal variations in pasture growth and with drainage conditions. The increased incidence of the disease which has been observed in the spring may be related to domination of the pasture by rapidly-growing grasses which have a lower cobalt content than legumes. There is also a great deal of variation between years in the severity of the losses encountered due to variations in the cobalt status of the animals. Forage grown on well drained soils has a greater cobalt content than that grown on poorly drained soils of the same cobalt status. Plant growth is not visibly affected by a low cobalt content of the soil but the addition of excessive quantities may retard growth.

Although the disease occurs most commonly in ruminants at pasture in severely deficient areas, sporadic cases occur in marginal areas especially after long periods of stable feeding. Bulls, rams and calves are the groups most commonly affected although dairy cows kept under the same conditions may develop a high incidence of ketosis.

Pathogenesis

Cobalt is peculiar as an essential trace element in ruminant nutrition in that it is stored in the body in limited amounts only and not in all tissues. In the adult ruminant its only known function is in the rumen and it must, therefore, be present continuously in the feed.

The effect of cobalt in the rumen is to participate in the production of vitamin B_{12} (cyanocobalamin) and compared to other species the requirement for vitamin B_{12} is very much higher in ruminants. In sheep the requirement is of the order of 11 μg. per day and probably 500 μg. per day are produced in the rumen, most being lost in the process (3). Animals in the advanced stages of cobalt deficiency are cured by the oral administration of cobalt or by the parenteral administration of vitamin B_{12}. On cobalt-deficient diets the appearance of signs is accompanied by a fall of as much as 90 per cent in the vitamin B_{12} content of the faeces, and on oral dosing with cobalt the signs disappear and vitamin B_{12} levels in the faeces return to normal. Parenteral administration of cobalt is without appreciable clinical effect although some cobalt does enter the alimentary tract in the bile and leads to the formation of a small amount of cobalamin.

The essential defect in cobalt deficiency in ruminants is an inability to metabolize propionic acid, which is accompanied by a failure of appetite and death from inanition (4). The efficiency of cobalt in preventing staggers in sheep grazing pasture dominated by *Phalaris tuberosa* (5), and possibly by canary grass (*Phalaris minor*) or Rhompa grass, a hybrid *Phalaris* spp. (6), is also unexplained.

Clinical Findings

No specific signs are characteristic of cobalt deficiency. A gradual decrease in appetite is accompanied by loss of body weight and final emaciation and weakness, and these are often observed in the presence of abundant green feed. Pica is likely to occur, especially in cattle. There is marked pallor of the mucous membranes and affected animals are easily fatigued. Growth, lactation and wool production are severely retarded and the wool may be tender or broken. Infertility, diarrhoea and lacrimation may be observed in the later stages. In sheep severe lacrimation with profuse outpouring of fluid sufficient to mat the wool of the face is one of the most important signs in advanced cases. Signs usually become apparent when animals have been on affected areas for about 6 months and death occurs in 3 to 12 months after the first appearance of illness, although severe wasting may be precipitated by the stress of parturition or abortion.

Clinical Pathology

Estimation of the cobalt or vitamin B_{12} content of the liver, as set down under necropsy findings, is the most valuable diagnostic test available. All tests suffer from the disadvantage that tissue cobalt levels will reflect the cobalt intake for a considerable time prior to the estimation and animals suffering from acute cobalt deficiency may be observed to have normal tissue levels of the element. Estimations of the cobalt content of soils and pasture have limited value because of the seasonal variations which occur (7).

Cobalt concentrations in the plasma of normal sheep are of the order of 1·0 ppm (1·0 to 3·0 μg. per 100 ml) and in deficient animals these are reduced to 0·2 to 0·8 ppm (7). Clinical signs of cobalt deficiency in sheep appear to be associated with serum vitamin B_{12} levels of less than 0·20 mg. per ml. (8). Although variable results are obtained, erythrocyte counts and estimations of haemoglobin and total blood volume may be useful aids to diagnosis. Affected animals are anaemic, but their haemoglobin and erythrocyte levels are often within the normal range because of an accompanying haemoconcentration. The anaemia is normocytic and normochromic. There is also a decrease in cellularity of the bone marrow in cobalt deficient sheep. It is not repaired by the administration of vitamin B_{12}, nor by the parenteral administration of cobalt (9).

Methylmalonic acid is ordinarily metabolized in ruminants by a vitamin B_{12} enzyme system. In a cobalt deficient animal the methylmalonic content of urine is abnormally high and this has some merit as a test for the presence of the deficiency. More work is required before the validity of the test is properly established (10, 3).

Necropsy Findings

At necropsy, emaciation is extreme. Heavy deposits of haemosiderin in the spleen, and to a less extent in the liver, cause pigmentation of these organs. Biochemical estimations reveal very high iron levels in the liver and spleen and low cobalt levels in the liver. In normal sheep cobalt levels in the liver are usually above 0·20 ppm DM and in affected sheep are less than 0·07 ppm DM (18), 0·05 ppm DM appearing to be the critical level. Normal levels of vitamin B_{12} in the liver are of the order of 0·3 ppm, falling to 0·1 ppm in deficient lambs (19). Comparable figures for cattle are: clinical signs occur with liver vitamin B_{12} levels of less than 0·1 μg. per g., and levels of more than 0·3 μg. per g. of liver are necessary for optimum growth (20). After oral dosing with cobalt the level of the element in the liver rises but returns to the pre-treatment level in 10 to 30 days.

Diagnosis

The chief difficulty encountered in the field is to differentiate the condition from other causes of 'illthrift' or 'enzootic marasmus'. In young animals, in which this situation is most often encountered, nutritional deficiencies of copper, selenium and vitamin D are possible causes but by far the most important cause is internal parasitism. Careful necropsy or faecal examination will determine the degree of worm infestation but cobalt-deficient animals are more susceptible to parasitism and the presence of a heavy parasite load should not rule out the diagnosis of primary cobalt deficiency (12). It is also common to have parasitic disease and cobalt deficiency occur together in the one animal. It is then necessary to make two diagnoses and conduct two control programmes. In sheep special care is needed to differentiate the disease from Johne's disease. The differential diagnosis of anaemia has been discussed elsewhere.

The response of animals to dietary supplementation with cobalt is generally accepted as a diagnostic test but laboratory analysis of tissues may be necessary to confirm the diagnosis, especially as ruminants with poor appetites due to many causes may show a marked response to dosing with cobalt.

Treatment

Affected animals respond satisfactorily to oral dosing with cobalt or the intramuscular injection of vitamin B_{12}. Oral dosing with vitamin B_{12} is effective but much larger doses are required. Oral dosing with cobalt sulphate is usually at the rate of about 1·0 mg. cobalt per day in sheep and can be given in accumulated doses at the end of each week. Intervals of two weeks between dosing are inadequate for the best possible response. On the other hand the monthly dosing of lambs with oral doses of 300 mg. of cobalt is sufficient to greatly reduce deaths and permit some growth at suboptimal levels (13). The response to dosing is very quick, significant elevation of serum vitamin B_{12} levels being evident within 24 hours. When large doses of cobalt are administered to some sheep, other undosed sheep on the same pasture may find sufficient additional cobalt on the pasture from the faeces of their flockmates to meet their needs (14). No exact data are available on dose rates for cattle but 10 times the prophylactic rate should be effective. Vitamin B_{12} should be given in 100 to 300 μg. doses for lambs and sheep at weekly intervals (12). Vitamin B_{12} therapy is not likely to be used generally because of the high cost and the comparable effect of oral cobalt administration.

Overdosing with cobalt compounds is unlikely but toxic signs of loss of weight, rough hair coat, listlessness, anorexia and muscular inco-ordination appear in calves at dose rates of about 40 to 55 mg. of elemental cobalt per 50 kg. body weight per day. Sheep appear to be much more resistant to the toxic effects of cobalt than are cattle (15).

Control

Cobalt deficiency in grazing animals can be prevented most easily by the top dressing of affected pasture with cobalt salts. The amount of top dressing required will vary with the degree of deficiency. Recommendations include 5 to 8 oz. cobalt sulphate per acre annually or 16 to 20 oz. per acre every 3 to 4 years. Supplementation of the diet with 0·1 mg. cobalt daily for sheep and 0·3 to 1·0 mg. cobalt daily for cattle should be aimed at and this can be accomplished by inclusion of the cobalt in salt or a mineral mixture.

The use of 'heavy pellets' containing 90 per cent cobalt oxide is an alternative means of overcoming the difficulty of maintaining an adequate cobalt intake in a deficient area. The pellet is in the form of a bolus (5 g. for sheep, 20 g. for cattle) which, when given by mouth, lodges in the reticulum and gives off cobalt continuously in very small but adequate amounts. Reports on their use in sheep and cattle indicate that they are effective (6, 16). Administration of the pellets to lambs and calves less than 2 months old is likely to be ineffective because of failure to retain them in the undeveloped reticulum. The problem of cobalt deficiency in sucking animals can be overcome in part if the dams are treated because of the increased vitamin B_{12} content of their milk (11), but the daily intake of the lambs will still be much below the minimal requirement. In about 5 per cent of animals the pellets do not lodge in the reticulum and approximately 20 per cent are rejected during the year after administration (17). If no response occurs retreatment is advisable. A further possible cause of failure is where pellets become coated with calcareous material, particularly if the drinking water is highly mineralized or if pasture top dressing is heavy. The effects of pellet coating can be overcome by simultaneous dosing with an abrasive metal pellet. The cost is relatively high and where top dressing of pastures is practised addition of cobalt to the fertilizer is the cheaper form of administration. Pellets are preferred in extensive range grazing where top dressing is impracticable and animals are seen only at infrequent intervals.

REVIEW LITERATURE

Robertson, W. W. (1971). *Vet. Rec.*, *89*, 5.

REFERENCES

(1) Pfander, W. H. *et al.* (1966). *Fed. Proc.*, *25*, 431.
(2) Lee, H. J. & Marston, H. R. (1969). *Aust. J. agric. Res.*, *20*, 905.
(3) Smith, R. M. & Marston, H. R. (1970). *Brit. J. Nutr.*, *24*, 615, 857.
(4) Marston, H. R. *et al.* (1961). *Nature* (*Lond.*), *190*, 1085.
(5) Bull, L. B. (1953). *Aust. vet. J.*, *29*, 2.
(6) Wessels, C. C. (1961). *J. S. Afr. vet. med. Ass.*, *32*, 289.
(7) Andrews, E. D. (1965). *N.Z. J. agric. Res.*, *8*, 788.
(8) Andrews, E. D. & Stephenson, B. J. (1966). *N.Z. J. agric. Res.*, *9*, 491.
(9) Ibbotson, R. N. *et al.* (1970). *Aust. J. exp. Biol. med. Sci.*, *48*, 161.
(10) Andrews, E. D. & Hogan, K. C. (1972). *N.Z. vet. J.*, *20*, 33.
(11) Skerman, K. D. & O'Halloran, M. W. (1962). *Aust. vet. J.*, *38*, 98.
(12) Andrews, E. D. *et al.* (1970). *N.Z. J. agric. Res.*, *13*, 950.
(13) Andrews, E. D. *et al.* (1966). *N.Z. vet. J.*, *14*, 191.
(14) Findlay, C. R. (1972). *Vet. Rec.*, *90*, 468.
(15) Andrews, E. D. (1965). *N.Z. vet. J.*, *13*, 101.
(16) Skerman, K. D. *et al.* (1961). *Aust. vet. J.*, *37*, 181.
(17) Millar, K. R. & Andrews, E. D. (1964). *N.Z. vet. J.*, *12*, 9.
(18) Russell, F. C. (1944). Minerals in pasture, deficiencies and excesses in relation to animal health. *Imp. Bur. Anim. Nutr. techn. Comm.*, 15.
(19) Andrews, E. D. & Hart, L. I. (1962). *N.Z. J. agric. Res.*, *5*, 403.
(20) Dewey, D. W. *et al.* (1969). *Aust. J. agric. Res.*, *20*, 1109.

Copper Deficiency

In ruminants a deficiency of copper causes interference with tissue oxidation resulting in a wide range of clinical manifestations including particularly those associated with anaemia and demyelination in the central nervous system.

Incidence

Copper deficiency causes diseases of economic importance in many parts of the world and may be sufficient to render large areas of otherwise fertile land unsuitable for grazing by ruminants. Although heavy mortalities occur in affected areas the major loss is due to failure of animals to thrive. Enzootic ataxia may affect up to 90 per cent of a lamb flock in badly affected areas and most of these lambs die of inanition. In falling disease up to 40 per cent of cattle in affected herds may die.

Aetiology

Copper deficiency may be primary, when the intake in the diet is inadequate, or secondary (conditioned) when the dietary intake is sufficient but the utilization of the copper by tissues is impeded. Apart from falling disease which occurs only in adult cattle, young animals are much more susceptible to primary copper deficiency than are adults. Calves on dams fed deficient diets may show signs at 2 to 3 months of age. As a rule the signs are severe in calves and yearlings, less severe in 2-year-olds and of minor degree in adults. Enzootic ataxia is primarily a disease of sucking lambs whose dams receive insufficient dietary copper. Ewes with a normal copper status take some time to lose their hepatic reserves of copper after transfer to copper-deficient pastures and do not produce affected lambs for the first 6 months. The occurrence of the disease in sucklings and its failure to appear after weaning point to the importance of foetal stores of copper and the inadequacy of milk as a source of copper. Milk is always a poor source of copper and when it is the sole source of nourishment the intake of copper will be low. Milk from normal ewes contains 0·2 to 0·6 mg. copper per litre but under conditions of severe copper deficiency this may be reduced to 0·01 to 0·02 mg. per litre (1).

Both primary and secondary copper deficiency occur most commonly in spring and summer coinciding with the time at which the copper content of the pasture is lowest. However, in some cases of secondary copper deficiency, the incidence may be highest at other times depending upon the concentration of the conditioning factor in the forage. For example the molybdenum content may be highest in the autumn when rains stimulate a heavy growth of legumes.

Occurrence

Primary copper deficiency. The amount of copper in the diet may be inadequate when the forage is grown on deficient soils or on soils in which the copper is unavailable. In general there are two types of soil on which copper-deficient plants are produced. Sandy soils, poor in organic matter and heavily weathered, such as occur on the coastal plains of Australia, and in marine and river silts, are likely to be absolutely deficient in copper as well as other trace elements, especially cobalt. The second important group of soils are 'peat' or muck soils reclaimed from swamps. These are the soils more commonly associated with copper deficiency in the U.S.A., New Zealand and Europe. Such soils may have an absolute deficiency of copper but more commonly the deficiency is relative in that the copper is not available and the plants growing on the soils do not contain adequate amounts of the element. The cause of the lack of availability of the copper is uncertain but is probably the formation of insoluble organic-copper complexes. An additional factor is the production of secondary copper deficiency on these soils due to their high content of molybdenum. A summary of the relevant levels of copper in soils and plants is given below.

For general purposes it may be assumed that pasture containing less than 3 ppm DM of copper will produce signs of deficiency in grazing ruminants. Levels of 3 to 5 ppm DM can be considered as dangerous and levels greater than 5 ppm DM (preferably 7 to 12) can be considered as safe unless complicating factors cause secondary copper deficiency. The extreme complexity of minimum copper requirements, affected as they are by numerous conditioning factors, necessitates examination under each particular set of circumstances.

The diseases caused by a primary deficiency of copper in ruminants are enzootic ataxia of sheep in Australia, New Zealand and the U.S.A., licking sickness, or liksucht of cattle in Holland, and falling disease of cattle in Australia. In pigs copper deficiency may cause anaemia in sucking pigs and on experimental diets an unusual abnormality of the limbs, characterized by lack of rigidity in the joints has been observed. Adult horses are unaffected but there have been reports of abnormalities of the limbs and joints of foals reared in copper deficient areas.

A concurrent deficiency of both copper and cobalt occurs in Australia (coast disease) and Florida, U.S.A. (salt sickness) and is characterized by the appearance of clinical signs of both deficiencies. All species of ruminants are affected. The disease is controlled by supplementation of the diet with copper and cobalt as set out under those specific headings.

Secondary copper deficiency. There are many disease states in ruminants in which clinical signs are caused by a deficiency of copper in tissues and in which the administration of copper is preventive and curative but in which the copper intake in the diet appears to be adequate. Such secondary copper

Copper Levels of Soils and Plants in Primary and Secondary Copper Deficiency

	Area	Soil Type	Soil Copper, ppm	Plant Copper, ppm, DM
Normal	—	—	18–22	11
Primary copper deficiency	West Aust.	Various	1–2	3–5
	New Zealand	Sand	0·1–1·6	3
	New Zealand	Peat	—	3
	Holland	Sand	—	< 3
Secondary copper deficiency	New Zealand	Peat	5	7
	Britain	Peat	—	7–20
	Britain	Limestone	—	12–27
	Britain	Stiff clay	—	11
	Holland	Sand	—	> 5
	Canada	Burned-over peat	20–60	10–25

deficiencies are summarized in the table below. The conditioning factor is known only in some instances, a dietary excess of molybdenum being most frequently incriminated. A high molybdenum intake can induce copper deficiency even when the copper content of the pasture is quite high, and a higher copper intake can overcome the effect of the molybdenum. Conversely, supplementation of the diet with molybdenum can be used to counteract the copper intake when its content in the diet is dangerously high. There are species differences in response to high copper and molybdenum intake; sheep are much more susceptible to copper poisoning, cattle to excess molybdenum (2).

Dietary inorganic sulphate in combination with molybdenum has a profound effect on the uptake of copper by ruminants. For example, an increase of sulphate concentration in a sheep diet from 0·1 to 0·4 per cent can potentiate a molybdenum content as low as 2·0 ppm to reduce copper intake below normal levels (22).

In general terms pastures containing less than 3 ppm DM of molybdenum are considered to be safe, but clinical signs may occur at 3 to 10 ppm if the copper intake is low. Pastures containing more than 10 ppm of molybdenum are dangerous unless the diet is supplemented with copper. And excess molybdenum may occur in soils up to levels of 10 and even 100 ppm. Perhaps more dangerous is the risk that over-zealous application of molybdenum to pasture to increase bacterial nitrogen fixation may have similar effects which are likely to be long lasting.

Swayback of lambs has been classed as a secondary copper deficiency but no conditioning factor has been determined. Lead has been suggested in this connection and does appear to reduce blood and liver concentrations of copper (3), but seems to have little effect on the incidence of swayback in the U.K. Recent work on swayback suggests that the naturally occurring disease is caused by a primary deficiency of copper but identical lesions are produced experimentally by feeding molybdenum and sulphate to the ewes (4). There is some evidence that heavy lime dressing of a pasture may predispose to swayback (23). Similar clinical and histopathological changes to those of enzootic ataxia of lambs have been observed in pigs with low levels of copper in their livers (5). A wasting disease similar to peat scours and preventable by the administration of copper, and pine of calves occur in the U.K. but in both instances the copper and molybdenum intakes are normal. Molybdenum appears to be the conditioning agent in enzootic ataxia in the U.S.A. A dietary excess of molybdenum is known to be the conditioning factor in the diarrhoeic diseases, peat scours in New Zealand, California and Canada, and teart in Britain.

Heavily limed pastures are often associated with a less than normal copper intake and a low copper status of sheep grazing them (6).

Pathogenesis

Primary copper deficiency. Copper plays an important role in tissue oxidation either by supplementing cytochrome-oxidase systems or entering into their formation. The pathogenesis of most of the lesions of copper deficiency has been explained in terms of faulty tissue oxidation because of failure of these enzyme systems (7). This role is exemplified in the early stages of copper deficiency by the changes in the wool of sheep. The straightness and stringiness of this wool is due to inadequate keratinization due probably to imperfect oxidation of free thiol groups. Provision of copper to such sheep is followed by oxidation of these free thiol groups and a return to normal keratinization within a few hours. In the later stages the impairment of tissue oxidation causes interference with intermediary metabolism and loss of condition or failure to grow. The known importance of copper

Secondary Copper Deficiency States

Disease	Country	Species Affected	Copper Level in Liver	Probable Conditioning Factor
Swayback	Britain, U.S.A.	Sheep	Low	Unknown
Renguerra	Peru	Sheep	Low	Unknown
Teart	Britain	Sheep and cattle	Unknown	Molybdenum
Scouring Disease	Holland	Cattle	Unknown	Unknown
Peat Scours	New Zealand	Cattle	Low	Molybdenum
Peat Scours	Britain	Cattle	Unknown, low level in blood	Unknown
Peat Scours	Canada	Cattle	Unknown	Molybdenum
Salt Sick	Florida, U.S.A.	Cattle	Unknown	Unknown
Pine	Scotland	Calves	Low	Unknown

in the formation of haemoglobin accounts for the anaemia that occurs in deficient animals. In view of the heavy haemosiderin deposits in tissues of copper-deficient animals, it is probable that copper is necessary for the re-utilization of iron liberated from the normal breakdown of haemoglobin. There is no evidence of excessive haemolysis in copper-deficiency states. Anaemia is common in primary copper deficiency but is not marked in the secondary form unless there is a marginal copper deficiency as occurs in peat scours in New Zealand. The osteoporosis which occurs in some cases of copper deficiency is caused by the depression of osteoblastic activity (8).

The myocardial degeneration of falling disease may be a terminal manifestation of anaemic anoxia or be due to interference with tissue oxidation. In this disease it is thought that the stress of calving and lactation contribute to the development of heart block and ventricular fibrillation when there has already been considerable decrease in cardiac reserve.

The mechanism by which copper deficiency halts the formation of myelin and causes demyelination in lambs has not been established although it appears probable that there is a specific relationship between copper and the maintenance of myelin sheaths. In experimental animals it has been shown that copper deficiency does interfere with synthesis of phospholipids (7). While anoxia is a cause of demyelination and an anaemic anoxia is likely to occur in highly deficient ewes, and anaemic ewes do produce a higher proportion of lambs with extreme ataxia, there is often no anaemia in ewes producing lambs with the more common subacute form of the disease. Experimentally produced copper deficiency has also caused sudden death due to rupture of the heart and great vessels in a high proportion of pigs fed a copper-deficient diet (20). The basic defect is degeneration of the internal elastic laminae (9). There is no record of a similar, naturally occurring disease.

A similar relationship appears to have been established between serum copper levels and fatal rupture of the uterine artery at parturition in aged mares (10).

Secondary copper deficiency. Molybdenum has been shown to interfere with copper metabolism, a high molybdenum intake reducing copper storage and utilization. This effect also operates in the foetus and interferes with copper storage in the foetal liver. The means by which molybdenum controls copper storage and the means by which

sulphate potentiates this control are unknown. However, it is known that clinical signs of hypocuprosis (viz. steely wool) can occur in sheep on diets containing high levels of molybdenum and sulphate even though blood copper levels are high. This suggests that under these circumstances copper is not utilizable in tissues and the blood copper rises in response to the physiological needs of the tissues for the element. Work with pigs has shown that a copper–molybdenum complex can exist in animals and that in this form the copper is unavailable (11). This would interfere with hepatic metabolism of copper and the formation of copper–protein complexes such as caeruloplasmin (12). Besides the relationship with molybdenum an interaction between the absorption of copper and selenium has been demonstrated, the administration of selenium to sheep on copper deficient pastures causing an improvement in copper absorption (13).

Clinical Findings

The general effects of copper deficiency are the same in sheep and cattle but in addition to these general signs there are specific syndromes more or less restricted to species and to areas.

Primary Copper Deficiency

Cattle. Primary copper deficiency causes unthriftiness, loss of milk production, anaemia and temporary infertility in adult cattle. The coat colour is affected, red and black cattle changing to a bleached, rusty red, and the coat itself becomes rough and staring. Calves grow poorly, and there is an increased tendency for bones to fracture, particularly the limb bones including the scapulae. In some cases ataxia develops after exercise, there being a sudden loss of control of the hind limbs with the animal falling or subsiding into a sitting posture. Normal control returns after rest. Itching and hair-licking is also recorded as a manifestation of copper deficiency in cattle (14).

In areas of severe copper deficiency sudden death due to acute heart failure (falling disease) may occur in adult cattle. Although diarrhoea occurs, persistent scouring is not characteristic of primary copper deficiency. In some affected areas calves have been observed to develop stiffness and enlargement of the joints and contraction of the flexor tendons causing the affected animals to stand on their toes. These signs may be present at birth or occur before weaning (1). Paresis and inco-ordination are not evident.

Sheep. Abnormalities of the wool are the first observed signs and may be the only sign in areas of marginal copper deficiency. Fine wool becomes limp and glossy and loses its crimp, developing a straight, steely appearance. Black wool shows depigmentation to grey or white, often in bands coinciding with the seasonal occurrence of copper deficiency. The straight, steely defect may occur in similar bands and the staple may break easily. There appear to be some differences between breeds in susceptibility to copper deficiency, merino sheep appearing to have a higher copper requirement than mutton sheep. The fleece abnormalities of merino sheep in Australia have not been observed in Romney Marsh sheep in copper-deficient areas in New Zealand but this may be due in part to the difficulty of detecting abnormality in wool which is normally rather straight and steely. Anaemia, scouring and unthriftiness may occur in conditions of extreme deficiency but in sheep the characteristic findings are in the lamb, the disease enzootic ataxia being the major manifestation. Osteoporosis with increased tendency of the long bones to fracture has also been recorded under conditions of copper deficiency insufficient to cause enzootic ataxia.

Other species. Enzootic ataxia is recorded rarely in goat kids (15) and is suspected to occur in red deer (16). Adult horses appear to be unaffected by copper deficiency but there are unconfirmed reports of abnormalities of limbs in foals. Foals in copper-deficient areas have been observed to be unthrifty and slow growing, with stiffness of the limbs and enlargement of the joints. Contraction of the flexor tendons causes the animal to stand on its toes. There is no ataxia or indication of involvement of the central nervous system. Signs may be present at birth or develop before weaning. Recovery occurs slowly after weaning and foals are unthrifty for up to 2 years.

Anaemia in young, growing pigs, which responded to treatment with copper has been observed to occur naturally and anaemia has been produced experimentally in young pigs by the feeding of diets deficient in copper. In experimentally produced cases there are abnormalities of the limbs, with lack of rigidity of joints and excessive flexion of the hocks, leading to the adoption of a sitting posture. The forelegs show varying types and degrees of crookedness. In extreme cases the use of the forelimbs is lost and the animal is recumbent. These abnormalities also respond to treatment with copper. Attempts to produce congenital copper deficiency syndromes in baby pigs have been unsuccessful although hypocuprosis is produced easily enough (17).

There is evidence that the addition of copper sulphate to the rations of fattening pigs improves the efficiency of food utilization and the rate of gain, particularly in the early post-weaning period. The amount used (150 to 250 ppm of copper in the ration) is greatly in excess of the accepted copper requirement of pigs and the mechanism by which growth is stimulated is unknown. In this connection copper appears to be more effective with low protein diets.

Secondary copper deficiency. The syndromes caused by secondary copper deficiency include the signs of primary copper deficiency except that anaemia occurs less commonly. This is probably due to the relatively better copper status in the secondary state, anaemia being largely a terminal sign in primary copper deficiency. For example anaemia occurs in peat scours of cattle in New Zealand but in this instance the copper intake is marginal. In addition to the other signs, however, there is a general tendency for scouring to occur, particularly in cattle. Because scouring is not a major sign in primary copper deficiency it is possible that it is due to the conditioning factor which reduces the availability of the copper. For example the severity of the scouring is roughly proportional to the level of intake of molybdenum.

ENZOOTIC ATAXIA AND SWAYBACK OF LAMBS

Enzootic ataxia affects only unweaned lambs. In severe outbreaks the lambs may be affected at birth but most cases occur in the 1 to 2 months age group. The severity of the paresis decreases with increasing age at onset. Lambs affected at birth or within the first month usually die within 3 to 4 days. The disease in older lambs may last for 3 to 4 weeks and survival is more likely, although surviving lambs always show some ataxia and atrophy of the hind quarters.

The first sign in enzootic ataxia is inco-ordination of the hind limbs appearing when the lambs are driven. Respiratory and cardiac rates are also greatly accelerated by exertion. As the disease progresses the inco-ordination becomes more severe and may be apparent after walking only a few yards. There is excessive flexion of joints, knuckling over of the fetlocks, wobbling of the hind-quarters and finally falling. The hind legs are affected first and the lamb may be able to drag itself about in a sitting posture. When the forelegs eventually become involved recumbency persists and the lamb dies of inanition. There is no true paralysis, the lamb being able to kick vigorously even in the recumbent stage. The appetite remains unaffected.

In swayback the lambs are affected at birth or in the first few weeks of life. They may be born dead, or weak and unable to stand and suck. Inco-ordination and erratic movements are more evident than in enzootic ataxia and the paralysis is spastic in type. Blindness also occurs occasionally. In the U.K. swayback is the only authentic manifestation of a primary nutritional deficiency of copper in sheep (18) but there is also a suggestion that a predisposition to swayback is inherited (19).

The few recorded cases of enzootic ataxia in pigs have occurred in growing pigs 4 to 6 months old. Posterior paresis progressed to complete paralysis in 1 to 3 weeks (5). Dosing with copper salts had no effect on the clinical condition but hepatic copper levels were 3 to 14 ppm.

FALLING DISEASE OF CATTLE

The characteristic behaviour in falling disease is for cows in apparently normal health to throw up their heads, bellow and fall. Death is instantaneous in most cases but some fall and struggle feebly on their sides for a few minutes with intermittent bellowing and running movements and attempts to rise. Rare cases show signs for up to 24 hours or more. These animals periodically lower their heads and pivot on the front legs. Sudden death usually occurs during one of these episodes.

PEAT SCOURS AND TEART OF CATTLE AND SHEEP

Persistent diarrhoea with the passage of watery, yellow-green to black faeces with an inoffensive odour occurs soon after the cattle go on to affected pasture, in some cases within 8 to 10 days. The faeces are released without effort, often without lifting the tail. Severe debilitation results although the appetite remains good. The hair coat is rough and depigmentation is manifested by reddening or grey flecking, especially around the eyes, in black cattle. The degree of abnormality varies a great deal from season to season and year to year and spontaneous recovery is common.

PINE OF CALVES

The earliest sign in pine of calves is a stilted gait, affecting particularly the hind limbs. Progressive emaciation follows, sometimes terminating fatally after 4 to 5 months. Greyness of the hair, especially around the eyes in black cattle, is apparent. Diarrhoea occurs in a few cases. Temporary infertility in adult cattle and swayback in lambs occur in the same area. Only young animals are affected and there is no anaemia. Skeletal lesions are absent and there is no apparent explanation of the abnormal gait.

Clinical Pathology

Anaemia is constant in advanced cases of primary copper deficiency, haemoglobin levels being depressed to 5 to 8 g. per cent and erythrocytes to 2 to 4 million per cmm. The levels of calcium and phosphorus in the blood are usually normal in spite of the increased tendency of bones to fracture. Estimations of copper in liver and blood may be of diagnostic value but should be interpreted with caution since clinical signs of copper deficiency may appear before there are significant changes in the levels of copper in the blood and liver. When liver biopsy samples are used specimens should be collected from at least 6 representative animals in the group. In general the levels are lower in the primary condition (see table below). Of the two estimations, that on liver is the most informative as

Levels of Copper in Body Tissues and Fluids

Species	Tissue	Normal Level	Primary Copper Deficiency	Secondary Copper Deficiency
SHEEP	Blood (mg. Cu per cent).	0·07 to 0·13	0·01 to 0·02	0·04 to 0·07
	Adult Liver (ppm DM).	More than 200 (usually 350+).	20	15 to 19
CATTLE	Blood (mg. Cu per cent).	0·07 to 0·17	0·01 to 0·02	0·05
	Adult Liver (ppm DM).	More than 100 (usually 200).	2 to 5	12
	Milk* (mg. per litre).	0·05 to 0·20	0·01 to 0·02	—
	Hair (ppm).	6·6 to 10·4	1·8 to 3·4	5·5

* Similar levels are found in ewes' milk.

levels in blood may remain normal for long periods after liver copper levels commence to fall and early signs of copper deficiency appear. Levels of copper in adult liver above 200 ppm DM in sheep, and above 100 ppm DM in cattle are usually considered to be normal. Levels of less than 80 ppm DM in sheep and less than 30 ppm DM in cattle are classed as low. In sheep blood levels of less than 0·07 mg. per cent are usually accompanied by significantly low liver levels (<25 ppm) but levels higher than this in the blood do not necessarily reflect levels in the liver. The levels of copper in milk and hair are also lower in deficient than in normal cattle. The levels in bovine hair are more markedly depressed when extra molybdenum is fed. It is necessary to be especially careful when collecting specimens for copper analysis to avoid contamination by needles, copper distilled water, vial caps, tins for liver specimens and so on.

The difficulty of getting uncontaminated samples, and of estimating blood copper levels, has led to an increasing dependence on the estimation of plasma levels of copper–protein complexes especially caeruloplasmin. Although it is possible to encounter low plasma caeruloplasmin levels which are due to a protein-losing enteropathy rather than a primary or secondary copper deficiency, the estimation can be used as a screening test. If it is subsequently supported by a liver biopsy or preferably autopsy examination of the whole organ, errors can be minimized and real copper deficiencies identified. Normal blood caeruloplasmin levels in sheep are in the region of 4·5 to 10 mg. per 100 ml. and the total plasma copper levels about 100 to 150 µg. per 100 ml. (24).

Necropsy Findings

The characteristic findings in copper deficiency are those of anaemia and emaciation. Extensive deposits of haemosiderin can be found in the liver, spleen and kidney in most cases of primary copper deficiency and in the secondary form if the copper status is sufficiently low. In cattle the bones appear normal in spite of the predisposition to fractures but in lambs there may be severe osteoporosis. In animals which have shown severe diarrhoea there are no obvious lesions in the alimentary tract. Necropsy examinations should include assay of copper in viscera. The levels of copper in liver are usually low (see table above) and in secondary copper deficiency there may be a high level of copper in the kidney and high levels of molybdenum in the liver, kidney and spleen.

The most significant finding in enzootic ataxia is demyelination of cerebellar tracts and the tracts of Lissauer in the spinal cord. In a few extreme cases and in most cases of swayback the demyelination also involves the cerebrum and there is destruction and cavitation of the white matter. There is marked internal hydrocephalus in these cases, the cerebrospinal fluid is increased in quantity and the convolutions of the cerebrum are almost obliterated. Acute cerebral oedema with marked brain swelling and cerebellar herniation, reminiscent of polioencephalomalacia, has been observed in lambs with hypocuprosis and the more typical lesions of nervous tissue (21). Although there is no anaemia in affected lambs haemosiderosis of the liver and pancreas may be observed.

In falling disease the heart is flabby and pale and on histological examination there is atrophy of the muscle fibres and considerable replacement with fibrous tissue. Venous congestion is marked and the liver and spleen are enlarged and dark. Deposits of haemosiderin are present in the liver, spleen and kidney and there is some glomerular destruction. Congestion of the abomasal and intestinal muscosae is evident.

Diagnosis

Field diagnosis depends on recognition of distinctive signs of copper deficiency and clinical response to treatment with copper. In contrast to supplementation with cobalt there is little improvement in most cases in the body weight of copper-deficient animals after supplementation. Depigmentation of hair and steeliness of wool are probably the most sensitive indicators of deficiency. Laboratory confirmation may be obtained by estimation of the copper content of tissues and body fluids, and of the diet. When the copper deficiency appears to be secondary, estimation of the content of molybdenum and inorganic sulphate in the feed and the molybdenum content of tissues, will aid in determining the aetiological significance of these substances. In specific instances such as enzootic ataxia, swayback and falling disease, histological evidence may assist in establishing the diagnosis.

Confusion may arise in differentiating the general syndrome of copper deficiency from that caused by internal parasitism. The general signs of scouring, emaciation and anaemia are common to both diseases which may also coexist. The response to the addition of copper to the ration is an adequate field test although a faecal examination for helminth eggs, or preferably a total worm count, should always be carried out.

Enzootic ataxia and swayback of lambs are seldom confused with other diseases because of their restricted occurrence in young lambs although cerebellar agenesis and poisoning by pea-vine ensilage cause similar syndromes in this age group. White muscle disease of lambs is characterized by typical lesions of muscular dystrophy.

Peat scours in cattle resembles Johne's disease but usually affects a much larger proportion of a group, with growing animals being more severely affected. Winter dysentery of cattle, salmonellosis, coccidiosis and mucosal disease are acute diseases characterized by diarrhoea but are accompanied by other signs and clinico-pathological findings which facilitate their identification. Many poisons, particularly arsenic, lead and salt, cause scouring in ruminants but there are usually additional diagnostic signs and evidence of access to the poison. Assay of feed and tissues helps to confirm a diagnosis of poisoning. A diagnosis of peat scours is usually made if there is an immediate response to oral dosing with a copper salt.

Falling disease occurs only in adult cattle whilst enzootic muscular dystrophy affects chiefly young calves. Poisoning by the gidgee tree (*Acacia georgina*) produces a similar syndrome in cattle.

Treatment

The treatment of copper deficiency is relatively simple but if advanced lesions are already present in the nervous system or myocardium complete recovery will not occur. Oral dosing with 4 g. of copper sulphate to cattle or 1·5 g. to sheep causes rapid disappearance of signs. Repetition of the treatment at weekly intervals is necessary to prevent recurrence. Parenteral administration of copper (e.g. 0·75 to 1 g. of copper sulphate in a dilute solution by intravenous injection to cattle) has the advantage that less frequent dosing is required but the injection is not without risk and should be given slowly.

Control

Copper can be supplied to livestock in several ways as outlined below. The dose rates given are those recommended for the control of primary copper deficiency and these may have to be increased or treatment given more frequently in some instances of secondary copper deficiency. In these circumstances it is often necessary to determine the most satisfactory procedure by trial and error.

Oral dosing with copper sulphate (4·0 g. to cattle, 1·5 g. to sheep weekly) is adequate as prophylaxis and will prevent the occurrence of ataxic lambs if the ewes are dosed throughout pregnancy. Lambs can be protected after birth by twice-weekly dosing with 35 mg. of copper sulphate.

Mineral mixtures or salt licks containing 0·25 to 0·5 per cent of copper sulphate for sheep and 2 per cent for cattle will supply sufficient copper provided an adequate intake of the mixture is assured. Iron preparations administered orally to pigs to prevent anaemia usually contain adequate amounts of copper.

In some deficient areas an effective method of administering copper is by the annual top dressing of pasture with 5 lb. copper sulphate per acre although the amount required may vary widely with the soil type and the rainfall. Top dressing may cause copper poisoning if livestock are turned onto pasture while the copper salt is still adherent to the leaves. Treated pasture should be left unstocked for 3 weeks or until the first heavy rain. It is also possible that chronic copper poisoning may result if the copper status of the soil increases sufficiently over a number of years.

Addition of copper salts to drinking water is usually impractical because the solution corrodes metal piping, and maintenance of the correct concentration of copper in large bodies of water is impracticable.

To overcome the difficulty of frequent individual dosing or top dressing of pasture, periodic parenteral injections of copper compounds which release copper gradually have given good results. Copper calcium ethylene diamine tetraacetate, copper amino-acetate or copper glycinate in a sterile cerate mixed with oil are suitable for use in cattle and sheep. The dose of copper in any of the compounds for cattle is 400 mg. and for sheep 150 mg. and one injection is thought to be sufficient to provide protection for about a year in sheep. The first-named preparation has the advantage of giving maximum copper storage very quickly—one week after injection and blood levels are elevated within a few hours (21). Young cattle probably require injections every 4 months and adult cattle at 6-month intervals. A marked local reaction occurs at the site of injection so that subcutaneous injection is preferable in animals to be used for meat although to avoid an unsightly blemish, breeding animals should receive an intramuscular injection. There may be some danger of precipitating blackleg in cattle on farms where this disease occurs. For sheep a single injection of 45 mg. of copper as copper glycinate in mid-pregnancy is sufficient to prevent swayback in the lambs. Subcutaneous injection is preferred in sheep, and to avoid the local reaction which occurs with the glycinate, an aqueous solution of a chelated copper compound (cupric-bis-8-hydroxyquinoline 5–7 disulphonic acid salt of tetra diethylamine) to give 30 mg. of copper is recommended. Some extensive mortalities have occurred in lambs (21) and calves after the parenteral injection of copper salts but the cause has not been determined.

As a final criterion it can be assumed that an intake of copper equivalent to 10 ppm DM of the diet will prevent the occurrence of primary copper deficiency in both sheep and cattle.

REFERENCES

(1) Bennets, H. W. & Beck, A. B. (1942). *Cwlth Aust. Counc. sci. ind. Res. Bull.*, 147.
(2) Pope, A. L. (1971). *J. Anim. Sci.*, *33*, 1332.
(3) Hemingway, R. G. *et al.* (1964). *Res. vet. Sci.*, *5*, 7.
(4) Fell, B. F. *et al.* (1961). *Proc. nutr. Soc.*, *20*, 27.
(5) McGavin, M. D. *et al.* (1962). *Aust. vet. J.*, *38*, 8.
(6) Macpherson, A. & Hemingway, R. G. (1968). *J. Sci. Fd Agric.*, *19*, 53.
(7) Gallagher, C. H. (1957). *Aust. vet. J.*, *33*, 311.
(8) Suttle, N. F. *et al.* (1972). *J. comp. Path.*, *82*, 93.
(9) Waisman, J. & Carnes, W. H. (1967). *Amer. J. Path.*, *51*, 117.
(10) Stowe, H. D. (1968). *J. Nutr.*, *95*, 179.
(11) Dowdy, R. P. & Matrone, G. (1968). *J. Nutr.*, *95*, 191, 197.
(12) Marcilese, N. A. *et al.* (1969). *J. Nutr.*, *99*, 177.
(13) Thomson, G. G. & Lawson, B. M. (1970). *N.Z. vet. J.*, *18*, 79.
(14) Haaranen, S. (1965). *Nord. Vet.-Med.*, *17*, 36.
(15) Owen, E. C. *et al.* (1965). *J. comp. Path.*, *75*, 241.
(16) Terlecki, S. *et al.* (1964). *Brit. vet. J.*, *120*, 311.
(17) Cancilla, P. A. *et al.* (1967). *J. Nutr.*, *93*, 438.
(18) Suttle, N. F. *et al.* (1970). *J. comp. Path.*, *80*, 151.
(19) Wiener, G. (1971). *J. comp. Path.*, *81*, 515.
(20) Waisman, J. *et al.* (1969). *Lab. Invest.*, *21*, 548.
(21) Ishmael, J. *et al.* (1971). *J. comp. Path.*, *81*, 455.
(22) Goodrich, R. D. & Tillman, A. D. (1966). *J. Nutr.*, *90*, 76.
(23) Kavanagh, P. J. *et al.* (1972). *Vet. Rec.*, *90*, 538.
(24) Srivastava, K. B. & Dwaraknath, P. K. (1971). *Ind. J. Anim. Sci.*, *41*, 471.

Iodine Deficiency

The cardinal sign of iodine deficiency is goitre. The major clinical manifestation is neonatal mortality, with alopecia and visible and palpable enlargement of the thyroid gland occurring in some animals.

Incidence

Iodine deficiency occurs in all of the continental land masses. It is not now of major economic importance because of the ease of recognition and correction but if neglected may cause heavy mortalities in newborn animals. The sporadic occurrence of the disease in marginal areas attracts most attention. All species including dogs, cats and humans are susceptible.

Aetiology

The iodine deficiency may be primarily due to deficient iodine intake or secondarily conditioned by a high intake of calcium, diets consisting largely of *Brassica* spp. or gross bacterial pollution of feedstuffs or drinking water. A continued intake of a low level of cyanogenetic glucosides is commonly associated with a high incidence of goitrous offspring. Linamarin, a glucoside in linseed meal is thought to be the agent producing goitre in newborn lambs from ewes fed the meal during pregnancy. Young animals are more likely to bear goitrous offspring than older ones and this may account for the apparent breed susceptibility of Dorset Horn sheep which mate at an earlier age than other breeds. An inherited tendency to goitre has been observed in certain strains of Merino sheep (1, 2), Boer goats (13) and Africander cattle (3).

Occurrence

A simple deficiency of iodine in diet and drinking water occurs and is related to geographical circumstances. Areas where the soil iodine is not replenished by cyclical accessions of oceanic iodine include large continental land masses and coastal areas where prevailing winds are off-shore. In such areas iodine deficiency is most likely to occur where rainfall is heavy and soil iodine is continually depleted by leaching. Soil formations rich in calcium or lacking in humus are also likely to be relatively deficient in iodine. The ability of soil to retain iodine under conditions of heavy rainfall is directly related to their humus content and limestone soils are in general low in organic matter. A high dietary intake of calcium also decreases intestinal absorption of iodine and in some areas heavy applications of lime to pasture are followed by the development of goitre in lambs. This factor may also be important in areas where drinking water is heavily mineralized.

Apart from these circumstances, there are a number of situations in which the relationship between iodine intake and the occurrence of goitre is not readily apparent. Goitre may occur on pasture which on analysis contains adequate iodine and is then usually ascribed to a secondary or conditioned iodine deficiency. The conditioning factors which produce secondary iodine deficiency have not been properly determined but there are some circumstances in which secondary iodine deficiency is known to occur. A diet rich in plants of the *Brassica* spp., including cabbages and brussels sprouts, may cause simple goitre and hypothyroidism in rabbits, which is preventable by administered iodine. Hypothyroidism has also been produced in rats by feeding rape seed and in mice by feeding rape seed oil meal. A heavy diet of kale to pregnant ewes causes a high incidence of goitre and hypothyroidism, also preventable by administered iodine in the newborn lambs (4). The goitrogenic substance in these plants is probably a thiocyanate (5). Some of these plants are excellent sources of feed, and in some areas it is probably economic to continue feeding them, provided suitable measures are taken to prevent goitre in the newborn. Although kale also causes mild goitre in weaned lambs this does not appear to reduce their rate of gain.

A diet high in linseed meal (20 per cent of ration) to pregnant ewes may also result in a high incidence of goitrous lambs, iodine or thyroxine being preventive in these circumstances (6). Under experimental conditions groundnuts are goitrogenic for rats, the goitrogenic substance being a glycoside—arachidoside. The goitrogenic effect is inhibited by supplementation of the diet with small amounts of iodine. Soyabean by-products are also considered to be goitrogenic. Gross bacterial contamination of drinking water by sewage is a cause of goitre in humans in countries where hygiene is poor. There is a record of a severe outbreak of goitrous calves from cattle running on pasture heavily dressed with crude sewage (7). Prophylactic dosing of the cows with potassium iodide prevented further cases.

Goitre in lambs may occur when permanent pasture is ploughed up and resown. This may be due to the sudden loss by decomposition and leaching of iodine-binding humus in soils of marginal iodine content. In subsequent years the disease may not appear. There may be some relation between this occurrence of goitre and the known variation in the iodine content of particular plant species especially if new pasture species are sown when the pasture is ploughed. The maximum iodine content of some plants is controlled by a strongly inherited factor and is independent of soil type or season. Thus, in the same pasture, perennial rye grass may contain 146 µg. iodine per 100 g. DM and Yorkshire fog grass only 7 µg. per 100 g. DM (8). Because goitre has occurred in lambs when the ewes are on a diet containing less than 30 µg. iodine per 100 g. DM the importance of particular plant species becomes apparent. A high incidence of goitre associated with heavy mortality has been observed in the newborn lambs of ewes grazing on pasture dominated by white clover (9) and by subterranean clover and perennial rye-grass (10).

Congenital goitre has been observed in foals born to mares fed an excessive amount of iodine during pregnancy (13).

Pathogenesis

Iodine deficiency results in a decreased production of thyroxine and stimulation of the secretion of thyrotropic hormone by the pituitary gland. This commonly results in hyperplasia of thyroid tissue and a considerable enlargement of the gland. Most cases of goitre of the newborn are of this type. The primary deficiency of thyroxine is responsible for the severe weakness and alopecia of the affected animals. A hyperplastic goitre is highly vascular and the gland can be felt to pulsate with the arterial pulse and a loud murmur may be audible over the gland. Colloid goitre is less common in animals and probably represents an involutional stage after primary hyperplasia.

Other factors, particularly the ingestion of low levels of cyanide, probably exert their effects by inhibiting the metabolic activity of the thyroid epithelium and restricting the uptake of iodine. Thiocyanates and sulphocyanates are formed during the process of detoxication of cyanide in the liver and these substances have a pronounced depressing effect on iodine uptake by the thyroid. Some pasture and fodder plants, including white clover, rape and kale are known to have a moderate content of cyanogenetic glucosides. These goitrogenic substances may appear in the milk and provide a toxic hazard to both animals and man. The inherited form in cattle appears to be due to the increased activity of an enzyme which de-iodinates iodotyrosines so rapidly that the formation of thyroxine is largely prevented.

Clinical Findings

Although loss of condition, decreased milk production and weakness might be anticipated these signs are not usually observed in adults. Loss of libido in the bull, failure to express oestrus in the cow and a high incidence of aborted, stillborn or weak calves have been suggested as manifestations of hypothyroidism in cattle whereas prolonged gestation is reported in mares (11), ewes and sows.

A high incidence of stillbirths and weak, newborn animals is the most common manifestation of iodine deficiency. Partial or complete alopecia, and palpable enlargement of the thyroid gland are other signs which occur with varying frequency in the different species. Foals show a normal hair coat and little thyroid enlargement but are very weak at birth. In most cases they are unable to stand without support and many are too weak to suck. Excessive flexion of the lower forelegs and extension of the lower parts of the hind legs have also been observed in affected foals. Enlargement of the thyroids also occurs commonly in adult horses in affected areas, thoroughbreds and light horses being more susceptible than draught animals.

In cattle the incidence of thyroid enlargement in adults is much lower than in horses and the cardinal manifestations are gross enlargement of the thyroid gland and weakness in newborn calves. If they are assisted to suck for a few days recovery is usual but if they are born on the range during inclement weather many will die. In some instances the thyroid gland is sufficiently large to cause obstruction to respiration. Partial alopecia is a rare accompaniment.

In pigs the major finding is the birth of hairless, stillborn or weak piglets often with myxoedema of the skin of the neck. Most affected piglets die within a few hours of birth. Thyroid enlargement may be present but is never sufficiently great to cause visible swelling in the live pig.

Adult sheep in iodine-deficient areas may show a high incidence of thyroid enlargement but are clinically normal in other respects. Newborn lambs manifest weakness, extensive alopecia and palpable, if not visible, enlargement of the thyroid glands. Goats present a similar clinical picture except that all abnormalities are more severe than in lambs.

Animals which survive the initial danger period after birth may recover except for partial persistence of the goitre. The glands may pulsate with the normal arterial pulse and may extend down a greater part of the neck and cause some local oedema. Auscultation and palpation of the jugular furrow may reveal the presence of a murmur and thrill, the 'thyroid thrill', due to the increased arterial blood supply of the glands.

Clinical Pathology

Estimations of iodine levels in the blood and milk are of considerable value in determining the thyroxine status of the animal. Organic or protein-bound iodine is estimated in serum or plasma and used as an index of circulating thyroid hormone provided access to exogenous iodine in the diet or as treatment is adequately controlled. There may be between-breed differences in blood iodine levels but levels of 2·4 to 4 μg. of protein-bound iodine per 100 ml. of plasma appear to be in the normal range. Blood cholesterol levels have been used as an indicator of thyroid function in humans but are not used in the investigation of goitre in animals.

In determining the iodine status of an area iodine levels in soil and pasture should be obtained but the relationship between these levels, and between them and the status of the grazing animal, may be complicated by conditioning factors.

Necropsy Findings

Macroscopic thyroid enlargement, alopecia and myxoedema may be evident. The weights of thyroid glands have diagnostic value. In full-term normal calves the average fresh weight is 6·5 g., in lambs 2·0 g. is average. The iodine content of the thyroid will also give some indication of the iodine status of the animal. At birth a level of 0·03 per cent of iodine on a fresh weight basis (0·1 per cent on dry weight) can be considered to be the critical level in cattle and sheep. On histological examination of the glands evidence of hyperplasia should be sought. Delayed osseous maturation, manifested by absence of centres of ossification, is also apparent in goitrous newborn lambs (10).

Diagnosis

Iodine deficiency is easily diagnosed if goitre is present but the occurrence of stillbirths without obvious goitre may be confusing. Abortion due to infectious agents in cattle and sheep must be considered in these circumstances. In stillbirths due to iodine deficiency gestation is usually prolonged beyond the normal period although this may be difficult to determine in animals bred at pasture. Inherited defects of thyroid hormone synthesis have already been noted.

Treatment

Treatment must be undertaken with care as overdosage will cause toxicity, the chief signs being anorexia and severe pityriasis. The recommendations for control can be adapted to the treatment of affected animals.

Control

Iodine can be provided as a fertilizer or in salt or a mineral mixture. The loss of iodine from salt blocks may be appreciable and an iodine preparation which is stable but which contains sufficient available iodine is required. Potassium iodate satisfies these requirements and should be provided as 5 oz. of potassium iodate per ton of salt. Potassium iodide alone is unsuitable but when mixed with calcium stearate (8 per cent of the stearate in potassium iodide) it is suitable for addition to salt—1 oz. to 300 lb. of salt.

Individual dosing of pregnant ewes, on two occasions during the fourth and fifth months of pregnancy, with 280 mg. potassium iodide or 370 mg. potassium iodate has been found to be effective in the prevention of goitre in lambs when the ewes are on a heavy diet of kale (4). For individual animals, weekly application of tincture of iodine (4 ml. cattle, 2 ml. pig and sheep) to the inside of the flank is also an effective preventive. The iodine can also be administered as an injection in poppy seed oil (containing 40 per cent bound iodine). One ml. given intramuscularly 7 to 9 weeks before lambing is sufficient to prevent severe goitre and neonatal mortality in the lambs. The gestation period is also reduced to normal. A similar injection 3 to 5 weeks before lambing is less efficient (12).

REFERENCES

(1) Falconer, I. R. (1966). *Biochem. J.*, *100*, 190.
(2) Rac, R. *et al.* (1968). *Res. vet. Sci.*, *9*, 209.
(3) Robbins, J. *et al.* (1966). *Endocrinology*, *68*, 1213.
(4) Sinclair, D. P. & Andrews, E. D. (1958). *N.Z. vet. J.*, *6*, 87.
(5) Wright, E. (1958). *Nature (Lond.)*, *181*, 1602.
(6) Care, A. D. (1954). *N.Z. J. Sci. Tech.*, *36*, 321.
(7) Jamieson, S. *et al.* (1945). *Vet. Rec.*, *57*, 429.
(8) Butler, G. W. & Johnson, J. M. (1957). *Nature (Lond.)*, *179*, 216.
(9) George, J. M. *et al.* (1966). *Aust. vet. J.*, *42*, 1.
(10) Setchell, B. P. *et al.* (1960). *Aust. vet. J.*, *36*, 159.
(11) Kalkus, J. W. (1920). A study of goitre and associated conditions in domestic animals, *State Coll. Wash. agric. exp. Sta. Bull.*, *156*, 1.
(12) Andrews, E. D. & Sinclair, D. P. (1962). *Proc. N.Z. Soc. Anim. Prod.*, *22*, 123.
(13) van Jaarsveld, P. *et al.* (1971). *J. S. Afr. vet. med. Ass.*, *42*, 295.

Iron Deficiency

A deficiency of iron in the diet causes anaemia and failure to thrive. It is most likely to occur in young piglets maintained under artificial conditions.

Incidence

More than one half of the iron in the animal body is found as a constituent of haemoglobin. A relatively small amount is found in myoglobin and in certain enzymes which play a part in oxygen utilization. Iron-deficiency states are rare in farm animals except in the very young confined to a milk diet. Sucking pigs are the only group in which the disease achieves economic importance and in some piggeries the incidence of the disease may be as high as 90 per cent. The losses that occur include those due to mortality, which may be high in untreated pigs, and to failure to thrive. Continued blood loss by haemorrhage in any animal may bring about a subclinical anaemia and an associated iron deficiency. Horses carrying heavy burdens of blood-sucking strongylid worms often have subnormal haemoglobin levels and respond to treatment with iron. On occasions veal calves, and possibly young lambs and kids, may also suffer from an iron deficiency.

Aetiology

Iron deficiency is usually primary and is most likely to occur in newborn animals whose sole source of iron is the milk of the dam, milk being a poor source of iron. Deposits of iron in the liver of the newborn are insufficient to maintain normal haemopoiesis for more than 2 or 3 weeks, and are particularly low in piglets.

Lack of access to the usual sources of iron may occur in veal calves reared intensively in crates on a milk or milk substitute diet but naturally occurring cases of anaemia have not been recorded in these circumstances. Asymptomatic iron deficiency anaemia also occurs in newborn calves and kids but there is debate as to whether the condition has practical significance (1). It is possible that suboptimal growth may occur during the period of physiological anaemia during early post-natal life. There is some evidence for this in calves in which haemoglobin levels of 11 g. per cent at birth fall to about 8 g. per cent between the 30th and 70th days and only begin to rise when the calves start to eat roughage. The daily intake of iron from milk is 2 to 4 mg. in calves and their daily requirement during the first 4 months of life is of the order of 50 mg. so that iron supplementation of the diet is advisable if the calves are fed entirely on milk. Even when hay and grain are fed to calves and lambs in addition to milk there is a marked growth response to the administration of iron-dextran preparations at the rate of 5·5 mg. per kg. body weight (2). The dietary iron requirement for fast-growing lambs is between 40 and 70 ppm and growth rate is sub-optimal on diets of less than 25 ppm iron (3).

The addition of calcium carbonate to the diet of weaned, fattening pigs is known to cause a conditioned iron deficiency and a moderate anaemia but this effect is not apparent in mature pigs. Manganese may exert a similar antagonistic effect.

Occurrence

Anaemia caused by iron deficiency occurs in those piglets confined in pens with concrete or other impervious floors and where the sole diet is the milk of the sow. The disease is of major importance in rearing units designed to control parasitic infestations, and in cold climates where indoor housing is essential. Access to earthen yards in most cases provides sufficient iron to overcome the deficiency in the sow's milk. On soils with an exceedingly low iron content the typical disease may occur (4, 5).

Signs may be present at birth but do not usually appear until the piglets are 3 to 6 weeks old. Considerable variation occurs in the incidence of cases between litters kept under identical conditions. Black pigs are more prone to the disease than white animals. There may be some difference in the age at which piglets begin to eat supplementary creep feed which may provide additional iron but under usual circumstances the amount of solid feed taken is not significant until about 5 weeks of age, by which time the disease may have already developed.

Pathogenesis

Piglets at birth have haemoglobin levels of about 9 to 11 g. per cent. A physiological fall to 4 to 5 g. per cent occurs in all pigs, the lowest levels occurring at about the 8th to 10th day of life. Levels of iron in the liver at birth are unusually low in this species and cannot be increased appreciably by supplementary feeding of the sow during pregnancy. The intramuscular injection of iron-dextran preparations to sows during late pregnancy does elevate the haemoglobin levels of the piglets during the first few weeks of life but not sufficiently to prevent anaemia in them (6). Piglets with access to iron show a gradual return to normal haemoglobin levels starting at about the 10th day of life but in pigs denied this access the haemoglobin levels continue to fall. One of the important factors in the high incidence of anaemia in piglets is the rapidity with which they grow in early post-natal life. The daily requirement of iron during the first few weeks of life is of the order of 15 mg. The average intake in the milk from the sow is about 1 mg. per day and the concentration in sow's milk cannot be elevated by feeding additional iron during pregnancy or lactation. Apart from the specific effect on haemoglobin levels, iron-deficient piglets consume less creep feed, and after the first 3 weeks of life make considerably slower weight gains than supplemented piglets. Although specific pathogen-free pigs show a less marked response to the administration of iron than pigs reared in the normal manner, it is obvious that they need supplementary iron to prevent the development of anaemia.

Clinical Findings

The highest incidence occurs at about 3 weeks of age although the disease can occur in pigs up to 10 weeks of age.

Affected pigs may be well grown and in good condition but the growth rate of anaemic pigs is significantly lower than that of normal pigs (8) and food intake is obviously reduced. Diarrhoea is very common, but the faeces are usually normal in colour and the diarrhoea usually stops spontaneously. The diarrhoea further reduces growth rate. Severe dyspnoea, lethargy and a marked increase in amplitude of the apex beat occur with exercise. The skin and mucosae are pale and often quite yellow in white pigs, and there may be oedema of the head and forequarters giving the animal a fat, puffed-up appearance. A lean, white, hairy look is probably more common. Death usually occurs suddenly, or affected animals may survive in a thin, unthrifty condition. A high incidence of infectious disease, especially enteric infection with *Escherichia coli* is associated with the anaemia and streptococcal pericarditis is a well recognized complication. Under experimental conditions similar signs occur in calves and there is, in addition, an apparent atrophy of the lingual papillae. A high incidence of stillbirths is recorded in the litters of sows suffering from iron-deficiency anaemia (5).

Clinical Pathology

Normal piglets show a post-natal fall of haemoglobin levels to about 8 g. per cent and sometimes to as low as 4 to 5 g. per cent during the first 10 days of life. In iron-deficient pigs there is a secondary fall to 2 to 4 g. per cent during the 3rd week. The haemoglobin level at which clinical signs appear in pigs is about 4 g. per cent (2). Erythrocyte levels also fall from a normal of 5 to 8 million down to 3 to 4 million per cmm. and are a better index of iron status than haemoglobin levels (8). Blood levels of iron considered to be normal in sheep and cattle are 100 to 200 μg. per 100 ml. In newborn calves the levels are 170 μg. per 100 ml. at birth and 67 μg. per 100 ml. at 50 days of age (7).

Necropsy Findings

The necropsy appearance is characterized by pallor, thin and watery blood, and moderate anasarca. The heart is always dilated, sometimes extremely so. The liver in all cases is enlarged, and has a mottled appearance and the greyish yellow colour of fatty infiltration. The mucosa of the gastric fundus in cases of the experimentally induced disease is characteristically shallower and less cellular and shows a pronounced decrease in parietal cells (8) and there is a greatly reduced capacity of the stomach to secrete acid.

Diagnosis

Confirmation of the diagnosis will depend upon haemoglobin determinations and curative and preventive trials with administered iron. The possibility that anaemia in piglets may be caused by copper deficiency should not be overlooked especially if the response to administered iron is poor. Iso-immunization haemolytic anaemia can be differentiated by the presence of jaundice and haemoglobinuria and the disease occurs in much younger pigs. Eperythrozoonosis occurs in pigs of all ages and the protozoan parasites can be detected in the erythrocytes.

Treatment

The recommendations for the prevention of the disease are set out below and can be followed when treating clinically affected animals.

Control

Preventive measures must be directed at the baby pigs because treatment of the sows before or after farrowing is generally ineffective, although some results are obtained if the iron preparations are fed at least two weeks before farrowing. Ferric choline citrate appears to have some special merit in this field (9). Allowing the suckers access to pasture or dirt yards, or periodically placing sods in indoor pens, offer adequate protection. Where indoor housing on impervious floors is necessary iron should be provided at the rate of 15 mg. per day until weaning either by oral dosing with iron salts of a commercial grade or the intramuscular injection of organic-iron preparations. These methods are satisfactory but the results are not usually as good as when piglets are raised outdoors. However, indoor housing is practised in many areas to avoid exposure to parasitic infestation and some bacterial diseases, especially erysipelas. If sods are put into pens care must be taken to ensure that these diseases are not introduced.

Oral dosing. Daily dosing with 4 ml. of 1·8 per cent solution of ferrous sulphate is adequate. Iron pyrophosphate may also be used (300 mg./day for 7 days). To overcome the necessity for daily dosing, several other methods of administering iron have been recommended. A single oral treatment with iron dextran has been recommended, provided an excellent creep feed is available (10) but the method seems unnecessarily expensive. Reduced iron (BVC) can be administered in larger doses because it does not cause irritation of the alimentary mucosa. A single dose of 0·5 to 1·0 g. once weekly is sufficient to prevent anaemia. Alternatively, the painting of a solution of ferrous sulphate on the sow's udder has been recommended (1 lb. ferrous sulphate, 2½ oz. copper sulphate, 1 lb. sugar, 2 litres water—applied daily) but has the disadvantage of being sticky and of accumulating litter. Excessive oral dosing with soluble iron salts may cause enteritis, diarrhoea and some deaths in pigs and high intakes of ferric hydroxide cause diarrhoea, loss of weight and low milk production in cattle (11). The presence of diarrhoea in a herd prevents absorption of orally-administered iron and treatment by injection is recommended in this circumstance.

Intramuscular injection of iron preparations. Suitable preparations must be used and are usually injected intramuscularly in pigs on one occasion only, on the 7th day of life. The dose rates should provide at least 100 mg. of elemental iron. Multiple injections give better haemoglobin levels but have not been shown to improve weight gains. Iron-dextran compounds are usually used and have very little toxicity even on repeated injection. These preparations are ideal for treatment because of the rapid response which they elicit and the absence of permanent discoloration of tissues after their use if given during the first month of life (12). Comparable doses have been used in the other species with excellent results. Slight local reactions may occur in the horse but are of little significance. Acute poisoning has occurred in large numbers of young pigs injected intramuscularly with certain organic iron preparations and this is discussed elsewhere.

REFERENCES

(1) Kolb, E. (1963). *Advanc. vet. Sci.*, *8*, 50.
(2) Carlson, R. H. *et al.* (1961). *J. Amer. vet. med. Ass.*, *139*, 457.
(3) Lawlor, M. J. *et al.* (1965). *J. Anim. Sci.*, *24*, 742.
(4) Venn, J. A. J. & Davies, E. T. (1965). *Vet. Rec.*, *77*, 1004.
(5) Moore, R. W. *et al.* (1965). *J. Amer. vet. med. Ass.*, *147*, 746.
(6) Pond, W. G. *et al.* (1961). *J. Anim. Sci.*, *20*, 747.
(7) Mollerberg, L. & Jacobsson, S. O. (1970). *Svensk Vet-Tidskr.*, *22*, 851.
(8) Hannan, J. (1971). *Vet. Rec.*, *88*, 181.
(9) Smithwick, G. A. *et al.* (1967). *Amer. J. vet. Res.*, *28*, 469.
(10) Blomgren, L. & Lannek, N. (1971). *Nord. Vet.-Med.*, *23*, 529.
(11) Coup, M. R. & Campbell, A. G. (1964). *N.Z. J. agric. Res.*, *7*, 624.
(12) Miller, E. R. *et al.* (1967). *J. Amer. vet. med. Ass.*, *150*, 735.

Sodium Chloride Deficiency

There is a lack of firm evidence that naturally occurring salt deficiency causes illness in grazing animals but it is also the consensus that it does occur in certain special circumstances. Of these the most commonly cited occurrences are on alpine pastures and heavily fertilized pasture leys. Pasture should contain at least 0·15 g. per 100 g. DM and animals begin to show signs after about one month on pasture containing 0·1 g. per 100 g. Milk yield falls first; craving for salt, licking dirt and each other's coats and drinking urine are other signs. Loss of appetite and weight are evident. Affected animals may develop salt poisoning if allowed unlimited access to it. Under experimental conditions lactating cows give less milk until the chloride deficiency is compensated. After a period of up to 12 months there is considerable deterioration in the animal's health and anorexia, a haggard appearance, lustreless eyes, rough coat and a rapid decline in body weight occur. Heavily producing animals are most severely affected and some of these may collapse and die. The oral administration of sodium chloride is both preventive and rapidly curative (1).

Good clinico-pathological evidence of deficiency is the level of sodium in the serum. The normal is 139 mEq/1. Licking begins when the level falls to 137 mEq/1 and signs are intense at 135 mEq/1.

In cattle a daily intake of 1·5 g. sodium and 5 g. chlorine is necessary for growth. For a mature cow giving 2 gallons of milk daily, a daily intake of 11 to 15 g. sodium and 14 to 23 g. chlorine is required. On normal daily dry matter intakes, the rations should contain for growth approximately 0·02 per cent sodium and 0·07 per cent chlorine, and for an adult cow producing 2 gallons of milk daily the rations should contain 0·15 per cent sodium and 0·19 per cent chlorine on a dry matter basis. Salt can be provided through salt-licks or in prepared feeds. A quick and easy method, which also tends to improve the palatability of the pasture, is to spray it with salt solution (14 lb. in 500 gal. per acre).

Experimentally induced sodium deficiency in young pigs causes anorexia, reduced water intake and reduced weight gains (2).

At one time it was suggested that salt deficiency was the cause of licking sickness, as it occurs in Europe, but this theory is no longer thought to be valid.

REFERENCES
(1) Russell, F. C. (1944). *Imp. Bur. anim. Nutr., tech. Comm.* No. 15, p. 56.
(2) Yusken, J. W. & Reber, E. F. (1957). *Trans. Ill. Acad. Sci.,* 50, 118.

Magnesium Deficiency

Although a nutritional deficiency of magnesium does play a part in causing lactation tetany in cows and hypomagnesaemic tetany of calves, these diseases are dealt with in the chapter on metabolic diseases (p. 702) because in both instances there are complicating factors which may affect the absorption and metabolism of the element.

Magnesium appears to be an essential constituent of rations for recently weaned pigs (1). Experimentally induced deficiency causes weakness of the pasterns, particularly in the forelegs causing backward bowing of the legs, sickled hocks, approximation of the knees and hocks, arching of the back, hyperirritability, muscle tremor, reluctance to stand, continual shifting of weight from limb to limb, and eventually tetany and death. A reduction in growth rate, feed consumption and conversion, and levels of magnesium in the serum also occur. The requirement of magnesium for pigs weaned at from 3 to 9 weeks of age is 400 to 500 ppm of the total ration.

REFERENCE
(1) Mayo, R. H. *et al.* (1959). *J. Anim. Sci., 18,* 264.

Zinc Deficiency
(*Parakeratosis of Swine*)

This is a chronic, afebrile, non-inflammatory disease affecting the epidermis and is characterized clinically by crusty proliferation and cracking of the skin.

Incidence

Recorded first in North America, the disease appears to have reached a level of incidence at which it assumes considerable economic importance in pigs. From 20 to 80 per cent of pigs in affected herds show lesions. The main economic loss is due to failure to put on weight since few animals die of the disease. In general the incidence is greater in pigs fed in dry lot or when pasture is not available. There are records of the natural disease in cattle and sheep and it has been produced experimentally in cattle, sheep and goats. A significant increase in rate of gain in feedlot steers after dietary supplementation has been reported (1) but there have been a number of negative trials.

The disease is well recognized in Europe, especially in calves (2). Naturally occurring cases are common in some families of cattle and an inherited increased requirement for zinc is suspected (3, 4).

Aetiology

The exact cause of parakeratosis in swine has not been determined although it is probably of nutritional origin because the disease occurs only in housed pigs fed on commercial rations. At least three factors which appear to play a part in the aetiology are an excess of calcium, a relative deficiency of zinc and a deficiency of unsaturated fatty acids in the diet. Diets high in calcium (0·5 to 1·5 per cent) and low in zinc (34 to 44 ppm) favour the appearance of the disease (5) and the addition of zinc to such diets at levels much higher (0·02 per cent zinc carbonate or 100 ppm zinc) than those normally required by animals prevents the occurrence of the disease. It has been suggested that parakeratosis occurs because very rapidly growing pigs outstrip their biosynthesis of essential fatty acids and, when the diet is high in calcium, the digestibility of fat in the ration is reduced at the same time. The net effect in rapidly growing pigs could be a relative deficiency of essential fatty acids (6). The level of copper in the ration seems to be of some significance, increased copper decreasing the requirement for zinc (7). Provision of a dietary supplement of soyabean oil containing 54 per cent linoleic acid prevents the development of the disease even when zinc supplementation is ineffective. The substitution of 20 per cent blood meal in a 'parakeratosis producing' ration has been shown to alleviate the skin lesions (22). It is postulated that this effect is related to its histidine content; blood meal is not a rich source of zinc.

The disease in cattle has been produced experimentally on diets low in zinc and naturally occurring cases have responded to supplementation of the diet with the element. Calves remain healthy on experimental diets containing 40 ppm zinc but parakeratosis has occurred in cattle grazing pastures with a zinc content of 20 to 80 ppm (normal 93 ppm) and a calcium content of 0·6 per cent (8). The suggestion that the natural disease may be caused by the immobilization of the zinc in the ration when it contains highly fibrous feeds is supported by the observation that phytic acid does interfere with the availability of zinc for swine. There is also an apparently improved response in cattle to zinc administration if copper is given simultaneously (9, 10). Parakeratosis has also been produced experimentally in goats (11) and sheep (12, 13). Clinical signs develop about 2 weeks after calves and lambs go onto a deficient diet so that there is no evident storage of zinc in tissues in these animals (14).

Occurrence

Parakeratosis occurs in rapidly growing pigs, particularly those fed on dry rations containing growth stimulants. The disease is most likely to occur during the period of most rapid growth, after weaning and between 7 and 10 weeks of age. The method of feeding is important. Self-feeding on dry feed is followed by more cases than occur with limited wet feeding twice daily. Pasture is preventive and curative.

Pathogenesis

Deficiency of unsaturated fatty acids is known to cause dermatitis whereas zinc deficiency or calcium excess are not known to affect skin metabolism. Experimental deficiency of essential fatty acids in pigs is characterized by a high incidence of skin lesions but they do not invariably occur. The typical histological lesion is impairment of the arteriolar walls (15). The cause of the depression of growth which is part of this disease is obscure.

Clinical Findings

Pigs. A reduced rate and efficiency of body weight gain is characteristic (14). Circumscribed areas of erythema appear in the skin on the ventral abdomen and inside the thigh. These areas develop into papules 3 to 5 mm. in diameter which are soon covered with scales followed by thick crusts. These crusts are most visible in areas about the limb joints, ears and tail, and are distributed symmetrically in all cases. The crusts develop fissures and cracks, become quite thick (5 to 7 mm.) and easily detached from the skin. They are crumbly and not flaky or scaly. No greasiness is present except in the depths of fissures. Little scratching or rubbing occurs. Diarrhoea of moderate degree is common. Secondary subcutaneous abscesses occur frequently but in uncomplicated cases the skin lesions disappear spontaneously in 10 to 45 days if the ration is corrected.

Ruminants. In the naturally occurring disease in cattle severe cases show parakeratosis and alopecia affecting about 40 per cent of the skin area. The lesions are most marked on the muzzle, vulva, anus, tail-head, ears, backs of the hind legs, the knee-folds, flank and neck. Most animals are below average condition and are stunted in growth. After treatment with zinc improvement is apparent in 1 week and complete in 3 weeks. Experimentally produced cases show poor growth, a stiff gait, swelling of the coronets, hocks and knees, soft swelling containing fluid on the anterior aspect of the hind fetlocks, alopecia and wrinkling of the skin of the legs and scrotum and on the neck and head, especially around the nostrils, haemorrhages around the teeth and ulcers on the dental pad (17). There is a marked delay in wound healing (18).

The natural disease in sheep is characterized by loss of wool and the development of thick, wrinkled skin. Induced cases in lambs have exhibited reduced growth rate, salivation, swollen hocks, wrinkled skin and open skin lesions around the hoof and eyes (11, 12, 13). The experimental disease in goats is similar to that in lambs.

One of the most striking effects of zinc deficiency in ram lambs is impaired testicular growth and complete cessation of spermatogenesis (16). Diets containing 2·44 ppm caused poor growth, impaired testicular growth and cessation of spermatogenesis and other signs of zinc deficiency within 20 to 24 weeks. A diet containing 17·4 ppm of zinc is adequate for growth but a content of 32·4 ppm is necessary for normal testicular development and spermatogenesis. On severely deficient experimental diets other clinical signs in young rams are drooling copious amounts of saliva when ruminating, parakeratosis around eyes, on nose, feet and scrotum, shedding of the hooves, dystrophy and shedding of wool, which showed severe staining, and development of a pungent odour.

Infertility in ewes and a dietary deficiency of zinc have not been officially linked but a zinc responsive infertility has been described in ewes. Again attention is drawn to the need for response trials when soil and pasture levels of an element are marginal (21).

Clinical Pathology

Laboratory examination of skin scrapings yields negative results but skin biopsy will confirm the diagnosis of parakeratosis. Serum-zinc levels may have diagnostic value. Normal levels are 80 to 120 µg. per 100 ml. in sheep and cattle. Calves and lambs on deficient diets may have levels as low as 18 µg. per cent. There is a general relationship between the zinc content of the hair and the level of zinc in the diet but until the various factors affecting the relationship are determined hair analysis must be used with caution (19). In the experimental disease in piglets there is a reduction in serum levels of zinc, calcium and alkaline phosphatase (20).

Necropsy Findings

Necropsy examinations are not usually performed but histological examination of skin biopsy sections reveals a marked increase in thickness of all the elements of the epidermis. Tissue levels of zinc differ between deficient and normal animals but the differences are statistical rather than diagnostic (19).

Diagnosis

Sarcoptic mange may resemble parakeratosis but is accompanied by much itching and rubbing. The parasites may be found in skin scrapings and treatment with appropriate parasiticides relieves the condition. Exudative epidermitis is quite similar in appearance but occurs chiefly in unweaned pigs. The lesions have a greasy character which is quite different from the dry, crumbly lesions of parakeratosis and the mortality rate is higher.

Treatment

The food intake of affected pigs should be reduced immediately and zinc added to the diet (0·02 per cent zinc carbonate). The injection of 1 to 2 mg. zinc per lb. body weight daily for 10 days is also effective (3). In cattle zinc sulphate (2 g. per week orally or 1 g. per week by injection) is an effective treatment.

Control

The calcium content of diets for growing pigs should be restricted to 0·5 to 0·6 per cent. However, rations containing as little as 0·5 per cent calcium and with normal zinc content (30 ppm) may produce the disease. Supplementation with zinc (to 50 ppm) as sulphate or carbonate has been found to be highly effective as a preventive and there appears to be a wide margin of safety in its use, diets containing 1000 ppm added zinc having no apparent toxic effect. The standard recommendation is to add 6½ oz. of zinc carbonate or sulphate to each ton of feed. Weight gains in affected groups are also appreciably increased by the addition of zinc to the diet. The addition of oils containing unsaturated fatty acids is also an effective preventive. Access to green pasture, reduction in food intake and the deletion of growth stimulants from rations will lessen the incidence of the disease but are not usually practicable.

For cattle the feeding of zinc sulphate (2 to 4 g. daily) is recommended as an emergency measure followed by the application of a zinc-containing fertilizer (8).

REFERENCES

(1) Beeson, W. M. *et al.* (1962). *Feedstuffs, 34,* 18, 54.
(2) van Adrichem, P. W. M. *et al.* (1970). *T. Diergeneesk., 95,* 1170.
(3) Brummerstedt, E. *et al.* (1971). *Acta path. vet. microbiol. scand., 79A,* 686.
(4) Stober, M. (1971). *Dtsch. tierärztl. Wschr., 78,* 257.
(5) Mills, C. F. & Dalgarno, A. C. (1967). *Proc. Nutr. Soc., 26,* xix.
(6) Hanson, L. J. *et al.* (1958). *Amer. J. vet. Res., 19,* 921.
(7) Ritchie, H. D. *et al.* (1963). *J. Nutr. Soc., 24,* 21.
(8) Grashuis, J. (1963). *Landbouwk. Tijdschr., 75,* 1127.
(9) Dynna, O. & Havre, G. N. (1963). *Acta vet. scand., 4,* 197.
(10) Haaranen, S. (1965). *Nord. Vet.-Med., 17,* 36.
(11) Miller, W. J. *et al.* (1964). *J. Dairy Sci., 47,* 556.
(12) Ott, E. A. *et al.* (1964). *J. Nutr., 82,* 41.

(13) Mills, C. F. *et al.* (1967). *Brit. J. Nutr.*, *21*, 751.
(14) Miller, E. R. *et al.* (1966). *Fed. Proc.*, *25*, 484.
(15) Hill, E. G. *et al.* (1957). *Proc. Soc. exp. Biol. Med.*, *95*, 274.
(16) Underwood, E. J. (1969). *Aust. J. agric. Res.*, *20*, 889.
(17) Ott, E. A. *et al.* (1965). *J. Anim. Sci.*, *24*, 735.
(18) Blackmon, D. M. *et al.* (1967). *Vet. Med.*, *62*, 265.
(19) Miller, W. J. *et al.* (1966). *J. Dairy Sci.*, *49*, 1446.
(20) Miller, E. R. *et al.* (1968). *J. Nutr.*, *95*, 278.
(21) Egan, A. R. (1972). *Aust. J. exp. Agric.*, *12*, 131.
(22) Dahmer, E. J. *et al.* (1972). *J. Anim. Sci.*, *35*, 1176, 1181.

Manganese Deficiency

There is no simple, single diagnostic test which permits detection of manganese deficiency in animals. Reproductive functions, male and female, are most sensitive to manganese deficiency and are affected before possible biochemical criteria, e.g. blood and bone alkaline phosphatase, liver arginase levels, are significantly changed. The only certain way of detecting moderate deficiency states is by measuring response to supplementation. Findings which may provide contributory evidence of manganese deficiency are set out below.

A primary soil deficiency is uncommon but can occur (1, 2, 3, 4). For example soils containing less than 3 ppm of manganese are unlikely to be able to support normal fertility in cattle (5). In areas where manganese responsive infertility occurs, soils on farms with infertility problems have contained less than 3 ppm of manganese, whereas soils on neighbouring farms with no infertility problems have had levels of more than 9 ppm. A secondary soil deficiency is thought to occur and one of the factors suspected of reducing the availability of manganese in the soil to plants is high alkalinity. Thus heavy liming is associated with manganese-responsive infertility. There are three main soil types on which the disease occurs:

(1) Soils low in manganese have low output even when pH is less than 5·5.
(2) Sandy soils where availability starts to fall at pH of 6·0.
(3) Heavy soils where availability starts to fall at pH of 7·0.

Many other factors are suggested as reducing the availability of soil manganese but the evidence is not conclusive.

Herbage on low manganese soils, or on marginal soils where availability is decreased (possibly even soils with normal manganese content), is low in manganese. A number of figures are given for critical levels. It is suggested (5) that pasture containing less than 80 ppm of manganese is incapable of supporting normal bovine fertility and that herbage containing less than 50 ppm is often associated with infertility and anoestrus. The Agricultural Research Council (7) feels that, although definite figures are not available, levels of 40 ppm in the diet should be adequate. Other authors state that rations containing less than 20 ppm may cause anoestrus and reduction in conception rates in cows (8, 9, 10) and the production of poor quality semen by bulls (24). Most pasture contains 50 to 100 ppm (11). Skeletal deformities in calves occur when the deficiency is much greater than the above; for example a diet containing more than 200 ppm is considered to be sufficient to prevent them (4).

There are important variations in the manganese content of seeds, an important matter in poultry nutrition (1). Maize and barley have the lowest content. Wheat or oats have 3 to 5 times as much, and bran and pollard are the richest natural sources with 10 to 20 times the content of maize or wheat. Cows' milk is exceptionally low in manganese.

Apart from a primary dietary deficiency of manganese the existence of factors which depress the availability of ingested manganese is suspected. An excess of calcium and/or phosphorus in the diet is known to increase the requirements of manganese in the diet of calves (12), and is considered to reduce the availability of dietary manganese to bovines generally (5).

Some years ago it was proposed that functional infertility occurred in cattle on diets with Ca:P ratios outside the range of 1:2 to 2:1 (8). This was not upheld on investigation but may have been correct if high Ca/P intakes directly reduced manganese (or copper or iodine) availability in diets marginally deficient in one or other of these elements.

Clinical Pathology

The blood of normal cattle contains 18 to 19 μg. per 100 ml. of manganese (13) although considerably lower levels are sometimes quoted (10). The livers of normal cattle contain 12 ppm of manganese and down to 8 ppm in newborn calves (14) which also have a lower content in hair. The manganese content of hair varies with intake. The normal level is about 12 ppm and infertility is observed in association with levels of less than 8 ppm (14). In normal cows the manganese content of hair falls during pregnancy from normal levels of 12 ppm in the first month of pregnancy to 4·5 ppm at calving (15). All of these figures require much more critical evaluation than they have had before they can be used as diagnostic tests.

Although tissue manganese levels in normal

animals have been described as being between 2 and 4 ppm in most tissues (1) there appears to be more variation between tissues than this (13). However tissue levels of manganese do not appear to be depressed in deficient animals except for ovaries in which levels of 0·6 ppm (3) and 0·85 ppm (9) are recorded in contrast to normal level of 2·0 ppm.

Manganese is necessary for the synthesis of cartilage ground substance and its absence is manifested in the bovine by the production of calves with congenital limb deformities (4, 10) and calves with manifest poor growth, dry coat and loss of coat colour. The deformities include knuckling over at the fetlocks (6), enlarged joints and possibly twisting of the legs (10). The bones of affected lambs are shorter and weaker than normal and there are signs of joint pain, hopping gait and reluctance to move (20). In cattle, manganese-responsive infertility is manifested by slowness to exhibit oestrus, and slowness to conceive, often accompanied by subnormal size of one or both ovaries. Suboestrus and weak oestrus have also been observed.

A manganese-responsive infertility has been described in ewes (19).

Rations fed to pigs usually contain more than 20 ppm of manganese and deficiency is unlikely unless there is interference with manganese metabolism by other substances. Experimental diets low in manganese cause reduction in skeletal growth, muscle weakness, obesity, irregular, diminished or absent oestrus, agalactia and resorption of foetuses or the birth of still-born pigs (21). Leg weakness, bowing of the front legs and shortening of bones also occur (22). Recent recommendations for dietary intakes are 24–57 mg. Mn per 100 lb. body weight (16). Expressed as a proportion of food intake the recommended dietary level is 40 ppm (40 mg. per kg.) in feed (7).

Young cattle have shown a general response in fertility to 2 g. MnSO$_4$ daily (3) but the general recommendation is daily supplementation with 4 g. manganese sulphate providing 980 mg. elemental manganese. This level of feeding is estimated to raise the dietary intake by 75 ppm (estimated on a daily intake of 27 lb. dry matter by a 1000 lb. cow). In some herds a full response was obtained only after doubling this rate of feeding (6). Although the feeding of 15 g. of manganese sulphate daily is reported to cause no signs of toxicity, manganese is known to interfere with the utilization of cobalt and zinc in ruminants (17). Very large levels of intake to calves can reduce growth rate and haemoglobin levels (18). The recommended procedure is to feed the supplement for 9 weeks commencing 3 weeks before the first service (6).

Excessive supplementation, up to 5000 ppm, of the diet with manganese for periods of up to three months appeared to cause only a reduction in appetite and weight gain (23).

REFERENCES

(1) Underwood, E. J. (1966). *The Mineral Nutrition of Livestock*. Reading, Berks.: Commonwealth Agricultural Bureaux.
(2) Cunningham, I. J. (1955). *Advanc. vet. Sci.*, 2, 138.
(3) Grashuis, J. *et al.* (1953). *De Schothorste*. Holland: Inst. Moderne Veevoeding, cited by Underwood, E. J. (1957). *Am. vet. J.*, 33, 282.
(4) Dyer, I. A. & Rojas, M. A. (1965). *J. Amer. vet. med. Ass.*, 147, 1393.
(5) Wilson, J. G. (1966). *Vet. Rec.*, 79, 562.
(6) Wilson, J. G. (1965). *Vet. Rec.*, 77, 489.
(7) Agricultural Research Council (1965). *The Nutrient Requirements of Farm Livestock No. 2, Ruminants. Technical Reviews and Summaries*. London.
(8) Hignett, S. L. (1956). *Proc. 3rd int. Congr. Animal Reprod.*, Cambridge, England, pp. 116–23.
(9) Bentley, O. G. & Phillips, P. H. (1951). *J. Dairy Sci.*, 34, 396.
(10) Rojas, M. A. *et al.* (1965). *J. Anim. Sci.*, 24, 664.
(11) Thompson, A. (1957). *J. Sci. Fd Agric.*, 8, 72.
(12) Hawkins, G. E. *et al.* (1955). *J. Dairy Sci.*, 38, 536.
(13) Sawhney, P. C. & Kehar, N. D. (1961). *Ann. Biochem. exp. Med.*, 21, 125.
(14) van Koetsveld, E. E. (1958). *T. Diergeneesk.*, 83, 229.
(15) Ushev, D. (1968). *Vet. Sbir. Sof. 65*, 57, in *Vet. Bull.* (1969). 39, 129.
(16) Littlejohn, A. & Lewis, G. (1960). *Vet. Rec.*, 72, 137.
(17) Pfander, W. H. *et al.* (1966). *Fed. Proc.*, 25, 431.
(18) Cunningham, G. N. *et al.* (1966). *J. Anim. Sci.*, 25, 532.
(19) Egan, A. R. (1972). *Aust. J. exp. Agric.*, 12, 131.
(20) Lassiter, J. W. & Morton, J. D. (1968). *J. Anim. Sci.*, 27, 776.
(21) Plumlee, M. P. *et al.* (1956). *J. Anim. Sci.*, 15, 352.
(22) Neher, G. M. *et al.* (1956). *Amer. J. vet. Res.*, 17, 121.
(23) Cunningham, G. N. *et al.* (1966). *J. Anim. Sci.*, 25, 532.
(24) Lardy, H. A. *et al.* (1942). *J. Anim. Sci.*, 1, 79.

Selenium Deficiency

Selenium is an essential nutrient for animals but its exact metabolic function is uncertain. Its functions are to a certain extent duplicated by those of vitamin E but it is not capable of replacing the vitamin in all situations, e.g. in the prevention of muscular dystrophy caused by cod liver oil, nor is the vitamin always capable of substituting for selenium, e.g. vitamin E does not have the growth promoting effect of selenium in animals on selenium-deficient diets (1).

Because of the large amount of information which indicates that natural cases of enzootic muscular dystrophy occur most commonly on selenium-deficient pastures, it may seem paradoxical to describe the disease under the heading of vitamin E deficiency. However present information suggests that the efficiency of selenium in this regard is due to its activity, when bound to protein, in enhancing activity and improving the transport and retention of vitamin E (2). On the other hand the absorption and retention of selenium is not affected by the vitamin E intake (3). The greater efficiency of selenium in the treatment and prevention of enzootic muscular dystrophy may depend upon inadequate dosage with the vitamin.

Soils, and therefore the pastures they carry, vary widely in their selenium content depending largely on their geological origin. In general, soils derived from rocks of recent origin, e.g. the granitic and pumice sands of New Zealand, are notably deficient in selenium (4). In U.S.A. the states of the Pacific north-west and of the north-eastern and south-eastern seaboard are generally low in selenium (5). A number of factors also reduce the availability of soil selenium to plants. The pH of the soil—alkalinity encourages selenium absorption—and the presence of a high level of sulphur which competes for absorption sites with selenium in both plants and animals, are two factors reducing availability. There is also much variation between plants in their ability to absorb selenium; 'selector' and 'converter' plants are listed under the heading of selenium poisoning; legumes take up much less selenium than do grasses. Seasonal conditions also influence the selenium content of pasture, the content being lowest in the spring and when rainfall is heavy. In this way a marginally deficient soil may produce a grossly deficient pasture if it is heavily fertilized with superphosphate, thus increasing its sulphate content, if the rainfall is heavy and the sward is lush and dominated by clover as it is likely to be in the spring months (6).

The role of selenium in the production of enzootic muscular dystrophy is described under the heading of vitamin E deficiency. As a result of work carried out on this disease it is now known that selenium has a much wider and less specific effect on the health of animals (7). Heavy neonatal mortality, unthriftiness in weaner calves, goats and lambs, chronic diarrhoea in calves, infertility due to foetal resorption in ewes and dietetic hepatosis in swine are the important non-specific diseases which often respond to dietary supplementation with the element. Although these diseases, and enzootic muscular dystrophy, occur extensively in areas where selenium levels in the soil are low, that they are caused by a dietary deficiency of selenium is not proven and it is common usage to refer to them as 'selenium-responsive' diseases. Apart from clinically recognizable disease there is also the gain

often obtained in some productivity index, e.g. wool production or body weight, after supplementation with selenium (8). Experiments under controlled conditions are equivocal with respect to these matters. Experiments with pigs showed no apparent effect on growth rate (9) but with ewes the appetite was improved by the administration of selenium (10). Selenium deficiency too has been shown to lead to abortion in sheep (11). A predisposition to retained placenta has also been noted in cows (12).

The most significant occurrence of these non-specific syndromes is in New Zealand (13) but limited occurrences are also recorded in the western United States (4), Finland (14), Australia (6) and the United Kingdom (15).

Although information on the critical levels of selenium in soil and plants is accumulating gradually, the estimations are difficult and expensive and most field diagnoses are made on the basis of the degree of improvement made in rate of gain of body weight by treatment with selenium. The existence of enzootic muscular dystrophy is accepted as presumptive evidence of selenium deficiency. Tentative critical levels of the element are:

Pasture. A content of 0·1 ppm is considered to be adequate (16).

Soil. Soils containing less than 0·5 ppm are likely to be dangerous.

Animal tissues. There is a good positive correlation between the selenium content of pastures and the selenium content of the tissues and blood of animals grazing the pastures (17). In sheep liver levels of less than 0·12 ppm on a wet matter basis suggest selenium deficiency (18) and levels of 0·21 ppm are considered to be the minimal safe level (19). A hair content of less than 0·25 ppm in cows is associated with a high incidence of muscular dystrophy in the calves produced (20). In pigs liver levels of selenium in normal animals are of the order of 10 to 11 ppm on a dry matter basis and in pigs affected with muscular or hepatic dystrophy levels of about 3·4 ppm (dry matter) are observed (21). On a wet matter basis normal levels are 0·220 ppm and levels in clinically affected pigs are of the order of 0·08 ppm (22).

Blood and milk levels of selenium are also used as indicators of selenium status. Dams of affected calves have had levels of 1·7 (blood) and 4·9 (milk) ng. per ml., their calves blood levels of 5 to 8 ng. per ml. Normal supplemented cows have 19 to 48 (blood) ng. per ml. and 10 to 20 (milk) ng. per ml. and their calves blood levels of 33 to 61 ng. per ml. (23). Mean selenium concentrations in the blood of normal mares have been 26 to 27 ng. per ml. (24).

Serum enzyme levels are also used to monitor degrees of hepatic damage and SGOT, SGPT and LDH (lactate dehydrogenase) levels are high in pigs on deficient diets (25).

Treatment and prevention of selenium deficiency should be carefully supervised because of the toxicity of the element. Recommended preventive procedures include pasture top dressing at the rate of 30 to 60 g. sodium selenite per acre per year (26) in severely deficient areas, the addition of selenium to prepared feeds to a concentration of 0·1 ppm selenium where animals are handfed, or oral dosing or parenteral injection. Injections are preferred to drenching (27) and either can be carried out intermittently at intervals of 1 to 3 months depending on the severity of the deficiency. For both methods the dose rate should approximate 0·02 mg. per lb. body weight, and although sodium selenite is in general use other less toxic preparations, such as barium selenite, may replace it (28). The infertility syndrome in ewes can be avoided by a single oral dose of 5·0 mg. of selenium (11 mg. sodium selenite) given one month before lambing (29). Vitamin E is ineffective in all of the above conditions. A routine programme in a badly deficient area comprises 3 doses of 5 mg. each to ewes, one before mating, one at mid-pregnancy and one 3 weeks before lambing, and 4 doses to the lambs. Selenium is transported across the placenta and treatment of the ewe before lambing provides protection for neonatal lambs (19). The first dose to lambs (of 1 mg.) is given at docking and the others (2 mg. each) at weaning and then at 3 month intervals. Oral doses are often combined with an anthelminthic, and injections with vaccines, particularly for enterotoxaemia. Pasture top dressing with selenium is too inefficient and wasteful to become a general practice. In small areas of severe deficiency it may be the only practicable procedure but is not without risks of causing poisoning (19, 30). When lactating cows are dosed with selenium milk levels rise but not to levels which can be considered hazardous to human health (31).

In situ pellets, similar to those used in cobalt deficiency, have produced satisfactory blood levels in sheep for up to 12 months (4). A satisfactory pellet is composed of elemental selenium and finely divided metallic iron (32). The technique is efficient but not completely so, due to wide variations between animals in the absorption rate of the selenium (33). The average delivery of selenium is 1·0 mg. per day and there is no danger of toxicity (34). Avoidance of high sulphate diets is desirable but provision of adequate selenium overcomes the sulphate effect (10). Little information is available on the need of horses for selenium but the optimum intake in this species is estimated to be 6 mg. per week (24) or 2·4 µg per kg. body weight daily (35). Serum selenium levels in this species vary from 7 in unweaned foals to 12 to 14 µg. per 100 ml. in weanlings and adults. The demonstration that the addition of arsenic (1 ppm) to a selenium deficient diet gives marked protection against myopathy to ewes (36) is a contribution to the study of the pathogenesis of the disease rather than to prophylaxis.

REVIEW LITERATURE

Andrews, E. D., Hartley, W. J., and Grant, A. B. (1968). Selenium-responsive diseases of animals in New Zealand. *N.Z. vet. J.*, *16*, 3.

REFERENCES

(1) Moore, T. (1962). *Proc. Nutr. Soc.*, *21*, 179.
(2) Desai, I. D. & Scott, M. L. (1965). *Arch. Biochem.*, *110*, 309.
(3) Ehlig, C. F. *et al.* (1967). *J. Nutr.*, *92*, 121.
(4) Pope, A. L. (1971). *J. Anim. Sci.*, *33*, 1332.
(5) Kubota, J. *et al.* (1967). *J. Agric. Fd Chem.*, *15*, 448.
(6) Gardiner, M. R. & Gorman, R. C. (1963). *Aust. J. exp. Agric.*, *2*, 261; *3*, 284.
(7) Andrews, E. D. *et al.* (1968). *N.Z. vet. J.*, *16*, 3.
(8) Gabbedy, B. J. (1971). *Aust. vet. J.*, *47*, 318.
(9) Ewan, R. C. *et al.* (1969). *J. Anim. Sci.*, *29*, 912.
(10) Whanger, P. D. *et al.* (1970). *Amer. J. vet. Res.*, *31*, 965.
(11) Buchanan-Smith, J. G. (1971). *Diss. Abstr. International*, *31B*, 4410.
(12) Trinder, N. *et al.* (1969). *Vet. Rec.*, *85*, 550.
(13) Robertson, T. G. & During, C. (1961). *N.Z. J. Agric.*, *103*, 306, 309.
(14) Westermarck, H. (1964). *Nord. Vet.-Med.*, *16*, 264.
(15) Blaxter, K. L. (1963). *Brit. J. Nutr.*, *17*, 105.
(16) Allaway, W. H. & Hodgson, J. F. (1964). *J. Anim. Sci.*, *23*, 271.
(17) Lindberg, P. & Jacobsson, S. O. (1970). *Acta vet. scand.*, *11*, 49.
(18) Andrews, E. D. *et al.* (1964). *N.Z. J. agric. Res.*, 7, 17.
(19) Allaway, W. H. *et al.* (1966). *J. Nutr.*, *88*, 411.
(20) Hidiroglou, M. *et al.* (1965). *Canad. J. Anim. Sci.*, *45*, 197.
(21) Lindberg, P. & Sirén, M. (1963). *Life Sci.*, *5*, 326.
(22) van Fleet, J. F. *et al.* (1970). *J. Amer. vet. med. Ass.*, *157*, 1208.
(23) Jacobsson, S. O. *et al.* (1970). *Acta vet. scand.*, *11*, 324.
(24) Bergsten, G. *et al.* (1970). *Acta vet. scand.*, *11*, 571.
(25) Ewan, R. C. & Wastell, M. E. (1970). *J. Anim. Sci.*, *31*, 343.
(26) Grant, A. B. (1965). *N.Z. J. agric. Res.*, *8*, 681.
(27) Oldfield, J. D. *et al.* (1963). *J. Agric. Fd Chem.*, *11*, 388.
(28) Kuttler, K. L. *et al.* (1961). *Amer. J. vet. Res.*, *22*, 422.
(29) Hartley, W. J. (1963). *Proc. N.Z. Soc. anim. Prod.*, *23*, 20.
(30) Pierce, A. W. & Jones, G. B. (1968). *Aust. J. exp. Agric.*, *8*, 277.
(31) Grant, A. B. & Wilson, G. F. (1968). *N.Z. J. agric. Res.*, *11*, 733.
(32) Kuchel, R. E. & Buckley, R. A. (1969). *Aust. J. agric. Res.*, *20*, 1099.
(33) Hidiroglou, M. *et al.* (1971). *Anim. Prod.*, *13*, 315.
(34) Handreck, K. A. & Godwin, K. O. (1970). *Aust. J. agric. Res.*, *21*, 71.

(35) Stowe, H. D. (1967). *J. Nutr.*, *93*, 60.
(36) Muth, O. H. *et al.* (1971). *Amer. J. vet. Res.*, *32*, 1621.

Potassium Deficiency

Naturally occurring dietary deficiency of potassium is thought to be rare. However, calves fed on roughage grown on soils which are deficient in potassium or in which the availability of potassium is reduced may develop a clinical syndrome of poor growth, anaemia and diarrhoea. Supplementation of the diet with potassium salts appears to be curative. A similar syndrome has been produced experimentally in pigs (1) which manifested poor appetite, emaciation, rough coat, inco-ordination and marked cardiac impairment as indicated by electrocardiographic examination. The optimum level of potassium in the diet of young growing pigs is about 0·26 per cent and in ruminants 0·5 per cent (i.e. 65 mg. per kg. body weight) (2). Electrocardiographic changes have also been observed in cattle on potassium-deficient diets and these are probably related to the degeneration of Purkinje fibres of the myocardium which occur on such diets. Similar changes have been recorded on diets deficient in magnesium or vitamin E.

An intake of potassium above requirement is more likely to occur than a deficiency, and although very large doses of potassium are toxic ruminants are capable of metabolizing intakes likely to be encountered under natural conditions (3). It seems probable, however, that potassium interferes with the absorption of magnesium and heavy applications of potash fertilizers to grass pastures may contribute to the development of the hypomagnesaemia of lactation tetany.

REFERENCES

(1) Cox, J. L. *et al.* (1966). *J. Anim. Sci.*, *25*, 203.
(2) Telle, P. P. *et al.* (1964), *J. Anim. Sci.*, *23*, 59.
(3) Ward, G. M. (1966). *J. Dairy Sci.*, *49*, 268.

Diseases caused by Dietary Deficiency of Phosphorus, Calcium and Vitamin D and to Imbalance of the Calcium:Phosphorus Ratio

A dietary deficiency or disturbance in the metabolism of calcium, phosphorus or vitamin D, including imbalance of the calcium:phosphorus ratio, is the principal cause of the osteodystrophies. The interrelation of these various factors is often very difficult to define and because the end result in all these deficiencies is so similar the precise aetiological agent is often difficult to determine in any given circumstance.

In an attempt to simplify this situation the diseases in this section have been dealt with in the following order:

Calcium Deficiency (Hypocalcicosis)
  (a) *Primary*—an absolute deficiency in the diet.
  (b) *Secondary*—when the deficiency is conditioned by some other factor, principally an excess intake of phosphorus.
Phosphorus Deficiency (Hypophosphatosis)
  (a) *Primary*—an absolute deficiency in the diet.
  (b) *Secondary*—when the deficiency is conditioned by some other factor. Although in general terms an excessive intake of calcium could be such a factor, specific instances of this situation are lacking.
Vitamin D Deficiency (Hypovitaminosis D)
  (a) *Primary*—an absolute deficiency in intake of the vitamin.
  (b) *Secondary*—when the deficiency is conditioned by other factors of which excess carotene intake is the best known.

In different countries with varying climates, soil types and methods of husbandry, these individual deficiencies are of varying importance. For instance in South Africa, northern Australia and North America the most common of the above deficiencies is that of phosphorus; vitamin D deficiency is uncommon. In Britain, Europe and parts of North America, a deficiency of vitamin D can also be of major importance. Animals are housed indoors for much of the year and they are exposed to little ultra-violet irradiation, and their forage may contain little vitamin D. Under such conditions the absolute and relative amounts of calcium and phosphorus in the diet need to be greater than in other areas if vitamin D deficiency is to be avoided. In New Zealand where much lush pasture and cereal grazing is used for feed, the vitamin D status is reduced not only by poor solar irradiation of the animal and plant sterols, but in addition an anti-vitamin D factor is present in the diet possibly in the form of carotene.

Now that the gross errors of management with respect to calcium and phosphorus and vitamin D are largely avoided, more interest is devoted to the marginal errors; in these, diagnosis is not nearly so easy and the deficiency can be evident only at particular times of the year (1). The conduct of a response trial in which part of the herd is treated is difficult unless they are hand-fed daily; there are no suitable reticular retention pellets or long-term injections of calcium or phosphorus because the daily requirement is so high. Two methods suggest themselves: analysis of ash content of samples of spongy bone from the tuber coxae (2) and the metabolic profile method (3). The latter programme has very great efficiency as a monitoring and diagnostic weapon in the fields of metabolic disease, nutritional deficiency and nutritional excesses.

REFERENCES
(1) Little, D. A. (1970). *Aust. vet. J.*, *46*, 241.
(2) Priboth, W. & Fritzsche, H. (1969). *Arch. exp. Vet.-Med.*, *23*, 653.
(3) Payne, J. M. *et al.* (1970). *Vet. Rec.*, *87*, 150.

Calcium Deficiency

Calcium deficiency may be primary or secondary, but in both cases the end result is an osteodystrophy, the specific disease depending largely on the species and age of the animals affected.

Incidence

Calcium deficiency is a sporadic disease which occurs in particular groups of animals rather than in geographically limited areas. Although death does not usually occur there may be considerable loss of function and disabling lesions of bones or joints.

Aetiology

A primary deficiency due to a lack of calcium in the diet seldom occurs, although a secondary deficiency due to a marginal calcium intake aggravated by a high phosphorus intake is not uncommon. In ponies such a diet depresses intestinal absorption and retention of calcium in the body, and the resorption of calcium from bones is increased (1). The effects of reduced calcium intake and parathyroidectomy are understandably additive in pigs (2) but parathyroid insufficiency seems an unlikely natural phenomenon.

Occurrence

Horses in training, cattle being fitted for shows, and valuable stud sheep are often fed artificial diets containing cereal or grass hays which contain little calcium, and grains which have a high content of phosphorus. The secondary calcium deficiency which occurs in these circumstances is often accompanied by a vitamin D deficiency because of the tendency to keep such animals confined indoors. Pigs are often fed heavy concentrate rations with insufficient calcium supplement. Dairy cattle may occasionally be fed similarly imbalanced diets the effects of which are exaggerated by high milk production. There are no well established records of a calcium deficiency in grazing sheep or cattle but there are records of low calcium intake in feedlots (3) accompanied by clinical osteodystrophy.

There is also a well recognized field occurrence of calcium deficiency in young sheep in south-east Australia (4). Outbreaks can affect many sheep and are usually seen in winter and spring, following exercise or temporary starvation. In most outbreaks the characteristic osteoporosis results from a long-term deprivation of food due to poor pasture growth. Occasional outbreaks occur on green oats used for grazing. The calcium intake in some cases is as low as 3 to 5 g. per week in contrast to the requirement of 3 to 5 g. per day.

In females there is likely to be a cycle of changes in calcium balance, a negative balance occurring in late pregnancy and early lactation and a positive balance in late lactation and early pregnancy and when lactation has ceased. The negative balance in late pregnancy is in spite of a naturally occurring increased absorption of calcium from the intestine at that time, at least in ewes (5).

Osteodystrophia fibrosa is the well-recognized manifestation of calcium deficiency in pigs. A further disease, slipped femoral head in sows, is considered by some to be a form of calcium deficiency because of the way it responds to heavy supplementation of the diet with calcium. Not all observers are convinced of the relationship (6). The more disturbing controversy centres around the suggestion that atrophic rhinitis is due to resorption of nasal turbinate bones as part of a general osteodystrophy (7).

Pathogenesis

The main physiological functions of calcium are the formation of bone and milk, participation in the clotting of blood and the maintenance of neuro-muscular excitability. In the development of osteodystrophies, dental defects and tetany the role of calcium is well understood but the relation between deficiency of the element and lack of appetite, poor growth, loss of condition, infertility, and reduced milk flow is not readily apparent. The disinclination of the animals to move about and graze and poor dental development may contribute to these effects.

It must be remembered that nutritional factors other than calcium, phosphorus and vitamin D may be important in the production of osteodystrophies which also occur in copper deficiency, fluorosis and chronic lead poisoning. Vitamin A is also essential for the development of bones, particularly those of the cranium.

Clinical Findings

The clinical signs, apart from the specific syndromes dealt with below, are less marked in adults than they are in young animals, in which there is decreased rate or cessation of growth and dental maldevelopment. The latter is characterized by deformity of the gums, poor development of the incisors, failure of permanent teeth to erupt for periods of up to 27 months and abnormal wear of the permanent teeth due to defective development of dentine and enamel, occurring principally in sheep (8, 9).

In spite of some evidence to the contrary it seems that calcium deficiency is followed, at least in sheep, by a profound fall in serum-calcium levels to as low as 3·5 mg. per cent. This occurs more readily in lactating ewes and sucking lambs, whose metabolic requirements for calcium are higher, than in dry and pregnant sheep. Tetany and hyperirritability do not usually accompany hypocalcaemia in these circumstances probably because it develops slowly. However, exercise and fasting often precipitate tetanic seizures and parturient paresis in such sheep. This is typical of the disease as it occurs in young sheep in south-east Australia (4). Attention is drawn to the presence of the disease by the occurrence of tetany, convulsions and paresis but the important signs are ill-thrift and failure to respond to anthelminthics. Serum calcium levels will be as low as 5·6 mg. per 100 ml. There is lameness but fractures are not common even though the bones are soft. A simple method for assessing this softness is compression of the frontal bones of the skull with the thumbs. In affected sheep the bones can be felt to fluctuate.

Pigs fed on heavy concentrate rations may develop a hypocalcaemic tetany which responds to treatment with calcium salts. Tetany may also occur in young growing cattle in the same circumstances.

Inappetence, stiffness, tendency of bones to fracture, disinclination to stand, difficult parturition, reduced milk flow, loss of condition and reduced fertility (10) are all non-specific signs recorded in adults.

Specific Syndromes

Primary calcium deficiency. No specific syndromes are recorded.

Secondary calcium deficiency. Rickets, osteomalacia, osteodystrophia fibrosa of the horse and pig, and degenerative arthropathy of cattle are the common syndromes in which secondary calcium deficiency is one of the specific causative factors. In sheep rickets is seldom recognized but there are marked dental abnormalities. Rickets has been produced experimentally in lambs by feeding a diet low in calcium (11).

Clinical Pathology

Because of the effect of the other factors listed above on body constituents, examination of specimens from living animals may give little indication of the primary cause of the disturbance. For example, hypocalcaemia need not indicate a low dietary intake of calcium. Data on serum-calcium and phosphorus and plasma phosphatase levels, roentgenological examination of bones and balance studies of calcium and phosphorus retention are all of value in determining the presence of osteodystrophic disease, but determination of the initial causative factor will still depend on analysis of feedstuffs and comparison with known standard requirements. In an uncomplicated nutritional deficiency of calcium in sheep there is only a slight reduction in the radiopacity of bone in contrast to sheep with a low phosphorus and vitamin D status which show marked osteoporosis (9). The response to dietary supplementation with calcium is also of diagnostic value.

Necropsy Findings

Severe osteoporosis and parathyroid hyperplasia are the significant findings. The ash content of the bone is low because the bone is resorbed before it is properly mineralized.

Diagnosis

A diagnosis of calcium deficiency depends upon proof that the diet is, either absolutely or relatively, insufficient in calcium, that the lesions and signs observed are characteristic and that the provision of calcium in the diet alleviates the condition. The diseases which may be confused with calcium deficiency are described under the diagnosis of each of the specific disease entities described below.

The close similarity between the dental defects in severe calcium deficiency of sheep and those occurring in chronic fluorosis may necessitate quantitative estimates of fluorine in the teeth or bone to determine the cause.

Treatment

The response to treatment is rapid and the preparations and doses recommended below are effective as treatment. Parenteral injections of calcium salts are advisable when tetany is present.

Control

The provision of adequate calcium in the diet, the reduction of phosphorus intake where it is excessive, and the provision of adequate vitamin D are the essentials of both treatment and prevention.

Daily Requirements of Calcium, Phosphorus and Vitamin D for Mature Animals

Species	Calcium	Phosphorus	Vitamin D (units per lb. body weight)
Cattle	10 g. dry cows to 40 g. for heavy milker	15 to 50 g.	3 to 5
Sheep (dry ewes) (100 lb. body weight)	3·2 g.	2·5 to 3·5 g.	3 to 5
Pigs (25–100 lb. body weight)	0·8% of ration	0·6% of ration	3 to 5
Pigs (100–200 lb. body weight)	0·7% of ration 16 g.	0·5% of ration 11 g.	3 to 5
Pigs (breeding sows)	0·8% to 1·0% of ration	0·6% to 0·7% of ration	3 to 5
Horses	14 to 15 g. 1·6% of ration	13 to 15 g. 1·4% of ration	3 to 5

Daily requirements of the three factors for the various species are set out in the table above.

Ground limestone is most commonly used to supplement the calcium in the ration, but should be prepared from calcite and not from dolomite. Variations in availability of the calcium in this product occur with variations in particle size, a finely ground preparation being superior in this respect. Bone meal and dicalcium phosphate are more expensive and the additional phosphorus may be a disadvantage if the calcium:phosphorus ratio is very wide. Alfalfa, clover and molasses are also good sources of calcium but vary in their content. The optimum calcium to phosphorus ratio is within the range of 2:1 to 1:1. In cattle absorption of both elements is better at the 2:1 ratio (12). For optimum protection against the development of urolithiasis in sheep a ratio of 2·0 to 2·5 Ca to 1 P is recommended (13).

The dustiness of powdered limestone can be overcome by dampening the feed or adding the powder mixed in molasses. Addition to salt or a mineral mixture is subject to the usual disadvantage that not all animals partake of it readily when it is provided free-choice, but this method of supplementation is often necessary in pastured animals. High-producing dairy cows should receive the mineral mixture in their ration as well as having access to it in boxes or in blocks. Pigs respond best to a mixture of four parts ground limestone, one part of salt sprinkled on the ration (30 g. daily for fattening pigs and 75 g. daily for heavily pregnant and lactating sows).

REFERENCES

(1) Schryver, H. F. et al. (1971). J. Nutr., 101, 259.
(2) Littledike, E. T. et al. (1968). Amer. J. vet. Res., 29, 635.
(3) Curtis, R. A. et al. (1969). Canad. vet. J., 10, 20.
(4) Palmer, N. C. (1969/70). Vict. vet. Proc., 28, 55.
(5) Braithwaite, G. D. et al. (1970). Brit. J. Nutr., 24, 661.
(6) Duthie, I. F. & Lancaster, M. C. (1964). Vet. Rec., 76, 263.
(7) Brown, W. R. et al. (1966). Cornell Vet., 56, Suppl. 1.
(8) Franklin, M. C. (1950). Cwlth Aust. sci. ind. Res. Org., Bull., 252, 34.
(9) McRoberts, M. R. et al. (1965). J. agric. Sci., Camb., 65, 1.
(10) Hignett, S. L. (1956). Proc. 3rd int. Congr. Anim. Reprod., Cambridge, England, 116–23.
(11) Dutt, B. & Sawhney, P. C. (1965). Ind. J. vet. Sci., 35, 345.
(12) Manston, R. (1967). J. agric. Sci., Camb., 68, 263.
(13) Pope, A. L. (1971). J. Anim. Sci., 33, 1332.

Phosphorus Deficiency

Phosphorus deficiency is usually primary and is characterized by pica, poor growth, infertility and, in the later stages, osteodystrophy.

Incidence

In contrast to calcium deficiency, a dietary deficiency of phosphorus is widespread under natural conditions. It has a distinct geographical distribution depending largely upon the phosphorus content of the parent rock from which the soils of the area are derived, but also upon the influence of other factors, such as excessive calcium, aluminium or iron, which reduce the availability of phosphorus to plants. Large areas of grazing land in many countries are of little value for livestock production without phosphorus supplementation. Animals in affected areas mature slowly and are inefficient breeders and additional losses due to botulism and defects and injuries of bones may occur. Apart from areas in which frank phosphorus deficiency is seen, it is probable that in many other areas a mild degree of deficiency is a limiting factor in the production of meat, milk and wool.

Aetiology

Phosphorus deficiency is usually primary under field conditions but may be exacerbated by a deficiency of vitamin D and possibly by an excess of calcium. Experimentally large doses of vitamin A decrease the absorption of phosphorus in cattle (1). and this may contribute to the development of nutritional osteodystrophies.

Occurrence

Heavy leaching by rain and constant removal by cropping contribute to phosphorus deficiency in the soil, and the low phosphorus levels of the plant cover may be further diminished by drought conditions. Pastures deficient in phosphorus are classically also deficient in protein.

Under range conditions milking cows are most commonly affected, but under intensive conditions it is the dry and young stock receiving little supplementation which suffer. The incidence of the disease varies: it is most common in animals at pasture during drought seasons but can also be a serious problem in housed cattle fed on hay only. The dietary requirements of phosphorus are given in the table below. Sheep and horses at pasture are much less susceptible to the osteodystrophy of phosphorus deficiency than are cattle and their failure to thrive on phosphorus-deficient pasture is probably due in part to the low protein content of the pasture. In fact there has been no clear demonstration of a naturally occurring phosphorus deficiency in sheep, nor is there any record of infertility in sheep caused by phosphorus deficiency.

A primary deficiency can occur in swine kept in confinement. Lactating sows are more commonly affected than growing pigs.

Secondary phosphorus deficiency is of minor importance compared with the primary condition. A deficiency of vitamin D is not necessary for the development of osteodystrophy although with suboptimal phosphate intakes deficiency of this vitamin becomes critical. Excessive intake of calcium does not result in secondary phosphorus deficiency although it may cause a reduction in weight gains, due probably to interference with digestion, and may contribute to the development of phosphorus deficiency when the intake is marginal. The presence of phytic acid in plant tissues, which renders phosphate unavailable to carnivora, is probably of less importance in pigs and of only minor importance in herbivora, except that increasing intakes of calcium may reduce the availability of phytate phosphorus even for ruminants. Rock phosphates which contain large amounts of iron and aluminium have been shown to be of no value to sheep as a source of phosphorus (2). A high intake of magnesium, such as that likely to occur when magnesite is fed to prevent lactation tetany, may cause hypophosphataemia if the phosphorus intake of dairy cows is already low (3).

Pathogenesis

Phosphorus is essential for the laying down of adequately mineralized bones and teeth and a deficiency will lead to their abnormal development. Inorganic phosphate, which may be ingested as such or liberated from esters during digestion or in intermediary metabolism, is utilized in the formation of proteins and tissue enzymes and is withdrawn from the plasma inorganic phosphate for this purpose.

Inorganic phosphate also plays an important role in the intermediary metabolism of carbohydrate and of creatine in the chemical reactions occurring in muscle contraction. This may be of importance in those cows which are recumbent after calving and have hypophosphataemia. The loss of phosphorus in the phospholipids of milk due to the onset of profuse lactation may be the crucial factor in the development of post-parturient haemoglobinuria. An increased susceptibility to bloat has been postulated as an effect of phosphorus deficiency.

Clinical Findings

Primary phosphorus deficiency is common only

Approximate Levels of Phosphorus in Soil and Pasture (Quoted as Phosphate Radical) at which Phosphorus Deficiency Occurs in Cattle

All figures quoted are on dry-matter basis and soil phosphate is citrate soluble

	Levels at which deficiency does not occur	Levels at which deficiency occurs
Soil	0·005%	0·002%
Pasture	0·3%	<0·2%—Osteophagia
		<0·01%—Rickets and Osteomalacia
Daily intake (cattle)	40 to 50 g.	25 g.

in cattle. Young animals grow slowly and develop rickets. In adults there is an initial subclinical stage followed by osteomalacia. Retarded growth, low milk yield and reduced fertility are the earliest signs of phosphorus deficiency. For example in severe phosphorus deficiency in range beef cattle the calving percentage has been known to drop from 70 per cent down to 20 per cent. Although it is claimed that relative infertility occurs in dairy heifers on daily intakes of less than 40 g. of phosphate, the infertility being accompanied by anoestrus, suboestrus and irregular oestrus and delayed sexual maturity (4, 5, 6), this has not been borne out by other experimental work which indicates that fertility is independent of the calcium or phosphorus content or the Ca:P ratio of the diet in cattle (7). The effects of malnutrition on fertility are likely to be general and the infertility may often be related to lack of total energy intake rather than to specific deficiency (8). The development and wear of teeth are not greatly affected, in contrast with the severe dental abnormalities which occur in a nutritional deficiency of calcium. However malocclusion may result from poor mineralization and resulting weakness of the mandible.

In a severely deficient area a characteristic conformation develops and introduced cattle revert to the district type in the next generation. The animals have a leggy appearance with a narrow chest and small girth, the pelvis is small and the bones are fine and break easily. The chest is slab-sided due to weakness of the ribs and the hair coat is rough and staring and lacking in pigment. In areas of severe deficiency the mortality rate may be high due to starvation especially during periods of drought when deficiencies of phosphorus, protein and vitamin A are exaggerated. Osteophagia is common and may be accompanied by a high incidence of botulism. Cows in late pregnancy often become recumbent and although they continue to eat are unable to rise. Such animals present a real problem in drought seasons because many animals in the area may be affected at the same time. Parenteral injections of phosphorus salts are ineffective and the only treatment which may be of benefit is to terminate the pregnancy by the administration of oestrogens or by Caesarian section.

Although sheep and horses in phosphorus-deficient areas do not develop clinically apparent osteodystrophy they are often of poor stature and unthrifty and may develop perverted appetites. An association between low blood phosphorus and infertility in mares has been suggested but the evidence is not conclusive. The principal sign in affected sows is posterior paralysis.

Clinical Pathology

Marked hypophosphataemia is a good indication of a severe phosphorus deficiency although a marginal deficiency may be accompanied by normal blood levels of inorganic phosphorus (9). As a rule clinical signs occur when blood levels have fallen from the normal of 4 to 5 mg. per cent to 1·5 to 3·5 mg. per cent and a response to phosphate supplementation in body weight gain can be anticipated in cattle which have blood inorganic phosphorus levels of less than 4 mg. per cent. Levels may fall as low as 1 mg. per cent or less in severe clinical cases. Serum levels of calcium are unaffected. Estimation of the mineral content in pasture and drinking water is a valuable aid in diagnosis. There is usually a marked deterioration in the radiopacity of the bones.

Necropsy Findings

The necropsy findings are those of the specific diseases, rickets and osteomalacia.

Diagnosis

A diagnosis of phosphorus deficiency depends upon evidence that the diet is lacking in phosphorus, that the lesions and signs are typical of those caused by phosphorus deficiency and can be arrested or reversed by the administration of phosphorus. Differentiation from those diseases which may resemble rickets and osteomalacia is dealt with under those headings (pp. 753 and 755).

Treatment

The preparations and doses recommended under control can be satisfactorily used for the treatment of affected animals. In cases where the need for phosphorus is urgent, as in post-parturient haemoglobinuria and in cases of parturient paresis complicated by hypophosphataemia, the intravenous administration of sodium acid-phosphate (30 g. in 300 ml. distilled water) is recommended.

Control

Under field conditions the difficulty usually encountered is that of providing phosphorus supplements to large groups of cattle running under extensive range conditions. The minimum daily requirement of cattle for phosphorus (as phosphate) is 15 g. and 40 to 50 g. is considered optimal.

Bone meal, dicalcium phosphate, disodium phosphate and sodium pyrophosphate may be provided in supplementary feed or by allowing free access to their mixtures with salt or more complicated mineral mixtures. The availability of the phosphorus in feed supplements varies and this needs to be taken into consideration when compounding rations. The relative biological values for young pigs in terms of phosphorus are; dicalcium phosphate or rock phosphate 83 per cent, steamed bone meal 56 per cent, and colloidal clay or soft phosphate 34 per cent (10). It is suggested that in deficient areas adult dry cattle and calves up to 300 lb. body weight should receive $\frac{1}{2}$ lb. bone meal per week; growing stock over 300 lb. body weight $\frac{3}{4}$ lb. per week and lactating cows 2 lb. weekly, but experience in particular areas may indicate the need for varying these amounts. The top dressing of pasture with superphosphate is an adequate method of correcting the deficiency and has the advantage of increasing the bulk and protein yield of the pasture but is often impractical under the conditions in which the disease occurs.

The addition of phosphate to drinking water is a much more satisfactory method provided the chemical can be added by an automatic dispenser to water piped into troughs. Adding chemicals to fixed tanks introduces errors in concentration, excessive stimulation of algal growth and precipitation in hard waters. Monosodium dihydrogen phosphate (monosodium orthophosphate) is the favourite additive and is usually added at the rate of 10 to 20 g. per 4 gallons of water. Superphosphate may be used instead but is not suitable for dispensers, must be added in larger quantities (50 g. to 4 gallons) and may contain excess fluorine. A reasonably effective and practical method favoured by Australian dairy farmers is the provision of a supplement referred to as 'super juice'. Five pounds of plain superphosphate is placed in a barrel with 10 gallons of water and stirred vigorously. When it has settled for a day the 'super juice' is ready for use and is administered by skimming off the supernatant and sprinkling 100 to 200 ml. on the feed of each cow.

REFERENCES

(1) Manston, R. (1964). *Brit. vet. J.*, *122*, 443.
(2) Reinach, N. & Louw, J. G. (1958). *Onderstepoort J. vet. Res.*, *27*, 611.
(3) McTaggart, H. S. (1959). *Vet. Rec.*, *71*, 709.
(4) Hignett, S. L. (1956). *Proc. 3rd int. Congr. Anim. Reprod.*, *Cambridge, England*, 116–23.
(5) Snook, L. C. (1964). *Proc. 5th int. Congr. Anim. Reprod.*, *Trento, Italy*, *5*, 148.
(6) Morrow, D. A. (1969). *J. Amer. vet. med. Ass.*, *154*, 761.
(7) Littlejohn, A. I. & Lewis, G. (1960). *Vet. Rec.*, *72*, 1137.
(8) Hart, B. & Michell, G. L. (1965). *Aust. vet. J.*, *41*, 305.
(9) Krook, L. (1968). *Cornell Vet.*, Suppl. 59.
(10) Morrison, S. H. (1964). *Proc. 101st ann. Mtg Amer. vet. med. Ass.*, *Chicago*, 41.

Vitamin D Deficiency

Vitamin D deficiency is usually caused by insufficient solar irradiation of animals or their feed and is manifested by poor appetite and growth, and in advanced cases by osteodystrophy.

Incidence

Although the effects of clinically apparent vitamin D deficiency have been largely eliminated by improved nutrition the subclinical effects have received little attention. For example retarded growth in young sheep in New Zealand and southern Australia during winter months has been recognized for many years as responding to vitamin D administration.

However, general realization of the importance of this subclinical vitamin D deficiency in limiting productivity of livestock has come only in recent years. This is partly due to the complexity of the relations between calcium, phosphorus and the vitamin and their common association with protein and other deficiencies in the diet. Much work remains to be done before these individual dietary essentials can be assessed in their correct economic perspective.

Aetiology and Occurrence

A lack of ultra-violet solar irradiation of the skin coupled with a deficiency of preformed vitamin D complex in the diet, leads to a deficiency of vitamin D in tissues. The lack of ultra-violet irradiation becomes important as distance from the equator increases and the sun's rays are filtered and refracted by an increasing depth of the earth's atmosphere. Cloudy, overcast skies, smoke-laden atmospheres and winter months exacerbate the lack of irradiation. The effects of poor irradiation are felt first by animals with dark skin (particularly swine and some breeds of cattle) or heavy coats (particularly sheep), by rapidly growing animals and those that are housed indoors for long periods. There is a marked difference in vitamin D status between sheep with a long fleece and those which have been recently shorn, especially in periods of maximum sunlight (1). The higher blood levels of vitamin D in the latter group is probably due to their greater exposure to sunlight. Pigs reared under intensive farming conditions and animals being prepared for shows are small but important susceptible groups.

The importance of dietary sources of preformed vitamin D must not be underestimated. Irradiated plant sterols with anti-rachitic potency occur in the dead leaves of growing plants or sun-cured hays but not in the green leaves of growing plants. Variation in the vitamin D content of hay can occur with different methods of curing. Exposure to irradiation by sunlight for long periods causes a marked increase in anti-rachitic potency of the cut fodder whereas modern haymaking technique with its emphasis on rapid curing tends to keep vitamin D levels at a minimum. Grass ensilage also contains very little vitamin D.

Information on the vitamin D requirements of housed dairy cattle is incomplete and contradictory. It appears, however, that in some instances natural foodstuffs provide less than adequate amounts of the vitamin for optimum reproductive performance in high producing cows (2).

The grazing of animals, especially in winter time, on lush green feed including cereal crops, leads to a high incidence of rickets in the young. An anti-vitamin D factor is suspected because calcium, phosphorus and vitamin D intakes are usually normal, but the condition can be prevented by the administration of calciferol. Carotene, which is present in large quantities in this type of feed, has been shown to have anti-vitamin D potency but the existence of a further rachitogenic substance seems probable (3). The rachitogenic potency of this green feed varies widely according to the stage of growth and virtually disappears when flowering commences. Experimental overdosing with vitamin A causes a marked retardation of bone growth in calves. Such overdosing can occur when diets are supplemented with the vitamin and may produce clinical effects (4).

The importance of vitamin D to animals is now well recognized and supplementation of the diet where necessary is usually performed by the livestock owner. Occasional outbreaks of vitamin D deficiency are experienced in intensive systems where animals are housed and in areas where specific local problems are encountered, e.g. rickets in sheep on green cereal pasture in New Zealand.

Pathogenesis

Vitamin D is a complex of substances with anti-rachitogenic activity. The important components are as follows:

Vitamin D_3 is produced from its precursor 7-dehydrocholesterol in mammalian skin and by natural irradiation with ultra-violet light.

Vitamin D_2 is present in sun-cured hay and is produced by ultra-violet irradiation of plant sterols. Calciferol or viosterol is produced com-

mercially by the irradiation of yeast. Ergosterol is the provitamin.

Vitamins D_4 and D_5 occur naturally in the oils of some fish.

AT-10 or Dihydrotachysterol is also produced in the commercial irradiation of yeast and is used in the prevention of parturient paresis. It has a powerful action in mobilizing calcium but has the least anti-rachitogenic potency of the D vitamins.

The mode of action of these vitamins in preventing rickets is incompletely understood. They facilitate the deposition of calcium and phosphorus in bones and increase the absorption of these minerals from the alimentary canal. A deficiency of vitamin D *per se* is governed in its importance by the calcium and phosphorus status of the animal. When the calcium:phosphorus ratio is wider than the optimum (1:1 to 2:1) vitamin D requirements for good calcium and phosphorus retention and bone mineralization are increased. A minor degree of vitamin D deficiency in an environment supplying an imbalance of calcium and phosphorus might well lead to disease, whereas the same degree of vitamin deficiency with a normal calcium and phosphorus intake could go unsuspected. For example, in growing pigs vitamin D supplementation is not essential provided calcium and phosphorus intakes are rigidly controlled but under practical circumstances this may not be possible.

The minor functions of the vitamin include maintenance of efficiency of food utilization and a calorigenic action, the metabolic rate being depressed when the vitamin is deficient. These actions are probably the basis for the reduced growth rate and productivity in vitamin D deficiency.

Clinical Findings

The most important effect of lack of vitamin D in farm animals is reduced productivity. A decrease in appetite and efficiency of food utilization cause poor weight gains in growing stock and poor productivity in adults. Reproductive efficiency is also reduced and the overall effect on the animal economy may be severe.

In the late stages lameness, which is most noticeable in the forelegs, is accompanied in young animals by bending of the long-bones and enlargement of the joints. This latter stage of clinical rickets may occur simultaneously with cases of osteomalacia in adults. An adequate intake of vitamin D appears to be necessary for the maintenance of fertility in cattle particularly if the phosphorus intake is low. In one study in dairy cattle, the first ovulation after parturition was advanced significantly in vitamin D supplemented cows (2).

Clinical Pathology

A pronounced hypophosphataemia occurs in the early stages and is followed some months later by a fall in serum-calcium. Plasma alkaline phosphatase levels are usually elevated. The blood picture quickly returns to normal with treatment, often several months before the animal is clinically normal.

Diagnosis

A diagnosis of vitamin D deficiency depends upon evidence of the probable occurrence of the deficiency and response of the animal when vitamin D is provided. Differentiation from clinically similar syndromes is discussed under the specific osteodystrophies.

Treatment

It is usual to administer vitamin D_2 in the dose rates set out under control. Affected animals should also receive adequate calcium and phosphorus in the diet.

Control

The administration of supplementary vitamin D to animals by adding it to the diet or by injection is necessary only when exposure to sunlight or the provision of a natural ration containing adequate amounts of vitamin D is impractical.

A total daily intake of 3 to 5 international units per lb. body weight is optimal. Sun-dried hay is a good source but green fodders are generally deficient in vitamin D. Fish liver oils are high in vitamin D but are subject to deterioration on storage particularly with regard to vitamin A. They have the added disadvantage of losing their vitamin A and D content in premixed feed, of destroying vitamin E in these feeds when they become rancid and of seriously reducing the butterfat content of milk. Stable water-soluble vitamin A and D preparations do not suffer from these disadvantages. Irradiated dry yeast is probably the simplest and cheapest method of supplying vitamin D in mixed grain feeds.

Single intramuscular injections of vitamin D_2 (calciferol) in oil protect ruminants for some months. A dose rate of 11,000 units per kg. body weight is recommended and should maintain an adequate vitamin D status for 3 to 6 months. Oral dosing with 20 to 45 units per kg. body weight is adequate provided treatment can be given daily. Massive oral doses can also be used to give long term effects, e.g. a single oral dose of 2 million units is an effective preventive for 2 months in lambs. Excessive doses may cause toxicity with signs of drowsiness, muscle weakness, fragility of bones and calcification in the walls of blood vessels. The latter finding has been recorded in cattle receiving 10 million units per day and in unthrifty lambs receiving a single dose of 1 million units, although larger doses are tolerated by healthy lambs. Severe toxicity in pigs occurs at a daily oral dose rate of 50,000 to 70,000 IU per kg. body weight. Signs include anorexia, diarrhoea, apathy, dyspnoea, aphonia, vomiting, emaciation and death (5).

REFERENCES

(1) Quarterman, J. et al. (1961). Proc. Nutr. Soc., 20, 28.
(2) Ward, G. et al. (1971). J. Dairy Sci., 54, 204.
(3) Grant, A. B. (1957). Proc. 7th int. Grasslands Congr., 1956, pp. 397–402.
(4) Grey, R. M. et al. (1965). Path. vet., 2, 446.
(5) Burgisser, H. et al. (1964). Schweiz. Arch. Tierheilk., 106, 714.

Rickets

Rickets is a disease of young growing animals characterized by defective calcification of growing bone. The essential lesion is a failure of provisional calcification with persistence of hypertrophic cartilage and enlargement of the epiphyses. The poorly mineralized bones are subject to pressure distortions.

Incidence

Clinical rickets is not as important economically as the subclinical stages of the various dietary deficiencies which produce it. The provision of diets adequate and properly balanced with respect to calcium and phosphorus, and sufficient exposure to sunlight are mandatory in good animal husbandry. Rickets is no longer a common disease because these requirements are widely recognized but the incidence can be high in extreme environments including purely exploitative range grazing, intensive feeding in fattening units and heavy dependence on lush grazing, especially in winter months.

Aetiology

The aetiology of rickets has been discussed under the headings of calcium, phosphorus and vitamin D deficiency. Deficiencies of one or more of these factors may be the cause of rickets in individual situations and the effects of the deficiency are likely to be exacerbated by a rapid growth rate.

An inherited form of rickets has been described in pigs (1). It is indistinguishable from rickets caused by nutritional inadequacy.

Occurrence

Rickets is a disease of young, rapidly growing animals and occurs naturally under the following conditions:

Calves. Primary phosphorus deficiency in phosphorus-deficient range areas, and vitamin D deficiency in calves housed for long periods are the common circumstances (2).

Lambs. Lambs are less susceptible to primary phosphorus deficiency than cattle but rickets does occur under the same conditions. Green cereal grazing and to a less extent pasturing on lush rye grass during winter months may cause a high incidence of rickets in lambs and this is considered to be a secondary vitamin D deficiency.

Pigs. Rickets in young pigs occurs in intensive fattening units where the effects of diet containing excessive phosphate (high cereal diets) are exacerbated by vitamin D and calcium deficiencies.

Foals. Rickets is uncommon in foals under natural conditions although it has been produced experimentally (3).

Pathogenesis

Dietary deficiencies of calcium, phosphorus and vitamin D result in defective mineralization of the osteoid and cartilaginous matrix of developing bone. There is persistence and continued growth of hypertrophic epiphyseal cartilage, increasing the width of the epiphyseal plate. Poorly calcified spicules of diaphyseal bone and epiphyseal cartilage yield to normal stresses resulting in bowing of long bones and broadening of the epiphyses with apparent enlargement of the joints. Rapidly growing animals on an otherwise good diet will be first affected because of their higher requirement of the specific nutrients.

Clinical Findings

The subclinical effects of the particular deficiency disease will be apparent in the group of animals affected and have been discussed previously. Clinical rickets will be evidenced by a stiffness in the gait, enlargement of the limb joints, especially in the forelegs, and enlargement of the costochondral junctions. The long bones show abnormal curvature, usually forward and outward at the knee in sheep and cattle. Lameness and a tendency to lie down are common. Arching of the back and contraction, often to the point of virtual collapse, of the pelvis occur and there is an increased tendency for bones to fracture.

Eruption of the teeth is delayed and irregular, and the teeth are poorly calcified with pitting, grooving and pigmentation. They are often badly aligned and wear rapidly and unevenly. These dental abnormalities, together with thickening and softness of the jaw bones may make it impossible for severely affected calves and lambs to close their mouths (4). As a consequence the tongue protrudes, and there is drooling of saliva and difficulty in feeding. In less severely affected animals dental malocclusion may be a significant occurrence (5). Severe deformity of the chest may result in dyspnoea and chronic ruminal tympany. In the final stages the animal shows hypersensitivity and tetany, recumbency and eventually dies of inanition.

Clinical Pathology

An elevation of plasma alkaline phosphatase is always evident but serum-calcium and phosphorus levels will depend upon the causative factor. If phosphorus or vitamin D deficiencies are the cause the serum-phosphorus level will usually be below the normal lower limit of 3 mg. per cent. Serum-calcium levels will be lowered only in the final stages.

Roentgenological examination of bones and joints is one of the most valuable aids in the detection of rickets. Rachitic bones have a characteristic lack of density compared to normal bones. The ends of long bones have a 'woolly' or 'moth-eaten' appearance and have a concave or flat, instead of the normal convex, contour. Surgical removal of a small piece of costochondral junction for histological examination has been used extensively in experimental work and should be applicable in field diagnosis.

Necropsy Findings

Apart from general poorness of condition the necropsy findings are restricted to abnormal bones and teeth. The bone shafts are softer and larger in diameter, due in part to the subperiosteal deposition of osteoid tissue. The joints are enlarged and on cutting, the epiphyseal cartilage can be seen to be thicker than usual. Histological examination of the epiphysis is desirable for final diagnosis and in sheep the best results are obtained from an examination of the distal cartilages of the metacarpal and metatarsal bones (6).

A valuable diagnostic aid is the ratio of ash to organic matter in the bones. Normally the ratio is 3 parts of ash to 2 of organic matter but in rachitic bone this may be depressed to 1:2, or 1:3 in extreme cases. A reduction below 45 per cent of the bone weight as ash also suggests osteodystrophy.

Because of the difficulty encountered in repeating the results of bone ash determinations, a standardized method has been devised in which the ash content of green bone is determined, using either the metacarpus or metatarsus, and the ash content related to the age of the animal, as expressed by the length of the bone. Although normal standards are available only for pigs (7) the method suggests itself as being highly suitable for all species.

Diagnosis

The diagnosis in clinical cases is relatively easy. It may be distinguished from infectious polyarthritis by the absence of a systemic reaction, pain and heat in the joints, and severe lameness. An hereditary form of rickets occurs in swine (1).

Subclinical and mild cases of rickets are more difficult to recognize and in these cases the diagnosis depends largely on laboratory examinations and response to therapy.

Treatment and Control

Recommendations for the treatment of the individual dietary deficiencies have been provided under their respective headings. Lesser deformities recover with suitable treatment but gross deformities usually persist. A general improvement in appetite and condition occurs quickly and is accompanied by a return to normal blood levels of phosphorus and alkaline phosphatase.

REFERENCES

(1) Plonait, H. (1969). *Zbl. Vet.-Med.*, *16A*, 271, 289.
(2) Spratling, F. R. *et al.* (1970). *Brit. vet. J.*, *126*, 316.
(3) Groenewald, J. W. (1949). Bone diseases in equines. *Rep. 14th int. vet. Congr.*, *3*, 34.
(4) Duckworth, J. *et al.* (1961). *Res. vet. Sci.*, *2*, 375.
(5) Nisbet, D. I. *et al.* (1968). *J. comp. Path.*, *78*, 73.
(6) Nisbet, D. I. *et al.* (1966). *J. comp. Path.*, *76*, 159.
(7) Pullar, E. M. (1960). *Aust. vet. J.*, *36*, 31.

Osteomalacia

Osteomalacia is a disease of mature animals affecting bones in which endochrondral ossification has been completed. The characteristic lesion is osteoporosis and the formation of excessive uncalcified matrix.

Incidence

Osteomalacia occurs under the same conditions and in the same areas as rickets in young animals but is recorded less commonly. Its main occurrence is in cattle in areas seriously deficient in phosphorus (1, 2). It is also recorded in sheep, again in association with hypophosphataemia (3).

Aetiology and Occurrence

Generally speaking the aetiology and occurrence of osteomalacia are the same as for rickets except that the predisposing cause is not the increased requirement of growth but the drain of lactation and pregnancy. Osteomalacia is most common in cattle, and sheep raised in the same area are less severely affected.

Pathogenesis

Increased resorption of bone mineral to supply the needs of pregnancy, lactation and endogenous metabolism leads to osteoporosis and weakness and deformity of the bones. Large amounts of uncalcified osteoid are deposited about the diaphyses.

Clinical Findings

In the early stages the signs are those of phosphorus deficiency, including lowered productivity and fertility and loss of condition. Licking and chewing of inanimate objects begins at this stage and may bring their attendant ills of oral, pharyngeal and oesophageal obstruction, traumatic reticuloperitonitis, lead poisoning and botulism.

The signs specific to osteomalacia are those of a painful condition of the bones and joints, and include a stiff gait, moderate lameness often shifting from leg to leg, crackling sounds while walking and an arched back. The hind legs are most severely affected and the hocks may be rotated inwards. The animals are disinclined to move, lie down for long periods, and are unwilling to get up. The colloquial names 'peg-leg', 'creeps', 'stiffs', 'cripples' and 'bog-lame' described the syndrome aptly. The names 'milk-leg' and 'milk-lameness' are commonly applied to the condition when it occurs in heavily milking cows. Fractures of bones and separation of tendon attachments occur frequently, often without apparent precipitating stress. In extreme cases deformities of bones occur, and when the pelvis is affected dystocia may result. Finally weakness leads to permanent recumbency and death from starvation.

Clinical Pathology

In general the findings are the same as those for rickets, including increased serum-alkaline phosphatase and decreased serum-phosphorus levels. Roentgenological examination of longbones shows decreased density of bone shadow.

Necropsy Findings

Lighter bones with a low ratio of ash to organic matter, and deposits of osteoid, as in rickets, are the characteristic findings. Epiphyseal enlargement is not apparent but severe erosions of articular cartilages have been recorded in cattle in primary phosphorus deficiency (2).

Diagnosis

The occurrence of non-specific lameness in animals with the attendant signs of poor condition, productivity and reproductive efficiency should arouse suspicion of osteomalacia. It is possible to confuse the condition with fluorosis but the typical mottling and pitting of the teeth in the latter condition is absent in osteomalacia. In some areas, e.g. northern Australia, where the water supply is obtained from deep subartesian wells, the two diseases may occur concurrently. Analysis of water supplies and feedstuffs for fluorine may be necessary in doubtful cases.

Detection of normal diet or vitamin D deficiency is necessary to confirm the diagnosis but field trials based on dietary supplementation may aid in determining the causative factor.

Treatment and Control

Recommendations for the treatment and control of the specific nutritional deficiencies have been described under their respective headings. Some weeks will elapse before improvement occurs and deformities of the bones are likely to be permanent.

REFERENCES

(1) Theiler, A. & Green, H. H. (1932). *Nutr. Abst. Rev.*, *1*, 359.
(2) Barnes, J. E. & Jephcott, B. R. (1955). *Aust. vet. J.*, *31*, 302.
(3) Nisbet, D. I. *et al.* (1970). *J. comp. Path.*, *80*, 535.

Osteodystrophia Fibrosa

Osteodystrophia fibrosa is very similar in its pathogenesis to osteomalacia but differs in that soft, cellular, fibrous tissue is laid down as a result of the weakness of the bones instead of the specialized uncalcified osteoid tissue of osteomalacia. It occurs in horses and swine.

Aetiology

A secondary calcium deficiency due to excessive phosphorus feeding is the common cause in horses and probably also in pigs. The disease can be readily produced in horses on diets with a ratio of calcium to phosphorus of 1:2·9 or greater, irrespective of the total calcium intake, and Ca:P ratios of 1:0·9 to 1:1·4 have been shown to be preventive and curative. With a very low calcium intake of 2 to 3 g. per day and a Ca:P ratio of 1:13 the disease may occur within 5 months. With a normal calcium intake of 26 g. per day and a

Ca:P ratio of 1:5 obvious signs appear in about 1 year but shifting lameness may appear as early as 3 months (1). The disease is reproducible in pigs on similar diets to those described above and also on diets low in both calcium and phosphorus (2). The optimum calcium phosphorus ratio is 1·2 to 1·0 and the intake for pigs should be within the range of 0·6 to 1·2 per cent of the diet.

Occurrence

Osteodystrophia fibrosa is principally a disease of horses and other Equidae, and to a lesser extent of pigs. Amongst horses, those engaged in heavy city work and in racing are more likely to be affected because of the tendency to maintain these animals on unbalanced diets. The major occurrence is in horses fed a diet high in phosphorus and low in calcium. Such diets include cereal hays combined with heavy grain or bran feeding. Legume hays, because of their high calcium content, are preventive.

The disease may reach enzootic proportions in army horses moved into new territories, whereas local horses, more used to the diet, suffer little. Although horses may be affected at any age after weaning it is the 2- to 7-years age group which suffer most, probably because they are the group most likely to be exposed to the rations which predispose to the disease.

Pathogenesis

Defective mineralization of bones follows the imbalance of calcium and phosphorus in the diet and a fibrous dysplasia occurs. This may be in response to the weakness of the bones or it may be more precisely a response to hyperparathyroidism stimulated by the excessive intake of phosphorus (1). The weakness of the bones predisposes to fractures and separation of muscular and tendinous attachments. Articular erosions occur commonly and displacement of the bone marrow may cause the development of anaemia.

Clinical Findings

As in most osteodystrophies the major losses are probably in the early stages before clinical signs appear or on diets where the aberration is marginal. In horses a shifting lameness is characteristic of this stage of the disease and arching of the back may sometimes occur. The horse is lame but only mildly so and in many cases no physical deformity can be found by which the seat of lameness can be localized. Such horses often creak badly in the joints when they walk. These signs probably result from relaxation of tendons and ligaments and appear in different limbs at different times. Articular erosions may contribute to the lameness. In more advanced cases severe injuries, including fracture and visible sprains of tendons, may occur but these are not specific to osteodystrophia fibrosa, although their incidence is higher in affected than in normal horses. Fracture of the lumbar vertebrae while racing has been known to occur in affected horses.

The more classical picture of the disease has largely disappeared because cases are seldom permitted to progress to this advanced stage. Local swelling of the lower and alveolar margins of the mandible are followed by soft, symmetrical enlargement of the facial bones, which may become swollen so that they interfere with respiration. Initially these bony swellings are firm and pyramidal and commence just above and anterior to the facial crests. The lesions are bilaterally symmetrical. Flattening of the ribs may be apparent and fractures and detachment of ligaments occur if the horse is worked. There may be obvious swelling of joints and curvature of long bones. Severe emaciation and anaemia occur in the final stages.

In pigs the lesions and signs are similar to those in the horse and in severe cases pigs may be unable to rise and walk, show gross distortion of limbs and enlargement of joints and the face. In less severe cases there is lameness, reluctance to rise, pain on standing, bending of the limb bones but normal facial bones and joints. With suitable treatment the lameness disappears but affected pigs may never attain their full size. The relationship of this disease to atrophic rhinitis is discussed under the latter heading (p. 912).

Clinical Pathology

There are no significant changes in blood chemistry in horses affected with severe osteodystrophia fibrosa. Normal levels of serum calcium (11·2 mg. per 100 ml.) and phosphorus (3·55 mg. per 100 ml.) have such a wide range that the levels observed in osteodystrophia are not significantly changed. Serum alkaline phosphatase estimations are obvious as a means of determining osteoclastic activity. Again there is the difficulty of assessing suspected variations from normality (3). Roentgenological examination reveals increased translucency of bones.

Necropsy Findings

The entire skeleton shows marked osteoporosis. The hard bone of the mandible, maxilla and nasal bones is replaced by soft fibrous tissue and there is characteristically replacement of red bone marrow with the same fibrous tissue.

Diagnosis

In the early stages diagnosis may be difficult because of the common occurrence of traumatic injuries to horses' legs. A high incidence of lameness in a group of horses warrants examination of the ration and determination of their calcium and phosphorus status. An identical clinical picture has been described in a mare with an adenoma of the parathyroid gland (5). Inherited multiple exostosis has been described in the horse (6).

In pigs osteodystrophia can be the result of hypovitaminosis A and experimentally as a result of manganese deficiency.

Treatment and Control

A ration adequately balanced with regard to calcium and phosphorus (Ca:P should be in the vicinity of 1:1 and not wider than 1:1·4) is preventive in horses and affected animals can only be treated by correcting the existing imbalance. Even severe lesions may disappear in time with proper treatment. Cereal hay may be supplemented with alfalfa or clover hay, or finely ground limestone (30 g. daily) should be fed. Dicalcium phosphate or bone meal are not as efficient because of their additional content of phosphorus.

REFERENCES

(1) Krook, L. & Lowe, J. E. (1964). *Path. vet.*, *1*, Suppl. 98.
(2) Storts, R. W. & Koestner, A. (1965). *Amer. J. vet. Res.*, *26*, 280.
(3) Krook, L. (1968). *Cornell Vet.*, *58*, 59.
(4) Joyce, J. R. *et al.* (1971). *J. Amer. vet. med. Ass.*, *158*, 2033.
(5) Bienfet, V. *et al.* (1964). *Ann. Méd. vét.*, *108*, 252.
(6) Morgan, J. P. *et al.* (1962). *J. Amer. vet. med. Ass.*, *140*, 1320.

'Bowie' or 'Bent-Leg'

This is a disease of lambs of unknown aetiology. There is a characteristic lateral curvature of the long bones of the front legs but the lesions differ from those of rickets. It has been observed only on unimproved range pasture in New Zealand (1). The cause is unknown although phosphorus deficiency has been suggested. Improvement of the pasture by top dressing with superphosphate and sowing improved grasses is usually followed by disappearance of the disease. Only sucking lambs are affected and cases occur only in the spring at a time when rickets does not occur. Up to 40 per cent of a group of lambs may be affected without breed differences in incidence. A similar syndrome has been produced by the feeding of wild parsnip (*Trachemene glaucifolia*).

Some tenderness of the feet and lateral curvature at the knees may be seen as early as 2 to 3 weeks of age and marked deformity is present at 6 to 8 weeks with maximum severity at weaning. The fore-limbs are more commonly affected than the hind. Medial curvature occurs in rare cases. The sides of the feet become badly worn and the lateral aspects of the lower parts of the limbs may be injured and be accompanied by lameness. The lambs grow well at first but by weaning affected lambs are in poor condition because of their inability to move about and feed properly. A rather similar syndrome has been observed in young Saanen bucks but the condition showed more tendency to recover spontaneously (2).

The levels of calcium and inorganic phosphate in serum are normal. At necropsy in spite of the curvature of the limbs there is no undue porosis, and although the epiphyseal cartilages are thickened they are supported by dense bone. There may be excessive synovial fluid in the joints and in the later stages there are articular erosions. Increased deposition of osteoid is not observed.

Supplementation of the diet with phosphorus or improvement of the pasture seems to reduce the incidence of the disease. Dosing with vitamin D or providing mineral mixtures containing all trace elements is ineffective (3).

REFERENCES

(1) Fitch, L. W. N. (1954). *N.Z. vet. J.*, 2, 118.
(2) Murphy, W. J. B. *et al.* (1959). *Aust. vet. J.*, 35, 524.
(3) Cunningham, I. J. (1957). *N.Z. vet. J.*, 5, 103.

Degenerative Joint Disease

A degenerative arthropathy occurs in cattle of all breeds but reaches its highest incidence as a sporadic affliction of young beef bulls (6). The occurrence of the condition in these animals is usually associated with rearing on nurse cows, housing for long periods, provision of a ration high in cereal grains and by-products (i.e. a high phosphorus: calcium ratio) and possibly with an inherited straight conformation of the hind legs. Although the disease occurs in all beef breeds there is a strong familial tendency which appears to be directly related to the rate of body weight gain and the straightness of the hind leg. If the potential for rapid weight gain is being realized in animals which are being force fed, the rate of occurrence appears to be dependent on their breeding (1) and animals in the same herd which are allowed to run at pasture under natural conditions are either not affected or are affected at a much later age. Thus, animals in a susceptible herd may show signs as

early as six months of age if they are heavily hand-fed and raised on dairy cow foster mothers. In the same herd signs do not appear until 1 to 2 years of age if supplementary feeding is not introduced until weaning, and not until 4 years if there is no significant additional feeding (5).

Clinically there is a more or less gradual onset of lameness in one or both hind legs, which becomes apparent in badly affected herds as early as 6 months of age. In less severely affected groups the onset may be delayed to 12 to 18 months, or to as late as 3 to 4 years in herds where intensive feeding is not practised. Almost invariably the disease progresses with the lameness becoming more severe over a period of 6 to 12 months. In some animals there is a marked sudden change for the worse, usually related to violent muscular movements as in breeding or fighting. In badly affected animals the affected limb is virtually useless and on movement distinct crepitus can often be felt and heard over the affected joints. The hip joints are always most severely affected but in advanced cases there may be moderate involvement of the stifles and minimal lesions in other joints. Affected animals lie down most of the time and are reluctant to rise and to walk. The joints are not swollen, but in advanced cases local atrophy of muscles may be so marked that the joints appear to be enlarged. There is an occurrence of the disease on record in which the lesions were confined mainly to the front fetlocks (7).

At necropsy the most obvious finding is extensive erosion of the articular surfaces, often penetrating to the cancellous bone, and disappearance of the normal contours of the head of the femur or the epiphyses in the stifle joint. The synovial cavity is distended with an increased volume of brownish, turbid fluid, the joint capsule is much thickened and often contains calcified plaques. Multiple, small exostoses are present on the periarticular surfaces. When the stifle is involved the cartilaginous menisci, particularly the medial one, are very much reduced in size and may be completely absent (2).

Adequate calcium, phosphorus and vitamin D intake, and a correct calcium–phosphorus ratio in the ration should be ensured. Supplementation of the ration with copper at the rate of 15 ppm has also been recommended for the control of a similar disease (3).

Degenerative joint disease of cattle is recorded on an enzootic scale in Chile (4) and is thought to be due to gross nutritional deficiency. The hip and tarsal joints are the only ones affected and clinical signs appear when animals are 8 to 12 months old. There is gross lameness and progressive emaciation. An inherited osteoarthritis is described under that heading. Sporadic cases of degenerative arthropathy, with similar signs and lesions, occur in heavy producing, aged dairy cows, and are thought to be caused by long-continued negative calcium balance. Rare cases also occur in aged beef cows but are thought to be associated with an inherited predisposition (1). In both instances the lesions are commonly restricted to the stifle joints.

REFERENCES

(1) Carne, H. R. *et al.* (1964). *Aust. vet. J.*, *40*, 382.
(2) Shupe, J. L. (1959). *Lab. Invest.*, *8*, 1190; (1961). *Canad. vet. J.*, *2*, 369.
(3) Washburn, L. E. (1946). *J. Anim. Sci.*, *5*, 395.
(4) Schulz, L. C. (1964). *Proc. int. Mtg Dis. Cattle, Copenhagen*, 284.
(5) Palmer, N. C. (1968–69). *Vict. vet. Proc.*, *27*, 68.
(6) Weaver, A. D. (1967). *Proc. 5th int. Meet Wld. Ass. Buiatrics, Zurich*, 1966, p. 489.
(7) Studer, E. & Nelson, J. R. (1971). *Vet. Med. small Anim. Clin.*, *66*, 1007.

DISEASES CAUSED BY DEFICIENCIES OF VITAMINS

Vitamin A Deficiency

(*Hypovitaminosis A*)

A deficiency of vitamin A may be caused by an insufficient supply of the vitamin in the ration, or its defective absorption from the alimentary canal. In young animals the manifestations of the deficiency are mainly those of compression of the brain and spinal cord. In adult animals the syndrome produced includes night blindness, corneal keratinization, pityriasis, defects in the hooves, loss of weight, and infertility. Congenital defects are common in the offspring of deficient dams.

Incidence

Vitamin A deficiency is of major economic importance in groups of animals on pasture or rations deficient in the vitamin or its precursors. Animals at pasture get adequate supplies of the vitamin, except during prolonged droughts, but animals confined indoors and fed on prepared rations may suffer from a severe deficiency if adequate precautions are not taken.

Aetiology

Primary vitamin A deficiency occurs most commonly because of lack of green feed or failure to add vitamin A supplements to deficient diets. The status of the dam is reflected in that of the foetus only in certain circumstances in that vitamin A in the alcohol form, as it occurs in green feed, does not pass the placental barrier and a high intake of green pasture before parturition does not increase the hepatic stores of vitamin A in newborn calves, lambs or kids and only to a limited extent in pigs. However, vitamin A in the ester form, as it occurs in fish oils will pass the placental barrier in cows and feeding of these oils before parturition will cause an increase in stores of the vitamin in foetal livers. Antepartum feeding of carotene and the alcohol form of the vitamin does, however, cause an increase in the vitamin A content of the colostrum. Young animals depend on the dam's milk for their early requirements of the vitamin which is always in higher concentration in the colostrum although it returns to normal levels within a few days of parturition. Pigs which are weaned very early—at 4 weeks—may require special supplementation.

Secondary vitamin A deficiency may occur in cases of chronic disease of the liver or intestines because much of the conversion of carotene to vitamin A occurs in the intestinal epithelium, and the liver is the main site of storage of the vitamin. Highly chlorinated naphthalenes interfere with the conversion of carotene to vitamin A and animals poisoned with these substances have a very low vitamin A status. The intake of inorganic phosphorus also affects vitamin A storage, low phosphate diets facilitating storage of the vitamin. This may have a sparing effect on vitamin A requirements during drought periods when phosphorus intake is low, and an exacerbating effect in stall-fed cattle on a good grain diet. On the other hand, phosphorus deficiency may lower the efficiency of carotene conversion. Vitamins C and E help to prevent loss of vitamin A in feedstuffs and during digestion. Additional factors which may increase the requirement of vitamin A include high environmental temperatures, a high nitrate content of the feed (1) which reduces the conversion of carotene to vitamin A, and rapid rate of gain. Both a low vitamin A status of the animal and high levels of carotene intake may decrease the biopotency of ingested carotene.

The continued ingestion of mineral oil (liquid paraffin), which may occur when the oil is used as a preventive against bloat in cattle, causes a severe depression of plasma carotene and vitamin A esters and the carotene levels in butter fat. The vitamin is fat-soluble and is probably absorbed by and excreted in the mineral oil. Deleterious effects on the cattle are unlikely under the conditions in which it is ordinarily used because of the short period for which the oil is administered and the high intake of vitamin A and carotene.

The addition of vitamin A supplements to rations may not always be sufficient to prevent deficiency. Carotene and vitamin A are readily oxidized particularly in the presence of un-saturated fatty acids. Oily preparations are thus less satisfactory than dry or aqueous preparations particularly if the feed is to be stored for any length of time. Pelleting of feed may also cause a serious loss up to 32 per cent of the vitamin A in the original feedstuff.

Occurrence

Primary vitamin A deficiency occurs in cattle and sheep on dry range country during periods of drought. Clinical vitamin A deficiency does not occur commonly under these conditions because hepatic storage is usually good beforehand and the period of deprivation not sufficiently long for these stores to reach a critically low level. Young sheep grazing natural, drought-stricken pasture can suffer serious depletion of reserves of the vitamin in 5 to 8 months but normal growth is maintained for 1 year at which time clinical signs develop. Adult sheep may be on a deficient diet for 18 months before hepatic stores are depleted and the disease becomes evident. Cattle subsist on naturally deficient diets for 5 to 18 months before clinical signs appear.

Pigs and poultry housed indoors, and feedlot cattle and sheep may be fed rations low in carotene and vitamin A. Grains, with the exception of yellow corn, contain negligible amounts of vitamin A, and cereal hay is often a poor source. Any hay which has been cut late, leached by rain, bleached by sun or stored for long periods loses much of its carotene content. The vitamin A activity of yellow corn also deteriorates markedly with long storage. Moreover, under conditions not yet completely understood, the conversion by ruminants of caro-tene present in feeds such as silage may be much less complete than was formerly thought. Young pigs on a deficient diet may show signs after several months but as in other animals the length of time required before signs appear is governed to a large extent by the status before depletion commences. As a general rule it can be anticipated that signs will appear in pigs fed deficient rations for 4 to 5 months, variations from these periods prob-ably being due to variations in the vitamin A status of the animal when the deficient diet is intro-duced. Congenital defects occur in litters from deficient sows but the incidence is higher in gilts with the first litter than in older sows. It is pre-

sumed that the hepatic stores of vitamin A in older sows are not depleted as readily as in young pigs. Adult horses may remain clinically normal for as long as 3 years on a deficient diet.

Pathogenesis

Vitamin A is essential for the regeneration of the visual purple necessary for dim-light vision, for normal bone growth and for maintenance of normal epithelial tissues. Deprivation of the vita-min produces effects largely attributable to dis-turbance of these functions. The same tissues are affected in all species but there is a difference in tissue and organ response in the different species and particular clinical signs may occur at different stages of development of the disease.

Night vision. Ability to see in dim light is reduced because of interference with regeneration of visual purple.

Bone growth. Vitamin A is necessary to maintain normal position and activity of osteoblasts and osteoclasts. When deficiency occurs there is no retardation of endochondral bone growth but there is inco-ordination of bone growth in that shaping, especially the finer moulding of bones, does not pro-ceed normally (2). In most locations this has little effect but may cause serious damage to the nervous system. Overcrowding of the cranial cavity occurs with resulting distortion and herniations of the brain and an increase in cerebrospinal fluid pres-sure up to 4 or 6 times normal. The characteristic nervous signs of vitamin A deficiency, including papilloedema, inco-ordination and syncope, fol-low. Compression, twisting and lengthening of cranial nerves and herniations of the cerebellum into the foramen magnum, causing weakness and ataxia (3), and of the spinal cord into inter-vertebral foraminae cause damage to nerve roots and localizing signs referable to individual peri-pheral nerves. Facial paralysis, and blindness due to constriction of the optic nerve (4), are typical examples of this latter phenomenon. The effect of excess vitamin A on bone development by its inter-ference with vitamin D has been discussed else-where.

Epithelial tissues. Vitamin A deficiency leads to atrophy of all epithelial cells but the important effects are limited to those types of epithelial tissue which have a secretory as well as a covering func-tion. The secretory cells are without power to divide and develop from undifferentiated basal epithelium. In vitamin A deficiency these secretory cells are gradually replaced by the stratified, kera-tinizing epithelial cells common to non-secretory epithelial tissues. This replacement of secretory epithelium by keratinized epithelium occurs chiefly in the salivary glands, the urogenital tract (including placenta but not ovaries or renal tubules) and the para-ocular glands and teeth (disappearance of odontoblasts from the enamel organ). The secretion of thyroxine is markedly reduced. The mucosa of the stomach is not markedly affected. These changes in epithelium lead to the clinical signs of placental degeneration, xerophthalmia and corneal changes.

Embryological development. Vitamin A appears to be essential for organ formation during growth of the foetus. Multiple congenital defects occur in pigs and rats and congenital hydrocephalus in rabbits on maternal diets deficient in vitamin A. In pigs administration of the vitamin to depleted sows before the 17th day of gestation prevented the development of eye lesions but administration on the 18th day failed to do so (5).

Clinical Findings

Generally speaking similar syndromes occur in all species but because of species differences in tissue and organ response some variations are observed. The major clinical findings are set out below (6).

Night blindness. Inability to see in dim light is the earliest sign in all species, except in the pig in which it is not evident until plasma vitamin A levels are very low. The inability of affected animals to see obstructions in half light (twilight or moonlit night) is an important diagnostic sign.

Xerophthalmia. True xerophthalmia, with thickening and clouding of the cornea, occurs only in the dog and calf. In other species a thin, serous mucoid discharge from the eyes occurs, followed by corneal keratinization, clouding and sometimes ulceration and photophobia.

Changes in the skin. A rough dry coat with a shaggy appearance and splitting of the bristle tips in pigs is characteristic but excessive keratinization such as occurs in cattle poisoned with chlorinated naphthalenes does not occur under natural conditions of vitamin A deficiency. Heavy deposits of bran-like scales on the skin are seen in affected cattle. Dry, scaly hooves with multiple, vertical cracks are another manifestation of skin changes and are particularly noticeable in horses. A seborrhoeic dermatitis may also be observed in deficient pigs but is not specific to vitamin A deficiency.

Body weight. Under natural conditions a simple deficiency of vitamin A is unlikely to occur and the emaciation commonly attributed to vitamin A deficiency may be largely due to multiple deficiencies of protein and carbohydrate. Although inappetence, weakness, stunted growth and emaciation occur under experimental conditions of severe deficiency, in field outbreaks severe clinical signs of vitamin A deficiency are often seen in animals in good condition. Experimentally sheep maintain their body weight under extreme deficiency conditions and with very low plasma vitamin A levels (7).

Reproductive efficiency. Loss of reproductive function is one of the major causes of loss in vitamin A deficiency. Both the male and female are affected. In the male libido is retained but degeneration of the germinative epithelium of the seminiferous tubules causes reduction in the number of motile, normal spermatozoa produced. In young rams the testicles may be visibly smaller than normal. In the female conception is usually not interfered with but placental degeneration leads to abortion and the birth of dead or weak young. Placental retention is common.

Nervous system. Signs related to damage of the central nervous system include paralysis of skeletal muscles due to damage of peripheral nerve roots, encephalopathy due to increased intracranial pressure, and blindness due to constriction of the optic nerve canal. These defects occur at any age but most commonly in young growing animals and they have been observed in all species except horses.

The paralytic form is ushered in by disturbances of gait due to weakness and inco-ordination. The hind legs are usually affected first and the forelimbs at a later stage. In pigs there may be stiffness of the legs initially with a stilted gait or flaccidity with knuckling of the fetlocks and sagging of the hind-quarters. Complete limb paralysis occurs terminally. Other manifestations of peripheral nerve injury include facial paralysis and rotation of the head in pigs and calves and curvature of the spinal column.

Encephalopathy, associated with an increase in cerebrospinal fluid pressure, is manifested by convulsive seizures which are common in calves and may occur in young pigs. Tonic or clonic convulsions occur and the animals are hypersensitive to touch. Such cases are usually paralysed between the convulsive episodes.

Papilloedema is the earliest sign of constriction of the optic nerve canal and can be detected ophthalmoscopically. It is common in young animals and occurs occasionally in adults in the terminal stages of the disease (6). It leads to complete blindness with degeneration of the retina. In calves and pigs there may be a gradual onset of blindness without obvious eye lesions although there is continuous pupillary dilatation and absence of the pupillary light reflex. Calves also show exophthalmos and excessive lacrimation (8).

Congenital defects. These have been observed in rabbits, rats, piglets (9) and calves. In calves the defects are limited to congenital blindness due to optic nerve constriction, and encephalopathy. In piglets complete absence of the eyes (anophthalmos) or small eyes (microphthalmos) occur. Other congenital defects attributed to vitamin A deficiency in pigs include cleft palate and hare-lip, accessory ears, malformed hind legs, subcutaneous cysts, abnormally situated kidneys, cardiac defects, diaphragmatic hernia, aplasia of the genitalia, internal hydrocephalus, herniations of the spinal cord and generalized oedema (10). Affected pigs may be stillborn, or weak and unable to stand, or may be quite active. Weak pigs lie on their sides, make slow paddling movements with their legs and squawk plaintively.

Oedema. Anasarca affecting particularly the legs and forequarters is often recorded in feedlot cattle fed on carotene-deficient diets for long periods.

Other diseases. Increased susceptibility to infection is often stated to result from vitamin A deficiency. The efficacy of colostrum as a preventive against scours in calves was thought at one time to be due to its vitamin A content but the high antibody content of colostrum is now known to be the important factor. A high incidence of otitis media and enteritis have often been reported in conjunction with vitamin A deficiency.

Clinical Pathology

Vitamin A levels in the plasma are used extensively in diagnostic and experimental work. Levels of 7 to 8 µg. per 100 ml. are considered to be critical with 10 µg. per 100 ml. necessary for normal growth. Clinical signs can be expected when the levels fall to 5 µg. per 100 ml. For complete safety optimum levels should be 25 µg. per 100 ml. or above (6, 7).

Plasma carotene levels vary largely with the diet. In cattle levels of 150 µg. per 100 ml. are optimum and in the absence of supplementary vitamin A in the ration, clinical signs appear when the levels fall to 9 µg. per 100 ml. In sheep carotene is present in the blood in only very small amounts even when they are on green pasture.

It is noteworthy that a direct relationship between plasma and hepatic levels of vitamin A need not exist since plasma levels do not commence to fall until the hepatic stores are depleted. A temporary precipitate fall occurs at parturition and in acute infections in most animals. The secretion of large amounts of carotene and vitamin A in the colostrum of cows during the last 3 weeks of pregnancy may greatly reduce the level of vitamin A in the plasma.

Hepatic levels of vitamin A and carotene can be estimated in the living animal from a biopsy specimen. Biopsy techniques have been shown to be safe and relatively easy provided a proper instrument is used. Hepatic levels of vitamin A and carotene should be of the order of 60 to 4·0 µg. per g. of liver respectively. These levels are commonly as high as 200 to 800 µg. per g. Critical levels at which signs are likely to appear are 2·0 and 0·5 µg. per g. for vitamin A and carotene respectively.

Cerebrospinal fluid pressure is also used as a sensitive indicator of low vitamin A status. In calves normal pressures of less than 100 mm. of water rise after depletion to more than 200 mm. In pigs normal pressures of 80 to 145 mm. rise to above 200 mm. in vitamin A deficiency. An increase in pressure is observed at a blood level of about 7 µg. vitamin A per 100 ml. plasma in this species. In sheep normal pressures of 55 to 65 mm. rise to 70 to 150 mm. when depletion occurs. In the experimentally induced disease in cattle, there is a marked increase in the number of cornified epithelial cells in a conjunctival smear and distinctive bleaching of the tapetum lucidum as viewed by an ophthalmoscope. These features may have value as diagnostic aids in naturally occurring cases (11, 12).

Necropsy Findings

Gross changes at necropsy are not characteristic of vitamin A deficiency. Careful dissection may reveal decrease in size of the cranial vault and of the vertebrae, and compression and injury of the cranial and spinal nerve roots, especially the optic nerve, may be visible. The lesions caused by secondary bacterial infections including pneumonia and otitis media are also common.

Squamous metaplasia of the interlobular ducts of the parotid salivary gland is considered to be pathognomonic of vitamin A deficiency in pigs, calves and lambs but the change is transient and may have disappeared 2 to 4 weeks after the intake of vitamin A is increased. The change is most marked and occurs first at the oral end of the main parotid duct (13). Focal necrotic hepatitis occurs in calves but no specific renal lesions are present. The anasarcous lesions which are recorded in vitamin A deficiency in feedlot cattle are associated with vascular damage and degeneration of muscles. Cattle also show hyperkeratinization of the epithelium of the prepuce, reticulum and rumen and a high incidence of pituitary cysts (14).

The abnormalities which occur in congenitally affected pigs have already been described. Generalized oedema is present to a marked degree.

Diagnosis

When the characteristic signs or lesions of vitamin A deficiency are observed a deficiency of the vitamin should be suspected if green feed or vitamin A supplements are not being provided. The detection of papilloedema and testing for night-blindness are the easiest methods of diagnosing early vitamin A deficiency in ruminants. Inco-ordination, paralysis and convulsions are the early signs in pigs. Increase in CSF pressure is the earliest measurable change in both pigs and calves. Laboratory confirmation depends upon estimations of vitamin A in plasma and liver, the latter being most satisfactory. Unless the disease has been in existence for a considerable time response to treatment is rapid. For confirmation at necropsy histological examination of parotid salivary gland, and assay of vitamin A in the liver are suggested.

The loss of condition, failure to grow and poor reproductive efficiency are general signs which are not limited to vitamin A deficiency. Convulsive seizures as occur in calves, and posterior paralysis as occurs in growing pigs on vitamin A deficient rations also resemble the syndromes which occur in many other diseases. Clinically it may be impossible to distinguish between encephalopathy caused by vitamin A deficiency and hypomagnesaemic tetany, polioencephalomalacia, enterotoxaemia caused by *Cl. perfringens* Type D, and acute lead poisoning. Rabies, however, is usually accompanied by a disturbance of consciousness and anaesthesia. Sporadic bovine encephalomyelitis is always accompanied by high fever and by serositis. Several other poisonings as listed below are more likely to occur in pigs than in calves and may cause clinical signs similar to those caused by vitamin A deficiency.

In pigs posterior paralysis is a more common observation in vitamin A deficiency than are convulsive episodes. The other diseases which may be confused with vitamin A deficiency in this species include pseudorabies and viral encephalomyelitis. A number of poisonings, including salt, organic arsenic and organic mercury also cause nervous signs. As in calves clinical differentiation is extremely difficult and a careful examination of the local environment and the feeding history is necessary to attempt to limit the diagnostic possibilities.

Congenital defects similar to those caused by vitamin A deficiency may be caused by deficiencies of other essential nutrients, by inheritance or by viral infections in early pregnancy. Final diagnosis often depends upon the necropsy findings although the clinical pathology may be of assistance.

Treatment

Animals which show clinical signs of vitamin A deficiency should be treated immediately with vitamin A at a dose rate equivalent to 10 to 20 times the daily maintenance requirement. As a rule 440 IU per kg. body weight is the dose rate used. Parenteral injection of an aqueous rather than an oily solution is preferred. The response to treatment in cases of severe, acute deficiency is often rapid and complete but the disease may be irreversible in chronic cases, especially when deficiency has continued over more than one generation.

Daily heavy dosing (about 100 times normal) of calves causes reduced growth rate, lameness, ataxia, paresis, exostoses on the plantar aspect of the third phalanx of the fourth digit of all feet and disappearance of the epiphyseal cartilage (15, 16, 17). Persistent heavy dosing in calves causes lameness, retarded horn growth and depressed cerebrospinal fluid pressure. At necropsy exostoses are present on the proximal metacarpal bones and the frontal bones are thin (18). Very high levels fed to young pigs may cause sudden death through massive internal haemorrhage and excessive doses during early pregnancy may result in foetal anomalies.

Control

The minimum daily requirement in all species is 30 international units of vitamin A or 75 IU of carotene per kg. body weight. To permit some hepatic storage optimum intakes should be 65 IU vitamin A or 155 IU carotene per kg. body weight. During pregnancy and lactation these doses should be increased by 50 per cent and those animals which are growing very rapidly also have a much greater requirement than those growing at a more normal rate. The supplementation of rations to groups of animals is governed by a number of factors, particularly their previous intake of the vitamin and its probable level in the diet being fed, and the rate of supplementation can vary from 0 to 110 IU per kg. body weight per day (1 international unit vitamin A ≡ 0·344 µg. or gamma of the vitamin. One IU of carotene ≡ 0·6 µg. carotene). In prepared rations for pigs 2·5 million units per ton of feed should be added for growing stock and 9 million units per ton for breed-stock. Cattle in feedlots are supplemented by the daily addition to their ration of 10,000 to 40,000 IU of vitamin A—the lower level being used for steers wintered mainly on roughage, the higher level for steers on full grain feed in hot weather.

Suitable dietary sources of vitamin A and caro-tene include fish oils and green feed. The former vary considerably in vitamin A content and only standardized preparations should be used. The potency of any oil preparation decreases rapidly with storage if the oil is exposed to the air, if it is stored in rusty metal containers, or if the container is only half-filled. There is some risk too in the addition of oils to rations because of their tendency to cause muscular dystrophy and reduce the yield of butter fat. Stabilized concentrates of vitamin A or products in which the vitamin is adsorbed on to paraffin wax crystals or coated in gelatin are preferred. These products have the advantages that they can be mixed with protein concentrates, high-moisture feeds, pelleted feeds and mineral mixtures and retain their potency for at least 3 months.

The prevention of vitamin A deficiency may be a particular problem in range cattle being moved from drought-stricken pastures into feedlots and in pregnant cows at range during long dry periods. Particularly in the latter group it may be less expensive to give vitamin A by parenteral injection during the latter stages of pregnancy than to feed a prepared ration containing supplemental vitamin A. Some economy can be effected by injecting crude preparations containing vitamin A intra-ruminally. Absorption and storage are good.

REVIEW LITERATURE

Clark, L. (1971). Hypervitaminosis A. A review. *Aust. vet. J.*, 47, 568.
Barnett, K. C. *et al.* (1970). Ocular changes associated with hypovitaminosis A in cattle. *Brit. vet. J.*, 126, 561.
Mitchell, G. E. (1967). Vitamin A nutrition of ruminants. *J. Amer. vet. med. Ass.*, 151, 430.

REFERENCES

(1) Hoar, D. W. *et al.* (1968). *J. Anim. Sci.*, 27, 1727.
(2) Davis, T. E. *et al.* (1970). *Canad. vet. J.*, 30, 90.
(3) Mills, J. H. L. *et al.* (1967). *Acta vet. scand.*, 8, 324.
(4) Hayes, K. C. *et al.* (1968). *Arch. Ophthal.*, 80, 777.
(5) Palludan, B. (1964). *Årsberetn. int. Sterilitetsforsk.*, 59.
(6) Eaton, H. D. *et al.* (1970). *J. Dairy Sci.*, 53, 1775.
(7) Franklin, M. C. *et al.* (1955). *Aust. J. agric. Res.*, 6, 324.
(8) Abrams, J. T. *et al.* (1961). *Vet. Rec.*, 73, 683.
(9) Goodwin, F. R. W. & Jennings, A. R. (1958). *J. comp. Path.*, 68, 82.
(10) Palludan, B. (1961). *Acta vet. scand.*, 2, 32.
(11) Huber, W. G. & Smith, G. S. (1963). *Vet. Med.*, 58, 875.
(12) Eaton, H. D. *et al.* (1970). *J. Dairy Sci.*, 53, 1775.
(13) Nielsen, S. W. *et al.* (1966). *Amer. J. vet. Res.*, 27, 223.
(14) Nielsen, S. W. *et al.* (1966). *Res. vet. Sci.*, 7, 143.
(15) Hazzard, D. G. *et al.* (1964). *J. Dairy Sci.*, 47, 391.
(16) Pryor, W. J. *et al.* (1969). *Aust. vet. J.*, 45, 563.
(17) Wolke, R. E. *et al.* (1968). *Amer. J. vet. Res.*, 29, 1009.
(18) Gallina, A. M. *et al.* (1970). *Arch. exp. Vet.-Med.*, 24, 1091.

Vitamin E Deficiency

(*Hypovitaminosis E*)

A deficiency of vitamin E occurs in most animal species and is characterized chiefly by hyaline degeneration of the skeletal muscle and myo-cardium.

Incidence

Muscular dystrophy, associated with vitamin E deficiency, has been reported from most countries but particularly from those in northern latitudes where animals are housed for long periods of the year. Scandinavia, Scotland, Northern Europe and Canada all report a high incidence. In the United States it is common in the north-east and north-west and uncommon on the relatively high selenium soils of the central plains. The disease appears to be increasing in incidence in young ruminants running on lush pastures and has recently been observed in New Zealand and Australia. The mor-bidity rate varies widely in affected groups, and under particularly adverse conditions may be as high as 50 per cent. Many affected animals die or fail to recover completely. The variation in inci-dence from year to year makes the disease par-ticularly troublesome as prophylactic measures are not practised consistently, resulting in severe losses in bad years. A high incidence in beef herds and fat lamb flocks is of major importance be-cause of the loss of potential productive units for the year.

Aetiology

Although there is a close association between muscular dystrophy and vitamin E deficiency, and myocardial failure has occurred following long-term, experimental feeding of deficient diets to cows, muscular dystrophy can occur despite an adequate intake of vitamin E. It appears that the vitamin acts in a protective capacity against agents which produce muscular dystrophy and that deficiency of vitamin E does not in itself produce the lesions, unless a primary myopathic agent is present (1). If one accepts this hypothesis the disease entities described below might be more accurately dealt with under the heading of myo-pathies, but because of common usage and because of the importance of vitamin E in their pathogenesis they are dealt with as a group under this heading.

Primary vitamin E deficiency occurs most commonly when animals are fed on poor hay or straw and on root crops. Cereal grains, green pasture, and well cured fresh hay contain adequate amounts of the vitamin. Pelleting of grains does not destroy vitamin E but a vitamin E deficiency occurs when mixed cereal rations containing cod liver or other oils are stored for more than a few days. Oxidation during rancidification of the oils causes destruction of the vitamin. Fish oils, lard, linseed, soyabean and corn oils have been implicated in the production of muscular dystrophy and a high proportion of coconut meal in the ration has been thought to have the same effect. The presence of myopathic agents in the oils may also contribute to the occurrence of the disease. A relative vitamin E deficiency can be said to occur when muscular dystrophy develops on rations containing vitamin E in amounts ordinarily considered to be adequate, but the disease is prevented by further supplementation with the vitamin. The lack of specificity of vitamin E in the prevention of muscular dystrophy in some circumstances is indicated by its failure, and by the efficiency of selenium, as a preventive agent in lambs on lush legume pasture.

The discovery of the high incidence of enzootic dystrophy on diets containing less than 0·1 ppm of selenium and the preventive effect of selenium has stimulated a good deal of investigation. The results so far suggest that although a primary deficiency of selenium in the diet may lead to the development of enzootic muscular dystrophy this is not always the case and a conditioned deficiency of selenium may arise, for example in the presence of a high sulphate content of the diet. Soils which have a selenium content of less than 0·5 ppm, and forages less than 0·1 ppm, are likely to be associated with a high incidence of the disease.

The myopathic agents concerned in the development of muscular dystrophy in farm animals have not all been identified. Unsaturated fatty acids in fish and vegetable oils appear to be important myopathic agents in many outbreaks of enzootic muscular dystrophy (white muscle disease of calves and stiff-lamb disease). In other circumstances the agent or agents have not been identified although a high content of unsaturated fatty acids in the milk of the dams has been suggested (1). It is difficult to conceive that even a relative vitamin E deficiency could be important in the muscular dystrophies which occur in lambs and calves on lush legume pasture, but there is some evidence that unsaturated

fatty acids may reach high levels in lush pasture herbage (1). The disease as it occurs on lush pasture has not been shown to be in any way associated with vitamin E deficiency and, at least in calves, cannot be prevented by the administration of the vitamin.

It is generally held that although enzootic muscular dystrophy can result from a dietary deficiency of selenium or vitamin E, a precipitating factor, such as myopathic agents in the feed, violent physical exercise, prolonged transport, exposure to other dietary or climatic stress or intercurrent disease, may convert an asymptomatic deficiency state to one of frank disease of the musculature.

Unaccustomed muscular activity is often the precipitating factor in the production of muscular dystrophy or its clinical manifestations in both myocardial and skeletal muscle forms. A dietary deficiency of phosphorus has been thought to exacerbate the myopathic effects of a vitamin E deficient diet in cattle.

The particularly high incidence in young animals is probably due to their poor vitamin E status as compared to that of adults. Newborn animals normally have some hepatic stores of the vitamin and this can be supplemented in lambs and kids by the feeding of extra tocopherols to the dams. The tocopherol content of milk, particularly colostrum, also varies with the intake but often appears to bear no relation to the incidence of muscular dystrophy. Muscular dystrophy has been observed in newborn lambs and in newborn calves but only in young from dams on lush pasture and without any apparent deficiency of vitamin E.

Occurrence

Green plants and cereal grains are good sources of vitamin E and a primary dietary deficiency is unlikely when animals are grazed on green pasture or fed on a high grain ration or good quality hay made while the plant is still green, cured well, and used during the following winter. Deficiency is likely to occur when animals are housed for long periods and fed on poor quality hay, straw and roots. Beef cows and ewes in breeding flocks are often subjected to these conditions. The disease is most common in their calves, particularly at 1 to 2 months of age, and occasionally up to 6 months, and lambs at 1 to 3 weeks of age. Clinical cases may occur while the animals are still housed but the highest incidence is seen in the two or three days immediately after they are let out in the spring. Unaccustomed activity while playing at pasture or upon being driven is commonly associated with the sudden appearance of clinical evidence of muscular dystrophy in a number of animals.

In sheep the disease may also occur on rations containing what appear to be adequate levels of vitamin E. Legume hays including alfalfa and clover, barley and beans appear to be the feedstuffs most commonly associated with a high incidence of muscular dystrophy in the lambs. Because supplementation of the diet with additional vitamin E is prophylactic this must be considered to be a relative deficiency state. The occurrence of muscular dystrophy on prepared rations supplemented with oils or fats containing unsaturated fatty acids, including fish, soya, corn and linseed oils, and lard can also be prevented by the administration of vitamin E. A particular occurrence of this disease is in calves fed on milk to which vegetable fats which are highly unsaturated, e.g. lard and corn oil, have been added. The effects of these milk substitutes are exaggerated if they are stored for a week after preparation.

The muscular dystrophy which occurs in calves and lambs, including the newborn, on lush pasture is mentioned here because of its similarity to the above mentioned diseases but there is no proven association with vitamin E in either case. It occurs most commonly on legume-dominant pasture and may be strictly limited in its distribution to certain farms. Cattle wintered entirely on alfalfa hay may show a much higher incidence of the disease in their calves when the hay is obtained from particular farms.

The incidence of enzootic muscular dystrophy on highly improved pasture appears to be increasing rapidly and varies from year to year depending on climatic conditions and productivity of the pasture. This form of the disease is also characterized by the ease with which it can be prevented by the administration of either selenium or vitamin E, results generally being better with selenium.

The occurrence of vitamin E deficiency in horses has been suggested in relation to paralytic myoglobinuria (azoturia) and a degenerative myopathy in foals (2). In foals the disease has been found to be associated with a subnormal intake of selenium and vitamin E and on clinico-pathological examination there were elevated serum levels of SGOT and SGPT (3). The purported effect of added alphatocopherol on the performance of thoroughbred horses has not been adequately tested.

In pigs, muscular dystrophy has been produced experimentally on vitamin E deficient rations (4) and is in some cases associated with hepatic injury and gastric ulceration. Natural occurrence of the disease has been recorded in pigs fed a diet containing about 50 per cent of coconut meal and in others fed a fish-liver oil emulsion. Feeding on fish scraps with a high content of unsaturated fatty acids, or flaxseed, produces yellow or brown discolouration of fat, preventable by the administration of adequate amounts of vitamin E.

Pathogenesis

Vitamin E occurs in nature as a mixture of alpha-, beta-, gamma- and delta-, and possibly other, tocopherols in varying proportions. The compounds vary widely in their biological activity so that chemical determination of total tocopherols is of much less value than biological assay. Alphatocopherol is the most potent and is available in a number of pharmaceutical forms which also vary in their biological activity. It has become necessary to express the unitage of vitamin E in terms of international units of biological activity (1 IU $\equiv$ 1 mg. synthetic racemic alpha-tocopheryl acetate. Natural *d*-alpha-tocopheryl acetate 1 mg. $\equiv$ 1 IU and natural *d*-alpha-tocopheryl 1 mg. $\equiv 0.92$ IU). The main biological function of vitamin E is to control the rate of tissue oxidation. Its sparing effect on vitamin A and essential unsaturated fatty acids are two important examples of this. How this physiological effect is translated into the prevention of muscular dystrophy is uncertain although prevention of the formation of abnormal phospholipids at cell surfaces which interfere with normal energy exchange has been suggested (1).

The role of vitamin E in preventing necrosis of the liver caused by a deficiency of sulphur-containing amino-acids is well known. This is probably related to the occurrence of hepatic dystrophy in pigs suffering from vitamin E deficiency but the gastric ulcers which also occur in these animals are not explained. 'Sawdust livers' in cattle are also described as nutritional hepatic necrosis due to a deficiency of selenium/vitamin E in the diet (5).

Selenium appears to have a sparing effect on vitamin E and is an efficient prophylactic against enzootic muscular dystrophy under certain conditions but does not prevent muscular dystrophy in animals fed on a diet containing cod liver oil. Selenium and vitamin E have an additive effect in reducing blood levels of SGOT, decreasing the ratio of urinary creatinine to creatine excretion and increasing the survival time of deficient lambs (6). Selenium has its sparing effect because it enhances the transport and retention of vitamin E.

The major clinical signs of vitamin E deficiency in calves, lambs and pigs are muscular weakness and dyspnoea. The first is evidently caused by the degeneration of skeletal muscle and the latter by either dystrophy of the diaphragmatic muscles or by the congestive heart failure resulting from myocardial involvement (7, 8). The skeletal muscle dystrophy which is so characteristic of the disease in calves, lambs, ducklings, dogs and adult sheep, is a true muscle degeneration and not a neurogenic atrophy. Acute muscular dystrophy results in the liberation of myoglobin into the blood stream, but the myoglobin content of muscle, and hence the tendency to myoglobinuria, varies between species and with age. Adult horses and pigs have a high content of myoglobin in their muscles, but in the other species myoglobin appears in the urine only in very small amounts after extensive muscle degeneration.

There is no firm evidence that a deficiency of vitamin E adversely affects the reproductive function of domestic animals, with the possible exception of the pig.

Clinical Findings

The presentation of a definite clinical picture is difficult because of the failure in many recorded outbreaks of muscular dystrophy to confirm the field diagnosis of vitamin E deficiency by curative and preventive tests and by laboratory examination. The following descriptions are subject to this deficiency and may include myopathies due to other causes.

There are two major syndromes, an acute form —myocardial dystrophy, and a subacute form— dystrophy of skeletal muscle, but the skeletal muscle lesions are present in varying degree in all forms of vitamin E deficiency, and cannot be considered to be pathognomonic of the deficiency. The common syndromes encountered in the field are described below.

Subacute enzootic muscular dystrophy. This form of the disease is most common in lambs and calves and occurs occasionally in pigs. In field cases the obvious signs are stiffness, weakness and trembling of the limbs and in many cases inability to stand. The gait in calves is accompanied by rotating movements of the hocks and in lambs a stiff, goose stepping action. Muscle tremor is evident if the animal is forced to stand for more than a few minutes. On palpation the muscles are hard and rubbery and often swollen. These abnormalities are always symmetrical. Most affected animals retain their appetite and will suck if held up to the dam. Major involvement of the diaphragm and intercostal muscles occurs in many cases and causes

dyspnoea with laboured and abdominal-type respiration. This may be the first sign in natural cases. The temperature varies widely from normal to as high as $41\cdot5\,^{\circ}C$ ($107\,^{\circ}F$).

Slow, spontaneous remission may occur but is always accompanied by marked residual atrophy of the affected muscles. Inability to move about and graze leads to inanition, and secondary bacterial infections are common.

In more severe and experimentally produced cases the upper borders of the scapulae protrude above the back line, and are widely separated from the chest, the toes are spread, there is relaxation of carpal and metacarpal joints or knuckling at the knees and standing on tip-toe, inability to raise the head, difficulty in swallowing, inability to use the tongue and relaxation of abdominal muscles. Choking may occur when the animals attempt to drink. The face has a drawn, haggard appearance.

Acute enzootic muscular dystrophy. Affected animals may die suddenly without premonitory signs especially after exercise. In calves under close observation a sudden onset of dullness and respiratory distress, accompanied by a frothy or blood-stained nasal discharge, may be observed in some cases. The heart rate is much faster than usual and often grossly irregular. Death ensues in 6 to 12 hours.

Although the emphasis in a particular case is often on skeletal muscle or myocardial dystrophy, lesions in the alternative site are usually present even though they are minimal. In sheep and lambs skeletal muscle dystrophy is the major lesion with some cases of myocardial dystrophy in lambs. In calves the major clinical signs are those due to involvement of skeletal muscles but myocardial dystrophy is more common than in lambs.

In pigs the defect is mainly myocardial with skeletal muscle lesions also present at necropsy. In this species the clinical signs are not diagnostic, comprising dullness followed by sudden death in most cases. Dyspnoea, vomiting and diarrhoea may occur in animals that survive for longer periods. Paralysis or paresis may also occur and if hepatic damage is present icterus may be observed. Reduction in litter numbers due to foetal death and resorption has also been recorded in sows fed on vitamin E deficient diets.

Foals with degenerative myopathy may die within 24 hours of the onset of signs but may survive for up to a week. Clinical signs include reluctance to move, hardness of the nuchal crest, gluteal muscles and abdominal wall, fever and increased heart and respiratory rates (2).

Clinical Pathology

The earliest test of any significance is the assessment of the quantity of glutamic oxalacetic transaminase present in serum. It is a sensitive indicator of the degree of muscle damage (9) although it is not necessarily specific for muscular dystrophy. In clinical cases of enzootic muscular dystrophy levels of 300 to 900 units per ml. in calves and 2000 to 3000 units per ml. in lambs have been observed. In normal animals of these species serum levels are usually less than 100 units per ml. The estimations have little value in predicting the development of muscular dystrophy, but the levels attained are directly proportional to the amount of muscle damage. Some clinically normal animals have high values (10). Other more tissue-specific enzymes have been used as clinico-pathological indicators of muscle damage. Some of these are lactate dehydrogenase (LDH), isocitrate dehydrogenase (ICD) and others in pigs (11) and these and creatinine phosphokinase in sheep (12). Serum ornithase carbamyl transferase levels are also elevated in vitamin E deficiency states in pigs (13), and aspartate aminotransferase and alanine aminotransferase in sheep (14).

Tocopherol levels in the blood and liver provide good information on the vitamin E status of the animal. Critical data are not available but plasma tocopherol levels of 0 to 100 µg. per 100 ml. of plasma occur in pigs and cattle on deficient diets and 500 to 1000 µg. per 100 ml. of plasma on pasture. Levels in plasma of less than 70 µg. per cent in calves and less than 150 µg. per cent in adult cattle are accepted as critical. Because there is considerable storage in liver the plasma may not be a true reflection of the current vitamin E intake. Tocopherol levels in the liver are a more accurate indication of vitamin E status than levels in the plasma. Critical levels of selenium in tissues and plants are given under the heading of selenium deficiency (p. 743).

Grossly abnormal electrocardiograms have been observed in some animals and may be of value in diagnosis (15). Similar changes are found in experimental and natural cases of enzootic muscular dystrophy and in many instances are detectable in the absence of clinical signs (16).

Creatine excretion increases markedly and is a useful method of diagnosing the disease and following its progress. The ratio of creatine to creatinine is most informative. Values of less than 0·7 occur in normal lambs, and values over 1 and as high as 5 are found in dystrophic lambs. In calves the normal excretion rate in the urine of 200 to 300 mg. per 24 hours may be increased to 1·3 g. per 24 hours, although in the late stages of the disease when much of the muscle mass has undergone degeneration the creatine excretion may be lower than normal.

Necropsy Findings

The macroscopic and histological appearance of the muscle lesions is quite constant but their distribution varies widely in different animals. Affected groups of skeletal muscle are always bilaterally symmetrical.

In skeletal muscle and the diaphragm there are localized white or greyish areas of degeneration which have an appearance of fish flesh. These areas may be in streaks, involving a large group of muscle fibres, running through the centre of apparently normal muscle or as a peripheral boundary around a core of normal muscle. In the diaphragm the distribution of dystrophic bundles gives the organ a radially striated appearance. The affected muscle is friable and oedematous and may be calcified. Secondary pneumonia often occurs in cases where the muscles of the throat and chest are affected.

In cases with myocardial involvement white areas of degeneration are visible particularly under the endocardium of the left ventricle in calves and both ventricles in lambs. The lesions may extend to involve the interventricular septum and papillary muscles. There may be cardiac hypertrophy and pulmonary congestion and oedema, and calcification of lesions has also been observed.

Histologically the muscle lesions are non-inflammatory. Hyaline degeneration is followed by coagulation necrosis. Biochemical analysis of affected muscle will indicate whether degeneration has occurred, as the creatine content of degenerate muscle falls markedly. A degeneration of Purkinje fibres in the myocardium has also been described but is reported also in calves fed diets deficient in potassium or manganese.

In pigs fed vitamin E deficient rations, additional necropsy findings are observed. There may be a massive generalized oedema similar to the exudative diathesis of chickens, a brown degeneration of fat depots, hepatic necrosis similar to that occurring in the vitamin E deficient rat, and ulceration in the cardial stomach. Abnormal red cells also occur in the bone marrow (13). The latter may lead to fatal internal haemorrhage. Extensive subendocardial haemorrhage may also be present in the left ventricle. Hepatic necrosis has also been observed in naturally occurring cases of enzootic muscular dystrophy in pigs (17). Yellowish brown discoloration of fat deposits is a feature of the disease in older (2 to 7 months) but not in young foals.

Diagnosis

Vitamin E deficiency should be considered when necropsy findings reveal a non-inflammatory, bilateral, hyaline degeneration of skeletal muscle or similar lesions in myocardium. A definite diagnosis must, however, depend upon curative and prophylactic trials with vitamin E. Analysis of feedstuffs for vitamin E potency may be of value but the possibility of a relative deficiency must be taken into consideration, particularly if there is a history of feeding of any fat or oil containing un-saturated fatty acids or access to lush pastures.

A great deal of interest has developed in recent years in the problem of myopathy in animals. This has been due largely to the complexity of the relations between vitamin E, selenium and myopathic agents, but also to the discovery of an unidentified, possibly inherited, myopathy associated with scrapie in sheep. Another unidentified myopathy has been observed at a high level of incidence in newborn lambs (18, 19). Affected lambs are unable to raise their heads and have flexed limb joints. The majority recover within a few weeks but permanent deformity caused by fibrous contracture of cervical muscles persists in a few. There are no lesions in the brain or spinal cord and although the clinical and necropsy findings resemble those of congenital myopathy ascribed to vitamin E deficiency, there has been no evidence of such a deficiency.

Enzootic muscular dystrophy may be easily confused with other diseases, particularly when the myocardial or diaphragmatic involvement is severe. Dyspnoea is evident and there may be a high fever so that the disease is often difficult to distinguish from pneumonia. However, severely affected calves are usually recumbent and unable to rise, and the heart rate is disproportionately high and irregular. Involvement of the atria in cases of lymphomatosis occurs usually in adult cows and acute heart failure (falling disease) caused by copper deficiency also occurs only in adult cows. Myocardial degeneration may also occur in foot-and-mouth disease.

Subacute enzootic muscular dystrophy, in which skeletal muscle lesions predominate, may be readily confused with other forms of paresis and paralysis, and in some areas commonly occurs concurrently with hypomagnesaemic tetany of calves. In lambs enzootic ataxia and swayback may be suspected and there is no simple method of differentiating the diseases other than by local experience of the deficiency most likely to occur. All three diseases occur most commonly in the spring and early summer, although enzootic muscular dystrophy is more closely associated with sudden exercise after release from confinement. A necropsy examination will usually serve to differentiate between the various conditions.

In lambs, calves and pigs arthritis caused by a number of bacterial infections is common and may be accompanied by endocardial involvement, but is usually manifested by fever and enlargement of joints as well as stiffness and lameness. Muscle lesions typical of enzootic muscular dystrophy are absent.

Treatment

In general terms the administration of selenium alone is more beneficial than vitamin E and the combination of the two is a superior treatment to either one alone.

Immediate treatment of affected cases by oral administration or the intramuscular injection of alpha-tocopheryl acetate is often followed by disappearance of signs in about 3 days provided lesions are not too extensive. Although clinical recovery occurs in such cases lesions will still be apparent at necropsy. Although recommended doses for the treatment of affected animals have been 300 to 500 mg. for lambs and 750 mg. for calves, daily for 3 or 4 days, much larger doses (four times) have been found to be advantageous in some areas. A proportion of animals recover spontaneously and this must be taken into consideration when evaluating the results of treatment. Oral treatment with a water dispersible preparation facilitates absorption of the vitamin, and is preferred to intramuscular injection in oil but experimental work with ruminants indicates much greater retention after administration by injection (20, 21). Because of the common association of phosphorus and vitamin E deficiency preparations containing phosphorus and vitamin E are often used for both treatment and prevention but phosphorus itself appears to have no preventive effect.

Selenium preparations are widely used as treatments and, combined with alpha-tocopherol, appear to be the best treatment available. For lambs a subcutaneous injection of 1·0 mg. of selenium and for pigs a similar injection of 0·2 mg. selenium per kg. body weight are recommended. The recommended mixture for injection contains 3 mg. selenium (as sodium selenite) and 150 IU of d-alpha-tocopheryl acetate per ml., and the dose rate for treatment is 2 ml. per 45 kg. body weight.

Control

In areas where legume pasture or hay from particular farms or areas is known to be dangerous, it may be possible to avoid this feed during the danger period.

It is not always possible to avoid the diets which cause the disease and the administration of protective substances, particularly alpha-tocopherol or selenium, is recommended.

Prophylactic dosing is usually by the addition of wheat germ oil or meal, wheat bran or alpha-tocopheryl acetate to the feed. Suggested doses of alpha-tocopherol are 1 g. daily before calving for cows and 150 mg. daily for the calves after birth. The corresponding doses for ewes and lambs are 75 mg. and 25 mg. respectively. Dosing of lambs and calves offers reasonably good protection and is the usual procedure but in exceptional circumstances it may be advisable to dose the dams before parturition. This method is not as effective as administration to the young and rather larger doses are required. It is the only method likely to be effective when the neonatal form of the disease is encountered. The prenatal dosing of the dam with selenium is more effective than dosing with vitamin E with respect to enhancing the status of the lamb (22).

To avoid the necessity of daily dosing a programme of intermittent dosing has been recommended (24). A dose of 3000 IU of *d*-alpha-tocopheryl acetate is given on the second day of life and repeated in 1 week. If the calves are to remain stabled for more than 3 weeks following the second dose a third, similar dose, is administered 1 week before they are turned out to pasture. Care must be taken to ensure that adequate doses of the correct unitage are used. The relative potencies of the available preparations and the relation between international units and mg. have been discussed previously.

The administration of selenium, in the feed or by injection, as a preventive has been a very popular research topic during the past few years and appears to have a modest advantage over vitamin E (9). It has proved to be highly effective in preventing enzootic muscular dystrophy in lambs on lush, legume pasture, in lambs turned out to pasture in spring, and calves of cows fed low-tocopherol diets, but not against the development of the disease in calves and lambs fed cod liver oil (24) even when the selenium is fed at the rate of 1·0 ppm in the diet. It has been suggested that the disease which occurs after the administration of cod liver oil is a vitamin E deficiency whilst that occurring on lush pasture is a selenium deficiency

(20). If the danger period in the area is in the first few weeks of life the selenium can be given to the dam; if it is later, at say 2 to 3 months of age, it is administered to the lamb or calf. The recommended dose rates are 0·1 to 0·5 ppm of selenium in the diet daily to young animals, or repeated injections at monthly intervals of 1·0 mg. of selenium to lambs, 5 mg. to ewes, 10 mg. to calves and 30 mg. to adult cattle. The injection is administered about a month before the anticipated danger period. Comparable dose rates of the various compounds in use are: 1 mg. selenium is equivalent to 2·2 mg. anhydrous sodium selenite, 2·4 mg. anhydrous sodium selenate or 4·7 mg. hydrated sodium selenate. These doses may be repeated without danger at monthly intervals. A mixture of selenium and vitamin E can also be used as a preventive at half the dose recommended under the heading of treatment above (23). It can be administered orally or by injection to the young or to the dam and can be repeated at 2- to 4-week intervals. Toxic reactions resulting from overdosing have been described under selenium poisoning. A slow release pellet (15 mg. selenium) implanted in calves soon after birth shows promise as a preventive measure (25).

A preliminary experiment has shown that the addition of sodium selenite (0·2 mg. per kg. of feed) prevents the occurrence of hepatic necrosis in recently-weaned pigs on a ration containing soya meal and possibly deficient in vitamin E. However, degeneration of skeletal muscle and deposits of ceroid in adipose tissue occurred in spite of the supplementation with selenium.

REFERENCES

(1) Blaxter, K. L. (1957). *Vet. Rec.*, *69*, 1150.
(2) Dodd, D. C. *et al.* (1960). *N.Z. vet. J.*, *8*, 45.
(3) Schougaard, H. *et al.* (1972). *Nord. Vet.-Med.*, *24*, 67.
(4) Lannek, N. *et al.* (1961). *Res. vet. Sci.*, *2*, 67.
(5) Todd, G. C. & Krook, L. (1966). *Path. vet.*, *3*, 379.
(6) Ewan, R. C. *et al.* (1969). *J. Anim. Sci.*, *27*, 751.
(7) Buchanan-Smith, J. G. *et al.* (1969). *J. Anim. Sci.*, *29*, 808.
(8) Nafstad, I. & Tollersrud, F. (1970). *Acta vet. scand.*, *11*, 452.
(9) Hopkins, L. L. *et al.* (1964). *J. Anim. Sci.*, *23*, 674.
(10) Hidiroglou, M. *et al.* (1967). *Canad. vet. J.*, *8*, 62.
(11) Tollersrud, S. & Nafstad, I. (1970). *Acta vet. scand.*, *11*, 495.
(12) Whanger, P. D. *et al.* (1970). *Amer. J. vet. Res.*, *31*, 965.
(13) Michel, R. L. *et al.* (1969). *J. Amer. vet. med. Ass.*, *155*, 50.
(14) Tollersrud, S. (1971). *Acta vet. scand.*, *12*, 365.
(15) Godwin, K. O. & Fraser, F. J. (1966). *Quart. J. exp. Physiol.*, *51*, 94.
(16) Godwin, K. O. (1968). *Nature (Lond.)*, *217*, 1275.
(17) Dodd, D. C. & Newling, P. E. (1960). *N.Z. vet. J.*, *8*, 95.
(18) Stamp, J. T. (1961). *J. comp. Path.*, *70*, 296.
(19) Nisbet, D. I. & Renwick, C. C. (1961). *J. comp. Path.*, *71*, 177.

(20) Hidiroglou, M. *et al.* (1970). *Brit. J. Nutr.*, *24*, 917.
(21) Caravaggi, C. *et al.* (1968). *N.Z. J. agric. Res.*, *11*, 313; *12*, 655.
(22) Paulson, G. D. *et al.* (1968). *J. Anim. Sci.*, *27*, 195.
(23) Nelson, F. C. *et al.* (1964). *Canad. vet. J.*, *5*, 268.
(24) Blaxter, K. L. (1962). *Proc. Nutr. Soc.*, *21*, 211.
(25) Hidiroglou, M. *et al.* (1972). *Anim. Prod.*, *14*, 115.

Vitamin K Deficiency

A primary deficiency of vitamin K is unlikely under natural conditions in domestic animals because of the high content of substances with vitamin K activity in most plants, and the substantial synthesis of these substances by microbial activity in the alimentary canal (1). Sporadic cases may occur when impairment of the flow of bile reduces the digestion and absorption of fat and concurrently the absorption of this fat-soluble vitamin. Experimentally produced vitamin K deficiency in piglets is manifested by hypersensitivity, anaemia, anorexia, weakness and a marked increase in prothrombin time (2). The minimum daily requirement for newborn pigs is 5 µg. per kg. body weight and the minimum curative injection dose is four times this.

The most important therapeutic use of vitamin K in domestic animals is in sweet clover poisoning where toxic quantities of coumarin severely depress the prothrombin levels of the blood and interfere with its clotting mechanism. Industrial poisons used in rodent control which contain anticoagulants of the coumarin type, e.g. warfarin, cause fatal hypothrombinaemia and vitamin K is an effective antidote. Menadione, the synthetic vitamin K, is used pharmaceutically.

A disease of young rapidly growing pigs characterized by spontaneous haemorrhage and failure of blood to clot has been observed in U.S.A. and England in recent years. There appears to be interference with normal vitamin K utilization but the exact cause has not been determined. Prevention and treatment can be accomplished by the addition of menadione sodium bisulphate, a synthetic vitamin K, to the feed or drinking water.

REFERENCES

(1) Kon, S. K. & Porter, J. W. G. (1947). *Nutr. Abst. Rev.*, *17*, 31.
(2) Schendel, H. E. & Johnson, B. C. (1962). *J. Nutr.*, *76*, 124.

DISEASES DUE TO DEFICIENCIES OF THE WATER-SOLUBLE VITAMINS

Water-soluble vitamins including vitamin C and the B complex are of little importance in herbivorous animals (except for vitamin B_{12}) because of their synthesis in the alimentary tract of these animals. Thiamine, nicotinic acid, riboflavine, pantothenic acid, pyridoxine, biotin and folic acid are all synthesized by microbial activity, and nicotinic acid and vitamin C are synthesized by other means. The young calf or lamb, in the period before ruminal activity begins, is likely to receive inadequate supplies of these vitamins and deficiency states can be produced experimentally. In the pre-ruminant stage colostrum and milk are good sources of the water-soluble vitamins, ewe's milk being much richer than cow's milk. The production of signs of deficiency of the B vitamins in horses by the feeding of deficient diets has raised some doubts as to the availability of the B vitamins synthesized in the large bowel in this species.

Vitamin C is synthesized by all species and is not an important dietary essential in any of the domestic animals. Synthesis occurs in tissues and although blood levels fall after birth in the newborn calf they begin to rise again at about 3 weeks of age. However, a dermatosis of young calves has been associated with low levels of ascorbic acid in their plasma and responds to a single injection of 3 g. of ascorbic acid (1). A heavy dandruff, followed by a waxy crust, alopecia and dermatitis commences on the ears and spreads over the cheeks, down the crest of the neck and over the shoulders. Some deaths have been recorded but spontaneous recovery is more usual.

Thiamine Deficiency

(*Hypothiaminosis*)

The disease caused by deficiency of thiamine in tissues is characterized chiefly by nervous signs.

Aetiology

Thiamine deficiency may be primary, due to deficiency of the vitamin in the diet, or secondary, because of destruction of the vitamin in the diet by thiaminase. A primary deficiency is unlikely under natural conditions because most plants, especially seeds, yeast and milk contain adequate amounts. Synthesis in the rumen of sheep is in excess of demand for both pregnant and non-pregnant animals, and cattle also are independent of dietary supplies. The degree of synthesis is governed to some extent by the composition of the ration, a sufficiency of readily fermentable carbohydrate causing an increase of synthesis of most vitamins of the B complex, and a high intake in the diet reducing synthesis (2). Microbial synthesis of thiamine also occurs in the alimentary tract of monogastric animals and in young calves and lambs but not in sufficient quantities to avoid the necessity for a dietary supply, so that deficiency states can be readily induced in these animals with experimental diets. Thiamine is relatively unstable and easily destroyed by cooking.

The coccidiostat, amprolium, is a thiamine antagonist and others are produced by certain plants, bacteria, fungi and fish.

Occurrence

Three major occurrences of secondary thiamine deficiency are recorded. The inclusion of excess raw fish in the diet of carnivores leads to destruction of thiamine because of the high content of thiaminase in the fish. In horses the ingestion of excessive quantities of bracken fern (*Pteridium aquilinum*) and horsetail (*Equisetum arvense*) causes nervous signs because of the high concentration of a thiaminase in these plants. The disease has been induced in a pig fed bracken rhizomes and the possibility exists of it occurring under natural conditions (21). It has also been reported in horses fed large quantities of turnips (*Beta vulgaris*) without adequate grain (22). The third important occurrence of thiamine deficiency is in the aetiology of polio-encephalomalacia and is discussed under that heading.

Pathogenesis

The only known function of thiamine is its activity as a cocarboxylase in the metabolism of fats, carbohydrates and proteins and a deficiency of the vitamin leads to the accumulation of endogenous pyruvates. Although the brain is known to depend largely on carbohydrate as a source of energy, there is no obvious relationship between a deficiency of thiamine and the development of the nervous signs which characterize it. Additional clinical signs do occur too in the circulatory and alimentary systems but their pathogenesis cannot be clearly related to the known functions of thiamine.

The efficiency of thiamine in the treatment of paralytic myoglobinuria in horses may be open to doubt but the high carbohydrate diet which precedes the attack, and the accumulation of lactic acid in the affected muscles suggest that its use is justified.

Clinical Findings

Bracken fern (*Pteridium aquilinum*) *and horsetail* (*Equisetum arvense*) *poisoning in the horse.* Incoordination to the point of falling, and bradycardia due to cardiac irregularity, are the cardinal clinical signs of bracken fern poisoning in the horse and these signs disappear after the parenteral administration of thiamine (3). Similar clinical effects occur with horsetail (4). Swaying from side to side occurs first, followed by pronounced inco-ordination, including crossing of the forelegs and wide action in the hindlegs. When standing the legs are placed well apart, and crouching and arching of the back are evident. Muscle tremor develops and eventually the horse is unable to rise. Clonic convulsions and opisthotonus are the terminal stage. Appetite is good until late in the disease when somnolence prevents eating. Temperatures are normal and the heart rate slow until the terminal period when both rise to above normal levels. Neither plant is palatable to horses and poisoning rarely occurs at pasture. The greatest danger is when the immature plants are cut and preserved in meadow hay.

Experimental syndromes. These syndromes have not been observed to occur naturally but are produced readily on experimental rations.

In pigs inappetence, emaciation and leg weakness, and a fall in body temperature, respiratory rate and heart rate occur. The electrocardiogram is abnormal and congestive heart failure follows. Death occurs in 5 weeks on a severely deficient diet (5).

In calves, weakness, inco-ordination, convulsions and retraction of the head occur and in some cases anorexia, severe scouring and dehydration (6).

Lambs 1 to 3 days old placed on a thiamine-deficient diet show signs after 3 weeks. Somnolence, anorexia and loss of condition occur first, followed by tetanic convulsions (7).

Clinical Pathology

Blood pyruvic acid levels in horses are raised from normal levels of 2 to 3 μg. per 100 ml. to 6 to 8 μg. per 100 ml. Blood-thiamine levels are reduced from normals of 8 to 10 μg. per 100 ml. to 2·5 to 3·0 μg. per 100 ml. Electrocardiograms show evidence of myocardial insufficiency. In pigs blood pyruvate levels are elevated and there is a fall in blood transketolase activity. These changes occur very early in the disease (27).

Necropsy Findings

No macroscopic lesions occur in thiamine deficiency other than non-specific congestive heart failure in horses. The myocardial lesions are those of interstitial oedema and lesions are also present in the liver and intestine.

In the experimental syndrome in pigs there are

no degenerative lesions in the nervous system but there is multiple focal necrosis of the atrial myocardium accompanied by macroscopic flabbiness and dilatation without hypertrophy of the heart.

Diagnosis

Diagnosis of secondary thiamine deficiency in horses must be based on the signs of paralysis and known access to bracken fern or horsetail. A similar syndrome may occur with poisoning by *Crotalaria* spp., perennial ryegrass, *Indigophera enneaphylla* and ragwort (*Senecio jacobea*) but is accompanied by hepatic necrosis and fibrosis. The encephalomyelitides are usually accompanied by signs of cerebral involvement, by fever and failure to respond to thiamine therapy.

Treatment

In clinical cases the injection of a solution of the vitamin produces dramatic results. In all species the dose rate is from 0·25 to 0·5 mg. per kg. body weight. In horses rather larger doses of up to 1·25 mg. per kg. body weight are used in the treatment of paralytic myoglobinuria. Excessive doses are toxic. Peripheral vasodilatation, cardiac arrhythmia, depression of respiration with asphyxial convulsions, and death due to respiratory failure occur with very large doses.

Control

The daily requirement of thiamine for monogastric animals is in general 30 to 60 µg. per kg. body weight. The addition of yeast, cereals, grains, milk, liver and meat meal to the ration usually provides adequate thiamine.

Riboflavine Deficiency

(*Hyporiboflavinosis*)

Although riboflavine is essential for cellular oxidative processes in all animals, the occurrence of deficiency under natural conditions is rare in domestic animals because actively growing green plants and animal protein are good sources, and some synthesis by alimentary tract microflora occurs in all species. Synthesis by microbial activity is sufficient for the needs of ruminants but a dietary source is required in these animals in the pre-ruminant stage. Milk is a very good source. Daily requirements for pigs are 60 to 80 µg. per kg. body weight and 2 to 3 g. per ton of feed provides adequate supplementation. The trend towards confinement feeding of swine has increased the danger of naturally occurring cases in that species.

On experimental diets the following syndromes have been observed:

In *pigs* slow growth, frequent scouring, rough skin and matting of the hair coat with heavy, sebaceous exudate are characteristic. There is a peculiar crippling of the legs with inability to walk and marked ocular lesions including conjunctivitis, swollen eyelids and cataract. The incidence of stillbirths may be high.

In *calves* anorexia, poor growth, scours, excessive salivation and lacrimation, and alopecia occur. Areas of hyperaemia develop at the oral commissures, on the edges of the lips and around the navel. There are no ocular lesions (7).

Nicotinic Acid Deficiency

(*Hyponiacinosis*)

Nicotinic acid or niacin is essential for normal carbohydrate metabolism. Because of the high content in most natural animal feeds deficiency states are rare in ordinary circumstances except in pigs fed rations high in corn. Corn has both a low niacin content and a low content of trytophane, a niacin precursor. A low protein intake exacerbates the effects of the deficiency but a high protein intake is not fully protective.

In ruminants, synthesis within the animal provides an adequate source. Even in young calves signs of deficiency do not occur and because rumen microfloral activity is not yet of any magnitude, extra-ruminal synthesis appears probable.

The daily requirements of niacin for mature pigs are 0·1 to 0·4 mg. per kg. body weight, but growing pigs appear to require rather more (0·6 to 1·0 mg. per kg. body weight) for optimum growth (8).

Experimentally induced nicotinic acid deficiency in pigs is characterized by inappetence, severe diarrhoea, a dirty yellow skin with a severe scabby dermatitis and alopecia. Posterior paralysis also occurs. At necropsy haemorrhages in the gastric and duodenal walls, congestion and swelling of the small intestinal mucosa and ulcers in the large intestine are characteristic and resemble closely those of necrotic enteritis caused by infection with *Salmonella* spp. Histologically there is severe mucoid degeneration followed by local necrosis in the wall of the caecum and colon.

The oral therapeutic dose rate of nicotinic acid in pigs is 100 to 200 mg. Ten to 20 g. per ton of feed supplies sufficient nicotinic acid for pigs of all ages (9). Niacin is low in price and should always be added to swine rations based on corn.

Pyridoxine (Vitamin B₆) Deficiency

(*Hypopyridoxinosis*)

A deficiency of pyridoxine in the diet is not known to occur under natural conditions. Experimental deficiency in pigs is characterized by periodic epileptiform convulsions, and at necropsy by generalized haemosiderosis with a microcytic anaemia, hyperplasia of the bone marrow and fatty infiltration of the liver. The daily requirement of pyridoxine in the pig is of the order of 100 μg. per kg. body weight or 1·0 mg. per kg. of solid food (10) although higher levels have been recommended on occasions. Certain strains of chickens have a high requirement for pyridoxine and the same may be true of swine.

Experimentally induced deficiency in calves is characterized by anorexia, poor growth, apathy, dull coat and alopecia. Severe, fatal epileptiform seizures occur in some animals (11). Anaemia with poikilocytosis is characteristic of this deficiency in cows and calves.

Pantothenic Acid Deficiency

(*Hypopantothenosis*)

Pantothenic acid is a dietary essential in all species other than ruminants, which synthesize it in the rumen. Deficiency under natural conditions has been recorded mainly in pigs on rations based on corn.

In pigs (5, 12, 13) a decrease in weight gain due to anorexia and inefficient food utilization occurs first. Dermatitis develops with a dark brown exudate collecting about the eyes and there is a patchy alopecia. Diarrhoea and inco-ordination with a spastic, goose-stepping gait are characteristic. At necropsy a severe, sometimes ulcerative, colitis is observed constantly, together with degeneration of myelin.

500 μg. per kg. body weight per day of calcium pantothenate is effective in treatment and prevention (14). As a feed additive 10 to 12 g. per ton is adequate (9).

Experimentally induced pantothenic acid deficiency in calves is manifested by rough-hair coat, dermatitis under the lower jaw, excessive nasal mucus, anorexia, and reduced growth rate and is eventually fatal. At necropsy there is usually a secondary pneumonia, demyelination in the spinal cord and peripheral nerves, and softening and congestion of the cerebrum (15).

Biotin Deficiency

(*Hypobiotinosis*)

Biotin is a vitamin of almost universal distribution in plant and animal materials and, being required in very small quantities, is unlikely to be deficient in diets under natural conditions especially as microbial synthesis occurs in the alimentary tract. Continual feeding of sulphonamide drugs or antibiotics may induce a deficiency. An antivitamin to biotin (avicidin) occurs in egg white and biotin deficiency can be produced experimentally by feeding large quantities of uncooked egg white.

Experimental biotin deficiency has been shown to cause paralysis of the hind quarters in calves (16). In pigs experimental biotin deficiency is manifested by alopecia, dermatitis and cracking of the soles and tops of the hooves. There is also inflammation of the oral mucosa (17).

Soymeal, dry whey, dry distiller's solubles and brewer's yeast are good sources of biotin.

Folic Acid Deficiency

(*Hypofolicosis*)

Folic acid (pteroylglutamic acid) is necessary for nucleic acid metabolism and its deficiency in humans leads to the development of pernicious anaemia. Under ordinary conditions domestic animals other than the pig produce sufficient folic acid by intestinal synthesis to make a dietary intake unnecessary. Although naturally occurring deficiencies have not been diagnosed positively in domestic animals, folic acid has numerous and complex interrelationships with other nutrients and the possibility of a deficiency playing a part in inferior animal performance should not be overlooked.

Choline Deficiency

(*Hypocholinosis*)

Choline is a dietary essential for pigs and young calves. Calves fed on a synthetic choline-deficient diet from the second day of life develop an acute syndrome in about 7 days (18). There is marked weakness and inability to get up, laboured or rapid breathing and anorexia. Recovery follows treatment with choline. Older calves are not affected. On some rations the addition of choline increases daily gain in feedlot steers, particularly during the early part of the feeding period. In pigs ataxia, fatty degeneration of the liver and a high mortality rate occur. Enlarged and tender hocks have been observed in feeder pigs. For pigs 1 kg. per ton of food is considered to supply sufficient choline (9).

Congenital splayleg of piglets has been attributed to choline deficiency but adding choline to the ration of the sows does not always prevent the condition (28).

Vitamin B$_{12}$ Deficiency

(*Hypocyanocobalaminosis*)

Vitamin B$_{12}$ deficiency is unlikely to occur under natural conditions other than because of a primary dietary deficiency of cobalt, which is an important disease in many countries of the world.

Although microbial synthesis of the vitamin occurs in the rumen in the presence of adequate cobalt, and in the intestines of other Herbivora such as the horse (25, 26), it is probably a dietary essential in the pig and young calf. Animal protein is a good source. A deficiency syndrome has been produced in young calves on a synthetic ration. Signs include anorexia, cessation of growth, loss of condition and muscular weakness. The daily requirement under these conditions is 20 to 40 μg. of vitamin B$_{12}$ (19). Sows vary in their ability to absorb the vitamin and those with poor absorption ability or on deficient diets show poor reproductive performance (23). For pigs 10 to 50 mg. per ton of feed is considered to be adequate (9). The vitamin is used empirically in racing dogs and horses to alleviate parasitic and dietetic anaemias in these animals at a dose rate of 2 μg. per kg. body weight. Cyanocobalamin zinc tannate provides effective tissue levels of vitamin B$_{12}$ for 2 to 4 weeks after one injection (20) and normal and abnormal blood levels have been established for all species (26). It is also used as a feed additive for fattening pigs usually in the form of fish or meat meal or as 'animal protein factor'. It is essential as a supplement if the diet contains no animal protein, and maximum results from the feeding of antibiotics to pigs are obtained only if the intake of vitamin B$_{12}$ is adequate.

REFERENCES

(1) Rydell, R. O. (1948). *J. Amer. vet. med. Ass.*, *112*, 59.
(2) Bugiassy, C. & Tribe, D. E. (1960). *Aust. J. agric. Res.*, *11*, 989 & 1002.
(3) Carpenter, K. J. *et al.* (1950). *Brit. vet. J.*, *106*, 292.
(4) Henderson, J. A. *et al.* (1952). *J. Amer. vet. med. Ass.*, *120*, 375.
(5) Goodwin, R. F. W. (1962). *J. comp. Path.*, *72*, 214.
(6) Johnson, B. C. *et al.* (1948). *J. Nutr.*, *35*, 137.
(7) Draper, H. H. & Johnson, B. C. (1951). *J. Nutr.*, *43*, 413.
(8) Powick, W. C. *et al.* (1947). *J. Anim. Sci.*, 6, 310.
(9) Cuthbertson, W. F. J. (1957). *Vet. Rec.*, *69*, 192.
(10) Miller, E. R. *et al.* (1957). *J. Nutr.*, *62*, 407.
(11) Johnson, B. C. *et al.* (1950). *J. Nutr.*, *40*, 309.
(12) Maclean, C. W. (1965). *Vet. Rec.*, *77*, 578.
(13) Sharma, G. L. *et al.* (1952). *Amer. J. vet. Res.*, *13*, 298.
(14) Ellis, N. R. (1946). *Nutr. Abst. Rev.*, *16*, 1.
(15) Sheppard, A. J. & Johnson, B. C. (1957). *J. Nutr.*, *61*, 195.
(16) Wiese, A. C. *et al.* (1946). *Proc. Soc. exp. Biol. Med.*, *63*, 521.
(17) Lehrer, W. P. *et al.* (1952). *J. Nutr.*, *47*, 203.
(18) Johnson, B. C. *et al.* (1951). *J. Nutr.*, *43*, 37.
(19) Lassiter, C. A. *et al.* (1953). *J. Dairy Sci.*, *36*, 997.
(20) Thompson, R. E. & Hecht, R. A. (1959). *Amer. J. clin. Nutr.*, *7*, 311.
(21) Evans, I. A. *et al.* (1963). *J. comp. Path.*, *73*, 229.
(22) Gratzl, E. (1960). *Wien. tierärztl. Mschr.*, *47*, 25.
(23) Frederick, G. L. (1965). *Canad. J. Anim. Sci.*, *45*, 22.
(24) Oakley, G. A. (1970). *Vet. Rec.*, *86*, 252.
(25) Davies, M. E. (1971). *Brit. vet. J.*, *1*, 34.
(26) Alexander, F. & Davies, M. E. (1969). *Brit. vet. J.*, *125*, 169.
(27) Evans, W. C. *et al.* (1972). *Vet. Rec.*, *90*, 471.
(28) Dobson, K. J. (1971). *Aust. vet. J.*, *47*, 587.

29

Diseases Caused by Physical Agents

Environmental Pollutants and Noise

ALTHOUGH there is now an extensive literature on this subject as it affects man it is not proposed to deal with it here in depth as a veterinary problem. The individual chemical agents which are likely to pollute the atmosphere, particularly fluorine, arsenic and lead, are dealt with under their headings as poisons. The significance and alleviation of the problems caused by the pollution of the atmosphere appears to us to be a subject for a textbook on preventive medicine. There remains the subject of air pollution by physical agents, of which smoke and dust are the most significant. In both instances the effects are most noticeable in the lungs after inhalation but ingestion after deposition on fodder can be important also. For definitive work on this form of animal disease it is necessary to use established techniques for measuring the degree of pollution and be aware of the composition of the polluting agent. For example, automobile fumes contain poisons such as carbon monoxide, fumes irritant to lungs and carbon particles capable of soiling animal exteriors. The subject has been extensively reviewed and annotated (1).

Pollution by noise, a matter of increasing importance for veterinarians who police codes of practice for animal welfare and for those who are called upon to act as expert witnesses in cases involving excessive noise and its effects on animals, is also an important subject. Unfortunately no extensive review is readily available.

Some examination has been made of the effects of the sonic bang produced by aircraft (2). Most of the effects are due to fear reactions and include injury due to sudden flight, killing of young by mink and rabbits, suffocation in panic-stricken chickens and reduced egg production. Cows appear to be unaffected. Experimentally, loud noises of 90 to 100 phons applied to horses cause an increase in heart rate (3).

REFERENCES

(1) Lillie, R. J. (1970). *Air Pollutants Affecting the Performance of Domestic Animals*. U.S. Dept. of Agriculture, Agricultural Research Service, Agriculture Handbook No. 380.
(2) Boutelier, C. (1967). *Rev. Corps vét. Armée*, **20**, 112.
(3) Sakurai, N. *et al.* (1967). *Exp. Rep. Eq. Hlth Lab. Japan Racing Association, Tokyo*, **4**, 14.

Radiation Injury

Animals exposed to radioactive materials may suffer radiation injury. They may also serve as reservoirs for radioactive material which could be passed to man in meat, milk and other animal products. This hazard to man is a problem of public health and the following discussion is restricted to the effects of irradiation on the health of animals exposed to it.

Aetiology

Radiation injury can be caused in a number of ways including atomic bomb injury and exposure to roentgen rays, but the effects on the tissues are the same, differences occurring only in depth of penetration and degree of injury caused.

The effects of atomic explosions on animals are due to the three major results of such explosions, blast, heat and irradiation. Irradiation is the main cause of animal mortality and studies of its effects have been extensively reviewed (1, 2).

There is considerable variation in the effects of an atomic explosion depending on the distance from and the time after the blast and whether the explosion occurs in the air or on the ground surface. Animals within the range of immediate irradiation are more severely affected than those exposed only to the 'fall-out' of fissionable material on pasture. However, grazing animals are exposed to very great risk because of this fall-out. Of the radioactive materials produced by an atomic explosion a number of radionuclides, including ^{131}I, ^{140}Ba, ^{89}Sr, ^{137}Cs and ^{90}Sr, are likely to enter biological systems. Of these radioactive iodine, barium and strontium 89 are of limited importance because of their short half-lives. On the other hand strontium 90 and caesium 137 are produced in very large quantities and have long half-lives and are therefore of greatest biological significance. If sufficient of these radionuclides is ingested and tissue levels of them reach critical points, injury similar to that produced by external irradiation will occur. The effects of exposure of animals to strontium 90 and iodine 131 have been exhaustively reviewed (3).

Pathogenesis

Veterinarians are concerned with the effects of radiation injury to animals at two levels, the somatic dose resulting from acute, direct exposure to irradiation, and the cumulative dose due to the gradual accumulation of radioactivity in tissues resulting from continued exposure to small but toxic levels of radioactive materials.

Somatic doses. With median lethal doses (500 roentgen, 'rem' or 'r' units received during a period of 24 hours is an approximate MLD for most domestic animals (4)) 'radiation sickness' develops, manifested by signs of acute irritation of the alimentary tract. With high lethal doses the animal may die at this stage but more commonly progresses to a second stage of apparent normality for a few days.

The third phase commences at the end of the first week due to profound depression of bone marrow activity. Initially there is a lymphopenia followed by a depression of granulocyte and platelet counts. The leucopenia permits invasion by bacteria from the alimentary tract and bacteraemia and septicaemia develop 1 to 4 weeks after irradiation. The clotting mechanism and antibody production are impaired and facilitate the invasion. Progressive necrosis of the gut wall without inflammation is characteristic. Thrombocytopenic haemorrhages into the lymphatic system and other tissues lead to the development of a profound anaemia.

The activity of germinative epithelium is also profoundly depressed and if the animal survives the early stages listed above, the hair commences to shed, the skin to ulcerate and a gross reduction in fertility occurs. Degenerative changes in the lens of the eye, particularly cataract, may also occur. Very long term effects of irradiation include a high rate of mutations and a high incidence of tumours, mostly of the haemopoietic system and particularly of the leukaemic series.

Chronic exposure. When 'fall-out' contaminates pasture there may be sufficient fissionable material on the leaves of the plants to produce the same effects as those which occur with direct irradiation with median lethal doses, except that radiation sickness does not occur. Two indexes are used to measure the chronic effects of low level exposure, the genetic and leukaemogenic indexes. The first depends on assessment of the increase in mutation

rate in the population and the second on the increase in leukaemia rate. Actual doses measured physically at this level are estimated in 'millirems' (one-thousandth of one 'rem' unit). With smaller doses the effects are quite different and depend on the radioactive substances formed, their solubilities and decay periods. Iodine and strontium are of importance when contamination of leaves occurs, but when the effects are due mainly to contamination of the soil and absorption by plants, strontium and caesium are the significant elements. Radioactive iodine causes damage to the thyroid gland and strontium causes destruction of bone tissue, depression of leucocyte and platelet production and a terminal depression of erythropoiesis. Both are excreted in the milk of animals and may cause deleterious effects in humans and animals drinking the milk. The maximum permissible concentration of radioactive substances in milk would be reached at much lower levels of pasture contamination than would be required to cause physical injury to the cattle.

Clinical Findings

Acute syndrome. After immediate irradiation with high doses, damage to the alimentary tract occurs and there is a resulting intense, refractory diarrhoea. Death occurs in a few days due to dehydration and salt depletion. Local contact of radioactive materials to skin causes changes within a few hours. Observable lesions vary from depilation and slight desquamation to extensive necrosis depending upon the irradiation dose.

Subacute syndrome. Immediately after irradiation with median doses there is an initial phase of 'radiation sickness' characterized by anorexia, vomiting and profound lethargy which lasts for from several hours to several days. The second phase is one of apparent normality lasting until 1 to 4 weeks after irradiation and is followed by a third phase in which most deaths occur. There is fever, knuckling at the fetlocks, swelling of one or more legs and diarrhoea developing to melaena and dysentery sometimes with tenesmus. Anorexia is complete but there is great thirst. Weakness, recumbency and hyperirritability are present. Respiration is rapid and panting and there is a profuse nasal discharge, sometimes blood stained. Severe anaemia and septicaemia occur in the terminal stages, death usually occurring about 20 days after irradiation.

In general if the animal survives this period, there is a long period of convalescence which is accompanied by failure to make normal weight gains, alopecia, sterility and lenticular defects. The sterility may be permanent or normal fertility may be restored by the end of 8 months in pigs and 2 years in cattle. During the ensuing years, recovered animals may produce mutant offspring. Tumours, especially of the haemopoietic system, and of areas of skin which suffer radiation injury (5) are also likely to occur. Experimental irradiation of pregnant animals causes foetal death and resorption, defects of individual organ and limb development, decreased survival of young born alive and depressed growth rate and fertility of surviving young, the type of abnormality depending upon the stage of pregnancy at which exposure is experienced (6).

These general statements do not apply to cows which survive one median somatic dose. Provided such cows survive for 40 days after irradiation they appear to recover quickly and conceive readily. Congenital anomalies appear to occur only rarely and only in calves which are irradiated in utero.

Chronic exposure to gamma and mixed neutron–gamma radiation for several years produces lenticular opacities (7). At levels of irradiation which cause lesions in the human lens similar opacities occur in the lens of cattle, but not pigs or burros.

Clinical Pathology

In cattle receiving median somatic doses the total leucocyte count falls precipitately during the first few days after irradiation with the peak of fall at the 15th to 25th post-irradiation (PI) day. In this species the most sensitive leucocyte is the neutrophil in contrast to the lymphocyte which is most seriously affected by irradiation in man. Platelet counts begin to decrease from a normal of 500,000 per cmm. on the 7th PI day to 40,000 per cmm. about PI day 21. Erythrocyte counts and haematocrit levels also fall and prothrombin times increase in parallel to the other changes mentioned.

Necropsy Findings

Gastroenteritis, varying from haemorrhagic to ulcerative, is constant, and ulceration of the pharyngeal mucosa and pulmonary oedema occur commonly. Haemorrhages into tissues are also characteristic and include all degrees from petechiae and ecchymoses to haematomas and large extravasations. Degeneration of bone marrow and lymphoid tissue is evident histologically. Many bacterial colonies are present in ulcerated areas and in parenchymatous organs.

Diagnosis

The subacute syndrome closely resembles poisoning by bracken fern in cattle and by trichlo-roethylene-extracted soyabean meal, but the diagnosis will usually depend upon a knowledge of exposure to irradiation.

Control

The problems of veterinary civil defence in the event of thermonuclear warfare are too extensive to discuss here and the necessary information is provided by most governments.

REVIEW LITERATURE

Garner, R. J. (1969). Radiation and radiation hazards. *Veterinary Annual*, 240. Bristol: Wright.

REFERENCES

(1) Trum, B. F. & Rust, J. H. (1958). *Advanc. vet. Sci.*, *4*, 51.
(2) Wilkins, J. H. (1963). *J. roy. Army vet. Corps*, 34, 64.
(3) McClellan, R. D. & Bustad, L. K. (1964). *Ann. N.Y. Acad. Sci.*, *111*, 793.
(4) Wilkins, J. H. (1962). *J. roy. Army vet. Corps*, 33, 74.
(5) Brown, D. G. *et al.* (1966). *Amer. J. vet. Res.*, 27, 1509.
(6) O'Brien, C. A. *et al.* (1966). *Amer. J. vet. Res.*, 27, 711.
(7) Brown, D. G. *et al.* (1972). *Amer. J. vet. Res.*, 33, 309.

Brisket Disease

(*Mountain Sickness*)

This is a sporadic disease of cattle, and possibly other species, kept at high altitudes. Clinically it is characterized by a syndrome of congestive heart failure.

Incidence

Brisket disease occurs sporadically in high mountainous areas in the U.S.A. and South America. The morbidity rate in indigenous cattle seldom exceeds 1 per cent, but may be much higher in newly introduced cattle. Recovery is rare.

Aetiology

At high altitudes the low density of the atmosphere results in environmental anoxia and this is presumed to be the predisposing cause of brisket disease. The fact that the incidence is greater in introduced than in indigenous cattle suggests that cattle reared at high altitudes may become adapted to the environment. Any additional factor such as myocardial dystrophy, anaemia, pulmonary disease, or hypoproteinaemia may exacerbate the primary cardiac decompensation and this probably accounts for the sporadic occurrence of the disease in herds kept at high altitudes. The additional effort required to obtain feed on sparse pasture may also be a predisposing cause. Cattle of all ages and breeds are susceptible but the disease occurs most commonly in yearlings. Goats, sheep, donkeys and horses are also reputed to be affected in that order of reducing susceptibility.

Occurrence

Brisket disease is recorded only in animals which have been maintained for some months at heights of over 1800 m. above sea level.

Pathogenesis

Anoxic anoxia at high altitudes causes pulmonary vasoconstriction and circulatory embarrassment because the oxygen requirements of tissues exceed the available oxygen supplies. In normal animals and man this is usually compensated by the development of polycythaemia, an increase in lung volume, and an increased volume of cardiac output. It has been shown that continued hypoxia can cause sufficient myocardial weakness to interfere with cardiac compensation and thus lead to congestive heart failure. This is most likely to occur if the animal has to walk long distances to get feed. The development of any additional factor, such as pneumonia or anaemia, which exacerbates the oxygen deficit will also increase the susceptibility to cardiac decompensation. Animals affected by these diseases can often exist satisfactorily at lower altitudes where their cardiac decompensation is compatible with the environment. That brisket disease can develop in the absence of these diseases has been proved experimentally. The removal of cattle from an altitude of 1100 m. to 3000 m. has been shown to cause hypertrophy of the right ventricle, an increase in pulmonary arterial pressure from 27 mm. Hg to from 45 to over 100 mm. Hg and the development of right heart failure (1, 2).

Clinical Findings

The animal has a dejected appearance, loses condition rapidly, has a rough, lustreless coat, and stands with the elbows abducted. Jugular vein engorgement is followed by the appearance of oedema of the brisket, spreading up the neck to the intermandibular space and back along the ventral aspect of the body. Abdominal enlargement due to the development of ascites is accompanied by diarrhoea. There is hyperpnoea at rest, and dyspnoea and weakness on slight exertion. The mucosae may be cyanotic, particularly after exercise, and the lung sounds vary from an increased vesicular murmur, to moist râles and an absence of breath sounds when pneumonia is present, and to crepitant râles in the presence of emphysema. Auscultation of the heart reveals tachycardia, increased absolute intensity of the sounds, or a

decrease when there is hydropericardium, and an increase in the size of the heart. A haemic murmur may also be present. The appetite is normal until the late stages and the temperature is normal unless secondary pneumonia develops.

Clinical Pathology

In affected cattle there is a significant reduction in the packed cell volume coincident with a fall in mean cell volume, and in haemoglobin levels. Hypocalcaemia, hyperphosphataemia and hyperpotassaemia also occur (3).

The effect of altitude on normal horses is of interest. In horses elevation from sea-level to 2200 m. causes elevation of heart rate, respiratory rate before and after exercise, ratio of heart to respiratory rate and an increase in red and white cell counts. A stabilization period of 21 to 28 days is considered necessary before horses perform at their best (4). In sheep and cattle elevations of 6000 to 11,500 feet cause rises in haemoglobin (35 per cent in sheep, 9 per cent in cattle) and packed cell volumes (27 per cent in sheep but no change in cattle) and haemoglobin concentration in red cells (8 to 9 per cent increase in cattle and sheep) (5).

Necropsy Findings

There is enlargement of the heart, with marked hypertrophy and dilatation of the right ventricle (3). There is an accompanying severe oedema of the pericardial, pleural and peritoneal sacs and subcutaneous tissues. The oedema may also involve the wall of the alimentary tract. Minor lesions are present on the heart valves and there may be areas of calcification in the large arteries. Typical congestive changes are evident in the liver—enlargement, rounding of the edges, dilatation of the hepatic veins, and a marked deposition of fibrous tissue around the central veins. In the lungs there is often severe alveolar emphysema, and in some cases bronchitis and pneumonia are also present.

Diagnosis

Congestive heart failure occurs in several diseases of cattle including traumatic pericarditis, lymphomatosis affecting the myocardium, congenital cardiac defects and valvular endocarditis. In these diseases there is cardiac involvement and care is necessary in differentiating the accompanying abnormal heart sounds. The occurrence of congestive heart failure in cattle at high altitudes should arouse suspicion of brisket disease.

Treatment

The cardiac reserve must be maintained and compensation encouraged. Avoidance of excessive exercise by the supplementary feeding of affected animals may cause temporary improvement and individual animals may be helped by the administration of digitalis or related glucosides but the drugs must be given parenterally and the improvement may be only temporary (5). Diuretics to promote fluid loss and antibiotics to combat secondary infection may be indicated in individual cases. Return of affected cattle to lower altitudes results in recovery in many cases.

Control

Control measures are difficult to implement. Restriction of grazing, hand feeding with particular emphasis on a high protein diet, and prompt treatment of cases of pulmonary disease are recommended as worthwhile procedures.

REFERENCES
(1) Guilbride, P. D. L. & Sillau, H. (1970). *Span*, *13*, 177.
(2) Wagenwoort, C. A. *et al.* (1969). *J. comp. Path.*, *79*, 517.
(3) Blake, J. T. (1966). *Amer. J. vet. Res.*, *26*, 68, 76.
(4) de Aluja, A. S. *et al.* (1968). *Vet. Rec.*, *82*, 368.
(5) Javed, A. H. & Washburn, L. E. (1968). *W. Pakist. J. agric. Res.*, *6*, 154.

Lightning Stroke and Electrocution

Exposure to high-voltage electric currents in the form of lightning stroke or electrocution causes sudden nervous shock with temporary unconsciousness or immediate death. Residual nervous signs may persist after recovery from nervous shock.

Incidence

The area incidence is never high but on individual farms heavy mortalities may occur when a barn or a group of animals sheltering under a tree is struck. As many as twenty head of cattle may be killed by one lightning flash. Faulty wiring in barns may kill occasional animals and lower production in others.

Aetiology

The three common causes are flashes of linear lightning during thunderstorms, broken overhead electrical transmission wires which usually carry very high voltages, and faulty electrical wiring in cowsheds and barns. In lightning stroke trees, fences, barns and pools of water may become electrified and it is not unusual for damp ground to act as a conductor for electricity passing along the roots of stricken trees. Animals electrocuted by standing on electrified earth are unlikely to show burn marks on the body. Oak trees are particularly prone to lightning stroke and because of their spreading foliage and extensive root system are common mediators of electrocution deaths in pastured animals. Poplar, elm, walnut, beech, ash and conifer are also highly susceptible (1). Transmission wires are most dangerous when they fall into pools of water, as they are likely to do during the storms which bring the wires down. In such cases the entire pool is electrified and animals passing through it may be killed instantly. In accidents caused by faulty wiring voltages of 110 to 220 volts are sufficient to kill adult cattle provided they make good contact with the source and the ground (2). Water pumps and milking machines are the common sources of electricity which may electrify water pipes or the milk line through the earth wire or a short circuit. The use of very heavy fuse wire (30 to 60 amps) may cause continuance of the trouble which could be avoided if lower capacity fuses were used.

Occurrence

Most fatalities caused by lightning stroke occur during the summer months when the cattle are at pasture. Deaths due to electrocution in barns may occur at any time.

Pathogenesis

Exposure to high-voltage electrical currents causes severe nervous shock with complete unconsciousness and flaccid paralysis. In some instances focal destruction of nervous tissue occurs and residual signs of damage to the nervous system persist after nervous shock disappears. Death when it occurs is usually due to paralysis of vital medullary centres. Ventricular fibrillation may also occur and contribute to the fatal outcome (1). Superficial burns may be evident at the site of contact with the current or along the path of flow from the point of contact to ground. The burn is produced by heat generated from the resistance of tissues to the passage of the electricity.

Clinical Findings

Varying degrees of shock occur. With high voltage currents and good earth contacts such as wet concrete floors, water, and damp earth, the animal may fall dead without a struggle. Singeing and burning are likely to occur because of the severity of the shock. The burns may be localized to the muzzle or feet and be in the form of radial deposits of carbon with or without disruption of tissue, or they may appear as tree-like, branching patterns of singeing running down the trunk and limbs.

In less severe shocks the animal falls unconscious but there is some struggling, followed by a period of unconsciousness varying from several minutes to several hours. When consciousness is regained the animal may rise and be perfectly normal, or show depression, blindness, posterior paralysis, monoplegia and cutaneous hyperaesthesia. In some cases there may be more local signs including nystagmus and unilateral paralysis (3, 4). Sloughing of the skin at the sites of burns may occur after a few days. These signs may persist or disappear gradually over a period of 1 to 2 weeks. In one severe episode of lightning stroke in pigs a large number of animals were affected by posterior paralysis due apparently to fracture of the ileum, ischium and the transverse processes of the lumbar vertebrae (5).

With minor shocks, especially as they occur in barns on low-voltage domestic current, the animal may be knocked down or remain standing. Consciousness is not lost and the clinical picture is one of restlessness and periodic convulsive episodes of short duration. In these episodes the animal may kick violently at the stanchion or the dividing rail. The attacks may be intermittent and occur only when the cattle supply a good ground contact such as standing in the gutter, when they are drinking, or when they are wet. In some cases the shock is so mild that no clear signs are evident but drinking may be interfered with and production lowered drastically (6). Dairy farmers are often unaffected in the same environment because their rubber boots provide effective insulation.

Clinical Pathology

Laboratory examinations are of no value in diagnosis.

Necropsy Findings

Diagnostic lesions are often minimal (7) but singe marks or damage to the environment, or both, occur in about 90 per cent of lightning deaths.

Rigor mortis develops but passes off quickly. Accumulation of gas in the alimentary tract is rapid and the carcase swells up and decomposes rapidly. Blood may exude from the external orifices and a blood-stained froth from the nostrils. The pupils are usually dilated and the anus relaxed. All viscera are congested and the blood is dark and unclotted. Petechial haemorrhages may occur throughout the body, including the trachea, endocardium, meninges and central nervous system. The superficial lymph nodes, particularly the prescapular and the interior cervical, are often haemorrhagic. Superficial singeing of the hair, burn marks on the feet or muzzle, and internal or subcutaneous extravasations of blood in arboreal patterns also occur. In some cases there are longitudinal fractures of long bones, and in one serious incident involving pigs extensive fractures of the bones in the pelvic area and local haemorrhage have been observed. Fractures of the ribs occurred in other pigs. If electrocution is suspected it is best to ensure that possible sources of electric power are shut off before proceeding with a post-mortem examination.

Diagnosis

Great care must be taken in accepting an owner's suggestion that an animal has been killed or injured by lightning stroke. Insurance against loss by lightning is commonly carried and the many other causes of sudden death or injury are seldom covered by insurance. To confirm a diagnosis there should be a history of exposure and evidence of sudden injury or death. In the latter case half-chewed food may still be present in the mouth. Burns on the skin, scorching of the grass and tearing of the bark on nearby trees are also accepted as contributory evidence. The possibility of electrocution caused by faulty wiring should be considered when sudden shocks or death occur in animals confined in stanchions. Snakebite, gunshot wound, acute heart failure and trauma of the brain may also result in sudden death without other signs and a careful necropsy examination may be necessary to determine the cause of death. There are very few agents other than electricity which can kill a number of animals within a few minutes. Hydrocyanic acid is the other common cause of such an incident.

Acute septicaemias including anthrax and blackleg, and some poisonings including hydrocyanic acid and nitrite may produce a similar syndrome but are detectable on necropsy or suitable laboratory examination. Unexpected outbreaks of bloat may need to be differentiated from electrocution because of the frequency with which ruminal tympany occurs rapidly after death in the latter.

Treatment

Central nervous system stimulants and artificial respiration should be provided for unconscious animals but in most instances the animals are dead or recovered before treatment can be instituted.

Control

Precautions taken to avoid lightning stroke in animals are largely ineffective, but proper installation of all electric equipment in barns and milking parlours is essential to prevent losses. All motors should be earthed to a special iron spike or pipe driven at least eight feet into the ground, preferably in a damp spot. Earthing to water pipes should not be permitted. A rubber connection between the pump of the milking machine and the vacuum line will prevent electrification of the line. Minimum amperage fuses should be used to provide protection in cases of short-circuiting.

REFERENCES

(1) Mills, J. H. L. & Kersting, E. J. (1966). *J. Amer. vet. med. Ass.*, *148*, 647.
(2) Fox, F. H. (1954). *Cornell Vet.*, *44*, 103.
(3) Holgado Rivas, D. E. (1970). *Gac. vet.*, *32*, 124.
(4) Barr, M. (1966). *Vet. Rec.*, *79*, 170.
(5) Best, R. H. (1967). *Canad. vet. J.*, *8*, 23.
(6) Salisbury, R. M. & Williams, F. M. (1967). *N.Z. vet. J.*, *15*, 206.
(7) Ramsey, F. K. & Howard, J. R. (1970). *J. Amer. vet. med. Ass.*, *156*, 1472.

Fleece Rot of Sheep

Fleece rot of sheep is a dermatitis caused by prolonged wetting of the skin and resulting in matting of the wool by exudate. A common accompaniment of the disease is discolouration produced by the growth of chromogenic bacteria in the matted wool.

Incidence

The disease is common in most parts of Australia during wet years and causes considerable financial loss because of the depreciation in the value of the damaged fleeces. The general health of the sheep is unaffected.

Aetiology

Experimentally, continued skin-wetting produces the disease and this is thought to be the main aetiological factor. When rainfall is sufficient to wet sheep to the skin for a week, fleece rot may occur. Young sheep are more susceptible than old, and heritable differences in fleece characters affect the susceptibility of individual sheep (1). These characters are probably related to the ease with which the skin can be wetted. The degree of 'grip' and skin wrinkling were found to be unimportant as factors affecting susceptibility. A long fleece dries slowly and for this reason predisposes to the condition. Fleeces with a high wax content are less susceptible probably because of the water-proofing effect of the wax. A dense fleece protects against wetting of the skin but during prolonged periods of wet weather such fleeces do become wet and predispose to fleece rot because of the slowness with which they dry out. The above factors are largely contributory, the fundamental factor affecting susceptibility being the sensitivity of the skin to continued wetness. Discolouration of the fleece may or may not occur depending upon the presence of chromogenic bacteria. The type of discolouration varies with the type of bacteria present. For example a blue discolouration can be produced by *Pseudomonas indigofera* (2).

Occurrence

Fleece rot occurs in sheep only in wet seasons and when the fleece is predisposed to wetting by its physical characters.

Pathogenesis

Dermatitis develops due to the wetness, the subsequent exudation causing a matting of the wool fibres and providing a suitable medium for the proliferation of chromogenic bacteria.

Clinical Findings

Lesions occur most commonly over the withers and along the back. The wool over the affected parts is always saturated and the tip is more open than over unaffected areas. The wool is leached and dingy and in severe cases can be plucked easily. Colouration of the skin changes from normal pink to purple, and a matted layer appears across the staple. Colouration of the wool by green, brown, orange, pink and blue bands occurs at any level in the staple, often separate from the matted layer.

Diagnosis

Fleece rot resembles mycotic dermatitis but there is no scab development and no skin ulceration.

Control

Treatment is unlikely to be of value but some degree of control may be effected by selection of sheep with suitable fleeces and skins for use in susceptible localities. In these same localities shearing before the wet season should facilitate drying of the fleece and lessen susceptibility.

REFERENCES

(1) Dunlop, A. A. & Hayman, R. H. (1958). *Aust. J. agric. Res.*, *9*, 260.
(2) Mulcock, A. P. *et al.* (1965). *Aust. J. agric. Res.*, *16*, 485.

30

Diseases Caused by Chemical Agents—I

WHEN animals are sick and the cause is not immediately apparent a diagnosis of suspected poisoning is often made. An analyst is faced with a hopeless task if he is provided with this information only. The examination of tissues and other materials is an expensive and laborious procedure and every effort should be made to provide information on the circumstances which have led to the diagnosis, some suggestion as to the poison or class of poisons suspected, and material for examination should be carefully selected and properly packed for transport.

The conditions which usually arouse suspicion of poisoning are illness in a number of previously healthy animals, affected at the same time, and showing the same signs and necropsy findings. These conditions of course may also apply to some infections, metabolic and nutritional deficiency diseases. It is only by acquaintance with the syndromes produced by the common poisons, particularly those likely to occur locally, that this primary differentiation can be made. Poisonous plants often show a geographical limitation in distribution; particular industrial enterprises may create poison hazards in local areas; certain agricultural practices, including the spraying of orchards, the dipping or spraying of cattle for ectoparasites and the use of prepared concentrate feed for pigs and cattle may also lead to poisoning in groups of animals. So many chemical agents are used in agriculture today that a section of miscellaneous farm chemicals likely to cause poisoning of animals has been included. The appearance of clinical illness soon after feeding, after a change of ration, after medication or spraying, or after change to new pasture is a common history in many outbreaks of disease caused by chemical agents.

The report which accompanies material for toxicological analysis should include a full record of history, clinical signs and necropsy findings and particularly the results of a search of the environment for access to a poison. If the animal has been treated, the drugs that were used and the dates of administration should be given as they may create difficulties for the analyst. The poison or group of poisons suspected should be defined.

Specimens for analysis should include a sample of the suspected source material. Next most important is a specimen of alimentary tract contents, so that ingestion of the material can be proven, and a sample of tissue, usually liver, to prove that absorption of the poison has occurred. Most toxic chemicals are ingested but percutaneous absorption and inhalation must be considered as possible portals of entry. One of the advantages of an examination of alimentary tract contents is that qualitative tests can be carried out and in many cases this determines whether or not further examination of tissues is necessary.

Additional specimens required other than liver and alimentary tract and contents, vary with the poison and the following list is suggested for the common chemicals:

Arsenic	Kidney, skin and hair
Lead	Kidney, bones and blood
Phosphorus	Kidney and muscle
Mercury	Kidney
Copper	Kidney and blood
Sodium Chloride	Alimentary tract and contents only
Fluorine	Bones, teeth and urine
Hydrocyanic Acid	Ingesta in a filled and airtight container, blood and muscle
Nitrate and Nitrite	Ingesta (plus chloroform or formalin) in an airtight, filled container, blood
Strychnine	Blood, kidney and urine

Careful packing of specimens is necessary to avoid loss of some poisons by escape as gas or conversion by bacterial fermentation, or to prevent contamination. No preservative should be added except in the case of suspected nitrite poisoning. If a preservative is necessary because of distance from the laboratory, packing in dry ice or ethyl alcohol (1 ml. per g. of tissue) is advisable but in the latter instance a specimen of the alcohol should also be sent. Ingesta and tissues must be kept separate as diffusion is likely to occur between the two. Specimens should be packed in glass or plastic to prevent contamination by lead in soldered joints of cans. Metal tops on jars should also be separated from the tissues by a layer of plastic or other impervious material. A suitable amount of material should be submitted for analysis. One kg. of ingesta, 1 kg. of liver and proportionate amounts of other viscera are suggested to cover all contingencies.

Poisoning is in most instances accidental although it may occasionally be deliberate. Deliberate or criminal poisoning is often suspected but is rarely proved. If there is a strong suspicion of criminal poisoning, or if litigation appears possible in accidental poisoning, specimens should be collected in duplicate and placed in sealed containers in the presence of witnesses. A complete set of specimens should be available to both plaintiff and defending parties for independent analysis.

PRINCIPLES OF TREATMENT IN CASES OF POISONING

There are certain principles which apply to all cases of poisoning and they are listed briefly below. The two main principles are the removal of the residual poison from the alimentary tract or skin, and the provision of chemical and physiological antidotes to the poison that has been absorbed.

In farm animals gastric lavage and emetics are of little or no practical value and the removal of residual poison from the alimentary tract depends largely upon the use of purgatives. The use of irritant purgatives is not advisable when the poison is an irritant and has already caused gastroenteritis, and oily purgatives are preferable in these cases. Saline purgatives are of value in the treatment of non-irritant poisons such as cyanogenetic glucosides. Neutralization of residual poison in the alimentary tract can be effected in some cases. For example oxidizing agents or tannic acid preparations are effective in precipitating alkaloids; proteins, including milk and eggs are effective chemical antidotes for poisons that coagulate proteins; lead is precipitated by the addition of sulphates to the alimentary tract contents.

Poison that has already been absorbed can in some instances be inactivated or its excretion facilitated by the provision of chemical antidotes. For instance sodium nitrite and sodium thiosulphate are effective systemic antidotes to hydrocyanic acid, and calcium versenate is an effective antidote against lead.

Treatment of the effects of a poison includes provision of physiological antidotes, for example the injection of a calcium salt in cases of overdosing with magnesium salts, and treatment of the effects of the poison. Ancillary treatment, including the provision of fluids in dehydration due to diarrhoea, demulcents in gastroenteritis, sedatives in excitement, stimulants in cases of central nervous system depression, all come under the latter heading.

REVIEW LITERATURE

Buck, W. B. (1969). Laboratory toxicological tests and their interpretation. *J. Amer. vet. med. Ass.*, **155**, 1928.

DISEASES CAUSED BY INORGANIC POISONS

Lead Poisoning
(*Plumbism*)

Incidence

Lead is one of the commonest causes of poisoning in farm animals, particularly sheep and cattle, in which the mortality rate approximates to 100 per cent.

Aetiology

Irrespective of the chemical form of the ingested lead only a small proportion is absorbed because of the formation in the alimentary tract of insoluble lead complexes which are excreted in the faeces. For example only 1 to 2 per cent of lead ingested as lead acetate or carbonate is absorbed from the alimentary tract of sheep (1). Of the lead absorbed some is excreted in the bile, milk and urine and the blood and urine levels of lead may give some indication of the lead status of the animal. Deposition in tissues occurs, particularly in the liver and renal cortex in acute poisoning and in the bones in chronic poisoning. In spite of the common occurrence of signs of nervous system involvement, the deposition of lead in brain is not high. The deposited lead is gradually liberated from tissues into the blood stream and excreted via the bile and urine. Consideration must be given to these aspects of lead metabolism when assessing the results of chemical analyses of tissues.

There is considerable variation between species in their susceptibility to lead, and the chemical composition of the compound containing lead may influence its toxicity. Also young animals are more susceptible than adults. A figure of 0·15 to 0·25 mg. lead per kg. body weight is often quoted as a lethal dose but doses of lead acetate accepted as being lethal are 500 g. for horses, 50 g. for cattle and 30 g. for sheep. In calves the ingestion of 0·2 to 0·4 g. per kg. body weight of lead acetate, basic carbonate or oxide in one day is known to be fatal (1) but deaths in cattle have also been caused by the ingestion of amounts as small as 4·8 mg. per kg. body weight of very finely ground lead oxide. Pigs are much more resistant to lead poisoning than are cattle and daily doses of 33 to 66 mg. per kg. body weight are required for periods of up to 14 weeks to have fatal effects (2).

Ruminants are most commonly affected and this may be due in part to the tendency for particulate material to settle in the reticulum and be converted to soluble lead acetate by the action of the acid medium of the forestomachs. In addition cattle in particular seem to be attracted to lead paint.

Occurrence

Lead poisoning occurs most commonly in cattle at pasture, particularly if the pasture is poor and the animals are allowed to forage in unusual places, such as rubbish dumps. Phosphorus deficiency may also be a predisposing cause in that affected animals will chew solid objects as a manifestation of osteophagia. However, cattle on lush pasture may also seek out foreign material to chew. Confined housing of calves with or without overcrowding is often followed by the appearance of pica which may be caused by boredom or by mineral deficiency.

The common sources of lead are lead-bearing paints and metallic lead. Discarded paint cans are particularly dangerous but fences, boards and the walls of pens, painted canvas and burlap are also common sources in calves (2). Painted silos may cause significant contamination of the ensilage.

Metallic lead in the form of car batteries, lead shot, solder or leaded windows has caused mortalities although under experimental conditions sheet lead does not cause toxic effects. Lead sheeting which has been exposed to the weather or subjected to acid corrosion appears to be more damaging, possibly because of the formation of a fine coating of a soluble lead salt. Lead poisoning appears to be a major hazard in the vicinity of oil fields and engine sump oil may contain over 500 mg. lead per 100 ml. (3). The palatability of automotive and other mineral oils to bovines is high. Less common but still potent sources of lead are linoleum, roofing felt, putty, automobile oil filters and aluminium paint. Some of the latter paints contain large quantities of lead, others none at all. Only lead-free aluminium paint should be used on fixtures to which animals have access.

Lead parasiticide sprays, particularly those containing lead arsenate, have caused heavy losses in cattle grazing in recently sprayed orchards or vegetable crops. Lead pipes carrying soft water may lead to the ingestion of excess lead, and pasture may be contaminated by fumes and residues from smelters at lead mines (4). Ruminants are able to withstand small doses of lead over very long periods. Chronic poisoning occurs in lambs, cattle and horses near old lead mines, and in the vicinity of foundries and smelters (5, 6, 7). Deaths have occurred in horses on pasture carrying 100 to 300 ppm of lead on the foliage (8). Tetraethyl lead may occur in dangerous concentrations on forage grown along major highways. Boiled linseed oil contains lead, and its accidental use as a laxative may result in lead poisoning. Although ingestion is by far the commonest mode of entry of lead, animals in the vicinity of lead smelters may inhale sufficient lead-laden fumes to produce toxic effects.

Although acute lead poisoning usually develops rapidly there may be a delay of several days after toxic material has been ingested before clinical signs appear.

Pathogenesis

The toxic effects of lead are manifested in three main ways, lead encephalopathy, gastroenteritis and degeneration of peripheral nerves. In general, acute nervous system involvement occurs following the ingestion of large doses in susceptible animals such as calves, alimentary tract irritation following moderate doses, and peripheral nerve lesions following long-term ingestion of small amounts of lead. The mechanism by which the nervous signs of encephalopathy and the lesions of peripheral nerve degeneration are produced appears to be related to the degenerative changes seen in nervous tissue (9). This may be a direct effect of the poison or be related to increased intracranial pressure because there is some increase in CSF pressure. Gastroenteritis is produced by the caustic action of lead salts on the alimentary mucosa. Ruminal atony occurs in cattle and sheep and causes an initial constipation later followed in some cases by diarrhoea due to gastroenteritis. Peripheral nerve degeneration occurs principally in horses.

The lesions, including degeneration of the liver and kidney, vary in their severity with the tissue levels of lead attained. Lead does not remain in tissues for long periods except in bone where it is deposited in an inert form, but from which it can be liberated at a later date in sufficient quantities to cause chronic lead poisoning. This is particularly likely to occur during periods of acidosis.

The blue 'lead-line' at the gum–tooth junction, which is seen in man and the dog does not commonly occur in ruminants because of failure to form tartar but may be present in the horse. The 'lead-line' is a deposit of lead sulphide formed by the combination of lead with sulphide from the tartar. Lead is transferred across the placental barrier and high liver levels occur in the lambs of ewes fed more than normal amounts of lead.

The mechanism by which osteoporosis is produced in young lambs affected by chronic lead poisoning has not been explained, nor has the paresis and paralysis of lambs which occurs in the same circumstances. The paralysis in the former condition is caused by compression of the spinal cord by collapsed lumbar vertebrae.

Clinical Findings

Cattle. Both acute and subacute syndromes occur in cattle, the former being more common in calves and the latter in adults. In the acute syndrome there is usually a sudden onset of signs and a short course of 12 to 24 hours so that many animals, especially those at pasture, are found dead without signs having been observed. Affected calves commence to stagger and show muscle tremor, particularly of the head and neck, with champing of the jaws and frothing at the mouth. There is snapping of the eyelids, rolling of the eyes and, in many cases, bellowing. The animal collapses and intermittent tonic-clonic convulsions develop and may continue until death occurs. Pupillary dilatation, opisthotonus and muscle tremor are marked and persist between the convulsive episodes. There is hyperaesthesia to touch and sound and the pulse and respiratory rates are increased. In some cases, particularly in adults, the cow remains standing and shows evidence of blindness and mania, charging into fences, attempting to climb walls and pressing strongly with the head against fixed objects. The general appearance of the animal is one of frenzy and on some occasions they will attack humans but the gait is stiff and jerky and progress is impeded. Death usually occurs during a convulsion and is due to respiratory failure.

In the subacute form the animal remains alive for 3 to 4 days. There is dullness, complete lack of appetite, blindness and some abnormality of gait including inco-ordination and staggering, and sometimes circling. The circling is intermittent and not always in the same direction. Muscle tremor and hyperaesthesia are present as in the more acutely affected animals. Salivation, grinding of the teeth, and abdominal pain as evidenced by kicking at the belly are other common signs. Alimentary tract dysfunction is one of the most common abnormalities. Ruminal atony is accompanied by constipation in the early stages. Later a foetid diarrhoea occurs in most cases. The animal presents a picture of extreme dullness, will not eat or drink, and stands immobile for very long periods. Death frequently occurs by misadventure, the animal walking blindly into a waterhole or being trapped in a fence or between trees. In other circumstances the animal becomes recumbent and dies quietly. In both syndromes the eye preservation reflex is diminished or absent and oedema of the optic disc is visible on ophthalmoscopic examination.

Sheep. Lead poisoning in sheep is usually manifested by a subacute syndrome similar to that seen in cattle. There is anorexia and an initial constipation followed by the passage of dark, foul smelling faeces. Weakness and ataxia follow, often with evidence of abdominal pain, but there is no excitement, tetany nor convulsions. Polyuria occurs when the intake of lead is small but with large amounts there is oliguria (1).

Although ruminants are supposed to be resistant to chronic lead intoxication, two syndromes of posterior paresis have been described in young lambs in old lead-mining areas and tissue levels of lead are abnormally high in both instances. In both of the paretic syndromes there is impairment of the gait. In one it is caused by osteoporotic changes in the skeleton but in the other there is no suggestion of skeletal changes (10). In the osteoporotic disease the signs occur only in lambs 3 to 12 weeks of age and never in adults. There is stiffness of gait, lameness and posterior paralysis. Affected lambs are unthrifty and the bones, including the frontal bones, are very fragile. The paralysis is caused by lesions of the vertebrae, usually affecting one or more of the lumbar bones, and resulting in compression of the spinal cord. In the second form of the disease, gait abnormalities occur in the same lamb age group and are manifested initially by incomplete flexion of the limb joints so that the feet drag while walking. In a later stage the fetlocks are flexed, the extensor muscles paretic, and the lamb soon becomes recumbent. Recovery is common although many lambs die of intercurrent disease.

Horses. Horses are not commonly affected by lead poisoning although chronic plumbism is sometimes seen, usually in the vicinity of lead mines and processing works. Inspiratory dyspnoea caused by paralysis of the recurrent laryngeal nerve is the commonest syndrome. This may be accompanied by pharyngeal paralysis in which recurrent choke and regurgitation of food and water through the nostrils occur. Aspiration pneumonia may result after inhalation of ingesta through the paralysed larynx. Paralysis of the lips occasionally accompanies the other signs. General muscle weakness and stiffness of the joints occur commonly and the coat is usually harsh and dry. When chronic poisoning with both lead and zinc occurs the signs of zinc poisoning predominate despite high lead levels in liver and kidney (16).

When large amounts of lead are ingested by horses a syndrome similar to that of the subacute form in cattle occurs. There is complete anorexia, severe nervous depression, partial paralysis of the limbs followed in most cases by complete paralysis and recumbency. Mild to severe abdominal pain and clonic convulsions may also occur.

Pigs. Early signs include squealing as though in pain, mild diarrhoea, grinding of the teeth and salivation. The disease is usually a prolonged one and listlessness, anorexia and loss of weight develop followed by muscle tremor, inco-ordination, partial or complete blindness, enlargement of the carpal joints and disinclination to stand on the front feet. Convulsive seizures occur in the terminal stages (2).

Clinical Pathology

In the living animal which has ingested lead the element can be recovered from faeces, urine, blood and milk. Because lead can be ingested in small doses over long periods without ill effects it is important that analyses be carried out on a number of specimens. Urine levels for example are variable and never high (0·2 to 0·3 ppm) and although elevated urine levels are usually associated with high blood levels this relationship does not necessarily hold. The estimation of blood levels is generally useful in determining the lead status of the animal. Normal milk levels in cattle (0·028 to 0·030 ppm) may be raised to as high as 2·26 ppm in severely poisoned cows (11). Faecal calves represent unabsorbed and excreted lead deriving from the bones, and are of limited value unless considered in conjunction with blood levels because the ingested lead may have been in an insoluble form and harmless to the animal. When faecal levels are high it can be assumed that the lead has been ingested in the preceding 2 or 3 weeks but high blood levels may be maintained for months after ingestion. Thus high blood and low faecal levels indicate that the lead was taken in some weeks previously but high blood and high faecal levels suggest recent ingestion and significant absorption. Because of the frequency with which lead appears in the environment as a pollutant there is often concern nowadays at the validity of the normal values for establishment of a diagnosis. However, in the average city polluted atmosphere it seems that

lead intake will be significantly elevated (12). The lead content of hair is reported to be raised significantly in poisoned animals (13) but hair is not routinely used in diagnosis. Representative data for normal and poisoned animals are given in the table below.

Levels of Lead in the Blood and Faeces of Normal and Poisoned Animals (12, 14, 4)

Specimen	Normal Animals, Lead ppm	Poisoned Animals, Lead ppm
Whole blood (ruminants and horses) (pigs)	0·05 to 0·25	0·25 to 2·5 (deaths commence at 1·0) 1·2
Faeces (DM) (cattle)	1·5 to 35	Up to 1000
Pasture		350 ppm

Necropsy Findings

In most acute cases there are no gross lesions at necropsy. In cases of longer standing there may be some degree of abomasitis and enteritis, diffuse congestion of the lungs and degeneration of the liver and kidney. Epicardial haemorrhages are common. Congestion of meningeal and cerebral vessels may also be observed and haemorrhages may be present in the meninges. An increase in cerebrospinal fluid is often recorded but is of minor degree in most cases. In chronic cases gross lesions are recorded in cattle (9). These include cerebrocortical softening, cavitation and yellow discoloration with most severe lesions in the occipital lobes. Histological lesions were most severe at the tips of the gyri. Similar lesions were produced experimentally. Acid-fast inclusion bodies deep in the renal cortex have diagnostic significance (17). Examination of the contents of the reticulum in ruminants for particulate lead matter is essential. Flakes of paint, lumps of red lead or sheet lead usually accumulate in this site. Their absence is not remarkable especially if animals have licked fresh paint but their presence does give weight to the provisional diagnosis.

The submission of alimentary tract contents and tissues for analysis forms an important part of the diagnosis of lead poisoning but results must be interpreted with caution. In cattle 25 ppm of lead in wet kidney cortex is diagnostic and is a more reliable tissue for assay than liver which may contain 10 to 20 ppm WM. Levels of 4 to 7 ppm of lead have been found in the livers of horses dying of chronic lead poisoning (8) but 25 to 250 ppm are more likely (4), and 40 ppm in the livers of affected pigs (2).

Diagnosis

Other nervous diseases of cattle which may require differentiation from lead poisoning are hypovitaminosis A, hypomagnesaemic tetany, nervous acetonaemia, tetanus, poisoning due to arsenic, mercury, *Claviceps paspali*, and rape, brain abscess, cerebral oedema and haemorrhage, and the encephalitides and encephalomalacias. In the nervous form of acetonaemia there is an absence of convulsions and excitation and ketonuria is present. Tetanus is characterized by the unrelieved tetany, prolapse of the third eyelid and a relatively long course. *Claviceps paspali* poisoning is apt to be anticipated when much ergot is present in a pasture. The course is long, tremor is marked and the syndrome is specifically one of cerebellar ataxia. Arsenic poisoning is usually accompanied by severe gastroenteritis, and mercury poisoning by acute nephrosis. Rape poisoning is sometimes manifested by depression, blindness and headpressing although acute haemolytic anaemia or pulmonary emphysema are more common.

Brain abscess or tumour can usually be recognized by the slow onset or the presence of signs of irritation accompanied by localizing signs of loss of function. Cerebral haemorrhage has a similar clinical appearance but is usually very sudden in onset and associated with trauma to the head. Hypovitaminosis A in calves may also produce a syndrome indistinguishable clinically from that of lead poisoning. Acute cerebral oedema, the encephalitides and encephalomalacias are also accompanied by signs of central nervous system derangement which closely resemble those of the acute and subacute syndromes of lead intoxication. Lactation tetany of cows, hypomagnesaemic tetany of calves and enterotoxaemia may also be confused with lead poisoning. Enzootic muscular dystrophy in calves in which myocardial lesions occur may cause sudden death and convulsions not unlike those of lead poisoning.

In all cases much importance must be attached to the possibility of access to lead and the environmental circumstances which may arouse suspicion of other poisonings or errors in management. Estimation of the lead content of blood and faeces should be carried out at the earliest opportunity and tissues from necropsy specimens submitted for analysis.

The chronic forms of lead poisoning in lambs require to be differentiated from other forms of posterior paralysis, particularly enzootic ataxia. Polyarthritis due to bacterial infection and enzootic muscular dystrophy may cause lameness and paresis similar in many ways to the paralysis of these forms of lead poisoning, but may be distinguished clinically by careful examination of the joints and skeletal muscles.

The occurrence of diarrhoea in lead poisoning may suggest the presence of a bacterial or viral enteritis but there is less fever and cultures of the faeces usually fail to reveal the presence of pathogenic organisms in any numbers. Bovine malignant catarrh may be manifested by severe enteritis and some signs of encephalitis.

Treatment

Acute lead poisoning of cattle is almost always fatal because of the nature of the material ingested and the susceptibility of members of this species. Sedation by intravenous injection of anaesthetic doses of pentobarbital sodium in calves and chloral hydrate in adults temporarily relieves the convulsions. Rumenotomy is often attempted but is seldom satisfactory because of the difficulty of removing particulate material from the recesses of the reticular mucosa. Oral dosing with small amounts of magnesium sulphate is often recommended on the grounds that soluble lead salts will be precipitated as the insoluble sulphate. The method is limited in value because the lead is often present in large quantities and in the form of particles which are only slowly dissolved.

Calcium versenate (calcium disodium ethylenediamine tetra-acetate) has been used successfully in cases of lead poisoning produced experimentally in calves and in natural cases in cattle. A 12·5 per cent solution should be used for intravenous injection but solutions of this strength given subcutaneously cause local pain and a more dilute solution (1 to 2 per cent in 5 per cent dextrose) is recommended. Repeated treatment is usually required and a dose rate of 70 mg. per kg. body weight per day should be aimed at, preferably given in two divided doses and the treatment repeated until general signs disappear. The optimum treatment is infusion intravenously by continuous drip to deliver 110 to 220 mg. per kg. over 12 hours or two rapid intravenous injections 6 hours apart and each of 110 mg. per kg. (15).

Blindness may persist for some days after general recovery and may continue indefinitely. Intermittent treatment on alternate days at double the dose rate has also been recommended (14). An increase in heart and respiratory rates and the development of muscle tremor during injection indicate a toxic reaction but can be avoided by injecting the material slowly. Recovery may take from 5 to 15 days and parenteral or stomach tube alimentation may be required. Dramatic improvement has also been reported in cases of chronic plumbism in horses after the use of calcium versenate (8). The drug is used orally in man with good results and in cases of long duration in animals the method has obvious advantages.

Control

Animals should be prevented from having access to lead paint. If the interior of barns or pens are to be painted care should be taken to avoid the use of a lead-bearing paint. Chewing of foreign objects by cattle and sheep may be minimized by appropriate feeding practices.

REFERENCES

(1) Harbourne, J. F. *et al.* (1968). *Vet. Rec., 83*, 515.
(2) Link, R. P. & Pensinger, R. R. (1966). *Amer. J. vet. Res., 27*, 759.
(3) Slatter, D. H. (1971). *Aust. vet. J., 47*, 461.
(4) Egan, D. A. & O'Cuill, T. (1970). *Vet. Rec., 86*, 736.
(5) Butler, E. J. *et al.* (1957). *J. comp. Path., 67*, 378.
(6) Stewart, W. L. & Allcroft, R. (1956). *Vet. Rec., 68*, 723.
(7) Schmitt, N. *et al.* (1971). *Arch. envir. Hlth, 23*, 185.
(8) Holm, L. W. *et al.* (1953). *J. Amer. vet. med. Ass., 123*, 383, 528.
(9) Christian, R. G. & Tryphonas, L. (1971). *Amer. J. vet. Res., 32*, 203.
(10) Clegg, F. G. & Rylands, J. M. (1966). *J. comp. Path., 76*, 15.
(11) Marshall, S. P. (1963). *J. Dairy Sci., 46*, 580.
(12) Willoughby, R. A. & Brown, G. (1971). *Canad. vet. J., 12*, 165.
(13) Russell, H. A. & Schoberl, A. (1970). *Dtsch. tierärztl. Wschr., 77*, 517.
(14) Hammond, P. B. & Sorenson, D. K. (1957). *J. Amer. vet. med. Ass., 130*, 23.
(15) Aronson, A. L. *et al.* (1958). *Toxicol. appl. Pharmac., 12*, 179.
(16) Willoughby, R. A. *et al.* (1972). *Vet. Rec., 91*, 382.
(17) Thomson, R. G. (1972). *Canad. vet. J., 13*, 88.

Arsenic Poisoning

Incidence

Arsenic is one of the more common causes of poisoning in livestock but the incidence varies widely with farm practices and industrial undertakings which cause exposure to the poison. The morbidity rate is variable but the mortality rate usually approximates 100 per cent except for poisoning by organic compounds in which recovery is more usual.

Aetiology

Arsenic poisoning usually occurs after ingestion of the toxic substance but percutaneous absorption can occur especially if the skin is abraded or hyperaemic and the percutaneous toxic dose is much lower than (probably one-tenth of) the oral toxic dose. The toxicity of arsenic compounds varies widely with their solubility and particle size. Soluble salts are highly poisonous; arsenic trioxide and sodium arsenate are much less soluble and thus less toxic than sodium arsenite. Organic arsenicals are quite rapidly absorbed but liberate their arsenic slowly.

Toxic doses vary with the animal species (1). The toxic doses of sodium arsenite are—horse 6·5, cattle 7·5, sheep 11 and pig 2 mg. per kg. body weight respectively. Toxic doses of arsenic trioxide are 7·5 to 11 mg. per kg. body weight for pigs and for horses, cattle and sheep 33 to 55 mg. per kg. body weight.

Occurrence

In cases of poisoning the commonest source of arsenic is in fluids used for the dipping and spraying of animals to control ectoparasites. Animals may swallow the solution whilst in the dip or in the draining yards after dipping. Animals that are not allowed to drain completely may contaminate the pasture, and faulty disposal of drainage from yards and dips may contaminate the environment. Opened containers of dipping solutions or powders may provide a source for accidental contamination of feed. An appreciable amount of arsenic is absorbed through the skin after dipping in sodium arsenite solution in both cattle and sheep. The absorption is increased if the animals are dipped when hot, if the fleece is long, if they are crowded too tightly in draining yards or driven too soon after dipping. However, in most outbreaks of poisoning some ingestion appears to occur and supplements the cutaneous absorption. There is some danger in dipping rams at mating time when erythema of the skin of the thighs and scrotum is present. Dipping immediately after shearing is also a predisposing cause and jetting at high pressure or with excessively strong solutions may also cause increased absorption. Most arsenical dipping and jetting solutions contain sodium arsenite.

Arsenical weed killers including sodium arsenite, arsenic pentoxide and monosodium acid methanearsonate sprays used to kill potato haulms prior to mechanical harvesting and containing sodium or potassium arsenite, and insecticidal sprays used in orchards, particularly lead arsenate, are less common causes of poisoning. In most instances poisoning occurs when animals accidentally gain access to recently sprayed areas although drifting of windblown spray may result in accidental contamination of pasture (1). Ash from timber treated with arsenicals may be toxic for several months.

With lead arsenate the major effects are usually ascribed to the effects of the lead but this does not always appear to be so. In several outbreaks of lead arsenate poisoning in cattle the clinical signs were primarily those of arsenic poisoning and the concentration of arsenic in tissues was greater than that of lead (2). Insect baits often contain Paris green (cupric acetoarsenite) mixed with bran and when these are laid over large areas of land in an attempt to control grasshopper plagues they constitute a major hazard to livestock. Arsenical preparations used as wood preservatives may cause poisoning when used in wooden calf pens.

Some metal-bearing ore deposits, including iron and copper ores, contain large quantities of arsenic which may be carried off in the fumes from smelters and contaminate surrounding pastures and drinking water supplies. Arsenic found in lake weed (including water hyacinths) in New Zealand is thought to be of geothermal origin. When fed continuously to sheep to provide a daily intake of 200 ppm of arsenic no apparent disease was produced (3).

Arsenic is still used therapeutically and overdosing may occur. Inorganic preparations are little used now although lead arsenate still has some devotees as an anthelminthic. At 88 mg. per kg. body weight a cumulative toxicity occurs after 7 doses at monthly intervals in sheep (4). Organic arsenicals, particularly arsanilic acid and sodium arsanilate, are used both as feed additives and in the control and treatment of vibrionic dysentery in animals, and as antidotes to selenium poisoning. Overdosage can accidentally occur when the administration is carried on for too long or when there is an error in mixing a batch of feed. In one outbreak in pigs the feed contained 450 to 650 ppm of arsenic (5). In another outbreak long-term feeding of feed containing 375 ppm of arsanilic acid caused poisoning (6). Experimentally the disease is reproduced by feeding food containing 611 ppm or more (7). The toxicity of feed containing arsanilic acid depends to a certain extent on the intake of drinking water but moderate water restriction does not make normal dose rates dangerous (8). Experimentally arsanilic acid at concentrations of 0·25 per cent produces clinical signs in pigs and levels of 0·2 to 0·4 per cent cause deaths in lambs.

Arsenic is, for the most part, excreted rapidly after absorption, chiefly in the urine. After the ingestion of non-toxic amounts by the cow there is no detectable excretion in the milk. When much larger doses are taken arsenic may be excreted in the milk, as well as urine and faeces, but the concentration is quite low (1).

Pathogenesis

Arsenic is a general tissue poison and exerts its toxic effect by combining with and inactivating the sulphydryl groups in tissue enzymes. Trivalent arsenicals are most toxic because of their greater affinity for these sulphydryl groupings. The efficiency of sulphur-containing compounds including BAL (dimercaptopropanol) as antidotes depends on the ability of these compounds to compete with sulphur-containing compounds of enzyme systems for the available arsenic. Although all tissues are affected, deposition and toxic effects are greatest in those tissues which are rich in these oxidation systems. Thus alimentary tract wall, liver, kidney, spleen and lung are most susceptible. When these organs are affected there is a general depression of metabolic activity. The alimentary tract lesion is the one which produces the most obvious clinical signs. The primary effect in this site is extensive damage to capillaries causing increased permeability and exudation of serum into tissue spaces. The mucosa is lifted from the underlying muscle coat and is shed with the resulting loss of large quantities of fluid from the body. A direct local effect of arsenic on alimentary tract mucosa is not likely to be important as indicated by the observation that the parenteral injection of arsenic produces lesions in the gut wall which are identical with those caused by the ingestion of arsenic. Moreover arsenic does not precipitate protein and does not thereby limit its own absorption, and there is a considerable timelag after ingestion, whereas corrosive substances produce lesions immediately.

When arsenic is absorbed from the skin it may cause local necrosis without systemic signs if the peripheral circulation is poor or the concentration of arsenic is excessively high, but if the cutaneous circulation is good the arsenic is quickly carried away and causes a systemic disease without skin necrosis. The chronic toxicity of arsenic at low levels of intake is due to its accumulation in particular organs especially the liver, kidney and alimentary tract wall. The epidermis, spleen and lung also have a special affinity for arsenic. Organic arsenicals appear to have a particular affinity for nervous tissue and cause only nervous signs.

Clinical Findings

In acute arsenic poisoning caused by the ingestion of large amounts of inorganic arsenic there is a severe gastroenteritis. Clinical signs do not appear until some time after the arsenic has been ingested, the time varying with the fullness of the stomach at the time of ingestion. There may be a delay of 20 to 50 hours in ruminants. Distress develops suddenly, the animal showing severe abdominal pain, restlessness, groaning, an increased respiratory rate, salivation, grinding of the teeth and vomiting, even in cattle. There is usually complete ruminal atony but a fluid and foetid diarrhoea develops especially in the late stages. The heart rate is greatly increased and the pulse small in amplitude. Many animals, especially cattle and sheep, show little except depression and prostration and die before signs of enteritis develop. There may be a fluid sound in the abdomen if the animal is shaken. Death occurs 3 to 4 hours after commencement of the illness and is usually preceded by clonic convulsions and diarrhoea. Additional signs in horses include marked congestion of the mucosae and a very sudden onset of severe colic which passes off in a few hours in horses which survive. Severe diarrhoea may be followed by a period of complete stasis of the alimentary tract with diarrhoea recurring just before death.

In less severe cases the course may extend over 2 to 7 days. The emphasis clinically is still on gastroenteritis manifested by vomiting in occasional animals, diarrhoea and sometimes dysentery, complete anorexia, absence of gut sounds, severe thirst and dehydration, and evidence of peripheral circulatory failure as indicated by a rapid heart rate and a rapid small pulse. Abdominal pain is evident and affected animals are stiff and reluctant to move. Nervous signs including muscle tremor and inco-ordination, and clonic convulsions occur quite commonly and terminally there is always coma.

In chronic cases the most commonly observed abnormalities are unthriftiness, poor growth, a dry, staring coat which is easily shed, and loss of vigour and spirit. The appetite is capricious, and unexplained bouts of indigestion occur. Reddening of the conjunctiva and visible mucosae is common and there may be oedema of the eyelids and conjunctivitis. Erythema of the buccal mucosa may be accompanied by ulceration which may extend to the muzzle. The milk yield in dairy cattle is seriously reduced and abortions and stillbirths may occur. When local skin lesions are the only manifestation there is an initial hyperaemia followed by necrosis and sloughing of the skin. The lesions are indolent and extremely slow to heal.

In chronic poisoning in swine and lambs resulting from overdosing with arsanilic acid the clinical signs are restricted to the nervous system. In one outbreak clinical signs of inco-ordination and blindness did not appear until 7 days after the contaminated diet was first fed. Consciousness, body temperature and appetite were unaffected.

The signs became gradually more severe over a period of 4 days but disappeared within a few days after the feed was changed. Some pigs remained permanently blind. In the experimental disease the clinical signs are tremor of the head, inco-ordination, blindness, ataxia and paresis (7).

Clinical Pathology

Arsenic can be detected in the urine, faeces and milk for periods of up to about 10 days beginning shortly after the toxic material is ingested. The most satisfactory material for laboratory examination from a living animal is a large volume (about 1 litre) of urine in which arsenic levels may be as high as 16 ppm (1). Levels in milk are low. Normal levels of up to 0·25 ppm in cows' milk may be elevated to 0·34 to 0·47 ppm in cases of acute poisoning and to 0·8 to 1·5 ppm in the milk of normal cows which graze arsenic-contaminated pasture for long periods. Deposition in the hair occurs and the arsenic persists there until the hair is shed making possible the detection of prior arsenic ingestion in the absence of arsenic from the blood and faeces. The hair of animals not exposed to arsenic should contain less than 0·5 ppm but that of normal animals may contain as much as 5 to 10 ppm. Estimations of the amount of arsenic present in suspected materials should be carried out, but if there is delay in sampling of herbage after a contaminating incident has occurred, the concentration of soluble compounds may be greatly decreased by leaching.

Necropsy Findings

In acute and subacute cases there is pronounced hyperaemia and patchy submucosal haemorrhage in the stomach, duodenum and caecum. In ruminants the forestomachs are unaffected but typical lesions are present in the abomasum. The gut contents are very fluid, and contain much mucus and shreds of mucosa. Profuse subendocardial haemorrhages are common and ulceration of gall-bladder mucosa is often observed in sheep. Macroscopic lesions may be minimal in cases which die after a very short course. Histologically there are severe degenerative lesions in the liver, kidney, myocardium and adrenal glands. Severe intravascular haemolysis has been observed in sheep. In chronic cases the gastroenteritis is not severe but there may be ulceration of the mucosa. Fatty degeneration of the liver and kidneys is characteristic.

The liver is the best source of arsenic and levels of over 10 to 15 ppm WM of arsenic trioxide in kidney or liver are considered to be diagnostic of arsenic poisoning. However, it is probable that many animals die of arsenic poisoning when their hepatic levels are much lower than this. Maximum concentrations of arsenic in tissues occur about 8 hours after ingestion and animals which survive for 2 or 3 days may have levels as low as 3 ppm and conversely normal animals which are dipped routinely in arsenical dips may have hepatic levels of the element as high as 8 ppm. The concentration in ingesta varies widely but is reported to average about 36 ppm (9).

Animals poisoned with organic arsenicals show no significant gross pathological changes although a distended urinary bladder has been noted as a frequent occurrence in pigs (7). Histologically degeneration of the optic nerves and tracts and peripheral nerves is apparent. The animals maintain tissue levels of arsenic for longer periods and although the levels fall rapidly during the first 7 days after feeding of the arsenic ceases, normal levels are not reached until a further 7 days. Levels of about 6 ppm arsenic trioxide on a fresh, wet-matter basis indicate poisonous levels of intake (7). A part of the lower alimentary tract including contents, and in chronic cases hair, should also be submitted for analysis. Because the stomach and intestinal wall appear to attain maximum concentrations of arsenic most rapidly after poisoning, the use of these tissues for quantitative assay has been recommended. Levels of 1 to 3 ppm are obtained in cattle dying from arsenic poisoning after percutaneous ingestion and levels of over 10 ppm in cattle which ingest arsenical dip (10).

Diagnosis

Arsenic poisoning presents a clinical syndrome of gastroenteritis with minor signs of nervous system involvement. This combination is not common in other diseases. Lead poisoning has some similarity but the emphasis is on nervous system signs with gastroenteritis an inconstant accompaniment. Bovine malignant catarrh develops in somewhat the same manner especially in the alimentary tract form but there are diagnostic lesions in the eyes and buccal mucosa. Mucosal disease is also characterized by erosions in the buccal and nasal mucosae. Of the bacterial enteritides salmonellosis is often confused with arsenic poisoning especially when the disease is seen in the later stages and the fever has subsided. There are several miscellaneous poison plants which cause nervous signs and gastroenteritis.

Chronic inorganic arsenical poisoning causes a syndrome not unlike that caused by inanition and internal parasitism and suspicion will probably only be aroused when a mining or smelting undertaking is in the vicinity.

The nervous syndrome in pigs poisoned by organic arsenicals may be confused with organic mercury poisoning, salt poisoning and the encephalitides but the mildness of the signs, the lack of effect on appetite and the absence of fever rather set it apart from the others.

Treatment

In acute cases treatment is of little value because of the large amounts ingested and the delay between ingestion and the appearance of illness. Nevertheless since affected animals are not suitable for human consumption treatment is usually undertaken. Residual arsenic in the gut should be removed by the administration of an oily demulcent. Dehydration is usually severe and drastic purgatives should be avoided. Several products are used in an attempt to precipitate arsenic in the gut lumen. Ferric hydrate is most commonly used but has little apparent effect on the course of the disease.

Compounds containing sulphur are theoretically the best antidotes and of these sodium thiosulphate is practicable and of some value. The compound is almost completely non-toxic and can be given in large amounts and without accurate measurement. Intravenous injection is desirable as an initial treatment using 15 to 30 g. of the salt in 100 to 200 ml. of water and this should be followed by oral dosing of 30 to 60 g. at 6-hour intervals. Treatment should be continued until recovery occurs which may require 3 to 4 days. BAL (2:3–dimercaptopropanol) is an efficient antidote for poisoning by organic arsenicals but is often disappointing in cases of poisoning by inorganic salts. Dosing at 4-hourly intervals is necessary and the oily injections cause some local pain. Although BAL has a general beneficial effect and is recommended as a treatment the drug is quite toxic itself and in the doses required may cause deaths in sheep (11).

Severe dehydration occurs and supportive treatment must include the provision of ample fluids preferably by parenteral injection. An adequate supply of drinking water containing electrolytes should be provided and the animals should be disturbed as little as possible and provided with shelter from the sun. Astringent preparations given by mouth may help to reduce the loss of body fluids.

After the treatment of pigs with arsanilic acid the arsenic content of their livers may exceed 1 ppm, the statutory level of arsenic in food for human consumption. At least 10 days should be permitted between ceasing to feed the arsanilate and slaughter to avoid poisoning of humans (12).

Control

Arsenical preparations must be handled and stored with care and contamination of feed and pasture avoided. Therapeutic preparations containing arsenic should be labelled 'Poison' and strict instructions given on dosage and particularly the length of time for which administration should continue. Farmers are sometimes inclined to overdose in the hope of expediting recovery and to continue treatment for long periods when the response to treatment is poor rather than call for further assistance. Animals to be dipped in arsenical solutions should be allowed to cool off before dipping, to drain properly afterwards and be allowed to dry before being driven. They should be watered before dipping to prevent them drinking the dip. Many mortalities have occurred when instructions for mixing dip solutions are not closely followed. Dipping solutions containing more arsenic than is safe usually occur when tanks which have lost water by evaporation are reconstituted by guesswork. The maximum safe concentration of arsenic trioxide in a dip for cattle is 0·20 per cent (10).

REFERENCES

(1) Weaver, A. D. (1962). *Vet. Rec., 74*, 249.
(2) McParland, P. J. *et al.* (1971). *Vet. Rec., 89*, 450.
(3) Lancaster, R. J. *et al.* (1971). *N.Z. vet. J., 19*, 141.
(4) Bennett, D. G. & Schwarz, T. E. (1971). *Amer. J. vet. Res., 32*, 727.
(5) Oliver, W. T. & Roe, C. K. (1957). *J. Amer. vet. med. Ass., 130*, 177.
(6) Menges, R. W. *et al.* (1970). *Vet. Med. small Anim. Clin., 65*, 565.
(7) Harding, J. D. J. *et al.* (1968). *Vet. Rec., 83*, 560.
(8) Vorhies, M. W. *et al.* (1969). *Cornell Vet., 59*, 3.
(9) Hatch, R. C. & Funnell, H. S. (1968). *Canad. vet. J., 10*, 117.
(10) Dingle, J. H. P. (1965). *Aust. vet. J., 41*, 369.
(11) White, I. G. *et al.* (1949). *Aust. vet. J., 25*, 8.
(12) Gitter, M. & Lewis, G. (1969). *Vet. Rec., 85*, 389.

Selenium Poisoning

Selenium poisoning occurs in specific areas where the selenium content of the soil is high. Acute cases show mainly signs of nervous system involvement with blindness and head-pressing. Chronic cases are manifested by emaciation, lameness and loss of hair.

Incidence

Selenium poisoning occurs in restricted areas in North America where the soils are derived from particular rock formations containing a high content of selenium. It has also been recorded in Ireland, Israel, Canada and Australia and is suspected of contributing to the development of 'geeldikkop' and toxaemic jaundice in South Africa. Losses are caused by failure of animals to thrive on pasture grown on seleniferous soils and some deaths occur.

Aetiology

The effective selenium is contained in the top 60 to 90 cm. of the soil profile, selenium at lower levels than this not being within reach of most plants. Selenium poisoning may occur on soils containing very little selenium—as low as 0·01 ppm (1)—but some soils may contain as much as 1200 ppm. Most pasture plants seldom contain selenium in excess of 100 ppm but several species, the so-called converter or indicator plants, take up the element in such large quantities that selenium levels may reach as high as 10,000 ppm (18). Such plants constitute a serious hazard in areas where the selenium content of the soil is high. *Astragalus* spp. and *Oxytropis* spp. are two of the common converter plants in North America. *Morinda reticulata*, *Neptunia amplexicaulis* and *Acacia cana* have been shown to be converter plants in Australia (1, 2).

Because of the number of factors which affect the toxicity of selenium there is much discrepancy between toxic doses quoted by different workers and the following information is subject to this limitation (3). There are many case reports of unexpected illness and mortality in animals dosed with selenium preparations and it is apparent that not all of the factors affecting selenium toxicity are known (4). Factors known to affect the toxicity of selenium compounds are the cobalt and protein status of the animal, deficiencies of either causing increased susceptibility (5), the length and rate of the ingestion period and the animal species, cattle being more tolerant than sheep. Organic selenium compounds, especially those occurring naturally in plants, are generally considered to be much more toxic than inorganic compounds but this difference may not be apparent in ruminants because of alterations in ingested compounds produced by digestive processes in the rumen. There is a difference of opinion as to whether the selenite or the selenate salts are more toxic but both are more damaging than selenium dioxide (3).

Selenium in feeds should not exceed 5 ppm DM if danger is to be avoided and feeding on pasture containing 25 ppm DM for several weeks can be expected to cause chronic selenium poisoning. Pasture may contain as much as 2000 to 6000 ppm of selenium and causes the acute form of the disease when fed for a few days (6). Daily intakes of 0·25 mg. per kg. body weight are toxic for sheep and cattle and feed containing 44 ppm selenium for horses and 11 ppm for pigs causes poisoning (3), the daily intake of a diet containing 2 ppm of selenium can be marginally toxic for sheep (7). Toxic single oral doses (as mg. per kg. body weight) are 2·2 for horses and sheep, 9 for cattle and 15 for pigs. An oral dose of 10 to 15 mg. of selenium has been known to kill lambs (4).

Because of the present popularity of selenium in the treatment of enzootic muscular dystrophy it has become necessary to determine toxic levels of selenium compounds administered by injection. In general the ratio between toxic and therapeutic doses is 50 to 100:1 and dosing accidents should not be common (3). The subcutaneous injection of selenium, as sodium selenite, causes poisoning in sheep at doses of 0·8 mg. per kg. body weight and doses of 1·6 mg. per kg. are lethal (8, 9). A single injection of 5·0 mg. of selenium may kill some lambs (4) and the toxic level for single injections in lambs has been reported as 455 μg. Se per kg. body weight (17). Lethal doses by injections are 1·2 mg. per kg. body weight for cattle (3) and pigs (10).

Occurrence

Selenium poisoning occurs chiefly when animals feed on plants grown on seleniferous soils which may be restricted to small, very distinct areas. The incidence of the disease is highest when selector plants are growing in the pasture. A low rainfall predisposes to selenium poisoning because soluble, available selenium compounds are not leached out of the top soil and lack of competing forage may force animals to eat large quantities of indicator plants. If the use of selenium in the prevention of enzootic muscular dystrophy becomes widespread induced selenium poisoning may increase in incidence.

Pathogenesis

Selenium occurs in plants in analogues of the sulphur-containing amino-acids and the probable mechanism of intoxication is by interference with enzyme systems which contain these amino-acids. Arsenic and antimony exert their toxic effects in the same way and both of these elements reduce the toxicity of selenium compounds. Selenium reduces the sulphur and protein content of sheep's liver and high protein diets have a protective effect against selenium poisoning (6). Selenium is deposited in greatest concentration in the liver, kidney and hair. It has a marked dystrophic effect on skeletal musculature and causes a marked rise in SGOT levels after subcutaneous administration.

It has not been possible to reproduce the chronic natural disease by the experimental administration of small amounts of selenium and it may be that a toxic action of the converter plant itself may contribute to the disease which is seen in the field. In the experimentally produced disease there is a gradual accumulation of selenium in tissues followed by the sudden onset of the acute form of the disease (11).

Clinical Findings

Acute selenium poisoning is known colloquially as 'blind staggers' because affected animals are blind, wander aimlessly and often in circles, and show head pressing. The appetite may be depraved and abdominal pain is evidenced. The terminal stage is one of paralysis with death due to respiratory failure. Essentially the same picture is produced by the experimental oral dosing of sheep with sodium selenite but dilation of the pupils and cyanosis are also present (12).

Chronic poisoning (alkali disease) is manifested by dullness, emaciation, lack of vitality, stiffness and lameness. In cattle, horses, and mules the hair at the base of the tail and switch is lost and in pigs there may be general alopecia. There are hoof abnormalities including swelling of the coronary band, and deformity or separation and sloughing of the hooves in all species. Lameness is severe. Congenital hoof deformities may occur in newborn animals whose dams have received diets containing an excess of selenium. Marginal levels of intake of selenium (10 ppm) are reported to lower the conception rate and increase neo-natal mortality in pigs.

Clinical Pathology

Selenium can be detected in the urine, milk and hair of affected animals but critical data are not available. Clinical illness is evident at blood levels of 3·0 ppm and at urine levels of more than 4 ppm of selenium. A moderate anaemia occurs in acute and chronic poisoning and a depression of haemoglobin levels to about 7 g. per cent is one of the early indications of selenium poisoning.

Necropsy Findings

In cases of acute selenium poisoning there is congestion and necrosis of the liver, congestion of the renal medulla, epicardial petechiation, impaction of the rumen, and hyperaemia and necrosis, sometimes with ulceration, in the abomasum and small intestine. The hooves are not involved but there may be erosion of the articular surfaces, particularly of the tibia. In acute poisoning of cattle with a massive accidental overdose of a selenium preparation there was histological evidence of extensive damage in liver, lungs and myocardium (13). Gross overdosage in sheep by overdrenching with sodium selenite has caused hydrothorax and pulmonary oedema (14).

In animals suffering from chronic selenium poisoning there is atrophy and dilatation of the heart, cirrhosis and atrophy of the liver, glomerulonephritis, mild gastroenteritis and erosion of articular surfaces (6). Deformities of the feet are usually apparent as described under clinical findings. In experimentally induced cases in sheep the significant lesions are degeneration and necrosis in the myocardium, and oedema and interstitial petechiation in the lungs (11, 15).

In chronic selenosis in sheep hepatic levels of selenium are about 20 to 30 ppm (10) and levels in wool are in the range of 0·6 to 2·3 ppm (5).

Diagnosis

The diagnosis of selenium poisoning rests largely on the recognition of the typical syndromes in animals in areas where the soil content of selenium is high. The acute form of the disease resembles subacute lead poisoning, encephalopathy due to liver insufficiency and many encephalitides and encephalomalacias. Chronic cases bear some resemblance to hypovitaminosis A.

Treatment

A number of substances have been tried in the treatment of selenium poisoning, including potassium iodide, ascorbic acid and beet pectin but without apparent effect. BAL is contraindicated (18).

Control

Protection against the toxic effects of selenium in amounts up to 10 ppm in the diet has been obtained by the inclusion in the ration fed to pigs of 0·01 to 0·02 per cent of arsanilic acid or 0·005 per cent of 3-nitro-4-hydroxyphenylarsonic acid (16). In cattle 0·01 per cent arsanilic acid in the ration or 550 mg. per day to grazing steers gives only slight protection. The addition of linseed oil to the ration improves the efficiency of this protection. A high protein diet also has a general protective effect.

REFERENCES

(1) Knott, S. G. & McCray, C. W. R. (1959). *Aust. vet. J.*, *35*, 161.
(2) McCray, C. W. R. & Hurwood, I. S. (1964). *Qld J. agric. Sci.*, *20*, 475.
(3) Muth, O. H. & Binns, W. (1964). *Ann. N.Y. Acad. Sci.*, *111*, 583.
(4) Gabbedy, B. J. (1970). *Aust. vet. J.*, *46*, 223.
(5) Gardiner, M. R. (1966). *Aust. vet. J.*, *42*, 442.
(6) Rosenfeld, I. & Beath, O. A. (1964). *Amer. J. vet. Res.*, *7*, 52, 57.
(7) Pope, A. L. (1971). *J. Anim. Sci.*, *33*, 1332.
(8) Caravaggi, C. & Clark, F. L. (1969). *Aust. vet. J.*, *45*, 383.
(9) Neethling, L. P. *et al.* (1968). *J. S. Afr. vet. med. Ass.*, *39*, 25.
(10) Kuttler, K. L. *et al.* (1961). *Amer. J. vet. Res.*, *22*, 422.
(11) Glenn, M. W. *et al.* (1964). *Amer. J. vet. Res.*, *23*, 1479, 1486.
(12) Morrow, D. A. (1968). *J. Amer. vet. med. Ass.*, *152*, 1625.
(13) Shortridge, E. H. *et al.* (1971). *N.Z. vet. J.*, *19*, 47.
(14) Lambourne, D. A. & Mason, R. W. (1969). *Aust. vet. J.*, *45*, 208.
(15) Gabbedy, B. J. & Dickson, J. (1969). *Aust. vet. J.*, *45*, 470.
(16) Wahlstrom, R. C. & Olsen, D. E. (1959). *J. Anim. Sci.*, *18*, 578.
(17) Caravaggi, C. *et al.* (1970). *Res. vet. Sci.*, *11*, 146.
(18) Harr, J. R. & Muth, O. H. (1972). *Clin. Toxicol.*, *5*, 175.

Phosphorus Poisoning

Phosphorus poisoning is characterized by severe inflammation of the alimentary mucosa and acute necrosis of the liver. Gastroenteritis and acute hepatic insufficiency are the clinical syndromes produced.

Incidence

Phosphorus poisoning is rare in farm animals because of lack of exposure. Small animals are rather more exposed to rat baits containing white phosphorus and amongst farm animals most cases are likely to occur in swine.

Aetiology

Phosphorus is rarely used as a rodent poison nowadays and this comprises the only likely source of phosphorus for animals. Toxic effects are most likely to occur when the phosphorus is finely divided and mixed with oils or fats which facilitate its absorption.

Occurrence

Rat or rabbit baits containing lumps of white phosphorus may be left about in barns or at pasture and be ingested accidentally by farm livestock. Phosphorus used for military purposes may cause extensive contamination of pasture.

Pathogenesis

Phosphorus has a local caustic action and on ingestion causes severe irritation of the alimentary mucosa with signs of gastroenteritis appearing within an hour or two. Some phosphorus may be absorbed and cause acute hepatic necrosis but signs do not appear for several days.

Clinical Findings

Violent gastroenteritis occurs with severe diarrhoea, acute abdominal pain, salivation and intense thirst. Pigs vomit violently and the vomitus is described as being luminous and having a garlic odour. The animal often dies of acute shock during this stage. If the animal survives this initial period of illness signs of hepatic and renal insufficiency appear 4 to 10 days later. There is jaundice, weakness and anorexia, oliguria and haematuria. Death may occur in coma or be accompanied by convulsions.

Clinical Pathology

Phosphorus can be detected in the vomitus and faeces of affected animals.

Necropsy Findings

Macroscopically there is congestion and haemorrhagic inflammation of the alimentary mucosa, enlargement of the liver with haemorrhage and yellowish pallor of lobules. Histologically there is acute hepatic necrosis and nephrosis. For analytical purposes liver, kidney and muscle should be supplied as well as a portion of the alimentary canal and its contents. The latter is most important as tissues are often negative for phosphorus. No preservative of any kind should be added to the specimens.

Diagnosis

Clinically phosphorus poisoning is characterized by acute gastroenteritis and differentiation from other causes requires evidence of access to the poison and the detection of large amounts of it in the alimentary tract.

Treatment

An emetic or purgative should be given immediately. Copper sulphate (1·0 per cent solution) given orally is an effective emetic in small animals and tends to reduce the solubility of the particles of phosphate by covering them with a coating of insoluble copper phosphide. In small animals 15 g. of the solution is given by mouth every 10 minutes until vomiting occurs and presumably this form of therapy could be instituted in the other species. A hydragogue cathartic is preferred for purgation, oils facilitating absorption of the phosphorus. Supportive treatment includes the administration of astringents to allay the gastroenteritis and parenteral electrolyte solutions to relieve the dehydration.

Mercury Poisoning

Poisoning by mercury causes inflammation of the alimentary mucosa and damage to the kidneys. It is manifested clinically by gastroenteritis and terminally by signs of uraemia.

Incidence

Mercury poisoning is not common in farm animals because of lack of exposure to mercury-bearing substances.

Aetiology

The toxicity of mercury compounds depends on their solubility and the susceptibility of the animals. Cattle are highly susceptible. Mercuric chloride and mercury biniodide are highly poisonous, the toxic dose for horses and cattle being about 8 g. and for sheep 4 g. Mercury is a cumulative poison because of its slow excretion from the intestines and kidney. Organic mercury taken regularly in the diet at a level of 1 ppm causes chronic poisoning in pigs (2). A level of 6 ppm has been recorded as causing deaths in pigs within five days (9).

Occurrence

Accidental administration of medicines containing mercury, licking of skin dressings and absorption from liberally applied skin dressings may cause sporadic cases. The continued administration of a strong mercuric ointment to horses has been shown to cause poisoning by inhalation of mercury vapour by cattle in the same stable (1). Seed grain which has been treated with antifungal preparations containing organic mercury compounds is one of the commonest sources of outbreaks of mercury poisoning in farm animals. The commonest agent used is Ceresan which contains 5·25 per cent methoxyethylmercury silicate or 1·75 per cent mercury. Methylmercury dicyandiamide is another common poisonous agent (2, 8). The seed is usually not harmful if it comprises only 10 per cent of the ration and must be fed in large amounts for long periods before clinical illness occurs (3). A single feeding even of large amounts of grain is thought to be incapable of causing mercury poisoning in ruminants but a fatal case has been reported in a horse.

A matter of vital interest in chronic poisoning by organical mercurials is the use of the meat from such animals for human consumption. There is one record of a family being poisoned in this way (4).

Pathogenesis

Inorganic mercury compounds cause coagulation of the alimentary mucosa and this caustic action results in the rapid development of gastro-enteritis. Animals that survive the alimentary tract disorder may show signs of systemic effects from absorbed mercury. This effect is largely one of damage to peripheral capillaries especially those at the sites where mercury is excreted, in the kidney, colon and mouth. Systemic involvement leads to the development of nephrosis, colitis and stoma-titis. Organic mercurials in small doses liberate their mercury slowly into tissues and cause degenerative changes in brain and peripheral nerves (5, 6) and in kidney. In larger doses there is stasis of the ali-mentary tract and with doses of 0·23 g. per kg. body weight there is general collapse (7). Toxic and lethal doses will vary with the compound used. Methylmercury dicyandiamide fed to pigs caused no apparent illness at a dose level of 2·5 mg. per kg. body weight. At dose levels of 5 to 15 mg. per kg. there were signs of illness and at 20 mg. per kg. deaths occurred. A delay of three weeks between dosing and illness was characteristic (8).

Clinical Findings

In very severe cases where large amounts of inorganic mercury are ingested there is an acute gastroenteritis with vomiting of blood-stained material and severe diarrhoea. Death occurs within a few hours due to shock and dehydration. In less acute cases salivation, a foetid breath and anorexia accompany the gastroenteritis and the animal sur-vives for several days. There is oliguria, an increase in heart and respiratory rates and in some cases posterior paralysis. Convulsions occur in the final stages.

The common form of the disease is chronic mercurialism where small amounts of mercury are ingested over long periods. There is depression, anorexia, emaciation, and a stiff stilted gait which may progress to paresis. Alopecia, scabby lesions around the anus and vulva, pruritis, petechiation and tenderness of the gums and shedding of the teeth are accompanied by chronic diarrhoea. Ner-vous signs are present and include weakness, inco-ordination and convulsions (10, 11). Poisoning of pigs by organic mercurial compounds causes blind-ness, staggering, continuous walking and inability to eat although the appetite appears to be good. Cattle poisoned in this way evidence a staggery gait, standing on tiptoes and paresis. The animals lie down most of the time but appear normal in other respects, often eating well. Clinical signs may not develop until 30 days after feeding is commenced. Cattle poisoned experimentally show marked nervous signs including inco-ordination, head-pressing, muscle tremor with twitching of the eye-

lids, tetanus-like spasms on stimulation, excessive salivation, recumbency and inability to eat or drink. These are followed by tonic-clonic convulsions with opisthotonus (7).

Clinical Pathology

Mercury can be detected in the faeces and urine of affected animals and in the toxic source material.

Necropsy Findings

In acute cases there is severe gastroenteritis with oedema, hyperaemia and petechiation of the ali-mentary mucosa. The liver and kidneys are swollen and the lungs are congested and show mul-tiple haemorrhages. There may be an accompany-ing catarrhal stomatitis. Histologically there are degenerative changes in the renal tubules. In chronic mercurialism caused by organic mercury compounds there are also degenerative changes in nerve cells in the cortex of cerebrum and cere-bellum. Mercury reaches its greatest concentration in kidney and this tissue should be submitted for assay. Levels of 100 ppm may be present in the kidney of animals poisoned with inorganic mercury (10). With chronic organic mercurial poisoning in swine levels of mercury up to 2000 ppm may be present in the kidney (12).

Diagnosis

Acute mercury poisoning is rare but should be suspected in animals which are exposed to inor-ganic mercury compounds and which show signs of gastroenteritis and nephritis. The occurrence of nervous signs results in a syndrome similar to that of poisoning by lead or arsenic. Pigs poisoned by organic mercury compounds manifest a syndrome similar to that caused by poisoning with organic arsenic preparations.

Treatment

In acute cases large amounts of coagulable protein such as eggs should be given by mouth immediately, followed by mild purgatives to facili-tate removal from the gut before digestion and absorption occur. Treatment with sodium thio-sulphate as described in arsenic poisoning is recom-mended. BAL has the same limitations here as in arsenic poisoning and delay in treatment of any sort is likely to be fatal. If the case can be treated early an injection of BAL (6.5 mg. per kg. body weight) should be given every 4 hours. Supportive treatment includes astringents given orally to con-trol the gastroenteritis and fluids given parenterally to correct the dehydration.

Control

Seed grains dusted with mercury compounds should not be fed to animals but the practice is reasonably safe if only small amounts are used.

REFERENCES

(1) Petrelius, T. (1953). *Proc. 15th int. vet. Congr.*, Pt. 1, pp. 506–12.
(2) Kahrs, R. F. (1968). *Cornell Vet.*, *58*, 67.
(3) Palmer, J. S. (1963). *J. Amer. vet. med. Ass.*, *143*, 1385.
(4) Curley, A. *et al.* (1971). *Science, N.Y.*, *172*, 65.
(5) Miyakawa, T. *et al.* (1971). *Acta neuropath.*, *17*, 6, 80.
(6) Tryphonas, L. (1971). *Diss. Abst. int.*, *31B*, 4423.
(7) Oliver, W. T. & Platanow, N. (1960). *Amer. J. vet. Res.*, *21*, 906.
(8) Piper, R. C. *et al.* (1971). *Amer. J. vet. Res.*, *32*, 263.
(9) Loosmore, R. M. *et al.* (1967). *Vet. Rec.*, *81*, 268.
(10) Reinders, J. S. (1972). *Neth. J. vet. Sci.*, *4*, 79.
(11) Herigstad, R. R. *et al.* (1972). *J. Amer. vet. med. Ass.*, *160*, 173.
(12) Alekseeva, A. A. (1969). *Veterinariya*, *5*, 58.

Fluorine Poisoning

Fluorosis is a chronic disease caused by the continued ingestion of small but toxic amounts of fluorine in the diet or drinking water, and is characterized by mottling and excessive wear of developing teeth and osteoporosis. Acute fluorine poisoning usually occurs as a result of the inhalation of fluorine-containing gases or accidental administration of large amounts of fluoride and is manifested by gastroenteritis.

Incidence

Fluorine intoxication has been observed in most countries, usually in association with specific natural or industrial hazards. In Europe and Great Britain losses are greatest on summer grazing of pastures contaminated by industrial fumes (1). Iceland is extensively affected by contamination from volcanic ash. Drinking water from deep wells, industrial contamination of pasture and the feeding of fluorine-bearing phosphatic supplements are the common causes in North America. Deep wells also are an important source in Australia and South America. In Africa the important cause is the feeding of phosphatic rock supplements. Some wood preservatives may contain large quantities of fluoride which may cause acute poisoning in some circumstances (20).

Death losses are rare and restricted largely to acute poisoning, the major losses taking the form of unthriftiness caused by chronic fluorosis.

Aetiology

The toxic effects of fluorine depend on the amount ingested, the solubility and availability of the fluorine compound, and the age of the animal. The intake may be expressed as parts per million in drinking water or feed, or as mg. per kg. body weight. The most satisfactory measure is the concentration in the total dry matter consumed.

Levels in excess of 100 parts of fluorine per million of dry ration consumed are likely to cause disease in cattle, sheep and pigs when the fluorine is contained in rock phosphate or cryolite. At this or lower levels minor teeth lesions may occur but not to such a degree that they will affect the animal's wellbeing during an ordinary commercial life span (2). If the fluorine is in the form of calcium fluoride much higher intakes are innocuous. Sodium fluosilicate is also relatively non-toxic, intakes of 400 mg. to 2 g. per kg. body weight being necessary for fatal effects (3). On the other hand sodium fluoride is approximately twice as toxic and a general level of 50 ppm of dry ration should not be exceeded. In experimentally induced fluorosis in cattle mottling of the tooth enamel occurs at intakes of 27 ppm but there is no pitting until levels of 49 ppm are fed, bony lesions are slight at intakes of 27 ppm, moderate at 49 ppm and marked at 93 ppm, and milk production in dairy cows is not affected by intakes of 50 ppm of fluorine in the diet until about the fourth lactation (4).

Contamination from industrial plants is a complex problem because of variation in the form of the contaminating compound. Two of the common effluent substances are hydrofluoric acid and silicon tetrafluoride, both of which are highly toxic. Hay contamination by these effluents is as toxic as sodium fluoride and dental lesions occur in 100 per cent of young ruminants on an intake of 14 to 16 ppm DM of these substances. Severe cases occur on pastures containing more than 25 ppm DM and similar lesions develop much more rapidly in cattle grazing on pasture containing 98 ppm DM (5). Fluoracetamide is also known to be a toxic factory effluent (6).

The available data for drinking water suggest that although minor teeth lesions occur at 5 ppm of fluorine it is not until levels of 10 ppm are exceeded that excessive tooth wear occurs and the nutrition of the animal is impaired. More serious systemic effects do not occur until the water contains 30 ppm. It seems highly unlikely that the fluoridation of water supplies to prevent human tooth decay would have any deleterious effect on animal health.

In terms of body weight daily intakes of 0·5 to 1·7 mg. per kg. body weight of fluorine as sodium fluoride produce dental lesions in growing animals without affecting general wellbeing. Intakes equal to twice these amounts are consumed by adult animals without ill-effect. In heifers an intake of 2·5 mg. per kg. body weight per day for two months was sufficient to cause severe dental fluorisis in one pair of incisors (7). An intake of 1 mg. per kg. body weight is the maximum safe limit for ruminants. An intake of 2 mg. per kg. body weight produces clinical signs after continued ingestion. The fluorine content of the bones of new-born calves depends on the dam's intake of fluorine in the last 3 to 4 months of pregnancy and not on her own bone composition. An uptake of up to 9 mg. F per g. body weight per day by the dam was not dangerous to the calf (8). In pigs an intake of 1 mg. per kg. body weight added fluorine for long periods has no deleterious effect and has no apparent beneficial effect on the formation of bone (9).

Occurrence

Fluorine occurs naturally in rock, particularly in association with phosphate, and these rocks, the soils derived from them and surface water leaching through the soils, may contain toxic quantities of fluorine. In such areas the soil content of fluorine may be as high as 2000 to 4000 ppm and the levels in water up to 8·7 ppm (10). Levels of fluorine likely to be toxic to animals are not usually encountered in natural circumstances, interference by man being necessary in most instances to increase fluorine ingestion above the critical level.

Plants, with few exceptions, do not absorb appreciable quantities of fluorine. Major outbreaks of intoxication occur as the result of the ingestion of pasture contaminated with fluorine, and drinking water and mineral supplements which contain excessive amounts of fluorine.

Pasture contamination. Top dressing of pasture with phosphatic limestone is a common cause of fluorosis. Most phosphatic limestones, particularly those from North Africa, are rich in fluorine (0·9 to 1·4 per cent). Non-phosphatic limestones contain insignificant amounts. Contamination of pasture by smoke, vapour or dust from industrial plants is also common, and such pasture may contain 20 to 50 ppm of fluorine. Factories producing aluminium by the electrolytic process, iron and steel with fluorine-containing fluxes, superphosphate, glazed bricks, copper, glass and enamels are likely to be potent sources and may cause toxic levels of contamination as far as 14 km. down wind from the factory. Industrial plants engaged in the calcining of ironstone have also been incriminated as sources of fluorine. Dust and gases from volcanic eruptions may cause acute fatal fluorine intoxication in the period immediately after the eruption, and contamination of pasture may be sufficient to cause subsequent chronic intoxication in animals eating the herbage. Iceland is particularly afflicted with fluorine intoxication deriving from this source.

Supplementary feeding of phosphates. The common occurrence of phosphorus deficiency in animals has led to the search for cheap phosphatic materials suitable for animal feeding. Rock phosphates are commonly used and many deposits contain dangerous amounts of fluorine (3 to 4 per cent).

Drinking water. Although surface drinking water varies considerably in its fluorine content the major occurrence of fluorine intoxication is from water obtained from deep wells or artesian bores. Chronic intoxication has occurred in sheep drinking bore water containing 12 to 19 ppm and in cattle drinking deep well water containing 16 ppm fluorine. Reported occurrences of fluoride poisoning in cattle at intakes of 1·5 to 4·0 ppm fluorine and with metacarpal fluorine levels of 4000 ppm must be open to some doubt with respect to aetiology (11).

Pathogenesis

Fluorine is a general tissue poison; its exact mode of action does not appear to have been closely examined. When large amounts of soluble inorganic fluorine compounds are ingested there is immediate gastrointestinal irritation due to the formation of hydrofluoric acid in the acid medium of the stomach. Nervous signs including tetany and hyperaesthesia may follow as a result of the fixation of serum calcium to form physiologically inactive calcium fluoride in the blood plasma. Blood clotting is inhibited for the same reason. Death occurs quickly. Organic fluorides, including sodium fluoracetate, also known as 1080, and fluoracetamide cause sudden death by poisoning the enzyme aconitase, leading to the accumulation of diagnostically significant levels of citrate in tissues and permanent damage to myocardium.

Chronic intoxication due to the ingestion of small amounts of inorganic fluorides over long periods of time is more common in animals. Under such conditions detoxication takes place by the deposition of fluorine in association with phosphate in the teeth and bones. Deposition in bone occurs throughout life but in teeth only in the formative stages. In bones the degree of deposition varies being greatest on the periosteal surface of the long bones where exostoses commonly develop. Thus lesions in teeth occur only if the intake is high before the teeth have erupted but bone lesions occur at any stage (7). When the tissue levels of fluorine are moderate characteristic lesions due to hypoplasia of the enamel appear in the teeth. At higher levels the storage capacity of these organs is exceeded and blood and urine levels rise. General signs of toxicity thus appear in tissues at the same time as bone lesions develop. The bone lesions of osteomalacia, osteoporosis and exostosis formation are caused by excessive mobilization of calcium and phosphorus to compensate for their increased urinary excretion in conjunction with fluorine. The other tissues particularly prone to fluorine intoxication and in which degenerative changes occur are bone marrow, kidney, liver, adrenal glands, heart muscle and central nervous system. A severe anaemia may occur as a result of toxic depression of bone marrow activity although this is not a constant sign. The facility of storage in bone explains the long latent period which occurs in animals subjected to chronic intoxication.

Fluorine does not pass the placental barrier nor does it occur in the colostrum or milk in appreciable amounts so that the newborn are not exposed to danger of intoxication until they begin to drink water. Temporary teeth are therefore not affected as they are formed before birth. After storage has occurred in bones a decrease in the intake of fluorine leads to lowering of blood levels and mobilization from bones and teeth commences. This is of importance when interpreting urine and blood levels of the element.

Clinical Findings

Acute intoxication. Gastroenteritis occurs with complete anorexia, vomiting and diarrhoea in pigs and dogs, and ruminal stasis with constipation or diarrhoea in ruminants. Affected animals are dyspnoeic. Vomiting acts as a protective mechanism and toxic doses in pigs may be eliminated in this way without the development of other signs. Nervous signs are characteristic and include muscle tremor and weakness, a startled expression, pupillary dilation, hyperaesthesia and constant chewing. Tetany and collapse follow and death usually occurs within a few hours.

Chronic intoxication—fluorosis. Lesions of the teeth and bones are characteristic of chronic fluorine intoxication and the signs are largely referable to these lesions. Teeth changes are the earliest and most diagnostic sign but may not produce clinical effects until other signs have developed. Consequently they are often missed until other clinical findings suggest that the teeth be examined. Because of the distinct clinical separation between animals with dental lesions and those which have in addition signs of lameness and general ill health it is customary to refer to two forms of the disease—dental fluorosis and damaging fluorosis. Lameness and unthriftiness are the signs usually observed first by farmers. These occur in animals of any age. There is lameness and stiffness with a painful gait, most marked in the loins, hip joints and hind legs. Pain is evinced on pressure over limb bones and particularly over the bulbs of the heels. The bones may be palpably and visibly enlarged. This is most readily observed in the mandible, sternum, metacarpal and metatarsal bones and the phalanges, all of which are increased in thickness. This overall thickness may be subsequently replaced by well defined exostoses. The bones are subject to easy fracture. These well-defined lesions occur only in advanced cases and are often accompanied by extensive tooth lesions in young animals. In addition to the generalized lameness there are cases which show a sudden onset of very severe lameness, usually in a forelimb, caused by transverse fracture of the third phalanx (12).

Only permanent teeth exposed to intoxication before eruption will be affected. The earliest and mildest sign is mottling with the appearance of pigmented (very light yellow, green, brown or black) spots or bands arranged horizontally across the teeth. Occasional vertical bands may be seen where pigment is deposited along enamel fissures. Mottling and staining occur on incisors and cheek teeth and are not evident when the affected tooth erupts and in fact may not appear until some months later. If the period of exposure to intoxication has been limited only some of the teeth may be affected but the defects will always be bilateral. Mottling may not progress any further but if the intoxication has been sufficiently severe defective calcification of the enamel leads to accelerated attrition or erosion of the teeth, usually in the same teeth as the mottling. The mottled areas become pits and the teeth are brittle and break and wear easily and unevenly. Patterns of accelerated attrition are dependent upon the chronological occurrence of the intoxication and the eruption time of the teeth (15). Uneven and rapid wear of the cheek teeth makes proper mastication impossible. Infection of the dental alveoli and shedding of teeth commonly follow. The painful condition of the teeth and the inability to prehend and masticate seriously reduce the food intake and cause poor growth in the young and unthriftiness and acetonaemia in adults. Affected cattle may lap cold drinking water to avoid the discomfort occasioned by normal drinking. Eruption of the teeth may be abnormal resulting in irregular alignment.

Reproduction, milk yield and wool growth are not usually considered to be adversely affected except indirectly by the reduced food intake. However there is a record of a significant increase in post-calving anoestrus in cows receiving a diet containing 8 to 12 ppm fluorine for a year with further declines in fertility with further exposure. Other signs of fluorine intoxication were not observed (13). Additional signs including diarrhoea in cattle and sheep and polydipsia and polyuria in pigs are recorded in the naturally occurring disease but cannot be considered as constant or pathognomonic.

In animals that are housed for part of the year and grazed on pasture contaminated by factory effluent during the summer there may be considerable clinical improvement during the winter and an annual recrudescence of signs when the animals are at pasture.

Horses with chronic fluorosis have a similar clinical picture to that of ruminants (14). There is lameness, dental lesions including excessive molar abrasion, hyperostotic lesions of the metatarsus, metacarpus, mandible and ribs.

Clinical Pathology

Laboratory examination of specimens from living animals can be of value in diagnosis. Normal cattle have blood levels of up to 0·2 mg. fluorine per 100 ml. of blood and 2 to 6 ppm in urine. Cattle on fluorine intakes sufficient to cause intoxication may have blood levels of 0·6 mg. per 100 ml., and urine levels of 16 to 68 ppm although blood levels are often normal. Such high levels may not be an indication of high intakes immediately preceding the examination as heavy deposits in bones may cause abnormally high blood and urine fluorine levels for some months after the intake has been reduced to normal. Urine levels should be corrected to a specific gravity of 1·040. Serum calcium and phosphorus levels are usually normal and there is a significant correlation between the amount of fluoride fed and the concentration of alkaline phosphatase in the serum. The increase in phosphatase activity is probably related to the abnormal formation of bone.

Significant changes can be detected by roentgenological examination of bones containing more than 4000 ppm of fluorine. These changes include increased density or abnormal porosity, periosteal feathering and thickening, increased trabeculation, thickening of the compact bone and narrowing of the marrow cavity. Spontaneous rib fractures show incomplete union. Good data are available for fluorine concentrations in rib bones and estimations of fluorine content in biopsy samples of ribs have been used in the clinico-pathological study of the disease (4). Tail bone biopsy has been used for the same purpose.

Necropsy Findings

Severe gastroenteritis is present in acute poisoning. In fluorosis the bones have a chalky, white appearance, are brittle and have either local or disseminated exostoses particularly along the diaphyses. Intra-articular structures are not primarily affected although there may be some spurring and bridging of the joints. Histologically there is atrophy of spongiosa, defective and irregular calcification of newly formed osseous tissue and active periosteal bone formation. Hypoplasia of the enamel and dentine are constant in young animals. Degenerative changes in kidney, liver, heart muscle, adrenal glands and central nervous system have been reported in severe cases. Degeneration of bone marrow and aplastic anaemia also occur.

Chemical examination of necropsy specimens is of considerable assistance in diagnosis. The fluorine content of bones is greatly increased. Levels of up to 1200 ppm are observed in normal animals but may be increased up to 3000 ppm in animals exposed to fluorine and showing only mottling of the teeth. Animals showing severe clinical signs have levels greater than 4000 ppm of bone on a dry, fat-free basis and after prolonged heavy feeding levels may be as high as 1·04 per cent (16). Care must be taken in selecting samples of bone because of the great variation in the concentration of fluorine which occurs between different bones. Good data are available for comparison between metacarpal, metatarsal, rib, pelvic and mandibular bones (4). Mandibles usually show the greatest concentrations and in the long bones the distal and proximal quarters are more sensitive indicators than the centre half (2).

The concentration of fluorine is greater in cancellous than in compact bone. Soft tissues are unreliable as a criterion for fluorosis because of their low levels of fluorine. In bone and teeth, ash levels of 0·01 to 0·15 per cent fluorine are found in normal animals. Levels up to 1·5 per cent fluorine indicate excessive intake but are not usually accompanied by anatomical changes. Where clinical signs of intoxication appear there is usually up to 2 per cent fluorine in bone ash and 1 per cent in teeth ash.

Diagnosis

Most confusion in the diagnosis of fluorine intoxication in the past has been in differentiating the disease from dietary deficiencies of phosphorus, calcium and vitamin D. The dental lesions of fluorosis are characteristic and the bone lesions are unlike those which occur in any of the deficiency diseases. Final diagnosis must depend upon fluorine assay of food and water, of blood and urine of affected animals, and bones and teeth at necropsy.

Treatment

The treatment of animals suffering from chronic fluorine intoxication, apart from removing them from the source of fluorine, is largely impractical. Acute cases require gastrointestinal sedatives, treatment to neutralize residual fluorine in the alimentary tract and calcium salts intravenously. Aluminium salts should be effective as neutralizers of the hydrofluoric acid produced in the stomach and because of their insolubility they are unlikely to have any deleterious effects even when given in large quantities. Doses of 30 g. of aluminium sulphate daily have been used in the prevention of chronic fluorosis and relatively larger doses may be useful in treatment. The calcium salts given intravenously to replace the precipitated calcium should be given to effect, using the disappearance of tetany and hyperaesthesia as a guide. This treatment will probably have to be repeated. The parenteral administration of glucose solutions is recommended at the same time because of the interference by fluorine with glucose metabolism. Irrespective of treatment used, no improvement in dental or osseous lesions can be anticipated but amelioration of the other clinical signs may occur.

Control

Phosphatic feed supplements should contain not more than 1000 ppm of fluorine and should not comprise more than 2 per cent of the grain ration if the fluorine content is of this order. In spite of this recommendation the feeding of rock phosphate containing 1 to 1·5 per cent fluorine to cattle for long periods has been recommended and appears to have no major deleterious effects on health in certain circumstances (17). Some deposits of rock phosphate have much higher contents of fluorine than others and commercial defluorination makes these toxic deposits safe for animal feeding. Bone meal in some areas may contain excessive quantities of fluorine and should be checked for its fluorine content. Access to superphosphate made from rock phosphate with a high fluorine content should be avoided. Water from deep wells and artesian bores should be assayed for fluorine content before use. Where levels are marginal careful husbandry including the watering of young, growing stock on fluorine-free supplies, and permitting only adults to be watered on the dangerous supplies, and rotating the animals between safe and dangerous waters at 3-month intervals may make it possible to utilize land areas otherwise unsuitable for stock raising. In some areas dairy herds may have to be maintained by the purchase of replacements rather than by the rearing of young stock. In areas where long-term ingestion of fluorine is likely to occur the aim should be to provide a diet of less than 50 ppm of the total diet of dairy cows.

Adequate calcium and phosphorus intakes should be ensured as these facilitate maximum bone storage of fluorine. Aluminium salts are the only substances used in an attempt to reduce the toxic effects of fluorine. They are relatively ineffective, reducing the accumulation of fluorine in bone by only 20 to 30 per cent, and are thus referred to as 'alleviators' (5). The sulphate and phosphate have been used but all the salts are unpalatable and can only be administered daily to animals being hand fed relatively large amounts of concentrates. It is presumed that highly insoluble aluminium fluoride is formed in the alimentary canal. An extensive field trial of aluminium as an alleviator has not justified its use as a practicable control measure. Best results are obtained by improvement in nutrition of the animals and better grassland management (1, 18).

The fluorine content of drinking water can be considerably reduced (from 10 down to 0·95 ppm) by adding freshly slaked lime to the water. 500 to 1000 ppm should be added and the water allowed to settle for 6 days. The method requires the use of large storage tanks (19).

REFERENCES

(1) Burns, K. N. & Allcroft, R. (1964). *M.A.F.F. Animal Disease Surveys*, Report 2, Pt. 1, p. 55; (1965). Report 2, Pt. 2, p. 58.
(2) Ammerman, C. B. *et al.* (1964). *J. Anim. Sci.*, *23*, 409.
(3) Egyed, M. & Rosner, M. (1969). *Refuah vet.*, *25*, 6.
(4) Shupe, J. L. *et al.* (1964). *Ann. N.Y. Acad. Sci.*, *111*, 618.
(5) Boddie, G. F. (1960). *Vet. Rec.*, *72*, 441.
(6) Allcroft, R. *et al.* (1969). *Vet. Rec.*, *84*, 399, 403.
(7) Suttie, J. W. & Faltin, E. C. (1971). *Amer. J. vet. Res.*, *32*, 217.
(8) Rosenberger, G. & Grunder, H. D. (1967). *Berl. Münch. tierärztl. Wschr.*, *80*, 41.
(9) Spencer, G. R. *et al.* (1971). *Amer. J. vet. Res.*, *32*, 1751.
(10) Merriman, G. M. & Hobbs, C. S. (1963). *Bull. Tenn. agric. Exp. Sta.*, *347*, 46.
(11) Obel, A. L. & Erne, K. (1971). *Acta vet. scand.*, *12*, 164.
(12) Burns, K. N. (1964). *Rep. 3rd int. Mtg Dis. Dairy Cattle, Copenhagen*, *2*, 292.
(13) van Rensburg, S. W. J. & de Vos, W. H. (1966). *Onderstepoort J. vet. Res.*, *33*, 185.
(14) Shupe, J. L. & Olson, A. E. (1971). *J. Amer. vet. med. Ass.*, *158*, 167.
(15) Garlick, N. L. (1955). *Amer. J. vet. Res.*, *16*, 38.

(16) Mortensen, F. N. *et al.* (1964). *J. Dairy Sci.*, *47*, 186.

(17) Snook, L. C. (1962). *Aust. vet. J.*, *38*, 42.

(18) Burns, K. N. & Allcroft, R. (1967). *4th int. Mtg World Ass. Buiatrics, Zurich*, 1966, p. 22.

(19) Mariakulandai, A. & Venkatamariah, M. A. (1955). *Indian J. vet. Sci.*, *25*, 183.

(20) Padberg, W. (1972). *Tierärztl. Umschau*, *27*, 428.

Molybdenum Poisoning

Molybdenum poisoning causes a secondary hypocuprosis and is manifested clinically by persistent scouring and depigmentation of the hair.

Incidence

Molybdenum poisoning is being recorded with increased frequency as the search for it is intensified. The disease is not highly fatal but severe stunting and loss of production occur.

Aetiology

Soil molybdenum levels in problem areas vary between 10 and 100 ppm. Illness may occur on pasture producing forage containing 3 to 10 ppm. Although levels of less than 3 ppm are usually considered to be safe, signs of toxicity may occur at levels as low as 1·0 ppm if the sulphate intake is high and the copper status low. Forage containing 10 ppm must be considered dangerous at all times and with aerial contamination levels of 10 to 200 ppm may be encountered. A daily intake of 120 to 250 mg. has proved to be toxic for cattle although the toxic dose varies widely with the intake of sulphate, copper and possibly other factors. Sheep and cattle are clinically affected in field outbreaks of the disease and signs are most marked in young growing animals. Cattle are much more susceptible than sheep. The concentration of molybdenum in forage varies with the season, being highest in the spring and autumn, and with the plant species, legumes, particularly alsike clover, taking up molybdenum in much greater quantities than grasses. On the basis of apparent increases in the digestibility of cellulose and improvement in weight gains in lambs fed added molybdenum it has been suggested that the element is an essential one for ruminants.

Occurrence

The major occurrence of molybdenum poisoning is on pasture growing on molybdenum-rich soils usually derived from particular geological formations. Such soils are those of the 'teart' pastures of Somerset, U.K., the U.S.A. and Canada. In addition excess molybdenum intake with or without a marginal deficiency of copper causes peat scours of cattle in New Zealand, Canada, Ireland and Australia. The use of molybdenum in fertilizer mixtures to increase nitrogen fixation by legumes may lead to excessive amounts of molybdenum in soils.

Aerial contamination of pastures by fumes from aluminium and steel alloy factories and oil refineries using molybdenum is also recorded (1). In these conditions simple contamination of the herbage may occur without an increase in soil molybdenum.

Pathogenesis

An extended discussion of the role of molybdenum in copper metabolism is provided in the section on secondary copper deficiency. Excess molybdenum intake interferes with the hepatic storage of copper and produces a state of copper deficiency. This situation is exacerbated by a high intake of sulphur or a low intake of copper. The syndrome of molybdenum intoxication resembles that of copper deficiency and treatment and prevention by the administration of copper is effective. However, some of the signs of molybdenum poisoning, particularly diarrhoea, are not characteristic of copper deficiency and may represent a specific toxic effect of molybdenum (2). The experimental feeding of molybdenum produces a syndrome identical with that seen in the naturally occurring disease in cattle (3) but liver and plasma levels of copper may not be depressed as is usual in naturally occurring cases (2). Experimental feeding of a large dose, up to 40 g., of molybdenum may cause only transient diarrhoea. Most of the molybdenum is rapidly absorbed and excreted, 90 per cent in the first week (4).

Clinical Findings

Persistent scouring commences within 8 to 10 days of the animals having access to the affected pasture. Emaciation and a dry, staring coat develop and there is profound depression of milk production. Depigmentation of black hair causes a red or grey tinge to appear. This may be particularly noticeable around the eyes giving a bespectacled appearance. Intense craving for copper supplement has been noted. Young cattle (3 months to $2\frac{1}{2}$ years) show in addition abnormalities of locomotion including marked stiffness of the legs and back, difficulty in rising and great reluctance to move. The gait is suggestive of laminitis but the feet appear normal. The appetite remains good (1).

Clinical Pathology

Blood copper levels are reduced from the normal of 100 µg. per 100 ml. to 16 to 60 µg. per 100 ml. Seasonal variations occur depending on the intake of molybdenum. Blood molybdenum levels in normal animals are of the order of 0·05 ppm and rise to above 0·10 ppm when excess molybdenum is ingested. Levels as high as 0·70 and 1·4 ppm have been recorded in cattle and horses grazing on pasture contaminated by smelter fumes (5). On very large intakes of molybdenum cattle which are clinically normal may have molybdenum levels of 1000 ppm in faeces, 45 ppm in urine, 10 ppm in blood and 1 ppm in milk (6).

Necropsy Findings

There are no gross or histological findings which characterize the disease, enteritis being conspicuously absent. The carcase is emaciated and dehydrated and there may be anaemia if there is an accompanying copper deficiency.

Diagnosis

The most effective method of confirming the diagnosis is to treat affected animals orally with copper sulphate (2 g. daily or 5 g. weekly for adult cattle and 1·5 g. for adult sheep). The diarrhoea ceases in 2 to 3 days and improvement in the other signs is rapid.

The persistence of the diarrhoea without other clinical signs, particularly in young cattle and sheep, may suggest internal parasitism and examination of faeces for worm eggs is necessary for differentiation. Johne's disease affects only adults and usually only one animal in a herd shows clinical signs at any one time. The acute enteridites including salmonellosis, winter dysentery and virus diarrhoea are acute diseases and are accompanied by other diagnostic signs.

Treatment and Control

In problem areas the administration of copper to large numbers of animals presents a number of problems. The methods available and their respective advantages are discussed under copper deficiency, but in general terms molybdenum toxicity can be controlled by increasing the copper content of the diet by 5 ppm (7).

REFERENCES

(1) Gardner, A. W. & Hall-Patch, P. K. (1968). *Vet. Rec.*, *82*, 86.
(2) Cook, G. A. *et al.* (1966). *J. Anim. Sci.*, *25*, 96.
(3) Lesperance, A. L. & Bohman, V. R. (1963). *J. Anim. Sci.*, *22*, 686.
(4) Tölgyesi, G. & Abd Elmothy, I. (1967). *Acta vet. hung.*, *17*, 39.
(5) Hallgren, W. *et al.* (1954). *Nord. Vet.-Med.*, *6*, 469.
(6) Tölgyesi, G. & Abd Elmothy, I. (1967). *Magy Allatorv. Lap.*, *22*, 123.
(7) Pope, A. L. (1971). *J. Anim. Sci.*, *33*, 1332.

Copper Poisoning

Copper poisoning is a complex problem because of the many factors which influence the metabolism of copper. Both acute and chronic copper poisoning occur under field conditions and although acute poisoning is relatively straightforward those diseases which are grouped under the general heading of chronic copper poisoning are difficult to define. Acute copper poisoning usually occurs because of the accidental administration of large quantities of soluble copper salts, but chronic copper poisoning is mainly a disease which occurs in certain areas where the soil is naturally rich in copper. The toxicity of the plants growing on these soils is governed not only by the absolute amount of copper in the soil but also by the interaction of a number of factors including the amount of molybdenum and probably of sulphate present in the diet and the presence or absence of specific plants and the level of protein in the diet. In fact either copper deficiency or copper poisoning can occur on soils with apparently normal copper levels, the syndrome depending on the particular conditioning factors present. The 'toxaemic jaundice' group of diseases result from the complex interactions of these factors (1). For convenience copper poisoning is dealt with here as primary and secondary copper poisoning. *Primary copper poisoning* includes acute copper poisoning caused by the accidental ingestion of large amounts of copper salts at one time and chronic poisoning caused by the continued ingestion of small amounts over a long period. *Secondary copper poisoning* includes *Phytogeneous chronic copper poisoning*, in which relatively small amounts of copper are ingested but excessive retention occurs because of the presence of specific plants which cause no apparent liver damage, and *Hepatogenous chronic copper poisoning* in which excessive retention of copper is caused by the ingestion of specific plants which cause liver damage. One of the plants which commonly contributes to hepatogenous chronic copper poisoning is *Heliotropum europaeum* which is also capable of causing uncomplicated toxipathic hepatitis without abnormality of copper metabolism. The toxaemic jaundice group of diseases includes all of these forms of secondary copper poisoning and toxipathic hepatitis caused by *Heliotropum europaeum*.

PRIMARY COPPER POISONING

Incidence

Sporadic outbreaks of primary copper poisoning occur in many circumstances. In both acute and chronic cases the mortality rate approximates 100 per cent.

Aetiology

Sheep are much more susceptible than adult cattle and single doses of 20 to 110 mg. of copper per kg. body weight produce acute copper poisoning in sheep and young calves. Sheep are peculiar in the way in which copper is handled metabolically. Increased absorption is not easily achieved but abnormally high excretion is more difficult still, so that there is the general tendency for copper to accumulate in the body of the sheep (2). In cattle a dose rate of 220 to 880 mg. per kg. body weight is necessary to cause death. Chronic copper poisoning occurs in sheep and calves with daily intakes of 3·5 mg. of copper per kg. body weight (3). Pasture containing 15 to 20 ppm DM of copper causes chronic copper poisoning in sheep but there are few records of cattle being affected by chronic copper poisoning while at pasture. Pelleted feeds containing 50 ppm and mineral mixtures containing 1400 ppm have caused fatalities in sheep and accidental feeding of 2 kg. daily of a pig-meal containing 250 ppm of copper to a heifer for 4 months has also been fatal. In lambs a concentrate ration containing 27 ppm fed for 16 weeks caused mortality (4). Copper is presently being used as a feed additive in pig rations and may result in poisoning of pigs. Concentrate feeds containing 20 ppm are dangerous for artificially fed lambs indoors and if the molybdenum content of the feed is very low, levels of 8 to 11 ppm can produce toxicity (5).

Copper by injection is being increasingly used to prevent copper deficiency in grazing ruminants when other cheaper methods are not applicable. The paste preparations, usually copper glycinate, appear to be non-toxic but the soluble preparations, e.g. copper edetate, when given at abnormally high levels, e.g. twice recommended dose levels, can cause heavy mortalities. In sheep (6, 7) and calves poisoned in this way death occurs in a few days with post mortem findings characterized by a massive accumulation of serous fluid in the body cavities, congestion of the liver and haemorrhages into the alimentary tract.

Occurrence

Most cases of acute poisoning are caused by the accidental administration of large quantities of soluble copper salts, by contamination of plants with fungicidal sprays containing copper, by overdosage with copper-containing parasiticide drenches, by contamination of drinking water when snail eradication programmes are in progress, by too liberal ingestion of mineral mixtures containing copper and when animals are grazed on pasture soon after it has been top dressed with a copper salt to correct a copper deficiency. In this circumstance the copper salt remains on the leaves and the pasture should not be grazed for at least 3 weeks or until heavy rain falls. Chronic poisoning may occur on soils rich in copper, or when pasture is contaminated by smelter fumes, by the feeding of seed grain which has been treated with antifungal agents containing copper and by the inclusion of excessive amounts of copper in licks and mineral mixtures.

Copper has achieved some prominence as a feed additive for pigs and is normally fed at levels of 125 to 250 ppm of copper in the total ration. However pigs will eat feed containing as much as 1000 ppm of copper and poisoning accidents in this species can easily occur especially if the feed is improperly mixed. In rations concentrations of copper greater than 250 ppm are toxic (8) and those greater than 500 ppm can cause deaths, but high levels of protein in, or supplementation of the diet with zinc and iron (9), exert some protective effect. If copper-supplemented rations are to be fed, great care should be taken to ensure that the recommended level is adhered to, mixing is adequate and that none of the supplemented ration is fed to sheep. The latter are more susceptible to copper poisoning than are pigs with cattle occupying an intermediate position (3).

Pathogenesis

Soluble copper salts in high concentrations are protein coagulants. The ingestion of large quantities causes intense irritation of the alimentary mucosa and profound shock. Severe intravascular haemolysis occurs if the animal survives long enough. The frequent ingestion of small amounts produces no ill effects while copper accumulates in the liver. When maximum hepatic levels are reached, after periods of exposure often as long as 6 months, the copper is released into the blood stream, the animal dying of acute intravascular haemolysis. Thus there is really no such thing as 'chronic' copper intoxication; syndromes so called are fatal as acute haemolytic crises. One of the dangers of cumulative copper poisoning is that animals show normal health until the haemolytic crisis when they become acutely ill and die very quickly. The liberation of the hepatic copper is incompletely understood. Various stresses including a fall in plane of nutrition, travelling and lactation, are considered to precipitate the liberation. On the other hand it is possible that the rise in concentration of copper in the blood may be due to inability of the liver to remove the copper from the blood, rather than to a sudden release of copper from the liver.

Clinical Findings

Acute intoxication. Severe gastroenteritis occurs accompanied by abdominal pain and severe diarrhoea and vomiting in some species. The faeces and vomitus contain much mucus and have a characteristic green to blue colour. Vomiting occurs in the pig and dog and intense thirst is apparent. Severe shock with a fall in body temperature and an increase in heart rate is followed by collapse and death usually within 24 hours. If the animal survives for a longer period dysentery and jaundice become apparent (19).

Chronic intoxication. In ruminants anorexia, thirst, haemoglobinuria, pallor and jaundice appear suddenly. There is no disturbance of alimentary tract function. Depression is profound and the animal usually dies 24 to 48 hours after the appearance of signs. The signs in toxaemic jaundice are identical with these. In pigs signs of illness are uncommon, most pigs being found dead without premonitory signs, although dullness, hyperaesthesia and muscle tremor may be observed occasionally (3).

Subclinical disease. Lambs receiving a high experimental intake of copper have shown a slight weight-gain loss on an intake of 27 µg. per g. DM of copper in the diet and a marked loss of weight-gain on an intake of 41 µg. per g. No clinical illness was apparent (10).

Clinical Pathology

Levels of copper in the blood and liver are markedly increased in chronic copper poisoning. In acute intoxications several days are required after ingestion before these levels rise appreciably. Faecal examination may show large amounts (8000 to 10,000 ppm) of copper. Liver biopsy is a satisfactory diagnostic technique and serves a most useful purpose in the detection of chronic copper poisoning as blood levels do not rise appreciably until the haemolytic crisis occurs just before death. Because of the greater concentration of copper in the caudate lobe as compared to other parts of the liver an autopsy specimen is to be preferred (11). Blood levels of copper during the haemolytic crisis are usually of the order of 500 to 2000 µg. per 100 ml., compared to about 100 µg. per 100 ml. in normal animals. Normal liver levels of less than 350 ppm DM rise to above

1000 ppm in the latter stages of chronic copper poisoning in sheep, to 6000 ppm in pigs (12), and to 2000 ppm in calves (13). In sheep liver values greater than 500 ppm and kidney values of greater than 80 to 100 ppm DM are diagnostic (5). After a massive single dose it is important to include kidney among specimens submitted for copper assay because levels may be high (more than 25 ppm DM) while liver copper levels have not yet risen (18).

The packed cell volume of the blood decreases sharply, from 40 down to 10 per cent in 48 hours, during an acute haemolytic episode. Methaemoglobinaemia may be present and the urine should be checked for haemoglobin.

Serum enzyme activity is greatly increased just before the haemolytic episode, and there is a significant reduction in the rate of bromsulphalein clearance during this period in sheep (14) and in calves poisoned experimentally (15). In sheep the SGOT levels may rise as high as 880 SF units per ml. up to 6 weeks before obvious clinical signs appear (16).

Necropsy Findings

In acute copper poisoning severe gastroenteritis is evident with erosion and ulceration particularly in the abomasum. Rupture of the abomasum may occur. If intravascular haemolysis has occurred the lesions characteristic of chronic intoxication may also be present.

In chronic copper poisoning a swollen, yellow liver, a friable spleen with soft pulp, swollen kidneys of a dark gun-metal colour, jaundice and haemoglobinuria are characteristic findings. Casts are present in the renal tubules and haemosiderin deposits in the liver and spleen. In both instances the analysis of tissues and alimentary tract contents is essential for confirmation of the diagnosis. Details of the critical copper levels of tissues are provided under clinical pathology. Although the lesions described above do occur in some outbreaks of the disease in pigs, they are not as pronounced as in ruminants and they are often accompanied by severe haemorrhage into the stomach, from ulcers in the *pars oesophagea*, or large intestine (9).

Diagnosis

Histological examination of liver tissue is necessary to determine whether or not liver damage is present. The history and the examination of feedstuffs and pastures are valuable aids in determining the cause. Acute haemolytic diseases which may be mistaken for chronic copper poisoning include leptospirosis, post-parturient haemoglobinuria, bacillary haemoglobinuria, rape poisoning and some cases of acute pasteurellosis. The bacterial infections are usually accompanied by fever and toxaemia but rape poisoning and post-parturient haemoglobinuria can only be diagnosed tentatively by an examination of the environment and consideration of the history. Acute copper poisoning can usually be differentiated from acute gastroenteritis caused by other agents by the blue-green colour of the ingesta.

Treatment

In acute cases gastrointestinal sedatives and symptomatic treatment for shock are recommended. BAL-intrav. increases copper excretion but there are no reports of its clinical use. Calcium versenate and penicillamine should be effective. Daily oral treatment of affected lambs with 100 mg. ammonium molybdate and 1 g. anhydrous sodium sulphate significantly reduced the copper content of tissues (17) and appears to prevent deaths in lambs known to have taken toxic amounts of copper.

Control

When chronic intoxication is occurring or appears probable the provision of additional molybdenum in the diet as described under the control of phytogenous chronic copper poisoning (see below) should be effective as a preventive. Ferrous sulphide is effective but difficulty is usually encountered in getting the animals to eat it. In pigs the administration of iron and zinc reduces the risk of copper poisoning on diets supplemented by this element and a diet high in calcium encourages the development of copper poisoning, probably by creating a secondary zinc deficiency (9).

SECONDARY COPPER POISONING

('Toxaemic Jaundice' Complex)

Phytogenous chronic copper poisoning occurs in sheep grazing pasture containing normal amounts of copper. Although the copper intake may be low liver copper levels are high and a haemolytic crisis typical of chronic copper poisoning occurs. The occurrence of this form of the disease is related to the domination of the pasture by subterranean clover (*Trifolium subterraneum*) which may contain lower than normal quantities of copper (15 to 20 ppm). British breeds of sheep and their crosses with merinos are most susceptible.

Control of copper poisoning of this type is aided by encouragement of grass growth in pastures. Outbreaks can also be avoided if sheep are prevented from grazing lush, clover-dominant pastures in the autumn. Avoidance of stress, particularly malnutrition, is also important in the prevention of outbreaks. Molybdenized superphosphate (4 oz. molybdenum per acre) is valuable to increase the molybdenum content of the pasture and reduce the retention of copper. Molybdenized licks or mineral mixtures (190 lb. salt, 140 lb. finely ground gypsum, 1 lb. sodium molybdate) can be used alternatively. When an outbreak occurs the administration of ammonium molybdate (50 to 100 mg. per head per day) together with sodium sulphate (0·3 to 1·0 g. per head per day) has stopped further deaths in sheep within 3 days. Solutions of the above salts may be sprayed onto hay and administration should be continued for several weeks. A number of other methods have been used with satisfactory results (5) but daily drenching of lambs for 3 to 13 weeks does not appeal as a practical procedure and administration in salt-lick and pellets is unsatisfactory.

Hepatogenous chronic copper poisoning. This form of the disease occurs most commonly following the ingestion of sufficient quantities of the plant *Heliotropum europaeum*, over a period of 2 to 5 months, to produce morphological and biochemical changes in liver cells without major impairment of liver function. Other plants containing hepatoxic alkaloids (*Senechio* spp. and *Echium plantagineum* may also cause this syndrome. After ingestion of these plants the liver cells have an increased affinity for copper and abnormally high amounts accumulate in the liver with an increased risk of a haemolytic crises. Sheep grazed on *H. europaeum* and then on subterranean clover are particularly prone to this form of the disease. Control depends upon preventing the ingestion of hepatoxic plants and restricting copper retention by the methods described above.

Poisoning by Heliotropum europaeum. Heliotrope contains hepatoxic alkaloids and continued ingestion of the plant causes liver damage. If a high copper storage occurs, hepatogenous chronic copper poisoning may develop. On the other hand if the sheep's copper status remains normal liver damage proceeds until the animal suffers from a simple toxipathic hepatitis. The effects of the plant are cumulative and grazing for one season may cause little apparent harm but further grazing in the subsequent year may cause heavy mortality. Control must aim at eradication of the plant.

REFERENCES

(1) Bull, L. B. *et al.* (1956). *Aust. vet. J.*, *32*, 229.
(2) Brown, J. M. M. (1968). *J. S. Afr. vet. med. Ass.*, *39*, 13.
(3) Todd, J. R. (1962). *Vet. Bull.*, *32*, 573.
(4) Tait, R. *et al.* (1971). *Canad. vet. J.*, *12*, 73.
(5) Pope, A. L. (1971). *J. Anim. Sci.*, *33*, 1332.
(6) Macleod, N. S. M. & Watt, J. A. (1970). *Vet. Rec.*, *86*, 375.
(7) Ishmael, J. *et al.* (1971). *Res. vet. Sci.*, *12*, 358.
(8) De Goey, L. W. *et al.* (1971). *J. Anim. Sci.*, *33*, 52.
(9) Suttle, N. F. & Mills, C. F. (1966). *Brit. J. Nutr.*, *20*, 135.
(10) Hill, R. & Williams, H. L. (1965). *Vet. Rec.*, *77*, 1043.
(11) Hogan, K. G. *et al.* (1971). *N.Z. J. agric. Res.*, *14*, 132.
(12) Allen, M. M. & Harding, J. D. J. (1962). *Vet. Rec.*, *74*, 173.
(13) Weiss, E. & Bauer, P. (1968). *Zbl. vet. Med.*, *15A*, 156.
(14) Ishmael, J. *et al.* (1971). *Res. vet. Sci.*, *13*, 22.
(15) Todd, J. R. & Thompson, J. R. (1965). *Brit. vet. J.*, *121*, 90.
(16) McPherson, A. & Hemingway, R. G. (1969). *Brit. vet. J.*, *125*, 213.
(17) Ross, D. B. (1970). *Res. vet. Sci.*, *11*, 295.
(18) Sharman, J. R. (1969). *N.Z. vet. J.*, *17*, 67.
(19) Cabadaj, R. & Gdovin, T. (1970). *Vet. Med. Praha*, *15*, 21.

Sodium Chloride Poisoning

The ingestion of excessive quantities of sodium chloride causes inflammation of the alimentary tract with the production of gastroenteritis and diarrhoea. The toxic effect produced when the salt intake is not excessive but the water intake is restricted is one of cerebral oedema with a clinical picture characterized mainly by nervous signs.

Incidence

Salt poisoning is of major importance in some areas where animals are kept under range conditions and have to depend on saline water supplies for drinking purposes. Many animals may be clinically affected and the mortality rate may be high. In animals kept under intensive conditions salt poisoning occurs only sporadically but most affected animals die and heavy losses may occur in groups of pigs.

Aetiology

Food and water containing excessive quantities of salt are usually unpalatable to animals but in certain circumstances listed below excessive quantities of salt are taken, especially in saline drinking waters. The problem of the degree of salinity of drinking water which is compatible with health in animals has received a great deal of attention, but specific details are difficult to provide because of the variation in the salts which occur in natural saline waters. Many of them contain appreciable amounts of fluorine and magnesium which exert a much greater effect on alimentary mucosa than does sodium. Variation also occurs in the relative proportions of the acid radicles, particularly sulphates, carbonates and chlorides. In Australia the two principal artesian basins provide waters of quite different composition. One which is classified as a 'chloride' water is safe for livestock up to a 1 per cent concentration of total salts; at 1·3 per cent concentration there is reduction in lambing percentage in ewes and weight gain in lambs and some increase in mortality rate. The other is classed as a 'bicarbonate' water, containing 0·5 per cent total salts, and has no apparent effect other than a reduction in lambing percentage (9).

Sheep, beef cattle and dry dairy cattle appear to be less susceptible than dairy cows in milk which are in turn less susceptible than horses. Heavy milking cows, especially those in the early stages of lactation are highly susceptible to salt poisoning because of their unstable fluid and electrolyte status. Environmental temperatures have an effect on toxicity, signs occurring in the summer on water containing levels of salt which appear to be non-toxic in the winter time. Australian recommendations (1) are that the maximum concentration for sodium chloride or total salts in drinking water should not exceed 1·3 per cent for sheep, 1·0 per cent for cattle and 0·9 per cent for horses. South African recommendations (2) are considerably lower than these and it is suggested that a concentration of 0·5 per cent total salts in drinking water is excessive for stock. Canadian data (3) recommend much lower levels than the above but there does not appear to be any proof that such low levels of total and individual salts are necessary to avoid poisoning of livestock. Apart from overt signs of toxicity which occur when too much salt is taken it is apparent that lower levels of intake can suppress growth. In cattle signs of toxicity occur in heifers drinking water containing 1·75 per cent NaCl, the animals only maintain weight at a level of 1·5 per cent and show suboptimal weight gains when the water contains 1·25 per cent NaCl. Saline waters often contain a mixture of salts and those containing high levels of fluorine may be quite toxic. Water containing 0·2 to 0·5 per cent magnesium chloride may cause reduced appetite and occasional diarrhoea in sheep, especially if the sodium chloride content is also high, but water containing similar quantities of sodium sulphate does not have any harmful effect.

Toxic doses quoted for acute sodium chloride poisoning are for pigs, horses and cattle 2·2 g. per kg. body weight and for sheep 6 g. per kg.

In the circumstances where animals are fed prepared feeds containing the standard recommendation of 2 per cent salt, disease does not occur unless the supply of drinking water is temporarily restricted. It is probable that the physiological disturbance in this instance is one of water intoxication rather than salt poisoning in the absolute sense. High salt intakes are extensively used in sheep to restrict food intake during drought periods and in the control of urolithiasis in feeder wethers but salt poisoning does not occur if there is free access to water. Rations containing up to 13 per cent of sodium chloride have been fed to ewes for long periods without apparent ill effects although diets containing 10 to 20 per cent and water containing 1·5 to 2·0 per cent sodium chloride do reduce food consumption (4). This may be of value when attempting to reduce feed intake but can be a disadvantage when sheep are watered on saline artesian water.

Occurrence

In animals at pasture salt poisoning can occur in a number of circumstances. A sudden change from fresh water to saline water may cause poisoning especially if the animals are thirsty when first allowed access to the saline water. Water accumulating in salt troughs during drought periods may also cause poisoning. Animals previously deprived of salt may eat excessive amounts if they are suddenly allowed access to unlimited quantities.

In animals kept in barns and small yards salt poisoning may occur if prepared feeds contain too much salt, if the salt is provided only at long intervals, and when trough space is limited and animals tend to gorge on swill or concentrate. Swill, fed to pigs, may contain excessive amounts of salt when it contains dough residues from bakeries, brine from butchers' shops, salt whey from cheese factories or salted fish waste. Excessive administration of sodium sulphate to pigs as a treatment for gut oedema also produces the disease if the water intake is restricted (5). Another rather special occurrence of salt poisoning is via environmental pollution by oil wells. Cattle are attracted to oil residues because of their salty flavour and may ingest toxic amounts (12).

One of the major occurrences in all species is when animals are being fed a high-normal salt intake but the water supply is temporarily restricted. Poisoning occurs when they are again allowed access to unlimited water. Pigs brought into new pens where drinking water is supplied in automatic drinking cups may not be accustomed to their use and be deprived of water for several days until they learn to operate the cups. Feeder lambs and cattle may also be deprived of water when their troughs are frozen over. This form of salt poisoning is recorded most commonly in pigs 8 to 12 weeks of age but does occur in lambs and calves. A similar occurrence has been recorded in wild life in the northern U.S.A. The source of salt was material deposited on road surfaces to reduce the hazards of ice.

A severe eosinophilic dermatitis has been observed at meat inspection in pigs transported in trucks which were salted to prevent slipping. The pigs were killed 48 hours after transport. The condition was reproduced experimentally by rubbing salt into the skin (13).

Pathogenesis

When excessive amounts of salt are ingested gastroenteritis occurs because of the irritating effects of the high concentrations of salt. Dehydration results and is exacerbated by the increased osmotic pressure of the alimentary tract contents. Some salt is absorbed and may cause involvement of the central nervous system as in chronic poisoning. Poisoning which occurs in these circumstances is described as acute poisoning in contradistinction to the chronic form in which sodium ions accumulate in tissues gradually.

In chronic poisoning where the defect is one of decreased water but normal salt intake there is an accumulation of sodium ions in tissues, including the brain, over a period of several days. When water is made available in unlimited quantities there is a sudden migration of water to the tissues to establish the normal salt–water equilibrium. In the brain this causes acute cerebral oedema and the appearance of signs referable to a sudden rise in intracranial pressure (6). The response is the same in all species but in pigs there is, in addition, an accumulation of eosinophils in nervous tissue and the meninges and before the cause of the disease was established it was known as eosinophilic meningo-encephalitis. The sodium ion is the one that accumulates in the tissues, identical syndromes being produced by the feeding of sodium propionate or sodium sulphate (5). It has also been observed that the feeding of soluble substances such as urea, which are excreted unchanged by the kidney, may cause anhydraemia and an increase in the sodium ion concentration in brain tissue and the development of encephalomalacia (7).

This form of salt poisoning is chronic only in the sense that the sodium ion accumulates gradually. The clinical syndrome is acute in much the same way as the syndrome is acute in chronic copper poisoning. There is an apparent relationship between this form of salt poisoning and polio-encephalomalacia in all species. Many outbreaks of this latter disease occur in circumstances which suggest chronic salt poisoning. Sheep become adapted to a continuous high salt intake (up to 1·3 per cent sodium chloride in the drinking water) by significant changes in numbers of microflora in the rumen but this is not usually accompanied by any change in total metabolic activity (8). The same levels of intake are reported to cause some mortality, chronic diarrhoea and reduction in fertility, weight gain and wool growth (9).

Clinical Findings

Acute salt poisoning in cattle is manifested largely by an alimentary tract disturbance. There is vomiting, diarrhoea with mucus in the faeces, abdominal pain and anorexia. Some nervous signs, including blindness, paresis and knuckling at the fetlocks, are evident. There may be a nasal discharge and polyuria occurs constantly. A period of recumbency follows and affected animals die within 24 hours of the appearance of clinical signs. In swine the syndrome suggests less alimentary tract involvement, the signs being largely referable to the nervous system (6). There is great weakness, and prostration, muscle tremor, clonic convulsions, coma and death after a course of about 48 hours.

Chronic salt poisoning in pigs is ushered in by the appearance of constipation, thirst and pruritus 2 to 4 days after exposure commences. A characteristic nervous syndrome follows within 12 to 24 hours. Initially there is apparent blindness and deafness, the pig remaining oblivious to normal stimuli and wandering about aimlessly, bumping into objects and pressing with the head. There may be circling or pivoting on one front leg. Recovery may occur at this stage or epileptiform convulsions may appear. These convulsive episodes recur at remarkably constant time intervals, usually 7 minutes, and commence with tremor of the snout and neck. Clonic contractions of the neck muscles may result in the jerky development of opisthotonus until the head is almost vertical and the pig walks backwards and assumes a sitting posture. This may be followed by a complete clonic convulsion with the pig laterally recumbent. During the convulsion there is champing of the jaws, salivation and respiratory distress. Death may occur due to respiratory failure or the pig relaxes into a state of coma for a few moments, revives and wanders about aimlessly until the next episode occurs. The pulse and temperature are normal except in convulsive pigs when both may be elevated. The course is variable and death may occur in a few hours or not for 3 or 4 days after the first appearance of illness.

A syndrome which is often described as chronic salt poisoning occurs in cattle and sheep on saline drinking water. There is a depression of appetite, loss of body weight, dehydration, depression of body temperature, weakness and occasional diarrhoea. If affected cattle are forced to take exercise they may collapse and have tetanic convulsions. In dairy cattle acetonaemia may occur in these circumstances.

Clinical Pathology

In pigs serum-sodium levels are elevated appreciably above normal levels (135 to 145 mEq. per litre), to about 180 to 190 mEq. per litre during the severe stage of chronic sodium salt poisoning (10). An eosinopenia is also evident during this stage and a return to normal levels usually indicates recovery. In cattle the same changes occur but there is no eosinopenia. Samples of feed and drinking water should be collected for salt assay.

Necropsy Findings

In acute salt poisoning of cattle there is marked congestion of the mucosae of the omasum and abomasum. The faeces are fluid and in some cases sufficiently dark in colour to suggest that they contain blood. Animals which have survived for several days show oedema of the skeletal muscles and hydropericardium. The blood appears to be thinner than normal. Gastroenteritis may be evident in some pigs poisoned with large doses of salt but in chronic poisoning there are no gross lesions. Histologically the lesions of chronic poisoning in the pig are quite diagnostic. There is acute cerebral oedema and meningo-encephalitis accompanied by an invasion by eosinophils of the meninges and perivascular spaces around the blood vessels of the brain. In pigs that survive the acute stages there may be residual polioencephalomalacia especially of the cerebral cortex. Chemical estimation of the amount of sodium and chloride in tissues, especially brain, may be of diagnostic value. Levels exceeding 150 mg. per cent of sodium in the brain and liver, and of chlorides in excess of 180 mg. in the brain, 70 mg. in muscle and 250 mg. per cent in the liver are considered to indicate salt poisoning (11).

Diagnosis

The appearance of typical signs in pigs which have been just moved to new quarters or subjected to change of ration during the preceding week, or which have not had access to water at all times, immediately suggests sodium salt poisoning. Other diseases of the nervous system in feeder pigs may resemble salt poisoning. If convulsions occur the temperature in pigs poisoned with salt may be sufficiently high to suggest encephalitis. Pseudorabies is restricted in its occurrence to young sucking pigs, viral encephalomyelitis occurs in pigs of all ages, but in both the syndrome may be very similar to that of salt poisoning. Polioencephalomalacia in pigs and ruminants is almost identical with chronic salt poisoning and occurs in many instances under the same set of circumstances. Gut oedema occurs in rapidly growing pigs in the same age group as chronic salt poisoning. There are some differences in the clinical syndromes as they occur in the field, particularly the periodicity of the convulsive episodes in salt poisoning and the altered squeal in gut oedema, but in many instances it will be impossible to decide on the diagnosis without reference to the history of salt and water intake. Mulberry heart disease may be accompanied by nervous signs similar to those of salt poisoning but the disease is usually restricted to older pigs and deaths occur quite suddenly

Gastroenteritis caused by excessive ingestion of saline drinking water has few diagnostic features and the diagnosis depends upon detection of the salinity of the water. A recent change in the source of drinking water is often a part of the history. Laboratory analysis of feed and water is necessary for confirmation.

Treatment

In both acute and chronic salt poisoning the toxic feed or water must be removed immediately. Initially access to fresh water should be restricted to small amounts at frequent intervals as unlimited access to water may result in a sudden increase in the number of animals affected. In advanced cases animals may be unable to drink and water may have to be administered by stomach tube.

Symptomatic treatment includes alimentary tract sedatives when gastroenteritis is present and the provision of isotonic fluids when dehydration has occurred. When there is evidence of cerebral oedema it may be necessary to administer a sedative and cerebral decompression may be attempted by the use of diuretics or hypertonic solutions injected parenterally.

Control

Drinking water for all classes of livestock should not contain more than 0·5 per cent sodium chloride or total salts although sheep and beef cattle can survive on water containing as much at 1·7 per cent sodium chloride or total salts. Waters containing a high concentration of fluoride or magnesium are particularly dangerous to livestock. Both salt and water should be freely available at all times. Diets fed to pigs should not contain more than 1 per cent salt. The way in which whey is fed to pigs—with minimum water intake—makes prevention difficult unless the whey can be kept free of salt at the cheese factory.

REFERENCES

(1) Pierce, A. W. (1963). *Aust. J. agric. Res.*, *14*, 815.
(2) Steyn, D. G. & Reinach, N. (1939). *Onderstepoort J. vet. Sci.*, *12*, 167.
(3) Ballantyne, E. E. (1957). *Canad. J. comp. Med.*, *21*, 254.
(4) Wilson, A. D. (1966). *Aust. J. agric. Res.*, *17*, 503.
(5) Dow, C. *et al.* (1963). *Vet. Rec.*, *75*, 1052.
(6) Smith, D. L. T. (1955). *Proc. 92nd ann. Mtg Amer. vet. med. Ass.*, 69.
(7) Done, J. T. *et al.* (1959). *Vet. Rec.*, *71*, 92.
(8) Potter, B. J. *et al.* (1972). *Brit. J. Nutr.*, *27*, 75.
(9) Pierce, A. W. (1968). *Aust. J. agric. Res.*, *19*, 577, 589.
(10) Smith, D. L. T. (1957). *Amer. J. vet. Res.*, *18*, 825.
(11) Bohosiewicz, M. (1962). *Weterynaria*, *11*, 3.
(12) Monlux, A. W. *et al.* (1971). *J. Amer. vet. med. Ass.*, *158*, 1379.
(13) Anderson, P. & Petaja, E. (1968). *Nord. Vet.-Med.*, *20*, 706.

Zinc Poisoning

Poisoning by zinc compounds occurs only rarely and the syndrome reported is poorly defined.

Incidence

Exposure to excessive quantities of zinc occurs very rarely and the element has relatively low toxicity.

Aetiology

Soluble zinc salts causing poisoning in animals usually originate from galvanized ironware used as piping or drinking utensils. Toxic doses are not well defined but drinking water containing 6 to 8 ppm of zinc has caused constipation in cattle (1), and 200 g. of zinc as lactate fed over a period of 2 months as a 0·1 per cent solution has caused arthritis in pigs (2). Zinc chromate used as a paste in joining electrical cables has caused poisoning in calves (3); the acute toxicity appears to be due to the chromic oxide content of the paste but chronic intoxication may be caused by the accumulation of zinc. Zinc ethylenebisdithiocarbamate, a fungicide, has proved toxic on experimental administration to sheep (4). Experimental zinc poisoning in sheep and cattle caused reduced weight gains and feed efficiency when zinc was fed at the rate of 1·0 g. per kg. body weight. At 1·5 to 1·7 g. per kg. body weight there was reduced feed consumption in both species and depraved appetite in cattle (5). The accidental inclusion of zinc oxide in a prepared feed for dairy cows led to the ingestion by some of 150 g. daily resulting in serious illness in many cattle and death in 7 per cent of them (6).

Occurrence

Zinc may be released from galvanized surfaces when subjected to electrolysis as occurs when galvanized and copper pipes are joined (1). An outbreak of poisoning has been recorded in pigs fed buttermilk from a dairy factory. The buttermilk was piped to the pig-pens each day through a long galvanized iron pipe. The buttermilk lay in pools in the pipe after each batch was run through, souring occurred and the lactic acid produced caused the formation of zinc lactate which was passed to the pigs in the next batch of buttermilk. The concentration of zinc in the milk (0·066 per cent) was slightly higher than the minimum toxic strength (0·05 per cent). The addition of zinc to pig rations as a preventive against parakeratosis is unlikely to cause poisoning because of the low toxicity of the element and the unpalatability of rations containing excessive amounts. The maximum amount tolerated by pigs is 0·1 per cent zinc (as zinc carbonate) in the diet. Levels greater than this cause decreased food intake, arthritis, haemorrhages in the axillae, gastritis and enteritis. Death may occur within 21 days (4).

Pathogenesis

The pathogenesis of zinc poisoning has not been determined.

Clinical Findings

Pigs fed buttermilk containing zinc show anorexia, unthriftiness, rough coat, stiffness and lameness. There is progressive weakness with enlargement of the joints, particularly the shoulder joint. Dairy cattle drinking contaminated water show chronic constipation and a fall in milk yield. Experimental dosing with large quantities of soluble zinc salts causes diarrhoea, dysentery, posterior weakness and death. A natural outbreak in cattle caused scouring and drastic reduction in milk yield.

Clinical Pathology

After experimental feeding high levels of zinc are detectable in tissues, especially liver, pancreas and kidney, and serum and liver levels of copper are reduced (5).

Necropsy Findings

Severe, acute poisoning in cattle has been accompanied by generalized pulmonary emphysema, pale flabby myocardium, haemorrhages in kidney and severe hepatic degeneration (6).

In chronic zinc poisoning in pigs there is a non-specific, degenerative arthritis affecting particularly the head of the humerus, the articular cartilage being separated from the underlying bone which has undergone extensive osteoporotic changes. There may be some renal damage. In more severe poisoning there is gastritis, enteritis, arthritis, haemorrhages under the skin, in the ventricles of the brain and in lymph nodes and spleen (4). Ingesta, liver, kidney, spleen and bone should be submitted for analysis. The zinc content of liver in normal animals is high (30 to 150 ppm WM in calves) and may reach levels of 400 to 600 ppm. WM after continued ingestion of zinc chromate paste without being accompanied by signs of zinc poisoning. In acute poisoning by zinc oxide in cattle levels of 2000 ppm DM in liver and 300 ppm DM in kidney may be achieved; tissue copper levels in these animals may be reduced to 10 to 20 ppm (6).

Diagnosis

Arthritis caused by zinc poisoning in pigs must be differentiated from rickets and erysipelas. Chronic constipation as a herd problem in cattle is most unusual and zinc poisoning should be considered as a possible cause when it occurs.

Treatment

Specific treatments have not been recommended and removal of the source of zinc and symptomatic treatment are suggested as the only measures available.

Control

Galvanized utensils and piping should be rinsed after each use in carrying milk. The addition of extra amounts of calcium to the diet of pigs does not prevent the toxic effects of large amounts of zinc (7).

REFERENCES

(1) Pickup, J. et al. (1954). Vet. Rec., 66, 93.
(2) Grimmett, R. E. R. et al. (1939). N.Z. J. Agric., 59, 140.
(3) Harrison, D. L. & Staples, E. L. J. (1955). N.Z. vet. J., 3, 63.
(4) Palmer, J. S. (1963). J. Amer. vet. med. Ass., 143, 994.
(5) Ott, E. A. et al. (1966). J. Anim. Sci., 25, 414, 419, 424, 432.
(6) Allen, G. S. (1968). Vet. Rec., 83, 8.
(7) Brink, M. F. et al. (1959). J. Anim. Sci., 18, 836.

Sulphur Poisoning

Elemental sulphur (flowers of sulphur) is often fed to livestock as a tonic and to control external parasites. It is also used in feed-lots to restrict the consumption of feed by lambs and thus reduce the incidence of enterotoxaemia. In small doses the substance is relatively non-toxic but excessive doses can cause fatal gastroenteritis and dehydration. Most deaths occur because of inadvertent over-dosing. The feeding of 85 to 450 g. per head to cattle has been fatal (1), as has 45 g. of sulphur in feed pellets to ewes (2), and the minimum lethal dose of a sulphur-protein concentrate for sheep is estimated to be 10 g. per kg. body weight. Continuous feeding of sulphur at the rate of 7 g. per day can be fatal to adult sheep (2). It is possible that sulphur is most toxic when fed in a ration containing a high level of protein. Sodium metabisulphite and sulphur dioxide gas are used in the preparation of ensilage but at the levels used are unlikely to have toxic effects in animals eating the ensilage. Hydrogen sulphide gas is often present in gases emanating from oil and natural gas wells, in cesspools and in wells but animals are not likely to be exposed to concentrations of the gas which are sufficiently high to cause illness (3) although a slatted floor system of manure disposal, if functioning imperfectly, might present problems.

Clinically the syndrome is characterized by dullness, abdominal pain, muscle twitching, black diarrhoea and a strong odour of hydrogen sulphide on the breath. Dehydration is severe and the animals soon become recumbent and dyspnoeic, develop convulsions and die in a coma. At necropsy the lungs are congested and oedematous, the liver is pale, the kidneys congested and black in colour and there is severe gastroenteritis with peritoneal effusion. Petechial haemorrhages have been observed to occur extensively in all organs and in musculature (2).

One of the early blows in the battle over pollution of animal environments has been struck in an examination of the effects of constant exposure of pigs to an atmosphere containing 35 ppm of sulphur dioxide for 1 to 6 weeks. Increased salivation was apparent and was accompanied by clinical and histological evidence of irritation of the conjunctiva and respiratory mucosa (4, 5).

REFERENCES

(1) McFarlane, D. F. (1952). Vet. Rec., 64, 345.
(2) White, J. B. (1964). Vet. Rec., 76, 278.
(3) O'Donaghue, J. G. (1961). Canad. J. comp. Med., 25, 217.
(4) Lawson, G. H. F. & McAllister, J. V. S. (1966). Vet. Rec., 79, 274.
(5) Martin, S. W. & Willoughby, R. A. (1971). J. Amer. vet. med. Ass., 159, 1518.

Poisoning by Organic Iron Compounds

Heavy fatalities have occurred in young piglets soon after the injection of organic iron compounds used to prevent anaemia. Death is due to acute iron poisoning (1). Within an hour or two of injection sudden deaths occur, sometimes accompanied by vomiting and diarrhoea. At necropsy examination there is severe myodegeneration (2) of skeletal but not cardiac muscle. The progeny of vitamin E deficient sows are most susceptible (3) and the most toxic compounds are those which contain a high proportion of their iron in ionic, and therefore readily absorbable form. In the absence of vitamin E the muscle cell membranes are damaged and extensive biochemical changes result. One of these is a great increase in extracellular potassium levels causing cardiac arrest and sudden death (1). Pigs at 2 days of age are much more susceptible to the toxic effects of these iron compounds than are 8-day-old pigs, apparently because of the older pigs' better renal functional ability to excrete iron. Another possible reason for this age difference in combating iron toxicity is the greater mobilization of calcium by older pigs in response to iron administration. This mobilization, or calciphylaxis, can be great enough to result in deposition of calcium in damaged tissues·or cause death. This effect appears to be precipitated by simultaneous or immediately preceding (within 24 hours) injection of vitamin D_3 (4) but the injection is not essential to it.

There is an additional possible damaging effect of iron injection in young pigs, the development of asymmetric hindquarters (1, 5). In this condition there is asymmetry but the muscles are normal in composition and appear to have asymmetric blood supplies.

REFERENCES

(1) Patterson, D. S. P. & Allen, W. M. (1972). Brit. vet. J., 128, 101.
(2) Arpi, T. & Tollerz, G. (1965). Acta vet. scand., 6, 360.
(3) Tollerz, G. & Lannek, N. (1964). Nature (Lond.), 201, 846.
(4) Penn, G. B. (1970). Vet. Rec., 86, 718.
(5) Hoorens, J. & Oyaert, W. (1970). Vlaams diergeneesk. Tijdschr., 39, 246.

31

Diseases Caused by Chemical Agents—II

DISEASES CAUSED BY ORGANIC POISONS

Hydrocyanic Acid Poisoning

ACUTE poisoning by hydrocyanic acid causes a histotoxic anoxia with a syndrome of dyspnoea, tremor, convulsions and sudden death. Chronic poisoning may lead to the development of goitre in newborn animals.

Incidence

Hydrocyanic acid poisoning occurs in most countries because of the common occurrence of plants which contain toxic quantities of cyanides. When the disease occurs most affected animals die and although the overall economic effects are not great, the losses may be heavy on individual farms.

Aetiology

Most outbreaks of hydrocyanic acid poisoning are caused by the ingestion of plants which contain cyanogenetic glucosides. In this form the acid is non-toxic but it may be liberated from the organic complex by the action of an enzyme which may also be present in the same or other plant, or by the activity of rumen micro-organisms. Horses and pigs are much less susceptible to the glucosides because the acidity of the stomach in monogastric animals helps to destroy the enzyme. Sheep are much more resistant than cattle, apparently because of differences between enzyme systems in the forestomachs of the two animals.

Many plants contain cyanogenetic glucosides and it is not proposed to list them all here. Many of them are weeds including native couch (*Brachyachne convergens*), Bermuda and blue couch grasses, arrowgrass, chokecherry, native fuchsia (*Eremophila maculata*) and particularly plants of the flax family. Reed sweet grass (*Poa aquatica*) can contain 1·52 mg. HCN per g. dry material and is thought to have caused heavy mortalities in hungry travelling stock (1). Some garden plants, including the cherry laurel tree, are potent sources. Of greatest importance, however, are a number of common pasture and cultivated plants. Johnson grass (*Sorghum halepense*), Sudan grass (*S. sudanense*) and sorghum (*S. vulgare*) are used extensively in some countries for forage and may cause heavy mortalities in particular circumstances. Hybrids of these three plants are usually much more toxic than the pure species. Sugar cane contains a cyanogenic glucoside from which hydrocyanic acid can be released. Release occurs through the action of an enzyme in algarrobo pods (*Prosopsis jubiflora*) when the two are fed together (2). Linseed in the form of cake or meal may also be highly toxic if eaten in large quantities. Some clovers, particularly white clover (*Trifolium repens*) and members of the *Brassica* genus may also contain significant amounts of cyanogenetic glucosides.

A number of specific glucosides have been isolated and include linamarin from linseed and flax, lotaustralin from white clover, dhurrin from sorghum, lotusin from *Lotus arabicus* and amygdalin from bitter almonds. The glucosides are by-products of plant metabolism and their concentration in the different plant species is variable depending upon climatic and other conditions which influence plant growth.

The minimum lethal dose of hydrocyanic acid (HCN) is about 2 mg. per kg. body weight for cattle and sheep when taken in the form of a glucoside. The MLD of lotaustralin for sheep approximates 4·0 mg. per kg. body weight (3). Plant material containing more than 20 mg. of HCN per 100 g. (200 ppm) is likely to cause toxic effects and highly poisonous samples may contain as much as 6000 ppm. The toxic doses quoted must be accepted with some reservation as the toxicity of a particular specimen varies with a number of factors including the concentration of the hydrolysing enzyme in the plant, the preceding diet of the animals and particularly the speed with which the material is eaten.

Occurrence

Poisoning is most likely to occur when the cyanide content of the material is high and it is eaten quickly. The glucoside content is highest when plants grow rapidly after a previous period of retardation. This is most likely to occur when autumn rains cause rapid growth after stunting during a summer drought, or when a crop is eaten back by livestock or grasshoppers, or following the application of herbicides. Wilted, frost-bitten and young plants are also likely to be more poisonous than normal, mature plants. The greatest danger exists when animals which are hungry are allowed access to heavy concentrations of the poisonous plants. Travelling or recently introduced animals may not be accustomed to local plants and thus may be poisoned on pastures that indigenous stock graze with impunity. There is evidence that animals become accustomed to the poison and can tolerate increasing doses with experience (3). Cattle or sheep may break out of dry, summer pastures into fields of immature sorghum or Sudan grass and gorge themselves. In these circumstances, heavy mortalities are likely to occur within an hour, sometimes within about 15 minutes. Toxic forage made into ensilage loses much of its cyanide content and on exposure to air may give off large quantities of free hydrocyanic acid.

Deaths due to the ingestion of excessive linseed meal or cake occur under the same circumstances. Sheep fed large quantities of linseed meal at the end of a period of starvation have died of HCN poisoning (4). Calves fed on milk replacer containing linseed which has been soaked but not boiled may also ingest lethal amounts of cyanogenetic linamarin. Occasional cases of HCN poisoning occur when animals are exposed to chemicals used for fumigation or the fertilizer, calcium cyanamide.

Pathogenesis

Acute cyanide intoxication causes a histotoxic anoxia, and a resultant tissue asphyxia, by paralysis of tissue enzyme systems. Oxygen exchange is suspended and oxygen is retained in the blood, giving it a characteristic bright red colour. If the course is prolonged the blood may be dark red due to inhibition of respiration and restriction of oxygen intake. Because of the severity of the anoxia the major manifestation of cyanide poisoning is that of cerebral anoxia with muscle tremor and convulsions, and dyspnoea. Cyanogenetic glucosides may be of importance as contributory causes of bloat in ruminants.

Doses which do not produce clinical effects appear to be well tolerated and the tolerance appears to increase with experience. Cyanides ingested in small amounts, however, are known to be goitrogenic and may be important in the pro-duction of clinical goitre in lambs on marginal intakes of iodine.

Hydrocyanic acid is normally detoxicated by its conversion to thiocyanate in the liver through the action of a specific enzyme system. After the administration of hydrocyanic acid to sheep the thiocyanate content of the liver may rise from 2·3 to 17·6 mg. per cent. Bovine liver also contains this enzyme system but thiocyanate levels do not rise after the administration of hydrocyanic acid in clover, suggesting that there may be more effective excretion or an alternate method of detoxication in cattle.

There is some interaction between hydrocyanic acid and vitamin B_{12} but its importance in farm animals is unknown. The vitamin has been used as an effective treatment for cyanide poisoning in mice and chronically poisoned rats have been shown to have a lowered level of vitamin B_{12} in the liver (5).

Clinical Findings

In its common form hydrocyanic acid poisoning is always acute and affected animals rarely survive for more than 1 to 2 hours. In the most acute cases animals become affected within 10 to 15 minutes of eating toxic material and die within 2 to 3 minutes of first showing signs. These include dyspnoea, anxiety, restlessness, moaning, recumbency and terminal clonic convulsions with opisthotonus. The mucosae are bright red in colour. In the more common, less acute cases the animals show depression, staggering, gross muscle tremor and dyspnoea. There may be hyperaesthesia and lacrimation. The muscle tremor is evident first in the head and neck but soon spreads to involve the rest of the body; the animal becomes weak and goes down. The pulse is small, weak and rapid. There is dilation of the pupils, nystagmus and cyanosis in the terminal stages, usually accompanied by clonic convulsions and in some cases by vomiting and aspiration of ingesta into the lungs (6). Vomition is not a typical sign in cyanide poisoning and, when it does occur, it may be the result of bloating in the recumbent animal and during the final convulsions. The course in these cases may be as long as 1 to 2 hours.

Clinical Pathology

The suspected plant material or ruminal contents may be tested for the presence of hydrocyanic acid (7, 8). The rumen sample, or shredded plant material, is placed in a test tube containing a little water and a few drops of chloroform and heated very gently in the presence of sodium picrate paper. A rapid change in the colour of the reagent paper from yellow to red indicates the presence of free hydrocyanic acid. Once started the colour change occurs rapidly although it may require 5 to 10 minutes of gentle warming before the change commences. The tube should be corked while being warmed and the paper hung from the top without touching the test material. Reagent papers are easily prepared by mixing 0·5 g. picric acid, 5·0 g. sodium carbonate in 100 ml. water. Filter paper is dipped in the reagent and allowed to dry in a dark place. The reagent is stable for at least 6 months if kept in a cool place but the papers deteriorate if kept for more than a week. Ruminal contents may also be tested by placing a drop of ruminal fluid on a test paper. A red discoloration is a positive reaction. The test is designed to detect free hydrocyanic acid and may not be positive even when cyanides are present if the gas is not liberated. Samples of suspected plant material sent to a laboratory for analysis should be immersed in a 1 to 3 per cent solution of mercuric chloride.

Necropsy Findings

In very acute cases the blood may be bright red in colour but in most field cases it is dark red due to anoxaemia. The blood clots slowly, the musculature is dark and there is congestion and haemorrhage in the trachea and lungs. Patchy congestion and petechiation may be evident in the abomasum and small intestines. Subepicardial and subendocardial haemorrhages occur constantly. A smell of 'bitter almonds' in the rumen is described as typical of hydrocyanic acid poisoning. It may occur with some plants but is not apparent with others. Specimens submitted for laboratory examination should include rumen contents, liver and muscle. Much hydrocyanic acid may be lost from specimens during transit and they should be immersed in a 1 to 3 per cent solution of mercuric chloride or despatched in a very tightly stoppered bottle. Muscle is least likely to lose its hydrocyanic acid and is the preferred tissue if the delay between death and necropsy has been long. To be satisfactory liver samples must be taken within 4 hours of death and muscle tissue within 20 hours. A level of hydrocyanic acid of 0·63 μg. per ml. in muscle justifies a diagnosis of poisoning (8).

Diagnosis

The development of an acute anoxic syndrome in ruminants pasturing on plants, or being fed on feeds, known to be cyanogenetic usually suggests the occurrence of hydrocyanic acid poisoning. Acute pulmonary oedema and emphysema may resemble it clinically but it is less acute and auscultation of the lungs usually indicates the presence of fluid and emphysema. Nitrite poisoning produces an almost identical syndrome but the blood is dark and tends to be coffee coloured. A similar syndrome may also occur in poisoning by algae. Occasional cases of anaphylaxis in cattle, particularly young calves, are manifested by acute dyspnoea but there are usually additional signs of an allergic reaction including bloat and sometimes urticaria or angioneurotic oedema, and, if the case is sufficiently severe, there is a profuse discharge of blood-stained froth from the nose. Cases occur only sporadically whereas hydrocyanic acid poisoning is likely to affect a number of animals at one time.

Treatment

A mixture of sodium nitrite and sodium thiosulphate is injected intravenously. The dose rates are 3 g. of sodium nitrite and 15 g. sodium thiosulphate in 200 ml. water for cattle; for sheep 1 g. sodium nitrite and 2·5 g. sodium thiosulphate in 50 ml. Treatment may have to be repeated because of further liberation of hydrocyanic acid. The sodium nitrite produces methaemoglobin which combines with the hydrocyanic acid to produce cyanmethaemoglobin which is not toxic. The acid is released gradually from this compound and is taken up by the thiosulphate to form thiocyanate which is also non-toxic and which is readily excreted. There is an upper limit of safe methaemoglobinaemia beyond which anaemic anoxia occurs and doses of nitrite greater than those recommended may exacerbate the tissue anoxia.

Alternative treatments include the use of sodium nitrite or sodium thiosulphate alone though neither is as effective as the combination of the two. The dose rate of sodium nitrite alone is the same as above but with sodium thiosulphate the amount is usually doubled. In all cases sodium thiosulphate should be given orally or intraruminally to fix the free hydrocyanic acid in the rumen. Doses of 30 g. are used in cattle and are repeated at hourly intervals. Animals that have been exposed showing no clinical signs may be treated similarly. Methylene blue also causes methaemoglobinaemia and is used in cattle for the treatment of hydrocyanic acid poisoning but is much less effective than sodium nitrite.

Non-specific treatment including respiratory stimulants and artificial respiration are unlikely to have any effect on the course of the disease.

Control

Hungry cattle and sheep should not be allowed access to toxic plants, especially cultivated *Sorghum* spp. when they are immature, wilted, frost bitten or growing rapidly after a stage of retarded growth. Plants of the sorghum family should be in flower before they are grazed or chopped to be fed green. If there is doubt as to the toxicity of a field of these plants a sample may be tested by the method described under clinical pathology. Linseed meal should be fed in small quantities without soaking and gruel containing linseed should be thoroughly boiled to drive off any free hydrocyanic acid.

REFERENCES

(1) Sharman, J. R. (1967). *N.Z. vet. J.*, *15*, 19.
(2) Seifert, H. S. H. & Beller, K. A. (1969). *Berl. Münch. tierärztl. Wschr.*, *82*, 88.
(3) Coop, I. E. & Blakeley, R. L. (1950). *N.Z. J. Sci. Tech.* (A), *31*, 44.
(4) Franklin, M. C. & Reid, R. L. (1944). *Aust. vet. J.*, *20*, 328, 332.
(5) Smith, A. D. M. *et al.* (1963). *Nature (Lond.)*, *200*, 179.
(6) Blood, D. C. & Steel, J. D. (1944). *Aust. vet. J.*, *20*, 338.
(7) Bergsten, M. L. (1964). *Vet. Med.*, *59*, 720.
(8) Terblanche, M. *et al.* (1964). *J. S. Afr. vet. med. Ass.*, *35*, 503, 199.

Nitrate and Nitrite Poisoning

Nitrates and nitrites are closely linked as causes of poisoning. Nitrates may cause gastroenteritis when ingested in large quantities but their chief importance is as a source of nitrite which may be formed before or after ingestion of the nitrate. The nitrites cause a syndrome of respiratory distress because of the formation of methaemoglobin which results in anaemic anoxia.

Incidence

Nitrate and nitrite poisoning are being diagnosed with increasing frequency as heavy fertilization with nitrogenous compounds becomes more widespread. While there is no doubt that the dangers have increased it is also evident that 'nitrate poisoning' is enjoying a vogue and that many cases so reported, particularly of chronic toxicity, rest on inadequate evidence.

Aetiology

The toxic principle as it occurs in growing plants is always nitrate, usually as potassium nitrate, and may be ingested as such in sufficient quantities to cause gastroenteritis. The nitrate may be reduced to nitrite in the plant before ingestion. This occurs in oaten hay in the stack, particularly if it is wet and hot, or if the hay is damp for some time before feeding. The gentle cooking of mangels may also convert nitrate to nitrite and cause poisoning of pigs. There is considerable variation between species in their susceptibility to nitrite poisoning, pigs being most susceptible followed by cattle, sheep and horses in that order. The susceptibility of cattle relative to sheep is due either to their ability to convert nitrate to nitrite in the rumen or because of the known greater ability of sheep to convert nitrite to ammonia. Pigs are highly susceptible to nitrite poisoning but are affected only if they ingest it preformed.

Cases that occur in sheep are caused either by the ingestion of preformed nitrite or by ruminal conditions which favour reduction of nitrate. A diet rich in readily fermentable carbohydrate reduces nitrite production in the rumen of the sheep. Also nitrite poisoning occurs in sheep fed an inadequate ration after dosing with nitrite at a level which is innocuous to sheep fed on a good ration. The degree of methaemoglobinaemia also varies with the quality of the diet.

The common sources of nitrate for farm animals include cereal crops, certain specific plants and water from deep wells. Oat hay may contain 3 to 7 per cent nitrate. Immature green oats, barley, wheat and rye hay, and Sudan grass, corn or sorghum fodder may contain toxic amounts. Freshly pulled mangels may also contain high concentrations. Turnip tops may contain 8 per cent nitrate, and sugar beet tops and rape have caused nitrite poisoning. Of the specific plants variegated thistle (*Silybum marianum*), redroot (*Amaranthus reflexus*) and mintweed (*Salvia reflexa*) are well known as causes of nitrite poisoning and these plants have caused heavy losses in cattle (1). Outbreaks of nitrite poisoning have occurred in sheep grazing heavy swards of capeweed (*Arctotheca calendula*) a normally safe plant, after a prolonged drought (2). In such circumstances some normally safe plants with a capacity for fast growth may become dangerous. It is presumed that high levels of nitrate accumulate in the soil during the drought and are absorbed in large amounts when the drought ends. Plants that accumulate more than 1·5 per cent by dry matter of nitrate are potentially toxic (3). Deep wells filled by seepage from highly fertile soils may contain levels as high as 1700 to 3000 ppm of nitrate and water of condensation in barns may trap ammonia and eventually contain 8000 to 10,000 ppm of nitrate (4).

Toxic doses are hard to compute because of variation in susceptibility, and in production of nitrite from nitrate. The lethal dose of sodium nitrite for pigs is 88 mg per kg. body weight.

Doses of 48 to 77 mg. per kg. cause moderate to severe but not fatal methaemoglobinaemia. Potassium nitrate in doses of 4 to 7 g. per kg. body weight causes fatal gastritis in pigs and the lethal dose of potassium nitrite is about 20 mg. per kg. (5). Measured as nitrate nitrogen the LD_{50} for pigs is 19 to 21 mg. per kg. body weight (6). At dose levels of 12 to 19 mg. clinical signs occur but the pigs recover (7). In cattle the minimum lethal dose of nitrite is 88 to 110 mg. per kg. body weight or about 0·6 g. of potassium nitrate per kg. body weight. Daily doses of about 0·15 g. potassium nitrate have caused abortion in cattle after 3 to 13 doses but continued low-level dosing does not appear to affect sheep (8). Drinking water containing 1000 ppm of nitrate nitrogen causes appreciable methaemoglobin formation in sheep but has no obvious clinical effect (9). Plants to be safe for feeding should contain less than 1·5 per cent potassium nitrate on a dry matter basis. Cattle can eat sufficient quantities of toxic plants to cause death in one hour.

Occurrence

Cereals and root crops are likely to contain high concentrations when heavily fertilized with nitrogenous manures and when growth is rapid during hot, humid weather. Ensiled material usually contains less nitrate than the fresh crop but juices draining from silos containing high-nitrate materials may be toxic. Heavily fertilized grass made into grass cubes may contain as much as 0·71 per cent nitrate (DM) and cause nitrite poisoning (10). Corn stalks in fields previously damaged by drought may be dangerous. Cereal hay, especially oat hay, grown under these conditions and cut when sappy may develop a high concentration of nitrite when the stacked material develops some heat. Dry oat hay which is damp for some time before it is eaten is also likely to contain a high concentration of nitrite. The nitrite is present chiefly in the leafy part of the hay. Weeds and sugar beet tops may contain toxic quantities of nitrate after spraying with the herbicide 2,4-D because of changes produced in the metabolism of the plants. Pigs are most likely to be poisoned when fed on cooked mangels which have not been thoroughly boiled, on whey to which potassium nitrate has been added in the cheese-making process, or on swill containing salt-brine from butchers' shops, or made with well water containing a high concentration of nitrate. Water containing 2300 ppm of nitrate and less than 10 ppm of nitrite when mixed into a swill, stored in tins and then cooked has resulted in the production of a mixture containing 1200 to 1400 ppm of nitrite (11).

Well waters containing 200 to 500 ppm of potassium nitrate equivalent may also cause poisoning in cattle and sheep, the nitrate being reduced to nitrite in the rumen.

Accidental poisoning with nitrates occurs sporadically when sodium or potassium nitrate is used in mistake for sodium chloride or magnesium sulphate. Poorly fed animals are more susceptible to nitrite poisoning than those on good diets and this probably influences the susceptibility of introduced and travelling cattle to this form of poisoning, although lack of acquaintance with the plants, and possibly adaptation, may also affect their susceptibility. Prior exposure to nitrate reduces susceptibility under experimental conditions but the practical significance of the observation is uncertain (12, 13). The most important factor influencing susceptibility appears to be the rate of ingestion of the nitrate-bearing plant (14).

Pathogenesis

Nitrates have a direct caustic action on alimentary mucosa and the ingestion of sufficiently large quantities causes gastroenteritis. Absorption of nitrites causes methaemoglobinaemia and the development of an anaemic anoxia. Nitrites are also vasodilators which may contribute to the development of tissue anoxia by causing peripheral circulatory failure, but this effect appears to be of little significance compared to that of methaemoglobin formation. When nitrite is ingested preformed the effects may be very rapid but when conversion of nitrate to nitrite occurs in the rumen there is a delay of some hours before clinical illness occurs. In cattle the maximum methaemoglobinaemia occurs about 5 hours after ingestion of nitrate. In pigs it is 90 to 150 minutes (6).

Death does not occur until a certain level of methaemoglobinaemia is attained. In farm animals lethal levels in cattle are about 9 g. methaemoglobin per 100 ml. blood (10); in pigs when 76 to 88 per cent of haemoglobin has been altered to methaemoglobin deaths occur (6).

In cattle abortion and a greatly increased requirement of vitamin A have been believed to result from the long-term ingestion of nitrite. Both have been discredited (15, 16, 17, 18) and prolonged ingestion of sublethal amounts of nitrite is not known to have any significant effect on productivity (7).

Clinical Findings

In animals poisoned by nitrate there is salivation, abdominal pain, diarrhoea and vomiting even in ruminants. The more typical syndrome is that caused by the anoxia of nitrite poisoning. Dyspnoea, with a gasping, rapid respiration is the predominant sign. Muscle tremor, weakness, staggering gait, severe cyanosis followed by blanching of the mucosae, a rapid, small, weak pulse, and a normal or subnormal temperature are other typical signs. The affected animals go down and there are terminal clonic convulsions. Death usually occurs within 12 to 24 hours of ingestion of the toxic plant, although in acute poisoning the duration of illness may be even shorter and clinical signs may not be observed.

In one report acute cardiac and circulatory failure without other observed clinical signs was much the most common syndrome in cattle (19).

Clinical Pathology

Methaemoglobinaemia may be detected by examination of the blood in a reversion spectrometer but it is not diagnostic of nitrite poisoning and results are not dependable unless the blood has been collected for less than an hour or two. An alternative method is the diphenylamine blue test (8) which is very sensitive to the presence of nitrite but not entirely specific. A satisfactory test can be conducted on a thick air-dried blood smear. Laboratory tests are available for the rough estimation of the nitrite or nitrate content of fodder but they are not sufficiently simple for field use nor accurate enough for critical assay. A modified diphenylamine reagent provides a qualitative test suitable for field use (20). The diphenylamine test does have disadvantages and can give inaccurate results. To avoid these errors it is recommended that the blood be diluted with phosphate buffer (1 part in 20). It is also worthwhile submitting a sample of urine as nitrite appears to pass unchanged into the urine (21).

Necropsy Findings

In nitrate poisoning there is gastroenteritis. In nitrite poisoning the blood is dark red to coffee brown in colour and clots poorly. Petechial haemorrhages may be present in the heart muscle and trachea and there is general vascular congestion and a variable degree of congestion in the rumen and abomasum. Specimens for laboratory examination should include blood for methaemoglobin estimation, ingesta and suspected plants or water, with added chloroform or formalin to prevent conversion of nitrates by bacterial fermentation. Post mortem specimens must be collected within 1 to 2 hours of death to be of any value.

Diagnosis

The acute dyspnoea, short course and nervous signs of tremor and convulsions resemble the signs of hydrocyanic acid poisoning but in acute cases the blood is dark red to brown in colour in contradistinction to the bright red colour of the blood in the latter poisoning. Caution should be exercised in interpreting this sign as a dark red appearance of the blood occurs commonly in the later stages of both poisonings. The source of the toxic material is also different. Analysis of tissues, ingesta and suspected material may be necessary to confirm the diagnosis, although the rapid response to treatment with methylene blue is a good criterion for field use. Acute pulmonary oedema and emphysema and anaphylaxis must also be considered in the differential diagnosis.

Treatment

Methylene blue is the specific treatment. The standard dose rate is 1 to 2 mg. per kg. body weight, injected intravenously as a 1 per cent solution. Treatment may have to be repeated when large amounts of toxic material have been ingested. Methylene blue in large amounts causes methaemoglobinaemia, hence its use in cyanide poisoning, but in small amounts causes rapid reconversion of methaemoglobin to haemoglobin.

Control

Ruminants likely to be exposed to nitrites or nitrates should receive adequate carbohydrate in their diet and travelling or hungry animals should not be allowed access to dangerous plants. Poisonous well water can be made safe by boiling. Haylage or silage suspected of dangerous levels of nitrate should be allowed to aerate overnight before feeding. If feed known to contain toxic quantities of nitrate has to be fed supplementation of the diet of sheep and cattle with chlortetracycline (22 mg. per kg. of feed) is partially effective for a period of about 2 weeks in suppressing the reduction of nitrate to nitrite (22).

REFERENCES

(1) Kendrick, J. W. *et al.* (1955). *J. Amer. vet. med. Ass., 126*, 53.
(2) Fairnie, I. J. (1969). *Aust. vet. J., 45*, 78.
(3) Harris, D. J. & Rhodes, H. A. (1969). *Aust. vet. J., 45*, 591.
(4) Andersen, H. K. (1962). *Nord. Vet.-Med., 14*, 16.
(5) London, W. T. *et al.* (1967). *J. Amer. vet. med. Ass., 150*, 398.
(6) Curtin, R. M. & London, W. T. (1967). *70th ann. gen. Mtg U.S. Live Stock sanit. Ass., Buffalo*, 339.
(7) London, W. T. *et al.* (1967). *J. Amer. vet. med. Ass., 150*, 398.
(8) Setchell, B. P. & Williams, A. J. (1962). *Aust. vet. J., 38*, 58.

(9) Seerley, R. et al. (1965). J. Anim. Sci., 24, 1014.
(10) Purcell, D. A. et al. (1971). Res. vet. Sci., 12, 598.
(11) Winks, W. R. et al. (1950). Qld J. agric. Sci., 7, 1.
(12) Diven, R. H. et al. (1964). Ann. N.Y. Acad. Sci., 111, 638.
(13) Sinclair, B. K. & Jones, D. I. H. (1964). J. Sci. Fd Agric., 15, 717.
(14) Crawford, R. F. et al. (1966). Cornell Vet., 56, 3.
(15) Sinclair, B. K. & Jones, D. I. H. (1964). Brit. vet. J., 120, 78.
(16) Winter, A. J. & Hokanson, J. F. (1964). Amer. J. vet. Res., 25, 353.
(17) Davidson, K. L. et al. (1964). J. Dairy Sci., 47, 1065.
(18) Dodd, D. C. (1967). 70th ann. gen. Mtg U.S. Live Stock sanit. Ass., Buffalo, 581.
(19) Johanssen, U. & Kuhnert, M. (1969). Arch. exp. vet. Med., 23, 375.
(20) Householder, G. T. et al. (1966). J. Amer. vet. med. Ass., 148, 662.
(21) Watts, H. et al. (1969). Aust. vet. J., 45, 492.
(22) Emerick, R. J. & Embry, L. B. (1961). J. Anim. Sci., 20, 844.

Oxalate Poisoning

The ingestion of excess oxalate causes some gastrointestinal irritation but the major effect is that of precipitation of blood calcium and the production of a hypocalcaemic syndrome of muscular weakness and paralysis. Continued ingestion of small amounts of oxalate may lead to renal damage or to the development of urinary calculi.

Incidence

Plants containing oxalates in dangerous quantities grow principally in specific areas. Heavy mortalities may occur in groups of animals which are not accustomed to grazing the toxic pasture.

Aetiology

Plants usually contain oxalate in the form of the potassium salt, and this is much less toxic than if it is given experimentally as the pure salt (1). High concentrations are present in Halogeton (*Halogeton glomeratus*), pigweed (*Amaranthus retroflexus*), fat hen (*Chenopodium album*), soursob (*Oxalis cernua*), greasewood (*Sarcobatus vermiculatus*), dock and orchard sorrell (*Rumex acetosella*), *Portulacca oleracea, Salsola Bali, Trianthema portulacastrum* and *Threlkeldia proceriflora*, and in the leaves of cultivated rhubarb, mangels and sugar beet, especially when the plants are in the green leafy stage. Young fresh plants may contain as much as 17 per cent potassium oxalate whilst old, dry plants rarely contain more than 1 per cent (2). On the other hand *Halogeton*, probably the most important of the above plants, becomes more toxic as the growing season advances and is most dangerous when frosted and dried. Grasses rarely contain significant amounts of oxalate but *Setaria sphacelata* has been shown to contain up to 7 per cent oxalate and cause poisoning in cattle (3). The oxalate is in the unusual form of ammonium oxalate and this may explain the toxicity which occurs at moderate levels of oxalate (4).

Large quantities of a toxic plant must be ingested to cause poisoning because not all the oxalate is absorbed and much is broken down in the alimentary tract. Up to 450 g. of sodium oxalate given by mouth is required to produce fatal effects in horses, and 6 g. of anhydrous oxalic acid per day is required to produce toxic effects in sheep. Cattle can eat as much as 685 g. of oxalic acid without harmful effect (2). Nephrosclerosis has been recorded in the horse as being due to chronic oxalate poisoning (5). Some fungi are capable of producing significant amounts of oxalate and their presence on mouldy feedstuffs may contribute to the occurrence of poisoning (5, 6).

Oxalate is normally metabolized in the rumen and the continued ingestion of oxalate in small quantities by sheep results in increased ability to decompose the oxalate to the point where relatively large quantities (up to 75 g. daily by sheep) can be ingested without toxic effects. This may explain the relative susceptibility of sheep and cattle when they are grazed for the first time on pasture containing the toxic plants, although it seems likely that other factors in the rumen will also affect the amount of oxalate rendered insoluble as calcium oxalate or digested to bicarbonate. Of these the level of calcium in the diet and the activities of bacteria in the rumen are considered to be important.

Occurrence

The disease occurs principally in sheep which are more likely to be grazed on the kind of pasture in which the toxic plants commonly occur. Pasture is at its most dangerous stage when there is a rapid growth of lush plants in a warm autumn after a dry summer. Travelling and recently introduced animals are more likely to be affected than indigenous animals and as a group pregnant and lactating animals are probably more susceptible than others. Clinical signs may appear within 2 to 4 hours of eating an oxalate containing plant. There is an increased susceptibility if the animals are hungry and consume large amounts of the plants. Salt hunger has been suggested as a predisposing factor in the aetiology of oxalate poisoning.

Cattle fed large amounts of *Oxalis cernua* containing high concentrations of oxalates, 85 per cent of it water-soluble, have been able to metabolize it without harmful effect. Calves drinking the milk from these cows exclusively are reputed to develop diarrhoea (2). However, oxalate poisoning and death have been observed in cattle eating *Setaria sphacelata*, a pasture grass grown in tropical areas (3).

Pathogenesis

Broadly speaking, three syndromes occur, depending on the amount of oxalate ingested. With large quantities the major effect is the absorption of free oxalate and precipitation of blood calcium as calcium oxalate to produce a hypocalcaemia. Immobilization of calcium in the alimentary tract may contribute significantly in the development of this hypocalcaemia. The resulting syndrome in sheep is indistinguishable from that caused by hypocalcaemia at parturition or on starving.

Continuous ingestion of soluble oxalates causes nephrosis due to precipitation of oxalate crystals in the lumen of the renal tubules. Up to 25 per cent of sheep may be affected in some flocks. Such damage is likely to be cumulative if the sheep are periodically exposed to oxalate-bearing plants (7). At intermediate levels of oxalate intake there is marked damage to vascular tissues especially in alimentary tract and lungs (4). Invasion of the chemical rumenitis that results may lead to an irreversible fungal or bacterial rumenitis or hepatitis.

Continued low level dosing in sheep may cause ruminal dysfunction due to changes in pH of its contents and interference with cellulose digestion (8). The importance of oxalate ingestion over long periods in the production of urinary calculi is discussed elsewhere.

Clinical Findings

In acute poisoning the clinical signs include paresis, muscle tremor, staggering and final recumbency and death in coma (9). The heart rate is rapid, ruminal movements are decreased, and the pupils dilated. There may be slight bloating, frequent getting up and lying down, eventual recumbency, frequent attempts to urinate, frothy blood-tinged nasal discharge and occasionally red-brown urine (10).

Clinical Pathology

Suspected plants should be assayed for oxalate content. Estimation of the level of calcium in serum is of debatable value as the levels of total calcium may be normal, the clinical illness being caused by depression of the ionizable fraction of the calcium. Albuminuria and sometimes haematuria may be observed.

Necropsy Findings

There are no gross findings at necropsy which are characteristic of oxalate poisoning although there may be deposition of crystals in the renal tubules and pelvis and even in the ureters and urethra. In experimental poisoning in the horse and sheep severe gastroenteritis and dehydration have been observed. Vesicular inflammation and necrosis of the epithelium of the oesophagus and rumeno-reticulum occurs in cattle poisoned by ammonium oxalate in the grass, *Setaria sphacelata* (3, 4).

Diagnosis

The hypocalcaemic syndrome is characteristic and oxalate poisoning must be differentiated from parturient paresis, hypocalcaemia due to starvation or forced exercise, and lactation tetany. Environmental conditions and the presence of known toxic plants give some indication of the cause. Acute indigestion due to overeating on grain may cause a similar syndrome but a history of free access to grain or concentrate is usually available in such cases.

Treatment

The parenteral injection of solutions of calcium salts is a specific treatment. Calcium borogluconate as a 25 per cent solution given intravenously or subcutaneously in doses of 300 to 500 ml. in cattle and 50 to 100 ml. in sheep usually effects recovery. Ancillary treatment should include the provision of ample fluids to decrease precipitation of oxalate crystals in the urinary tract.

Control

Hungry sheep and cattle should not be allowed to feed on large quantities of the toxic plants. The water intake of sheep also affects the oxalate intake. Halogeton poisoning is more likely to occur when sheep are watered and then allowed to graze (11). Prophylactic feeding of dicalcium phosphate is effective, other calcium salts and bone meal being ineffective and adequate salt should be made available.

REFERENCES

(1) James, L. F. *et al.* (1968). *J. Anim. Sci.*, *27*, 718.
(2) Lai, P. & Cosseddu, A. M. (1967). *Arch. vet. ital.*, *18*, 171.
(3) Seawright, A. A. *et al.* (1970). *Aust. vet. J.*, *46*, 293.
(4) James, M. P. *et al.* (1971). *Aust. vet. J.*, *47*, 9.
(5) Andrews, E. J. (1971). *J. Amer. vet. med. Ass.*, *159*, 49.
(6) Wilson, B. J. & Wilson, C. H. (1961). *Amer. J. vet. Res.*, *22*, 961.
(7) Gardiner, M. R. & Royce, R. D. (1963). *J. Agric. W. Aust.*, *4*, 153.
(8) James, L. F. *et al.* (1967). *J. Anim. Sci.*, *26*, 1438.
(9) James, L. F. (1970). *J. Amer. vet. med. Ass.*, *156*, 1310.

(10) Shupe, J. L. & James, L. F. (1969). *Cornell Vet.*, *59*, 41.
(11) James, L. F. *et al.* (1970). *J. Range Mgmt*, *23*, 123.

Strychnine Poisoning

Strychnine poisoning is an uncommon occurrence in farm animals and is usually caused by accidental overdosing with strychnine preparations. Cattle are particularly susceptible to parenteral administration (30 to 60 mg. of strychnine hydrochloride may be fatal) but less susceptible to oral administration because of destruction of the drug in the rumen. Lethal doses by parenteral injection are 200 to 250 mg. in horses, 30 to 400 mg. in cattle and 15 to 50 mg. in pigs.

In strychnine poisoning there is greatly increased reflex excitability and, after an initial period of muscle stiffness and tremor, tetanic convulsions occur. These can be provoked by the application of minor external stimuli. In these convulsive episodes there is extension of the limbs, opisthotonus and protrusion of the eyeballs. Respiratory arrest may lead to death from respiratory paralysis. The seizures may last for 3 to 4 minutes and are followed by periods of partial relaxation which become progressively shorter as the disease develops.

Strychnine is rapidly excreted and detoxicated and sedation of the animal with barbiturate anaesthetics or chloral hydrate for a sufficiently long period may result in recovery. Tannic acid preparations administered orally precipitate the alkaloid in the alimentary tract and interfere with further absorption.

DISEASES CAUSED BY FARM CHEMICALS

With the increasing application of a great variety of chemicals to agricultural undertakings the subject of poisoning caused by farm chemicals has grown very rapidly in recent years and has been the basis of a complete new literature. It is not possible to review all the known toxic compounds in a few pages and only the more common substances are dealt with here. The reader is referred to the more exhaustive treatises below for more detailed descriptions.

REVIEW LITERATURE

O'Brien, J. J. (1970). Toxicological aspects of some modern anthelminthics. *Aust. vet. J.*, *46*, 297.
Palmer, J. & Radeleff, R. D. (1964). *Ann. N.Y. Acad. Sci.*, *111*, 729.
Radeleff, R. D. (1964). *Veterinary Toxicology*. Philadelphia: Lea & Febiger.
Scott, W. N. (1964). *Vet. Rec.*, *76*, 964.

Anthelminthics

Carbon Tetrachloride Poisoning

The ingestion of toxic amounts of carbon tetrachloride causes acute toxipathic hepatitis and death from liver insufficiency. The inhalation or ingestion of a gross overdose of carbon tetrachloride causes acute anaesthetic depression of the central nervous system.

Incidence

The mass dosing of sheep with standard doses of carbon tetrachloride as an anthelminthic may occasionally cause severe death losses. In individual outbreaks up to 25 per cent of the sheep dosed may die and many others may be seriously affected.

Aetiology

Carbon tetrachloride is used commonly for the treatment of fascioliasis in sheep. A standard dose of 2 ml. is used and in most instances produces no toxic effects but in certain circumstances this dose is highly toxic. There are probably a number of metabolic states which make animals more susceptible to poisoning. One of these is known to be a high rumenal level of ammonia which occurs after the ingestion of a high protein diet (1). Plant poisoning, e.g. with stinkwort (*Inula graveolens*) (2), with heliotrope (*Heliotropum europaeum*) (3) and with sorrel (*Rumex acetosa*) and soursob (*Oxalis* spp.) which are rich in oxalate (4) also predisposes to poisoning with carbon tetrachloride in sheep. Prolonged moderate dosing with selenium does too, but small doses of selenium near the time of administration of carbon tetrachloride reduces this susceptibility (5). Cold stress in shorn sheep also appreciably increases susceptibility (7). Hypocalcaemia or a calcium deficiency have been suggested but these, with the exception of oxalate poisoning, have not been satisfactorily shown to be predisposing causes. Protection against the toxic effects of carbon tetrachloride by nicotinic acid and tryptophane has been observed in rats and sheep.

The method of administration, into the rumen or the abomasum or by intramuscular injection, appears to have no effect on blood levels of carbon tetrachloride, nor does fasting for 48 hours or administration of the compound neat or in mineral oil, although peak levels are reached at different times with each route of administration.

Cattle are more susceptible than sheep at all times and for this reason hexachloroethane and tetrachlorethylene are commonly used for the treatment of fascioliasis in this species. Chronic carbon tetrachloride poisoning is an industrial hazard in man but in normal circumstances repeated dosing in sheep at the rate of 1 to 3 ml. at monthly intervals produces no ill effects.

Occurrence

Accidental administration of the drug into the respiratory tract, or the oral administration of a massive dose, causes immediate collapse. Failure of the animal to swallow a normal dose because of faulty placement of the dose, may have the same effect. The occurrence of outbreaks of hepatic necrosis in sheep due to dosing with standard dose rates is recorded when sheep are kept overlong without food at drenching time. This is particularly likely to happen when drenching is combined with other operations. Outbreaks also occur during inclement weather when the sheep are not grazing, when they are put out into new pastures immediately after drenching, and when pastures are lush or growing rapidly. Lactating ewes may also be more susceptible than dry sheep.

Pathogenesis

Inhalation of carbon tetrachloride causes immediate and acute depression of the central nervous system and peripheral and central circulatory collapse. Sheep which survive show marked pulmonary, as well as hepatic and renal damage (7). Ingestion of toxic doses has a delayed effect after 3 to 4 days. The major effect is on the liver where acute hepatitis develops caused probably by severe restriction of the intralobular circulation which produces a typical centrilobular necrosis. Extensive damage to the renal tubules may also occur and appears to be the critical lesion in sheep (8). The rapidity with which liver regeneration occurs in surviving animals after an attack of carbon tetrachloride poisoning makes chronic poisoning unlikely.

Clinical Findings

With gross overdosing or after inhalation there is an immediate onset of staggering, falling, progressive narcosis, collapse, convulsions, and death due to respiratory failure. Animals that survive this stage or, as in the most common form of carbon tetrachloride poisoning in which animals absorb insufficient to produce narcosis, additional signs may be manifested in 3 to 4 days. These comprise anorexia, depression, muscle weakness, diarrhoea and jaundice. After a further 2 or 3 days affected sheep go down and mild to moderate clonic convulsions may occur, but death is always preceded by a period of coma. Those that survive

are emaciated and weak, and are prone to develop photosensitization or shed their wool. They are very susceptible to environmental stresses, particularly inclement weather, and isolated deaths may occur for several months.

Clinical Pathology

In the first 3 days after dosing liver dysfunction is suggested by a pronounced elevation of SGOT levels and renal dysfunction by an elevation of blood urea levels. After four days from dosing the SGOT levels return to normal but blood urea levels remain high (9).

Necropsy Findings

Animals dying after inhalation of the drug show marked pulmonary, hepatic and renal damage. Those dying of massive oral overdosing may show abomasitis and inflammation of the duodenum in addition to the hepatic and renal lesions observed in animals which die after the ingestion of small doses. In the latter animals there is acute hepatitis with swelling, pallor and mottling of the liver. The lobules are more obvious than usual and histologically there is centrilobular necrosis in animals which die within 3 days of dosing and fatty degeneration in sheep dying more than 4 days afterwards (10). The renal lesions comprise extensive degeneration and necrosis of the tubular epithelium on histological examination. Animals that die weeks or months later show hepatic fibrosis and nodular regeneration of the liver, often confined to the right lobe with the left lobe of the liver completely destroyed and replaced by a small tag of fibrous tissue.

Diagnosis

The history of deaths commencing in sheep 3 to 4 days after drenching with carbon tetrachloride usually suggests the diagnosis. When poisoning from inhalation is suspected pulmonary lesions should be sought. Acute hepatitis affecting a number of sheep may occur in animals grazing on perennial rye-grass or following access to some poison plants including ragwort, Crotalaria spp., and heliotrope.

Treatment

In inhalation poisoning, artificial respiration and respiratory centre stimulants are indicated. There is no specific treatment for the hepatitis but supportive treatment should include the parenteral administration of calcium solutions and the provision of readily digestible carbohydrate. In valuable and seriously affected animals the latter are probably best provided by the repeated parenteral injection of glucose and protein hydrolysate solutions.

Control

The general recommendations for the prevention of toxicity after standard doses of carbon tetrachloride include the provision of a diet high in calcium and readily digestible carbohydrate prior to drenching, avoidance of starvation at drenching time and of drenching shorn sheep in cold, wet weather. A diet rich in protein is to be particularly avoided. Treated sheep should not be placed on new pastures, especially if they are lush or growing rapidly. The prophylactic effect of vitamin B_{12} in laboratory animals suggests that an adequate intake of cobalt should be ensured. If there is any suspicion that an outbreak of poisoning may occur a small group of sheep should be dosed as a pilot test. The drenching method used must ensure that the administered dose is swallowed immediately; the dose should be deposited into the pharynx but not against the back of it (11).

REFERENCES

(1) Kondos, A. C. & McClymont, G. L. (1965). *Aust. vet. J.*, *41*, 349.
(2) Setchell, B. P. *et al.* (1964). *Aust. vet. J.*, *40*, 30.
(3) Hunt, E. R. (1972). *Aust. vet. J.*, *48*, 57.
(4) Setchell, B. P. (1962). *Aust. vet. J.*, *38*, 487.
(5) Kondos, A. C. & McClymont, G. L. (1967). *Aust. J. agric. Res.*, *18*, 667.
(6) Kondos, A. C. & McClymont, G. L. (1966). *Aust. J. agric. Res.*, *17*, 363.
(7) Gallagher, C. H. (1964). *Aust. vet. J.*, *40*, 229.
(8) Setchell, B. P. (1961). *Aust. J. agric. Res.*, *12*, 944.
(9) Setchell, B. P. (1962). *Aust. vet. J.*, *38*, 580.
(10) Gallagher, C. H. (1963). *Aust. vet. J.*, *39*, 49.
(11) Gallagher, C. H. (1962). *Aust. vet. J.*, *38*, 575.

Phenothiazine Poisoning

Several modes of poisoning are recorded after the use of phenothiazine in animals and the more common ones are set out below. There are many more recorded occurrences of phenothiazine poisoning in animals but they are not generally well defined and are open to criticism in that other specific causes of illness were not satisfactorily eliminated. So little phenothiazine is used currently that what follows begins to assume an historical complexion.

PHOTOSENSITIZATION KERATITIS

This condition has been recorded most commonly in calves and to a less extent in pigs, goats and possibly in sheep. Phenothiazine sulphoxide is produced in the alimentary tract but is normally detoxicated in the liver. At high dose rates detoxication is not sufficiently rapid to prevent accumulation of the sulphoxide in the aqueous and the development of light sensitization of the cornea. Other photosensitizing substances do not usually reach the aqueous humour from the blood stream and corneal photosensitization is characteristic of phenothiazine poisoning. With standard doses toxicity probably arises because of hepatic insufficiency and the resulting interference with detoxication. Sheep are not commonly affected because of their greater efficiency in converting the sulphoxide to phenothiazine in the liver.

Outbreaks occur most commonly in poorly nourished calves less than 8 months old during the late summer. Individual calves or entire groups may be affected after treatment with standard dose rates of 10 to 15 g. Profuse lacrimation usually commences 12 to 36 hours after dosing and is followed by the development of a white opacity of the cornea lateral to the pupil. The lesion occurs on that part of the cornea which has maximum exposure to the sun's rays. There is marked blepharospasm and photophobia. Ulceration may occur in severe cases where shade is not available but most cases recover in a few days and residual opacity is rare. Affected animals should be kept indoors or in the shade for several days and an antiseptic eye ointment applied. Prior treatment with 500,000 units vitamin A orally is reported to prevent the occurrence of the condition (1).

HAEMOLYTIC ANAEMIA

Phenothiazine given in doses of more than 30 g. may provoke a severe haemolytic anaemia in horses, especially in those that are poorly nourished or suffering severely from a heavy parasitic infestation. Smaller doses (20 g.) of micronized phenothiazine may produce a similar effect (2, 3). One to 2 days after dosing there is depression, anorexia, pallor of the mucosae, jaundice, haemoglobinuria and in some cases abdominal pain. At necropsy, jaundice, anaemia and enlargement of the liver, kidneys and spleen are evident. Treatment should include blood transfusions and the provision of ample fluids, if necessary administered parenterally.

ABORTION

Abortion has been recorded in ewes dosed with phenothiazine during the last 3 weeks of pregnancy. Dosing of mares during pregnancy is not recommended.

PHENOTHIAZINE AND THE THYROID GLAND

The administration of commercial phenothiazine may reduce the uptake of iodine from natural sources by the thyroid gland. This was originally ascribed to a thyrotoxic effect of the substance but it has since been determined to be due to the presence of iodine in the commercial phenothiazine.

ATAXIA AND PARALYSIS

Phenothiazine is not commonly used as an anthelminthic in pigs because of the efficiency of a number of other drugs for this purpose. Occasional outbreaks of poisoning occur in this species due to overdosing or idiosyncrasy. The clinical signs include inco-ordination, circling, posterior paralysis, running movements, prostration and coma, but fatalities are rare. Corneal opacity may occur during the convalescent period.

Very young lambs are highly susceptible to phenothiazine poisoning, manifesting a syndrome of opisthotonus, nystagmus, circling and ataxia. The mortality rate is high.

RENAL PAPILLARY NECROSIS

In sheep deprived of water, or otherwise dehydrated, the administration of normal doses of phenothiazine can cause fatal necrosis of the papillae in the kidney. Similar lesions can be produced in cattle but only with above-normal doses (4).

REFERENCES

(1) Snyder, H. A. (1965). *Vet. Med.*, *60*, *166*.
(2) McSherry, B. J. *et al.* (1966). *Canad. vet. J.*, 7, 3.
(3) Baird, J. D. *et al.* (1970). *Aust. vet. J.*, *46*, 496.
(4) Salisbury, R. M. *et al.* (1969). *N.Z. vet. J.*, *17*, 187, 227.

Poisoning Caused by Miscellaneous Anthelminthics

TETRACHLORETHYLENE POISONING

Tetrachlorethylene rarely produces toxic effects in cattle or sheep. The signs are similar to those of carbon tetrachloride poisoning and in calves inco-ordination may be evident for an hour or two after dosing. Treatment is not usually necessary.

HEXACHLOROETHANE POISONING

Hexachloroethane is preferred to carbon tetrachloride for the treatment of fascioliasis in cattle but it is not completely without danger. Emaciated animals may show narcosis and recumbency after administration of the standard dose (15 g. per 6 months of age up to a maximum of 60 g.) and

such animals should be given half this dose on two occasions at 48-hour intervals.

Occasional animals show an idiosyncrasy to the drug, the reaction taking the form of ataxia, dullness, anorexia and sometimes abdominal pain, diarrhoea and dysentery. In severe cases the signs are identical with those of parturient paresis. Outbreaks of poisoning also occur in certain areas under certain dietary conditions and possibly when the liver damage caused by fluke infestation is severe. High protein diets, rape and kale are reported to predispose to toxicity. Parturient or heavily lactating cows may also show increased susceptibility. Animals that die show acute abomasitis and enteritis, with oedema of the abomasal mucosa, and hepatic centrilobular necrosis. Deaths are rare in cattle (1 in 20,000 treated), and in sheep (1 in 40,000) but non-fatal illness is not uncommon.

Hexachloroethane poisoning in sheep may occur at a dose level of 0·4 g. per kg. body weight and the clinical signs include narcosis, staggering and falling. There is muscle tremor, a weak pulse and shallow respiration. In cattle and sheep there is a rapid response to treatment with calcium borogluconate as used in parturient paresis.

HEXACHLOROPHENE

At high dose rates (25 to 50 mg. per kg. body weight) hexachlorophene causes atrophy of seminiferous epithelium of the testis of the young adult ram (1). Repeated dosing causes periportal fatty changes in liver.

NICOTINE POISONING

Nicotine poisoning seldom occurs in animals except in lambs and calves where nicotine sulphate is still incorporated in some vermifuges. Doses of 0·2 to 0·3 g. nicotine sulphate have been toxic for lambs weighing 14 to 20 kg. Animals in poor condition are more susceptible than well nourished animals. Animals are affected within a few minutes of dosing and show dyspnoea with rapid shallow respirations, muscle tremor and weakness, recumbency and clonic convulsions. Death is due to respiratory failure. At necropsy there may be abomasitis and inflammation of the duodenum, and animals that survive the depression of the respiratory centre may show abdominal pain, salivation and diarrhoea.

Treatment should include artificial respiration and the administration of respiratory centre stimulants. Oral dosing with tannic acid preparations will precipitate the alkaloid and retard further absorption.

TOLUENE

Toluene has wide applicability as an anthelminthic but its use may be followed by toxic effects. It causes severe irritation of mucous membranes and has a depressant effect on the central nervous system. Repeated exposure causes depression of bone marrow activity and anaemia. With overdosing vomiting and slight purgation may occur, and in young animals inco-ordination and muscle tremor may appear transiently soon after treatment.

CADMIUM SALTS

Cadmium oxide and cadmium anthranilate are of considerable value for the treatment of ascariasis in swine. However, these compounds are quite toxic and should be administered only once because of their marked tendency to accumulate in tissues. Gastroenteritis with vomition is the most obvious sign of toxicity but deaths due to uraemia may occur some days later. BAL is an effective antidote because of the mode of action of cadmium, which inhibits tissue enzyme systems containing sulphydryl groups.

The clinical picture produced by chronic experimental poisoning in calves is similar to that of zinc deficiency and the effect can be partially offset by added zinc (2). In an outbreak of suspected cadmium poisoning in ponies, caused by the consumption of paint, the principal signs were colic, disorientation and ataxia (3).

PIPERAZINE

Piperazine compounds are relatively non-toxic and occasional vomiting, diarrhoea and transitory inco-ordination are the only signs likely to be encountered with moderately large doses. Very large doses cause increased peristalsis, convulsions and respiratory depression.

THIABENZOLE
(2-(4' Thiazolyl)-Benzimidozole)

At an oral dose rate of 800 mg. per kg. body weight in sheep transient signs of salivation, anorexia and depression appear. There are similar signs at larger dose rates and death is likely at a dose rate of 1200 mg. per kg. body weight (4).

TETRACHLORODIFLUORETHANE
('Freon-112')

Tetrachlorodifluorethane is an effective anthelminthic against mature liver flukes but some samples of the product are highly toxic to sheep and cattle and its use in treatment is not recommended. The degree of toxicity appears to depend on the concentration of the asymmetric isomer of the compound in the sample. Fatal poisoning, including marked prolongation of the blood clotting time, widespread haemorrhages, kidney, liver and myocardial damage, venous congestion and anasarca, occur at recommended therapeutic levels for cattle (200 mg. per kg. body weight) and at levels of 1000 mg. per kg. body weight for sheep (5).

REFERENCES
(1) Thorpe, E. (1969). *J. comp. Path.*, 79, 167.
(2) Powell, G. W. *et al.* (1964). *J. Nutr.*, 84, 205.
(3) Sass, B. *et al.* (1972). *Vet. Med. small Anim. Clin.*, 67, 745.
(4) Bell, R. R. (1964). *Ann. N.Y. Acad. Sci.*, 111, 662.
(5) Gallagher, C. H. (1965). *Aust. vet. J.*, 41, 167.

Insecticides
Chlorinated Hydrocarbons

This group includes DDT, benzene hexachloride (and its pure gamma isomer—lindane), aldrin, dieldrin, chlordane, toxaphene, methoxychlor, DDD, isodrin, endrin and heptachlor. The toxic effects produced by the members of this group include increased excitability and irritability followed by muscle tremor, weakness and paralysis and terminal convulsions in severe cases. Salivation and teeth grinding occur in large animals and vomiting in pigs. Complete anorexia occurs constantly. Most of the substances accumulate in the fat depots, may be excreted in the milk in dangerous amounts, and may be concentrated still further in butter and cream. Fat depots are a potential source of danger in that sudden mobilization of the fat may result in liberation of the compound into the blood stream and the appearance of signs of toxicity.

To produce systemic signs these insecticides must enter the blood stream and ingestion, inhalation, aspiration and percutaneous absorption are all possible portals of entry. Dipping is the most hazardous method of application because entry may occur through all portals. Spraying is safer, percutaneous absorption and inhalation being the only portals of entry. Small particle size of the compound and concentration of animals in confined spaces while spraying increase the possibility of poisoning. Although oily preparations are not usually used for animal treatment they may be used inadvertently and in this form are readily absorbed through the skin. Concentrations used for spraying barns are usually much higher than those used for animals. Of the usual spray preparations simple solutions are most dangerous followed by emulsions and least of all suspensions of wettable powder. Dusting is safest and is preferred to other methods. Although the treatment of pastures to control their insect pests is usually, with an occasional notable exception, safe to animals grazing the treated pasture or hay made from it, contamination of animal products occurs often. This contamination can be avoided by incorporating the insecticide into superphosphate granules ('prills') instead of applying it as sprays or dusts. The use of chlorinated hydrocarbons to protect stored seeds provides a hazard to animals if they are fed on the treated seed.

The compounds vary in their ability to pass the skin barrier. BHC, aldrin, dieldrin and chlordane are readily absorbed. Species susceptibility to skin absorption also varies widely. Very young animals of any species are more susceptible than adults and lactating and emaciated animals also show increased susceptibility. General toxicity data for the more common compounds are given in the table below. Methoxychlor is less toxic than DDT, and isodrin and endrin are more toxic than aldrin and dieldrin.

When these compounds were first used in dips, skin and foot infections occurred frequently because of contamination of the dip in the absence of a bactericidal agent. Cases of otitis media occurred for the same reason but more rarely.

At necropsy there are no specific lesions and specimens of hair, if the portal is percutaneous, and of the ingesta, if oral intake is probable, should be sent to the laboratory for assay. If possible the specimens should be deep frozen and the suspected compound should be nominated as assay procedures are long and involved.

DDT AND METHOXYCHLOR

DDT and methoxychlor cause initial stimulation of the central nervous system followed by terminal depression and death due to respiratory failure. Chronic poisoning causes liver damage, and a fall in blood sugar and liver glycogen levels and elevation of blood lactate and potassium.

At necropsy there are no lesions in the nervous system but in chronic cases there is focal centrilobular necrosis in the liver. Treatment comprises sedation with pentobarbital sodium, intravenous injections of glucose and calcium and the administration of a non-oily purgative. Residual DDT should be removed from the coat.

BHC, LINDANE, CHLORDANE, TOXAPHENE, DIELDRIN, ALDRIN AND HEPTACHLOR

Poisoning with these compounds has been recorded in dogs, lambs, calves and steers (2). Clinical signs resemble those of DDT poisoning but to a more extreme degree. Muscle tremors are not evident but there is excitement with grinding of the teeth, dyspnoea, tetany, snapping of the eyelids and frequent micturition. Movements are frenzied and include walking backwards, climbing walls, violent somersaults and aimless jumping. In steers salivation, inco-ordination and muscle tremor are recorded (3). Recovery may occur but with smaller

Toxic Oral Doses and Maximum Safe Spray Concentrations of Common Insecticide Sprays
(Adapted from McGirr (1)).

Compound	Method of Application	Calves to 2 weeks	Cattle	Sheep	Pig	Goat	Horse
DDT	Oral single dose: mg./kg. bw.	—	450	200	200	200	200
	Maximum safe spray: %			In general above 5%			
BHC	Oral single dose: mg./kg. bw.	—	1000	1000	1000	1000	1000
Lindane	Oral single dose: mg./kg. bw.	5	25	25	—	—	—
	Maximum safe spray: %	0·025	0·1	1·0	1·0	—	0·5
Aldrin	Oral						
	a. Single dose: mg./kg. bw.	2·5–5·0	10–25	>10	—	—	—
	b. Daily dose: mg./kg. bw.	—	2–5	2–5	—	—	—
Dieldrin	Oral single dose: mg./kg. bw.	5–10	10–25	<25	25–50	—	<25
	Maximum safe spray: %	0·1–0·25	1–2	0·2–0·3 (lambs)	4·0	4·0	100
Toxaphene	Oral single dose: mg./kg. bw.	5·0	—	25	—	50	—
	Maximum safe spray: %	0·5	2·0	1·5	4·0	—	—
Chlordane (and Heptachlor)	Oral single dose: mg./kg. bw.	25	—	100	—	—	—
	Maximum safe spray: %	0·5	2–3	2–3 (1·0 lambs)	—	—	—

animals paralysis follows and finally collapse and death ensue. Repeated doses of pentobarbital sodium are recommended until signs disappear. Similar clinical effects are produced by poisoning with chlordane, toxaphene, dieldrin, aldrin and heptachlor. In one outbreak in lambs in which undiluted aldrin was applied to oral lesions of contagious ecthyma 105 to 107 lambs died. Deaths began soon after application of the aldrin and 45 per cent of the lambs were dead within 36 hours. Although histological changes were evident in the brain, they were mild and probably reversible. The significant lesions appeared to be an acute toxic hepatitis and an acute tubular nephritis (4). An outbreak of benzene hexachloride (Gammexane) poisoning has been observed in horses which ate contaminated bran. Grasshopper baits containing toxaphene and chlordane have caused poisoning in cattle which ate large quantities of the bait.

The chlorinated hydrocarbons are still under a great deal of pressure because of their persistence in nature and the dangers which they create for wildlife, man and the domestic animals. As a result of a survey in the United Kingdom it has been recommended that aldrin, dieldrin and heptachlor be withdrawn from agricultural use and that the usefulness of DDT be reviewed. No restriction on the use of BHC was recommended (5).

REDUCTION OF TISSUE RESIDUES

Cows fed DDT prepartum have required an average of 189 days from parturition for the level in the milk fat to decline to 125 ppm (6). Contamination in other species and with other chlorinated hydrocarbon compounds also tends to be persistent. After the source of contamination is removed it is recommended that cows be drenched with up to 5 lb. of activated charcoal and that 3 lb. be incorporated in their feed daily for two weeks. Sodium phenobarbital has been shown to increase the excretion rate of chlorinated hydrocarbons significantly when fed to dairy cows at the rate of 5 g. per day for up to a month. Charcoal and phenobarbital have a similar effect on contaminated swine (7).

REVIEW LITERATURE

Harrison, D. L. (1971). Veterinary aspects of insecticides: Organochlorines. *N.Z. vet. J.*, *19*, 227.

REFERENCES

(1) McGirr, J. L. (1956). *Vet. Rec.*, *68*, 902.
(2) Alsupp, T. N. & Wharton, M. H. (1967). *Vet. Rec.*, *80*, 583.
(3) Rothenbacher, H. (1963). *Vet. Med.*, *58*, 734.
(4) Bacter, J. T. (1959). *J. comp. Path.*, *69*, 185.
(5) Cook, J. (1964). *Vet. Rec.*, *76*, 400.
(6) Miller, D. D. (1967). *J. Dairy Sci.*, *50*, 1444.
(7) Dobson, R. C. *et al.* (1971). *Bull. environ. Contam. Toxicol.*, *6*, 189.

Organophosphatic Compounds

Organophosphates inactivate cholinesterase and produce a syndrome of salivation, diarrhoea, and muscle stiffness indicative of stimulation of the parasympathetic nervous system.

Incidence

Poisoning by organophosphates does not occur commonly but the substances are highly poisonous and heavy mortalities can occur in animals accidentally exposed to toxic amounts. Their toxic effect is purely functional and no residual defects persist in recovered animals. The introduction of these compounds into animal therapeutics as treatments for nematode, bot-fly, sheep nasal bot and warble-fly infestations has increased their importance as possible causes of poisoning.

Substances in the organophosphate (OP) group are included in the instruments of modern biological warfare as 'nerve gases'. Their use in war would be expected to have effects similar to those described here. The famous 'Utah sheep kill' phenomenon is thought to have been due to an accidental release of an OP from a defence forces proving ground (1).

Aetiology

A number of compounds are included in the group and there is a great deal of variation in their toxicity for animals, those used for the direct treatment of animals having been selected for their low toxicity. A tremendous volume of information has become available on the relative toxicities of the many compounds which are now commercially available. It is not possible to provide details here and the information does not lend itself to summarization.

The compounds are readily absorbed after ingestion, inhalation and application to the skin and conjunctiva. Young animals are usually much more susceptible than adults but with some compounds the reverse is the case. Brahman and Brahman-cross cattle appear to be more susceptible to some compounds than other cattle (2) and there is a suggestion of a higher than normal susceptibility of Dorset Down sheep (3). Restriction of water intake renders animals more susceptible to the toxic effects especially after oral treatment with these compounds to control warble-fly infestations. The toxicity of some compounds appears to increase with storage.

Occurrence

Accidental exposure may occur when animals are allowed to graze in recently sprayed areas, particularly orchards where the most toxic compounds are frequently used. Accidental contamination of pasture may occur when spray used on cereal crops and in orchards is carried by wind on to pasture fields. Many accidents occur as a result of improper use of sprays, either because of too high a concentration of the insecticide or, more commonly, because of the application to animals of products containing oily bases and designed specifically for spraying on walls and other inanimate objects. In the race for supremacy with anthelminthics a number of compounds have been released which are not safe in all circumstances. The reasons for outbreaks of toxicity with these compounds are often not understood. On the other hand with proper care these compounds can be safe. In Australia it has been recorded that in 17.5×10^6 cattle dippings there were 563 deaths—an incidence of 0.003 per cent (5).

An unexpected side effect of the use of organophosphate anthelminthics in the horse is their effect in potentiating the action of succinylcholine chloride for up to one month after the administration of the organophosphate (4). The administration of the relaxant to a sensitized horse can be followed by persistent apnoea and death.

Pathogenesis

The inactivation of cholinesterase by these organophosphatic compounds causes an increase in acetylcholine in tissues and increased activity of the parasympathetic nervous system and of the post-ganglionic cholinergic nerves of the sympathetic nervous system. The toxic effects thus reproduce the muscarinic and nicotinic responses of acetylcholine administration. The muscarinic effects are the visceral responses of increased peristalsis, salivation, bronchial constriction, increased mucous secretion by bronchiolar glands, pupillary constriction and sweating. The nicotinic effects are the skeletal muscle responses of twitching, tremor and tetany initially followed by weakness and flaccid paralysis. There is a difference in the relative muscarinic and nicotinic responses between species, the visceral effects being more marked in ruminants and the muscular effects more evident in pigs.

Effects additional to those quoted include terminal effects on the nervous system, particularly drowsiness, convulsions and coma.

Organophosphatic compounds do not usually cause any permanent effects in recovered animals but with some compounds, especially coumaphos and Ronnel, the recovery period may be quite long, up to 3 months in the case of Ronnel, because of slow excretion of the compound. Also the fluid diarrhoea which is a transient sign in moderate intoxication in foals may be expanded to a severe gastroenteritis with heavier dose rates. Although the organophosphates act largely by destroying cholinesterase the levels of cholinesterase in the blood are not in any way indicative of the presence or absence of these compounds. Many poisoned animals die with normal blood cholinesterase levels.

Clinical Findings

In cattle the premonitory signs in acute cases, and the only signs in mild cases, are salivation, dyspnoea, diarrhoea and muscle stiffness with staggering. In the acute cases additional signs include protrusion of the tongue, constriction of the pupils with resulting impairment of vision, muscle tremor commencing in the head and neck and spreading over the body, bloat, collapse, and death without convulsions or severe respiratory distress. In sheep the signs are similar and include also abdominal pain.

In pigs visceral effects are less pronounced and salivation, muscle tremor, nystagmus and recumbency are characteristic. In some instances, the syndrome is an indefinite one with muscle weakness and drowsiness the only apparent signs. Respiratory distress and diarrhoea do not occur. In horses signs of toxicity include abdominal pain and grossly increased intestinal sounds, a very fluid diarrhoea, muscle tremor, ataxia, circling, weakness and dyspnoea. Increased salivation occurs rarely (6, 7).

Illness may occur within minutes of inhalation or ingestion of solutions of the more toxic compounds and deaths may commence 2 to 5 minutes later. With less toxic compounds in solid form signs may not appear for some hours and deaths may be delayed for 12 to 24 hours.

Clinical Pathology

Although levels of cholinesterase activity in the blood are depressed the degree of depression is often unrelated to the severity of the clinical signs. For example in cattle dying of OP poisoning blood cholinesterase levels were reduced to 6 to 16 per cent of prior levels but some surviving animals had levels below 16 per cent (5). The estimation of cholinesterase, not usually welcomed by diagnostic laboratories, is the only technique available for diagnosing OP poisoning (6, 8, 9). Suspected food material can be assayed for its content of organophosphatic compounds but assay of animal tissues or fluids is virtually valueless and may be misleading.

Necropsy Findings

There are no gross or histological lesions at necropsy, but tissue specimens should be collected for toxicological analysis. Material sent for laboratory analysis for cholinesterase should be refrigerated but not deep frozen.

Diagnosis

Dyspnoea, salivation and muscle stiffness after exposure to organic phosphorus insecticides suggest intoxication with these compounds. Occasional animals may show a similar syndrome when affected by anaphylaxis, and groups of cattle affected by fog fever may show a sudden onset of dyspnoea but pulmonary oedema is obvious on auscultation, and salivation and muscle stiffness are absent. In pigs the signs are less diagnostic and may suggest arsenic, rotenone, salt or mercury poisoning, or avitaminosis A. In pigs the recovery rate is good and all pigs may recover if the intake has been low and access is stopped. With the other poisons listed above death is much more common and residual defects including blindness and paralysis occur in a proportion of the survivors. The history of exposure to the various poisons or of nutritional deficiency may give the clue to the diagnosis but it is usually necessary to depend on assay of the food material for confirmation. It should be remembered that reactions following OP treatment for grubs may be due either to the drug or to the damaged grub and treatment with atropine would be contraindicated in the latter.

Treatment

Atropine in large (about double the normal) doses is the rational and approved treatment. Recommended doses are 0·25 mg. per kg. body weight in cattle and 1·0 mg. per kg. body weight in sheep. In very sick animals about one-third of this dose should be given very slowly intravenously in a dilute (2 per cent) solution and the remainder by intramuscular injection (9). Injections may have to be repeated at 4- to 5-hourly intervals as signs return, and continued over a period of 24 to 48 hours.

A group of compounds known as oximes have some efficiency in treatment. The oxime TMB is superior to 2-PAM and DAM. Recommended dose rates for 2-PAM are 50 to 100 mg. per kg. body weight given intravenously and for TMB 10 to 20 mg. per kg. body weight (10). These dose rates can also be used for subcutaneous and intraperitoneal injection. Administration by any route is as a 10 per cent solution in normal saline. In horses 2-PAM at doses of 20 mg. per kg. body weight has given good results. Combination of an oxime and atropine is recommended (11). Treatment with PAM may need to be repeated for up to 10 days to counteract slower acting compounds such as coumaphos (10). Atropine appears to have low efficiency in sheep. This is not a serious drawback as sheep are much less susceptible than cattle to larger doses of atropine.

Animals that have been dipped or sprayed should be washed with water to which soap, soda or a detergent is added to remove residual organic phosphorus material.

Control

Most outbreaks occur after accidental access to compounds and this cannot always be avoided. Animals to be treated orally with organic phosphorus insecticides should be permitted ample fresh drinking water beforehand.

REVIEW LITERATURE

Solly, S. R. B. (1971). Veterinary aspects of insecticides: Organophosphates. *N.Z. vet. J.*, *19*, 233.

REFERENCES

(1) Van Kampen, K. R. *et al.* (1969). *J. Amer. vet. med. Ass.*, *154*, 623.
(2) Palmer, J. S. & Danz, J. W. (1964). *J. Amer. vet. med. Ass.*, *144*, 143.
(3) Smith, I. D. (1970). *Vet. Rec.*, *86*, 284.
(4) Himes, J. A. *et al.* (1967). *J. Amer. vet. med. Ass.*, *151*, 54.
(5) Roe, R. T. (1969). *Aust. vet. J.*, *45*, 332, 411.
(6) Bello, T. R. & Torbert, B. J. (1972). *Amer. J. vet. Res.*, *33*, 329.
(7) Younger, R. L. (1965). *Amer. J. vet. Res.*, *26*, 776.
(8) Anderson, P. H. *et al.* (1969). *Res. vet. Sci.*, *10*, 29.
(9) Anderson, P. H. & Machin, A. F. (1969). *Vet. Rec.*, *85*, 484.
(10) Younger, R. L. & Wright, F. C. (1971). *J. Amer. vet. med. Ass.*, *32*, 1053.
(11) Younger, R. L. & Radeleff, R. D. (1964). *Amer. J. vet. Res.*, *25*, 981.

Rotenone

Rotenone is relatively non-toxic when taken orally but toxic effects have been observed in pigs fed a ration containing 2·5 per cent of rotenone. In this instance assay of ingesta at necropsy revealed the presence of 2130 ppm of rotenone. Clinically there was salivation, muscle tremor, vomiting, ascending paralysis accompanied by inco-ordination, followed by paralysis of all four limbs. Respiratory depression and coma preceded death which occurred in all of the ten pigs exposed (1).

REFERENCES

(1) Oliver, W. T. & Roe, C. K. (1957). *J. Amer. vet. med. Ass.*, *130*, 410.

Herbicides

DINITROPHENOL COMPOUNDS

Dinitrophenols find considerable use in agriculture because of their versatility as herbicides and fungicides. Animals can be poisoned accidentally by inhalation, ingestion or percutaneous absorption of these compounds which have the effect of increasing the basal metabolic rate. Poisoning is manifested by an acute onset of restlessness, sweating, deep, rapid respiration, fever and collapse. Death may occur 24 to 48 hours later.

Dinitrophenol (DNP) and dinitro-orthocresol (DNOC) are the commonest members of this group (1). In all species doses of 25 to 50 mg. per kg. body weight are usually toxic but much smaller doses produce toxicity when environmental temperatures are high. There is no accumulation of the drug within the body.

HORMONE WEED KILLERS

2,4-D, Silvex, MCPA and 2,4,5-T are reputed to be non-toxic in the concentrations used on crops and pasture but dosing with 300 to 1000 mg. per kg., as a single dose, causes deaths in 50 per cent of cattle. Reversible toxic effects are produced with single doses of 2,4-D in calves with doses of 200 mg. per kg. and in pigs with 100 mg. per kg. (2). Repeated administration of 50 mg. per kg. is toxic to pigs. In calves the clinical signs are dysphagia, tympanites, anorexia and muscular weakness; in pigs there is in addition inco-ordination, vomiting and transient diarrhoea. In very long-term experiments with pigs (500 ppm in the diet for 12 months) moderate degenerative changes in kidney and liver were produced. 2,4-D may cause poisoning indirectly by its effect on the metabolism of weeds and sugar beets, resulting in a significant increase in the nitrate content of the leaves. A commonly used mixture of 2,4-D, 2,4,5-T and a brushwood killer, monosodium methyl arsenate, is very toxic by mouth or after application to the skin; the chief clinical signs are anorexia, diarrhoea, loss of weight and death in most cases (3). Repeated dosing of sheep with Silvex causes death after dosing for about 30 days at dose rates of 150 mg. per kg. body weight. Single doses of 250 mg. per kg. body weight of other compounds used as herbicides (carbamate, triazine, propionanilide and diallylacetomide) are fatal to sheep. Repeated smaller doses of carbamate A caused marked alopecia. Acute poisoning with any of these compounds is unlikely unless large amounts are ingested accidentally (4). Paraquat causes fibrosing pneumonitis in pigs but this does not develop in sheep or cattle with doses large enough to be fatal (5).

SODIUM CHLORATE

This substance is still widely used as a weed killer and constitutes a potential hazard to grazing stock. Animals seldom ingest sufficient sprayed plant material to produce clinical illness and the principal danger is from accidental dosing or permitting salt-hungry cattle to have access to the chemical.

The lethal oral dose is 2 to 2·5 g. per kg. body weight for sheep, 0·5 g. per kg. for cattle and 3·5 g. per kg. for dogs. Irritation of the alimentary tract causes diarrhoea and deep, black erosions of the abomasal and duodenal mucosae. Methaemoglobinaemia results and somnolence and dyspnoea are characteristic. At necropsy the blood, muscles and viscera are very dark. No specific treatment is available. Sodium thiosulphate and methylene blue appear to have little effect on the course of the disease but copious blood transfusions have been recommended.

DELRAD

Delrad is an algaecide used to control the growth of algae on ponds and other water reservoirs. Cattle and sheep are unharmed by the ingestion of water containing 100 ppm of the compound (6). Dose rates of 250 g. per kg. body weight in adult cattle, 150 mg. per kg. in calves and 500 mg. per kg. in sheep cause toxic effects.

DEFOLIANTS

Substances used to remove the leaves from plants used for harvesting seed may represent a toxic hazard if the residual stalks are fed to livestock. Monochloroacetate is commonly used for this purpose and although it is unlikely to cause poisoning unless very large quantities of the stalks are fed, animals which gain access to recently sprayed fields may be seriously affected. Toxic signs in cattle include diarrhoea, colic, muscular tremor and dyspnoea (7).

REVIEW LITERATURE

McIntosh, I. G. (1967). Herbicides and their toxicity to livestock. *N.Z. vet. J.*, *15*, 70.

REFERENCES

(1) Scott, W. N. (1964). *Vet. Rec.*, *76*, 964.
(2) Bjorklund, N. E. & Erne, K. (1966). *Acta vet. scand.*, *7*, 364.
(3) Libke, K. G. *et al.* (1971). *Mod. vet. Pract.*, *52*, 37.
(4) Palmer, J. S. (1964). *J. Amer. vet. med. Ass.*, *145*, 787, 917.

(5) Smalley, H. E. & Radeleff, R. D. (1970). *Toxicol. appl. Pharmac.*, *17*, 305.
(6) Radeleff, R. D. (1958). *Advanc. vet. Sci.*, 265.
(7) Dalgaard-Mikkelsen, S. & Rasmussen, F. (1961). *Nord. Vet.-Med.*, *13*, 271.

Rodenticides

The commonly used rodenticides are sodium fluoroacetate, ANTU (alphanaphthylthiourea), warfarin (3-(acetonylbenzyl)-4-hydroxycoumarin) and zinc phosphide. They are all toxic to domestic animals and may cause deaths when ingested accidentally (1).

SODIUM FLUOROACETATE

Two actions are manifest, myocardial depression with ventricular fibrillation, and stimulation of the central nervous system producing convulsions. In cattle the predominant effect is on myocardium; in dogs it is the nervous system (2). Observations on experimental animals suggest that sedation with barbiturates and procaine injection into the cardiac chambers may be of value in treatment. A dose rate of 0·3 mg. per kg. body weight seems to have been established as a toxic dose level for domestic species and 0·4 mg. per kg. is lethal for sheep (1) and cattle (3). Sublethal doses may be cumulative if given at sufficiently short intervals. The fluoroacetate ion is present in sufficient quantities in the leaves of the gidgee tree and the plant *Gastrolobium grandiflorum* to cause poisoning of livestock.

ANTU

Horses, pigs, calves and dogs are susceptible as well as rats. Tolerance develops after the ingestion of sublethal doses. Death occurs within 24 to 48 hours after ingestion due to marked pleural effusion, pulmonary oedema, and to a less extent pericardial effusion. The toxic dose rate is of the order of 20 to 40 mg. per kg. body weight in a single dose.

WARFARIN

This anticoagulant is in very widespread use as a rodenticide because it causes no poison shyness. Although most deaths occur because of misuse by farmers, contamination of feedstuffs at the milling plant is not unknown and may cause death when the history of warfarin use is negative. Calves and poultry are not usually affected, most outbreaks being recorded in pigs, cats and dogs. Single doses, unless massive, are unlikely to cause poisoning but repeated ingestion for some days may do so. Daily doses of 0·2 to 0·5 mg. per kg. body weight are fatal to pigs in 6 to 12 days. In cattle dose rates of up to 200 mg. per kg. daily for 5 days cause 50 per cent mortality. At a dose rate of 0·25 mg. per kg. for 10 days prothrombin times are depressed 20 per cent and at 0·1 to 0·3 mg. per kg. abortions occur (4). Sudden massive haemorrhage into body cavities or brain may cause sudden death, or death may occur slowly with accompanying lameness due to haemorrhage into subcutaneous tissues. Massive or multiple haemorrhages are characteristic at necropsy. Vitamin K is the antidote and blood transfusions are also indicated in treatment.

RED SQUILLS

Poisoning by red squills seldom occurs because the material is extremely unpalatable and when eaten is usually vomited (5). In all species large doses (100 to 500 mg. per kg. body weight) must be administered to produce toxic effects. Young calves are most susceptible and goats least. Experimental poisoning causes convulsions, gastritis and bradycardia.

ZINC PHOSPHIDE

Zinc phosphide is also unpalatable to domestic animals (5). Experimental poisoning with doses of about 40 mg. per kg. body weight causes death in most species. A general toxaemia with depression of appetite, dullness and some increase in respiratory rate occurs but there are no diagnostic signs. Necropsy lesions include congestion and haemorrhages in all organs, fatty degeneration of the liver and inflammation in the small intestine. Chemical assay is necessary to establish a diagnosis.

REFERENCES

(1) Annison, E. F. *et al.* (1960). *J. comp. Path.*, *70*, 145.
(2) Allcroft, R. *et al.* (1969). *Vet. Rec.*, *84*, 399, 403.
(3) Robison, W. H. (1970). *J. Wildl. Mgmt*, *34*, 647.
(4) Pugh, D. M. (1968). *Brit. J. Pharmac. Chemother.*, *33*, 210P.

Wood Preservatives

Lumber used in the construction of barns, stables, pens and yards is often treated with wood preservatives, chiefly pentachlorophenol, dinitro-orthophenols, dinitrophenol, and coal tar creosote, or mixtures of these, and animals which have access to freshly treated material or the neat preservative may be poisoned. A high mortality may be encountered in newborn pigs and there may be a greater than normal incidence of stillbirths when sows are farrowed in treated crates. Weaned pigs may show depression, skin irritation and occasionally death. The toxic cresols may be imbibed orally or absorbed percutaneously and contact with freshly treated wood may cause local cutaneous necrosis (1). Acute fatal doses in all species are in the range of 120 to 140 mg. per kg. body weight for pentachlorophenol and chronic fatal doses range from 30 to 50 mg. per kg. body weight. Fatal doses for coal tar creosote are 4 to 6 g. per kg. body weight as a single dose and 0·5 g. per kg. body weight daily (2). Creosote, applied as a treatment for ringworm, has shown marked toxic effects in cattle (3).

Other wood preservatives including arsenicals, naphthalenes and fluorides are dealt with under those headings.

REFERENCES

(1) Schipper, I. A. *et al.* (1964). *N. Dak. Farm. Res.*, *23*, No. 3, p. 4.
(2) Harrison, D. L. (1959). *N.Z. vet. J.*, 7, 89, 94.
(3) Blandford, T. B. *et al.* (1968). *Vet. Rec.*, *82*, 323.

Additives in Feeds

Many substances including antibiotics, fungistatics, vermicides, oestrogens, arsenicals, urea, iodinated casein and copper salts are added to prepared feed mixes to improve food utilization and hasten growth and fattening. Many of these substances may be toxic if improperly used. The toxic effects of arsanilic acid are described under arsenic poisoning (p. 764). Copper sulphate has recently been introduced as an additive to rations for pigs and feeding of the treated material for long periods to cattle has caused chronic copper poisoning.

IODINATED CASEIN

Iodinated casein has been used as a feed additive to increase milk production in dairy cows but its use is not without risk (1), particularly in hot weather. The feeding of 20 g. per day for 6 weeks has caused illness in dairy cows although the milk yield is significantly increased in the early stages. Clinical signs of toxicity include abnormality of cardiac rhythm, high respiratory rate, nervousness, digestive disorders and scouring.

OESTROGENIC SUBSTANCES

Improvement in fattening and weight gains occur when oestrogenic substances are fed to growing animals or injected in a repository form. Toxicity occurs with overdosage and has been observed in animals grazing particular pasture plants including lucerne, subterranean clover, red clover and ladino clover, and in some cases mixed pasture (2) and green forage crops (3) in which the oestrogen-rich plants have not been identified. Small quantities of oestrogens are also present in rye grasses during the spring (4). White clover does not usually contain detectable amounts but plants heavily infested with fungi may contain significant amounts (5). Oestrogens may also be present in large amounts in mouldy corn and produce toxic effects when fed to pigs. An outbreak of poisoning in pigs has been recorded in which the source was probably hexoestrol implants in capon necks fed to the pigs (6). Cattle treated orally or by subcutaneous implants with oestrogenic substances pass significant amounts in the faeces, especially when the substance is fed and there is one record of abortions in heifers fed on ensilage contaminated by the manure of steers fed hexoestrol (7). In all these circumstances the clinical findings and necropsy lesions are referable to the urogenital system.

Standard recommendations are for the feeding of 5 to 10 mg. of stilboestrol daily to fattening cattle of 180 to 270 kg. body weight. The feeding of up to 20 mg. per day to cattle has no visible effect on the reproductive tract. Larger doses of stilboestrol to cattle may cause prolapse of the rectum and vagina with relaxation of the pelvic ligaments, elevation of the tail-head and susceptibility to fracture of the pelvic bones and dislocation of the hip. Nymphomaniac behaviour in such animals invites skeletal injury.

Heavy mortalities have occurred in feeder lambs after the use of 12 mg. implants of oestrogens. Prolapse of the rectum, vagina and uterus occurred together with urethral obstruction. In another outbreak 20 per cent of 300 feedlot wethers died within 35 days of implantation with pellets containing 30 mg. of stilboestrol whereas none of 150 control wethers was affected (8). In these outbreaks the calculi consisted largely of desquamated epithelial and pus cells which formed a nidus for the deposition of mineral, the desquamation probably being stimulated by the oestrogen. The possibility also exists that partial urethral obstruction caused by the oestrogen facilitated complete obstruction by the calculi.

The daily feeding of 0·75 mg. per kg. body weight of stilboestrol has also caused poisoning in pigs; clinical signs included straining, prolapse of the rectum, incontinence of urine, anuria and death. At necropsy there was inflammation and necrosis of the rectal wall, enlargement of the kidneys, thickening of the ureters and distension of the bladder, and gross enlargement of the prostate and seminal vesicles.

A number of specific pasture plants may contain large amounts of oestrogenic substances but increased oestrogenic activity has also been observed in mixed pasture. This activity may be apparent only at certain times and is often restricted to particular fields (2). Clinically the effects are those of sterility, some abortions, swelling of the udder and vulva in pregnant animals and in virgin heifers, and endometritis with a slimy, purulent vaginal discharge in some animals. Oestrus cycles are irregular. In milking cows there is depression of the milk yield, reduction in appetite and an increase in the cell count of the milk.

UREA

Urea has been introduced as a feed additive for ruminants to provide a cheap protein substitute. Poisoning occurs when cattle accidentally gain access to large quantities of urea, or are fed large quantities when they are unaccustomed to it, or when feeds are improperly mixed. Some care is required in bringing the animals on to urea gradually and an adequate proportion of carbohydrate must be included in the ration. The toxic effects are due to the sudden production of large quantities of ammonia and signs occur within 20 to 30 minutes of feeding. The severity of signs is related to blood ammonia levels and not to levels of ammonia in the rumen (9). The rapidity with which the ammonia is released in the rumen may be increased if soya bean meal is being fed—soya beans containing urease which facilitates the breakdown of urea to ammonia.

Toxic dose levels vary but in cattle which have been starved beforehand dose levels up to 0·33 g. per kg. body weight cause increases in blood levels of ammonia and dose levels of 0·44 g. per kg. body weight produce signs of poisoning within 10 minutes of dosing (10). Animals unaccustomed to urea may show clinical illness when fed 20 g. per 100 lb. body weight, but by gradually increasing the quantity fed this amount can be tolerated. This tolerance is lost rapidly and animals which receive no urea for 3 days are again susceptible. Tolerance is also reduced by starvation and by a low protein diet. Sheep can eat 6 per cent of their total ration as urea provided it is well mixed with roughage and fed throughout the day, preferably by spraying the urea mixed with molasses onto the roughage. Much more urea is tolerated if given to sheep in molasses (18 g.), than if given as a drench (8 g.) and prior feeding on lucerne further increases the tolerance (9) and fasting for 24 hours reduces it. In general, urea should not constitute more than 3 per cent of the concentrate ration of ruminants. Horses appear to be tolerant to relatively large doses of urea but the disease has been produced experimentally in ponies by administering 450 g.

by stomach tube. The clinical picture is similar to that in cattle, being largely related to the central nervous system (11).

Clinical signs of toxicity in cattle include severe abdominal pain, muscle tremor, inco-ordination, weakness, dyspnoea, bloat, and violent struggling and bellowing. The death rate in affected animals is high. There are no lesions visible at necropsy.

Treatment is unlikely to be effective but the oral administration of a weak acid such as vinegar (1 to 2 pints to a sheep) may reduce the amount of ammonia absorbed. The administration of 5 per cent acetic acid is recommended as an antidote but repeated dosings may be necessary as clinical signs tend to recur about 30 minutes after treatment (10). Intravenous administration of gamma-aminobutyric acid is not an effective preventive (14). The relationship between high rumen ammonia levels and hypomagnesaemia suggests that treatment with calcium and magnesium solutions may be of value. Encephalomalacia has been produced in pigs by feeding a ration containing 15 per cent urea (12). The clinical picture and histopathological findings were similar to those of salt poisoning except that no eosinophilic aggregations were present in the cerebral lesions.

PROPYLENE GLYCOL

Propylene glycol is an unlikely poison but it is used extensively in veterinary practice and can cause poisoning if it is accidentally administered to horses. Dose rates of 3 litres to horses of 500 kg. by stomach tube can cause severe ataxia, depression and a foetid odour of the faeces. Much larger doses (8 litres) can be fatal. Moderate to severe inflammation of the lining of the gut and oedema of the brain are noticeable at necropsy examination (13).

REFERENCES

(1) Blaxter, K. L. (1964). *J. agric. Sci.*, *36*, 117.
(2) Schoop, G. & Klette, H. (1952). *Rep. 2nd int. Congr. Physiol. Path. Anim. Reprod. art. Insem., Copenhagen*, *2*, 87.
(3) Sanger, V. L. & Bell, D. S. (1959). *J. Amer. vet. med. Ass.*, *134*, 237.
(4) Cunningham, I. J. & Hogan, K. C. (1954). *N.Z. vet. J.*, *2*, 128.
(5) Wong, E. *et al.* (1971). *N.Z. agric. Res.*, *14*, 639.
(6) Ranby, P. D. & Ramsay, W. R. (1959). *Aust. vet. J.*, *35*, 90.
(7) Rankin, J. E. F. (1959). *Vet. Rec.*, *71*, 924.
(8) Udall, R. H. & Jensen, R. (1958). *J. Amer. vet. med. Ass.*, *133*, 514.
(9) McBarron, E. J. & MacInnes, P. (1968). *Aust. vet. J.*, *44*, 90.
(10) Word, J. D. *et al.* (1969). *J. Anim. Sci.*, *29*, 786.
(11) Hintz, H. F. *et al.* (1970). *J. Amer. vet. med. Ass.*, *157*, 963.
(12) Done, J. T. *et al.* (1959). *Vet. Rec.*, *71*, 92.

(13) Myers, V. S. & Usenik, E. A. (1969). *J. Amer. vet. med. Ass.*, *155*, 1841.
(14) Morris, J. G. & Payne, E. (1970). *J. agric. Sci. (Camb.)*, *74*, 259.

Miscellaneous Farm Chemicals

Poisoning by Highly Chlorinated Naphthalenes

The local application or ingestion of highly chlorinated naphthalenes to cattle produces a disease characterized by thickening and scaliness of the skin, due to hyperkeratosis, emaciation and eventual death. The toxic compounds interfere with the conversion of carotene to vitamin A and, in effect, cause hypovitaminosis A. The naphthalenes were extensively used in industry as lubricants, insulants and wood-preserving agents. Recognition of their toxicity has resulted in their exclusion from the farm environment and virtual elimination of the disease.

REVIEW LITERATURE

Olson, C. (1968). *Advanc. vet. Sci.*, *13*, 101.

Coal Tar Pitch Poisoning

Pigs may be exposed to coal tar pitch and its toxic cresols when housed in pens with tarred walls or floors, or when they have access to 'clay pigeons' used as targets by gun clubs (1). Bitumen and asphalt appear to be non-toxic. Affected pigs nibble the tarred material in pens or ingest fragments of the 'clay pigeons' at pasture. Young pigs 6 to 20 weeks of age are most commonly affected and the incidence in this group may be as high as 20 per cent. Clinically there may be an acute illness or the disease may run a chronic course of some weeks. In the acute illness there are non-specific signs of inappetence, rough coat, tucked-up abdomen, weakness and depression. The chronic illness is characterized by anorexia, depression, weakness, anaemia and jaundice, and pigs affected subclinically may manifest only a reduction in growth rate of up to 20 to 30 per cent (2). A severe reduction in haemoglobin concentration and erythrocyte count is detectable on examination of the blood. Vitamin A storage is also reduced.

At necropsy there may be jaundice, ascites and anaemia but the characteristic finding is a red and yellow mottling of the hepatic surfaces. On histological examination there is severe centrilobular necrosis of the liver and the necrotic zones are suffused with blood (3, 4). Cresols can be detected in the ingesta and liver of affected pigs.

REFERENCES

(1) Graham, R. *et al.* (1940). *J. Amer. vet. med. Ass.*, *96*, 135.

(2) Maclean, C. W. (1969). *Vet. Rec.*, *84*, 594.
(3) Libke, K. G. & Davis, J. W. (1967). *J. Amer. vet. med. Ass.*, *151*, 426.
(4) Davis, J. W. & Libke, K. G. (1968). *J. Amer. vet. med. Ass.*, *152*, 382.

Methaldehyde

Methaldehyde is in common use as a molluscicide in domestic gardens and because it is usually dispensed in a bran base and is toxic to animals it represents a poisoning hazard to farm livestock. Clinical signs include inco-ordination, dyspnoea, unconsciousness, cyanosis and death due to respiratory failure. An outbreak of poisoning has been observed in sheep and experimental cases have been produced in a donkey and in a goat (1).

REFERENCE

(1) Egyed, M. N. & Brisk, Y. L. (1966). *Vet. Rec.*, *78*, 753.

DISEASES CAUSED BY
POISONOUS PLANTS

Algae

Many green or blue-green algae (water bloom) of the *Microcystis* spp. (*Anacystis cyanea*) contain toxic substances but outbreaks of poisoning in farm animals are uncommon, occurring chiefly when the algae are concentrated by on-shore winds so that large quantities may be ingested by animals while drinking. Smaller animals who drink near the edge of the lake get more toxin because it is concentrated in the superficial layers at the edge (1). The disease has been recorded in the U.S.A., Canada, South Africa, Australia and New Zealand and affects all animals and birds. In New South Wales the algae occur seasonally in most dams in the area but deaths do not necessarily occur, especially if animals are able to avoid large concentrations. Heavy growth occurs in the late summer to autumn period (2).

The toxic effects of algae vary widely depending on the strains of algae present, the types of bacteria growing in association with the algae, the conditions of growth, accumulation and decomposition and the amounts of toxic material consumed. In general the algae, on decomposition, liberate an endotoxin which is highly poisonous and kills quickly—the fast-death factor (3). Commonly associated with the algae are bacteria which produce substances capable of causing gastroenteritis and hepatitis—the slow-death factor (4). Clinical signs may become apparent within half-an-hour after exposure. In acute cases the affected animals show muscle tremor, stupor, staggering, recumbency, and in some cases hyperaesthesia to touch so that slight stimulation provokes a convulsion with opisthotonus. After experimental dosing death may occur within a few minutes of the first appearance of clinical signs (5) but in field cases the course may be prolonged for several hours. Necropsy lesions which occur in animals that die suddenly include generalized petechiation, plasma transudates in body cavities and congestion of most viscera.

When the poisoning is due to bacterial toxins there is severe liver damage accompanied by jaundice and photosensitization in cattle and sheep (6). Severe gastroenteritis with intestinal haemorrhage has also been observed in some outbreaks (7). The photosensitization is caused by the presence of a photodynamic pigment, phyocyan, the excretion of which is retarded by the liver damage.

The intravenous injection of a mixture of sodium nitrite and sodium thiosulphate as recommended for cyanide poisoning is credited with curative properties. Excessive growth of algae is favoured by the presence of large quantities of organic matter in the water and by hot weather. Algal growth can be controlled by the use of copper sulphate or other algaecides such as Delrad.

REFERENCES

(1) Hammer, U. T. (1968). *Canad. vet. J.*, 9, 221.
(2) May, V. (1970). *Contr. N.S.W. natn. Herb.*, 4, 84.
(3) Gorham, P. R. (1960). *Canad. vet. J.*, 1, 235.
(4) Flint, E. A. (1966). *N.Z. vet. J.*, 14, 181.
(5) Stewart, A. G. *et al.* (1950). *Canad. J. comp. Med.*, 14, 197.
(6) Steyn, D. G. (1943). *Fmg S. Afr.*, 18, 489, 510.
(7) Senior, V. E. (1960). *Canad. J. comp. Med.*, 24, 26.

Poisoning by Fungi

(*Mycotoxicosis*)

The importance of fungi as poisonous agents has been appreciated for many years but it is only recently that the scope and magnitude of the losses that they cause have become apparent. Partly this has come about because of the greater accuracy of definition of other diseases with which mycotoxicoses have been confused. There has also been a significant improvement in the investigational effort used to identify fungi. The one problem that remains is the experimental production of the subject diseases. The cultivation of fungi in large quantities is difficult and it seems that on many occasions the fungi become poisonous because of their conditions of growth, especially the composition of the substrate on which they are growing.

Moulds grow on any stored feeds, the highest incidence being on feeds with high moisture content. Thus a common fungal poisoning is on mouldy corn or maize, which is a high moisture grain and difficult to harvest or store at the correct stage of maturity and moisture content. A degree of spoilage must be expected in corn grain with a moisture content in excess of 20 per cent.

Many of the moulds on feeds are non-toxic, many are toxic only at certain times and many have an as yet undetermined status. Many syndromes generally considered to be caused by fungal toxins, e.g. the haemorrhagic diathesis which occurs on feeding mouldy lespedeza hay (1), corn grain (2), hay, chaff and bedding (3), have no recognized specific mycotoxic origin.

REVIEW LITERATURE

Forgacs, J. (1962). *Proc. 66th ann. gen. Mtg U.S. Live Stock sanit. Ass.*, 426.
Crawford, M. (1962). *Vet. Bull.*, 32, 415.

REFERENCES

(1) Muhrer, M. E. *et al.* (1946). *J. Anim. Sci.*, 5, 420.
(2) Albright, J. L. *et al.* (1964). *J. Amer. vet. med. Ass.*, 144, 1013.
(3) Bruins, B. (1953). *T. Diergeneesk.*, 78, 787.

Poisoning by *Fusarium* spp.

Fusarium spp. fungi produce toxins capable of causing a great variety of clinical signs. *F. graminearum* (*Giberella zea*) growing on maize has produced oestrogenic substances and when fed to pigs has produced vulvovaginitis (1) and to cattle has increased services per conception from 1·2 to 4 (2). The oestrogenic substance has been identified as zearalenone (3). *F. moniliforme* fed to cattle cause an oestrogenic syndrome (4) and *F. culmorum* is also reputed to have oestrogenic effects (5). As well as its oestrogenic toxin *F. culmorum* causes inappetence, scouring, ataxia and a fall in milk yield when an infected standing crop of maize is fed to cattle (6). *F. sporotrichiella* var. *poae* fed at low dose rates to cattle produces changes in electrocardiographic patterns, and mild neurological signs when given at higher dose rates (7). *F. sporotrichiella*, growing on stored grain, has also produced haemorrhagic enteritis, renal hyperaemia and death in 24 hours, up to 4 to 5 days in less severe cases in cattle (8). In rabbits the toxin of this species and of *F. sporotrichoides* and *F. sambucinum* shows a powerful, cumulative neurotoxic effect. There is depression of nerve impulse transmission and cardiovascular collapse. At necropsy haemorrhages and oedema are characteristic (9).

Fusarium tricinctum, a fungus of ear corn, produces a toxin whose effects are manifested by necrotic lesions and haemorrhages in the intestines, liver and kidneys (10). The toxin can be absorbed through the alimentary mucosa or through the skin. *Fusarium javanicum* growing on sweet potato tubers is associated with the presence of a number of toxins, but the toxins occur with a number of fungi and are probably dependent on the chemical composition of the sweet potato.

F. moniliforme infestation of corn grain is thought to be the cause of leucoencephalomalacia of horses and is described under that heading below.

REFERENCES

(1) Bristol, F. M. & Djurickovic, M. (1971). *Canad. vet. J.*, *12*, 132.
(2) Mirocha, C. J. *et al.* (1968). *Appl. Microbiol.*, *16*, 797.
(3) Hald, B. & Krogh, P. (1970). *Proc. 11th nordic vet. Congr.* *Bergen*, 279.
(4) Mirocha, C. J. *et al.* (1968). *Biotechnol. Bioengng*, *10*, 469.
(5) Roine, K. *et al.* (1971). *Nord. Vet.-Med.*, *23*, 628.
(6) Fisher, E. E. *et al.* (1967). *Nature (Lond.)*, *215*, 322.
(7) Kurmanov, I. A. (1968). *Veterinariya*, *9*, 53.
(8) Ogurtsov, A. F. & Kurmanov, I. A. (1969). *Trudÿ vses. Inst. Vet. Sanit.*, *27*, 142, 149.
(9) Kurmanov, I. A. (1970). *Trudÿ vses. Inst. Vet. Sanit.*, *36*, 34, 50.
(10) Kosuri, N. R. *et al.* (1971). *Amer. J. vet. Res.*, *32*, 1843.

Vulvovaginitis of Swine

Not infrequently oestrogens are produced by moulds on grain in sufficient concentration to cause signs when the grain is consumed. Among farm animals swine are most frequently affected, the syndrome being characterized by swelling of the vulva and prolapse of the vagina and caused by the feeding of mouldy barley or corn.

An oestrogenic substance is produced by *Fusarium graminearum* (*Giberella zea*) growing on barley (1) and other fungi also produce oestrogenic substances. All the female pigs exposed may be clinically affected and the mortality rate is high due to the secondary development of cystitis, uraemia and septicaemia.

Signs appear 3 to 6 days after feeding of the mouldy grain commences and disappear soon after the feeding is stopped. The basic lesion is an engorgement of the genital mucosa. Signs may appear in pigs of all ages including sucking pigs but are most common in gilts of 6 weeks to 7 months old. The vulva is swollen to 3 to 4 times normal size and the lips are oedematous and congested. These abnormalities extend only as far as the external urethral opening. There may be a thin catarrhal exudate from the vulva and moderate enlargement of the mammary glands. Prolapse of the vagina occurs commonly (up to 30 per cent of affected pigs) and prolapse of the rectum in some (5 to 10 per cent). In males there may be enlargement of the prepuce and enlargement and erythema of the rudimentary teats and mammary glands.

Necropsy findings are limited to engorgement of the genitalia, and vaginal prolapse and its complications. Assay of the feed for oestrogenic activity by feeding it to laboratory animals may be attempted. A high incidence of rectal and vaginal prolapse is also recorded in pigs fed stilboestrol as a feed additive. Outbreaks of rectal prolapse, without vaginal prolapse, occur in swine with diarrhoeic diseases.

Complete recovery follows when the feeding of the affected grain is stopped and no treatment other than surgical repair of the prolapsed organs is attempted.

REFERENCE

(1) McErlean, B. A. (1952). *Vet. Rec.*, *64*, 539.

Leuco-encephalomalacia of Horses

This is an afebrile, non-infectious disease of horses (1) and donkeys (2, 3) caused by the ingestion of mouldy corn grain. It occurs chiefly when a wet autumn permits heavy mould growth on the corn ears while it is standing in the field or when it is harvested and stored. Clinically it is manifested by muscle tremor and weakness, staggering, circling, inability to swallow and marked depression of consciousness. Jaundice may occur in some cases. Death occurs in 48 to 72 hours. At necropsy there are macroscopic areas of softening, accompanied by haemorrhages, in the white matter of the cerebral hemispheres. The disease has been produced experimentally by feeding mouldy corn grain on which *Fusarium moniliforme* was the predominant fungus (2) and the disease is generally considered to be a manifestation of *Fusarium* spp. poisoning.

REFERENCES

(1) Biester, H. E. *et al.* (1940). *Vet. Med.*, *35*, 636.
(2) Wilson, B. J. & Maronpot, R. R. (1971). *Vet. Rec.*, *88*, 484.
(3) Badiali, L. *et al.* (1968). *Amer. J. vet. Res.*, *29*, 2029.

Poisoning Caused by *Claviceps purpurea* (Ergot of Rye)

(*Ergotism*)

Poisoning caused by the ingestion of large quantities of the naturally occurring ergots of *Claviceps purpurea* is manifested by derangement of the central nervous system, constriction of arterioles and damage to capillary endothelium. Two distinct syndromes occur, one in which there is gangrene of the extremities and the other characterized by signs of central nervous system stimulation.

Incidence

Ergot of rye is widespread in its distribution but it is seldom that sufficient is ingested in its toxic stage to cause poisoning.

Aetiology

Claviceps purpurea is a fungus which under natural conditions infests cereal rye and less commonly other cereals, rye-grasses, tall fescue grass, timothy, cocksfoot, Yorkshire fog, crested dogstail and tall oat grasses and bulrush millet. It is harvested commercially for the manufacture of pharmaceutical ergot preparations. Ingestion of large quantities of seed heads infested with the fungus causes ergotism in cattle, sheep, pigs, horses, dogs and birds. The ergots contain a number of alkaloids and amines with pharmacological activity and these vary in concentration with the maturity of the ergot. There is some evidence that corn smut may have pharmacological activity similar to that of *Cl. purpurea*.

Occurrence

Ergotism occurs commonly only in cattle and usually in stall fed animals feeding on heavily contaminated grain over a considerable period of time. Other species are not usually exposed to the infested grain. Ergot-infested pasture may cause the disease (1). Cows may show early signs of lameness in as short a period as 10 days after going onto an infested pasture, but most animals do not become affected until 2 to 4 weeks after exposure.

Pathogenesis

The alkaloids of ergot, particularly ergotamine, cause central nervous system stimulation with the production of convulsions when taken in large amounts, and arteriolar spasm and capillary endothelial damage with restriction of the circulation and gangrene of the extremities when small amounts are taken over long periods. Chronic ergotism is much more common in animals because of the circumstances in which the disease occurs. In spite of the known abortifacient action of *Cl. purpurea*, abortion does not usually occur in poisoned animals.

The experimental feeding of ergots (1 to 2 per cent of ration) caused severe reduction in feed intake and growth rate in young pigs without producing overt signs of ergotism (2).

Clinical Findings

Chronic ergotism. The extremities, particularly the lower part of the hind limbs, the tail and ears are affected. There are reddening, swelling, coldness and lack of sensation of the parts initially, followed by the development of a blue-black colour, dryness of the skin and its separation from normal tissues. The gangrene usually affects all local tissues and after the lapse of some days the affected part becomes obviously separated and may eventually slough. The lesions are not painful but some lameness is evident even in the early stages and the animal may remain recumbent most of the time. Severe diarrhoea is often an accompanying sign. Although the gangrenous form of the disease is most common in cattle acute poisoning with nervous signs has been recorded (3).

Long-term low-level feeding of ergot to fattening beef cattle can result in reduced feed intake and weight gain, increased water intake and urination, failure to shed winter coat and increased susceptibility to heat stress (10).

In sheep under experimental conditions there is no gangrene of the limbs but ulceration and necrosis occur on the tongue, and the mucosae of the pharynx, rumen, abomasum and small intestine. In pigs the chronic syndrome is manifested by lack of udder development and agalactia in sows and the birth of small pigs which suffer a heavy neonatal mortality. A specific ergot, *Claviceps fusiformis*, which grows on bulrush millet (*Pennisetum typhoides*), is known to be a cause of agalactia in sows in Rhodesia (4).

Acute ergotism. Convulsive episodes are the major manifestations of this form of the disease but may be preceded by signs of nervous depression (5). These signs, which may be transient, include drowsiness, staggering and a tendency to fall. There may be intermittent blindness and deafness and the skin may also show alternating periods of increased and decreased sensitivity. In mild cases these may be the only signs observed but in severe cases they are followed by convulsions which are usually generalized but may be restricted to one limb or other part of the body. The generalized convulsions are epileptiform in type, are followed by temporary paralysis and coma, and appear to cause pain, the animals crying out during the period of muscular activity.

Apparent recovery may occur between convulsions but there is usually cardiac irregularity, and diarrhoea and vomiting occurs in some species. The appetite is often good, although some animals show pharyngeal paralysis and eating may precipitate a convulsion. The course of the disease is very irregular, some animals dying during the first convulsions and others only after several days. Some animals persist in a state of chronic ill-health for several months. Gangrene of the extremities may occur in this form of the disease.

Clinical Pathology

Samples of fungus-infested material may be submitted for assay or test feeding.

Necropsy Findings

Gangrene of the extremities is the principal gross lesion. There may be evidence of congestion, arteriolar spasm and capillary endothelial degeneration in the vicinity of the gross lesions and in the central nervous system. Ulceration and necrosis of the oral, pharyngeal, ruminal and intestinal mucosae are recorded in sheep.

Diagnosis

Gangrene of the extremities may occur after trauma or exposure to extreme cold or possibly, in calves, following infection with *Salmonella* spp. (9). The nervous signs of the acute form, which is rare in farm animals, are not diagnostic and may be confused with those of many other diseases in which convulsions occur. A number of poisonous fungi produce similar nervous signs as does poisoning with nematode larvae which infest the seedheads of some grasses. The galls produced by the larvae are not unlike the sclerotia of ergot but are much harder in consistency (6). A high prevalence of this disease has been recorded in sheep and cattle grazing mature Wimmera rye grass (*Lolium rigidum*) in which the seeds were heavily infected with nematodes and bacteria. The clinical syndrome seen naturally, and produced experimentally, includes inco-ordination, abortion, multiple haemorrhages and death (7). The inco-ordination, collapse and tetanic convulsions which occur on driving are reminiscent of poisoning with perennial rye-grass (*L. perenne*). The disease has been recorded widely in Australia and the nematode has been identified as *Anguina* sp. accompanied by a bacterium, *Corynebacterium* sp. (8).

Treatment

Treatment is not usually attempted although vasodilator drugs may have some beneficial effect. The infested grain should be withdrawn from the ration immediately.

Control

Heavily ergotized grain or pasture fields containing ergotized grasses should not be used for animal feeding. Pasture fields may be grazed if the seed-heads are mowed with the mower blade set high.

REFERENCES

(1) Woods, A. J. et al. (1966). *Vet. Rec.*, 78, 742.
(2) Friend, D. W. & MacIntyre, T. M. (1970). *Canad. J. comp. Med.*, 34, 198.
(3) Dillon, B. E. (1955). *J. Amer. vet. med. Ass.*, 126, 136.
(4) Loveless, A. R. (1967). *Trans. Brit. mycol. Soc.*, 50, 18.
(5) Guilhon, J. (1955). *Rev. Path. gen.*, 55, 1467.
(6) Galloway, J. H. (1961). *J. Amer. vet. med. Ass.*, 139, 1212.
(7) McIntosh, G. H. et al. (1967). *Aust. vet. J.*, 43, 349.
(8) Gwynn, R. & Hadlow, A. J. (1971). *Aust. vet. J.*, 47, 408.
(9) O'Connor, P. J. et al. (1972). *Vet. Rec.*, 91, 459.
(10) Dinnusson, W. E. et al. (1971). *N. Dak. Fm Res.*, 29, 20.

Poisoning Caused by *Claviceps paspali* (Ergot of Paspalum or Dallas Grass)

Claviceps paspali is an ergot which parasitizes paspalum or dallas grass (*Paspalum dilatatum*), Argentine bahia grass (*Paspalum notatum*) and water-couch grass (*P. distichum*). The degree of infestation of pastures varies widely with climatic conditions, being heaviest after wet, humid summers. Outbreaks of the disease occur in winter when animals at pasture graze the seed-heads because of a shortage of other feed. The ergots are most toxic when they are passing from the sticky 'honey-dew' (sphacelial) stage to the hard, black (sclerotical) stage. Illness can occur when mature ergots are eaten but the disease is not so severe. Cattle are most commonly affected but sheep and horses are less susceptible (1). A very similar syndrome is produced by *Claviceps cinerea* (2). The husk of the seeds of *Paspalum scrobiculatum*, when fed to buffalo calves, causes severe tremors without other signs of ergotism (3).

The clinical signs are all manifestations of nervous system derangement. There is hypersensitivity to noise or movement but not to touch. Muscle tremor is at first only noticeable on exercise but is later continuous, even at rest, and is sufficiently severe to cause shaking of the limbs and trunk and nodding of the head. Involuntary movements may prevent grazing. There is a severe ataxia with gross inco-ordination of movement, sideways progression and frequent falling into unusual postures. Animals which fall paddle violently in attempts to rise. After a period of rest they can usually rise unassisted.

The appetite is always unaffected but there may be scouring, salivation and some loss of condition. Abortion does not occur. Some deaths are caused by misadventure but recovery occurs quickly in most cases if the animals are removed from affected pastures. At necropsy there are no gross changes, except for some increase in cerebro-spinal fluid volume, and histological examinations are negative. No treatment is necessary but live-stock should be removed from the affected pasture, which may, however, be used by permitting only intermittent grazing or after mowing and raking of the seed-heads.

REFERENCES

(1) Ehret, W. J. et al. (1968). J. S. Afr. vet. med. Ass., 39, 103.
(2) Dollahite, J. W. (1963). SWest. Vet., 16, 295.
(3) Gupta, I. & Bhide, N. K. (1967). Indian vet. J., 44, 787.

Poisoning Caused by the Fungus
Pithomyces chartarum (Sporidesmium bakeri)
(Facial Eczema)

Facial eczema is a disease characterized by hepatitis and photosensitization in sheep and cattle, caused by the ingestion of a fungus which grows on dead and damaged plant material in pasture.

Incidence

The disease has been recorded most commonly in New Zealand and occurs to a limited extent also in Australia. The incidence varies widely depending on climatic conditions; in some years the disease does not occur, in others the morbidity rate in affected flocks of sheep may be 70 to 80 per cent and 5 to 50 per cent of these may die (1). In cattle the morbidity rate is much lower and rarely exceeds 50 per cent.

Aetiology

Facial eczema is caused by a hepatoxic agent—sporidesmin—present in the fungus Pithomyces chartarum (Sporidesmium bakeri) which infests dead plant material on pastures. Sporidesmin has been isolated and identified as a resinous sub-stance. The environmental factors which encour-age the growth of the fungus and the production of sporidesmin have been accurately determined. Although the disease is commonly associated with rye-grass pastures, the causative fungus is capable of growing on all kinds of dead leaf material and facial eczema has been observed in sheep fed on cereal hay which was heavily infested with P. chartarum (2).

Of the farm animals only sheep and cattle are affected.

Occurrence

Facial eczema occurs extensively only when pas-ture is short and contains recently killed plant material in abundance, and under climatic condi-tions, warm, humid weather, which favour a heavy infestation with the fungus. This is most likely to be a problem in autumn when the summer has been hot and dry, the pasture well eaten back and good rains fall when the ground is still warm. In such circumstances the grass and the fungus grow rapidly. This is a different set of conditions to those which favour the appearance of rye-grass staggers, the other disease occurring on this type of pasture, and the two diseases are not usually seen together.

Pathogenesis

Sporidesmin causes acute toxipathic hepatitis and biliary obstruction and a resulting severe hepatic insufficiency manifested by loss of condi-tion, obstructive jaundice and photosensitization (3, 4). Sporidesmin administered by mouth is excreted unchanged in high concentrations in urine and bile, especially the latter where it reaches 100 times the concentration in serum (5). The resulting inflammation of the bile ducts and progressive obliterative cholangiolitis slow down the rate of bile flow to negligible levels over a period of about 14 days (6). The photodynamic agent is phyllo-erythrin, a normal metabolic product of chloro-phyll, which is retained in tissues because of failure of its excretion through the damaged liver and bile ducts. The frequent observation that only part of the liver is involved is probably explained by the deposition of toxin in particular parts of the liver, due to portal streaming, on its first passage through hepatic sinusoids: the toxin which reaches the general circulation is probably destroyed.

Clinical Findings

In cattle and sheep the disease starts suddenly with the appearance of lethargy, dullness, ano-rexia, jaundice and photosensitive dermatitis. The skin lesion and jaundice are both variable in occurrence and sheep may die without either hav-ing been observed. Many animals die during this acute stage but some survive and pass into a state of chronic ill-health manifested by poor bodily condition and a susceptibility to minor environ-mental stresses. A moderate fall in the plane of nutrition, parasitic infestation and pregnancy may cause further mortalities, and photosensitive dermatitis may recur if the animals are fed on lush green pasture. Cattle are not as commonly affected by the chronic form of the disease as are sheep but dermatitis of the teats may lead to the development of mastitis. Details of the clinical findings in photosensitive dermatitis are given under the head-ing of photosensitization.

Clinical Pathology

Tests of hepatic function and serum transaminase tests should be of value in determining the presence of hepatic insufficiency.

Necropsy Findings

In the acute stages of facial eczema there is jaundice and a swollen, mottled liver with thickened bile-duct walls. In the chronic phase there is extensive hepatic fibrosis, the liver is tough and contracted and the left lobe is almost completely atrophic. Areas of regeneration are usually apparent macroscopically. Histologically there is perilobular fibrosis with obliteration of the bile ducts and pressure atrophy of hepatic cells. The changes are much more marked in the left than the right lobe.

Diagnosis

Facial eczema must be differentiated from those other diseases in which photosensitization and hepatitis occur. It bears a marked resemblance to a disease of cattle of southern U.S.A. believed to be caused by the ingestion of dead forage on which a fungus (*Periconia* spp.) is growing.

Treatment

General, supportive treatment for hepatitis and photosensitization, as outlined under those headings, and the administration of antibiotics and antihistamines to control secondary infection and shock may be applicable in animals of sufficient economic value.

Control

One of the major difficulties in the control of the disease is that of predicting the occurrence of an outbreak. Meteorological observation can be of value but the counting of spores by a mobile spore catcher is now routinely used in danger areas.

In bad seasons the incidence of facial eczema can be reduced by alternating grazing between native and improved pastures or by reducing the intake of the fungus in any other way. Because of the proclivity of the fungus for dead grass two acceptable management procedures for prevention are summer irrigation and hard grazing, both of which reduce the amount of foliar substrate available for fungal growth. Avoidance of sandy soils in bad seasons is also advisable because of the greater tendency for grass death on this kind of soil. Allowing pasture to flower, the sward to grow long, the pasture to be damaged by diseases and

pests, and frequent mowing, encourage facial eczema (7).

The application of a fungistatic agent to pasture to limit the growth of toxic fungi has received attention. Thiabendazole (one spraying in January at 113 g. per acre), Belnate (same application) controlled the development of facial eczema in New Zealand (8, 9) and Benomyl controls *P. chartarum* growth (10).

REFERENCES

(1) Clare, N. T. (1952). *Photosensitization in Diseases of Domestic Animals.* Farnham Royal, England: Commonwealth Agriculture Bureaux.
(2) Gardiner, M. R. & Nairn, M. (1962). *J. Dept. Agric. W. Aust.*, *3*, 85, 90.
(3) Leaver, D. D. (1968). *Res. vet. Sci.*, *9*, 255, 265.
(4) Mortimer, P. H. (1963). *Res. vet. Sci.*, *4*, 166.
(5) Mortimer, P. H. & Stanbridge, T. A. (1968). *J. comp. Path.*, *78*, 505.
(6) Mortimer, P. H. & Stanbridge, T. A. (1969). *J. comp. Path.*, *79*, 267.
(7) Brook, P. J. & Mutch, G. C. (1964). *N.Z. J. agric. Res.*, *7*, 138.
(8) Sinclair, D. P. & Howe, M. W. (1969). *N.Z. J. agric. Res.*, *11*, 59.
(9) Parle, J. M. & di Menna, M. E. (1972). *N.Z. J. agric. Res.*, *15*, 48, 54, 64.
(10) McKenzie, E. H. C. (1971). *N.Z. J. agric. Res.*, *14*, 379.

Aflatoxicosis

A restricted number of strains of *Aspergillus* spp. produce a series of hepatoxins, the aflatoxins, of which aflatoxin B_1 is the most important. The first observed and most common source of the toxin was groundnuts infested by *A. flavus* but cotton seed meal (1, 2), sorghum grain (3, 4) and corn can also be sources. All animal species are susceptible. The toxigenicity of 392 strains of *Aspergillus* spp. has been determined (5). A carcinogen, aflatoxin M_1, has also been identified (6). *A. clavatus* has produced similar effects to *A. flavus* in cattle (7) but *A. fumigatus* administered to sheep has produced erosive mucosal lesions and renal cortical necrosis (8).

The aflatoxins are not related to the pyrrolizidine alkaloids but produce almost identical effects. Aflatoxin B_1 has been isolated and its toxic properties accurately calibrated. At a dose rate of 4 mg. per kg. to wethers death occurs at 15 to 18 hours due to acute hepatic insufficiency; at dose rates of 2 mg. per kg. there is increased respiratory rate, a rise in temperature of $1.5°C$ and diarrhoea with blood and mucus; at a dose rate of 0.23 mg. per kg. there is anorexia and diarrhoea (9). Similar dose relationships have been established for calves (10) and for pigs (17).

In cattle the clinical signs include blindness,

walking in circles, frequent falling, ear-twitching, teeth grinding, diarrhoea, severe tenesmus and anal prolapse. Terminally there are convulsions, and abortion is common. Affected animals usually die within 48 hours, calves in the 3 to 6 months group being most susceptible (11, 12). Aflatoxicosis is also reputed to interfere with clotting of the blood in cattle leading to the development of haematomas (3). Amounts of toxin insufficient to cause overt disease in cows may be sufficient to reduce food intake, weight gains, and milk production (13).

In pigs the period between when the toxin is ingested and when signs appear is thought to be quite long, at least 6 weeks, and varies with the toxicity of the batch of feed (14). In pigs a pronounced lower enterocolitis with diarrhoea and dysentery is common. Abortion is a commonly reported sequel but there is doubt about the relationship (4, 15). Also described in pigs after feeding on *A. flavus* is a syndrome of depression, fever, reduced liver function and marked elevation of serum GOT and OCT levels (16). At necropsy there is icterus, ascites, swelling of the liver, and mesenteric oedema.

Another toxin (ochratoxin A) has been isolated from *A. ochraceus* and is thought to cause foetal death and resorption in cattle (18).

The aflotoxin level in corn can be markedly reduced by treatment with ammonia.

REFERENCES

(1) Hald, B. & Krogh, P. (1970). *Nord. Vet.-Med.*, *22*, 39.
(2) Loosmore, R. M. *et al.* (1964). *Vet. Rec.*, *76*, 64.
(3) Aust, S. D. (1964). *Illinois vet.*, 7, 10.
(4) Connole, M. D. & Hill, M. W. M. (1970). *Aust. vet. J.*, *46*, 503.
(5) Semeniuk, G. *et al.* (1971). *Mycopath. Mycol. appl.*, *43*, 137.
(6) Stoloff, L. *et al.* (1971). *Food Cosmet. Toxicol.*, *9*, 839.
(7) Abadjieff, W. *et al.* (1966). *Mh. Vet.-Med.*, *21*, 452.
(8) Thornton, R. H. *et al.* (1968). *N.Z. J. agric. Res.*, *11*, 1.
(9) Armbrecht, B. H. *et al.* (1970). *Nature (Lond.)*, *225*, 1062.
(10) Lynch, G. P. *et al.* (1970). *J. Dairy Sci.*, *53*, 63; *54*, 1688.
(11) Allcroft, R. & Lewis, G. (1963). *Vet. Rec.*, *75*, 487, 493.
(12) Kremlev, E. D. (1970). *Veterinariya*, *10*, 83.
(13) Duthie, I. F. *et al.* (1966). *Vet. Rec.*, *79*, 621.
(14) Loosmore, R. M. & Harding, J. D. J. (1961). *Vet. Rec.*, *73*, 1362.
(15) Blevins, D. L. *et al.* (1969). *J. Amer. vet. med. Ass.*, *154*, 1043.
(16) Cysewski, S. J. *et al.* (1968). *Amer. J. vet. Res.*, *29*, 1577, 1591.
(17) Duthie, I. F. *et al.* (1968). *Vet. Rec.*, *82*, 427.
(18) Still, P. F. *et al.* (1971). *Nature (Lond.)*, *234*, 563.

Myrotheciotoxicosis

Myrothecium spp. are fungi isolatable from growing rye-grass and white clover plants and from stored roughages.

Experimental oral dosing of cultured fungus to calves and sheep caused death in 24 hours with haemorrhages in the alimentary tract, especially the abomasum, hepatitis and pulmonary congestion and oedema. With smaller doses the same signs and lesions were produced but the course was 7 to 10 days before death. Very small doses for 30 days caused weight loss and growth retardation in lambs without histological lesions (1).

The principal toxic species are *M. roridum* and *M. verrucaria* and their toxins have been identified (2).

REFERENCES

(1) Menna, M. E. di. & Mortimer, P. H. (1971). *N.Z. vet. J.*, *19*, 246.
(2) Mortimer, P. H. *et al.* (1971). *Res. vet. Sci.*, *12*, 508.

Stachybotrytoxicosis

Forage moulded by *Stachybotrys alternans* produces the disease known as stachybotrytoxicosis, a favourite subject in Russian literature (1). Horses, cattle, sheep and pigs may be affected and the disease is characterized by fever, ruminalatony, diarrhoea, necrotic ulceration of the mucosae and skin, haemorrhages into tissue and agranulocytosis (2, 3, 4). The important lesion appears to be depression of leucocyte formation which produces a disease not unlike that caused by bracken poisoning in cattle (5).

REFERENCES

(1) Spesiwzewa, N. A. (1963). *Proc. 17th Wld vet. Congr. Hanover*, *1*, 305.
(2) Izmailov, I. A. & Moroshkin, B. F. (1962). *Veterinariya*, 4, 27.
(3) Stankushev, K. *et al.* (1965). *Vet.-Med. Nauk., Sof.*, *2*, 11.
(4) Szabo, I. & Szeky, A. (1970). *Magy Allatorv. Lap.*, *25*, 633.
(5) Moroshkin, B. F. *et al.* (1954). *Veterinariya*, *41*, 98.

Poisoning by *Rhizoctonia leguminicola*

Profuse salivation is a characteristic sign produced by the ingestion (1) or experimental dosing (2) of the fungus *Rhizoctonia leguminicola* in cattle and goats. Anorexia and diarrhoea also occur. The salivation is at its peak at 5 to 6 hours after ingestion and disappears at about 24 hours.

The fungus infests clover hay.

REFERENCES

(1) Crump, M. H. *et al.* (1967). *Amer. J. vet. Res.*, *28*, 871.
(2) Isawa, K. *et al.* (1971). *Bull. natn. Inst. Anim. Ind., Summaries*, *24*, 10.

Poisoning by *Penicillium* spp.

Penicillium spp. fungi are known to produce toxins with serious effects on animals (1). An extract of *P. rubrum* causes frothing at the mouth, champing of the teeth, jaundice, cutaneous erythema and collapse in goats and pigs; in experimental horses inco-ordination, clonic spasms, jaundice, diarrhoea, abdominal pain and vomiting are produced. *P. islandicum* is known to cause hepatic necrosis in rats (2). *Penicillium* spp. are also associated with haemorrhagic syndromes in birds (3). *P. viridicatum* has been isolated from barley fed to pigs which developed chronic renal degenerative disease and was thought to be the cause (4). Nephropathy and oedema have been produced experimentally in miniature swine by feeding cultures of this fungus (6). *P. cyclopium* and *P. frequentans* produce toxins capable of causing renal or hepatic lesions in experimental animals (5). *P. palitans* is reported to produce a tremorgen causing marked nervous signs of ataxia and convulsions in mice; the fungus has been associated with deaths in cattle (7).

REFERENCES

(1) Burnside, J. E. *et al.* (1957). *Amer. J. vet. Res.*, *18*, 817.
(2) Payne, J. B. & Newberne, P. M. (1967). *Proc. 70th ann. gen. Mtg U.S. Live Stock sanit. Ass., Buffalo*, 554.
(3) Mirocha, C. J. *et al.* (1968). *Biotechnol. Bioengng*, *10*, 469.
(4) Krogh, P. *et al.* (1970). *Proc. 11th nordic vet. Congr., Bergen*, 280.
(5) Carlton, W. W. & Tuite, J. (1971). *Toxicol. appl. Pharmac.*, *20*, 538.
(6) Carlton, W. W. & Tuite, J. (1970). *Pathologia vet.*, *7*, 68.
(7) Ciegler, A. (1969). *Appl. Microbiol.*, *18*, 128.

Poisoning caused by Other Miscellaneous Fungi

A number of aberrations of reproductive function in animals are caused by fungal intoxications. The production of oestrogenic substances by *Fusarium* spp. fungi has been described above. White clover does not normally contain oestrogens but when heavily infested with fungi it may contain significant amounts (1). Barley smut fungus (*Ustilago hordei*) is thought to be toxic to farm animals; feeding it to experimental animals has caused infertility and stillbirths (2). In south-eastern Australia a common infertility–abortion–mummified foetus syndrome has been ascribed to an onion-like weed, *Romulea rosea*. There is now a suspicion that the disease may be due to a toxin produced by a fungus, *Helminthosporium biseptatum*, growing on the weed (3).

A fungus, *Periconia* sp., which grows on forage in the field is also suspected of causing hepatic damage and photosensitization in cattle in the southern U.S.A. (4): there is a close resemblance in clinical signs and circumstances of occurrence to facial eczema and myrotheciotoxicosis.

Ngaione, a hepatotoxic ketone, is found in sweet potato tubers infested with black rot due to the fungus *Ceratostomella fimbriata* (5). Three other toxins have been isolated from sweet potatoes infested by fungi, especially *Fusarium javanicum*, which caused serious mortality when fed to beef cattle (6). The toxins were present in tubers with only minor blemishes. One of the toxins produces pulmonary oedema and respiratory distress, another is a specific hepatotoxin; renal lesions are also produced. The respiratory form of the disease has been produced experimentally by feeding sweet potatoes and the mould (13).

Phomopsis leptostromiformis has been found as a fungal infection of lupins causing lupinosis in sheep (7). Typical hepatic injury was produced experimentally by feeding sheep on pure cultures of the fungus. *P. rossiana* has been similarly identified (12).

Nervous signs predominate in the toxic effects ascribed to the ingestion of *Trichothecium roseum* (8). Sterigmatocystin is a fungal toxin capable of causing hepatic carcinoma. It has been isolated from *Bipolaris* spp. (9) and *Aspergillus nidulans* (10) growing on groundnuts.

Dendrochium toxicum is reported to produce a great variety of disorders when fed to pigs (11). A haemorrhagic diathesis, a thrombocytopenia, leucocytosis and necrotic, ulcerative and degenerative lesions in viscera are only some of the effects.

REFERENCES

(1) Wong, E. *et al.* (1971). *N.Z. J. agric. Res.*, *14*, 633.
(2) Ibragimov, Kh.Z. & Khabiev, M. S. (1970). *Veterinariya*, *8*, 77.
(3) Fisher, E. E. & Finnie, E. P. (1967). *Nature (Lond.)*, *215*, 1276.
(4) Kidder, R. W. *et al.* (1961). *Fla agric. Exp. Stn Bull.*, *630*, 21.
(5) Denz, F. A. & Hanger, W. G. (1961). *J. Path. Bact.*, *81*, 91.
(6) Wilson, B. J. *et al.* (1970). *Nature (Lond.)*, *227*, 521.
(7) van Warmelo, K. T. *et al.* (1970). *J. S. Afr. vet med. Ass.*, *4*, 235.
(8) Richard, J. L. *et al.* (1969). *Mycopath. Mycol. appl.*, *38*, 313.
(9) Purchase, I. F. H. & van der Watt, J. J. (1969). *Fd Cosmet. Toxicol.*, *7*, 135.
(10) Holzapfel, *et al.* (1966). *S. Afr. med. J.*, *40*, 1100.
(11) Stepushin, E. A. & Chernov, K. S. (1969). *Veterinariya*, *7*, 60, 62.
(12) Gardiner, M. R. & Petterson, D. S. (1972). *J. comp. Path.*, *82*, 5.
(13) Peckham, J. C. *et al.* (1972). *J. Amer. vet. med. Ass.*, *160*, 2, 169.

Mushroom and Toadstool Poisoning

Reports of poisoning caused by mushrooms and toadstools in animals are rare. *Amanita verna* has been shown to cause fatal poisoning in cattle (1) but large quantities must be eaten before toxic effects occur. Severe pain at defaecation and matting of the perianal region with faeces is caused by vesicular and necrotic eruption about the anus and vulva (1, 2). At necropsy there is severe inflammation of the alimentary mucosa.

A large cauliflower-like toadstool (*Ramaria* sp.) is credited with causing death in cattle (3). Clinical signs include salivation, mucosal erosions, ocular lesions, abortion and anorexia. Similar signs plus loosening of the hair and hooves and nervous signs have been observed in sheep and cattle and attributed to consumption of fungi of genus *Clavaria* (4).

REFERENCES

(1) Piercy, P. L. *et al.* (1944). *J. Amer. vet. med. Ass.*, *105*, 206.
(2) Burton, H. A. (1944). *Vet. Med.*, *39*, 290.
(3) Bauer, A. G. *et al.* (1966). *Arch. Inst. Pesq. vet. Desiderio Finamor*, *3*, 85.
(4) de Freitas, J. *et al.* (1967). *Proc. 5th panam. Congr. vet. med. Zootech.*, (*Caracas 1966*), *2*, 818.

Ferns

Bracken Fern *(Pteridium aquilina)* Poisoning

Bracken fern poisoning in horses and pigs causes a conditioned thiamine deficiency and has been described under that heading (p. 771). In ruminants the defect is one of depression of bone marrow activity with pancytopenia expressed primarily as ecchymotic haemorrhages and often followed by bacterial invasion of tissues. There is also a relationship between bracken and the disease enzootic haematuria which is discussed under that heading. Benign adenomatous polyps have also been produced in the small intestine of rats fed high levels of bracken for long periods (1).

Incidence

Bracken fern poisoning occurs in most countries as a sporadic disease. The disease is highly fatal in cattle. Although the losses due to the disease are usually small because of the high intake of the fern required to produce illness, heavy mortalities have been observed in some outbreaks.

Aetiology

The toxic factor in bracken fern which causes poisoning in ruminants has not been identified. Thiaminase or toxopyrimidine administered to cattle do not produce the disease and thiamine, vitamin B_{12} and folic acid do not prevent the occurrence of the disease (1). Most field outbreaks of the disease occur in cattle but it can be produced in sheep by feeding bracken fern over a much longer period and natural outbreaks have been recorded (2). Large amounts of bracken fern must be eaten before poisoning occurs but the toxicity of the plant varies with the stage of growth, younger plants being more toxic. The underground stems (rhizomes) of the fern also contain the toxic principle, in approximately five times the concentration of that found in the fronds, and have been used to produce the disease experimentally in cattle (3). Cattle allowed access to recently ploughed fields of bracken eat the rhizomes avidly and may suffer heavy mortalities.

Occurrence

Animals do not eat bracken fern readily but samples of meadow hay may contain toxic amounts and animals at pasture may eat large quantities, especially when young, green fronds appear after drought or burning off or when other forage is sparse. Bracken used as bedding may also be ingested in dangerous amounts by animals with a poor nutritive status. The toxin is excreted in the milk in significant quantity (4).

Pathogenesis

Bracken fern poisoning in ruminants is caused by the depression of bone marrow activity, an increased capillary fragility, prolonged bleeding time and defective clot retraction but with normal clotting and prothrombin times. The clotting defect in calves appears to be due to the formation of heparinoid substances and the presence of toxic amines in the blood.

In the bone marrow the myeloid cells are particularly affected leading to a severe reduction in blood platelets and granular leucocytes. The erythrocyte series in bone marrow is affected but only in the terminal stages. It has been suggested that haemorrhage into the alimentary mucosa or submucosa occurs as the result of the thrombocytopenia and ulcers develop at these haemorrhage sites. Bacterial invasion follows and the resulting bacteraemia may cause infarction in the liver if small vessels are blocked by clumps of bacteria, or the organisms may be carried into the systemic circulation and cause infarction in other organs including the kidneys, lungs and heart.

The capillary fragility, intestinal ulceration and laryngeal oedema which occur in some cases are thought to be due to damage to tissue mast cells and the liberation of histamine.

Clinical Findings

Signs characteristic of bracken fern poisoning may not appear in cattle until there has been access to bracken for from 2 to 8 weeks. Initially there is loss of condition and dryness and slackness of the skin. Clinical signs occur suddenly and include high fever (40·5 to 43°C or 105 to 109°F), dysentery or melaena, bleeding from the nose, eyes and vagina, and drooling of saliva. Nasolabial ulcers and haematuria may be observed. Petechial and ecchymotic haemorrhages may be visible under mucosae and skin and in the anterior chamber of the eye. An increase in respiratory and heart rates occurs at this stage. Death usually follows in 1 to 3 days.

Cattle may continue to become ill for up to 6 weeks after being taken off the bracken fern. Calves 2 to 4 months of age show essentially the same clinical and necropsy picture as adult animals except that marked bradycardia and death from heart failure are common, and a laryngitic form, with marked dyspnoea due to laryngeal oedema, is not uncommon. Although only a few animals in a group are affected most of those showing clinical signs die.

A syndrome known as 'bright-blindness' in sheep has been observed to occur on pastures heavily infested with bracken and the disease has been produced experimentally in sheep fed bracken nuts (5, 6, 7). Affected sheep are blind, the pupils are dilated and show a poor light reflex and on ophthalmoscopic examination there is retinal degeneration. This degeneration may be observable in many more sheep than those clinically blind. Affected sheep are always more than 18 months old. The number of sheep affected is increasing and there is concern that the cause should be positively identified. An association between blindness and leucopenia (a hallmark of bracken poisoning) has been established but little else.

A carcinogenic action has also been ascribed to bracken because of the high incidence of malignant adenocarcinoma in the ileum of sheep and rats on diets high in bracken (8, 1). Many of the signs and lesions of enzootic haematruia have been produced by the prolonged feeding of bracken (9) but the role of bracken in the aetiology of this disease is unknown.

Clinical Pathology

Estimations of the occurrence of platelets in blood smears appear to be the most valuable laboratory test in diagnosis and prognosis of the disease. Platelet counts fall gradually from normals of about 500,000 per cmm. to about 40,000 per cmm. just before death. Total leucocyte levels fall gradually at first and then precipitously to about 1000 per cmm. in the terminal stages. Polymorphonuclear leucocytes are the most profoundly depressed and often none are visible in a smear.

Haematological changes may not be sufficiently marked to enable prophylactic treatment to be undertaken in clinically normal animals.

Bone marrow biopsy is valuable as an indication of the status of the platelet and granulocyte series. Increase in capillary fragility is detectable and defective clot retraction is also a feature of this disease. A fall in erythrocyte count and haemoglobin content may be detectable in the late stages. Depression of erythropoiesis is more marked in sheep than in cattle (10). Urine examination may reveal the presence of erythrocytes and many epithelial cells.

Necropsy Findings

Death is due to the combined effects of multiple internal haemorrhages and bacteraemia. Multiple haemorrhages, varying in size from petechiae to large extravasations occur in all tissues. In some organs, particularly the alimentary tract, necrosis and sloughing occur over the haemorrhages. Areas of oedema are also common in the gut wall. The bone marrow is paler than normal. Multiple small, pale or red areas representing infarcts and areas of necrosis are present in the liver, kidney and lungs.

Diagnosis

Bracken fern poisoning may be readily confused with many of the acute septicaemias of cattle, including anthrax, blackleg, septicaemic pasteurellosis and leptospirosis, but bacteriological findings are negative for these specific infections except for the occasional occurrence of a pasteurella septicaemia. Haemorrhages are not a common finding in babesiasis and anaplasmosis and the causative protozoa can usually be demonstrated. Exposure to a high intake of bracken fern is usually sufficient reason for a presumptive diagnosis of poisoning when the characteristic lesions are present.

Several other poisonings including sweet clover and some moulds produce similar lesions and signs to those caused by bracken fern but there is no fever or leucopenia. Trichloroethylene-extracted soyabean meal causes aplasia of bone marrow and produces a syndrome indistinguishable on clinical, haematological and necropsy grounds from that produced by bracken fern. The clinical, pathological and haematological findings also closely resemble those of radiation sickness.

Treatment

DL-batyl alcohol, a known bone-marrow stimulant, has been recommended as a treatment but has not always been successful (11). It should be combined with an antibiotic. One g. of the alcohol is injected intravenously or subcutaneously daily for 4 to 5 days. Treatment is not likely to be successful in advanced cases when the leucocyte count is below 2000 per cmm. and the platelet count is less than 50,000 to 100,000 per cmm. because of the effects of secondary bacterial invasion and haemorrhage.

Additional supportive treatment may include blood transfusions in those animals in which serious depression of erythrocyte and leucocyte counts have occurred. The transfusions should be large and 4·5 litres is considered to be a minimum dose in adult cattle.

Control

Fields containing large quantities of bracken fern should not be harvested for hay, and animals forced to graze affected areas should be supplied with a supplementary diet when the pasture is short.

REFERENCES

(1) Schacham, P. *et al.* (1970). *Amer. J. vet. Res.*, *31*, 191.
(2) Parker, W. H. & McCrea, C. T. (1965). *Vet. Rec.*, *77*, 861.
(3) Evans, W. C. *et al.* (1961). *Vet. Rec.*, *73*, 852.
(4) Evans, I. A. *et al.* (1972). *Nature* (*Lond.*), *237*, 107.
(5) Watson, W. A. *et al.* (1972). *Vet. Rec.*, *91*, 665.
(6) Watson, W. A. & Barnett, K. C. (1970). *Brit. vet. J.*, *126*, 482.
(7) Barnett, K. C. & Watson, W. A. (1970). *Res. vet. Sci.*, *11*, 287.
(8) Evans, I. A. & Mason, J. (1965). *Nature* (*Lond.*), *208*, 913.
(9) Rosenberger, G. (1965). *Wien. tierärztl. Mschr.*, *52*, 415.
(10) Moon, F. E. & McKeand, J. M. (1953). *Brit. vet. J.*, *109*, 321.
(11) Dalton, R. G. (1964). *Vet. Rec.*, *76*, 411.

Poisoning Caused by Miscellaneous Ferns

HORSETAIL (*Equisetum* spp.)

This plant contains thiaminase and causes a syndrome of thiamine deficiency in horses which is described under that heading.

BURRAWANG PALM (*Macrozamia* spp.)

The leaves of plants of this species cause inco-ordination of the hindquarters when eaten. Many members of the species are toxic, particularly the young shoots of *Macrozamia spiralis*, *Zamia integrifolia* and *Z. media*, and *Cycas* and *Bowenia* spp. (1). Initial signs include uncontrolled extension and flexion of the hind-limbs, the hindquarters tending to sag or sway when moving. In the early stages over extension of the lower joints gives rise to a 'goose-stepping gait', and this is followed in the later stages by flexion of the fetlocks and walking on the anterior aspect of the foot. The gait worsens with exercise and the hindquarters sag or sway, the animal either falling or dragging itself along on its forelegs with the hind-legs trailing behind. Some recovery occurs if ingestion ceases but is never complete. The experimental feeding of leaves of *Bowenia serrulata* and *Macrozamia lucida* to cattle produced degenerative lesions in the nerve fibres of the fasciculus gracilis and dorsal spinocerebellar pathways. Similar lesions are found in natural cases (5). Cattle and sheep are affected and cattle may show some addiction to the plant particularly when other forage is not available.

The seeds of this plant contain a toxic alkaloid, macrozamin, which has caused gastroenteritis and jaundice in sheep. Experimental feeding with the nuts has caused hepatic cirrhosis, proliferative gastroenteritis, myocarditis, pancreatitis, pneumonitis and arteriosclerosis in pigs, cattle, horses (2, 3) and sheep (4).

GRASS TREE
(*Xanthorrhoea hastile* syn. *X. resinosa*)

Ingestion of the flower spikes of this plant causes poisoning in cattle and there is some evidence that a dietary deficiency of phosphorus predisposes to the disease. In some cases the appearance of clinical signs may be delayed for 2 or 3 weeks after consumption of the plant has ceased. Inco-ordination is the cardinal sign, the affected animal lurching to one side while walking and swinging laterally or spinning around, often falling heavily. The hind-legs are most seriously affected and there is lateral flexion of the spine and incontinence of urine. Even severely affected animals recover if fed and watered and prevented from eating the plant.

ROCKFERNS

Cheilanthes tenuifolia and *Notholoena distans* cause a slow stumbling gait and severe depression of consciousness in sheep in Australia. Affected sheep appear to be blind.

REFERENCES

(1) Hall, W. T. K. & McGavin, M. D. (1968). *Path. vet.*, *5*, 26.
(2) Mugera, G. M. *et al.* (1964). *Fed. Proc.*, *23*, 106.
(3) Gardiner, M. R. (1970). *Aust. J. agric. Res.*, *21*, 519.
(4) Healey, P. J. (1968). *Clinica chim. Acta*, *22*, 603.
(5) Mason, M. M. & Whiting, M. G. (1968). *Cornell Vet.*, *58*, 541.

Grasses

Poisoning Caused by Canary Grasses
(*Phalaris* spp.)

(*Phalaris Staggers*)

The ingestion of *Phalaris* spp. grasses causes two distinct syndromes: sudden death and inco-ordination, in sheep, and inco-ordination in cattle. The oral administration of cobalt prevents the nervous form of the disease.

Incidence

The disease has been recorded in many parts of Australia and in New Zealand, and South Africa where these grasses are in common use as pasture plants. Thirty per cent of a flock may be affected.

Aetiology

Toowoomba Canary Grass (*Phalaris tuberosa*) is known to cause this disease and it is possible that Canary grass (*P. minor*) and a hybrid species, Rhompa grass, can also cause it. *P. arundinacea* is assumed to cause the staggers and acute death syndromes. As in *P. tuberosa* poisoning there is a slate grey discoloration of the brain stem and diencephalon (1). Provision of cobalt appears to stimulate the proliferation in the rumen of micro-organisms which are capable of destroying the causative agent. Sheep affected with phalaris staggers do not usually show any of the signs of cobalt deficiency. Sheep of all ages are affected and mild cases may occur among cattle. The acute form of the disease is also recorded in cattle on irrigated *Phalaris* sp. pasture in hot humid weather (2).

Occurrence

The disease occurs only when the *P. tuberosa* dominates the pasture or is preferentially grazed, and toxicity is greatest when the plants are young and growing rapidly especially after a break in a dry season. On lightly stocked pastures the acute syndrome, with signs appearing within 4 hours but usually between 12 and 72 hours after going on to the pasture, is most likely to occur. Hungry animals are understandably most commonly affected. Deaths are most common in the early morning or in foggy or cloudy weather. The nervous form of the disease occurs in similar circumstances but in sheep which have protracted or repeated exposure (3). In this case clinical signs appear 2 to 3 weeks after sheep are put on to pasture showing new growth, usually in the autumn or early winter. Both forms may occur in the one flock of sheep.

Pathogenesis

Three tryptamine alkaloids, structurally similar to serotonin, are present in the grass under certain conditions and are thought to be the causative toxins (4). The alkaloids are capable of interfering with the functions of serotonin, a chemical transmitter in the autonomic nervous system with functions analogous to those of acetylcholine. As such

the alkaloids are capable of causing both neurological signs and the cardiac abnormalities of tachycardia and ventricular block. The nervous disturbance appears to be functional initially but anatomical changes may occur in advanced cases.

The relevant tryptomine alkaloids vary significantly in their toxicity so that plants in a pasture can vary greatly in the danger they present (5). Other factors which affect the concentration of tryptomines, and hence the toxicity of the grass, are high environmental temperature and growing in shade (6).

Clinical Findings

The 'sudden death' or cardiac syndrome is manifested by sudden collapse, especially when excited, a short period of respiratory distress with cyanosis, and then death or rapid recovery (8). During the stage of collapse there is arrhythmic tachycardia followed by ventricular fibrillation and cardiac arrest. Consciousness is retained.

In the initial stages of the nervous form of the disease in sheep signs appear only when the animals are disturbed. Hyperexcitability and generalized muscle tremor, including nodding of the head, occur first. On moving, the limb movements are stiff and there is inability to bend the hocks causing dragging of the hind feet. Inco-ordination and swaying of the hindquarters follow. In the most severe cases tetanic convulsions occur with lateral recumbency, paddling movements of the legs, muscle tremor of the trunk, nodding of the head, salivation, and irregular involuntary movements of the eyeballs. There is rapid respiration and irregular tachycardia. The sheep may die at this stage but if left undisturbed it may recover from the convulsion and walk away apparently unaffected. If the sheep are left on the pasture the condition worsens in individual cases, the animal becoming recumbent and manifesting repeated clonic convulsions until death occurs.

There is a great deal of variation from day to day in the number of sheep which show signs and in the severity of the signs observed. Even after sheep are removed from the pasture the clinical state may deteriorate and, although some appear to recover, clinical signs can usually be elicited by forcing them to exercise. Deaths are reported to continue for 1 week after removal of sheep from toxic pasture and clinical signs of the nervous form of the disease may persist for as long as 2 months. The extraordinary situation is recorded where new cases continued to occur for as long as 12 weeks after sheep were moved onto pasture which contained no *Phalaris* spp. In cattle the signs are usually restricted to stiffness of the hocks and dragging of the hind toes but severe cases similar to the common syndrome in sheep occur occasionally.

Clinical Pathology

Laboratory tests on ante-mortem material are of no value in diagnosis.

Necropsy Findings

Exhaustive histological examinations have not been carried out and gross lesions are absent. Degeneration of spinal cord tracts and of the ventral portion of the cerebellum has been observed in the nervous form of the disease but is not a consistent finding (3). Abnormal greenish pigmentation of tissues occurs in the renal medulla and the brain stem and mid-brain.

In the 'sudden death' or cardiac syndrome sheep are usually found dead on their sides with their heads strongly dorsiflexed and legs rigidly extended. Some sheep have blood-stained nasal discharges and many have been frothing at the mouth (7). Abdominal visceral congestion, epicardial and duodenal haemorrhages are present and indicate acute heart failure.

Diagnosis

The association between the disease and the plants should suggest the diagnosis. The appearance of signs only on exercise is significant, suggesting a functional rather than a physical lesion. Poisoning caused by *Claviceps paspali*, perennial rye-grass, marshmallow, stagger weed and other plants produces a very similar syndrome and the diagnosis must depend on the identification of the toxic plant.

Treatment

Flocks of affected sheep should be removed immediately from the toxic pasture.

Control

No preventive measures are available against the acute form of the disease but the nervous form can be prevented by the oral administration of cobalt.

Affected pastures may be grazed if sheep are dosed with cobalt (at least 28 mg. per week) at intervals of not more than a week, or if alternative grazing is provided in rotation. Dosing at too long intervals or with inadequate amounts may account for some failures in prevention. The parenteral administration of cobalt or vitamin B_{12} is not effective. The additional cobalt can be provided by drenching the sheep individually or spreading it on the pasture mixed with fertilizer as described under cobalt deficiency.

REFERENCES

(1) Simpson, B. H. *et al.* (1969). *N.Z. vet. J.*, *17*, 240.
(2) Kerr, D. R. (1972). *Aust. vet. J.*, *48*, 421.
(3) Gallagher, C. H. *et al.* (1966). *Aust. vet. J.*, *42*, 279.
(4) Gallagher, C. H. *et al.* (1964). *Nature (Lond.)*, *204*, 542.
(5) Rendig, V. V. *et al.* (1970). *Crop Sci.*, *10*, 682.
(6) Moore, R. M. *et al.* (1967). *Aust. J. biol. Sci.*, *20*, 1131.
(7) Gallagher, C. H. *et al.* (1967). *Aust. vet. J.*, *43*, 495.

Poisoning Caused by Perennial Rye-grass
(*Lolium perenne*)
(*Rye-grass Staggers*)

Two distinct syndromes occur in animals on rye-grass-dominant pastures, one of liver damage and photosensitization, and one of inco-ordination. The former is caused by a fungus growing on the rye-grass and is dealt with under the heading of poisoning caused by *Pithomyces chartarum*.

Incidence

Rye-grass staggers occurs chiefly in New Zealand but occurs to a limited extent in Australia and Great Britain. The incidence is extremely variable depending on climatic conditions. Rye-grass staggers affects a variable number of animals (5 to 75 per cent) but causes few, if any, deaths.

Aetiology

Sheep, cattle and horses grazing pastures dominated by *L. perenne* can be affected. In young shoots and seedlings the alkaloid content is very high and in mature grass fluctuates wildly depending on meteorological conditions. In mature grass the principal alkaloid is perloline which produces clinical signs of rye-grass staggers when given parenterally. In young grass halostachine is the principal alkaloid. It has sympathomimetic properties. It seems likely that these alkaloids are related to the occurrence of the disease (1).

Occurrence

Rye-grass staggers occurs most commonly in the autumn but when the grass is dry and making only a small amount of slow growth. A sudden fall of rain and rapid growth of the grass is followed by disappearance of the disease. For this reason facial eczema and rye-grass staggers do not occur together in the same flocks at the same time. A high degree of infestation of the grass with ergot (*Claviceps purpurea*) is commonly associated with outbreaks of staggers but is not thought to have direct aetiological significance (2).

Pathogenesis

Because of the transient nature of the disease, the nervous signs in rye-grass staggers are presumed to be caused by a functional derangement of nervous tissue.

Clinical Findings

In sheep the disease occurs commonly in animals in very good bodily condition. In mild cases signs are observed only on driving, the limbs being moved without flexion of the joints. In severe cases the animal is unable to make any movement without the legs becoming extended and abducted causing it to fall. Tetanic convulsions follow. If the sheep are left undisturbed they appear to recover, get up and move off, only to repeat the performance within a few yards. In extreme cases the sheep are permanently prostrate.

In cattle the syndrome is similar to that which occurs in sheep but the convulsions are more severe and flexion of the limbs is more marked than extension. In horses there is a reeling, drunken gait which may proceed to posterior paralysis. Recovery occurs in a few days when the animals are moved to new pasture. Horses and cattle affected mildly are unable to move quickly because of limb and trunk stiffness and a tendency to fall. Turning is achieved only with difficulty. The signs are not apparent when the animals are grazing, occurring only when they are disturbed.

Clinical Pathology

There are no tests available which aid in the diagnosis of rye-grass staggers. Heinz-body anaemia is common in cattle grazing rye-grass but its significance in relation to rye-grass staggers is unknown.

Necropsy Findings

The necropsy findings in rye-grass staggers include macroscopic pallor of skeletal muscles and focal areas of hyaline necrosis on histological examination. Degenerative lesions of Purkinje cell neurones are described in long-standing cases (4, 5).

Diagnosis

Rye-grass staggers resembles many other functional diseases of the nervous system especially those caused by poisonous plants. Nervous syndromes caused by *Claviceps paspali*, *Phalaris tuberosa* and rough-bearded grass (*Echinopogon ovatus*) are very similar to rye-grass staggers.

Treatment

Livestock should be immediately removed from affected pasture but no treatment is required since spontaneous recovery is rapid.

Control

Sheep and cattle should not be allowed to graze potentially toxic pasture for more than 2 to 3 hours a day unless it is more than 12 inches high. Supplementation of the diet with vitamin E, vitamin A and minerals has had no effect on the incidence of the disease.

REFERENCES

(1) Aasen, A. J. *et al.* (1969). *Aust. J. agric. Res.*, *20*, 71.
(2) Thornton, B. H. (1964). *N.Z. vet. J.*, *12*, 13.
(3) Clegg, F. G. & Watson, W. A. (1960). *Vet. Rec.*, *72*, 731.
(4) Mason, R. W. (1968). *Aust. vet. J.*, *44*, 428.
(5) Munday, B. L. & Mason, R. W. (1967). *Aust. vet. J.*, *43*, 598.

Poisoning Caused by Miscellaneous Grasses

MILLET AND PANIC GRASSES (*Panicum* spp.)

Panicum effusum, *P. miliaceum* and possibly *P. decompositum* (native millet) and other *Panicum* spp. (cereal millet) contain hepatoxic substances which cause liver damage and photosensitization in sheep. Photosensitive dermatitis is the major manifestation but it may be accompanied by jaundice and other signs of liver insufficiency in severe cases giving rise to the colloquial name of 'yellow big-head'. The plants are most toxic when young and growing rapidly.

TALL FESCUE GRASS (*Festuca arundinacea*)

The grazing of pasture dominated by this grass causes the disease known as 'fescue foot' in cattle. Clinical signs may appear within 10 to 14 days after animals are turned on to the pasture. Cattle permanently pastured on the field do not appear to be susceptible and horses appear to be able to graze on affected areas with impunity. The usual incidence in an affected herd is around 10 per cent. The lesions and clinical signs are similar to those caused by poisoning with the ergot of rye (*Claviceps purpurea*) and comprise initial lameness followed 2 weeks or more later by dry gangrene of the extremities. As in ergotism the lesions are thought to be caused by vasoconstrictive agents in the grass and contributed to by low environmental temperatures (1). Under freezing temperatures, frostbite may be a complicating factor (2). New cases may continue to appear up to 1 week after removal from the pasture (3). The grass heads are commonly infested with *Cl. purpurea* but the disease may occur in its absence and the toxic principle is distinct from ergot (1). It may be a metabolite of the plant itself but it seems more probable that it should be a toxin produced by a parasitic disease of the plant. Fungi other than *Claviceps* spp., *Fusarium* spp., have been isolated and are capable of producing relevant toxins (4). The disease has also been observed in animals fed on hay made from affected pasture.

There are field reports that mares grazing on fescue grass may suffer from agalactia after foaling. There is no adverse effect on the udder and milk production may be normal in subsequent lactations.

BERMUDA OR COUCH GRASS (*Cynodon dactylon*) AND BLUE COUCH GRASS (*Cynodon incompletus*)

Both of these grasses have been known, in some circumstances, to cause hydrocyanic acid poisoning. A disease of cattle characterized chiefly by nervous signs has also been attributed to the consumption of Bermuda grass. Bermuda grass is a common pasture grass and is eaten readily and without danger under most conditions.

ROUGH-BEARDED GRASS (*Echinopogon ovatus*)

Ingestion of this grass when it is in the early, flowering stages causes inco-ordination and convulsions in lambs and calves. Affected animals nod their heads continuously while standing still. The limbs are stiff, the animals bounding rather than running. On exercise they go down and have clonic convulsions during which they bawl with pain. The respiration rate is rapid and there is marked sweating and hypersensitivity. Recovery occurs if the animals are moved from the pasture for a few days.

YELLOW BRISTLE GRASS (*Setaria lutescens*)

This grass carries heavy bristles which cause mechanical stomatitis in cattle and horses.

Setaria sphacelata is an Australian grass which contains sufficient oxalate to cause oxalate poisoning under which heading the disease is described.

REFERENCES

(1) Jacobsen, D. R. *et al.* (1963). *J. Dairy Sci.*, *46*, 416.
(2) Williams, G. F. (1965). *J. Dairy Sci.*, *48*, 1135.
(3) Hore, D. (1961). *Aust. vet. J.*, *37*, 312.
(4) Yates, S. G. *et al.* (1970). *Appl. Microbiol.*, *19*, 103.

Pasture and Cultivated Legumes

Sweet Clover Poisoning

Sweet clover poisoning is caused by the ingestion of mouldy sweet clover hay which contains dicoumarol. It is characterized by extensive haemorrhages into tissues and severe blood loss after injury or surgery.

Incidence

The disease is recorded most commonly in North America where sweet clover is grown fairly extensively as a fodder crop. The occurrence of the disease has brought the plant into some disfavour and the incidence of the disease has been greatly reduced for this reason. Severe losses may occur when affected animals are dehorned or castrated.

Aetiology

Coumarol is a normal constituent of sweet clover (*Melilotus alba*) and is converted to dicoumarol (dicoumarin or bishydroxycoumarin) through the action of moulds. Not all mouldy sweet clover hay contains dicoumarol and the degree of spoilage is no indication of the toxicity of the hay sample. Varieties of sweet clover differ in their content of coumarol and thus in their potential toxicity. For example the Cumino variety has a low, and the Arctic variety a high, coumarol content (1). The disease can occur in all species but is most common in cattle. Sheep are less susceptible, clinico-pathological evidence of toxicity occurring on diets containing 10 ppm of dicoumarol. However, significant changes in clotting time do not occur on diets containing less than 20 to 30 ppm. Similar changes commence to occur in lambs and calves when the dietary intake of dicoumarol rises to above 2 mg. per kg. body weight (1). The disease can occur in all species but, is most common in cattle. *Melilotus indica*—Hexham Scent or King Island Melitot—also contains a dicoumarol-like substance and hay containing the plant can be highly toxic (2).

Occurrence

It is difficult to make sweet clover hay without the development of mould because of the succulent nature of the plant and the heaviness of the stems and the degree of spoilage is directly related to the moisture content of the cut material. Grazing the crop is not dangerous but the presence of dicoumarol in mouldy sweet clover ensilage has been reported (3). Clinical signs may appear without apparent precipitating cause but trauma and surgery are often followed by deaths from haemorrhage. Migrating warble larvae are also suspected of precipitating fatal haemorrhages (4). New-born calves may die of the disease during the first few days of life when their dams have been fed affected hay without the dams being clinically affected (5).

Pathogenesis

Dicoumarol interferes with the formation of prothrombin in the liver probably because of its competition with substances having vitamin K potency (6). Because of the deficiency of prothrombin, clotting is interfered with and affected animals are subject to internal and external haemorrhage resulting in severe anaemia. Large extravasations of blood into tissues may cause secondary signs by the pressure they exert on internal organs.

Clinical Findings

Extensive haemorrhages into subcutaneous tissues, intermuscular planes and under serous surfaces cause pain and discomfort. The haemorrhages may be visible and palpable but are not painful or hot and do not crepitate. They may cause stiffness and disinclination to move. There are no signs of toxaemia, the affected animal continues to eat well and the temperature, respiration and heart rate are normal until the terminal stages. Accidental and surgical wounds cause severe bleeding but haemorrhages in the mucosae and from the orifices seldom occur except for nosebleed in an occasional animal.

When the loss of whole blood is severe signs of haemorrhagic anaemia appear. The animal is weak, the mucosae pallid, the heart rate increases, and the absolute intensity of the heart sounds increases markedly.

Clinical Pathology

Severe anaemia with greatly increased clotting and prothrombin times are characteristic of the disease. Extension of prothrombin times occurs before there is any increase in clotting time and the former is therefore a useful prognostic test (7). Experimental feeding of the suspected hay to rabbits and using prothrombin times as a measure of toxicity is a satisfactory diagnostic test.

Necropsy Findings

Extensive extravasations of blood or small haemorrhages may be present in any tissue or organ, particularly in the subcutaneous tissue as a result of mild trauma, and in the pericardium and myocardium. There is no intravascular haemolysis, jaundice, haemoglobinuria or haemosiderosis.

Diagnosis

A similar syndrome has been recorded after poisoning by some moulds which occur on feeds. Extensive subcutaneous extravasations of blood and serum also occur in purpura haemorrhagica but this disease is uncommon except in the horse and rarely affects more than one animal in a group. The clotting and prothrombin times are not abnormal, the defect being one of vascular damage. Other extensive subcutaneous swellings such as those caused by angioneurotic oedema are not usually accompanied by anaemia. There is some similarity between sweet clover poisoning and poisoning by bracken fern and trichloroethylene-extracted soyabean meal.

Treatment

Feeding of the damaged hay should be stopped immediately but cases may continue to occur for about 4 days afterwards unless positive steps are taken to correct the prothrombin deficiency. Vitamin K_1 is an effective antidote to poisoning with either sweet clover or *Melilotus indica*. A single massive dose, 2000 mg. administered intravenously, restores prothrombin time to nearly normal within 24 hours in cattle (8). Additional treatment may be necessary to counteract the dicoumarol present in the alimentary tract. Vitamin K is superior to menadione preparations (synthetic vitamin K). Another effective treatment is a transfusion of defibrinated or whole blood, taking care that the donor has not recently been exposed to sweet clover hay. Defibrinated blood can be prepared by collecting blood into a bottle containing sterile glass beads, shaking vigorously during the collection. One or two pints is sufficient but if the animal is clinically affected and showing evidence of anaemia a dose rate of 9 ml. per kg. body weight should be used.

Control

Sweet clover hay must be carefully prepared and not fed if it is damaged or spoiled during curing. Dilution of spoiled clover one part to three parts of unspoiled material is considered to be safe (7).

REFERENCES

(1) Williams, G. F. (1965). *J. Dairy Sci.*, *48*, 1135.
(2) Wignall, W. N. *et al.* (1961). *Aust. vet. J.*, *37*, 456.
(3) White, W. J. *et al.* (1954). *Canad. J. agric. Sci.*, *34*, 601.
(4) Meads, E. B. *et al.* (1964). *Canad. vet. J.*, *5*, 65.
(5) Fraser, C. M. & Nelson, J. H. (1959). *J. Amer. vet. med. Ass.*, *135*, 283.
(6) Quick, A. J. (1944). *Physiol. Rev.*, *24*, 297.
(7) Linton, J. H. (1963). *Canad. J. Anim. Sci.*, *43*, 344, 353; *44*, 76.
(8) Goplen, B. P. & Bell, J. M. (1967). *Canad. J. Anim. Sci.*, *47*, 91.

Poisoning Caused by Miscellaneous Legumes

SUBTERRANEAN CLOVER
(*Trifolium subterraneum*)

A special form of infertility has been observed in sheep grazing pasture dominated by subterranean clover. The infertility is caused by the high content of oestrogenic substances in the leaves of the plant. Of the isoflavones or phyto-oestrogens which occur it is formononetin which is the most active biologically and the risk of a pasture can be determined by its chemical assay. The various strains of the clover vary greatly in their oestrogenic activity. Thus Dinninup, Dwalganup and Yarloop are very active while Clare, Mt Barker, Bacchus Marsh, Daliak, Northam A and Woogenellup are poorly active and Geraldton occupies an intermediate position (1). Pastures containing the first three varieties cannot be considered as safe if they comprise more than 30 per cent of the pasture. A number of environmental factors affect the concentration of the important isoflavones in the pasture. They are much higher when the soil is deficient in phosphorus (2). In the search for other factors affecting oestrogenic potency it has been observed that clover leaves that are entirely red or have red margins have a much higher content of oestrogenic isoflavones than green leaves (3). It is assumed that the leaf redness is due to a viral infection.

One of the difficulties encountered in research work on phyto-oestrogens in ruminants has been the different results obtained by chemical analysis, by laboratory biological assay and by assay in ruminants in long-term grazing experiments. Ruminants are now known to develop ruminal detoxication mechanisms against some phyto-oestrogens and not others (4).

Plants which have matured in the field and set seed have no oestrogenic potency, but the making of potent fodder into hay causes little depression of oestrogen content (5). There is no direct evidence relative to ensilage but it is known that clover ensilage can contain high levels of oestrogens (6). The disease is most severe in spring, especially in exceptionally good growing seasons but it occurs also in normal years and is most common in sheep. Although cattle are generally considered to be unaffected (7), an infertility syndrome has been described in them when they graze pastures dominated by subterranean and other clovers (8) and on pastures which have a high oestrogen content (9). The subject is still a controversial one. Horses appear to be able to graze the toxic pasture without ill effects.

The most commonly observed abnormality is a failure to conceive even with multiple matings, and the flock breeding status worsens progressively, with the lambing percentage falling from a normal 80 per cent down to 30 per cent. Under these conditions sheep farming becomes unprofitable and large areas of country have been made unsuitable for sheep raising by this disease. The infertility is permanent and affected sheep moved to other pastures do not recover. At necropsy there is severe cystic degeneration of the endometrium. Similar clinical and histopathological changes have been produced by the daily injection of 0·03 mg. of diethylstilboestrol per ewe for a period of 6 months.

In affected flocks there may also be a high incidence of maternal dystocia due to uterine inertia. Affected ewes show little evidence of impending parturition and many full-term foetuses are born dead. The mortality rate in lambs may be as high as 40 per cent, and 15 per cent to 20 per cent of ewes may die of metritis and toxaemia. Uterine prolapse may also occur in unbred and virgin ewes and in mature ewes some months after lambing. The incidence of prolapse is usually 1 to 2 per cent but may be as high as 12 per cent. There is marked udder development and copious milk secretion in the ewes. Wethers may also secrete milk, and metaplasia of the prostate and bulbo-urethral glands is evident. These can be detected at an early stage of development by digital rectal palpation. Continuing hyperplasia and cystic dilation of these glands causes their prolapse in a subanal position, followed by rapid weight loss and fatal rupture of the bladder (10). Rams usually show no clinical abnormality and their fertility is not impaired. However there is one record of lactation in rams grazing subterranean clover dominated pasture, without apparent effect on fertility (11).

It is possible that a good deal of the infertility seen in ewes on improved clover pasture may be caused by its high oestrogen content, in spite of the absence of the more dramatic evidence of hyperoestrogenism described above. Because of the necessity to utilize this pasture a great deal more needs to be known about the seasonal occurrence of the oestrogenic substances and the management of sheep grazing the pasture so that the effects of the disease can be minimized. One of the major difficulties in field investigations has been the absence of a suitable method of oestrogen assay. Increase in the length of the teats of wethers has been used as a method (12).

The syndrome seen in cattle is manifested clinically by anoestrus and by swelling of the vulva and lactation in maiden heifers.

Another syndrome caused by subterranean clover and unrelated to the infertility syndrome is that of obstructive urolithiasis in sheep, discussed under that heading. This disease occurs in outbreaks in spring in Merino wethers grazing oestrogenic strains of the clover. As the isoflavone concentrations in the plants rise the daily excretion of phenols and acid-precipitable material in the urine increases, and so does the occurrence of obstruction by the characteristic soft yellow calculi containing benzocoumarins (13).

WHITE CLOVER (*Trifolium repens*)

This clover is in widespread use as a pasture plant and although it may contain significant amounts of hydrocyanic acid, acute poisoning due to this substance does not occur on pastures dominated by the clover. However, the high cyanide content may contribute to a high incidence of bloat, and of goitre in lambs. The plant, in contradistinction to Ladino clover, does not have a high content of oestrogens. However when heavily infested with fungi it can contain significant amounts (14). It is believed that the production of oestrogens is a byproduct of the plant's mechanism of resistance to the fungal infection.

LADINO CLOVER (*Trifolium repens*)

Ladino clover, a large-growing variety of white clover, may contain large quantities of a highly active oestrogen (coumestrol), and when it dominates a pasture and is grazed when the pasture is lush it may cause cornification of vaginal epithelium and functional infertility in ewes (15).

RED CLOVER (*Trifolium pratense*)

Three oestrogenic compounds have been isolated from red clover and where this plant dominates the pasture a clinical syndrome similar to that caused by subterranean clover may be observed. One of the features of the infertility which occurs in ewes is its reversibility, ewes which have grazed oestrogenic red clover pasture for 21 to 33 days returning to normal fertility 3 weeks or more after being removed from the pasture (16). However, permanent sterility due to cystic hyperplasia of the endometrium can result from prolonged exposure (17).

LUPINS (*Lupinus angustifolius* and *L. varius*)

Several disease entities are caused by eating the ripe seeds of lupins which are grown extensively in many countries as a source of protein-rich feed for livestock in winter months. The green plants are usually safe to feed but the dried, mature plants, especially the seeds, are highly toxic although variation in toxicity occurs from year to year and between the members of the lupin family. This variation may be explicable in terms of the possibility that seedheads infested with the fungi *Phomopsis leptostromiformis* (7) and *P. rossiana* (30) are rendered toxic by their presence (18, 19). Differences between animals in their copper status also appear to cause variations in susceptibility, sheep with high copper intakes being more susceptible. The relationship is also explicable in terms of the sudden release of copper from the liver as a result of toxic damage to the liver (20), or that the copper intake itself produces the hepatic damage (21). Cattle and sheep are most commonly affected probably because of their greater exposure. An outbreak of poisoning in pigs fed on the ground seeds has also been reported (22). Poisoning of horses has occurred on rare occasions (23). The disease occurs commonly in Europe, Australia, New Zealand and South Africa.

The two major syndromes produced are a nervous syndrome caused by alkaloids in the plant and an hepatic syndrome, lupinosis. In the nervous form of the disease convulsive episodes occur in which there is staggering, falling, clonic convulsions, dyspnoea and frothing at the mouth, the signs often appearing only with exercise. There is no liver damage and the mortality rate varies from very low to as high as 50 per cent.

Lupinosis is the commoner of the two syndromes. It is characterized clinically by anorexia, depression, loss of body weight and jaundice. Photosensitization is not uncommon. Death may occur within a few days of first illness or be delayed for months, affected animals standing immobile for long periods or wandering aimlessly, often dying from misadventure. Recovery may occur if animals in the early stages of the disease are taken off the dangerous pasture but severely affected animals usually die. At necropsy there is jaundice and the liver is mottled, friable and bright yellow in colour in acute cases, and small and fibrotic in chronic cases (24). Prevention of the disease is assisted by restricting grazing on mature dry lupins during warm, humid conditions which favour fungal growth, by avoiding copper supplementation near danger periods and by encouraging the administration of cobalt.

In recent years evidence has accumulated to incriminate consumption of lupins, particularly *Lupinus sericeus*, as the causative factor in a 'crooked calf' syndrome in western U.S.A. (24).

Affected calves show arthrogryposis or torticollis and scoliosis or both, and occasionally cleft palate. The dam is most susceptible between the 40th and 70th day of gestation. Affected calves bear a marked similarity to those reported under the heading of manganese deficiency. A lathyrogen, amino-acetonitrile, or an extract of *Lupinus caudatus* both produce foetuses with excessive flexure, malpositioning, malalignment and rotation of limbs. It is suggested that there is a similarity of action (25).

LUCERNE OR ALFALFA (*Medicago sativa*)

Lucerne may, in certain circumstances, produce photosensitization in all animal species due probably to the transient occurrence of a photodynamic agent (26). It has also a high bloat-producing potential and may contain sufficient oestrogens to cause infertility (27).

BURR TREFOIL (*Medicago denticulatum*)

Natural pastures may be dominated by this plant especially in the spring when luxuriant growth occurs. Large amounts of the plant may be eaten by all animal species and photosensitization may result. Skin lesions disappear quickly when animals are taken off the pasture and there is no liver damage nor permanent after effects. The photosensitive dermatitis was thought at one time to be due to the aphids which commonly infest the plant in very large numbers. Aphids do contain large amounts of a photodynamic agent and may be important in some outbreaks of the disease. Medics, particularly annual varieties, may also contain significant amounts of oestrogens. *Medicago littoralis* and *M. truncatula* are the most active varieties and the most potent portions of the plants are the mature leaves of dry pasture (28).

ALSIKE CLOVER (*Trifolium hybridum*)

Alsike clover causes photosensitization in all animals but whether this is due to the presence of a photodynamic agent in the plant or to liver damage and accumulation of phylloerythrin is not clear. In horses alsike clover poisoning is associated with signs of liver disease including jaundice, dullness, staggering and blindness and gross enlargement of the liver.

Alsike clover is a converter plant for molybdenum and, in areas where the molybdenum content of the soil is above normal, grazing on the clover may contribute to the development of clinical molybdenosis in animals.

KALEY-PEA OR WILD WINTER PEA (*Lathyrus hirsutus*)

This plant is often sown with grasses to provide early spring grazing. In late spring signs of toxicity may occur in cattle grazing mature plants bearing seed pods. Pain in the feet is the most evident sign, affected animals being lame, standing with the feet under the body and showing a marked disinclination to rise (29).

REVIEW LITERATURE

Bickoff, E. M. (1968). *Oestrogenic Constituents of Forage Plants*, Commonwealth Agricultural Bureaux Review Series, No. 1.
Gardiner, M. R. (1967). Lupinosis. *Advanc. vet. Sci.*, 11, 85.

REFERENCES

(1) Rossiter, R. C. (1970). *Aust. vet. J.*, 46, 141.
(2) Rossiter, R. C. & Beck, A. B. (1966). *Aust. J. agric. Res.*, 17, 447.
(3) Thain, R. I. & Robinson, E. C. (1968). *Aust. J. Sci.*, 31, 121.
(4) Lindsay, D. R. & Kelly, R. W. (1970). *Aust. vet. J.*, 46, 219.
(5) Davies, H. L. & Dudzinski, M. L. (1965). *Aust. J. agric. Res.*, 16, 937.
(6) Lotthammer, K. H. et al. (1970). *Berl. Münch. tierärztl. Wschr.*, 83, 353.
(7) van Warmelo, K. T. et al. (1970). *J. S. Afr. vet. med. Ass.*, 4, 235.
(8) Thain, R. I. (1965). *Aust. vet. J.*, 41, 277.
(9) Rankin, J. E. F. (1963). *Brit. vet. J.*, 119, 30.
(10) Seddon, H. D. (1968). *Aust. vet. J.*, 44, 309.
(11) Meyer, E. P. (1970). *Aust. vet. J.*, 46, 305.
(12) Braden, A. W. H. et al. (1964). *Aust. J. agric. Res.*, 15, 142.
(13) Parr, W. H. et al. (1970). *Aust. J. agric. Res.*, 21, 933.
(14) Wong, E. et al. (1971). *N.Z. J. agric. Res.*, 14, 633.
(15) Sanger, V. L. et al. (1958). *Amer. J. vet. Res.*, 19, 288.
(16) Morley, F. H. W. et al. (1966). *Aust. vet. J.*, 42, 204.
(17) Barrett, J. F. et al. (1965). *Aust. J. agric. Res.*, 16, 189.
(18) Gardiner, M. R. (1966). *Brit. vet. J.*, 122, 508.
(19) Petterson, D. S. & Parr, W. S. (1970). *Res. vet. Sci.*, 11, 282.
(20) Gardiner, M. R. (1966). *J. comp. Path.*, 76, 107.
(21) Gardiner, M. R. (1967). *Aust. vet. J.*, 43, 243.
(22) Marczewski, H. (1955). *Méd. vét. Varsovie*, 11, 738.
(23) Gardiner, M. R. & Seddon, H. D. (1966). *Aust. vet. J.*, 42, 242.
(24) Shupe, J. L. et al. (1967). *J. Amer. vet. med. Ass.*, 151, 191, 198.
(25) Keeler, R. F. et al. (1969). *Canad. J. comp. Med.*, 33, 89.
(26) Clare, N. T. (1952). *Photosensitization in Diseases of Domestic Animals.* Farnham Royal, England: Commonwealth Bureaux of Animal Health.
(27) Adler, J. H. & Trainin, D. (1960). *Refuah vet.*, 17, 115.
(28) Francis, C. M. & Millington, A. J. (1965). *Aust. J. agric. Res.*, 16, 927.
(29) Gibbons, W. J. (1959). *Mod. vet. Pract.*, 40, 43.
(30) Gardiner, M. R. & Petterson, D. S. (1972). *J. comp. Path.*, 82, 5.

Weeds

Poisoning by

Crotalaria	*Crotalaria* spp.
Ragwort	*Senecio jacobaea*
Tarweed	*Amsinckia intermedia*
Caltrops or Puncture Vine	*Tribulus terrestris*

Lantana   *Lantana camara*
Heliotrope   *Heliotropum europaeum*
Sacahuiste   *Nolina texana*
Horsebrush   *Tetradymia* spp.
Paterson's Curse or
   Salvation Jane   *Echium plantagineum*
Ganskweed   *Lasiospermum*
        bipinnatum (1)

All of the above plants contain hepatoxic substances and cause a syndrome of hepatic insufficiency plus photosensitization and, in many instances, marked signs of central nervous system derangement.

Incidence

Disease caused by the ingestion of these plants occurs in many countries. Ragwort and tarweed poisoning have been recorded most commonly in the U.S.A. as a cause of 'walking disease' in horses and cattle. Ragwort causes 'Winton disease' of horses and cattle in New Zealand and, with *Crotalaria* spp. causes 'dunsiekte' of horses in South Africa. *Crotalaria retusa* and *C. crispata* are causes of the disease known as 'walkabout' or 'Kimberley horse disease' in northern Australia and *C. sagittalis* is suspected as the cause of hepatic fibrosis of horses which occurs commonly in the south-eastern United States. *Crotalaria mucronata* has been shown to be poisonous for sheep (3). Experimental feeding of the leaves of the plant cause sudden death with pulmonary lesions the only prominent finding at necropsy. Heliotrope causes severe losses in sheep in Australia and is commonly associated with 'toxaemic jaundice' in this species causing hepatitis and playing a part in the development of hepatogenous chronic copper poisoning. Provided the heliotrope is in a sufficient concentration in the pasture, young cattle can also be affected but the disease is much less common in cattle than in sheep (2). Caltrops poisoning is common in South Africa and lantana poisoning in Australia (4), the Indian sub-continent (5, 6), Florida, the U.S.A. and Mexico (7). *Echium plantagineum* poisoning has occurred in sheep, and possibly cattle and pigs, in Australia (8) and poisoning by *Myoporum* spp. in Australia and New Zealand (9). The morbidity rate with all plants is often high and the majority of affected animals die.

Aetiology

Toxic substances are present in all of the above plants, and in all parts of these plants. *Senecio* spp. contain an alkaloid, retrorsine; heliotrope contains two alkaloids, lasiocarpine and heliotrine, and monocrotaline, fulvine and crispatine are present in *Crotalaria* spp. They are all pyrrolizidine alkaloids. Lantana contains a hepatoxic substance lantadene A, a terpene compound (11). Other toxic principles are present in *Crotalaria* spp. and cause erosion of the oesophageal and gastric mucosae of horses. Affected animals are unable to swallow and may die of starvation (12).

Occurrence

Crotalaria spp. have some value as soil improvers and have been introduced to some areas for this purpose but usually become a pest. These weeds are for the most part not readily eaten by animals, except heliotrope which is not unpalatable, but when other feed is short they may be consumed in quantities sufficient to cause toxic effects. Outbreaks have occurred in animals feeding on silage, hay (13) and pelleted feeds contaminated by *Senecio jacobaea*, and wheat screenings contaminated by the seeds of *Amsinckia intermedia*. Although sheep which eat these plants, especially *Heliotropum europaeum* and *S. jacobaea*, suffer a chronic hepatopathy they are much less susceptible than cattle (8). Pigs have been poisoned experimentally with *S. jacobaea*, the chief clinical signs being dyspnoea and fever (14).

Pathogenesis

The pyrrolizidine alkaloids of *Senecio* spp. and *Crotalaria* spp. have a primary toxic effect on liver parenchyma causing a megalocytosis (8), and secondarily on centrilobular and hepatic veins causing proliferation of the endothelium and occlusion of the vessels. This veno-occlusive effect is characteristic of these alkaloids and does not appear to occur in sheep poisoned by *Heliotropum* spp. Clinical signs do not occur until there is sufficient liver damage to impair its function. Thus, the development of lesions occurs gradually but the onset of clinical signs is usually quite sudden and often some time after the animals have stopped ingesting the toxic material. The relationship between disease of the liver and the nervous signs which are a major manifestation in these diseases is difficult to explain. It is suggested that the hepatic damage interferes with the animal's ability to synthesize urea with a resulting ammonia intoxication of the central nervous system. It is known that some pyrrolizidine alkaloids have severe toxic effects on lung (15).

In poisoning by *Tribulus terrestris* there is a concurrent hepatic and renal dysfunction and a low-grade intra-vascular haemolysis. A subclinical intoxication by selenium is also thought to contribute to the disease (16).

One of the difficulties with this poisoning is the high level of confusion between it and geeldikkop and enzootic icterus.

Lantana poisoning causes hepatic insufficiency and renal tubular lesions, neither of which are specific (11). Triterpenes are considered to be the principal toxic agents in this plant.

Clinical Findings

Disturbances of consciousness, muscle weakness, jaundice and, to a less degree, photosensitization, are the major clinical abnormalities in these diseases. In severe cases of poisoning by *S. jacobaea* in cattle there is dullness with occasional periods of excitability and frenzy, severe diarrhoea with straining, staggering and partial blindness. Abdominal pain may be evident and the straining may be sufficiently severe to cause rectal prolapse. The staggering gait is most noticeable in the hind-legs and the feet are dragged rather than lifted. Walking in circles may also occur. The excitability may be extreme, with animals charging moving objects. Jaundice may be present but pallor of the mucosae is more usual. Most acute cases die within a few days but occasional animals linger on for several weeks. In less severe cases of poisoning by *Senecio* spp. there is little or no excitability, and jaundice and photosensitization are more common. In horses poisoned by *Senecio* spp. there is profound dullness and depression, the animal standing with the head held down and often ceasing to eat half way through a mouthful. There is muscle tremor, particularly of the head and neck, frequent yawning and difficulty in swallowing, sometimes to the point where food and water are regurgitated through the nose or aspirated into the lungs. Blindness is apparent and the horse may walk compulsively in circles, or in a straight line for long distances, bumping into objects, becoming wedged in inaccessible situations and being unable to back out, falling into streams and often walking into houses and outbuildings. Head-pressing is common and there may be sudden attacks of frenzy with violent, uncontrollable galloping. Most affected horses die after a period of illness varying from a week to several months.

The clinical picture in poisonings caused by other hepatoxic plants is in general the same as those described above for poisoning by *Senecio* spp. *Lantana* spp. has secondary toxic effects on kidneys causing a terminal nephrotoxicosis, nephrosis and uraemia and on alimentary tract smooth muscle causing chronic constipation (17). The disease pro-

duced experimentally with this plant in Mexico showed all the signs of hepatic insufficiency including jaundice and photosensitization (7, 18).

Clinical Pathology

Liver function tests, liver biopsies and serum transaminase activity have been used to try to predict the outcome of the disease in individual animals (18, 19). The bromsulphalein test is too laborious to be practical and does not become positive until the late stages of poisoning by *Senecio* spp. in cattle but liver biopsy may be of value as a prognostic aid in this disease.

Necropsy Findings

A necropsy picture of progressive destruction of liver cells and replacement fibrosis is common to poisonings by this group of plants.

In acute cases of poisoning there may be inflammation of the abomasum with acute hepatic degeneration and petechial haemorrhages scattered through the subcutaneous tissue and viscera. In more chronic cases there is fibrosis and shrinkage of the liver, ascites, anasarca and inconstantly, jaundice and photosensitization.

Diagnosis

This group of plants produces a syndrome which is similar in many ways to primary disease of the nervous system, particularly the encephalomyelites. In the horse the disease may be mistaken for infectious equine encephalomyelitis except that fever is not present and there may be signs of liver dysfunction. Leucoencephalomalacia caused by eating mouldy corn is also similar and may be accompanied by jaundice. Nigropallidal encephalomalacia caused by the ingestion of yellow star thistle is another similar disease but affects only the nervous system.

In cattle rabies, lead and coal tar pitch poisoning, herring meal poisoning, and poisoning by other plants may resemble poisoning by these hepatoxic plants and again the differentiation depends on diagnosis of the presence of primary liver disease and recognition of the toxic plant. In sheep the difficulties in diagnosis are similar except that photosensitization is a frequent sign in these diseases and they must be differentiated from the other causes of photosensitive dermatitis.

Treatment

Treatment is of uncertain value but the provision of a high intake of carbohydrate by forced oral or intravenous feeding may help to tide the animal over the period of severe liver dysfunction.

Control

These plants are toxic at all times and their eradication from grazing areas is the only satisfactory method of controlling the disease. If *Crotalaria* spp. are to be used as soil-improvers *C. giant striata* is preferred to other species because of its lower toxicity (20). A high carbohydrate diet may aid in preventing the disease in horses and the feeding of molasses and sugar is recommended as a prophylactic measure. With some of these plants significant damage occurs only after prolonged grazing. Thus it is possible, for example with *H. europaeum*, to utilize the plants as fodder provided sheep are grazed on them for only one season. Sheep are relatively resistant to *Senecio* spp. and stocking infested pastures with sheep is suggested as a control measure (21).

REFERENCES

(1) Fair, A. E. *et al.* (1970). *J. S. Afr. vet. med. Ass.*, *41*, 231.
(2) Kinnaird, P. J. *et al.* (1968). *Aust. vet. J.*, *44*, 39.
(3) Laws, L. (1968). *Aust. vet. J.*, *44*, 453.
(4) Seawright, A. A. (1965). *Aust. vet. J.*, *41*, 235.
(5) Sastry, M. S. & Mahadevan, V. (1963). *Indian vet. J.*, *40*, 78.
(6) Dhillon, K. S. *et al.* (1970). *J. Res. Ludhiana*, 7, 262.
(7) Aluja, A. S. (1970). *Vet. Rec.*, *86*, 628.
(8) Bull, L. B. (1961). *Aust. vet. J.*, *37*, 37, 126.
(9) Denz, F. A. & Hanger, W. G. (1961). *J. Path. Bact.*, *81*, 91.
(10) Dick, A. T. *et al.* (1963). *Nature* (*Lond.*), *197*, 207.
(11) Seawright, A. A. & Allen, J. G. (1972). *Aust. vet. J.*, *48*, 323.
(12) Hall, W. T. K. (1964). *Aust. vet. J.*, *40*, 176.
(13) Fowler, M. E. (1968). *J. Amer. vet. med. Ass.*, *152*, 1131.
(14) Harding, J. D. J. *et al.* (1964). *Path. vet.*, *1*, 204.
(15) McLean, E. K. (1970). *Pharmac. Rev.*, *22*, 429.
(16) Brown, J. M. M. (1968). *Ondersterpoort J. vet. Res.*, *35*, 319.
(17) Seawright, A. A. (1963). *Aust. vet. J.*, *39*, 340.
(18) Aluja, A. S. de & Skewes, H. R. (1971). *Proc. 19th Wld vet. Congr.*, *Mexico City*, *1*, 327.
(19) Sippel, W. L. (1964). *Ann. N.Y. Acad. Sci.*, *111*, 563.
(20) Bierer, B. W. (1960). *J. Amer. vet. med. Ass.*, *136*, 318.
(21) Muth, O. H. (1968). *J. Amer. vet. med. Ass.*, *153*, 310.

Poisoning by *Solanum malacoxylon*

(*Enteque Seco, Manchester Wasting Disease, Naalehu*)

Manchester wasting disease occurs in cattle in Jamaica, W.I. (1), and similar diseases are recorded as 'enteque seco' in South America and 'naalehu', in Hawaii. In Argentina sheep and possibly horses are also reported to be affected. Clinically there is progressive wasting and stiffness of the joints with reluctance to rise or lie down. The stiffness is most severe in the forelegs and the animal stands for long periods with stiff legs and an arched back, the thorax fixed and distended. Heart murmurs are audible and severe distress develops with exercise. Cattle aged 15 months and over may be affected.

Regression of the disease occurs when affected animals are hand fed or are moved to a 'clean' area.

At necropsy the carcase is emaciated and shows anasarca and ascites. Calcification of small blood vessels, patchy oedema and pale discoloration of skeletal musculature are evident. Calcification of the coronary arteries, endocardium and aorta occurs commonly and may extend into the large arteries. Calcification is also present in the pleura and in the emphysematous parenchyma of the lung and, in varying degrees, in most other viscera. Degenerative arthritis occurs in the limb joints, and calcification of tendons and ligaments is also present.

The cause of the disease has been identified in South America as the ingestion of the weed *Solanum malacoxylon* (2). Blood levels of calcium and phosphorus are 20 to 25 per cent above normal. The disease has been produced experimentally (3) and the mode of action of *S. malacoxylon* determined to be a dramatic increase in calcium absorption from the diet (4).

A very similar disease has been described in Europe in recent years under the name of 'enzootic calcinosis' (5, 6). On affected farms many animals become affected at about 3 years of age and introduced animals are affected about $1\frac{1}{2}$ years after introduction to the alpine pastures on which the disease occurs. The disease is chronic and may take several years to run its course, and is worst when the animals are at pasture. There is chronic wasting, reluctance to walk, constant shifting of weight from foot to foot. Calcification of vessels is palpable, especially on rectal examination. Serum calcium (up to 13·4 mg. per 100 ml.) and phosphorus (up to 12 mg. per 100 ml.) levels are elevated.

At necropsy examination the calcification of endocardium, vessels generally, lungs and tendons is very evident in advanced cases.

It occurs on alpine pastures which have been heavily fertilized with phosphorus (6) and there is suggestive evidence that consumption of the grass *Tricetum flavescens* may be the cause (7).

REFERENCES

(1) Arnold, R. M. & Bras, G. (1956). *Amer. J. vet. Res.*, *17*, 630.
(2) Worker, N. A. & Carillo, B. J. (1967). *Nature* (*Lond.*), *215*, 72.
(3) Camberos, H. R. (1971). *Gac. vet.*, *33*, 120.
(4) Sansom, B. F. *et al.* (1971). *Res. vet. Sci.*, *12*, 604.
(5) Dirksen, G. *et al.* (1970). *Dtsch. tierärztl. Wschr.*, *77*, 321.
(6) Liebetseder, J. *et al.* (1971). *Dtsch. tierärztl. Wschr.*, *78*, 603.
(7) Dirksen, G. *et al.* (1972). *Dtsch. tierärztl. Wschr.*, *79*, 77.

Miscellaneous Poison Weeds

Many weeds which occur in cultivation and pasture land are thought to be poisonous in certain circumstances and it is impossible to include them all here. Many countries publish bulletins dealing with the common poison plants of the area and a list of these is provided at the end of this section. In the following list an attempt has been made to group the plants according to the disease syndromes that they produce.

WEEDS WHICH CAUSE PRINCIPALLY NERVOUS SIGNS

Darling pea (*Swainsonia galegifolia*). A native of Australia, this plant causes nervous signs including stiffness of the limbs, inco-ordination and muscle tremor. Unusual postures, particularly a 'stargazing' attitude, are adopted. Terminally, sheep, which are the species most commonly affected, are unable to rise and may die of starvation. Addiction to the pea is common. Necropsy findings are restricted to microscopic lesions of vacuolation of cytoplasm in neurones throughout the central nervous system (1). Vacuolations in cells occur in other organs also. Their presence in circulating lymphocytes may have diagnostic value (2). These have been produced experimentally in guinea-pigs (3). Identical lesions and clinical signs are produced by *S. canescens* (4). The disease is very similar to that caused by *Astragalus* sp. (see below). Poisoning with Darling pea has also been recorded in cattle in which there are neurological signs similar to those which occur in sheep but in addition there is emaciation and a poor breeding performance (5). The disease is also recorded in a horse (6).

Amaranthus retroflexus or reflexus (*redleg, pigweed, red amaranth, Prince of Wales' feather*) *and Chenopodium album* (*lambsquarters, fat hen*). Consumption of these weeds, commonly found in pig yards, by feeder pigs unaccustomed to them has been related to a syndrome characterized by trembling, inco-ordination of the hindquarters, coma and a high mortality (7). A consistent finding on post-mortem examination is perirenal oedema. There are also degenerative changes in the brain and kidneys (8). In cattle tubular nephrosis causes terminal uraemia (9). *C. album* also contains large amounts of oxalate and may produce hypocalcaemia (10). *A. retroflexus* is also often high in oxalate.

Loco weed or poison vetch (*Astragalus and Oxytropis spp.*) A number of these leguminous plants are known to be poisonous to all domestic animals. They act as 'converter' plants for selenium and on seleniferous soils contain very high concentrations of the element. These plants are also toxic, independently of their role as selenium 'converters',

due to the presence of a toxic substance, miserotoxin (11). Part of their importance as poisonous plants depends on their palatability and the concentration they can achieve in pasture. The disease is most common in spring on desert range in the western U.S.A. Acutely poisoned animals may die quickly but in most cases the course of the disease is prolonged. The more common form of the disease includes abortion, congenital deformities and nervous signs including holding the head high, nervousness, stiffness, loss of directional sense, inco-ordination, head-pressing and recumbency (12). There is also constipation, emaciation, long rough coat and blindness. There is a mild nephritis and liver damage is indicated by the sulfabromophthalein liver function test. Cytoplasmic vacuolation of proximal renal tubular epithelium and of neurones, proceeding to neuronolysis of most of the central and autonomic nervous systems, have been produced by experimental feeding in sheep and appear to be the critical lesions (13). The similarity between the clinical signs and lesions produced by *Swainsonia* sp. and *Astragalus* sp. has already been noted. However, sheep fed the latter have aborted and produced congenitally deformed lambs, neither of which occurred after feeding on *Swainsonia* sp. (14). The principal deformities in affected lambs and calves (12) include lateral rotations of forelimbs, contracted tendons, anterior flexure and hypermotility of hock joints and flexure of the carpus.

A similarity between the abortifacient and teratological effects of *Astragalus* sp. and of *Lathyrus* and *Vicia* spp. has led to the suggestion that lathyrogens such as aminoacetonitrile may be present in the former (15). A similarity to the teratological effect of extracts of lupins is also noted (16). Addiction to the plants is thought to occur.

Sneezeweed (*Helenium autumnale*). This is a common weed of wet pastures in eastern North America. Sheep, cattle and horses may be affected, the flowering heads being the most toxic part of the plant. Clinical signs of toxicity include hypersensitivity, inco-ordination, dyspnoea and tachycardia. *Smallhead sneezeweed* (*H. microcephalum*) is also poisonous (17). Clinical signs in sheep include salivation, nasal discharge, bloat, severe abdominal pain and diarrhoea.

Hemlock water dropwort (*Oenanthe crocata*). The roots of this plant contain a poisonous substance which causes severe convulsions similar to those of acute lead poisoning in cattle. Most affected animals die and at necropsy there is hyperaemia of the oral and ruminal mucosae and a celery-like odour in the rumen.

Perennial broomweed (Gutierrezia microcephala). This plant is most toxic when growing rapidly on sandy soils. In the U.S.A. it is known to cause acute illness and rapid death but more commonly it is associated with abortion or the birth of premature, weak calves and retention of the placenta.

Birdsville indigo (Indigophera dominii or ennea-phylla). Birdsville indigo causes poisoning in horses in desert areas of Australia. All ages and classes of horses are affected and most cases occur in spring and summer with variation in incidence from year to year.

The clinical syndrome, known locally as 'Birdsville disease', is ushered in by inappetence, segregation and somnolence, the animal often standing out in the open in the hot sun when unaffected horses have sought the shade. There is marked inco-ordination, the front legs being lifted and extended in an exaggerated manner. The hocks are not flexed causing the fronts of the hind hooves to be dragged on the ground. The head is held in an unnaturally high position and the tail is held out stiffly. There is difficulty in changing direction and inco-ordination increases as the horse moves. The horse commences to sway and at the canter there is complete disorientation of the hind legs so that the animal moves its limbs frantically but stays in the one spot with the legs becoming gradually abducted until it sits down and rolls over. Rapid emaciation and laboured respiration are commonly seen in acute cases. Terminally there is recumbency with intermittent tetanic convulsions which may last for up to 15 minutes and during which death usually occurs.

A chronic syndrome may develop in some animals subsequent to an acute attack. Affected animals can move about but there is inco-ordination and dragging of the hind feet with wearing of the toe, and inspiratory dyspnoea may also occur. Detailed necropsy findings have not been recorded but liver changes have been suggested. Supplementation of the diet with arginine-rich protein feeds prevents development of the disease (18). Peanut meal and gelatin provide readily available and cheap sources of arginine. *E. dominii* contains two toxic alkaloids, indospicine, an analogue of arginine, and canavanine.

Hemlock (Cicuta spp.). Many water hemlocks are poisonous. They occur in most countries of the northern hemisphere and have caused heavy losses, particularly in cattle. Initially there is frothing at the mouth and uneasiness followed by tetanic convulsions during which the animal bellows as though in pain. Diarrhoea may occur and there may be bloating and spasmodic contractions of the diaphragm. The course is extremely short and death may occur within a few minutes.

Rubber vine (Cryptostegia grandiflora). This poisonous vine causes sudden death in cattle and sheep in north Queensland. After experimental ingestion of the plant sudden death occurs after short periods of vigorous exercise (19).

Albizia tanganyicensis. The disease occurs naturally in cattle and has been produced experimentally in sheep. Hyperthermia, hypersensitivity, tetanic convulsions and dyspnoea are the important clinical signs and at necropsy petechiation in many tissues, pulmonary oedema, degenerative changes in myocardium and other organs and in some cases in the brain (22).

Papaver nudicaule (iceland poppy). This elegant member of many winter gardens is blamed for causing ataxia and muscle tremor in horses (23) and other species. To their credit is the apparent restriction of their toxicity to the post-flowering stage.

White snakeroot (Eupatorium rugosum). A toxic alcohol, tremetol, is present in this plant which is common in North America (20). The alcohol is excreted in the milk of cattle which ingest the plant and may cause clinical illness and even death in humans drinking the milk. Severe muscle tremor is characteristic of the disease and is accompanied by salivation, nasal discharge, vomiting and dyspnoea. The animal becomes progressively weaker and is finally unable to stand, lapsing into a coma before death.

Yellow star thistle (Centaurea solstitialis) and Russian knapweed (C. repens) (21). The disease nigropallidal encephalomalacia of horses is caused by the continued ingestion of large quantities of yellow star thistle and has been recorded only in the United States (24). There is a sudden onset with difficulty in eating and drinking, varying from complete inability to less obvious defects such as difficulty in prehension, in moving feed back to the molars or in swallowing. A fixed facial expression is common, the mouth being held half open or the lips drawn into a straight line. Wrinkling of the skin of the lips and muzzle and protrusion of the tongue are present in many cases. Tongue and lip movements are often awkward and persistent chewing movement without food in the mouth, and rhythmic protrusion of the tongue occur. Yawning and somnolence are evident but the horse is easily aroused. Some horses show aimless, slow walking and, in the early stages, transient circling. The gait is not grossly abnormal, a slight stiffness at the walk being the only abnormality except for weakness in the terminal stages. Signs fluctuate in severity for 2 to 3 days and then remain static until the animal dies or is destroyed.

No major liver lesions are present at necropsy but areas of necrosis or softening are visible macroscopically in the brain, in the globus pallidus and substantia nigra. The lesions are bilateral in most cases. The disease occurs in summer and late autumn in horses on weedy pasture and experimental feeding with thistle plants produces the disease. The plant does not appear to be toxic to ruminants, rodents or monkeys, and is thought to contain an antimetabolite which is specific to the horse (25).

Gomphrena celosioides. Ingestion of this weed causes extensive outbreaks of inco-ordination in horses in northern Australia. When moving the hindquarters sway and the toes are dragged. The horse is dull, eats little and stands with the feet bunched well underneath the body. If the disease progresses the horse stands with the legs spread wide apart. When movement is attempted the head is pushed forward and the limbs moved uncertainly, and the animal may rear backwards or collapse forward and fall heavily. Completely inco-ordinated movements are made in attempts to rise. Recovery occurs if ingestion of the plant ceases.

Marshmallow (*Malva parviflora*), *Stagger-weed* (*Stachys arvensis*). In Australia these plants cause abnormalities of gait in sheep. Signs do not appear until the sheep have grazed affected pasture for some weeks. Exercise provokes the abnormal gait which commences with muscle tremor, weakness and inco-ordination in the hind-limbs and frequent urination. If the animals are forced to move they go down with extension of the limbs but without convulsions. After a short rest they get up and walk normally again. Removal from the affected pasture usually results in recovery within 3 or 4 days.

Ipomoea muelleri is a straggling prostrate vine which contains hallucinogenic compounds of the lysergic acid type and causes poisoning of sheep, and probably cattle, in Australia. Clinical signs include ataxia, posterior weakness, rapid fatigue accompanied by dyspnoea, loss of weight and death after a long period of illness. There are no significant lesions at necropsy (26).

Sarcostemma viminale and *Euphorbia mauritanica* in Africa (27) and *Sarcostemma australe* (28)

produce marked nervous signs in sheep, including hypersensitivity, stiffness, inco-ordination, recumbency, tremor and convulsions. There is also hyperglycaemia and a post-mortem picture resembling that of *Clostridium perfringens* (type D) poisoning.

WEEDS WHICH CAUSE GASTROENTERITIS AND NERVOUS SIGNS

A very large number of plants cause gastroenteritis manifested by salivation, grinding of the teeth, abdominal pain, vomiting and diarrhoea, usually accompanied by muscle tremor, inco-ordination and convulsions. There are some differences between the syndromes caused by individual plant species but for brevity the common plants are listed below. For greater detail the reader is referred to the extended reading list at the end of the section.

Spurges	*Euphorbia* spp.
Castor Oil Bean	*Ricinus communis* (29)
Black Nightshade	*Solanum nigrum*
Silver-leafed	
Nightshade	*S. elaeagnifolium*
Cape Tulip	*Homeria collina*
Cockleburr	*Xanthium orientale*
Death Camas	*Zygadenus gramineus*
Tall and Low	
Larkspur	*Delphinium* spp.
Timber Milk Vetch	*Astragalus* spp.
Monkshood	*Aconitum* spp.
Pokeweed	*Phytolacca americana* (30)
	P. dodecandra (31)
Cockles	*Agrostemma* spp. and *Saponaria* spp.
Buttercup	*Caltha palustris* and *Ranunculus* spp.
Dutchman's Breeches	*Dicentra cucularia*
Squirrel Corn	*D. canadensis*
Indian Tobacco	*Lobelia inflata*
Dogbane	*Apocymum* spp.
Laurel	*Kalmia* spp.
Whorled Milkweed	*Asclepias verticillata*
Short-crown	
Milkweed	*A. brachystephana* (32)
Meadow Saffron	*Colchicum autumnale* (33)
Alfombrilla	*Drymaria arenarioides*
Pingue (Colorado	
Rubber Weed)	*Hymenoxis richardsonii*

WEEDS CAUSING MISCELLANEOUS CLINICAL SIGNS

Crofton weed (*Eupatorium glandulosum* and *E. riparium*). Poisoning by these plants is reputed to cause acute pulmonary consolidation of horses, 'Numinbah horse sickness', in Australia.

Halogeton (*Halogeton glomeratus*), *Greasewood* (*Sarcobatus vermiculatus*), *Docks and Sorrels* (*Rumex spp.*), *Soursob* (*Oxalis cernua*), *Portulacca oleracea, Salsola kali, Trianthema portulacastrum and Threlkeldia proceriflora*. The leaves of these plants may contain sufficient oxalate to cause oxalate poisoning.

Variegated thistle (*Silybum marianum*), *Mintweed* (*Salvia reflexa*). Both plants are known to cause nitrite poisoning in ruminants when the plants are lush and growing rapidly but on many occasions cattle can eat them in large quantities without ill effects.

Seaside or Marsh arrowgrass (*Triglochin maritima*). These plants cause cyanide poisoning in parts of North America.

St. John's Wort or *Klamath weed* (*Hypericum perforatum*), *Lecheguilla* (*Agave lecheguilla*) *and Lady's thumb* (*Polygonum* spp.). These plants contain photodynamic agents (hypericin in St. John's Wort) which cause photosensitive dermatitis when ingested by animals. Sheep and cattle are most commonly exposed. All parts of the plant are toxic when eaten in large quantities. They are not very palatable and most outbreaks occur when the plants are in the young stage and dominate the pasture. Clinical signs may appear within a few days of stock going on to affected fields and usually disappear within 1 or 2 weeks after removal from the fields.

Veratrum californicum (*Skunk cabbage, Western hellebore, False hellebore or Wild corn*) is unique among poisonous plants in that its ingestion by ewes on the 14th day of pregnancy causes severe congenital cyclopean deformities of the head, absence or displacement of the pituitary gland with prolonged gestation, and giantism in the foetus. Leg deformities, including overextension of the pasterns, and supernumerary claws also occur. Foetal resorption is also a common phenomenon. The plant grows naturally in alpine pastures in the U.S.A. (34) and contains a number of toxic amines, some of which have been shown to produce the relevant defects if fed to ewes on the 14th day of pregnancy (36). The plant is also toxic for adult sheep causing salivation, purgation, diuresis, vomiting, weakness, cardiac irregularity, dyspnoea, cyanosis and terminal convulsions (35).

Cassia occidentalis, coffee senna (37, 38), and *Karwinskia humboldtiana* coyotillo (39) have attrac-

ted attention because of their capacity to cause degenerative lesions in skeletal muscle. In both plants the mature fruits contain the most toxin. Reports of outbreaks of poisoning by these plants come chiefly from Texas, U.S.A. Empirical treatment with selenium and vitamin E has been thoroughly discredited by the finding that either preparation, especially vitamin E, enhances the poisonous effect of the plant (40). An axonal dystrophy has been observed in the cerebellum and spinal cord and the lesions have a close correlation with clinical signs (41). The clinical picture of coyotillo poisoning in goats includes increased alertness, hypersensitivity, tremor and disturbances of gait such as stiff, stilted movements, hypermetria and terminal recumbency. Patellar and gastrocnemius reflexes disappear. These clinical findings suggest decreased function of peripheral nerves and cerebellum (42).

In coffee senna poisoning the early signs are anorexia and diarrhoea and these are followed by hyperpnoea, tachycardia and progressive muscular malfunction. The muscle lesion is accompanied by marked elevations of SGOT and CPK levels (48).

Desert rice flower, flaxweed, wild flax, mustard weed, broom bush (*Pimelea trichostachya, P. simplex*). The disease caused in cattle by this plant has been known in Queensland for many years under the name of 'St George Disease', but the cause has only recently been identified. The findings are oedema under the jaw and down the brisket, intermittent diarrhoea and death. The causative substance in the plant causes construction of pulmonary venules and right heart failure. Inhalation of the powdered plant causes the pulmonary lesion only, ingestion causes the congestive heart failure/pulmonary lesions plus diarrhoea. The usual field picture is that cattle graze looking for feed between old dry flaxweed plants and inhale it so that the pulmonary cardiac form is the common one and the commonest occurrence is in summer (43).

The disease is recorded only in cattle. Sheep are resistant under experimental conditions. Fatal necrotic gastroenteritis is produced by feeding *Pimelea* spp. to horses but it is unlikely that they would eat the plant in natural circumstances (44).

Whiteheads (*Sphenosciadium capitellatum*). This alpine pasture plant has caused disease in horses and cattle. It acts in a manner similar to an anaphylactic reaction with pulmonary oedema and photosensitization (49).

Mercurialis spp. Dog's mercury (*M. perennis*) causes gastritis and haemolytic anaemia in sheep (45).

Allium validum (46) or wild onion also causes haemoglobinuria, and a severe haemolytic crisis.

Isotropis spp. are plants confined in their distribution to Australia. They cause serious kidney damage and fatal uraemia in sheep and cattle (47).

REVIEW LITERATURE

Campbell, J. B. *et al.* (1956). *Poisonous Plants of the Canadian Prairies.* Canada Dept. Agric., Pub. 900, Ottawa, Canada.
Connor, H. E. (1951). *The Poisonous Plants of New Zealand.* Dept. Sci. Ind. Res., Bull. 99, Wellington, N.Z.
Kingsbury, J. M. (1958). Plants poisonous to livestock. *J. Dairy Sci.,* 41, 875.
Hall, W. T. K. (1964). Plant toxicoses of tropical Australia. *Aust. vet. J.,* 40, 176.
Muenscher, W. C. (1951). *Poisonous Plants of the United States.* New York: Macmillan.
Simmonds, F. J. (1967). Biological control of pests of veterinary importance. *Vet. Bull.,* 37, 71.

REFERENCES

(1) Laws, L. & Anson, R. B. (1968). *Aust. vet. J.,* 44, 447.
(2) Huxtable, C. R. & Gibson, A. (1970). *Aust. vet. J.,* 46, 446.
(3) Huxtable, C. R. (1969). *Aust. J. exp. Biol.,* 47, 339.
(4) Gardiner, M. R. *et al.* (1969). *Aust. J. agric. Res.,* 20, 87.
(5) Hartley, W. J. & Gibson, A. J. F. (1971). *Aust. vet. J.,* 47, 301.
(6) Hartley, W. J. (1971). *Acta neuropath.,* 18, 342.
(7) Buck, W. B. *et al.* (1966). *J. Amer. vet. med. Ass.,* 148, 1525.
(8) Osweiler, G. D. *et al.* (1969). *Amer. J. vet. Res.,* 30, 557.
(9) Cursack, H. A. & Romano, L. A. (1967). *Gac. vet.,* 29, 69.
(10) Herweijer, C. H. & Den Houter, L. F. (1971). *Netherlands J. vet. Sci.,* 4, 52.
(11) Williams, M. C. *et al.* (1969). *Amer. J. vet. Res.,* 30, 2185.
(12) James, L. F. *et al.* (1969). *Amer. J. vet. Res.,* 30, 377.
(13) van Kampen, K. R. & James, L. F. (1970). *Path. vet.,* 7, 503.
(14) James, L. F. *et al.* (1970). *Path. vet.,* 7, 116.
(15) Keeler, R. F. & James, L. F. (1971). *Canad. J. comp. Med.,* 35, 332, 342.
(16) Keeler, R. F. *et al.* (1969). *Canad. J. comp. Med.,* 33, 89.
(17) Dollahite, J. W. *et al.* (1964). *J. Amer. vet. med. Ass.,* 145, 694.
(18) Hooper, P. I. *et al.* (1971). *Aust. vet. J.,* 47, 326.
(19) McGavin, M. D. (1969). *Qd J. agric. Anim. Sci.,* 26, 9.
(20) Christensen, W. T. (1965). *Econ. Bot.,* 19, 293.
(21) Farrell, R. K. *et al.* (1971). *J. Amer. vet. med. Ass.,* 158, 1201.
(22) Basson, P. A. *et al.* (1970). *J. S. Afr. vet. med. Ass.,* 41, 117.
(23) de Malmanche, I. (1970). *N.Z. vet. J.,* 18, 96.
(24) Fowler, M. E. (1965). *J. Amer. vet. med. Ass.,* 147, 607.
(25) Mettler, F. A. & Stern, G. M. (1963). *J. Neuropath.,* 22, 164.
(26) Gardiner, M. R. *et al.* (1965). *Brit. vet. J.,* 121, 272.
(27) Terblanche, M. *et al.* (1966). *J. S. Afr. vet. med. Ass.,* 37, 3, 311, 317.
(28) Hall, W. T. K. (1964). *Aust. vet. J.,* 40, 76.
(29) Fowler, M. E. (1964). *Ann. N.Y. Acad. Sci.,* 111, 577.
(30) Kingsbury, J. M. & Hillman, R. B. (1965). *Cornell Vet.,* 55, 534.
(31) Mugera, G. M. (1970). *Bull. epizoot. Dis. Afr.,* 18, 41.
(32) Rowe, L. D. *et al.* (1970). *SWest. Vet.,* 23, 219.
(33) Tribunskii, M. P. (1970). *Veterinariya,* 6, 71.
(34) Binns, W. *et al.* (1966). *J. Amer. vet. med. Ass.,* 147, 839.
(35) Binns, W. *et al.* (1964). *Ann. N.Y. Acad. Sci.,* 111, 571.
(36) Keeler, R. F. & Binns, W. (1968). *Teratology,* 1, 5.
(37) Henson, J. B. & Dollahite, J. W. (1966). *Amer. J. vet. Res.,* 27, 947.
(38) Mercer, H. D. *et al.* (1967). *J. Amer. vet. med. Ass.,* 151, 735.
(39) Dewan, M. L. *et al.* (1965). *Amer. J. Path.,* 46, 215.
(40) O'Hara, P. J. *et al.* (1970). *Amer. J. vet. Res.,* 31, 2151.
(41) Charlton, K. M. *et al.* (1970). *Path. vet.,* 7, 385, 408, 420, 435.
(42) Charlton, K. M. *et al.* (1971). *Amer. J. vet. Res.,* 32, 1381.
(43) Clark, I. A. (1971). *Aust. vet. J.,* 47, 285.
(44) Hill, M. W. M. (1970). *Aust. vet. J.,* 46, 287.
(45) Baker, J. R. & Faull, W. B. (1968). *Vet. Rec.,* 82, 485.
(46) van Kampen, K. R. *et al.* (1970). *J. Amer. vet. med. Ass.,* 156, 328.
(47) Gardiner, M. R. & Royce, R. D. (1967). *Aust. J. agric. Res.,* 18, 505.
(48) O'Hara, P. J. *et al.* (1969). *Amer. J. vet. Res.,* 30, 2173.
(49) Fowler, M. E. *et al.* (1970). *J. Amer. vet. med. Ass.,* 157, 1187.

Trees and Shrubs

Oak (Quercus spp.). Young oak leaves and acorns are sometimes browsed by animals and cause no illness when they form only a small part of the diet but if little else is eaten they may cause polyuria, ventral oedema, abdominal pain and constipation followed by the passage of faeces containing mucus and blood. At necropsy there is severe gastroenteritis and a characteristic nephrosis. The toxic principle has not been identified. All species of animals are affected, losses in sheep and cattle being reported most commonly, with occasional cases occurring in horses. Extensive areas of oak-brush range in the United States can be utilized for cattle grazing but require careful management if losses are to be avoided (1). All parts of the sand shin oak (*Quercus havardi*), a low shrub common in southwest U.S.A., are toxic to cattle causing emaciation, oedema and constipation. The toxic agent is a tannin (2). Other species of oak are also toxic and cause signs similar to those listed above (3). Calcium hydroxide (15 per cent of the ration) is an effective antidote under experimental conditions.

Laburnum (Cystisus laburnum) and Broom (Cytisus scoparius). Cytisine, a toxic alkaloid, is present in both laburnum and broom trees, particularly the flowers and seeds. Ingestion results in excitement, inco-ordination, convulsions and death due to asphyxia.

Cherry laurel (Prunus laurocerasus), Choke cherry (Prunus demissa). A cyanogenetic glucoside, amygdalin, is present in the leaves of the cherry laurel tree, and hydrocyanic acid poisoning may result if large quantities of the leaves are eaten. The leaves of choke cherry also cause hydrocyanic acid poisoning.

Mountain laurel (*Kalmia spp.*). Leaves of this plant are not ordinarily palatable but poisoning of ruminants can occur when other feed is scarce. Clinical signs in cattle include hyperexcitability, inco-ordination and paralysis.

Rhododendron (*Andromeda spp.*). A toxic glucoside, andromedotoxin, present in the leaves of rhododendron, causes abdominal pain, weakness, staggering and collapse. Vomiting is common even in ruminants. Death follows after several days of illness.

Oleander (*Nerium oleander*). This decorative shrub is very poisonous and there are many records of deaths due to feeding prunings to animals, usually cattle, or when animals break into gardens. Death is sudden and due to ventricular fibrillation. Treatment is not usually possible but atropine is recommended (4).

Cestrum (*Cestrum aurantiacum and C. laevigatum*). This hedge and windbreak bush causes mortality in goats and cattle (5). It causes a haemorrhagic gastroenteritis and degenerative lesions in the liver, kidney and brain.

Sapium sebiferum (*chinese tallow tree*). This ornamental tree causes gastroenteritis in cattle (6).

Yew (*Taxus baccata*). All parts of the yew tree contain a highly poisonous alkaloid, taxine, which has a strong depressive effect on the heart. Commonly there is sudden death without obvious clinical signs. Signs, if they appear, include dyspnoea, muscle tremor, weakness and collapse. Sudden death is recorded in a horse which ate foliage from a Japanese yew tree (7).

Yellow-wood tree (*Terminalia oblongata*). The leaves of this tree may be eaten when other food is scarce and cause some losses in cattle and sheep in north-east Australia. In an acute form of the disease there is a sudden onset of profuse diarrhoea, dullness, anorexia, dyspnoea and dryness of the muzzle. Marked oedema of the jowl, neck and brisket occurs constantly. At necropsy there is ascites, anasarca and a toxic nephrosis. A more chronic syndrome is manifested by scouring, emaciation, photophobia, a purulent ocular discharge, keratitis and blindness. There may be incontinence of urine with frequent straining and continuous dribbling. At necropsy the bladder wall is thickened and the bladder much enlarged. Renal tubular damage is also present. Bromsulfalein clearance tests indicate that there is also a serious depression of liver function present (8). The mortality rate is 100 per cent, most deaths occurring after an illness of less than 6 weeks (9).

Ironwood tree (*Erythrophloeum chlorostachys*). This is a common tree in Australia and the leaves contain a highly toxic alkaloid, erythrophleine. All animal species seem to be affected, clinical signs including anorexia, a staring expression, partial blindness, contraction of abdominal muscles, increased heart sounds, mucosal pallor, and terminal dyspnoea (9).

Gidgee or Gidyea tree (*Acacia georgina*). In northern Australia poisoning by this tree has caused heavy mortalities in sheep and cattle and seriously reduced the productivity of large areas of grazing land (9). The toxic principle has been identified as the fluoroacetate ion which is present in the leaves and seed pods, particularly the latter (10). The toxicity of the plant varies and in some areas may be eaten with no apparent ill-effects. Clinically there is a sudden onset of tachycardia with heart rates up to 300 per minute, dyspnoea, cyanosis, convulsions and death within a few minutes to several hours. Cardiac irregularity, moderate bloat and frequent micturition are also observed in some cases. Signs commonly appear when affected animals are driven. At necropsy there is congestion of the alimentary mucosa, flabbiness of the myocardium and multiple subendocardial and subepicardial haemorrhages. There may be oedema and congestion of the lungs. The plants *Gastrolobium grandiflorum* and *Oxylobium* sp. also cause poisoning because of their content of monofluoroacetic acid (11). Similarly to other organic fluorides fluoroacetate is known to exert its effect by poisoning the enzyme aconitase leading to the accumulation of significant amounts of citrate in tissues and to irreversible cardiac damage (19).

Ngaio tree (*Myoporum laetum*). The leaves of this New Zealand tree, and other *Ngaio* spp., in Australia, contain ngaione, a hepatoxic ketone which causes jaundice, photosensitization and death in all animal species which ingest them.

Yellow pine tree (*Pinus ponderosa*). It is commonly held by farmers that the ingestion of the needles of this tree causes abortion in cattle (12).

Jumbey (*Bahamas*), *Lamtoro* (*Indonesia*) *or Koa Haole* (*Hawaii*) (*Leucaena leucocephala*). This leguminous tree is used as fodder in many tropical countries and contains a toxic amino-acid—mimosine. Horses are most commonly affected, signs including loss of the hair of the mane and tail and occasionally around the hocks and knees, emaciation and ring formation of the hooves. Inco-ordination, temporary blindness and occasionally alopecia occur in cattle when the tree is dominant in the diet. Experimental feeding to pregnant cattle has produced goitre, stillbirths and low birth weight (14). In sheep neonatal goitre and shedding of the fleece are recorded after feeding on *L. leucocephala* but the absence of these abnormalities on some occasions suggests that substances other than mimosine may be responsible for them (15). The feeding of diets containing up to 15 per cent of dried *L. leucocephala* leaves to pregnant gilts caused a high proportion of foetuses to be resorbed and some foetuses to have limb deformities. The feeding of 1 per cent ferrous sulphate reduced these effects (16).

Stinkwood (*Zieria arborescens*). This tall shrub or small tree occurs in areas of over 30 in. annual rainfall in Tasmania and eastern Australia. Cattle eat it when other food is scarce. The natural disease is reproducible by feeding 30 to 60 lb. of the herbage during a period of 2 to 4 weeks. The clinical signs appear as tachypnoea up to 80 per minute, grunting, extension of the head, mouth breathing, abdominal respiration and a nasal discharge. In bad cases the temperature and pulse are elevated. Death occurs after an illness of 1 to 21 days; some cases survive. At necropsy examination there is massive pulmonary oedema and emphysema (17). The disease resembles closely atypical interstitial pneumonia as it occurs in western U.S.A.

Supple Jack (*Ventilago viminalis*). This tree is a palatable and valuable fodder tree but if it is used as the major part of the diet of sheep for about 3 weeks (an unlikely field occurrence) toxicity appears. The principal signs are hypersensitivity to external stimuli, resulting in repeated tetanic convulsions. Autopsy findings include abomasal ulceration and hepatic and renal degenerative lesions (18).

REFERENCES

(1) Fowler, M. E. & Richards, W. P. C. (1965). *J. Amer. vet. med. Ass.*, *147*, 1215.

(2) Dollahite, J. W. *et al.* (1962). *Amer. J. vet. Res.*, *23*, 1264, 1268, 1271.

(3) Dollahite, J. W. *et al.* (1966). *J. Amer. vet. med. Ass.*, *148*, 908.

(4) Szabuniewicz, M. *et al.* (1971). *Arch. int. Pharmacodyn. Ther.*, *189*, 12.

(5) Mugera, G. M. & Nderito, P. (1968). *Bull. epizoot. Dis. Afr.*, *16*, 501.

(6) Russell, L. H. *et al.* (1969). *Amer. J. vet. Res.*, *30*, 1233.

(7) Lowe, J. E. *et al.* (1970). *Cornell vet.*, *60*, 36.

(8) Hunt, S. E. & McCosker, P. J. (1968). *Amer. J. vet. clin. Path.*, *2*, 161.

(9) Hall, W. T. K. (1964). *Aust. vet. J.*, *40*, 176.

(10) Denz, F. A. & Hanger, W. G. (1961). *J. Path. Bact.*, *81*, 91.

(11) Aplin, T. E. H. (1968). *J. Dept. Agric. West Aust.*, *9*, 356.

(12) Allen, M. R. & Kitts, W. D. (1961). *Canad. J. Anim. Sci.*, *41*, 1.

(13) Hegarty, M. P. *et al.* (1964). *Aust. J. agric. Res.*, *15*, 153.

(14) Hamilton, R. I. *et al.* (1968). *Aust. vet. J.*, *44*, 484.

(15) Little, D. A. (1971). *Aust. vet. J.*, *47*, 457.

(16) Wayman, O. *et al.* (1970). *J. Anim. Sci.*, *30*, 583.

(17) Munday, B. L. (1968). *Aust. vet. J.*, *44*, 501.

(18) Pryor, W. J. *et al.* (1972). *Aust. vet. J.*, *48*, 339.

(19) Allcroft, R. *et al.* (1969). *Vet. Rec.*, *84*, 403.

Fodder Crops

Many crops grown to provide feed for livestock may cause poisoning in some circumstances.

Rape *(Brassica napus)* Poisoning

Also Kale or Cole (Brassica oleracea), Chou Moellier, Turnips and Swedes

Plants of all the Brassica species cause several syndromes including haemolytic anaemia, blindness, pulmonary emphysema, and digestive disturbances which may occur separately or in combination.

Incidence

The diseases have been recorded where the plants are grown extensively as fodder or pasture crops for autumn and winter. The incidence is not great but on individual farms a number of animals may be affected and the outcome is fatal in most cases.

Aetiology

Attempts at isolation of toxic factors have been unsuccessful. In the haemolytic form of the disease there is a close association between the feeding of the plants and the existence of hypophosphorosis and this form of the disease is closely related to post-parturient haemoglobinuria. In the haemolytic form of the disease most attention has been focused on toxic thioglucosides, at least in kale. The pulmonary emphysema associated with grazing on rape and allied plants also occurs at the same time of the year on other types of pasture and there may be no direct causal relationship between rape and the disease.

The seeds and leaves of these plants may contain significant quantities of cyanogenetic substances and this may be related to their capacity to produce goitre in lambs and occasional outbreaks of bloat in cattle. Rape seed meal has also been shown to cause goitre in pigs when fed in the proportion of 10 to 20 per cent in the diet but the goitrogenic substance in the meal is an organic substance other than cyanide.

The toxicity of the plants appears to vary from year to year and on rape grazing most outbreaks occur in wet years when early frosts occur and the plants assume a purple colour. Nitrate and nitrite poisoning have also been recorded on rape. The toxicity of kale has been reported to increase markedly after the seeds develop and it is suggested that the toxic material is in maximum concentration in the seeds. With the development of the rapeseed oil industry rape-seed cake is becoming more commonly available for feeding purposes and one might expect records of poisoning. Severe haemorrhagic gastroenteritis has been recorded in cattle fed rape-seed cake containing crotonyl isosulphocyanate (1). However, the haemolytic disease does occur in cattle feeding on the leaves and stems. The haemolytic toxicity of kale varies widely between varieties (2) but all varieties have some toxicity. The important factor precipitating outbreaks of disease is the amount of kale eaten (3).

Occurrence

Poisoning may occur in cattle and sheep grazed on the crops, and goitre in lambs may develop when the ewes are fed on kale. Frosted, wilted and discoloured leaves may be more toxic than others and the diseases are more likely to occur in low-lying, poorly drained areas. The haemolytic syndrome occurs more frequently when the phosphorus status of the animals is low and possibly also during cold weather (4).

Both marrowstem and thousandhead kale are toxic and the apparent toxic, haemolytic principle in the plant is destroyed in heat-dried or ensiled kale, but it is still present in frozen material (5).

Pathogenesis

Little is known of the mode of development of the various syndromes. Kale has been shown to cause a haemolytic anaemia in sheep and cattle, and heavily pregnant and recently parturient animals have increased susceptibility to this haemolytic effect (4, 6, 7). One notable characteristic of the anaemia is that in goats and sheep continued feeding after the anaemia develops is followed by a return to normal of haemoglobin levels (5, 8). The association between the haemolytic anaemia and hypophosphataemia has already been mentioned.

Allergy has been proposed as a possible cause of the emphysema syndrome by analogy with similar diseases caused by pulmonary invasion with lungworm larvae in sensitized cattle—the so-called 'fog fever'. Paralysis of rumen musculature can result from the ingestion of cyanogenetic substances and the same compounds reduce the uptake of iodine by the thyroid.

Clinical Findings

Bloat and goitre are discussed as clinical entities in other sections and only the more specific syndromes of haemolytic anaemia, 'rape blindness', pulmonary emphysema and digestive disturbances are described here.

Haemolytic anaemia has been observed in cattle and sheep on rape and kale, in cattle on drumhead cabbage and brussels sprouts (4) and in sheep on chou moellier. Lactating cows are most commonly affected but the disease has been seen in steers. The onset in severe cases may be so sudden that no signs are observed before the animal collapses and dies. If clinical illness is apparent haemoglobinuria is observed first and is soon followed by weakness and dejection. Pallor of the mucosae, moderate jaundice, tachycardia and a slight increase in respiratory rate and depth are also observed. Diarrhoea occurs commonly and, although body temperatures are usually normal to low, there may be fever up to $40.5°C$ ($105°F$). Death is common unless effective treatment is provided and surviving animals require a long period of convalescence. A normal haematological status may not be regained for up to 6 weeks. In an affected herd it is common to find a number of animals which are not seriously ill but which have a subclinical anaemia.

'*Rape blindness*' is manifested by the sudden appearance of blindness in cattle and sheep grazing on rape. More severe nervous signs including headpressing and mania have been observed in steers. The eyes are normal on ophthalmoscopic examination, the pupils show some response to light and may or may not be dilated. Complete recovery usually occurs but may take several weeks.

Pulmonary emphysema has been observed only in cattle. Affected animals show severe dyspnoea, with stertorous rapid respiration, mouth breathing and subcutaneous emphysema. The temperature may or may not be elevated. Affected animals may survive but often remain chronically affected and do poorly.

Digestive disturbances in steers on rape are usually accompanied by anorexia, the passage of small amounts of faeces, absence of ruminal sounds and the presence of a solid, doughy mass in the rumen. Only a small quantity of sticky, black material is present on rectal examination.

Clinical Pathology

In the haemolytic anaemia syndrome the erythrocyte count, haemoglobin level, haematocrit and leucocyte levels are reduced and Heinz–Ehrlich bodies are present in up to 100 per cent of erythrocytes. They are significantly increased in numbers before anaemia appears (9). The anaemia is macrocytic and may be of very severe degree. Haemoglobin is present in the urine. There is often a concurrent hypophosphataemia.

Necropsy Findings

In the haemolytic syndrome there is pallor, jaundice, haemoglobinuria, thin, watery blood, dark colouration of the kidney, and accentuation of the lobular appearance of the liver. Histologically there is moderate hepatic necrosis in the liver. In the emphysema syndrome there is emphysema and oedema, sometimes accompanied by the hepatic lesions of the anaemic syndrome, and the accumulation of dark-coloured ingesta and patchy congestion of the alimentary mucosa which characterize the digestive form of the disease.

Diagnosis

The occurrence of the disease when cattle or sheep are grazing on plants of the *Brassica* spp. suggests the presumptive diagnosis. There are many other causes of haemolytic anaemia including postparturient haemoglobinuria, which is limited to cows which have calved recently, leptospirosis, bacillary haemoglobinuria, anaplasmosis, and babesiasis all of which are accompanied by fever and toxaemia. Chronic copper poisoning can only be proved by estimation of blood and liver copper levels.

Acute pulmonary oedema and emphysema occur in 'fog fever' and other allergies. 'Rape blindness' has some clinical signs in common with poisoning by lead, *Senecio* spp. and other hepatoxic plants as well as rabies and other encephalitides.

Treatment

In severe cases of anaemia immediate blood transfusion is necessary if the animal is to be saved. Ancillary treatment includes the use of haematinic preparations and the provision of a highly nutritious diet. 'Rape blindness' and pulmonary emphysema respond poorly to treatment but antihistamines are recommended and in violent cases sedatives may be of value. The treatment of acute pulmonary oedema and emphysema is discussed in detail under atypical interstitial pneumonia (p. 878). In the digestive form it is usual to treat the animal with mild rumenatorics over a period of 7 to 10 days but the response is poor.

Control

The provision of ample hay either daily before the animals are pastured on the rape, or as a stack in the rape field, or allowing access to a field of rough grass are recommended to reduce the consumption of rape. Rape showing purple discolouration should be regarded with suspicion and only limited grazing permitted until doubts as to its safety are satisfied. Cattle and sheep grazing on these plants should be kept under close observation so that affected animals can be treated in the early stages of the disease. An adequate phosphorus intake is particularly necessary when ruminants are grazed on plants of this species.

REFERENCES

(1) Debackere, M. *et al.* (1966). *Vlaams Diergeneesk. Tijdschr.*, *35*, 393.
(2) Greenhalgh, J. F. D. *et al.* (1970). *Res. vet. Sci.*, *11*, 232.
(3) Greenhalgh, J. F. D. *et al.* (1972). *Res. vet. Sci.*, *13*, 15.
(4) Clegg, F. G. (1967). *4th int. Mtg Wld Ass. Buiatrics, Zurich, 1966*, p. 11.
(5) Greenhalgh, J. F. D. *et al.* (1969). *Res. vet. Sci.*, *10*, 64.
(6) Penny, R. H. C. *et al.* (1964). *Vet. Rec.*, *76*, 1053.
(7) Williams, H. L. *et al.* (1965). *Brit. vet. J.*, *121*, 2.
(8) Tucker, E. M. (1969). *Brit. vet. J.*, *125*, 472.
(9) Grant, C. A. *et al.* (1968). *Acta vet. scand.*, *9*, 126, 141.

Miscellaneous Fodder Crops

Sorghum (*Sorghum vulgare*), Johnson Grass (*S. halepense*), Sudan Grass (*S. sudanense*) and their hybrids, and Common Flax (*Linum usitatissimum*).

The sorghums are commonly used to provide green fodder, ensilage, or grain. Flax is grown commercially for fibre and linseed oil and meal. The plants may contain high concentrations of cyanogenetic glucosides, especially when growing rapidly after a period of retarded growth, and cause heavy mortalities due to cyanide poisoning. The nitrate content of the plants may be sufficiently high to cause nitrite poisoning in cattle.

In recent years a syndrome characterized by cystitis, urinary incontinence, loss of hair due to scalding and ataxia, which is most marked in the hind-legs when the horse is backed or turned, has been reported as occurring in horses grazing Sudan or hybrid Sudan grass pastures in southwestern U.S.A. (1). Foetal deformities are also recorded after ingestion of the plant (2) and death in adult horses is usually due to pyelonephritis (3). Only the growing plant produces this effect and the factors responsible are unknown. Lathyrogenic nitriles have been suggested because suitable precursors are present in the plants and the clinical signs have a considerable resemblance to lathyrism in man (3). Focal axonal degeneration and demyelination are present in lumbar and sacral parts of the spinal cord (1). The foetal deformities comprise fixation of all joints causing dystocia (2).

SUGAR BEETS, MANGELS AND FODDER BEETS (*Beta vulgaris*)

These roots are in common use as feeds for animals but they may cause toxic effects in some circumstances. When frozen they may cause indigestion and when fed in excessive amounts mangels, sugar and fodder beet may cause acute rumen impaction with lactic acidaemia in cattle. The latter disease is not identical with that caused by overeating on grain because dehydration is not always present and deaths occur irrespective of the degree of haemoconcentration. Hypocalcaemia and hypermagnesaemia also occur. The recommended maximum intake of fodder beet is 30 kg. daily for adult cattle and 3 kg. for sheep. Recently lifted or partly cooked mangel roots may cause nitrite poisoning. The tops of the growing plants may contain large amounts of oxalates and may cause oxalate poisoning and in some circumstances blindness and haemolytic anaemia similar to the diseases caused by ingestion of plants of the *Brassica* spp.

POTATO (*Solanum tuberosum*)

Potatoes are toxic only if they are green and sprouted and the toxic alkaloid solanin is concentrated in the sprouts and green skin. Pigs are most commonly affected but all species are susceptible. Potatoes must constitute more than 50 per cent of the diet before toxicity occurs. Clinical signs appear several days after feeding commences. In pigs there is dullness, copious diarrhoea, anorexia and a subnormal temperature, and coma in the terminal stages. The mortality rate in groups of affected pigs may be high. In horses the signs include depression and prostration but usually there are no signs of alimentary tract irritation. In cattle a dermatitis, manifested by vesicles and scabs, appears on the legs. At necropsy in all species there is a moderate hyperaemia of the alimentary mucosa.

Treatment should include central nervous system stimulants and alimentary tract astringents. Recovery follows when the potatoes are omitted from the diet of pigs. Sprouted or diseased potatoes can be fed safely if they are boiled and the amount fed restricted to less than 25 per cent of the diet.

CORNSTALK POISONING

Cornstalk poisoning is an all-inclusive term which may include nitrite poisoning, bloat or various fungal intoxications but not all of the reported outbreaks can be so classified.

Poisoning is reported in cattle fed on corn plants which are stunted by drought conditions or early frosts. Although the incidence is usually low, the morbidity rate may reach 50 per cent in affected herds and the mortality rate approximates 100 per cent. Clinical signs usually commence 7 to 10 days after the cattle are turned on to the stalk field and include dullness, recumbency and muscle tremor affecting the ears, thorax and abdomen. If the animal is forced to rise the gait is weak and staggery. The pulse, temperature and respiration are normal but there is atony of the rumen, complete closure of the iris, so that the animal is unable to see, and dribbling of urine. Clonic convulsions may precede death. At necropsy petechial haemorrhages are present under most serous surfaces and striped zones of haemorrhage are present in the mucosa of the terminal portion of the large bowel. The liver and kidneys are swollen. No effective treatment has been found, although dextrose solutions administered intravenously may cause temporary improvement.

CEREAL CROP POISONING

Grazing of cereal crops when in the young growing stages often results in a condition allied to lactation tetany and known colloquially as 'wheat poisoning'. Heavily fertilized crops may contain sufficient nitrate to cause nitrite poisoning in cattle but clinical illness does not usually occur unless the crop is made into hay and undergoes heating or wetting. Stunted mature crops are sometimes grazed when they are too short to harvest. The crops may contain sufficient grain to cause acute rumen impaction.

BUCKWHEAT (*Fagopyrum sagittatum*)

Buckwheat is grown for its seeds and they and the vegetation contain photodynamic substances which may cause photosensitive dermatitis in all species of animals.

PEA VINE ENSILAGE

Pea vines salvaged from pea-canning factories are made into ensilage, usually in stacks, and when fed out to ewes in the winter have produced a nervous disorder in 90 per cent of the young lambs (4). Silage which has turned black rather than the normal dark green is most frequently involved. The lambs are normal at birth but signs appear at 1 to 3 days of age. While standing the lambs show tetany and either walk backwards or run forwards with the head lowered and back depressed. After a period of activity they become recumbent, limp and unable to stand but after a few minutes can get up and appear normal. The nervous syndrome reappears with exercise or excitement. Normal growth occurs if the lambs are confined. Dietary supplementation with added minerals and vitamins does not prevent the condition. At necropsy there is degeneration of Purkinje cells in the cerebellar cortex and vacuolar degeneration of cerebral neurones.

REFERENCES

(1) Adams, L. G. *et al.* (1969). *J. Amer. vet. med. Ass.*, 155, 518.
(2) Prichard, J. T. & Voss, J. L. (1967). *J. Amer. vet. med. Ass.*, 150, 871.
(3) Van Kampen, K. R. (1970). *J. Amer. vet. med. Ass.*, 156, 629.
(4) Whiting, F. *et al.* (1957). *Canad. J. comp. Med.*, 21, 77.

Miscellaneous Plant By-products Used as Feed

TRICHLOROETHYLENE-EXTRACTED SOYABEAN MEAL

Soyabean meal prepared by the trichloroethylene extraction of soyabeans contains an unidentified toxic substance which causes aplastic anaemia, leucopenia and damage to vascular endothelium. The disease has been known for many years but is now of historic interest only, other methods of extracting soyabean oil having been introduced. The disease produced has a striking resemblance to radiation sickness and the ruminant form of bracken poisoning. All farm animal species other than pigs are susceptible.

REVIEW LITERATURE

Strafuss, A. C. & Sautter, J. H. (1967). *Amer. J. vet. Res.*, 28, 1805.

LINSEED CAKE

Linseed cake is a common constituent of animal feeds. In certain circumstances it may cause toxic effects because of its high content of cyanide present in the form of the glucoside linamarin. Hydrocyanic acid poisoning may occur when large quantities of the cake are fed to hungry sheep, or calves are fed on cake which has been soaked. A high incidence of goitre in new-born lambs may result when large quantities are fed to ewes during late pregnancy. The cake can be detoxicated by soaking and then boiling for 10 minutes to eliminate the hydrocyanic acid.

COTTONSEED CAKE

Gossypol, a poisonous phenolic substance present in variable amounts in cottonseed cake, causes damage to the myocardium and liver parenchyma and significant changes in the electrocardiographs of treated pigs (1). Most recorded outbreaks of gossypol poisoning refer to pigs. Sheep are susceptible if the toxin is injected but appear to be unaffected when it is fed (2). Clinical signs do not appear until animals have been fed on rations containing cottonseed cake for 1 to 3 months. Anorexia, dyspnoea and weakness are the characteristic signs and death occurs after an illness of several days. Cottonseed cake may be fed with safety to pigs provided it constitutes less than 10 per cent of the ration, or in larger quantities if the material is detoxified. Cooking of the cake or the addition of 1 per cent calcium hydroxide or 0·1 per cent ferrous sulphate to it are efficient methods of detoxification (3). In experimental trials the addition of iron in equal proportions to gossypol up to 600 ppm of the ration will protect pigs (4). At necropsy there is generalized oedema due to congestive heart failure, and histologically there is degeneration of the myocardium and skeletal musculature. Centrilobular necrosis in the liver is also a characteristic lesion.

Many of the outbreaks of disease ascribed to the feeding of cottonseed cake have probably been due to deficiencies of essential nutrients, especially vitamin A.

BREWERS' GRAIN

Wet brewers' grain may develop high concentrations of lactic acid especially when kept in a heap rather than being spread out. If large amounts are fed, especially to cows on heavy grain rations, lactic acid poisoning, similar to that caused by overeating on grain, may result. Important clinical signs include ataxia, dehydration, sinking of the eyes, and sticky, foul-smelling faeces. Treatment by the oral administration of sodium bicarbonate is recommended (5).

HERRING MEAL

Certain batches of herring meal have been reported as causing widespread poisoning of ruminants in Norway (6). The toxic principle is thought to be dimethylnitrosamine (7) and the essential lesion is liver necrosis. Clinical signs appear after feeding the meal 2 to 3 weeks and include depression, loss of appetite and milk yield and ruminal atony, sometimes progressing to complete anorexia, ataxia of the hind limbs and abdominal pain with marked contractions of the abdominal muscles. There is a characteristic unpleasant odour on the breath and milk. Convulsions are observed occasionally but more often severe cases develop a 'dummy' syndrome followed by coma and death. The bromsulfalein clearance test appears to be of diagnostic value in both cattle and sheep.

REFERENCES

(1) Albrecht, J. E. *et al.* (1968). *J. Anim. Sci.*, 27, 976.
(2) Danke, R. J. *et al.* (1965). *J. Anim. Sci.*, 24, 1199.
(3) Jarquin, R. *et al.* (1966). *J. agric. Food Chem.*, 14, 275.

(4) Ullrey, D. E. (1966). *Mich. State Univ. Vet.*, *26*, 109.
(5) Owens, E. L. (1959). *N.Z. Vet. J.*, 7, 43.
(6) Hansen, M. A. (1964). *Nord. Vet.-Med.*, *16*, 323.
(7) Sakshaug, J. *et al.* (1965). *Nature, Lond.*, *206*, 1261.

DISEASES CAUSED BY ANIMAL AND INSECT BITES AND TOXINS

Snakebite

The bites of venomous snakes may cause serious effects in farm animals, but mortalities are rare. Nervous signs occur and there may or may not be local swelling depending on the type of snake.

Incidence

The incidence of snakebite is controlled by the geographical distribution of the snakes and their numbers. Asia, India, Africa, Central and South America, Australia and the southern United States are areas in which snake populations are large. In general the morbidity rate in farm animals is not high although a mortality rate of 20 per cent has been recorded in a small group of bitten animals (1).

Aetiology

At least four toxic actions can result from snake venoms and different snakes have varying combinations of toxins in their venoms. The toxins include necrotizing and coagulant fractions as well as neurotoxic and haemolytic fractions. Although there is often insufficient toxin injection to cause death in large animals a serious secondary bacterial infection may be set up in the local swelling and cause the subsequent death of the animal.

Occurrence

Most snakebite accidents occur during the summer months and bites are mainly about the head because of the inquisitive behaviour of the bitten animal. Pigs are not highly susceptible but not, as generally believed, because of their extensive subcutaneous fat depots (2). Sheep may be bitten on the udder but their long wool coat is generally effective as a protective mechanism on other parts of the body. Large animals tend to be resistant because of their large size and the large dose rate required to cause death. However horses appear to be much more susceptible to venom than any other species.

Pathogenesis

The effects of snakebite (envenomation) depend upon the size and species of the snake, the size of the bitten animal and the location of the bite, particularly with reference to the thickness of the hair coat and the quantity of subcutaneous fat. As a general rule the venom is injected by fangs which leave a bite mark comprising a row of small punctures with two large punctures outside them. An exception is the coral snake which must chew to inoculate the venom. The bites may be visible on hairless and unpigmented skin but can only be seen on reflection of the skin at necropsy in many instances. Non-poisonous snakes may bite animals but the bite mark is in the form of two rows of small punctures.

The neurotoxins cause initial stimulation of the central nervous system followed by paralysis. Effects of the other toxins include local tissue necrosis, capillary damage and haemolysis.

Clinical Findings

Bites by adder-type snakes cause a local swelling which develops very rapidly and causes severe pain, usually sufficient to produce signs of excitement and anxiety. Bites about the head may be followed by swellings of sufficient size to cause dyspnoea. If sufficient neurotoxin has been injected a secondary stage of excitement occurs and is followed by marked dilation of the pupils, salivation, hyperaesthesia, tetany, depression, recumbency and terminal paralysis. In small animals death may occur due to asphyxia during convulsions in the excitement stage of the disease. In animals that recover there is usually local sloughing at the site of the swelling.

Bites by cobra-type snakes cause no local swelling except in animals that survive the effects of the neurotoxin. These commonly develop local swellings due to bacterial infection 3 to 4 days later. The major effects after bites of cobra-type snakes are excitement with convulsions, and death due to asphyxia. The signs appear quickly and death occurs usually within 1 to 10 hours in dogs and in up to 48 hours in horses. In calves the effects of the neurotoxin are manifested by marked pupillary dilation, excitement, inco-ordination and later paralysis (3).

Necropsy Findings

Local swellings at the site of the bite are due to exudation of serous fluid which is often deeply bloodstained. Fang marks are usually visible on the under surface of the reflected skin.

Diagnosis

In acute cases death has usually occurred by the time the animal is seen. If the actual bite is observed the diagnosis is made on the history. Bacterial infection of bite-wounds may be confused with blackleg, anthrax or non-specific phlegmonous infections.

Treatment

Local treatment should include the application of a tourniquet above the bite to restrict the circulation and the application of suction if possible. The tourniquet should be released for a few minutes at 20-minute intervals. If the bite area is incised the incision should reach the site of deposition of the venom but does not require to be more than 0·5 cm. in depth. If it can be carried out very quickly after the bite has occurred, excision of the part is recommended for the bites of snakes which cause a serious local reaction (4). If possible the bitten area should be rested and immobilized.

Systemic treatment should include antivenin, antibiotics and antitoxin (5). Antivenin containing antibodies against the venoms of all the snakes in the area can usually be obtained locally, often in highly purified form. It is expensive to use but highly effective. Speed is essential and the intravenous route is preferred. A portion of the antivenin should be injected locally around the bite. The dose rate varies widely with the size of the animal, one unit often being sufficient for animals weighing 70 kg. or more, but smaller animals of 9 to 18 kg. body weight require about 5 units. A broad spectrum antibiotic should also be administered to control the local infection at the site of the bite. The occurrence of clostridial infections after snakebite suggests the administration of antitoxins against tetanus and gas gangrene. Supportive fluid treatment may be advisable when shock is severe and the administration of a sedative may be necessary to control pain and excitement.

Many other treatments have been used in snakebite including particularly ACTH, cortisone and antihistamines. These drugs have been found to be valuable as a protection against possible anaphylaxis after treatment with antivenin but in cases where local tissue damage is evident they are without value and in many cases exert deleterious effects (5, 6). Adrenaline or epinephrine have little or no value and calcium salts do not significantly reduce mortality. The application of chemicals to the incised bite area is also of no value and may exacerbate tissue damage. Attention has been drawn to the need to appreciate the mode of action of one's local snakes before attempting a general programme of treatment—what may be effective in one country may very well be lethal in another (4, 7).

REVIEW LITERATURE

Clarke, E. G. C. & Clarke, M. L. (1969). Snakes and snakebite. *Veterinary Annual*, Bristol: Wright.
Garnet, J. R. (1968). *Venomous Australian Animals Dangerous to Man*. Commonwealth Serum Laboratories, Melbourne.

REFERENCES

(1) Parrish, H. M. & Scatterday, J. E. (1957). *Vet. Med., 52*, 135.
(2) Araujo, P. *et al.* (1963). *Arch. Inst. biol. S. Paulo, 30*, 43, 49.
(3) Couttie, P. M. (1969). *Aust. vet. J., 45*, 384.
(4) Liefman, C. E. (1970). *Aust. vet. J., 46*, 182.
(5) Horak, I. G. (1964). *J. S. Afr. vet. med. Ass., 35*, 343.
(6) Parrish, H. M. *et al.* (1957). *J. Amer. vet. med. Ass., 130*, 548.
(7) Snyder, C. C. (1967). *J. Amer. vet. med. Ass., 151*, 1635.

Bee Stings

Multiple stings by bees may cause severe local swelling in animals. Pain may result in pronounced excitement and in severe cases in horses there may be diarrhoea, haemoglobinuria, jaundice, tachycardia and prostration. Animals attacked about the head may show dyspnoea because of severe local swelling. In rare cases the attack may be fatal (1). Treatment includes the local application of a weak solution of ammonia or sodium bicarbonate, nervous system stimulants if prostration is severe and tracheotomy if asphyxia threatens.

REFERENCE

(1) Wirth, D. (1943). *Wien. tierärztl. Mschr., 30*, 129.

Tick Paralysis

Infestations with a variety of species of ticks (see table on p. 668) cause paralysis of animals (1, 2). Dogs are most commonly affected but losses can occur in lambs, calves, goats and foals and even children (3). The ticks under natural conditions parasitize wild fauna, and infestations of other species occur accidentally. The disease is limited in its distribution by the ecology of the ticks and the natural host fauna. The paralysis which is characteristic of the disease is caused by a toxin secreted by the salivary glands of female ticks and which is present in much greater concentration in the glands of adults than in other stages. The severity of the paralysis is independent of the number of ticks involved; susceptible animals may be seriously affected by a few ticks. The toxin of *Dermacentor andersoni* interferes with liberation or synthesis of acetylcholine at the motor end-plates of muscle fibres (4). The disturbance is functional and paralysis of the peripheral neurones is the basic cause (5). Continuous secretion of toxin by the ticks is necessary to produce paralysis, recovery occurring rapidly as soon as the ticks are removed.

Clinically there is an ascending, flaccid paralysis commencing with inco-ordination of the hind-legs, followed by paralysis of the fore limbs and chest muscles. The respiration is grossly abnormal because of its diaphragmatic form; there is a double expiratory effort and the rate is slow but deep. All limb reflexes are absent, the pupils dilate widely and death is due to respiratory paralysis. In dogs there are additional signs including vomiting, absence of voice and secondary aspiration pneumonia. Death, due to respiratory failure, may occur in 1 to 2 days but the course is usually 4 to 5 days. The mortality rate may be as high as 50 per cent in dogs but is usually much lower in farm animals. Since tick-borne diseases, such as tularaemia, often coexist with tick paralysis, this possibility should always be considered in arriving at a diagnosis (6).

Hyperimmune serum is used in the treatment of dogs but in farm animals removal of the ticks in the early stages is usually followed by rapid recovery. Control necessitates eradication of the ticks or host fauna. The use of appropriate insecticides is an effective preventive.

REFERENCES

(1) Clunies-Ross, I. (1935). *Counc. sci. ind. Res. J., Aust.*, *8*, 8.

(2) Neitz, W. O. (1963). *Rep. 2nd. meet. FAO/OIE Panel Tick-borne Dis. Cairo 1962*, p. 24.
(3) Bootes, B. W. (1962). *Aust. vet. J.*, *38*, 68.
(4) Emmons, P. & McLennan, H. (1959). *Nature, Lond.*, *183*, 474.
(5) Abbott, K. H. (1943). *Proc. Mayo Clin.*, *18*, 39, 59.
(6) Jellison, W. *et al.* (1965). *Proc. 68th. ann. gen. Mtg U.S. Livestock san. Ass.*, pp. 60–64.

Cantharides Poisoning

Poisoning of horses by consumption of the beetle, *Epicauta vittata*, has been recorded in southern U.S.A. (1). The beetle, which contains cantharidin, is found in lucerne hay. Administration of 1 g. of ground beetles by stomach tube is fatal to a pony. Cattle are not affected.

Signs include irritation in the mouth, frequent urination and colic. On necropsy there is severe enteritis.

REFERENCE

(1) Bahme, A. J. (1968). *SWest. Vet.*, *21*, 147.

32

Diseases Caused by Allergy

Iso-immune Haemolytic Anaemia of the Newborn

THIS is a haemolytic disease of newborn animals caused by an incompatible blood group reaction between the serum antibodies of the mother and the erythrocytes of the newborn.

Incidence

The disease in horses occurs in most parts of the world. Both horse and mule foals are affected. In one area in France an incidence of 10 per cent in mule foals was recorded, apparently due to sensitization of mares to donkey red cells. In England, six cells were observed in a series of 1200 thoroughbred foalings. In the United States in a group of 65 thoroughbred mares observed over a 4-year period, nine affected foals were born to four mares.

The incidence of the disease in pigs after hog cholera vaccination has assumed some importance in Britain, and it has also occurred in the United States. Although the area incidence is small serious losses may occur in individual piggeries. In affected litters all piglets are affected, and many die of the disease.

Aetiology

In horses and mules the disease is caused by the natural occurrence of inherited blood groups. The foal inherits erythrocyte antigens from the sire and these pass through the placenta into the dam's circulation. If the antigens are not also part of the dam's normal complement, antibodies are produced in the dam's circulation against the foal's erythrocytes. The antibodies are usually produced in large quantities by the 8th to 10th month of pregnancy but do not affect the foetus because they are unable to pass the placental barrier. Thus, no reaction occurs until the foal is born and ingests colostrum which contains the antibodies in high concentration. Experimental immunization of mares against donkey erythrocytes has resulted in the birth of affected mule foals, suggesting that placental transmission of antibodies can occur (1).

Not all incompatible pregnancies result in sensitization of the mare. It has been suggested that abnormality of the placenta permits passage of the foetal red-cell antigen into the mare's circulation in some instances only. Vaccination of mares against equine viral rhinopneumonitis using foetal tissue vaccines has been considered as a possible cause of the disease. A rise in haemagglutination titre does occur after such vaccination but in most cases there are no clinical effects in the foals, probably because of the disappearance of the antibodies by foaling time. If vaccination is carried out twice during pregnancy the clinical syndrome may occur and the danger is greatest when the mares are vaccinated during the last 3 months of pregnancy.

Although the disease is recorded as occurring spontaneously in pigs (2, 3) the main occurrence is related to repeated vaccination against hog cholera, using the crystal-violet vaccine. The vaccine contains erythrocytes, and iso-antibodies to the cells are produced in the sows and transmitted to the piglets in the colostrum. This may cause iso-agglutination if the piglets have blood groups to which the sow has become sensitized. The disease is much more common in the litters produced by mating Large White boars with Essex or Wessex sows than in litters produced by Large White sows, and the variation is thought to be due to a differential inheritance of erythrocyte antigens (4). In pigs the high antibody titres may persist for several years causing losses in successive litters, or recede rapidly with no piglets affected at subsequent farrowings (5, 6). The occurrence of the disease has been related to the immunization of the sow against the boar's erythrocyte antigens via the foetus at parturition (7). If the breeding were repeated a significant antibody level could develop.

The disease has also occurred in calves whose dams had been vaccinated against babesiosis (8) or anaplasmosis (10) using a vaccine containing bovine blood. The calves had inherited blood group antigens from the sire that were not present in the dam's blood. As a result of vaccination the dam had developed lytic antibodies against the same sire antigens, and the presence of these antibodies in the colostrum provided the mechanism for the acute haemolytic anaemia in the calves. Attempts to produce the disease experimentally in lambs have been unsuccessful (9).

Pathogenesis

At parturition the antibody is concentrated in the dam's colostrum and soon after ingestion it is absorbed into the suckling's circulation. The interaction between the antibody and the red cells of the newborn is followed by intravascular haemolysis with resultant anaemia, haemoglobinuria and jaundice. Permeability of the intestine of the newborn foal to antibody disappears at about 36 hours and hourly milking of the mare rapidly reduces the antibody content of the colostrum. The duration of the alimentary permeability in piglets has not been determined.

The cause of death is usually the acute anaemia, although neonatal hypoglycaemia may also play a part in piglets with only moderate anaemia. It has been pointed out that many cases in pigs may be subclinical and be unobserved (5).

Clinical Findings

In the mare, pregnancy and parturition are uneventful and the foal is normal for some hours after birth. Signs appear only if colostrum is taken, and vary a great deal in severity.

Peracute cases develop within 8 to 36 hours of birth, show severe haemoglobinuria and pallor but little jaundice. The first observed abnormality may be complete collapse. The mortality rate is high. In acute cases signs do not develop until 2 to 4 days after birth and jaundice is marked, with only moderate pallor and haemoglobinuria. Subacute cases may not show signs until 4 to 5 days after birth. Jaundice is marked, there is no haemoglobinuria and only mild pallor of mucosae. Many subacute cases recover.

General signs include lassitude, weakness and disinclination to suck and the foal lies down in sternal recumbency for long periods and yawns frequently. There is no febrile reaction but the heart rate is increased up to 120 per minute. The cardiac impulse is readily palpable over a wide area and may be visible. Cardiac sounds are increased in amplitude and the area of auscultation is increased. The sounds have a metallic quality and a systolic thrill is audible over the left base of the heart and posteriorly. The arterial pulse has a very small amplitude and there is a well-marked positive jugular pulse in severe cases. Respiration is normal until severe anaemia develops when hyperpnoea, dyspnoea (respiratory rate up to 80 per minute) and yawning are observed. Peripheral oedema does not occur and there are no signs of involvement of the central nervous system. Constipation may occur late in the syndrome.

Piglets show essentially the same syndrome, being normal at birth but developing jaundice at 24 hours, and weakness at 48 hours with most affected pigs dying by the fifth day. Peracute cases occur and piglets may die within 12 hours of birth, showing acute anaemia but no jaundice or haemoglobinuria. A proportion of subclinical cases also occurs in which haemolysis can be detected only by haematological examination.

In calves clinical signs develop within 24 to 48 hours after birth and the calves die during the first week of life (10). Surviving calves are returned to normal health in 2 to 3 weeks. Peracute cases die within 24 hours, and at necropsy examination are characterized by pulmonary oedema and splenomegaly.

Clinical Pathology

Erythrocyte counts, packed cell volumes and haemoglobin levels are low and although the blood cells appear normal there is greatly increased erythrocyte fragility and sedimentation rate. In piglets, the erythrocyte count may be as low as 1 million per cmm. and the haemoglobin level below 2 g. per cent. Leucocyte counts are normal and immune iso-antibodies to the red cells of the foal or piglet and the sire are present in the dam's serum, colostrum and milk. The vital test is the direct sensitization test between the mare's serum and the foal's erythrocytes (11). The same test is of course applicable to all species. It has been found that careful drying of a few drops of blood from affected piglets on a glass slide shows marked erythrocyte agglutination. The slide is rocked gently to wash the cells in the plasma. A positive result is indicated by the appearance of the erythrocytes in clumps rather than as a homogeneous smear on the drying slide (12).

Necropsy Findings

In affected foals, marked pallor is evident but jaundice is slight in peracute cases. No gross change is observable in the liver but there is splenomegaly with soft pulp. In less severe cases jaundice is marked but pallor is only moderate in degree. Bacteriological examination is negative and histopathological changes are not marked. In piglets haemoglobinuria is an important sign, and jaundice or port wine colouration of tissues occur constantly (12). The presence of blood-stained peritoneal fluid and an enlarged spleen is also typical of the disease in piglets.

Diagnosis

There are no diseases of the newborn which present the same clinical picture as that of iso-immune haemolytic anaemia. Physiological icterus of the newborn may occur occasionally but rarely causes clinical illness. An iso-immune haemorrhagic anaemia has been recorded in newborn pigs, but gross haemorrhages were evident at necropsy and the age incidence was 5 to 14 days (13, 14).

Treatment

The aims of treatment are to repair the anaemia and prevent damage from anaemic anoxia and haemoglobinuric nephrosis. A transfusion of compatible blood causes a marked and rapid improvement. Because of the possibility of transfusion reactions in horses compatibility tests should be performed (11). If the necessity for rapid action makes this impossible any donor other than the dam may be used. It is also possible to select a donor by testing the donor's blood against the dam's serum. The blood of the dam, or other animal in which incompatibility appears probable, may be used after separating the cells, washing them free of plasma and resuspending them in saline or preferably donor plasma. The procedure has obvious practical limitations.

Whole blood may be stored for 5 days at 4°C (30°F) before use but haemolysis is likely if resuspended blood is stored. The intravenous injection of 500 to 600 ml. of blood into the saphenous vein is recommended. The transfusion should be repeated in 12 to 24 hours but phlebitis, thrombosis and embolism are likely to occur after multiple venepunctures. The transfusion should take 30 minutes as overdosage or too rapid injection may cause circulatory embarrassment. Exchange transfusion appears to overcome this danger and a highly efficient method has been devised which makes this technique simple and economical (11). Four litres of whole blood and 500 ml. of blood concentrated by sedimentation is recommended as a suitable dose.

In cases occurring in the first 3 days of life, the foal should be placed on a foster mother or on reconstituted cows' milk. After 48 hours it is safe to permit sucking of the mare. In pigs the prevention of sucking for periods of up to 24 hours does not prevent the disease. If the fluid intake is low 200 to 400 ml. of normal saline containing 4 per cent glucose and 3 per cent sodium bicarbonate, should be administered to foals by stomach tube twice daily.

In piglets the safest procedure is to remove them from the sow, feed them artificially for 48 hours and then return them to the sow. Frozen bovine colostrum collected as soon as possible after calving is a satisfactory substitute for sow colostrum but is improved by the addition of pig serum. When transfusion is necessary the intraperitoneal is a practical and safe route (15). In both species it is also advisable to use penicillin or other antibiotics to prevent secondary infection if colostrum is not provided.

Control

In horses the only method available at present is to test the mare's serum against the sire's cells during the last 2 weeks of pregnancy. A positive agglutination reaction will suggest fostering or hand-rearing the foal. If the test can be repeated on several occasions at 2-week intervals a rapid rise in titre of the mare's serum suggests the probability of an incompatible mating. After birth the foal's erythrocytes may be submitted to an agglutination test with the mare's serum. If the test is positive (at titres of 1:32 or above), in either case, the foal should be muzzled for 48 hours and fed cows' milk and lime water (2:1) or colostrum from a nonsensitized dam. Addition of vitamins A and C to the milk improves its nutritive value. Suckling is permitted for five minutes at the end of this time and if after 12 hours there is no apparent reaction the foal is put back on the dam. Hourly milking of the dam in the meantime will reduce the haemagglutination titre of the milk from 1:64 to less than 1:2.

The frequent occurrence of the disease after the use of crystal-violet vaccine against hog cholera in the litters of Essex and Wessex sows has given rise to the suggestion that vaccine for use in these breeds should be prepared from homologous blood rather than from blood of another breed (4).

REFERENCES

(1) Girard, O. et al. (1956). Ann. Inst. Pasteur, 90, 96.
(2) Goodwin, R. F. W. & Coombs, R. R. A. (1956). J. comp. Path., 66, 317.
(3) Nansen, P. et al. (1970). Nord. Vet.-Med., 22, 1.
(4) Goodwin, R. F. W. & Saison, R. (1956). J. comp. Path., 66, 163.
(5) Goodwin, R. F. W. (1957). Vet. Rec., 69, 1290.
(6) Goodwin, R. F. W. & Saison, R. (1957). J. comp. Path., 67, 126.
(7) Linklater, K. A. (1968). Vet. Rec., 83, 203.
(8) Dimmock, C. K. & Bell, K. (1970). Aust. vet. J., 46, 44.
(9) Tucker, E. M. (1961). Nature (Lond.), 189, 847.
(10) Dennis, R. A. et al. (1970). J. Amer. vet. med. Ass., 156, 1861.
(11) Roberts, E. J. & Archer, R. K. (1966). Vet. Rec., 79, 61.

(12) Goodwin, R. F. W. (1957). *Vet. Rec.*, 69, 505.
(13) Stormorken, H. *et al.* (1963). *Nature (Lond.)*, 198, 1116.
(14) Nordstoga, K. (1965). *Path. vet.*, 2, 601.
(15) Edwards, B. L. (1965). *Vet. Rec.*, 77, 268.

Purpura Haemorrhagica

This is an acute, non-contagious disease, occurring chiefly in the horse, and characterized by extensive, oedematous and haemorrhagic swellings in subcutaneous tissues, accompanied by haemorrhages in the mucosae and viscera.

Incidence

Purpura haemorrhagica occurs only sporadically and usually as a sequel to upper respiratory infections in the horse. It achieves its highest incidence in large groups of horses used for military purposes, or during and after shipment. Most affected animals die of the disease.

Aetiology

The cause of the disease is uncertain. Its common association with streptococcal infection of the upper respiratory tract has led to the suggestion that it is caused by an allergic reaction to streptococcal protein. However, in some instances there is no history of prior occurrence of streptococcal infection. Purpura haemorrhagica is most common in horses although it has been recorded in pigs and is observed occasionally in cattle. A similar condition has been observed in newborn pigs. The purpura was thrombocytopenic and there were isoantibodies against the piglet thrombocytes in the dam's serum. Bleeding commenced at 5 days of age and continued for more than 7 days (1, 2, 3). A haemorrhagic disease which is similar in many respects to purpura haemorrhagica affects Charolais cattle in France (4).

Pathogenesis

Damage to capillary walls with extravasation of plasma and blood into the tissues is the basis of the disease process (3). It is not known whether the capillary damage is toxic or allergic in origin.

Occurrence

Most commonly the disease occurs as a sequel to strangles in horses, or in association with infectious equine arteritis or infectious equine rhinopneumonitis. Only a small proportion of horses become affected but the incidence is highest when extensive outbreaks of strangles occur, possibly because of reinfection with streptococci of horses already sensitized by previous infection.

Clinical Findings

Extensive subcutaneous, oedematous swellings are the characteristic sign of the disease. They occur most commonly about the face and muzzle, but are often present on other parts of the body and are not necessarily symmetrical in distribution. The swellings may appear suddenly or develop gradually over several days. They are cold and painless and pit on pressure and merge gradually in normal tissue without a definite line of demarcation between. There is no discontinuity of the skin although it may be tightly distended and even ooze serum. Swellings about the head may cause pressure on the pharynx and dyspnoea and difficulty in swallowing. Extensive oedema of the limbs, with a sharply defined upper margin, may occur but typical, discrete swellings do not develop below the knees or hocks.

Submucous haemorrhages occur in the nasal cavities and mouth, and petechiae may be present under the conjunctiva. Haemorrhage and oedema of the gut wall may cause severe, fatal colic but in most cases there is no diarrhoea or constipation. The temperature is normal or slightly elevated but the heart rate is frequently raised (90 to 100 per minute) probably because of loss of plasma or blood. The course of the disease is usually 1 to 2 weeks and many animals die at the end of this time from blood loss and secondary bacterial infections. Relapses occur commonly during convalescence.

Clinical Pathology

In severe cases there is a fall in the erythrocyte count and haemoglobin level, a marked neutrophilia but no marked depression of platelet counts. A leucocytosis occurs in less severe cases. There is no defect in the clotting mechanism. There may be oligocythaemia or polycythaemia depending upon the degree of loss of the plasma or whole blood. The urine is normal although there may be oliguria.

Necropsy Findings

Petechial haemorrhages are present generally throughout the body. The subcutaneous swellings contain plasma which may be bloodstained, or whole blood and plasma, and blood may be present in the body cavities. The intestines, lungs and spleen may be congested and there may be oedematous thickening of the intestinal wall. Details of the histopathology are available (5).

Diagnosis

In horses purpura haemorrhagica may be mistaken for congestive heart failure but in the latter the oedema is of the dependent parts only and haemorrhages are not present in the mucosae. Angioneurotic oedema is accompanied by large subcutaneous swellings but again there are no haemorrhages and the lesions disappear quickly after treatment. There is also some resemblance between purpura haemorrhagica and infectious equine arteritis and, to a less extent, infectious equine rhinopneumonitis but both of these diseases spread rapidly whilst purpura haemorrhagica affects only occasional animals and the oedema in the viral diseases is restricted to the limbs. Petechial haemorrhages of the mucosae and anaemia also occur in infectious equine anaemia but this disease is characterized by a regional distribution, a chronic recurrent course, jaundice, and restriction of oedema to dependent parts. Dourine is a venereal disease, and although oedematous swellings occur they originate in the external genitalia. 'Blue nose' is a photosensitization which occurs in the U.K. in horses on spring grass. Purplish colouration of the unpigmented skin around the muzzle and urticarial swellings in other parts of the body may create a resemblance to purpura haemorrhagica (6).

In cattle, haemorrhagic septicaemia, poisoning by bracken fern and sweet clover, and some other septicaemias are more likely causes of a haemorrhagic syndrome than is purpura haemorrhagica.

Treatment

Many treatments have been tried, including blood transfusions, antihistamine drugs, and formalin and calcium administered parenterally, but with variable results. Blood transfusions give the greatest chance of recovery and are usually supported by full and continuous doses of corticosteroids. At least 4 litres of blood should be given every 48 hours. Calcium gluconate (100 to 200 ml. of a 7·5 per cent solution), or calcium lactate (600 ml. of a 10 per cent solution), intravenously daily have also been found useful. Adrenaline (10 ml. of 1:1000) given daily as a subcutaneous injection may have some value. The intravenous injection of 10 ml. of 40 per cent formalin in 100 ml. of saline is an old-fashioned remedy with little to recommend it.

Control

The control and prevention of upper respiratory tract infections in horses should lead to a reduction in the incidence of purpura haemorrhagica.

REFERENCES

(1) Stormorken, H. *et al.* (1963). *Nature (Lond.)*, *198*, 1116.
(2) Nordstoga, K. (1965). *Path. vet.*, *2*, 601.
(3) Saunders, C. N. *et al.* (1966). *Vet. Rec.*, *79*, 549.
(4) Cottereau, P. (1965). *Encycl. vet. period.*, *22*, 33.
(5) King, A. S. (1949). *Brit. vet. J.*, *105*, 35.
(6) Greatorex, J. C. (1969). *Equine vet. J.*, *1*, 157.

Laminitis

Laminitis is a disease of all species, particularly the horse, characterized by damage to the sensitive laminae of the hooves. Clinically it is manifested by severe lameness with heat and pain around the coronets.

Incidence

Laminitis occurs only sporadically but a number of cases may occur at one time in a group of animals in special circumstances. It is of most importance in horses and cattle on heavy concentrate feed and has attracted particular attention in young cattle ($4\frac{1}{2}$ to 6 months of age) being fattened on heavy grain diets—the 'barley beef' calves—in the U.K. (11). Death is unusual but the severe lameness may cause a great deal of inconvenience and affected horses may develop permanent deformities of the feet.

Aetiology

Laminitis appears to be caused by an allergic reaction to protein, particularly that in grain feeds. The occurrence of the disease in mares which retain the placenta may also be a manifestation of allergy to protein derived from tissue breakdown or from streptococci which invade the uterus. Other factors are probably of importance also and predisposing causes may include obesity and standing for long periods during transport.

In cattle the disease is reported to occur after metritis, retained placenta, mastitis and mammary oedema (1) but the incidence is never very high. It is not uncommon to come upon herds of cattle which appear to be having a special problem with laminitis. The disease usually develops soon after calving and seems to be associated with a high incidence of metritis. It is possible that the disease, or rather a susceptibility to it, is inherited, especially as it occurs more frequently in Guernseys and in Jerseys (2). Laminitis has been recorded in pigs but the disease is difficult to diagnose in this species and many cases secondary to other diseases, e.g. postparturient fever, may be missed (3, 4). The disease is also recorded in this species when pigs are fed very heavy concentrate diets.

Pathogenesis

Until recently, it has been considered that laminitis is caused by engorgement of the vascular bed in the structures of the foot and that histamine is the causative mechanism of the engorgement.

An increase in blood histamine in horses affected with laminitis has been observed in contradistinction to the absence of histamine in the blood of normal horses (5). The histamine content of the ingesta of affected horses is also increased, and the intravenous injection of histamine does cause some of the clinical signs of laminitis.

The pathogenesis of the disease must be reconsidered in the light of more recent observations. For example, it has been suggested that the vascular changes are secondary and that the primary defect is one of epidermal horn formation resulting in weakening of the bond between hoof and laminae (6). On the evidence it seems more likely that the disease is primarily vascular and that the disappearance of the onychogenic substance is the result of hypoxia (8). On the other hand the study of the experimentally produced disease has shown that the arterial blood supply to the terminal arch in the hoof is markedly decreased or completely destroyed (7) rather than increased.

Occurrence

Laminitis is most common in horses which engorge moderately on grain feeds; it seldom occurs in those which eat sufficient to cause acute dilatation of the stomach. There seems to be a predisposition to laminitis in individual animals. Mares which retain the placenta are often affected. Fat ponies running at pasture and getting little exercise commonly develop the chronic form of the disease. Horses standing for periods of several days during transport may develop the acute form.

In ruminants, the disease is uncommon and occurs only as a result of overfeeding. Cattle and lambs introduced too quickly to heavy grain rations in feedlots may be affected and occasionally individual dairy cows which overeat develop the disease. Beef cattle being prepared for shows are often grossly overfed on high grain rations and become affected with a chronic form of the disease which markedly affects their gait and may cause permanent foot deformity. This is a serious matter to owners of show cattle because they have difficulty in regulating the food intake to achieve fatness and yet avoid laminitis. As in horses there appears to be a variation in susceptibility between individual animals, one or two animals in a group kept under identical conditions often developing the disease.

Clinical Findings

Laminitis may develop as an acute disease and be followed by recovery or persistence of a chronic state, or it may develop in a mild form from the beginning. In acute cases there is severe pain in all four feet; in occasional cases only the hind-feet are affected. The clinical signs are all manifestations of pain and include an expression of great anxiety, muscle shivering, sweating, a marked increase in heart rate, rapid, shallow respiration and a moderate elevation of temperature. The posture is characteristic, all four feet being placed forward of their normal position, the head held low and the back arched. There is usually a great deal of difficulty in getting the animal to move and when it does so the gait is shuffling and stumbling and the animal evidences great pain when the foot is put to the ground. The act of lying down is accomplished only with difficulty, often after a number of preliminary attempts. There is also difficulty in getting the animal to rise and some horses may be recumbent for long periods. It is not unusual for horses to lie flat on their sides. The diagnostic sign in laminitis is pain on palpation around the coronet, light palpation causing a marked pain reaction. In cattle and sheep the clinical picture is similar to but less marked than that observed in the horse. In calves 4 to 6 months of age an acute syndrome similar to that seen in the horse has been described. In sows the clinical signs are similar and include arching of the back, bunching of the feet, awkwardness of movement, increased pulsation in the digital arteries and pain when pressure is applied to the feet (4).

In the chronic stages of the disease there is separation of the wall from the sensitive laminae and a consequent dropping of the sole. The hoof wall spreads and develops marked horizontal ridges, and the slope of the anterior surface of the wall becomes accentuated and concave. Eventually the lameness may disappear but the animal is clumsy, goes lame easily with exercise and may suffer repeated, mild attacks of laminitis. In occasional cases the separation of the wall from the laminae is acute and the hoof is shed. A long-term study of the effects of an acute attack of laminitis on the subsequent performance of the horn has been conducted in cattle (10) and has shown that the solar horn of affected animals was thinner and more soft and waxy than that of normal animals. Also previously affected animals were much more susceptible to injury to the sole.

Clinical Pathology

Blood histamine levels and eosinophil counts may be raised but are often within the normal range and other haematological findings are normal (11). Radiological examination is an essential part of the diagnosis of laminitis, especially chronic laminitis in the horse. The downward tilting of the toe of the third phalanx and the ventral displacement of the whole phalanx are characteristic. In cattle rarefaction of the pedal bone, particularly the toe, and the development of osteophytes at the heel and on the pyramidal process are recorded (12).

Necropsy Findings

The disease is not usually fatal but if a necropsy examination is carried out on an acute case the stomach contents usually contain excessive amounts of grain, have a pasty, mealy consistency and an odour suggestive of putrefaction of protein. Retained placenta and metritis may be present in post-parturient laminitis in mares. No other gross findings are visible although there may be perceptible engorgement of the vessels of the sensitive laminae. Histological examination reveals disappearance of some of the keratogenic structures of the inner zone of cornification in the epidermal laminae. This is followed by vascular engorgement and some necrosis of laminar tissues. In subacute and chronic laminitis there are obvious gross changes in the shape of the foot (9).

Diagnosis

Laminitis is easily missed unless a typical history is available. The animal's distress, immobility and increased pulse and respiration always suggest severe pain but it is only when the posture and gait and pain in the feet are taken into consideration that it is possible to localize the lesion. Cases of laminitis in horses have been mistaken for tetanus, azoturia, rupture of the stomach or bladder, or colic, but in none of these diseases is the pain localized in the feet and there are other differentiating signs. In cattle and lambs recumbency after overeating is usual and the presence of laminitis may be difficult to detect. A clinically similar condition in young Hereford bulls appears to be genetic in origin. There is epiphysitis at the distal metacarpus and first phalanx and calcium deposits in the testes and kidneys (13).

Treatment

In acute cases antihistamine drugs give good results if administered during the first 24 hours of the onset of signs. Maximum doses should be given and repeated at 12-hour intervals for at least three injections. Corticosteroids have given good results in acute cases of the disease but should not be used beyond the second day because of the possibility of further reducing the protein status of the hoof horn (7). Excellent recoveries are reported after the treatment of acute and chronic cases with methionine. The treatment is based on the known requirement for methionine in the chondroitin complex of collagen (14). Ancillary treatment should include an analgesic in severe cases (Butazolidin, chloral hydrate or an ataractic drug), cold packs to the feet (either ice packs or standing the horse in mud or a water bath), and a mild purgative to hasten elimination of the toxic ingesta. If the animal will walk, forced exercise for short periods at frequent intervals is recommended in order to increase movement of blood through the foot. This could be improved further by locally anaesthetizing the volar nerves in the affected leg (7).

Additional non-specific treatments which have been used include venesection either from the jugular vein or from the sole of the foot, and autogenous blood therapy. In the latter 50 ml. of whole blood collected from the jugular vein is injected immediately in a deep intramuscular site. Excellent results are claimed for the procedure in both horses and cattle. Many recommended treatments have little justification. Spontaneous recovery from the acute disease does occur, often very rapidly and after an illness of only 24 hours. The acute disease in intensively fed calves does not appear to respond to any of these recommended treatments.

Medical treatment of chronic cases is seldom satisfactory and surgical procedures are recommended. Reduction of weight by a high quality protein, low-calorie diet may be advisable, along with Butazolidin when pain persists.

Control

The disease is not readily subject to control because of its sporadic nature. Heavily fed or fat horses should be given some exercise when not working; if possible horses in transit should be removed from the transport vehicle, given light exercise and rested for several hours at the end of each day; retained placenta in mares should be completely removed and early metritis treated promptly. Cattle and lambs which are brought into feedlots should be gradually introduced to grain feeds.

REFERENCES

(1) Nilsson, S. A. (1963). *Acta vet. scand.*, *4*, Suppl. 1, 304.
(2) Merritt, A. M. & Riser, W. H. (1968). *J. Amer. vet. med. Ass.*, *153*, 1074.
(3) Nilsson, S. A. (1964). *Nord. Vet.-Med.*, *16*, 128.
(4) Maclean, C. W. (1968). *Vet. Rec.*, *83*, 71.
(5) Akerblom, E. (1943). *Svensk vet. Tidskr.*, *48*, 10.
(6) Obel, N. (1948). Studies on the histopathology of acute laminitis. *Coll. Pap. vet. Inst.*, Stockholm, 63.
(7) Coffman, J. R. *et al.* (1970). *J. Amer. vet. med. Ass.*, *156*, 76.
(8) Maclean, C. W. (1971). *J. comp. Path.*, *81*, 563.
(9) Maclean, C. W. (1966). *Vet. Rec.*, *78*, 223.
(10) Maclean, C. W. (1971). *Vet. Rec.*, *89*, 34.
(11) Maclean, C. W. (1970). *Vet. Rec.*, *86*, 710.

(12) Maclean, C. W. (1970). *Vet. Rec.*, *86*, 457.
(13) Brown, C. J. *et al.* (1967). *J. Anim. Sci.*, *26*, 201, 206.
(14) Urmas, P. (1968). *Finsk VetTidskr.*, *74*, 11.

Allergic Dermatitis

(*Queensland Itch*)

This is an intensely itchy dermatitis of horses caused by hypersensitivity to insect bites.

Incidence

The disease is quite common in Australia, particularly in hot, humid coastal areas and similar conditions are recorded in Japan, North America, the Philippines, India and France. Only a proportion of horses in a group will be affected. Deaths do not occur but badly affected horses may be of little use as working animals because of the intense pruritus.

Aetiology

Hypersensitivity to the bites of a sandfly *Culicoides robertsi* has been shown to be a cause (1). Occasional cases in areas where sandflies do not exist suggest that other allergens may cause the disease. *Stomoxys calcitrans* has been identified as a causative insect in Japan (2).

Most cases occur during the hot humid months of summer and disappear during cooler weather. Only horses are affected and characteristic lesions have been observed in animals of all ages. Lesions disappear when the horses have been stabled for several weeks or are moved to an unaffected area.

Pathogenesis

Local accumulations of eosinophils and a general eosinophilia, together with a significant, seasonal increase in blood histamine levels occur and are suggestive of hypersensitivity (3).

Clinical Findings

Lesions are usually confined to the butt of the tail, rump, along the back, withers, crest, poll and ears. In severe cases the lesions may extend down the sides of the body and neck and on to the face and legs. Itching is intense, especially at night, and the horse scratches against any fixed object for hours at a time. In the early stages slight, discrete papules, with the hair standing erect, are observed. Constant scratching may cause severe inflammatory lesions and loss of hair. Scaliness and loss of hair on the ears and tail-butt may be the only lesions in mildly affected horses.

The general condition of the horse is unaffected except for some loss of condition due to interference with grazing.

Clinical Pathology

Affected animals have significantly elevated blood eosinophil and platelet counts. In early lesions, before trauma masks the true picture, oedema, capillary engorgement and eosinophil infiltration can be observed in a biopsy specimen.

Diagnosis

The intense scratching, the dorsal distribution of the dermatitis and the seasonal occurrence of the disease in association with biting insects are characteristic of this form of dermatitis.

A very similar disease occurs in cattle in Japan. It is thought to be due to an allergy to the bite of an external parasite (4).

Treatment

Local and parenteral application of antihistamine drugs may have some transient value.

Control

Prevention of the disease necessitates protection against sandfly bites by stabling in insect-proof quarters. Continuous spraying of the horses with insecticides or repellents may be of some value.

REFERENCES

(1) Riek, R. F. (1953). *Aust. vet. J.*, *29*, 177, 185.
(2) Ishihara, T. & Ueno, H. (1958). *Bull. natn. Inst. Hlth*, *Japan*, *34*, 105.
(3) Riek, R. F. (1955). *Aust. J. agric. Res.*, *6*, 161.
(4) Arisawa, M. (1971). *Bull. Nippon vet. zootch. College*, *19*, 46.

Milk Allergy

Signs of allergy, principally urticaria, are often manifested by cows during periods of milk retention (1). Most of these occur as the cow is being dried off. Cattle of the Channel Island breeds are most susceptible and the disease is likely to recur in the same cow at subsequent drying off periods; it is almost certainly inherited as a familial trait.

The important clinical signs relate to the skin. There is urticaria which may be visible only on the eyelids or be distributed generally. Local or general erection of the hair may also be seen. A marked muscle tremor, respiratory distress, frequent coughing, restlessness to the point of kicking at the abdomen and violent licking of themselves and even maniacal charging with bellowing may occur. Other cows may show dullness, recumbency, shuffling gait, ataxia and later inability to rise. The temperature and pulse rates are usually normal or slightly elevated but the respiratory rate may be as high as 100 per minute.

Diagnosis of milk allergy can be made by the intradermal injection of an extract of the cow's own milk. A positive reaction occurs with milk diluted as much as 1 in 10,000 and the oedematous thickening is present within minutes of the injection. Other clinico-pathological observations include the development of eosinopenia neutrophilia and hyperphosphataemia during an attack.

Spontaneous recovery is the rule but antihistamines are effective, especially if administered early and repeated at short intervals for 24 hours. Prevention is usually a matter of avoiding milk retention in susceptible cows but in many cases it is preferable to cull them.

REFERENCE

(1) Campbell, S. G. (1970). *Cornell Vet.*, *60*, 684.

33

Diseases Caused by
The Inheritance of Undesirable Characters

THE occurrence of congenital and other defects in one or more animals in a group may lead to the suspicion that the defect is inherited. Such defects may be lethal when they are incompatible with life, debilitating when the animal can survive but in an impaired state, or aesthetic when the animal is normal except in appearance. The majority of inherited defects are congenital but many congenital defects arise because of causes other than inheritance, including nutritional deficiency, viral infection in early pregnancy and the administration of some drugs. Differentiation of the causes or groups of causes is often difficult because the genesis of the defect and the administration of the causative insult will have occurred some months prior to the recognition of the disease.

Most inherited defects are conditioned by recessive genes and the final diagnosis of inheritance as the cause of a defect can only be made on the results of test matings in which the occurrence of the defect matches the statistically predicted occurrence. Test matings are in many instances impossible and a tentative diagnosis is usually made on the basis of contributory evidence. The appearance of the defect in a small proportion (about 25 per cent) of a litter or a group of animals sired by one male and out of a number of females related to each other, although not necessarily to the male, should arouse suspicion of inheritance as a cause. When a defect occurs suddenly in a high percentage of a litter or a group, environmental influences are probably involved and the same is true when multiple defects occur in one animal.

The widespread use of artificial insemination in cattle may lead to an apparent increase in the incidence of inherited undesirable characters, particularly when a popular bull is used extensively in a population of cows which carry an undesirable factor which is also present in the bull's genetic make-up. Such an occurrence can only be prevented by strong action on the part of breed societies which should refuse to register the sons of known carriers unless they are test-mated with other known carriers and shown not to be carriers of the undesirable factor. Satisfactory evidence of freedom from the factor is accepted when normal calves are born from matings with 10 known carriers or 20 daughters of carriers. The practical application of this procedure has been described in the control of 'bulldog' calves in the Guernsey breed (3).

Only the more common inherited defects are described here and for greater detail more comprehensive works are recommended (1, 2, 4, 5, 6, 7).

REFERENCES

(1) Stormont, C. (1958). *Advances in Veterinary Science*, Vol. 4, pp. 137–163, New York: Academic Press.
(2) Koch, P., Fischer, H. & Schumann, H. (1957). *Erbpathologie der landwirtschaftlichen Haustiere*, Berlin & Hamburg: Paul Parey.
(3) Jones, W. A. (1961). *Vet. Rec.*, *73*, 937.
(4) Filkins, M. E. (1965). *The Veterinarian*, *3*, 255.
(5) Young, G. B. (1967). *Vet. Rec.*, *81*, 606.
(6) Anonymous (1971). *Vet. Rec.*, *Members Info*. Suppl. No. 74.
(7) Priester, W. A. *et al.* (1967). *Amer. J. vet. Res.*, *31*, 1871.

INHERITED METABOLIC DEFECTS

Inherited Congenital Porphyria

This is a congenital defect of porphyrin metabolism in cattle and swine characterized by excessive excretion of porphyrins in urine and faeces and deposition of porphyrins in tissues, especially bones and teeth. Photosensitization occurs in affected cattle.

Incidence

The disease occurs rarely and as yet is of little economic importance. It has been recorded in Shorthorn, Holstein, Black and White Danish (1) and Jamaica Red and Black cattle (2). Affected cattle suffer from incapacitating photosensitization when exposed to sunlight and must be kept indoors.

In countries where sunlight hours are limited the disease may go unnoticed. The disease is also recorded in pigs, which appear to suffer little harm (3).

Aetiology

Most cases of porphyria in cattle are due to the inheritance of a single recessive factor, heterozygotes being clinically normal (1). Although there is no strict sex linkage in the mode of inheritance, the incidence is higher in females than in males. In pigs the pattern of inheritance is uncertain but may be due to one or more dominant genes (3). Porphyria in man is of three types and must be differentiated from the porphyrinuria which occurs in liver insufficiency and which is the result of deficient conversion rather than excess production of porphyrins. Cattle and pigs are the only domestic species in which congenital porphyria has been recorded.

Occurrence

Congenital porphyria occurs rarely and is of importance only when affected animals with relatively light coloured skins are exposed to sunlight.

Pathogenesis

The porphyrins are natural pigments but in this disease they are present in larger than normal concentrations in the blood, urine and faeces. The metabolic defect is probably one of abnormal synthesis of haem due to enzymatic insufficiency at the stage of conversion of pyrrol groups to series 3 porphyrins. Excess series 1 porphyrins are produced as a result and there is flooding of the tissues with these colouring and photosensitizing substances. Thus this disease is one of overproduction of physiologically inactive porphyrins. Photosensitivity occurs in cattle because the high tissue levels of porphyrins sensitize the skin to light.

Clinical Findings

The passage of amber to port-wine coloured urine, a pink to brown discolouration of the teeth and bones, and severe photosensitization are characteristic of the disease in cattle. Additional signs include pallor of the mucosae and retardation of growth. The health of affected pigs is usually normal and photosensitivity does not occur but the disease can be recognized by the red-brown discolouration of the bones and teeth which is present even in the newborn.

Clinical Pathology

The urine is amber to port-wine colour when voided due to the high content of porphyrins. The colour darkens to brown on exposure to light. Spectroscopic examination is necessary to identify the pigment as porphyrin. Erythrocyte survival time is reduced considerably. A macrocytic, normochromic anaemia occurs and its severity appears to be related to the level of uroporphyrins in the erythrocytes (4). Cattle with the highest erythrocyte uroporphyrin levels are also the most sensitive to sunlight (5).

Necropsy Findings

The teeth and bones are stained brown or reddish purple, the pigment occurring chiefly in the dentine in teeth and often in concentric layers in the bones. Affected bones and teeth show a red fluorescence under illumination with ultra-violet light.

Diagnosis

The disease must be differentiated from photosensitization due to other causes and symptomatic porphyrinuria caused by liver insufficiency. Affected cattle and pigs can be detected at birth by the discolouration of the teeth. Breeding trials are necessary to detect heterozygous, normal carrier animals (5).

Treatment

Non-specific treatment for photosensitization may be necessary. Affected cattle should be reared indoors.

Control

Elimination of affected carrier animals from the breeding programme is the only control measure available. Periodic examination of the urine and faeces for excessive quantities of coproporphyrin is carried out on bulls used for artificial insemination in breeds in which the disease occurs (1).

REFERENCES

(1) Jorgensen, S. K. (1961). *Brit. vet. J.*, *117*, 1, 61.
(2) Nestel, B. L. (1958). *Cornell Vet.*, *48*, 430.
(3) Jorgensen, S. K. (1959). *Brit. vet. J.*, *115*, 160.
(4) Kaneko, J. J. & Mills, R. (1970). *Cornell Vet.*, *60*, 52.
(5) Wass, W. M. & Hoyt, H. H. (1965). *Amer. J. vet. Res.*, *26*, 654, 659.

Familial Polycythaemia

This inherited defect has been observed only in Jersey cattle. Attention is drawn to the presence of the disease by early calfhood deaths and a clinical syndrome including congestion of mucosae, dyspnoea and poor growth. Haematologically there is marked elevation of erythrocyte count, haemoglobin concentration and packed cell volume (1, 2). The disease appears to be a primary polycythaemia inherited as a simple autosomal recessive.

REFERENCES

(1) Tennant, B. *et al.* (1969). *Cornell Vet.*, *49*, 594.
(2) Kaneko, J. J. *et al.* (1968). *Amer. J. vet. Res.*, *29*, 949.

Inherited Goitre

This disease is recorded in Merino sheep (1, 2) and appears to be inherited as a recessive character. The essential defect is in the synthesis of thyroid hormone leading to increased production of thyrotropic factor in the pituitary gland, causing in turn a hyperplasia of the thyroid gland. Clinically there is a high level of mortality, enlargement of the thyroid above the normal 2·8 g., but varying greatly up to 222 g., and the appearance of 'lustrous' or 'silky' wool in the fleeces of some lambs. Other defects which occurred concurrently were oedema and floppiness of ears, enlargement of, and outward or inward bowing of, the front legs at the knees, and dorso-ventral flattening of the nasal area.

REFERENCES

(1) Rac, R. *et al.* (1968). *Res. vet. Sci.*, *9*, 209.
(2) Mayo, G. M. E. & Mulhearn, C. J. (1969). *Aust. J. agric. Res.*, *20*, 533.

Chediak–Higashi Syndrome

This inherited disease occurs in man, in mink and in Hereford and possibly other breeds of cattle. Affected animals are incomplete albinos and have a defect in immune defence mechanisms so that they often die of septicaemia. The average life-span of affected cattle is 12·4 months. It is readily diagnosed by the detection of anomalous enlarged cytoplasmic granules in neutrophils, lymphocytes, monocytes, and eosinophils (1). The disease is conditioned by a factor inherited as a single autosomal recessive.

Non-lethal albinism also occurs in cattle (2) and a lethal dominant form has been recorded in horses (3).

REFERENCES

(1) Padgett, G. A. (1968). *Advanc. vet. Sci.*, *12*, 240.
(2) Winzenreid, H. U. & Lauvergne, J. J. (1968). *Proc. XII int. Congr. Genet.*, *Tokyo*, *1*, 280.
(3) Pulos, W. L. & Hutt, F. B. (1969). *J. Hered.*, *60*, 59.

INHERITED DEFECTS OF THE ALIMENTARY TRACT

Inherited Harelip

Harelip in cattle often has a distinct familial tendency but little work appears to have been done on the mode of inheritance (1).

REFERENCE

(1) Wheat, J. D. (1960). *J. Hered.*, *51*, 99.

Inherited Atresia of Alimentary Tract Segments

Atresia ani occurs quite commonly in pigs, sheep and to a less extent in cattle. Affected animals may survive for up to 8 days but develop marked abdominal distension. Surgical repair is possible in some cases but in others a large segment of rectum is missing and creation of a colonic fistula in the inguinal region is necessary. The condition is thought to be inherited in pigs and calves; the evidence is less clear in sheep (1, 4).

Inherited atresia coli with complete closure of the ascending colon at the pelvic flexure, has been recorded in Percheron horses (2). Death occurs during the first few days of life. The defect appears to be inherited as a simple recessive character.

Inherited atresia ilei has been recorded in Swedish Highland cattle (3). Affected calves manifest marked abdominal distension causing foetal dystocia. The distension is caused by accumulation of intestinal contents. Inheritance of a single recessive gene conditions the occurrence of the defect.

REFERENCES

(1) Dennis, S. M. & Leipold, H. W. (1972). *Vet. Rec.*, *91*, 219.
(2) Hutt, F. B. (1946). *Cornell Vet.*, *36*, 180.
(3) Nihleen, B. & Eriksson, K. (1958). *Nord. Vet.-Med.*, *10*, 113.
(4) Norrish, J. G. & Rennie, J. C. (1968). *J. Hered.*, *59*, 186.

Smooth Tongue

(*Epitheliogenesis imperfecta linguae bovis*)

A defect of Holstein-Friesian and Brown Swiss cattle, this condition is inherited as an autosomal recessive factor (1, 2). The filiform papillae on the tongue are small, there is hypersalivation and poor haircoat and the calves do not fare well. The heterozygote is normal.

REFERENCES

(1) Weisman-Hamerman, Z. M. (1970). Proefschrift Vet. Fak. Rijksuniv. Utrecht, 135.
(2) Huston, K. *et al.* (1968). *J. Hered.*, *59*, 65.

INHERITED DEFECTS OF THE CIRCULATORY SYSTEM

Inherited Lymphatic Obstruction of Ayrshire Calves

This defect has been recorded in Ayrshire calves in New Zealand (1), Scotland (2), Australia (3), the United States (4) and Finland (5). Males are more often affected than females; it has been suggested that some affected females may not be detected. The defect appears to be inherited as a single, autosomal recessive character.

The degree of oedema varies from slight to severe, severe cases causing dystocia to the point where embryotomy or Caesarean section is necessary. Some mortality occurs among the dams. Many calves are dead at birth and those born alive may be reared but the oedema persists. Before parturition the cow may show evidence of hydrops amnii and have difficulty in rising. In calves the oedema may be generalized or, more commonly, be localized to the head, neck, ears, legs and tail. Drooping of the ears caused by increased weight is characteristic and accessory lobes are commonly situated behind and at the base of the ears.

The oedema is caused by a developmental abnormality of the lymphatic system. The lymph nodes are small and contain cystic dilatations and the lymphatic vessels are enlarged, tortuous and dilated. Oedema of the subcutaneous tissues and body cavities varies in degree; the skin is usually thickened and there is oedema of the stomach wall. A cyst has been described in the pituitary gland of one animal (4). The liver is usually small. A similar condition is observed in newborn pigs born to sows vaccinated with attenuated hog cholera virus during the first 30 days of pregnancy.

REFERENCES

(1) Hancock, J. (1950). *Proc. 10th ann. Conf. N.Z. Soc. Anim. Prod.*, p. 91.
(2) Donald, H. P. *et al.* (1952). *Brit. vet. J.*, *108*, 227.
(3) Morris, B. *et al.* (1954). *Aust. J. exp. Biol. Med. Sci.*, *32*, 265.
(4) Herrick, E. H. & Eldridge, F. E. (1955). *J. Dairy Sci.*, *38*, 440.
(5) Korkman, N. (1940). *Nordisk Jordbrugsforsk.*, *22*, 225.

Ventricular Septal Defect

There is one report of the occurrence of ventricular septal defect in Hereford cattle in such a way as to suggest that the condition is inherited (1).

REFERENCE

(1) Belling, T. H. (1962). *Vet. Med.*, *57*, 965.

Inherited Aortic Aneurysm

An inherited defect of the abdominal aorta, resulting in a high mortality from intra-abdominal haemorrhage, has been observed in cattle in Holland (1). The breed of cattle is not recorded.

REFERENCE

(1) Schuiringa-Sybesma, A. M. (1961). *T. Diergeneesk.*, *86*, 1192.

INHERITED DEFECTS OF THE NERVOUS SYSTEM

Inherited Idiopathic Epilepsy of Cattle

Idiopathic epilepsy has been reported as an inherited condition in Brown Swiss cattle (1) and appears to be inherited as a dominant character. Typical epileptiform convulsions occur especially when the animals become excited or are exercised. Attacks do not usually commence until the calves are several months old and disappear entirely between the ages of 1 and 2 years.

REFERENCE

(1) Atkeson, F. W. *et al.* (1944). *J. Hered.*, *35*, 45.

Familial Convulsions and Ataxia in Cattle

A new neurological disease is recorded as being inherited in Aberdeen-Angus cattle (1). In young calves there are recurrent attacks of convulsions and in older animals these are replaced by a residual ataxia. It is conditioned by a character inherited in a dominant fashion. The first signs appear within a few hours of birth up to several months later. There are single or multiple tetanic convulsions lasting for 3 to 12 hours. As these episodes disappear a spastic 'goose-stepping' gait is apparent in the forelegs and difficulty in placing the hindlegs. The characteristic necropsy lesion is a very selective cerebellar cortical degeneration.

REFERENCE

(1) Barlow, R. M. *et al.* (1968). *Vet. Rec.*, *83*, 60.

Inherited Congenital Hydrocephalus

Congenital hydrocephalus without abnormality of the frontal bones occurs sporadically but is also known to be an inherited defect in Holstein and Hereford and possibly in Ayrshire (1) cattle. There is obstruction to drainage of the cerebro-spinal fluid from the lateral ventricles which become distended with fluid and may cause bulging of the forehead, often sufficient to cause foetal dystocia. Hereford calves with this defect have partial occlusion of the supra-orbital foramen, a domed skull and poorly developed teeth and at necropsy the cerebellum is found to be small. They are usually born a few days prematurely and are small in size. In some cows the amniotic fluid is increased in volume. Another form of inherited hydrocephalus due to malformation of the cranium and with a variable degree of enlargement of the cranium has also been observed in Hereford cattle (2, 3). Affected calves may be alive at birth, are blind and unable to stand but do not usually survive for more than a few days. At necropsy there is internal hydrocephalus of the lateral ventricles with marked thinning of the overlying cerebrum. Other lesions include constriction of the optic nerve, detachment of the retina, cataract, coagulation of the vitreous humour, and a progressive muscular dystrophy (3). The condition is inherited as a recessive character.

Congenital hydrocephalus in Yorkshire and European pigs (4) has been recorded. The abnormality varies from a small protrusion of dura (meningocele) to an extensive brain hernia in which the cerebral hemispheres protrude through the frontal suture, apparently forced there by increased fluid pressure in the lateral and third ventricles. The condition is thought to be inherited in a recessive manner, but exacerbated in its manifestation by a coexisting hypovitaminosis A.

REFERENCES

(1) Barlow, R. M. & Donald, L. B. (1963). *J. comp. Path.*, *73*, 410.
(2) Baker, M. L. *et al.* (1961). *J. Hered.*, *52*, 135.
(3) Urman, H. K. & Grace, O. D. (1964). *Cornell Vet.*, *54*, 229.
(4) Meyer, H. & Trautwein, G. (1966). *Path. vet.*, *3*, 529, 543.

Inherited Congenital Achondroplasia with Hydrocephalus

(*Bulldog Calves*)

First recorded in Dexter cattle this inherited defect has since been observed in a variety of forms in other breeds, including Jerseys, Guernseys and Holsteins. Affected calves are often aborted but some reach full term and cause foetal dystocia because of the extreme hydrocephalus (1). The forehead bulges tremendously over a foreshortened face with a depressed, short nose. The tongue protrudes, the palate is cleft or absent, the neck is short and thick and the limbs are shortened. Accompanying defects are foetal anasarca and hydrops amnii in the dam.

The defect is primarily a chondrodystrophy rather than an achondroplasia and the nasal bones and maxillae do not grow. Hydrocephalus develops because of the deformed cranium. In most breeds the condition is inherited as a simple recessive character but a dominant form has occurred in Jerseys (2). The heterozygous form in Dexters is easily recognized by the shortness of the limbs. The heterozygote in other breeds is normal in appearance.

REFERENCES

(1) Jones, W. A. (1961). *Vet. Rec.*, *73*, 937.
(2) Innes, J. R. M. & Saunders, L. Z. (1957). *Advanc. vet. Sci.*, *3*, 35.

Inherited Congenital Cerebellar Defects

Three inherited cerebellar defects occur congenitally in farm animals; cerebellar hypoplasia of calves, cerebellar atrophy of lambs and hereditary ataxia of calves. They all need to be differentiated from similar defects known to be caused by viral infections such as swine fever, bovine mucosal disease/virus diarrhoea and bluetongue in early pregnancy.

Cerebellar hypoplasia occurs in Herefords, Guernseys, Holsteins (1), Shorthorns (2) and Ayrshires (3) and appears to be conditioned by a factor inherited in a recessive manner. Most calves are obviously affected at birth. While lying down there is no marked abnormality although a moderate lateral tremor of the neck occurs, causing a gentle side-to-side swaying of the head. Severely affected calves are blind, have widely dilated pupils and their pupils do not react to light. Such calves are unable to stand, even when assisted, because of flaccidity of limb muscles. When less severely affected animals attempt to rise the head is thrown back excessively and the limb movements are exaggerated in force and range and are grossly inco-ordinated, and many calves are unable to rise without assistance. If they are placed on their feet the calves adopt a straddle-legged stance with the feet wide apart and the legs and neck extended excessively. On attempting to move, limb movements are inco-ordinated and the calf falls, sometimes backwards because of over-extension of the forelimbs. Affected animals drink well but have great difficulty in getting to the teat or pail, attempts usually being wide of the mark. There are no defects of consciousness and no convulsions. Tremor may be evident while standing and post-rotational nystagmus after rapid lateral head movements may occur. Sight and hearing are unimpaired and, although complete recovery does not occur, the calf may be able to compensate sufficiently to enable it to be reared to a vealing weight.

At necropsy the most severe defect comprises complete absence of the cerebellum, hypoplasia of the olivary nuclei, the pons and optic nerves and partial or complete absence of the occipital cortex. Less severe defects include a reduction in size of the cerebellum and absence of some neuronal elements in a cerebellum of normal size.

An occurrence of cerebellar hypoplasia has been recorded in Arabian foals. On one farm 6 to 8 per cent of foals were affected over several years. Signs, which include head tremors and erratic gait, can be present at birth or appear up to 4 months later (5). The aetiology is uncertain.

Cerebellar atrophy of lambs has been recorded in many breeds in Britain and in Corriedales in Canada. Affected lambs are normal at birth but are unable to walk properly. There is severe incoordination of limb movement, opisthotonus, tremor, and a straddle-legged stance. At necropsy the cerebellum may be of normal size but on histological examination there is gross atrophy of cerebellar neurons. The disease appears to be conditioned by a recessive gene but not as a simple homozygous recessive.

Inherited ataxia of calves. This is a true cerebellar ataxia inherited as a recessive character in Jerseys, Shorthorns and Holsteins. Clinically the condition resembles cerebellar hypoplasia except that signs may not occur until the calves are a few days to several weeks old. At necropsy the cerebellum is normal in size but histologically aplasia of neurones is evident in the cerebellum and also in the thalamus and cerebral cortex. An inherited condition, manifested by cerebellar ataxia which did not develop until calves were 6 weeks to 5 months old has also been recorded (4) but the cerebellum was small and macroscopically abnormal. Conspicuous degeneration of cerebellar Purkinje cells was evident on histological examination.

Inherited congenital spasms of cattle. This condition has been recorded only in Jersey cattle and appears to be conditioned by a factor inherited in a recessive manner. Affected calves show intermittent, vertical tremor of the head and neck and there is a similar tremor of all four legs which prevents walking and interferes with standing. Although the calves are normal in all other respects they usually die within the first few weeks of life. No histological examinations have been reported but a cerebellar lesion seems probable. A similar condition, described as being inherited as a single recessive character, has been described in horses in Europe.

REFERENCES

(1) Innes, J. R. M. & Sunders, L. Z. (1957). *Advanc. vet. Sci.*, *3*, 35.
(2) Finnie, E. P. & Leaver, D. D. (1965). *Aust. vet. J.*, *41*, 287.
(3) Howell, J. McC. & Ritchie, H. E. (1966). *Path. vet.*, *3*, 159.
(4) Johnson, K. R. *et al.* (1958). *J. Dairy Sci.*, *41*, 1371.
(5) Sponseller, M. L. (1968). *Mod. vet. Pract.*, *49*, 40.

Inherited Spastic Paresis of Cattle

(*Elso-Heel*)

This disease occurs in the Holstein, Aberdeen Angus, Red Danish, Ayrshire, Beef Shorthorn (1) and several Dutch and German breeds of cattle and probably in many others. It has been observed in an Ayrshire × Beef Shorthorn crossbred steer (2). The disease occurs principally in calves with signs appearing from several weeks to 6 months or more after birth. Occasional cases are reported as developing in adult European cattle and there is one report of the occurrence of the disease in adult Indian cattle (3). It is suggested that different time appearances represent a single disease entity with varying expressivity, the late forms being affected by cumulative environmental factors (4). In both diseases there is excessive tone of the gastrocnemius muscle and straightness of the hock, usually more marked in one hind-leg. If only one leg is affected it may be thrust out behind while the calf is walking and advanced with a restricted, swinging motion often without touching the ground. There is no resistance to passive flexion of the limb. The gastrocnemius and perforatus muscles are rigid and in a state of spastic contraction. There is a characteristic elevation of the tail. The lameness becomes progressively worse and affected animals spend much time lying down. Much body weight is lost and the animal is usually destroyed between 1 and 2 years of age. Minor lesions described as regressive changes in the neurones of the red nucleus, in the reticular substance and the lateral vestibular nucleus (5) are of doubtful significance (1). There are demonstrable lesions on radiological examination of the tarsus. The disease is conditioned by an inherited factor, but the precise mechanism of inheritance is arguable (6). It seems extraordinary that the continued use of affected animals for breeding purposes should be condoned. This is done in Europe on the basis of the efficacy of the curative surgical operation (6, 7) and in view of the high incidence of double muscling in such calves. In the Holstein breed, and several German breeds, bulls which sire affected calves have been observed to have very straight hocks and to suffer from various forms of stifle and hock lameness early in life.

REFERENCES

(1) Leipold, H. W. *et al.* (1967). *J. Amer. vet. med. Ass.*, *151*, 598.
(2) Love, J. & Weaver, A. D. (1963). *Vet. Rec.*, *75*, 394.
(3) Gadgil, B. A. *et al.* (1970). *Vet. Rec.*, *86*, 694.
(4) Lojda, L. (1967). *Veterinarstvi*, *17*, 256.
(5) Chomiak, M. & Szteyn, S. (1970). *Schweiz. Arch. Tierheilk.*, *112*, 397.
(6) Schonmuth, G. *et al.* (1971). *Mh. Vet.-Med.*, *26*, 17, 24.
(7) Bouckaert, J. H. & de Moor, A. (1966). *Vet. Rec.*, *79*, 226.

Inherited Periodic Spasticity of Cattle

This disease has been observed in Holstein and Guernsey cattle and usually does not appear until the animals are adults (1). It is a particular problem in mature bulls maintained in artificial insemination centres. In the early stages the signs are apparent only on rising, the hind-legs being stretched out behind and the back depressed. Marked tremor of the hind-quarters may be noted. Initially the attacks persist for a few seconds only but are of longer duration as the disease progresses and may eventually last for up to 30 minutes. Movement is usually impossible during the attacks. The tetanic episodes fluctuate in their severity from time to time but there is never any abnormality of consciousness. Lesions of the vertebrae have been recorded but no lesions have been found in the nervous system. The disease is familial and the mode of inheritance appears to be by inheritance of a single recessive factor with incomplete penetrance (2).

Administration of the spinal cord depressant, mephenesin (3 to 4 g. per 100 kg. body weight given orally in 3 divided doses and repeated for 2 to 3 days) controls the more severe signs. A single course of treatment may be effective for some weeks.

REFERENCES

(1) Roberts, S. J. (1965). *Cornell Vet.*, *55*, 437.
(2) Becker, R. B. *et al.* (1961). *J. Dairy Sci.*, *44*, 542.

Inherited Neonatal Spasticity

The defect is recorded in Jersey and Hereford cattle (1). Affected calves are normal at birth but develop signs 2 to 5 days later. The signs commence with inco-ordination and bulging of the eyes and a tendency to deviation of the neck causing the head to be held on one side. Subsequently the calves are unable to stand and on stimulation develop a tetanic convulsion in which the neck, trunk and limbs are rigidly extended and show marked tremor. Each convulsion is of several minutes duration. Affected calves may survive for as long as a month if nursed carefully. There are no gross or histological lesions at necropsy. Inheritance of the defect is conditioned by a single, recessive character.

REFERENCE

(1) Gregory, K. E. *et al.* (1962). *J. Hered.*, *53*, 130.

Hereditary Neuraxial Oedema

This congenital defect of the nervous system has been reported only in Polled Hereford cattle (1, 2) and appears to be transmitted by inheritance in an autosomal recessive pattern. At birth affected calves are unable to sit up or rise and are very sensitive to external stimuli, manifested by extreme extensor spasm, including fixation of thoracic muscles and apnoea, especially if lifted and held upright. The intellect of the calves seems unaffected, vision is normal, they drink well and can be reared but at great cost in time. Intercurrent disease is common and calves usually die of pneumonia or enteritis before they are a month old.

There are no gross lesions at necropsy examination but in some cases there is widespread vacuolation, interpreted as oedema, in terminal portions of myelinated nerve bundles and in gray substance containing heavily myelinated fibres.

REFERENCES

(1) Cordy, D. R. *et al.* (1969). *Path. vet.*, *6*, 487.
(2) Blood, D. C. & Gay, C. C. (1971). *Aust. vet. J.*, *47*, 520.

Inherited Congenital Posterior Paralysis

Two inherited forms of congenital posterior paralysis are recorded in cattle (1). In Norwegian Red Poll cattle posterior paralysis is apparent in affected calves at birth. Opisthotonus and muscle tremor are also present. No histological lesions have been found. The disease is conditioned by an inherited recessive factor. In Red Danish cattle a similar condition occurs but there is spastic extension of the legs, particularly the hind-legs, and tendon reflexes are exaggerated. Histological examination has revealed degenerative changes in mid-brain motor nuclei. Both defects are lethal because of prolonged recumbency.

An inherited posterior paralysis has been recorded in several breeds of swine in Europe (1). Affected pigs are able to move their hind-legs but are unable to stand on them. They are normal in other respects. Degeneration of neurones is evident in cerebral cortex, mid-brain, cerebellum, medulla and spinal cord. The disease is conditioned by the inheritance of a recessive character.

REFERENCE

(1) Innes, J. R. M. & Saunders, L. Z. (1957). *Advances in Veterinary Science*, Vol. 3, pp. 35–196. New York: Academic Press.

Inherited Congenital Myotonia of Goats

This disease has been observed in goats and possibly in a horse (1) and because of its great similarity to Thomsen's disease (myotonia congenita) of humans, affected goats have been used in experimental studies to determine the nature of the disease in man. There is no apparent defect of the nervous system and the condition is thought to be due to abnormality of the muscle fibres. Affected animals run when startled but quickly develop extreme rigidity of all four limbs and are unable to move. Relaxation occurs in a few seconds and the animal can then move again. Signs are not usually present until some time after birth and may vary from day to day for no apparent reason (3). They tend to diminish immediately before and after parturition. When water is withheld from affected goats for 2 to 3 days clinical signs disappear but reappear when drinking is permitted (2). The disease is inherited but the mode of inheritance is unknown.

REFERENCES

(1) Steinberg, S. & Botelho, S. (1962). *Science, N.Y.*, *137*, 979.
(2) Hegyeli, A. & Szent-Gyorgi, A. (1961). *Science, N.Y.*, *133*, 1011.
(3) Bryant, S. H. *et al.* (1968). *Amer. J. vet. Res.*, *29*, 2371.

Exophthalmos with Strabismus of Cattle

This disease has been recorded in Shorthorn (1) and Jersey cattle. In the former it is not manifested until the first pregnancy or lactation but in the latter may appear at 6 to 12 months of age. Defective vision is the first sign and is followed by severe protrusion and antero-medial deviation of both eyeballs. The defects may get worse over a long period. It appears to be inherited in a recessive manner.

REFERENCE

(1) Holmes, J. R. & Young, G. B. (1957). *Vet. Rec.*, *69*, 148.

INHERITED DEFECTS OF THE MUSCULO-SKELETAL SYSTEM
Inherited Osteoarthritis of Cattle

There are strong indications from field evidence that both degenerative arthropathy, in which the hip joint is principally involved (1), and degenerative osteoarthritis affecting particularly the stifle joint, are inherited in cattle. In both diseases other factors, particularly nutritional deficiency and the stress of lactation, exert an important influence on the appearance of the clinical disease and in degenerative arthropathy there is no clear evidence that it is in fact inherited. On the other hand there is good evidence that osteoarthritis can be inherited, at least in Holstein-Friesian and in Jersey cattle (2).

In inherited degenerative osteoarthritis in which the stifle joints are most severely affected there is usually a gradual onset of lameness in both hind-legs in aged animals of both sexes. Occasionally only one leg appears to be involved. Progression of the disease proceeds over a period of 1 to 2 years and is evidenced by failure to flex the limb resulting in the foot not being lifted high from the ground. Crepitation in the stifle joint can be heard and felt,

the muscles of the limb atrophy and the joints are enlarged. Movement is slow, the hind-legs at rest are placed further forward than normal, the stifles are abducted and the feet held together. Joint fluid can be aspirated and is clear and straw-coloured. Appetite and milk yield remain normal until the late stages, except in cattle running at pasture.

At necropsy there is severe osteoarthritis involving particularly the stifle, with extensive erosion of the articular cartilages, great increase in synovial fluid and the development of many osteophytes around the edges of the articular surfaces. Less severe changes are evident in other joints. It is suggested that the disease is conditioned by the inheritance of a single autosomal recessive character.

An inherited defective development of the acetabulum occurs in Døle horses. There is no clinical evidence of the disease at birth but osteoarthritis of the joint and disruption of the round ligament develop subsequently (3).

REFERENCES

(1) Carnahan, D. L. (1968). *J. Amer. vet. med. Ass.*, *158*, 1150.
(2) Kendrick, J. W. & Sittmann, K. (1966). *J. Amer. vet. med. Ass.*, *149*, 17.
(3) Sokoloff, L. (1960). *Advanc. vet. Sci.*, 6.

Inherited Multiple Ankylosis of Cattle

Multiple ankylosis affecting all limb joints has been recorded as an inherited congenital defect in Holstein calves (1). The abdomen of the dam shows marked enlargement at the 6th to 7th month of pregnancy and this may occasion some respiratory distress. Excessive foetal fluids are present and insertion of the hand per rectum is impeded by the distended uterus. Abortion during the last month of pregnancy is a common occurrence. Affected foetuses have a very short neck, ankylosed intervertebral joints and varying degrees of ankylosis of all limb joints. The limbs are fixed in flexion and there is some curvature of the spine. Foetal dystocia always occurs and embryotomy or Caesarean section is necessary to deliver the calf.

Ankylosis of limb joints combined with cleft palate occurs occasionally in Charolais cattle and is suspected of being inherited (2). Ankylosis of the coffin joint, developing at several weeks of age, has been reported in Simmental calves. The aetiology of the condition is not clear (3).

REFERENCES

(1) Murray, M. D. (1951). *Aust. vet. J.*, *27*, 73, 76.
(2) Lauvergne, J. J. & Blin, P. C. (1967). *Annl. Zootech.*, *16*, 291.
(3) Martig, J. *et al.* (1972). *Vet. Rec.*, *91*, 307.

Inherited Multiple Tendon Contracture

This disease has been recorded in Shorthorn calves and is thought to be inherited as a single recessive character. It resembles closely the non-inherited disease of calves, arthrogryposis. The limbs of affected calves are fixed in flexion or extension and cause dystocia due to abnormal positioning and lack of flexibility. There is no involvement of joint surfaces and the joints can be freed by cutting the surrounding tendons or muscles. There is atrophy of limb muscles and those calves which are born alive are unable to stand and usually die or are destroyed within a few days. Clinically similar defects have been observed to be inherited amongst Døle cattle in Norway and merino sheep. Contracture of appendicular joints also occurs congenitally in foals but appears not to be inherited (1).

A defect similar in some respects to the above syndrome has been recorded in cattle (2) and appears to be inherited in a dominant manner. The front legs are straight and rigid down to the fetlock which is permanently flexed. The hind-legs are sickle-shaped but the joints are freely movable in all directions. The teeth are soft, fleshy and easy to bend. There is no defect of bones or joints other than marked softness and the presence of excess cartilage at the epiphyses. There is abnormal ossification of the cartilage. The calves are of normal size, do not cause dystocia and although they are unable to stand because of the excessive flexibility of the limbs, they can suck. Hypostatic pneumonia usually develops and causes death of the calf.

REFERENCES

(1) Rooney, J. R. (1966). *Cornell Vet.*, *56*, 172.
(2) Johnston, W. G. & Young, G. B. (1958). *Vet. Rec.*, *70*, 1219.

Inherited Reduced Phalanges

This defect has been recorded in cattle and appears to be inherited as a single recessive character. The limbs are normal down to the metacarpal and metatarsal bones, which are shorter than usual, but the first two phalanges are missing and the normal hooves and third phalanges are connected to the rest of the limb by soft tissues only. The calves are unable to stand but can crawl about on their knees and hocks.

An even more serious defect, in which the mandible and all the bones below the humerus and stifle were vestigial or absent has been reported in British (1), French (2) and German (3) Friesians. It appears to be conditioned by the inheritance of a single recessive gene. Similar 'amputates' have been shown not to be inherited (4).

REFERENCES

(1) Bishop, M. W. H. & Cembrowicz, H. J. (1964). *Vet. Rec.*, *76*, 1049.
(2) Lauvergne, J. J. & Cu, Q. P. (1963). *Ann. Zootech.*, *12*, 181.
(3) Rieck, G. W. & Bähr, H. (1967). *Dtsch. tierärztl. Wschr.*, *74*, 356.
(4) Harbutt, P. R. *et al.* (1965). *Aust. vet. J.*, *41*, 173.

Inherited Defects of Claws

Extra claws (polydactylism) and fusion of the claws (syndactylism) are known hereditary defects of cattle, the former in the Normandy breed (1) and the latter in Holsteins (2). In most cases they cause no more than inconvenience.

REFERENCES

(1) Lauvergne, J. J. (1962). *Ann. Zootech.*, *11*, 151.
(2) Leipold, H. W. *et al.* (1969). *J. Dairy Sci.*, *52*, 1422.

Inherited Multiple Exostosis

Multiple exostosis affecting both cortical and medullary bone of the limbs and ribs has been described as an inherited condition in Quarter horses and Thoroughbreds in the U.S.A. The lesions are visible externally but cause little apparent inconvenience (1, 2).

REFERENCES

(1) Morgan, J. P. *et al.* (1962). *J. Amer. vet. med. Ass.*, *140*, 1320.
(2) Shupe, J. L. (1970). *Mod. vet. Pract.*, *51*, 34.

Inherited Thick Forelegs of Pigs

This defect is thought to be caused by the inheritance of a simple recessive character (1). Affected piglets show obvious lesions at birth and although many of them die or are destroyed immediately a proportion of them may survive. The forelegs are markedly enlarged below the elbows and the skin is tense and may be discoloured. There is difficulty in standing and moving about and starvation and crushing contribute to the mortality rate. There is extensive oedema of the subcutaneous tissues, thickening of the bones and roughness of the periosteum.

REFERENCE

(1) Kaye, M. M. (1962). *Canad. J. comp. Med.*, *26*, 218.

Osteogenesis Imperfecta in Lambs

Affected lambs are of normal size at birth but, although bright and alert, are unable to stand. The main feature of the condition is bone fragility with multiple fractures particularly of the limbs and ribs. The bones are of normal length and thickness and, in contrast to a similar disease in cats, the thyroid appears normal. The essential change appears to be a defect in the formation of bone matrix. Affected lambs may show a temporary response to calcium therapy. A genetic aetiology appears certain although the mode of inheritance is not clear (1).

REFERENCE

(1) Holmes, J. R. et al. (1964). Vet. Rec., 76, 980.

Inherited Rickets in Pigs

The disease is indistinguishable from rickets due to nutritional inadequacy. The pigs are healthy at birth. Subsequently there is hypocalcaemia, hyperphosphataemia and increased serum alkaline phosphatase. The defect is failure of active transport of calcium through the wall of the small intestine (1).

REFERENCE

(1) Plonait, H. (1969). Zbl. vet. Med., 16A, 271, 289.

Inherited Achondroplastic Dwarfism

Achondroplastic dwarfs are short-legged with short, wide heads and protruding lower jaws. The mandibular teeth may protrude 2 to 4 cm. beyond the dental pad preventing effective grazing and necessitating hand feeding if the animal is to survive. There is protrusion of the forehead and distortion of the maxillae, and obstruction of the respiratory passages results in stertorous respiration and dyspnoea. The tip of the tongue usually protrudes from the mouth and the eyes bulge. There is some variation between affected animals in their appearance at birth. In most cases the defects are as described above but they become more exaggerated as the calf grows. In addition abdominal enlargement and persistent bloat develop. The head is disproportionately large. The calves fail to grow normally and are about half the weight of normal calves of the same age.

The predominant form of the condition appears to be inherited as a simple recessive character although the relationship of the 'comprest' types to the total syndrome is more complex (1). Heterozygotes vary widely in conformation but some of them show minor defects which may be attractive to cattle breeders who are seeking a chunkier, short-legged type of animal. For this reason, unconscious selection towards the heterozygote has undoubtedly occurred, resulting in widespread dissemination of the character. Herefords and Aberdeen Angus are the breeds most commonly affected but similar dwarfs occur also in Holstein and Shorthorn cattle, and typical dwarf animals have been produced by mating heterozygous Aberdeen Angus and Herefords.

The detection of the heterozygous carrier animals is of first importance and many tests have been proposed to effect this differentiation. Careful examination of the head using a special 'profilometer' has been widely used. Radiographic examination of the lumbar vertebrae during the first 10 days of life may reveal compression of the vertebrae, disappearance of the concavity in the ventral surface of the vertebral body and bending forward of the lumbar transverse processes in affected animals (2). It is claimed that carrier, heterozygous animals have these defects in less, but recognizable, degree. Premature closure of the spheno-occipital synchondrosis is characteristic of dwarfism. Closure is reported to occur at $5\frac{1}{2}$ months compared to 24 to 36 months in normals and can be detected by roentgenological examination (3). Other characteristics of dwarf calves which are detectable by radiographic examination are the presence of two intracranial projections and shortening of the shafts of the long bones of the limbs (4).

Physiological tests have also been used. Because of a possible relationship between the disease and hypothyroidism, tests of thyroid function have been carried out and dwarf calves may have significantly lower plasma cholesterol levels than normal calves. Tests of pituitary and adrenal cortical function have also been studied. It is reported that after an injection of insulin the blood sugar level falls to a greater degree and returns to normal more slowly in dwarf animals and that there is a much smaller leucocytic response. Heterozygotes react in an intermediate manner but the variation in degree of abnormality in this group makes the test impractical as a means of selecting them. Serum protein, calcium, phosphorus and magnesium levels are within the normal limits in affected calves. There is a significant difference between the cerebrospinal fluid pressure in normal and dwarf animals, but the estimation of cerebrospinal fluid pressure is not a feasible method of differentiating between carrier and non-carrier animals.

The margin of error in all indirect tests is too great for general acceptance and the testing of animals with unknown genetic constitution by mating them with known carriers is still the most efficient method of detecting dwarf genes. This has the obvious disadvantage of requiring the maintenance of a carrier herd but is thought to be worth while by some breeders of valuable cattle.

Other types of dwarfs have been described (3) and include 'comprest' and 'compact' cattle in

Herefords and Shorthorns and various other forms of proportionate dwarfs. Other forms of chondrodystrophy, including 'bulldog calves' and one which causes fatal nasal obstruction in the German Black Spotted breed of cattle have also been recorded. In the latter there are multiple deformities of limb bones and the condition appears to be inherited due to the influence of a single recessive gene (5).

REFERENCES

(1) Gregory, P. W. et al. (1964). Growth, 28, 191.
(2) Emmerson, M. A. & Hazel, L. N. (1956). J. Amer. vet. med. Ass., 128, 381.
(3) Julian, L. M. et al. (1959). J. Amer. vet. med. Ass., 135, 104.
(4) Tyler, W. S. et al. (1961). Amer. J. vet. Res., 22, 693.
(5) Weber, W. (1962). Schweiz. Arch. Tierheilk., 104, 67.

Inherited Displaced Molar Teeth

Inherited as a simple recessive character this defect usually results in the death of affected calves within the first week of life. The six premolars of the lower jaw are impacted or erupted in abnormal positions, often at grotesque angles. The mandible is shorter and narrower than normal. There is no abnormality of the incisors or upper jaw (1).

REFERENCE

(1) Heizer, E. E. & Hervey, M. C. (1937). J. Hered., 28, 123.

Inherited Mandibular Prognathism

Defective apposition of upper and lower incisors, or lower incisors and dental pad in ruminants, may result in inefficient grazing and malnutrition. This is of most importance in ruminants and there is good evidence that abnormal length of the mandible is inherited. Among British breeds the defect is more common in beef than in dairy breeds (3). In Herefords the inheritance is thought to be conditioned by a single recessive gene (1). Underdevelopment of the mandible has also been recorded in Dairy Shorthorn, Jersey, Holstein and Ayrshire cattle, with the defect so severe in some cases that the animals are unable to suck (2). Inheritance of the defect is probably conditioned by a recessive gene. A less severe degree of mandibular underdevelopment has been recorded in Merino and Rambouillet sheep and designated as brachygnathia. The mode of inheritance is suggested to be by the interaction of several pairs of genes. Mandibular prognathism occurs as a part of other more general defects including achondroplastic dwarfism and inherited displaced molar teeth.

REFERENCES

(1) Gregory, K. E. et al. (1962). J. Hered., 53, 168.
(2) Grant, H. T. (1956). J. Hered., 47, 165.
(3) Wiener, G. & Gardiner, W. J. F. (1970). Anim. Prod., 12, 7.

Congenital Osteopetrosis

This inherited defect is recorded in Aberdeen-Angus calves. The major manifestations are shortening of the mandible, impaction of lower molars, a patent fontanelle, small body size and absence of bone marrow cavity in the long bones (1). Radiographic examination makes ante-mortem diagnosis simple.

REFERENCE

(1) Leipold, H. W. et al. (1970). Canad. vet. J., 11, 181.

Inherited Probatocephaly
(Sheepshead)

This defect is inherited in Limousin cattle (1). The cranial bones are deformed so that the head resembles that of a sheep. The accompanying defects in heart, buccal cavity, tongue and abomasum increase the chances of an early death.

REFERENCE

(1) Blin, P. C. & Lauvergne, J. J. (1967). Annl. Zootech., 16, 65.

Inherited Umbilical and Scrotal Herniae, Cryptorchidism and Hermaphroditism

Umbilical herniae in cattle and scrotal herniae and cryptorchidism in pigs have been considered to be inherited defects for many years. Umbilical hernia of Holstein cattle has been shown to occur because of the influence of either one or more pairs of autosomal recessive factors of rather low frequency (1). It is unlikely that the responsible genes are sex-linked, in spite of the apparent greater incidence in females. Umbilical hernia in Holstein-Friesian cattle can also be conditioned by a dominant character with incomplete penetrance, or be due to environmental factors (2). Scrotal herniae of pigs have also been shown to be inherited and evidence suggesting the inheritance of cryptorchidism in swine, horses and Hereford cattle (3) and hermaphroditism in swine (4) has also been presented. Hernias of various types are seen in lambs but their aetiology is uncertain (5).

REFERENCES

(1) Gilman, J. P. W. & Stringham, E. W. (1953). J. Hered., 44, 113.
(2) Angus, K. & Young, G. B. (1972). Vet. Rec., 90, 245.
(3) Wheat, J. D. (1961). J. Hered., 52, 244.
(4) Pond, W. G. et al. (1961). Cornell Vet., 51, 394.
(5) Dennis, S. M. & Leipold, H. W. (1968). J. Amer. vet. med. Ass., 152, 999.

Inherited Taillessness and Tail Deformity

Complete absence of the tail or deformity of the appendage occurs relatively commonly as a congenital defect and is thought to be inherited in Holstein cattle and in Landrace and Large White pigs.

Muscular Hypertrophy

(Double Muscling, Doppellender, Culard)

An inherited form of muscular hypertrophy has been observed occasionally in many breeds of cattle but appears to be most common in the Charolais, Piedmont and South Devon breeds. Severely affected animals show a marked increase in muscle mass most readily observed in the hindquarters, loin and shoulder, an increase in the muscle/bone ratio and a decrease in body fat (1). Since these changes are in the direction of the current demand for lean, meaty carcasses, there is interest, especially in Europe, in the exploitation of this anomaly for meat production (2).

Affected calves demonstrate above average weight gains during the first year of life if well fed and managed, although mature size is somewhat reduced. Well-marked grooves along the intramuscular septa in the hind-quarters are a distinguishing feature as is an apparent forward positioning of the tail head. The skin tends to be thinner than normal. These features vary widely in their expression. The muscle mass appears to be normal and to be due to a disproportionate number of glycolytic fibres (3).

The condition often gives rise to dystocia, possibly due to increased gestation length, and affected females are said to be less fertile than normal. Macroglossia, prognathism and a tendency toward muscular dystrophy and rickets have been observed in affected calves. Blood lactate is increased as is susceptibility to stress (4). There is also a very high incidence of Elso-heel in affected cattle and this interferes greatly with their economic value. The mode of inheritance has not been established but heterozygotes usually show some degree of hypertrophy.

Pietrain pigs exhibit many of the characteristics of double-muscled cattle, including large muscle mass and susceptibility to stress.

REFERENCES

(1) Butterfield, R. M. (1966). *Aust. Vet. J.*, *42*, 37.
(2) Lauvergne, J. J. *et al.* (1963). *Annl. Zootech.*, *12*, 133.
(3) Ashmore, C. R. & Robinson, D. W. (1969). *Proc. Soc. exp. Biol. Med.*, *132*, 548.
(4) Holmes, J. H. G. *et al.* (1972). *J. Anim. Sci.*, *35*, 1011.

Inherited Entropion

Entropion is inherited in sheep and this is known to occur in the Suffolk breed (1). Affected lambs are not observed until about 3 weeks of age when attention is drawn to the eyelids by the apparent conjunctivitis. A temporary blindness results but even without treatment there is a marked improvement in the eyelids and the lambs do not appear to suffer any permanent harm.

REFERENCE

(1) Crowley, J. P. & McCloughlin, P. (1963). *Vet. Rec.*, *75*, 1104.

INHERITED DEFECTS OF THE SKIN

Inherited Symmetrical Alopecia

This is an inherited skin defect of cattle in which animals born with a normal hair coat lose hair from areas distributed symmetrically over the body. It has been observed in Holstein cattle (1) as a rare disease but its appearance among valuable pure bred cattle has economic importance. It appears to be inherited as a single autosomal recessive character.

Affected animals are born with a normal hair coat but progressive loss of hair commences at 6 weeks to 6 months of age. The alopecia is symmetrical and commences on the head, neck, back and hind-quarters, and progresses to the root of the tail, down the legs and over the forelimbs. The affected skin areas become completely bald. Pigmented and unpigmented skin is equally affected; there is no irritation and the animals are normal in other respects. Failure of hair fibres to develop in apparently normal follicles can be detected by skin biopsy.

The disease is similar to congenital hypotrichosis which is, however, present at birth or very soon afterwards.

REFERENCE

(1) Holmes, J. R. & Young, G. B. (1954). *Vet. Rec.*, *66*, 704.

Inherited Congenital Hypotrichosis

In this congenital disease there is partial or complete absence of the hair coat with or without other defects of development. The disease is inherited in pigs and is associated with low birth weights, weakness and high mortality (1). It has also been reported in Poll Dorset sheep (2). There are six known forms of congenital hypotrichosis in cattle (3). One form, recorded in North America in Guernsey cattle (4), is usually viable provided the calves are sheltered. They grow normally but are unable to withstand exposure to cold weather or hot sun. In most instances hair is completely absent from most of the body at birth but eyelashes and tactile hair are present about the feet and head. Occasionally hair may be present in varying amounts at birth but is lost soon afterwards. There is no defect of horn or hoof growth. The skin is normal but has a shiny, tanned appearance and on section no hair follicles are present in the skin. The condition is inherited as a single, recessive character. A similar form of hypotrichosis has been observed in Jersey cattle. A non-viable form of complete hypotrichosis occurs in British Friesian cattle (5). In this form there is an abnormally small and hypofunctional thyroid and the calves die shortly after birth. The third form of the disease is hypotrichosis with anodontia. The calves are born hairless and without teeth (3). Inheritance of the defect is conditioned by a sex-linked recessive gene.

In Holsteins a sex-linked semi-dominant gene causes development of a streaked hairlessness in which irregular narrow streaks of hypotrichosis occur. The defect is present only in females (6). A partial hypotrichosis has also been observed in Hereford cattle (7). At birth there is a fine coat of short, curly hair which later is added to by the appearance of some very coarse, wiry hair. The calves survive but do not grow well. The character is inherited as a simple recessive. Hypotrichosis also occurs in adenohypophyseal hypoplasia in Guernseys and Jerseys.

REFERENCES

(1) Meyer, H. & Drommer, W. (1968). *Dtsch. tierärztl. Wschr.*, 75, 13.
(2) Dolling, C. H. S. & Brooker, M. G. (1966). *J. Hered.*, 57, 86.
(3) Hutt, F. B. (1963). *J. Hered.*, 54, 186.
(4) Becker, R. B. (1963). *J. Hered.*, 54, 3.
(5) Shand, A. & Young, G. B. (1964). *Vet. Rec.*, 76, 907.
(6) Eldridge, F. W. & Atkeson, F. W. (1953). *J. Hered.*, 44, 265.
(7) Young, J. G. (1953). *Aust. vet. J.*, 29, 298.

Baldy Calves

This is an inherited defect of calves characterized by alopecia, skin lesions, loss of bodily condition and failure of horns to grow.

The disease has so far been observed only in the Holstein breed. The calves are normal at birth but at one to two months of age begin to lose condition in spite of good appetites, and develop stiffness of the joints and abnormalities of the skin. These include patches of scaly, thickened and folded skin especially over the neck and shoulders, and hairless, scaly and often raw areas in the axillae and flanks and over the knees, hocks and elbow joints. There is usually alopecia about the base of the ears and eyes. The tips of the ears are curled medially. The horns fail to develop and there is persistent slobbering although there are no mouth lesions. Gross overgrowth of the hooves and stiffness of joints cause a shuffling, restricted gait. Severe emaciation leads to destruction at about 6 months of age. The similarity of this condition to inherited parakeratosis, described below, and to experimental zinc deficiency suggests an error in zinc metabolism. There is no record of this having been investigated.

There is a definite familial incidence and inheritance is of the autosomal recessive type (1).

Another disease has been described in this breed which has much in common with 'baldy calves' and inherited parakeratosis of calves (2). The hooves are not affected as they are in 'baldy calves' and there are ulcerative lesions in the mouth, oesophagus and forestomachs.

REFERENCES

(1) Gilman, J. P. W. (1956). *Proc. 92nd ann. Mtg vet. med. Ass.*, pp. 49–53.
(2) McPherson, E. A. *et al.* (1964). *Nord. Vet.-Med.*, 16, Suppl. 1, 533.

Inherited Parakeratosis of Calves

This defect is recorded in Black Pied Danish cattle (1) but probably occurs in a number of European breeds of cattle (2, 3), including Friesian-type cattle. It is inherited as an autosomal recessive character. Calves are normal at birth and signs appear at 4 to 8 weeks of age; untreated animals die at about 4 months of age. There is exanthema and loss of hair, especially on the legs, parakeratosis in the form of scales or thick crusts around the mouth and eyes, under the jaw, and on the neck and legs and a very poor growth rate. At necropsy the characteristic lesion is hypoplasia of the thymus.

There is a significant response to oral treatment with zinc (0·5 g. zinc oxide per day) and an apparently complete recovery can be achieved in a few weeks if treatment is continued. The disease reappears if treatment is stopped. The dose rate needs to be increased as body weight increases. It is thought that the disease is an inherited excessive requirement for zinc and that the thymic hypoplasia is due to the dietary deficiency.

REFERENCES

(1) Brummerstedt, F. *et al.* (1971). *Acta path. microb. scand.*, 79A, 686.
(2) Stober, M. (1971). *Dtsch. tierärztl. Wschr.*, 78, 257.
(3) Trautwein, G. (1971). *Dtsch. tierärztl. Wschr.*, 78, 265.

Inherited Congenital Absence of Skin

(*Epitheliogenesis Imperfecta*)

Absence of mucous membrane, or more commonly, absence of skin over an area of the body surface has been recorded at birth in pigs (1), calves (2) and foals (3). There is complete absence of all layers of the skin in patches of varying size and distribution. In cattle the defect is usually on the lower parts of the limbs and sometimes on the muzzle and extending onto the buccal mucosa. In pigs the skinless areas are seen on the flanks, sides, back and other parts of the body. The defect is usually incompatible with life and most affected animals die within a few days. Inheritance of the defect in cattle is conditioned by a single recessive gene.

REFERENCES

(1) Sailer, J. (1955). *Tierärztl. Umsch.*, *10*, 215.
(2) Dyrendahl, S. (1956). *Nord. Vet.-Med.*, *8*, 953.
(3) Butz, H. & Meyer, H. (1957). *Dtsch. tierärztl. Wschr.*, *64*. 555.

Inherited Photosensitization

An inherited photosensitization has been observed in Southdown sheep in New Zealand and U.S.A. (1).

The lambs are normal at birth but severe, persistent photosensitization develops at 5 to 7 weeks, that is, as soon as they commence to eat a chlorophyll-containing diet. Blindness is apparent. Death follows in 2 to 3 weeks if the lambs are left without shelter.

Liver insufficiency is present but the liver is histologically normal. Phylloerythrin and bilirubin excretion by the liver is impeded and the accumulation of phylloerythrin in the blood stream causes the photosensitization. There is also a significant deficiency in renal function (2). The disease is conditioned by a single recessive gene. Symptomatic treatment of photosensitization and confining the animals indoors may enable the lambs to fatten to market weight.

A similar photosensitivity is inherited in Corriedales (3).

REFERENCES

(1) Cornelius, C. E. & Gronwall, R. R. (1968). *Amer. J. vet. Res.*, *29*, 291.
(2) Mia, A. S. *et al.* (1971). *Proc. Soc. exp. Biol.*, *137*, 1237.
(3) Gronwall, R. R. (1970). *Amer. J. vet. Res.*, *31*, 2131.

Inherited Congenital Ichthyosis

(*Fish Scale Disease*)

Congenital ichthyosis is a disease characterized by alopecia and the presence of plates of horny epidermis covering the entire skin surface. It has been recorded only in Holstein (1) and Norwegian Red Poll and probably in Brown Swiss calves among the domestic animals, although it occurs also in man.

The newborn calf is either partly or completely hairless and the skin is covered with thick, horny scales separated by fissures which follow the wrinkle lines of the skin. These may penetrate deeply and become ulcerated. A skin biopsy section will show a thick, tightly adherent layer of keratinized cells. The disease is incurable and although it may be compatible with life most affected animals are disposed of for aesthetic reasons. The defect has been shown to be hereditary and to result from the influence of a single recessive gene.

REFERENCE

(1) Julian, R. J. (1960). *Vet. Med.*, *55*, 35.

Inherited Dermatitis Vegetans of Pigs

This disease appears to be conditioned by the inheritance of a recessive, semi-lethal factor (1). Affected pigs may show defects at birth but in most instances lesions appear after birth and up to 3 weeks of age. The lesions occur at the coronets and on the skin. Those on the coronets consist of erythema and oedema with a thickened, brittle, uneven hoof wall. Lesions on the belly and inner surface of the thigh commence as areas of erythema and become wart-like and covered with grey-brown crusts. Many affected pigs die but some appear to recover completely. Many of the deaths appear to be due to the giant-cell pneumonitis which is an essential part of the disease. It is known to have originated in the Danish Landrace breed (3).

REFERENCES

(1) Flatla, J. L. *et al.* (1961). *Zbl. vet. Med.*, *8*, 25.
(2) Percy, D. H. & Hulland, T. J. (1968). *Path. vet.*, *5*, 419 & (1969). *Canad. J. comp. Med.*, *33*, 48.
(3) Done, J. T. *et al.* (1967). *Vet. Rec.*, *80*, 292.

Dermatosparaxia

This is an extraordinary fragility of skin and connective tissue in general, with or without oedema, which occurs in Belgian cattle. It is probably inherited as a recessive character (1). A similar disease of calves has been recorded in U.S.A. (2). The skin is hyperelastic, as are the articular ligaments and marked cutaneous fragility, delayed healing of skin wounds and the development of papyraceous scars are also characteristic.

REFERENCES

(1) Hanset, R. (1971). *Hoppe-Seyler's Z. physiol. Chem.*, *352*, 13.
(2) O'Hara, P. J. *et al.* (1970). *Lab. Invest.*, *23*, 307.

MISCELLANEOUS INHERITED DEFECTS

Inherited Multiple Eye Defects

Iridiraemia (total or partial absence of iris), microphakia (smallness of the lens), ectopia lentis and cataract have been reported to occur together in Jersey calves. The mode of inheritance of the characters is as a simple recessive (1).

The calves are almost completely blind but are normal in other respects and can be reared satisfactorily if they are hand fed. Although the condition has been recorded only in Jerseys similar defects, possibly inherited, have also been seen in Holsteins and Shorthorns.

An inherited, congenital opacity of the cornea occurs in Holstein cattle. The cornea is a cloudy blue colour at birth and both eyes are equally affected. Although the sight of affected animals is restricted they are not completely blind, and there are no other abnormalities of the orbit or the eyelids. Histologically there is oedema and disruption of the corneal lamellae (2).

Although the vision appears unaffected a large number of congenital defects of the eye have been observed in cattle, including Herefords, affected by partial albinism (3). The defects include iridal heterochromia, tapetal fibrosum and colobomas. Congenital blindness is also seen in cattle with white coat colour, especially Shorthorns (4, 7). The lesions are multiple including retinal detachment, cataract, microphthalmia, persistent pupillary membrane and vitreous haemorrhage. Internal hydrocephalus is present in some, and hypoplasia of optic nerves also occurs.

Complete absence of the iris in both eyes is also recorded as an inherited defect in Belgian horses (5). Affected foals develop secondary cataract at about two months of age. Total absence of the retina in foals has also been recorded as being inherited in a recessive manner (6).

REFERENCES

(1) Saunders, L. Z. & Fincher, M. G. (1951). *Cornell Vet.*, *41*, 351.
(2) Deas, D. W. (1959). *Vet. Rec.*, *71*, 619.
(3) Gelatt, K. N. *et al.* (1969). *Amer. J. vet. Res.*, *30*, 1313.
(4) Leipold, H. W. *et al.* (1971). *Amer. J. vet. Res.*, *32*, 1019.
(5) Eriksson, K. (1955). *Nord. Vet.-Med.*, *7*, 773.
(6) Koch, P. (1952). *Rep. 2nd int. Congr. Physiol. Path. Anim. Reprod. artif. Insem.*, *2*, 110.
(7) Willoughby, R. A. (1968). *Mod. vet. Pract.*, *49*, 36.

Inherited Prolonged Gestation

Prolonged gestation occurs in cattle and sheep in several forms and is usually, although not always, inherited. The two recorded forms of the disease are prolonged gestation with foetal giantism and prolonged gestation with deformed foetuses of normal or small size. The latter form is accompanied by adenohypophyseal hypoplasia.

Prolonged gestation with foetal giantism. This disease is recorded in Holstein, Ayrshire and Swedish cattle and in Karakul sheep (1). The cause of the disease in the sheep is unknown. A similar condition of prolonged gestation with foetal giantism in sheep has been found to be caused by the ingestion of *Veratrum californicum* or of the shrub *Salsola tuberculata* (2). The disease in cattle is familial in most instances.

The usual clinical picture in this form of the disease is prolongation of pregnancy for periods of from 3 weeks to 3 months. The cows may show marked abdominal distension but in most cases the abdomens are smaller than one would expect. Parturition when it commences, is without preparation in that udder enlargement, relaxation of the pelvic ligaments and loosening and swelling of the vulva do not occur. There is also poor relaxation of the cervix and a deficiency of cervical mucus. Dystocia is usual and Caesarean section is usually advisable in Holstein cattle but the Ayrshire calves have all been reported as having been born without assistance. The calves are very large (48 to 80 kg. body weight) and show other evidence of post-term growth, with a luxuriant hair coat and large, well-erupted teeth which are loose in their alveoli, but the birth weight is not directly related to the length of the gestation period. At birth the calves exhibit a laboured respiration with diaphragmatic movements more evident than movements of the chest wall. They invariably die within a few hours in a hypoglycaemic coma. At necropsy there is adenohypophyseal hypoplasia and hypoplasia of the adrenal cortex (3). The progesterone level in the peripheral blood of cows bearing affected calves does not fall before term as it does in normal cows.

Prolonged gestation with adenohypophyseal hypoplasia. This form of the disease has been observed in Guernsey (4) and Jersey cattle (5) and differs from the previous form in that the foetuses are dead on delivery, show gross deformity of the head and are smaller than the normal calves of these breeds born at term. In Guernseys the defect has been shown to be inherited as a single recessive character and it is probable that the same is true in Jerseys. The gestation period varies widely, with a mean of 401 days.

Clinical examination of the dams carrying defective calves suggests that no development of the calf or placenta occurs after the seventh month of pregnancy. Death of the foetus occurs and is followed in 1 to 2 weeks by parturition unaccompanied by relaxation of the pelvic ligaments or vulva or by external signs of labour. The calf can usually be removed by forced traction because of its small size. Mammary gland enlargement does not occur until after parturition.

The calves are small and suffer varying degrees of hypotrichosis. There is hydrocephalus and in some cases distension of the gut and abdomen due to atresia of the jejunum. The bones are immature and the limbs are short. Abnormalities of the face include cyclopian eyes, microphthalmia, absence of the maxilla and the presence of only one nostril. At necropsy there is partial or complete aplasia of the adenohypophysis. The neural stalk is present and extends to below the diaphragm sellae. Brain abnormalities vary from fusion of the cerebral hemispheres to moderate hydrocephalus. The other endocrine glands are also small and hypoplastic.

The disease has been produced experimentally in ewes by severe ablation of the pituitary gland, or destruction of the hypothalamus, or section of the pituitary stalk in the foetus (6) and by adrenalectomy of the lamb (7). Infusion of ACTH into ewes with prolonged gestation due to pituitary damage produces parturition but not if the ewes have been adrenalectomized beforehand.

A third form of prolonged gestation, which occurs in Hereford cattle and is thought to be inherited, is accompanied by arthrogryposis, scoliosis, torticollis, kyphosis and cleft palate (8).

REVIEW LITERATURE

Holm, L. W. (1967). *Advanc. vet. Sci.*, *11*, 159, 206.

REFERENCES

(1) De Lange, M. (1962). *Proc. 4th int. Congr. anim. Reprod.*, *The Hague*, 1961, *3*, 590.
(2) Basson, P. A. *et al.* (1969). *Onderstepoort J. vet. Res.*, *36*, 59.
(3) Holm, L. W. & Short, R. V. (1962). *J. Reprod. Fertil.*, *4*, 137.
(4) Kennedy, P. C. *et al.* (1957). *Cornell Vet.*, *47*, 160.
(5) Blood, D. C. *et al.* (1957). *Aust. vet. J.*, *33*, 329.
(6) Liggins, G. C. *et al.* (1966). *J. Reprod. Fertil.*, *12*, 419.
(7) Drost, M. & Holm, L. W. (1968). *J. Endocrin.*, *40*, 293.
(8) Shupe, J. L. *et al.* (1967). *J. Hered.*, *58*, 311.

34

Specific Diseases of Unknown or Uncertain Aetiology

It was anticipated that as time went on this chapter would shrink in succeeding editions and eventually disappear. It is true that diseases are removed from it to other chapters as their causes are demonstrated, but the net effect on the chapter is negligible since other diseases are added. The process could be hastened by moving diseases when the consensus of opinion, short of proof, is that the cause is identified. For the present, at least, we think it preferable to leave those diseases here and also those in which the combination of causes is complex: thus 'weaner ill-thrift', and 'metritis–mastitis–agalactia'.

It is with a good deal of reluctance that, for reasons of space, we have excluded the diseases of the newly discovered domestic animal species *Brunus edwardii* (n.s.), better known to our American readers as *Ursinella theodori*, or perhaps *Ursus deodatus nurserii* (1, 2, 3). For the most part its diseases are obscure as to cause, so much so that the consensus of opinion is that the commonly used veterinary phrase, 'the fairies did it', arose in association with this animal. Adding to this uncertainty is a general doubt about identity (3) and, in some quarters, the importance of these animals to a learned profession (4). The confused status of the species is perhaps best exemplified by two apparently irreconcilable observations, one that the species must reproduce parthenogenetically because no conception, pregnancy or parturition has been recorded and, moreover, there are apparently no diseases of the reproductive tract of *Brunus* (syn. *Ursinella* or *Ursus*) *edwardii* (syn. *theodori* or *deodatus nurserii*), the other that diseases of other systems, particularly those of the integument, the limbs and the abdomen, are recorded voluminously (5). In spite of these contradictions questions have been raised about the genetic future of the species (6). Obviously there are problems in relation to *Brunus* sp. on which the efforts of our research colleagues should be brought to bear.

REFERENCES

(1) Blackmore, D. K., Owen, D. G. & Young, C. M. (1972). *Vet. Rec.*, *90*, 382.
(2) Bone, J. F. (1972). *Vet. Rec.*, *90*, 642.
(3) Howard, E. C. (1972). *Vet. Rec.*, *90*, 521.
(4) Noel-Smith, A. (1972). *Vet. Rec.*, *90*, 541.
(5) Barwick, M. W. (1972). *Vet. Rec.*, *90*, 521.
(6) Francis, P. G. (1972). *Vet. Rec.*, *90*, 428.

DISEASES CHARACTERIZED BY SYSTEMIC INVOLVEMENT

Bovine Leucosis

(Lymphomatosis, Lymphocytoma, Lymphoid Leucosis, Leucaemia)

This is a highly fatal malignant neoplasia characterized by the development of aggregations of neoplastic lymphocytes in almost any organ, with a corresponding variety of clinical signs. In cattle the disease occurs in two forms, one sporadic and relatively rare, the other enzootic and with a high morbidity.

Incidence

It is generally accepted that the enzootic form of the disease—enzootic bovine leucosis—is infectious. It occurs in specific herds in restricted areas in Holland, Denmark, Germany and Sweden and possibly in the U.S.S.R. and the U.S.A. There is a recent report of its occurrence in Australia (1). New Zealand and the U.K. (2) appear to be free of the disease. In affected herds in Europe the animal mortality due to the disease may be as high as 2 to 5 per cent. In enzootic areas the morbidity rate may reach 60 per 100,000 head per year compared with an incidence of 4 per 100,000 in other areas. In Denmark the disease is thought to be of sufficient importance to warrant an eradication programme, which in its first 10 years of existence has lowered the occurrence of the disease to one third of its original prevalence (3). The losses in East

Germany are estimated to be 10,000 head annually at a cost of 24 million marks (4).

Sporadic leucosis occurs in all species but is relatively rare. It is probably the commonest neoplasm in pigs (5) and has been recorded in sheep (6, 7), goats, horses (8), roe deer (9) and Indian buffalo (10).

Aetiology

Because of the apparent spread of enzootic bovine leucosis to new farms and areas by the movement of cattle and the transmissibility of a similar disease in this and other species (11), an infective agent has been postulated as the cause (12). Transmission experiments have been equivocal if the criterion for a positive test is the subsequent development of tumours (13), but if the criterion used is the occurrence of a lymphocytosis after inoculation the evidence is more impressive (14, 15). The long incubation periods reported make transmission experiments difficult and expensive. There are a number of records of transmission between cattle (12, 16, 18) and one record of experimental transmission from cattle to sheep (19).

A number of environmental influences have been suggested as predisposing causes and inherited susceptibility in local strains or breeds of cattle and swine (17) has received much support. There is a marked familial tendency to the disease and although susceptibility to an infectious agent may be conditioned by inheritance, the observed incidence is also explainable in terms of the vertical transmission of an infective agent through the parents (20). The exact nature of the infective agent is uncertain but it is thought to be a virus.

All breeds of cattle are susceptible to enzootic bovine leucocis. It occurs very rarely in animals less than 2 years of age and increases in incidence with increasing age (21). Large herds appear to have a much greater incidence than smaller herds and the incidence in dairy cattle is higher than in beef cattle, due probably to the higher average age in the dairy group and to their closer confinement. The possibility of the spread of the disease from cattle to man has often been proposed. An epidemiological survey has shown that there were no significant differences between farms that did have and farms that did not have the disease with respect to death rate and cancer and leukaemia–lymphoma occurrence in humans (22).

Sporadic bovine leucosis is considered to be aetiologically different from the enzootic disease and no causative agent has been proposed. A few cases may occur in adults but most occur in young calves, sometimes newborn, and yearlings.

Transmission

Enzootic bovine leucosis is usually brought into a herd by the introduction of subclinical cases from affected herds. Although horizontal transmission occurs the means by which it occurs is unknown (23). Suspected means include contaminated hypodermic needles, blood transfusions and vaccinations. Horizontal transmission from infected dams or newborn calves to other susceptible newborn calves appears to have occurred (24). The principal route is vertical from dam to offspring via the placenta (18) or milk (25, 26). Although there is good evidence of dissemination from the sire via the spermatozoa (27) there is no satisfactory information on the transmission of the infective agent by artificial insemination and it is generally accepted that it does not occur.

Pathogenesis

Lymphomatosis is essentially a neoplasia of the whole lympho-reticular system. It is never benign, the lesions developing at varying rates in different animals so that the course may be quite short or protracted over several months. However, a number of animals in infected herds develop no tumours and may remain in this preclinical (precancerous) stage for periods of years. These animals can be indentified by the detection of lymphocytosis. In some animals the lymphocytosis has receded by the time tumours develop.

In adult cattle, almost any organ may be the site of lesions, but the abomasum, heart, and visceral and peripheral lymph nodes are the organs most commonly affected. In calves, the visceral lymph nodes and spleen and liver are the common sites. Depending upon the organ which is most involved, a number of clinical syndromes occur. With major involvement of the abomasal wall, the syndrome is one of impaired digestion resulting in persistent diarrhoea. When the atrial wall is affected, congestive heart failure may supervene. Involvement of the spinal meninges and nerves is followed by the gradual onset of posterior paralysis. In nervous tissue, the primary lesion is in the roots of peripheral nerves and grows along the nerve to involve meninges and cord. Other common localizations of the disease are in the skin, genitalia and periorbital tissues. In the cutaneous form, intradermal thickenings develop which persist but do not cause discontinuity of the epithelium. Oesophageal obstruction may result from mediastinal lymphnode involvement in calves.

The exact nature of the tumour is open to question. The tumours consist of aggregations of neoplastic lymphocytes but in many cases they may be more accurately described as reticulosarcoma. Certainly, they are highly malignant and metastasize widely. The blood picture is variable and, although there may be an accompanying lymphocytosis, the presence of large numbers of immature lymphocytes in the blood smear is a more reliable indication of the presence of the disease. Some degree of anaemia is almost always present.

Clinical Findings

Because there are in general two patterns of development of the disease in cattle as suggested in the discussion of aetiology they are described as separate entities here. The relative incidence of the two forms has been determined only in Denmark (80 per cent enzootic, 20 per cent sporadic) and whether both forms occur in other countries is undecided.

Enzootic bovine leucosis. The usual incubation period appears to be 4 to 5 years. At least cases tend to occur 4 to 5 years after the original case was introduced or a blood transfusion from an outside herd was given. This form is rarely seen in animals under 2 years of age and is most common in the 4- to 8-years age group. Lymphocytosis without clinical signs occurs earlier but again rarely before 2 years of age. Many cows remain in this preclinical stage for years, often for their complete productive lifetime, and without any apparent reduction in performance, but in a proportion clinical disease appears. The clinical signs and the duration of the illness vary with the number and importance of the sites involved and the speed with which the tumour masses grow.

A proportion (5 to 10 per cent) run a peracute course and the affected animals often die without showing prior signs of illness. Involvement of the adrenal glands, rupture of an abomasal ulcer and rupture of an affected spleen followed by acute internal haemorrhage are known causes of such terminations. Such animals are often in good bodily condition.

Most cases run a subacute (up to 7 days) to chronic (several months) course and are initiated by loss of condition and appetite, anaemia and muscular weakness. The heart rate is not increased unless the myocardium is involved and the temperature is normal unless tumour growth is rapid and extensive when it rises to 39·5 to 40 °C (103 to 104 °F). Although the following specific forms of the disease are described separately, in any one animal any combination of them may occur. In many cases clinical illness sufficient to warrant the attention of the veterinarian is not observed until extensive involvement has occurred and the possibility of slaughter of the animal for meat purposes cannot be considered. On the other hand many cases are examined at a time when diagnostic clinical signs are not yet evident. Once signs of clinical illness and tumour development are detectable the course is rapid and death is usually only 2 to 3 weeks away.

Enlargement of the superficial lymph nodes is common (75 to 90 per cent of cases show it) and is often an early sign. This is usually accompanied by small (1 cm. in diameter), subcutaneous lesions, often in the flanks and on the perineum. These skin lesions are probably enlarged haemolymph nodes and are of no diagnostic significance, often occurring in the absence of other signs of the disease. In many cases with serious visceral involvement, peripheral lesions may be completely absent. Enlargement of visceral lymph nodes is common but these are usually symptomless unless they press on other organs such as intestine or nerves. However, they may be detected on rectal examination. Special attention should be given to the deep inguinal and iliac nodes. In advanced cases extensive spread to the peritoneum and pelvic viscera makes diagnosis easy.

Although the enlargement of lymph nodes is often generalized many cows have only a proportion of their nodes involved. Thus the enlargements may be confined to the pelvic nodes or to one or more subcutaneous nodes. Involvement of the symphysis of the mandible and the nodes of the head is sometimes observed. The affected nodes are smooth and resilient and in dairy cattle are easily seen. Their presence may be marked by local oedema. Occasional cases are seen in which the entire body surface is covered with tumour masses 5 to 11 cm. in diameter in the subcutaneous tissue.

Digestive form. With involvement of the abomasal wall there is a capricious appetite, persistent diarrhoea, not unlike that of Johne's disease and, occasionally, melaena due to bleeding from the not infrequent abomasal ulcer. Tumours of the mediastinal nodes may cause chronic, moderate bloat.

Cardiac form. Lesions in the heart usually invade the right atrial wall primarily and the signs are referable to right-sided congestive heart failure. There is hydropericardium with muffling of the heart sounds, hydrothorax with resulting dyspnoea, engorgement of the jugular veins and oedema of the brisket and sometimes of the intermandibular space. The heart sounds, besides being muffled, show a variety of abnormalities. There may be tachycardia due to insufficiency and there is often irregularity due to heart block. A systolic murmur is also common as is an associated jugular pulse. The liver may be enlarged and portal stasis may lead to diarrhoea.

Nervous form. Neural lymphomatosis is usually manifested by the gradual onset over several weeks of posterior paralysis. The cow begins to knuckle at the hind fetlocks while walking; sometimes one leg is affected more than the other. She then has difficulty getting up and is finally unable to do so. At this stage, sensation is retained but movement is limited or absent. There may be a zone of hyperaesthesia at the site of the lesion which is usually at the last lumbar or first sacral vertebra. Appetite and other functions, apart from the effects of recumbency, are usually normal. Metastases in the cranial meninges produce signs of space-occupying lesions with localizing signs referable to the site of the lesion.

Respiratory form. Enlargement of the retropharyngeal lymph nodes may cause snoring and dyspnoea.

Less commonly, clinically detectable lesions occur in the periorbital tissues causing protrusion of the eyeball, and in limb muscles, ureter, kidney and genitalia. Involvement of the uterus may be detectable as multiple nodular enlargement on rectal examination. Periureteral lesions may lead to hydronephrosis with diffuse enlargement of the kidney while tumours in renal tissue cause nodular enlargements. In either case terminal uraemia develops.

Sporadic bovine leucosis. In adults this is manifested by cutaneous plaques (1 to 5 cm. diameter) which appear on the neck, back, croup and thighs. The plaques become covered with a thick grey-white scab and the hair is shed; then the centre becomes depressed and the nodule commences to shrink. After a period of weeks or months hair grows again and the nodules disappear as does the enlargement of the peripheral lymph nodes. Relapse occurs in 1 or 2 years with reappearance of cutaneous lesions and signs of involvement of internal organs as in the enzootic form of the disease.

The disease in calves up to 6 months of age is manifested primarily by gradual loss of weight and the sudden enlargement of all lymph nodes, accompanied by depression and weakness (28). Fever, tachycardia and posterior paresis are less constant signs. Death occurs in 2 to 8 weeks from the first obvious illness. There may be signs of pressure on internal organs, including bloat and congestive heart failure. Infiltration of the thymus is a common finding in animals 1 to 2 years of age and is characterized by massive thymic enlargement and lesions in bone marrow and regional lymph nodes. Jugular engorgement and local oedema usually result (29).

The clinical picture in pigs is poorly defined, non-specific emaciation, limb weakness and anorexia being most commonly observed (5). One outbreak in sheep has been observed, with clinical and necropsy findings similar to those of enzootic bovine leucosis (2). In horses the disease occurs most commonly in animals over 6 years of age. The chief clinical manifestations are subcutaneous enlargements which may ulcerate, enlargement of internal and external lymph nodes, jugular vein engorgement, cardiac irregularity, exophthalmia and anasarca. The course varies from acute to chronic but most affected horses die within a month of first showing signs (8). In Indian buffalo (10) the lesions predominantly involve serous surfaces with large volumes of turbid peritoneal or other fluid.

Clinical Pathology

Some degree of anaemia, due to bone-marrow necrosis, is present but the major pathological change observable antemortem is in the leucocyte picture. In some advanced cases there is a considerable increase in the percentage of lymphocytes, particularly immature lymphocytes. The total leucocyte count may vary from normal to high (6000 to 150,000/cmm.). An increase in the lymphocytes from a normal of 50 per cent to 65 per cent or more and the presence of 25 per cent or more of atypical, immature lymphocytes is usually considered to be significant. Haematological examination may provide a clear diagnosis but, in many cases, the results are equivocal. A common observation is that haematological changes are most obvious in the early stages, the blood picture returning to normal as the condition progresses, so that by the time obvious clinical signs are evident, no abnormality of the blood picture may be detectable. A much better indication can be obtained by biopsy of a subcutaneous lesion or haemolymph node (30) or exploratory laparotomy.

In a high proportion of affected animals there is massive involvement of bone marrow and leucaemic and erythropoenic changes may be apparent in biopsy specimens but the method is less dependable than a haematological examination (31). Chromosomal changes have been reported in cells from lymph nodes or in leucocytes from peripheral blood in some affected animals (20, 32). Interesting observations have been made on electrocardiographic changes in affected animals (33), but these are unlikely to be of value in differential diagnosis.

Major interest in recent years has been devoted to the early detection of cases of enzootic bovine leucosis by haematological examination. The criteria provided by Bendixen (see table below) allow cattle in known leucosis herds to be graded as normal, suspicious or positive. In such herds

Total Lymphocyte (per cmm.) Values Used to Classify Cattle in Herds with Enzootic Bovine Leucosis

Age in years	Group 1 Normal	Group 2 Suspicious	Group 3 Leucaemic
0–1	< 10,000	10,000–12,000	> 12,000
1–2	< 9,000	9,000–11,000	> 11,000
2–3	< 7,500	7,500– 9,500	> 9,500
3–4	< 6,500	6,500– 8,500	> 8,500
> 4	< 5,000	5,000– 7,000	> 7,000

most positive animals remain clinically normal and almost all animals which die of the disease pass through this phase. The proportion of positive cases increases markedly with age and at 3 to 4 years 50 per cent of cows in leucosis herds are positive. Detection of a positive animal in a herd where clinical leucosis has not occurred does not necessarily indicate the presence of the disease (1), and herds apparently affected with enzootic leucosis do not always give evidence of lymphocytosis (34). Repeated samplings are probably necessary if the method is expected to select cattle for culling (35). There seems to be no reason why meat from haematologically-positive animals which have no gross lesions should not be used for human consumption (36).

Necropsy Findings

In cattle firm white tumour masses may be found in any organ although two rather different patterns of distribution are apparent. In newborn and young animals the common sites are kidney, thymus, liver, spleen and peripheral and internal lymph nodes (37, 28). This may or may not be a characteristic of the 'sporadic' form of the disease. In adults the heart, abomasum and spinal cord are often involved. In the heart, the tumour masses invade particularly the right atrium, though they may occur generally throughout the myocardium and extend to the pericardium. The frequency of early changes in the subepicardial tissue of the right atrium suggests that this is an area from which tissues should be selected in latent or doubtful cases (38). The abomasal wall, when involved,

shows a gross, uneven thickening with tumour material in the submucosa, particularly in the pyloric region. Deep ulcerations in the affected area are not uncommon. Involvement of the nervous system usually includes thickening of the peripheral nerves coming from the last lumbar or first sacral cord segment or more rarely in a cranial cervical site. This may be associated with one or more circumscribed thickenings in the spinal meninges. Affected lymph nodes may be enormously enlarged and be composed of both normal and neoplastic tissue. The latter is firmer and whiter than normal lymphoid tissue and often surrounds foci of bright yellow necrosis. Less common sites include the kidney, the ureters, usually near the renal pelvis, the uterus, either as nodular masses or diffuse infiltration, mediastinal, sternal, mesenteric and other internal lymph nodes, and mandibular ramus. Histologically the tumour masses are composed of lymphocytic cells. Similar lesions occur in the lymph nodes, spleen, kidney, liver and bone marrow of affected pigs and horses (8).

Diagnosis

Because of the very wide range of signs, a positive diagnosis of lymphomatosis is often difficult. Enlargement of peripheral lymph nodes without fever or lymphangitis is unusual in other diseases, with the exception of tuberculosis which can be differentiated by the tuberculin test. In the absence of these enlargements, the digestive form may easily be confused with Johne's disease or even mucosal disease. However, there are no oral lesions and the johnin test and examination of faecal smears for typical acid-fast bacilli are negative. The cardiac form closely resembles traumatic pericarditis and endocarditis but there is an absence of fever and toxaemia, and the characteristic neutrophilia of these two diseases is usually absent. Involvement of the spinal nerves or meninges may be confused with spinal cord abscess or with the dumb form of rabies. An examination of cerebrospinal fluid may be of value in determining the presence of an abscess and rabies has a much shorter course and other diagnostic signs. Multiple lymph node enlargements in the abdominal cavity, and nodular lesions in the uterine wall may be confused with fat necrosis but the nature of the lesion can usually be determined by careful rectal palpation. Snoring caused by enlargement of the retropharyngeal lymph nodes is also commonly caused by tuberculosis and actinobacillosis. A definitive diagnosis of lymphomatosis requires either positive haematological evidence or examination of lymphoid tissue by biopsy.

Treatment

Treatment has not been attempted in large numbers of animals. The use of nitrogen-mustard (30 to 40 mg. daily for 3 to 4 days) has resulted in temporary remissions of signs in affected cattle. Triethylenemelamine has also been reported to cause some improvement.

Control

Because of the uncertainty about the cause of the disease, control measures are not usually undertaken in North America. In Europe, the high incidence in individual herds has led to the trial of complete slaughter of affected herds of cattle, and the less drastic method of segregation of cattle showing evidence of the disease on haematological examination, as methods of control. Both methods are claimed to be effective. Families of cattle which evidence predisposition to the disease should be avoided and this is probably the most positive step to take in a country where the prevalence is low.

The Danish control programme depends on detection of infected herds on the basis of clinical cases and a high incidence of animals positive to the haematological criteria listed above. Such herds are placed under the leucosis control programme and are subject to the following regulations: (i) Sale of animals other than for slaughter is prohibited; (ii) contact of animals with those in free herds is prohibited; (iii) spread of contagious material is controlled. Herds which have clinical enzootic-type cases but negative haematological findings are kept under observation, retested twice at yearly intervals during which quarantine is maintained and if still negative at the end of this time, are released. Herds which have sporadic-type cases are not controlled in any way. Results of the Danish control programme look promising but a final judgement must await a longer period of observation (39).

Eradication of leucosis herds by total slaughter has been attempted and is recommended but prompt disposal of animals positive on blood test, and raising calves in a separate unit until first calving has reduced the herd incidence greatly. It is unlikely that the latter procedure will be economic. Eradication on an area basis seems impractical at the present time but control measures to prevent the introduction of the disease into known free areas appear desirable in countries where the incidence is high.

REVIEW LITERATURE

Bendixen, H. J. (1965). *Advanc. vet. Sci.*, *10*, 129.
Jarrett, W. F. H. *et al.* (1966). *Vet. Rec.*, *79*, 693.
Marshak, R. R. (1968). *J. natn. Cancer Inst.*, *41*, 243.

REFERENCES

(1) Clague, D. C. & Granzien, C. K. (1966). *Aust. vet. J.*, *42*, 177.
(2) Weipers, W. L. *et al.* (1964). *Rep. Brit. Emp. Cancer Campaign*, *42*, 682.
(3) Bendixen, H. J. & Gaede, T. (1969). *Dtsch. tierärztl. Wschr.*, *76*, 645.
(4) Mieth, K. *et al.* (1970). *Mh. Vet.-Med.*, *25*, 929.
(5) Logger, J. C. L. *et al.* (1966). *T. Diergeneesk.*, *91*, 842.
(6) Paulsen, J. *et al.* (1971). *Zbl. vet. Med.*, *18B*, 33.
(7) Ulbrich, F. *et al.* (1970). *Tierärztl. Umsch.*, *25*, 277, 283.
(8) Theilen, G. H. & Fowler, M. E. (1962). *J. Amer. vet. med. Ass.*, *140*, 923.
(9) Woodford, M. (1966). *Vet. Rec.*, *79*, 74.
(10) Singh, C. M. (1968). *Proc. 3rd int. Symp. comp. Leucaemia Res.*, *Paris, 1967*, pp. 237–43.
(11) Jarrett, W. F. H. *et al.* (1964). *Nature (Lond.)*, *202*, 566.
(12) Rosenberger, G. (1968). *Proc. 3rd int. Symp. comp. Leucaemia Res.*, *Paris, 1967*, pp. 136–9.
(13) Hatziolos, B. C. *et al.* (1966). *Amer. J. vet. Res.*, *27*, 489.
(14) Bindrich, H. & Gensel, C. (1963). *Rindertuberk. Brucellose*, *12*, 169.
(15) Bederke, G. & Tolle, A. (1964). *Zbl. vet. Med.*, *11B*, 433.
(16) Theilen, G. H. *et al.* (1967). *Amer. J. vet. Res.*, *28*, 373.
(17) McTaggart, H. S. *et al.* (1971). *Nature (Lond.)*, *232*, 557.
(18) Straub, O. C. (1969). *Dtsch. tierärztl. Wschr.*, *76*, 365.
(19) Wittman, W. *et al.* (1971). *Arch. exp. Vet. Med.*, *25*, 587.
(20) Marshak, R. R. *et al.* (1964). *Canad. vet. J.*, *5*, 180.
(21) Anderson, R. K. *et al.* (1964). *Proc. 68th ann. gen. Mtg U.S. Live Stock sanit. Ass.*, 52.
(22) Priester, W. A. *et al.* (1970). *Lancet, i*, 367.
(23) Straub, O. C. (1971). *Arch. ges. Virusforsch.*, *33*, 145.
(24) Larson, V. L. *et al.* (1970). *Amer. J. vet. Res.*, *31*, 1533.
(25) Straub, O. C. & Weinhold, E. (1971). *Dtsch. tierärztl. Wschr.*, *78*, 441.
(26) Bederke, G. *et al.* (1970). *Zbl. vet. Med.*, *17B*, 701.
(27) Ritter, H. (1965). *Dtsch. tierärztl. Wschr.*, *72*, 56.
(28) Hugoson, G. (1967). *Acta vet. scand.*, Suppl. *22*, 108.
(29) Dungworth, D. L. *et al.* (1964). *Path. vet.*, *1*, 323.
(30) Labelle, J. A. & Conner, G. H. (1964). *J. Amer. vet. med. Ass.*, *145*, 1107.
(31) Weber, W. T. & Marshak, R. R. (1963). *Amer. J. vet. Res.*, *24*, 515.
(32) Hare, W. C. D. & McFeely, R. A. (1966). *Nature (Lond.)*, *209*, 108.
(33) Karge, E. & Werner, E. (1963). *Mh. Vet.-Med.*, *18*, 849.
(34) Marshak, R. R. *et al.* (1963). *Ann. N.Y. Acad. Sci.*, *108*, 1284.
(35) Hare, W. C. D. *et al.* (1963). *Amer. J. vet. Res.*, *24*, 98.
(36) Kruger, K. E. & Rabl, R. (1965). *Zbl. vet. Med.*, *12A*, 161.
(37) Theilen, G. H. & Dungworth, D. L. (1965). *Amer. J. vet. Res.*, *26*, 696.
(38) Järplid, B. (1964). *Path. vet.*, *1*, 366.
(39) Bendixen, H. J. (1964). *Int. Mtg Dis. Cattle, Copenhagen*, *2*, 420.

Mulberry Heart Disease of Pigs

(*Dietetic Microangiopathy*)

The cause of mulberry heart disease of pigs is unknown. Clinically the disease is characterized by acute heart failure and sudden death and there are typical lesions at necropsy.

Incidence

Mulberry heart disease (MHD) has been known for many years but appears to be increasing in incidence and assuming greater economic importance. The morbidity rate in an affected group is not usually high but the mortality rate is virtually 100 per cent. The economic loss in these herds may be great because affected pigs are usually approaching market weight.

Aetiology

The cause is unknown but the common occurrence of the disease in close association with outbreaks of gut oedema suggests that it is an enterotoxaemia. MHD is often grouped with gut oedema as a separate form of that disease and although haemolytic strains of *Escherichia coli* are sometimes incriminated (1), the association between the bacteria and the disease is not as clear-cut as it is in gut oedema. There is a relationship with hepatitis dietetica in that both diseases occur on the same kind of diet. The suspected role of unsaturated fatty acids and some evidence that the disease can be prevented by the administration of vitamin E suggests that a dietary factor may be concerned in the aetiology (2). Some breeds (especially Landrace) are considered to be more susceptible than others (3). There appears to be a relationship between stress susceptibility and intensified breeding for meat-type pigs but the association with this disease is not clear.

Occurrence

Although MHD occurs most commonly in fattening pigs over 100 lb. weight it also occurs in young weaned pigs. There is no general husbandry or feeding practice which seems to be related to the occurrence of the disease although most outbreaks occurs in pigs with a high food intake.

Pathogenesis

Death appears to be caused by acute heart failure although the lesions suggest that the initial disturbance is one of congestive heart failure further exacerbated by hydropericardium. The general distribution of the oedema suggests damage to vascular endothelium by a circulating toxin.

Clinical Findings

The disease is acute and the course short. Affected pigs usually show a subnormal temperature, anorexia, dyspnoea, muscular tremor, incoordination and muscle weakness, which is sometimes so severe that the animal may be unable to rise. Lethargy, dullness and, in the terminal stages, cyanosis occur, and death usually follows after a course of up to 24 hours. A number of pigs survive with residual nervous signs of blindness and ataxia and reduced weight gains.

Clinical Pathology

Laboratory procedures of diagnostic value are not available.

Necropsy Findings

The carcase is usually in good condition. All body cavities contain excessive amounts of fluid and shreds of fibrin. In the peritoneal cavity, the fibrin is often in the form of a lacy net, covering all the viscera. The liver is enlarged, mottled and has a characteristic nutmeg appearance on the cut surface. Excessive fluid in the pleural cavities is accompanied by collapse of the ventral parts of the lungs. The lungs are oedematous and the interlobular septa are distended with gelatinous material. The pericardial sac is filled with gelatinous fluid interlaced with bands of fibrin. Beneath the epicardium are multiple haemorrhages of various size. The haemorrhages often run in a linear fashion in the direction of the muscle fibres. Similar haemorrhages are present under the endocardium, and local oedema is often present over the face and elsewhere. Marked reddening of the gastric mucosa is also common. Histologically the characteristic lesion is widespread myocardial congestion, haemorrhage and parenchymal degeneration and there is lysis of cerebral white-matter in some cases (4).

Diagnosis

It is possible that MHD and gut oedema are different manifestations of the one disease but the clinical picture in MHD is one of circulatory failure whilst that of gut oedema is primarily one of depression of function of the central nervous system and the two diseases do not occur together in the one animal. The acute course in MHD offers little opportunity for clinical diagnosis but necropsy findings are characteristic. Erysipelas and streptococcal endocarditis may cause acute heart failure but the lesions are those of verrucose endocarditis and, in chronic cases, typical endocardial bruits are audible on auscultation. There is some similarity to fatal syncope (Herztod) except that this disease becomes apparent and causes death only after exercise and at necropsy there is marked degeneration of skeletal muscle. Glasser's disease is characterized by a fibrinous pericarditis and pleurisy but there is also involvement of the joints and meninges and there is absence of the typical subepicardial haemorrhages of MHD.

The common causes of sudden death in pigs include coliform enteritis, mulberry heart disease, intestinal accident, swine dysentery, gastric ulcer and pneumonia (5).

Treatment

The administration of broad spectrum antibiotics, parenteral diuretics and central nervous stimulants is usually instituted but there is no evidence that they influence the course of the disease.

Control

Control measures are difficult to outline because of the uncertainty as to the cause. The usual recom-. mendations are to reduce the food intake and supply high levels of broad spectrum antibiotics in the feed or drinking water.

REFERENCES

(1) Terpstra, J. I. (1958). *T. Diergeneesk.*, *83*, 1078.
(2) Nafstad, I. (1969). *Tierärztl. Umsch.*, *24*, 158.
(3) Oakley, G. A. (1963). *Vet. Rec.*, *75*, 148.
(4) Harding, J. D. J. (1960). *Res. vet. Sci.*, *1*, 129.
(5) Wilson, M. R. (1970). *Canad. vet. J.*, *11*, 178.

Metritis–Mastitis–Agalactia Syndrome in Sows

This disease has been in evidence for many years but it appears to have increased markedly in prevalence in recent years, especially in highly intensive herds where high capital costs and close surveillance make it a disease of very great economic importance and one which is likely to be recognized.

Affected sows are normal immediately after parturition and remain so for 12 to 48 hours. Then suddenly there is a rapid fall-off in milk production. There is an absence of milk in the teats and the piglets quickly become gaunt, and are restless and shivering. There is a severe toxaemia, the sow is depressed, does not eat, is disinclined to get up, has a fever of 39·5 to 41 °C (103 to 106 °F), is constipated and has a stiff gait and usually a creamy vaginal discharge. The course of the disease varies from a minimum of 3 days to a much longer period so that many baby pigs die of hypoglycaemia. The sow may die too, but this is rare.

In an affected piggery there is a tendency for the disease to appear suddenly and affect a series of sows as one would expect a specific infectious disease to do. A common diagnosis is mastitis but the decision is made mostly on clinical grounds and there is a pronounced lack of laboratory supported diagnoses. In one series of sows examined carefully, many of the quarters diagnosed clinically as having mastitis, had only a few small foci of inflammation, and many were only congested and non-functional (1). Although a vaginal discharge was evident in almost all sows, only 1 in 10 had had metritis.

There were similar results in another series (2) and it is apparent that accurate identification of the degree of mastitis is not possible clinically and that mastitis and metritis were only loosely related to a primary agalactia. The determination of a single cause for this poorly defined amorphous entity has so far eluded investigators. *E. coli* has been a firm favourite for many years (3) but other infectious agents, including *Klebsiella aerogenes* (4) are frequently advanced as specific causes. The most likely candidate as the cause of the mastitis–metritis is a *Mycoplasma* sp. (5) but as is so often the case in animal diseases of uncertain aetiology the front-running mycoplasmosis is hotly pursued by an adrenocortical malfunction (6).

Because of the uncertainty about the cause of the disease (7), and the probable multiplicity of causes, it is difficult to make simple recommendations about treatment which will cover all situations. The commonest form of therapy is a combination of an antibiotic or sulphonamide, systemically or intrauterine or both, and oxytocin or ergometrine, or both, to contract the uterus and cause let-down of available milk (8). All of the broad-spectrum antibiotics have been used and recommended (5) and perhaps tylosin should be tried also. Corticosteroids appear to be of no value as treatment or prevention (9). Our recommended treatment is penicillin–streptomycin combination or chloramphenicol for 3 days plus repeated small doses of oxytocin. The recovery rate is not high, but is much higher if treatment is begun very early. Without artificial rearing the entire litter is often lost and the mortality in a piggery may be 50 per cent.

In prevention overfatness and lack of exercise in the sow are regarded as important and constipation is considered to be a necessary precursor of the disease. Good management is certainly desirable and to be recommended but purgation, starvation and forced exercise seem an unlikely triad of prophylaxes. Prophylactic injection of the selected antibiotic just before farrowing gives much the best results in our hands.

REVIEW LITERATURE
Penny, R. H. C. (1970). The agalactia complex in the sow. A Review. *Aust. vet. J.*, *46*, 153.

REFERENCES
(1) Martin, C. E. *et al.* (1967). *J. Amer. vet. med. Ass.*, *151*, 1629.

(2) Swarbrick, O. (1968). *Vet. Rec.*, 82, 241.
(3) Ross, R. F. *et al.* (1969). *J. Amer. vet. med. Ass.*, 155, 1844, 1860.
(4) Luke, S. G. & Jones, J. E. T. (1970). *Vet. Rec.*, 87, 484.
(5) Moore, R. W. *et al.* (1966). *Vet. Med.*, 61, 883.
(6) Nachreiner, R. F. *et al.* (1971). *Amer. J. vet. Res.*, 32, 1065.
(7) Jones, J. E. T. (1971). *Vet. Rec.*, 89, 72.
(8) Keller, H. (1968). *Dtsch. tierärztl. Wschr.*, 75, 501.
(9) Martin, C. E. & Threlfall, W. R. (1970). *Vet. Rec.*, 87, 768.

Unthriftiness in Weaner Sheep
(*Weaner Ill-Thrift*)

Loss of weight at weaning and failure to make satisfactory weights subsequently, in spite of the presence of ample feed and when adult sheep are faring well, has been a problem in sheep for many years (1). The problem has seemed to be most severe in the Southern hemisphere but this may be because sheep are so prevalent there. It may also be due partly to the predominance of Merino and Merino-type sheep; the disease is most common in these breeds which have their own particular timorous nature and this makes weaning and the need to shift for themselves more traumatic than in most other breeds. This trait is particularly noticeable if there is overcrowding on pasture. Other management factors likely to lead to un-thriftiness are multibirth lambs, small ewes, ewes with little milk and lambs born late in the season (2).

Apart from the need for more gentle and considerate handling of the young at weaning to ensure a smooth transition a number of less abstract measures are often practised. Supplementation of the diet to replace deficient items is most common and of the deficiencies the most likely one in many environments is protein, especially at the end of a dry summer. Diagnosis by response to cobalt, selenium, perhaps copper or vitamin D, the latter in areas far from the equator, is often used in situations where such trace elements or vitamins are suspect (3). Clinical or subclinical infestations with nematodes are also common occurrences at this time in the sheep's life before immunity is properly developed and infections with coccidia or *Eperythrozoon ovis* are probably significant causes of ill-thrift (3).

Examination of the above-mentioned possible causes is time-absorbing and costly and, if there is a residuum of unsolved cases, they are likely to remain undiagnosed. One additional factor which might be taken into consideration is the villous atrophy seen in ruminal epithelium in young sheep grazing on pasture composed of a pure stand of one pasture plant species, especially perennial rye grass (4, 5). The change in the epithelium is similar to that which occurs in sheep fed heat-treated pellets. It has been pointed out (3) that this lesion, with its attendant malabsorption, can arise by virtue of trauma by coccidia or nematodes which are no longer in evidence at the time of post-mortem examination or response trial.

In bad years there may be many deaths; in any circumstance there is a gross delay in maturation so that maiden lambing may be delayed to as late as three years of age (5). The economic effects can be disastrous.

REFERENCES

(1) Pulsford, M. R. *et al.* (1966). *Aust. vet. J.*, 42, 165, 169, 388.
(2) Findlay, G. R. & Heath, G. B. S. (1969). *Vet. Rec.*, 85, 547.
(3) Pout, D. D. & Harbutt, P. (1968). *Vet. Rec.*, 83, 373.
(4) Lancashire, J. A. & Keogh, R. G. (1966). *N.Z. J. agric. Res.*, 9, 916.
(5) McLoughlin, J. W. (1967). *Vict. vet. Proc.*, 25, 60.

Thin Sow Syndrome

The 'thin sow syndrome' must be classified as a problem rather than as a disease because of its probable multiple aetiology. Admittedly it has been recorded much more in recent years (1) but it is by no means new. At one time it was possible to evade the problem but in today's cost- and waste-conscious agriculture, the 'thin sow syndrome' needs to be admitted, quantified and examined. Its effects on fertility and overall farm productivity can be formidable (2).

Affected sows lose more than the usual amount of weight during pregnancy and after farrowing, the latter being more noticeable. No abnormalities are evident on clinical examination but the sow fails to regain weight after weaning and the most critical period for weight loss is the first two weeks after weaning. Affected sows have a poor appetite but often show pica and excessive water intake and are anaemic. The most important characteristic of the disease is the failure to respond to treatment and culling is usually advisable.

In some instances the problem is parasitic and accompanied by high egg counts and a significant population of *Oesophagostomum* spp. and *Hyostronglus rubidus* and this group is discussed under those headings. In others the problems appear to arise because of errors in management which are likely to be exaggerated and multiplied on farms where intensive management is practised. The most common errors are cold or draughty housing, low-level feeding to avoid obesity and low fertility, wet bedding and lack of drinking water. Modern-day rapid re-mating of sows and very early weaning increase the chances of metabolic breakdown, especially if nutrition is inadequate. The latter is most likely when sows are run in large groups with different stages of pregnancy present and where timid sows are likely to be bullied out of their fair share of food. When breeds are mixed it is often the Landrace, Saddleback and their crossbreds which are the most timid and most likely to become affected (2). Individual stalls give an opportunity for individual feeding and tend to avoid this problem. A satisfactory level of feed intake must be maintained during lactation because most affected sows fail to respond to improved nutrition after weaning.

REFERENCES

(1) Maclean, C. W. (1968). *Vet. Rec.*, *83*, 308.
(2) Maclean, C. W. (1969). *Vet. Rec.*, *85*, 675.

Hyperlipaemia of Ponies

This condition could have been included in the section on systemic states because it can only be a systemic manifestation of some other disease such as hepatic insufficiency. However, its occurrence is limited to ponies, especially Shetlands, and it has a peculiarity of manifestation that sets it apart as a disease entity. It is recorded principally from Holland (1, 2) but it has occurred in Australia and elsewhere. Hyperlipaemia occurs almost always in pregnant mares or mares which have recently foaled or aborted. It is therefore most common in spring. Affected ponies are anorectic and mostly constipated, a few showing severe diarrhoea. Lethargy, stumbling gait and coating of the oral mucosa are evident. Most (over 65 per cent) affected animals die.

The probable pathogenesis of the condition is that a primary disease causes anorexia, followed by massive fat mobilization causing hyperlipaemia and the extraordinary fattiness of the liver which are diagnostic characteristics. It may well be that death occurs because of fatty infiltration of the liver to the point of causing hepatic insufficiency. The hyperlipaemia can be readily seen in the serum after the cells have sedimented; the serum has a milk-like opacity.

Treatment is difficult and must be related to the primary disease, especially worm infestations, sand in the intestines causing enteritis, and viral infections of the respiratory tract. Correction of the hyperlipaemia is a formidable task if the pony is fat, pregnant and not eating, as they usually are. Many therapeutic agents have been used with indifferent results (2).

REFERENCES

(1) Schotman, A. J. H. & Wagenaar, G. (1969). *Zbl. vet. Med.*, *16A*, 1.
(2) Schotman, A. J. H. & Kroneman, J. (1969). *Neth. J. vet. Sci.*, *2*, 60.

Post-Vaccinal Hepatitis of Horses

This disease has been recorded chiefly as a sequel to infectious encephalomyelitis, occurring 1 to 3 months after an outbreak of this disease. An outbreak was recorded recently in the U.K. where IEE does not occur (1). Although the hepatitis is thought to be related to the use of serum and vaccine used in the control of IEE, cases have occurred in horses which do not appear to have received any biological preparation in the period of several months prior to the development of the disease. This form of hepatitis bears some resemblance to infectious hepatitis of man and its possible method of spread on hypodermic needles further heightens the resemblance. However, attempts to transmit the disease have been unsuccessful and it is thought that a hepatotoxic agent may be present in any equine serum or tissue extract used as vaccine. Occurrence of the disease in horses is recorded after vaccination against IEE, African horse sickness, anthrax, enterotoxaemia and influenza (1). A third possibility is that a hepatotoxic agent is combined with an infectious agent not capable of transmitting the disease without the intervention of the toxin. A mild case of the disease appears to have been produced by the injection of IEE anti-serum and the feeding of ragwort (*Senecio latifolius*).

Clinically the disease is characterized by intense icterus, cessation of alimentary tract movement and oliguria, absence or rare occurrence of fever, and severe nervous signs including stupor and mania.

There may be a straddle-legged posture with continuous head-pressing, violent, uncontrolled movement and walking in circles. Haemoglobinuria occurs in some cases. Most affected animals die within 12 to 48 hours. Some animals recover without apparent after-effects whilst others manifest imbecility and an intractable disposition.

At necropsy the most significant changes are seen in the liver which, although normal in size, is light or greenish in colour and soft and friable in texture (2, 3). Degenerative changes may also be seen in the kidneys. There is hyperaemia or submucosal haemorrhage of the small intestine and petechial and ecchymotic haemorrhages are present under the serous membranes and in the musculature. Icterus is present throughout the carcass.

Treatment with antibiotics, glucose and electrolyte solutions and B-complex vitamins may be of some value (2).

REFERENCES

(1) Thomsett, L. R. (1971). *Equ. vet. J.*, *3*, 15.
(2) Hjerpe, C. A. (1964). *J. Amer. vet. med. Ass.*, *144*, 734.
(3) Panciera, R. J. (1969). *J. Amer. vet. med. Ass.*, *155*, 408.

DISEASES CHARACTERIZED BY ALIMENTARY TRACT INVOLVEMENT

Grass Sickness of Horses

Grass sickness is a non-infectious disease of horses of unknown aetiology. It is characterized clinically by alimentary stasis, emaciation and severe mental depression. Degenerative lesions are detectable on histological examination of the sympathetic ganglia.

Incidence

Grass sickness is not common and appears to be restricted in occurrence to Scotland and Northern England and to Sweden. Most affected horses die or are destroyed because of weakness and emaciation.

Aetiology

The cause is unknown. Viral infection has been suggested because of the nature of the lesions in the sympathetic ganglia but the disease has not been transmitted. Cases do tend to occur close together and if an infectious agent is involved an incubation period of about 7 days is suggested (1). Intoxication has also been suggested as a cause because most cases occur in horses at pasture. Intoxication caused by *Clostridium perfringens* Type D was suggested but vaccination with an anaculture of the organism, while producing antibodies, did not prevent the disease (2). Horses are the only species affected and all breeds and age groups, other than sucking foals, are susceptible, but the incidence is highest in the 3- to 6-years age group.

Occurrence

Most cases develop while horses are at pasture but sporadic cases occur in stabled animals (3). Cases occur throughout the year but the highest incidence is in the summer months. In Scotland the occurrence of the disease is dependent on rain and on an increasing environmental temperature (4) with a high point of prevalence in May and a peak incidence in horses 3 years of age, but the disease is common in horses of 2 to 8 years of age.

Pathogenesis

The early hypothesis of sympatheticotonia (5) has not been refuted and the clinical picture is, apart from the absence of pupillary dilatation, one of increased sympathetic tone. The alimentary signs are those of paralytic ileus due to functional stasis. The lesions in the sympathetic ganglia bear out the suggestion that the sympathetic nervous system is the site of the important defect. However, one might expect that the degenerative nature of the lesions would cause a decrease in sympathetic tone, rather than the observed sympathetic dominance, and the presence of identical lesions in clinically normal control horses suggests that the lesions may be secondary.

Peristalsis stops, contents of the large intestine become dehydrated, digestive tract becomes distended with decomposing ingesta and gas and rupture is the usual termination (1).

Clinical Findings

Acute, subacute and chronic cases occur. In all cases, there is lethargy and difficulty in swallowing, resulting in drooling of saliva and trickling of ingesta from the nose. Bowel movements cease, peristaltic sounds are absent and there may be tympanites. Abdominal discomfort may suggest the presence of subacute impaction of the large intestine. On rectal examination, the faeces are hard, dry pellets covered with sticky mucus. Urination is frequent and may be accompanied by tenesmus. Affected horses may wander about in a restless manner and a fine muscle tremor occurs constantly, especially in the upper forelimb. Periodic attacks of patchy sweating occur commonly.

The course of the disease varies. Acute cases die in 1 to 5 days and may or may not show signs of colic. In subacute cases, the course is usually 2 to 3 weeks and, during this time, the animal loses much condition and becomes extremely gaunt. The skeletal muscles appear to be stretched tight and are very hard to the touch. Chronic cases may appear to recover but are incapable of hard work.

Clinical Pathology

All haematological and biochemical examinations on affected horses have failed to show any significant abnormalities.

Necropsy Findings

In cases of short duration, the stomach and small intestines are distended with an excess of fluid and gas, and the colon contains small, hard, black pellets of manure. The spleen is always enlarged. In chronic cases, the alimentary tract is empty and of very small calibre. Histologically there is extensive degeneration of neurones in the sympathetic ganglia without evidence of inflammation (6) and neuronal necrosis in the central nervous system; the lesions are present in oculomotor, facial, lateral vestibular, hypoglossal and vagal nuclei (7).

Diagnosis

Grass sickness is strictly limited in its geographical distribution. Early acute cases may resemble subacute impaction of the colon except for difficult swallowing and the accumulation of fluid in the alimentary tract. Failure of cases of grass sickness to respond to treatment for colonic impaction may serve as a further aid in diagnosis.

Treatment

All attempts at treatment have been without effect. Decompression of the stomach by drainage and the administration of large quantities of isotonic solutions parenterally prolong the life of affected animals but do not influence the final outcome of the disease (8).

Control

Successful measures have not been satisfactorily established and no recommendations can be made.

REFERENCES

(1) Limont, A. G. (1971). *Vet. Rec.*, *88*, 98.
(2) Gordon, W. S. (1946). *Vet. Rec.*, *58*, 516.
(3) Lannek, N. *et al.* (1961). *Vet. Rec.*, *73*, 601.
(4) Anonymous (1971). *Vet. Rec. Members Info. Suppl.* No. 78.
(5) Greig, J. R. (1928). *Vet. Rec.*, *8*, 31.
(6) Brownlee, A. (1965). *Vet. Rec.*, *77*, 323.
(7) Barlow, R. M. (1969). *J. comp. Path.*, *79*, 407.

Colitis-X

This disease of horses has come to public attention only during the past decade and although it is known to occur in the U.S.A. (1), Canada, the West Indian Federation and Australia, there are few written reports on which to base an accurate description. Because of its highly fatal nature, most affected horses dying within 24 hours of first illness, and because it sometimes occurs as an 'outbreak' with a number of horses in a group (up to 20 per cent) becoming affected within a space of 1 to 2 weeks, this disease is of major economic importance. Most cases occur in adult horses but affected animals may be in the range of 1 to 10 years. The

cause is unknown and no treatment appears to have any effect on the course of the disease. Cases may occur sporadically or as 'outbreaks' but no infectious agent has been isolated nor are the lesions suggestive of viral, bacterial or other infection. Two causes have been suggested, endotoxaemia due to a bacterial toxin (2) and exhaustion shock (3). *E. coli* endotoxin, infused rapidly intravenously into ponies, produces a similar clinical and pathological picture (4). Although the histories of many cases of colitis-X suggest that the animals were subjected to stress including transport, deprivation of food or water or disease prior to the development of the disease, many horses are affected without such a history. On the other hand the lesions seen do suggest that spontaneous exhaustion shock is the cause of death.

Clinically there is a very sudden onset of enteritis, or occasionally intestinal distension with gas, and death in 3 to 24 hours (5). The horse suddenly becomes depressed, shows muddy, discoloured mucosae, a very fast (100 per minute) small amplitude pulse, patchy sweating, moderate dyspnoea and abdominal pain. In the early stages the temperature may rise to $39 \cdot 5 \,^{\circ}$C ($103 \,^{\circ}$F) but soon falls to become subnormal terminally, and the skin feels cold and clammy almost from the first signs of illness. The horse becomes very weak and is inclined to collapse where it stands, lie over on its side and die quietly a few minutes later. The pupils are dilated. Profuse diarrhoea may or may not occur, animals surviving for less than 3 or 4 hours tending to have normal faeces even on rectal examination. There is a complete absence of intestinal sounds. Dehydration is evident in animals which survive for longer periods. On haematological examination elevation of the blood urea nitrogen (over 60 mg. per cent) and haemoconcentration are evident. A marked acidosis develops and there may be a leucopenia.

There are extensive lesions at necropsy examination (4) the most dramatic being in the large intestine, especially the caecum and ventral colon. These lesions vary from hyperaemia with petechiation to an intense, greenish black, haemorrhagic necrosis. The contents are fluid, often foamy and evil smelling and may be blood-stained. Lesions in the small intestine are minimal (6).

From the clinical and necropsy examinations it is possible to confuse the disease with enteritis due to salmonella infection or arsenic poisoning and before death difficulty may be encountered in distinguishing between colitis-X and acute intestinal obstruction or acute arterial occlusion by *Strongylus vulgaris* larvae. Even though treatment with massive infusions of balanced electrolyte infusions and with adrenal corticosteroids is indicated, the disease is usually so acute that death is inescapable. Infusion therapy must be intensive and 10 litres of Ringer's lactate solution, to which is added 40 to 60 g. sodium bicarbonate and 500 ml. of 50 per cent dextrose, should be given intravenously. A similar dose by stomach tube is recommended as a minimal level of treatment. Because of the peracute nature of the disease the initial dose of corticosteroids should be given intravenously followed by further doses at 8-hour intervals (7).

REFERENCES

(1) Teighland, M. B. (1960). *Proc. 6th ann. Mtg Amer. Assoc. equine Pract.*, pp. 81–92.
(2) Carroll, E. J. *et al.* (1965). *J. Amer. vet. med. Ass.*, 146, 1300.
(3) Rooney, J. R. *et al.* (1966). *Cornell Vet.*, 56, 220.
(4) Burrows, G. E. & Cannon, J. (1970). *Amer. J. vet. Res.*, 31, 1967.
(5) Pickrell, J. W. (1968). *Mod. vet. Pract.*, 49, 63.
(6) Hudson, R. S. (1968). *Auburn Vet.*, 24, 92.
(7) Olson, N. E. (1966). *J. Amer. vet. med. Ass.*, 148, 418.

Equine Intestinal Trichomoniasis

This is a chronic disease of horses characterized by persistent diarrhoea. In many cases the disease is irreversible and the horses are destroyed.

Incidence

The disease is rarely recorded but veterinarians in most countries are quite familiar with it. The incidence is very low and is usually restricted to one horse in a group but the disease is an important one because it is chronic and often fatal. An additional form of loss is the cost of treatment, often for long periods and with expensive remedies.

Aetiology

Literally nothing is known of the cause. *Trichomonas faecalis* (or *T. equi*) has been nominated as a possible cause (1) but the nomination has not been received enthusiastically (2). One of the principal difficulties encountered in any investigation of the disease is that of defining it pathologically. There is no lesion, macroscopically or histologically, and no constant pathogenic agent, only a constant clinical picture.

There is no suggestion of an infectious agent but stress is often recorded and frequently implicated. It certainly is common for affected animals to have a history which includes illness, an upper respiratory tract infection, trauma, surgery, etc., plus in almost every case treatment with an antibiotic. The infection and treatment occur about two weeks before the illness commences. Horses have died

after the experimental administration of 15 g. oxytetracycline i.v. but the disease was much more acute and the intestinal lesions more distinct than is the case in this disease (3).

When trichomonads are present, they are present in large numbers, and are readily identified by their motility, their large size and flagellated structure. They are not usually detectable in the faeces of normal horses.

Pathogenesis

No lesion has been identified, even in the myoneural plexuses of the intestinal wall. The disease appears to be a functional hypermotility. One would expect to see lesions in the sympathetic ganglia or parasympathetic nerves, as in grass sickness. This disease is not unlike Johne's disease of cattle.

Clinical Signs

There is a sudden onset of profuse watery diarrhoea, with large amounts of faeces passed frequently. There is a characteristic smell and there is absence of blood, mucus, mucosa or other abnormal constituents. The horse is not otherwise sick. There is no fever, the appetite remains fair to good. However, the animal loses weight rapidly and is chronically dehydrated. There is no colic but large intestinal sounds are exaggerated.

Complete recovery may occur at any time. Partial recovery, with the persistence of semi-soft faeces of the consistency of cow manure, is common enough. In many cases the horse becomes so thin that on humane grounds euthanasia is performed.

Clinical Pathology

Faeces taken fresh from the rectum should be examined immediately under the microscope for the presence of trichomonads. Further examination should be made by culture of the faeces.

Necropsy Findings

No significant lesions have been observed.

Treatment

No specific treatment is possible although the administration of metronidazole (1·25 to 2·5 g. per day for 5 days) has been recommended on the assumption that *Trichomonas faecalis* is the causative agent (3). Iodochlorhydroxyquinoline (Vioform) 15 g. daily by nasal tube initially, reducing to 10 g. daily as the diarrhoea improves, for a total treatment period of 30 to 36 days is recommended (1, 2, 4). Tincture of opium, tincture of chloroform and morphine, bismuth subnitrate and catechu mixture all have their value in reducing fluid loss. Broad-spectrum antibiotics are not recommended.

In early, acute cases dehydration may occur and affected animals may require treatment for dehydration. One of the principal treatments used is an infusion of faecal material from a horse abattoir but it must be administered by stomach tube and in large volume (1). Administration via an enema is unsatisfactory. A good general practice is to administer 3 gallons of this daily for 3 days.

REFERENCES

(1) Laufenstein-Duffy, H. (1969). *J. Amer. vet. med. Ass., 155*, 1835.
(2) Manahan, F. F. (1970). *Aust. vet. J., 46*, 231.
(3) Miller, J. M. (1969). *Proc. 15th ann. Conv. Amer. Ass. equine Pract.*, Houston, Texas.
(4) Stoner, J. C. (1966). *Vet. Med., 61*, 660.

Acute Intestinal Haemorrhage in Pigs

This disease has been present for some years, known as 'bloodyguts', in pigs in fattening units associated with dairy factories (1). It was recorded originally as reaching its highest incidence in 2- to 5-month-old pigs fed heavily on whey (2), although older pigs can also be affected. On affected farms the occurrence is very sporadic with an occasional pig dying in a pen or group. Pigs with the disease are usually found dead. Clinical signs are rarely seen but include sudden collapse, rolling from side to side with their backs against the floor and screaming with pain.

At necropsy examination there is very marked skin pallor, gross abdominal distension, marked hyperaemia of the intestine and uniform extensive blood staining of the contents of the small intestine. Extensive subendocardial haemorrhages in the left ventricle are characteristic. The cause is not known but acute anaphylaxis after ingesting milk, or as a result of toxin of *E. coli* or *Cl. perfringens* is suspected.

Heavy doses of framomycin appeared to control the disease in at least one instance. Treatment of all animals of breeding age with promethazine hydrochloride (3 to 5 ml. of 5 per cent solution intramuscularly daily for 5 successive days) has also been recommended (3).

REFERENCES

(1) Kinnaird, P. J. (1964–65). *Vict. vet. Proc.*, p. 45.
(2) Jones, J. E. T. (1967). *Brit. vet. J., 123*, 286.
(3) Rowntree, P. G. M. (1972). *Vet. Rec., 91*, 347.

Muzzle Disease

(*Mycotic Stomatitis*)

A disease condition described as muzzle disease bears much similarity to mucosal disease. It has been observed in the southern and eastern United States, in Canada and in Australia (1) in herds with varying grades of management and in different seasons but particularly in the later summer and early autumn. Usually, only a few animals in each herd are affected but the incidence may reach 50 per cent.

Erosions on the nasal mucosa, muzzle, dental pad, gums, tongue, lateral aspects of the teats, scrotum, vulva and coronary bands are characteristic. There is some mucoserous, nasal discharge and an offensive odour emanates from the mouth when oral lesions are extensive. Anorexia, excessive salivation and lameness develop and there is local pain on palpation of the coronet. Diarrhoea is absent except just before death in the uncommon fatal case. The cause of the disease is unknown and no specific treatment is available. Extensive attempts to transmit the disease have been unsuccessful (2). Although many cases occur in cattle being fed forage heavily contaminated by mould a direct relationship has not been established. The most significant opinions are that the disease is a chronic form of either mucosal disease or of bluetongue.

REFERENCES

(1) Hutchins, D. R. *et al.* (1964). *Aust. vet. J., 40*, 269.
(2) Pritchard, W. R. & Wassenaar, P. W. (1959). *J. Amer. vet. med. Ass., 135*, 274.

Necrotic Glossitis

Another member of the group of bovine diseases characterized by oral lesions is necrotic glossitis (1, 2). The disease has been recorded only in the U.S.A. in feedlot steers on a diet of corn, concentrate and hay. It has a very high morbidity (75 to 100 per cent) but causes no deaths and although affected steers are off feed for a few days there is little loss of weight. The cause is unknown. At first glance the disease resembles vesicular stomatitis in many ways but serological examination has shown no evidence of this disease and in one outbreak there was no evidence of disease in pigs running with cattle (1).

The syndrome includes salivation, protrusion of the tongue, reluctance to eat, chewing movements, lapping at water and elevation of the head to swallow. The anterior 2 to 5 cm. of the tip of the tongue is black and necrotic and is separated from normal lingual tissue by a definite line of demarcation. Sloughing of the necrotic portion may follow. Some crusting of the muzzle and obstruction of the external nares with exudate may be present. Spontaneous recovery occurs in a few days but the course of the disease in a herd may be as long as 45 to 90 days. Recovery usually occurs without treatment.

A similar disease which is preceded by respiratory involvement and by contact with swine has been described (3).

REFERENCES

(1) Wake, W. L. (1961). *J. Amer. vet. med. Ass.*, *138*, 7.
(2) Hill, J. K. & Herrick, J. B. (1961). *Vet. Med.*, *56*, 190.
(3) McDaniel, H. A. & Sherman, K. C. (1968). *Proc. 71st ann. gen. Mtg U.S. Live Stock sanit. Ass.*, 547.

Oesophago-Gastric Ulceration of Swine

Oesophago-gastric ulceration of swine has become a disease of major proportions during recent years. Examination of pigs' stomachs at abattoirs shows that a very high proportion of young pigs have ulcers, or potential or healed ulcers, without having shown signs of clinical illness. For example in a series of 24,000 stomachs of slaughter pigs examined at abattoirs 34 per cent showed lesions and 8 per cent showed severe lesions (1). The incidence of clinical disease is not very high but the mortality rate is so great that individual farmers may suffer significant losses (2).

The cause of the disease has not been fully determined but largely by inference from the suspected causes of gastric ulcer in other species many agents, including rough feed and conversely the absence of sufficient fibre in the ration, high concentrations of irritant mineral mixtures improperly mixed with the grain ration, hyperacidity due to stress, and erosion of the mucosa by keratolytic fungi encouraged by a high sugar content of the diet, have been advanced as aetiological agents (1, 3).

The occurrence is limited to penned pigs and particularly to those receiving a heavy grain diet and growing rapidly, although the disease also occurs in pigs being fed large quantities of whey (4). On grain rations there is a much higher incidence on diets containing a higher proportion of corn (maize) than other grains (5). The tendency is greater still if the corn is finely ground (6) or is gelatinized or expanded (7). The size of particles in the feed is significant whatever feed is used, even straw; coarsely ground barley straw at 5 to 10 per cent of the ration gives almost complete protection (8). On the other hand pelleting of feed seems to increase the number of ulcers occurring (9). Oat hulls in the diet are also highly effective, 25 per cent coarsely ground oats in a corn ration being protective (10).

Of the suspected causes there is good evidence, from the administration of histamine and reserpine, that gastric hyperacidity is an important factor (11, 12). This is probably related to the effects of psychological stress, including noise, excessive disturbing and overcrowding of pigs, which is known to be a significant contributor to the development of gastric ulcer in pigs (2). It is probably safe to assume that a dietary factor and a management factor (psychological stress) are capable, either singly or together, of causing the disease (2, 13).

Oesophago-gastric ulceration is most common in pigs of 45 to 90 kg. body weight but there is also a significant occurrence as early as 2 months and as late as gilts near the end of pregnancy (2). All breeds are affected but the disease is more common in farrows than in gilts (14). There is evidence of an inherited susceptibility (21).

Clinical signs are often not observed, affected pigs being found dead from acute haemorrhage into the stomach. A few subacute cases survive for 12 to 48 hours with signs of marked pallor, weakness, anorexia and black pasty faeces changing to mucous-covered pellets in small amounts. The weakness may be sufficient to cause recumbency. Animals that survive are often unthrifty, usually due to anaemia from chronic blood loss with a few cases affected by chronic peritonitis. When the disease is occurring careful observation may detect early cases. Suggestive signs are a darkening of the faeces and the development of pallor.

At necropsy the ulcers are confined to the oesophageal region of the stomach. They may be acute or chronic with the latter often showing signs of recent exacerbation, and fresh blood may be found in the stomach and intestines. Early lesions in clinically unaffected animals include hyperkeratinization of the mucosa and epithelial denudation without actual ulceration. Affected stomachs consistently have more fluid contents than unaffected ones (15). Evidence of bile staining in some affected stomachs has led to the suggestion that duodenal regurgitation of bile into the stomach may cause ulceration (16).

Differentiation from other causes of sudden death is necessary, particularly acute anaemia caused by diffuse haemorrhage into the lumen of the colon.

Supplementation of the diet with vitamin E (18 mg. per kg. of feed), with or without selenium, has given mixed results as a prophylactic in field cases (17, 18, 19). Supplementation of the diet with antibiotics, copper sulphate, vitamins A and E, antihistamines or tranquillizers failed to prevent ulceration in pigs fed rations high in corn (20). On present knowledge the prevention of losses could include restriction of the corn content of the diet, avoidance of psychologically stressful situations and perhaps the inclusion of some roughage in the diet. Any procedure which keeps food in the stomach for long periods will provide a buffer against gastric hyperacidity and reduce the occurrence of the disease. Addition of antacid substances would have the same buffering effect.

REVIEW LITERATURE
Kowalczyk, T. (1969). *Amer.'J. vet. Res.*, 30, 393.
O'Brien, J. J. (1969). *Vet. Bull.*, 39, 75–82.

REFERENCES
(1) Hoorens, J. *et al.* (1965). *Vlaams Diergeneesk. Tijdschr.*, 34, 112.
(2) Kowalezyk, T. *et al.* (1971). *Vet. Med. small Anim. Clin.*, 66, 1185.
(3) Kadel, W. L. *et al.* (1969). *Amer. J. vet. Res.*, 30, 401.
(4) O'Brien, J. J. (1968). *Vet. Rec.*, 83, 245.
(5) Reese, N. E. *et al.* (1966). *J. Anim. Sci.*, 25, 14.
(6) Bjorklund, N. E. *et al.* (1970). *Proc. 11th nordic vet. Congr. Bergen*, 1970, 274.
(7) Mason, D. W. *et al.* (1968). *J. Anim. Sci.*, 27, 1006.
(8) Baustad, B. & Nafstad, I. (1969). *Path. vet.*, 6, 546.
(9) Chamberlain, C. C. *et al.* (1967). *J. Anim. Sci.*, 26, 72, 214, 1054.
(10) Maxwell, C. V. (1970). *Diss. Abstr. int.*, 31B, 777.
(11) Muggenburg, B. A. *et al.* (1966). *Amer. J. vet. Res.*, 27, 292, 1663.
(12) Huber, W. G. & Wallin, R. F. (1967). *Amer. J. vet. Res.*, 28, 1455.
(13) Reese, N. A. *et al.* (1963). *J. Anim. Sci.*, 22, 1129.
(14) Muggenburg, B. A. *et al.* (1964). *Amer. J. vet. Res.*, 25, 1673.
(15) Muggenburg, B. A. *et al.* (1964). *Amer. J. vet. Res.*, 25, 1354.
(16) Reed, J. H. & Kidder, D. E. (1970). *Res. vet. Sci.*, 11, 438.
(17) Kinnaird, P. J. (1964–65). *Vict. vet. Proc.*, 23, 45.
(18) Hannan, J. & Nyhan, J. F. (1962). *Irish vet. J.*, 16, 196.
(19) Dobson, K. J. (1967). *Aust. vet. J.*, 43, 219.
(20) Nuwer, A. J. *et al.* (1965). *J. Anim. Sci.*, 24, 113.
(21) Berruecos, J. M. & Robinson, O. W. (1972). *J. Anim. Sci.*, 35, 20.

Diverticulitis and Ileitis of Pigs

(Proliferative Ileitis)

In this disease there is thickening of the wall of the ileum, particularly in the terminal portion, so that the intestine becomes thick and rigid. There is a close clinical similarity to Crohn's disease in man and the aetiology of both conditions is obscure. Familial predisposition is probable in man and has been suggested in pigs.

The signs are those of acute peritonitis due to ulceration and, sometimes, perforation of the affected ileum. Illness occurs suddenly with loss of appetite, excessive thirst, dullness and disinclination to rise. The temperature is subnormal, the respiration is distressed and there is a bluish discolouration of the skin. Death occurs in 24 to 48 hours.

Acute cases occur in young pigs up to 3 months of age, and chronic cases, due to ulceration and chronic peritonitis, in the 7- to 8-months age group.

At necropsy there may be diffuse peritonitis due to leakage of alimentary tract contents through perforating ileal ulcers. Gross thickening of the ileal wall with nodular proliferation of the ileal mucosa (1) and enlargement of the mesenteric lymph nodes are common accompaniments. Although the macroscopic findings are similar to those of Crohn's disease in man, the histopathological findings differ markedly (2, 3, 4).

REFERENCES
(1) Dodd, D. C. (1968). *Path. Vet.*, 5, 333.
(2) Field, H. I. *et al.* (1953). *J. comp. Path.*, 63, 153.
(3) Nielsen, S. W. (1955). *J. Amer. vet. med. Ass.*, 127, 437.
(4) Rahkot, T. & Saloniemi, H. (1972). *Nord. Vet.-Med.*, 24, 132.

DISEASES CHARACTERIZED BY RESPIRATORY TRACT INVOLVEMENT

Atrophic Rhinitis

Atrophic rhinitis is a disease affecting primarily young pigs but causing anatomical lesions which may persist for life. The cause has not been identified but the disease is characterized clinically by an initial attack of acute rhinitis followed by chronic atrophy of the turbinate bones and deformity of the face.

Incidence

Atrophic rhinitis appears to have originated in Scandinavia and spread to western Europe and to North America and the U.K. The disease is important because of its probable infectious nature and the inadequacy of known control measures. The morbidity rate varies but may reach as high as 50 per cent in individual herds. The mortality rate is very low but there is severe financial loss because of the adverse effects of the disease on rate of gain and the efficiency of food utilization. Under good husbandry conditions, the depression of weight gains may be negligible (1), but under adverse conditions, the effects appear to be much greater.

Aetiology

In the past many agents and influences have been indicted as causes of atrophic rhinitis and the position has not been completely clarified even yet (2, 3, 4). Of the many suggested causes, inherited susceptibility, dusty feed and bedding and poor hygiene have been generally rejected as major influences, although it is accepted that they may play a part as predisposing or exacerbating factors.

The general belief for many years has been that the disease is infectious, but in the light of the evidence at present available the only assumption which seems reasonable is that atrophic rhinitis can be caused by an infectious agent or by a dietary deficiency of calcium or possibly by a combination of both factors.

Infectious agents including bacteria, viruses and trichomonads have all been proposed as important causative agents. The virus of inclusion body rhinitis was strongly supported when that disease was first identified but it has been shown not to be necessary for the production of the disease. Trichomonads are often present in large numbers in the nasal cavities of infected pigs but do not appear to be capable of causing the disease (4). In recent years most attention has turned to bacteria, especially *Haemophilus bronchisepticus* (*Bordetella bronchiseptica*) (5, 6, 7) and to a less extent *Pasteurella multocida* type B as the important pathogenic agents (4). A combination of *B. bronchiseptica* and *P. multocida* has also been proposed as a significant agent (8). *Corynebacterium pyogenes*, *Sphaerophorus necrophorus*, *Haem. suis* and *Pseudomonas pyocyaneus* are often present in large numbers but are probably only secondary invaders.

Nutritional deficiency of calcium. There is evidence that atrophic rhinitis can be a manifestation of osteodystrophia fibrosa (2). Naturally occurring and experimentally produced cases have been shown to have an absolute or relative deficiency of calcium in the diet and inflammation was not a characteristic lesion. On the other hand, pigs on a diet sufficiently low in Vitamin D to cause rickets do not develop atrophic rhinitis (9) and calcium deficiency is not generally accepted as a major cause of the disease.

It is probable that the disease is not entirely infectious and that other factors such as diet and dusty feed do affect the severity of the disease but it seems very likely that the virus of inclusion body rhinitis is the common primary agent and that *B. bronchiseptica* is a necessary secondary agent. At least it can be recommended that the best way to control the disease would be eradication of inclusion body rhinitis from genetic nucleus herds (10).

Transmission

Experimentally the disease is transmissible to very young pigs by the intranasal instillation of material obtained from the nasal cavities of affected animals. Because of the severe sneezing that occurs in the early stages of the disease, it is probable that any infectious agent is spread naturally by the inhalation of infective droplets. It is unlikely that the infection spreads readily on inanimate objects and, in most field outbreaks of the disease, there is a history of introduction of pigs into the herd. Other species of animals are not known to act as carriers of the disease. Although very young piglets are the only ones readily susceptible to the disease, infected animals probably persist as carriers for long periods.

Pathogenesis

Many agents, both infectious and chemical, are capable of causing rhinitis in young pigs but it is only in this specific disease that decalcification of the turbinate bones and their subsequent atrophy occur. The disappearance of these structures and the involvement of the bones of the face lead to deformity of the facial bones with the appearance of dishing and bulging of the face and, if the lesion is unilateral, to lateral deviation of the snout. The appreciable effect on the growth and thriftiness of the pig has not been explained but is probably due to the chronic irritation, interference with prehension and digestion, and inefficiency of protection against inhalation infections usually afforded by the nasal mucosa.

Clinical Findings

In many instances the disease is manifested by severe clinical signs as set out below, but under ideal conditions of management, the signs may be restricted to sneezing and a slight decrease in efficiency of food utilization. In acute cases, swelling of the nasal mucosa causes obstruction to breathing, a watery nasal discharge, sneezing and rubbing of the nose against objects or on the ground. A watery ocular discharge usually accompanies this and may result in the appearance of dried streaks of dirt under the eyes. In severe cases, respiratory obstruction may increase to the point of dyspnoea and cyanosis, and sucking pigs may have great difficulty in nursing. The nasal secretions become thicker and nasal bleeding may also occur. In the more chronic stages, inspissated material may be expelled during paroxysms of sneezing. During this chronic stage, there is often pronounced deformity of the face due to arrested development of the bones, especially the turbinates, and the accumulation of necrotic material in the nasal cavities. The nasal bones and premaxillae turn upwards and interfere with approximation of the incisor and, to a less extent, the molar teeth.

Prehension and mastication become difficult with a resulting loss of body condition. Facial distortion in the final stages takes the form of severe 'dishing' of the face with wrinkling of the overlying skin. If the condition is unilateral, the upper jaw may be twisted to one side. These visible distortions develop most commonly in pigs 8 to 10 weeks old but may occur in younger pigs.

The most serious effects of the disease are depression of growth rate and unthriftiness. The appetite may be unaffected but much food is lost by spillage and the weight gains per kg. of food may be reduced in some instances.

Clinical Pathology

Ante-mortem laboratory examinations are of little diagnostic value and, in most instances, one resorts to necropsy examination of sample pigs to confirm the diagnosis. Nasal swabs and washings may be used in transmission experiments but the source material is usually more readily obtained from necropsy specimens. Transmission experiments are not usually undertaken in field work because clinical and necropsy examinations are usually sufficient for a herd diagnosis.

Necropsy Findings

The typical lesions of atrophic rhinitis are restricted to the nasal cavities although concurrent diseases, especially virus pneumonia of pigs, may produce lesions elsewhere. In the early stages, there is acute inflammation, sometimes with the accumulation of pus but, in the later stages, there is evidence only of atrophy of the mucosa, and decalcification and atrophy of the turbinate and ethmoid bones, which may have completely disappeared in severe cases. The inflammatory and atrophic processes may extend to involve the facial sinuses. There is no evidence of interference with the vascular supply to the affected bones. The changes in the nasal cavities are most readily seen if the head is split in the sagittal plane but for accurate diagnosis the degree of atrophy should be assessed by inspection of a vertical cross-section of the skull made at the level of the second premolar tooth (4).

Diagnosis

The occurrence of sneezing in the early stages and of facial deformity in the later stages are characteristic of this disease. In the early acute stages, atrophic rhinitis may be mistaken for swine influenza which, however, usually occurs as an outbreak affecting older pigs and is accompanied by a severe systemic reaction without subsequent involvement of facial bones. Necrotic rhinitis is manifested by external lesions affecting the face, and virus pneumonia of pigs is characterized by coughing rather than sneezing. The inherited prognathic jaw of some breeds of pigs has been mistaken for the chronic stage of atrophic rhinitis.

Treatment

The prophylactic intranasal instillation or intramuscular injection of streptomycin is known to reduce the severity of the disease (11). A more practicable procedure for large-scale use is the administration of sulphamezathine in the feed (100 g. per ton of feed) or sodium sulphathiazole in the drinking water (15 mg. per litre) for 4 weeks in young pigs or 2 weeks in adults. The treatment is considered to be effective in atrophic rhinitis caused by *Bordetella bronchiseptica* but not when *Pasteurella multocida* is the causative agent (4, 12).

Control

The control of atrophic rhinitis is a difficult problem because of the lack of knowledge of the causative agent. Vaccines and sera have not been satisfactory preventive agents and, although the prophylactic injection of streptomycin reduces the incidence of the disease, it is not widely applicable as a control measure. Any attempt at limiting the spread or at eradicating the disease must, therefore, depend upon hygienic precautions to prevent contact between infected and non-infected animals.

Area control. In some enzootic areas, attempts have been made to reduce the incidence of the disease by a system of notification and quarantine. Pigs are permitted to leave the farm only if going for immediate slaughter, the farm is left unstocked for 3 months and restocking is permitted only when the premises have been properly cleaned and disinfected (11). The greatest stumbling block in this scheme is the difficulty in obtaining disease-free pigs for restocking. The same difficulty applies when restrictions are placed on the entry of pigs into a control area and the scheme must be reinforced by the establishment and annual certification of individual atrophic rhinitis-free herds.

Herd control. Much the same difficulty is encountered in the control of the disease in a herd as in an area. The radical method, involving the sale of all pigs, leaving the farm unstocked for several months, and disinfecting the premises is of little value unless a source of disease-free pigs is available. The more conservative procedure of attempting to select disease-free animals from within the herd and to raise them in isolation is tedious and may fail on individual farms but is sometimes recommended. Diagnosis in the sow herd by nasal swabbing and clinical examination and culling of infected animals may be the most practicable procedure in some circumstances. The use of SPF pigs obtained by Caesarean section has been much more widely used but has not been entirely satisfactory (7).

A combined attempt to eradicate enzootic pneumonia and atrophic rhinitis in the one operation suggests itself as a worth while and practicable procedure except in herds where the incidence is very high. It may be advisable in such herds to institute improvements in hygiene and nutrition before attempting eradication.

In the light of the possible effect of nutrition on the disease it would be unwise to neglect the calcium and phosphorus status of the diet, especially in pregnant and lactating sows and in young pigs (1). The recommended levels of intake are 1·2 per cent calcium and 1·0 per cent phosphorus in the ration. The high intake of calcium necessitates the intake of more zinc than is usually recommended. A level of 100 parts zinc per million of total diet is suggested as adequate. It is also recommended that attention be given to the control of any infectious disease, particularly enteric disease, which might limit the assimilation of minerals in the diet.

REFERENCES

(1) Pearce, H. G. & Roe, C. K. (1967). *Canad. vet. J.*, 8, 186.
(2) Brown, W. R. *et al.* (1966). *Cornell Vet.*, 56, Suppl. 1, 1.
(3) Pearce, H. G. & Roe, C. K. (1966). *Canad. vet. J.*, 7, 243.
(4) Switzer, W. P. (1965). *J. Amer. vet. med. Ass.*, 146, 348.
(5) Cross, R. F. & Claflin, R. M. (1962). *J. Amer. vet. med. Ass.*, 141, 1467.
(6) Duncan, J. R. *et al.* (1966). *Amer. J. vet. Res.*, 27, 457.
(7) Dunn, J. W. *et al.* (1964). *Proc. 68th ann. gen. Mtg U.S. Live Stock sanit. Ass.*, 266.
(8) Harris, D. L. & Switzer, W. P. (1968). *Amer. J. vet. Res.*, 29, 777.
(9) Baustad, B. *et al.* (1967). *Acta vet. scand.*, 8, 369.
(10) Done, J. T. (1971). *Proc. 19th Wld vet. Congr. Mexico City*, 2, 408.
(11) Gwatkin, R. (1958). *Advanc. vet. Sci.*, 4, 211.
(12) Ross, R. F. *et al.* (1963). *Vet. Med.*, 58, 562, 566, 571.

Atypical Interstitial Pneumonia of Cattle

This disease has been known for many years and under many names, including pulmonary adenomatosis, acute alveolar emphysema and oedema, bovine pulmonary emphysema, 'panters', 'lungers', bovine asthma, pneumoconiosis and 'fog fever'. On clinical grounds there are two forms of the disease, the acute and the chronic, but most descriptions are confined to the acute form.

The introduction of a new name, atypical interstitial pneumonia, may appear to further confound the nomenclature of the disease, but it is suggested because the names listed above do not adequately describe the condition. Pulmonary adenomatosis is already an accepted name for a specific viral disease of sheep; emphysema is a secondary lesion in this disease, as it is in many others; bovine asthma is a much rarer disease and differs markedly from atypical interstitial pneumonia, both clinically and at necropsy; pneumoconiosis is characterized by granulomatous lesions of the lung, quite unlike those of this disease; 'lungers', 'panters' and 'fog fever' have local significance only.

There appear to be a number of probable causes of atypical interstitial pneumonia, and there are two clinical forms of the disease, but pathologically there is sufficient similarity between all of these aetiological and clinical forms to justify grouping them as one disease (1).

Incidence

Insufficient has been written about this disease to indicate its true incidence but the acute form is recorded very commonly in the U.S.A. (1, 2); in Canada, the acute and chronic forms both occur (3); in Switzerland, only the chronic form is recognized (4). In Great Britain, the acute form of the disease, known locally as 'fog fever', is common (5); and the acute form has been recognized in Holland and New Zealand (6). In the acute form the morbidity is often 50 per cent, sometimes 100 per cent, and the mortality rate is usually about 35 per cent (7). The chronic form occurs only sporadically and most affected animals die. Although by definition the disease belongs to cattle it is evident that the disease could occur in sheep and it has in fact been recorded in that species (7, 8). Extensive alveolar epithelialization is present, as it is in pulmonary adenomatosis.

Aetiology

A number of specific causes of atypical interstitial pneumonia are known, but in many outbreaks the cause cannot be determined, although suspicious agents are often suggested. The reaction in the lungs is not inflammatory and those transmission studies which have been carried out have been negative (4, 9), suggesting that the disease is not infectious.

It is known that a massive infestation of the lungs by large numbers of lungworm larvae in a sensitized animal can cause an allergic reaction resulting in the development of atypical pneumonia. However, in many cases lungworms do not appear to be present, at least a search for lungworm larvae in the pasture, in the faeces of affected and in-contact animals, and in the lungs of animals at necropsy is often negative. The migration of abnormal parasites, particularly ascarids, has been observed to cause the disease, but is unlikely to occur commonly.

The inhalation of nitrogen dioxide gas is capable of causing atypical interstitial pneumonia in cattle and severe alveolar oedema and emphysema in pigs (10) but it seems unlikely that animals of either species would be exposed to a significant concentration of the gas for a sufficiently long period to produce any lesions. Pigs which survive experimental exposure to silo gas do not show the lesions seen in 'silo-filler's' disease in man and experimental exposure of cattle to nitrogen dioxide gas produces lesions which do not occur in natural fog fever (11). During the stabling period, cattle may be briefly exposed to an agent which causes bronchial irritation and coughing if large amounts of ensilage are fed (12). There is a strong correlation between the occurrence of the disease and pasturing on rape or turnip tops or the ingestion of algae, but the specific causative agent has not been determined.

Another probable cause of atypical interstitial pneumonia is exposure to moulds, either by inhalation or ingestion. Many mouldy feeds, including corn stalks and sweet potatoes, have been implicated by field observers (2). Again, the specific cause is not determined, but the nature of the lesions and the rapidity of development of the acute form of the disease suggest allergy as the basic mechanism. If this is so, the inhalation or ingestion of allergens such as moulds or hay dust and pollen could cause the disease. A high incidence of precipitin reactions to 'farmer's lung hay' (FLH) antigens has been observed in cows with respiratory disease after exposure to mouldy hay. The antigens derive largely from the thermophilic actinomycetes, especially *Thermopolyspora polyspora* (13) and *Micropolyspora faeni* and *Thermoactinomyces vulgaris* (14). Although it is apparent that there is a relation between inhaled fungal spores and respiratory tract disease, it is obvious that all cases of fog fever are not due to the intrinsic allergic alveolitis caused by fungal spore inhalation. This is evidenced by the absence of specific serum precipitins in some affected cows (15).

The high incidence of the disease in early autumn, when many legumes and other pasture plants are in flower, and the common occurrence at this time of allergic rhinitis in cattle, suggest that the inhalation of pollen may cause an allergic response of the alveolar epithelium. Also, the tendency for the disease to occur about 10 days after the cattle have been moved on to a new pasture suggests that sensitization may occur initially with an allergic reaction at a later date. However, in many autumn outbreaks the cattle are on pure grass pasture with no flowers visible; in housed animals hay dust is more likely to be inhaled than is pollen. Intradermal tests of sensitivity to many pasture plants and to the ruminal contents of affected animals have been negative and blood histamine levels are within the normal range (9).

One relationship which is thought to be of importance in Canada is the occurrence of the disease in cattle standing near the hay chute from which hay and bedding are thrown down from the mow to the barn floor. It is not uncommon to have a selective distribution of the disease so that only animals which stand near the chute, and are thus more exposed to the inhalation of the dust, become affected. In barns where measures have been taken to cut down dust, the development of the chronic form of the disease appears to have been reduced. In Switzerland a high incidence of precipitins against *Micropolyspora faeni* (60 per cent) and mouldy hay antigen (80 per cent) was demonstrated in exposed but apparently healthy cattle from an area where 'allergic pneumonia' is common. Many animals lost their precipitins during the pasture season and regained them during winter housing (26).

An additional important occurrence of the disease is when cattle are fed sweet potato tubers which are heavily infested with *Fusarium javanicum* fungus (24), and ingestion of 'stinkwood' (*Zieria arborescens*) produces a similar syndrome (27).

Other less likely causes of the disease have been suggested, including a nutritional deficiency of phosphorus and *Clostridium perfringens* intoxication. Tests for the presence of *Cl. perfringens* toxin in the intestinal contents of cows have been negative (9). A disease, which is identical clinically and histopathologically with naturally occurring atypical interstitial pneumonia, has been produced experimentally in cattle by the oral administration of the amino-acid tryptophan (16, 18, 25). The disease occurs in cattle, but not in sheep, and only after oral administration of the DL form of tryptophane. Injection produced similar levels of tryptophane in plasma but no disease suggesting that the toxic agent is a rumen metabolite (17). Amongst five common cattle breeds, Jersey, Holstein, Shorthorn, Angus and Hereford, the latter appear to be most sensitive to trypto-phane (18). The exact relationship of these observations to field cases of the disease remains to be determined.

Because of the number and variety of the circumstances in which the disease occurs, it is difficult to suggest a basic underlying cause. It is admitted that the particular reaction of the pulmonary parenchyma in atypical interstitial pneumonia is a non-specific reaction to injury and may be caused by exposure to agents other than exogenous allergens or nitrogen dioxide. The possibility that the reaction may be one of irritation by an endogenous allergen, such as the bronchial exudate of a bronchopneumonia, cannot be discarded. It may be that those chronic cases, in which lesions of atypical pneumonia and bronchopneumonia occur concurrently, may be explainable in these terms rather than in terms of secondary bacterial invasion of tissues devitalized by a primary allergic reaction.

Occurrence

Beef and dairy cattle are equally susceptible and the disease is most common in adults, particularly cows which have recently calved, although it can occur in yearlings and in ordinary circumstances only rarely in calves. However a high incidence (up to 38 per cent) has been observed in calves 2 to 6 months of age, especially those in the 4- to 6-months age group, in veal-fattening feedlots in the U.K. (19). In this group the disease is always acute although some may survive with persistent, chronic emphysema. Cattle at pasture, in feedlots and in barns may be affected. Seasonally the incidence appears to be highest in the pasture season—particularly the acute form which often affects a number of animals at one time—but the acute and chronic forms can occur at any time of the year. In areas where cattle are housed, the chronic form is more common in the winter (4), and possibly in the Channel Islands breeds (1).

There are some differences between the occurrence of the two forms of the disease. In the acute form, the call is often an urgent one; sometimes a number of cows become affected suddenly and, in many instances, deaths may occur within 24 hours. In the chronic form, although several animals may become affected during the course of a week, it is more usual to have sporadic cases, often at intervals of several months, and it may only be with the second or third animals that the veterinarian and the farmer realize that they are confronted by an atypical pneumonia.

The acute form is also commonly associated with a change of pasture, usually a change from poor to good pasture. Many veterinarians in mountain areas have observed a high incidence when cattle are brought down to lowland pastures in the autumn (20). Change from one field to another can have the same effect and the new pasture may be dominated by either legumes or grasses. Turning cattle on to rape or kale, or on to a field where turnips have been pulled and the cattle allowed access to the tops, may have the same effect. In all of these instances, the outbreak usually occurs sharply, about 10 (2 to 12) days after the change. The field disease in sheep is recorded after grazing on wheat or barley stubble or *Phalaris canariensis* pasture (8).

An uncommon occurrence of a similar clinical condition has been described in fat cattle exposed to a very foggy atmosphere. Pigs and sheep in the same environment were unaffected (21).

Pathogenesis

That the primary cause in many instances is an allergic reaction is corroborated by the sudden gross outpouring of a protein-rich fluid, often with a high level of eosinophiles, into the alveoli throughout a large part of the lung, the common occurrence after a change of environment 10 days before, and the good response in early acute cases to the administration of adrenaline and anti-histamines. An additional supporting observation is that there is, in acute cases, a marked increase in serum gamma-globulin levels (22). The concurrent occurrence of ruminal atony and tympany in some cases is also in accord with an allergic aetiology. The physical occupation of alveolar space by fluid is no doubt the primary cause of the dyspnoea, and the failure to respond to treatment is due to the nature of this fluid and its immovability. Alveolar and interstitial emphysema, and epithelialization and fibrosis of the alveolar walls, follow and confer irreversibility on the lesion.

Clinical Findings

Acute form. The onset is sudden. Laboured breathing, often with grunting, mouth breathing and frothing at the mouth, is the most obvious sign. There may be associated bloat and diarrhoea and ruminal atony is characteristic of severe cases. Although the animal shows anxiety, there is no apparent toxaemia and moderately affected animals will attempt to eat and drink. Coughing, if it occurs, is not frequent, but there may be a frothy nasal discharge. The temperature is usually about $39 \cdot 5\,°C$ (103°F) but varies from 38 to 41°C (101 to 106°F), the more severely affected animals having higher temperatures. There is a similar variation in the heart rate (80 to 150 per minute) and those with a rate of more than 120 per minute are usually in the terminal stages of the disease.

Auscultation of the lungs may be disappointing if one is not accustomed to listening for consolidation without bronchial involvement. Loud bronchial tones, indicating consolidation but a clear airway, are heard over the ventral parts of the lungs. There may be an absence of breath sounds over the dorsal parts if involvement is severe, but in animals that live for several days the loud friction rubs and dry râles characteristic of interstitial emphysema are signs of diagnostic significance. There may be emphysema under the skin. Death may occur in as short a time as 12 hours, but most fatal cases survive until the 2nd or 3rd day. The average mortality rate is about 30 per cent. Those which survive often have chronic emphysema and are unthrifty.

Chronic form. In most cases, 3 or 4 days elapse after the appearance of signs before the owner is sufficiently worried to call for veterinary assistance. There is an increase in the rate and depth of respiration, frequent deep coughing, a fall in milk yield and a loss of weight. It is probable that the disease develops for some time before these signs are evident. A secondary bacterial pneumonia often develops and it is probably this, together with interference with heat loss, which causes the usual moderate elevation of temperature to 39·5 to 40°C (103 to 104°F). For the same reason, there may be a moderate mucopurulent nasal discharge and toxaemia. The heart rate is usually elevated, the degree depending upon the amount of lung involved.

On auscultation gross abnormality of the pulmonary sounds is evident. There is the grating friction sound of interstitial emphysema over the dorsal part of the chest and loud bronchial tones ventrally, particularly on the right side. To these may be added the moist râles of a purulent bronchopneumonia.

Complete recovery occurs rarely, if at all. Death may not occur for weeks or months and there may be periods of partial recovery during this time. Most affected animals are disposed of because of ill-health, but death may occur as a result of toxaemia or congestive heart failure.

Clinical Pathology

In this disease there are no clinico-pathological findings which have any diagnostic significance, although bacteriological examination of a nasal swab may indicate the cause of the secondary bronchopneumonia which is so often present. Examination of faeces and herbage for lungworm larvae should also be carried out. The observed high levels of 'farmers' lung hay' antibodies in serum are not of much value diagnostically because of the similar levels found in many clinically normal cows (23). And many cases of classical fog fever have negative serum precipitin levels (15).

Necropsy Findings

In both forms, the lungs are enlarged and firm and do not collapse on cutting. In the early stages of acute cases they contain much fluid which is more viscid than usual oedema fluid. The pleura is pale and opaque and appears to be thickened. In very acute cases, the entire lungs are homogeneously affected in this way. Such cases usually have oedema of the larynx. In the more common acute case, the lung has a marbled appearance. Adjacent lobes may be affected with any one of four abnormalities. Areas of normal, pink lung are restricted to the dorsal part of the diaphragmatic lobes. There are areas of pale tissue indicative of alveolar emphysema, areas of a dark pink colour affected by early alveolar exudation, yellow areas in which the alveoli are filled with coagulated protein-rich fluid and dark red areas where epithelialization has occurred. The latter two lesions are firm on palpation and resemble thymus or pancreas. They are more common in the ventral parts of the anterior lobes. In chronic cases, the obvious differences in the age of the lesions suggests that the disease progresses in steps by the periodic involvement of fresh areas of tissue. In all cases there is usually a frothy exudate, sometimes containing flecks of pus in the bronchi and trachea and the mucosa of these passages is markedly hyperaemic.

Histologically, the characteristic findings are an absence of inflammation, except in the case of secondary bacterial invasion, and the presence of an eosinophilic, protein-rich fluid which coagulates in the alveoli, or may subsequently be drawn out into a hyaline membrane. This is more apparent in acute cases, and, if animals live for a few days, there is evidence of epithelialization of the alveolar walls, the interstitial pneumonia which gives the disease its name. In long-standing cases, there is extensive epithelialization and fibrosis. A hyaline degeneration of the walls of small pulmonary arteries is a common finding and is considered to be typical of this disease.

Bacteriological examination of the lungs is often negative, although in cases of long standing in which secondary bacterial pneumonia has developed *Past. multocida, Past. haemolytica, Streptococcus* spp., and *Cory. pyogenes* may be found. A careful search should be made for nematode larvae.

Diagnosis

The justification for the use of the word 'atypical' in the name of the disease is that the reaction of the pulmonary tissue is quite unlike that in any of the standard forms of pneumonia and there is little or no response to standard treatments for pneumonia. One stumbles on to the diagnosis, particularly of the chronic form, in this way. However, there are some clinical characteristics which set the cases of atypical pneumonia apart from other pneumonias. In the acute form, the very rapid onset of deep, laboured respiration in the absence of signs of toxaemia, and often with no fever, differentiates it from bacterial pneumonias. Pneumonic pasteurellosis (shipping fever) might warrant consideration in the differential diagnosis, especially if the animals have been moved in the preceding 2 weeks, but in pasteurellosis there is usually only moderate dyspnoea and the signs of toxaemia are marked. The closest resemblance to acute atypical pneumonia can be caused by poisoning with organophosphatic insecticides. The differential features are the pupillary constriction, mucoid diarrhoea, muscular tremor and stiffness of the limbs in the latter. Infectious bovine rhinotracheitis, 'summer snuffles' and bovine malignant catarrh all resemble this disease only slightly.

Enzootic (viral) pneumonia may be difficult to differentiate from either acute or chronic atypical pneumonia, but in our experience it is almost entirely restricted to animals less than 6 months of age and is a very mild disease in older animals. Cough is usually marked and there is some response to treatment with broad spectrum antibiotics. When enzootic calf pneumonia is accompanied by a bacterial bronchopneumonia it is virtually impossible to distinguish it from a similarly complicated chronic atypical pneumonia, except on an age basis and the probability that the enzootic pneumonia will affect a number of animals at one time. One tends to choose chronic atypical pneumonia, rather than a chronic bacterial bronchopneumonia, in an adult when the subject is one of the Channel Island breeds, when the disease appears during the housing period and when there is gross change in pulmonary sounds heard on auscultation over most of the lung. It is impossible to differentiate clinically between atypical and verminous pneumonia except by the identification of *Dictyocaulus viviparus* larvae in

the faeces of other animals in the herd or in a necropsy specimen. A similar difficulty is encountered in differentiating the disease from that caused by invasion of *Ascaris suis* larvae.

Treatment

Cases of acute atypical pneumonia must be treated as urgent and, although controlled experiments have not been carried out, a combined double dose of adrenalin and antihistamine appears to give excellent results in very early cases. Both are given subcutaneously to avoid excitement, which may prove fatal, and are repeated at 8-hour intervals as required. Grazing cattle should be removed from the pasture immediately and, if necessary, fed hay in a barn or yard. If an acute outbreak occurs in housed cattle every effort must be made to minimize dust, and, if possible, the hay supply should be changed.

Chronic cases present a much more difficult task. In most instances the animals are not seen, or the diagnosis is not made, until the damage to lung tissue is irreversible. It is therefore wisest in most cases to advise slaughter. If treatment is attempted, a broad spectrum antibiotic is usually used to treat or prevent concurrent bronchopneumonia. Although it appears to be desirable to remove the hyaline material from the alveoli, parenteral treatment with enzymes, diuretics and corticosteroids appears to exert little of this desired effect, even when continued, together with the antibiotics, for 4 to 7 days.

Control

Control measures depend upon a knowledge of the cause, but in all cases the herd should be removed from the pasture.

The control of lungworm infestations is essential in areas where the infestation occurs. Cattle which have been previously exposed to infestation should not be allowed unlimited access to pasture or stubble fields which are likely to carry very large numbers of larvae, particularly fields which have heavily manured with barnyard manure. If these areas need to be grazed, the cattle should be allowed in for only a short time daily for the first 2 weeks to desensitize them. If the disease appears, the cattle should be removed immediately. Further cases may occur up to 3 weeks after the cattle are removed. Trouble may be avoided, when grazing rape, if hay or straw is provided or there is access to a suitable field.

For housed cattle, the feeding of mouldy hay or other feeds and the use of mouldy bedding should be avoided, and every effort should be made to keep down dust. This can be done by wetting the hay, by using a slide from the mow or by hanging a burlap curtain around the chute. Damping the hay will also reduce the amount of dust created by the cattle searching through the hay. Farmers are encouraged to use harvesting techniques which reduce the amount of dust created. Some forage harvesters, for example, tend to crumble legume leaves to powder. If there has been an increase in incidence of the disease in housed cattle in recent years, it may be because of the changes in the composition of pasture and in hay-making methods.

REFERENCES

(1) Blood, D. C. (1962). *Canad. vet. J.*, *3*, 40.
(2) Vickers, C. L. *et al.* (1960). *J. Amer. vet. med. Ass.*, *137*, 507.
(3) O'Donoghue, J. G. (1960). *Canad. vet. J.*, *1*, 482.
(4) Fankhauser, R. & Luginbuhl, H. (1960). *Schweiz. Arch. Tierheilk.*, *102*, 47, 146.
(5) Pirie, H. M. *et al.* (1971). *Vet. Rec.*, *88*, 346.
(6) Bennell, D. G. (1966). *N.Z. vet. J.*, *14*, 73.
(7) Stamp, J. T. & Nisbet, D. I. (1963). *J. comp. Path.*, *73*, 319.
(8) Pascoe, R. R. & McGavin, M. D. (1969). *Vet. Rec.*, *85*, 376.
(9) Moulton, J. E. (1961). *J. Amer. vet. med. Ass.*, *139*, 669.
(10) Giddens, W. E. *et al.* (1970). *Amer. J. vet. Res.*, *31*, 1779.
(11) Cutlip, R. C. (1966). *Path. vet.*, *3*, 474.
(12) Haynes, N. B. (1963). *J. Amer. vet. med. Ass.*, *143*, 593.
(13) Jenkins, P. A. & Pepys, J. (1965). *Vet. Rec.*, *77*, 464.
(14) Lacey, J. (1968). *J. gen. Microbiol.*, *51*, 173.
(15) Pirie, H. M. *et al.* (1971). *Res. vet. Sci.*, *12*, 586.
(16) Dickinson, E. O. *et al.* (1967). *Vet. Rec.*, *80*, 487.
(17) Carlson, J. R. *et al.* (1968). *Amer. J. vet. Res.*, *29*, 1983.
(18) Monlux, W. S. *et al.* (1970). *Cornell Vet.*, *60*, 547.
(19) Omar, A. R. & Kinch, D. A. (1966). *Vet. Rec.*, *78*, 766.
(20) Blake, J. T. & Thomas, D. W. (1971). *J. Amer. vet. med. Ass.*, *158*, 2047.
(21) Barber-Lomax, J. W. (1961). *Vet. Rec.*, *73*, 1321.
(22) Moulton, J. E. *et al.* (1963). *J. Amer. vet. med. Ass.*, *142*, 133.
(23) Harbourne, J. F. *et al.* (1970). *Vet. Rec.*, *87*, 559.
(24) Peckham, J. C. *et al.* (1972). *J. Amer. vet. med. Ass.*, *160*, 169.
(25) Eyre, P. (1972). *Vet. Rec.*, *91*, 38.
(26) Nicolet, J. *et al.* (1972). *Infect. Immun.*, *6*, 38.
(27) Stephens, W. H. (1967). *Tasm. J. Agric.*, *38*, 84.

Enzootic Nasal Granuloma of Cattle

Of the three known clinical types of chronic nasal obstruction in cattle two have been identified. One recorded in beef cattle appears to be caused by a fungus *Rhinosporidium* sp. Another is caused by the parasite *Schistosoma nasalis*. The third type, enzootic nasal granuloma, occurs commonly in southern Australia and remains unidentified (1, 2). An allied condition has been described in the U.S.A. as maduromycosis (3) and

an enzootic nasal adenocarcinoma occurring in sheep has been recorded (4).

Enzootic nasal granuloma occurs sporadically in some herds but may reach an incidence of 30 per cent. In an area as many as 75 per cent of herds may have the disease. Animals aged between 6 months and 4 years are most commonly affected and the chronic disease may or may not be preceded by an attack of acute rhinitis. Most cases commence in the autumn months. The cause is not known but an allergy, probably to fungi, is suspected. Transmission experiments have not been successful and, although there may be an inherited predisposition to the disease, this has not been conclusively demonstrated.

Established cases of enzootic nasal granuloma have lesions, consisting of granulomatous nodules 1 to 4 mm. in diameter and height, in both nostrils. The lesions extend from just inside the nostril posteriorly for 5 to 8 cm. They may be few in number or packed closely together. Their texture is firm and the mucosa over them appears to be normal. A mucopurulent discharge occurs in many animals. The predominant clinical sign is respiratory stertor and dyspnoea caused by obstruction to the air flow. The severity of these signs may fluctuate but in general they progress slowly over several months and then remain static. Although the respiratory distress may be sufficiently severe to cause a loss of condition and marked reduction in milk yield, affected animals do not die. A good proportion of them have to be culled as uneconomic units.

REFERENCES

(1) Hore, D. E. (1966). *Aust. vet. J.*, *42*, 273.
(2) O'Connor, P. F. & Gorrie, C. J. R. (1961). *Vict. vet. Proc.*, pp. 10, 11.
(3) Roberts, E. D. *et al.* (1963). *J. Amer. vet. med. Ass.*, *142*, 42.
(4) Duncan, J. R. *et al.* (1967). *J. Amer. vet. med. Ass.*, *151*, 732.

DISEASES CHARACTERIZED BY URINARY TRACT INVOLVEMENT

Enzootic Haematuria

Enzootic haematuria is a chronic, non-infectious disease of cattle characterized by the development of haemangiomatous lesions of the wall of the urinary bladder and clinically by intermittent haematuria and death due to anaemia.

Incidence

Enzootic haematuria occurs as an area problem on all continents. The overall incidence is not great but the disease may cause heavy losses in affected areas. It is usually fatal.

Aetiology

The specific cause is still undecided but the great bulk of evidence points to chronic poisoning with bracken as the principal cause. A high incidence has been observed where bracken fern is growing (1) and the disease has been reproduced by the experimental feeding of bracken, either green or dried or as hay (2, 3). On the other hand cases are seen in cattle which have no access to bracken. Many other plants have been incriminated from time to time but their aetiological significance remains unproved. Research workers have gone to extraordinary lengths to establish the presence of carcinogens in bracken fern (4). Neoplasms histologically indistinguishable from natural lesions of enzootic haematuria have been produced experimentally by feeding cattle on fresh bracken from an area where enzootic haematuria was common (5). A high incidence of vesicular carcinomas, similar to the bladder lesions of enzootic haematuria in cattle, has been recorded in sheep grazing bracken for 18 months (6). Rats fed bracken develop a high frequency of urinary bladder carcinoma and this is greatly increased by the supplementation of the diet by thiamine (7). Multiple intestinal tumours also developed and tumours have been observed affecting the upper digestive tract of cattle in field cases in Brazil (12). Attempts at transmission by the oral administration or infusion into the bladder of urine and bladder tissue extracts have not been successful. It is generally agreed that some irritant substance is present in the urine of affected animals although its nature has not been determined. A similar lesion has been produced experimentally by the submucosal injection into the bladder of a suspension of bovine cutaneous papilloma (8), but repeated vaccination with partly-inactivated papilloma virus does not prevent the development of lesions (9). Many other possible causes have been considered but evidence is lacking to incriminate any particular agent. Cows affected with the disease excrete large quantities of tryptophan metabolites in their urine and one tryptophan metabolite, 3-hydroxy-L-kynurenine, is a known bladder carcinogen. It is possible that abnormal metabolism of tryptophan could occur in cattle in specific dietary circumstances (10, 11). The disease is sometimes associated with a high content of molybdenum in pasture and its incidence appears to be reduced by heavy applications of gypsum. Cattle over 1 year of age are most com-

monly affected and the disease has also been recorded in water buffalo.

Occurrence

The disease is confined mainly to poor, neglected or recently opened up land and tends to disappear as soil fertility and land management improves. It is not closely associated with a particular soil type although it is recorded most commonly on lighter soils.

Pathogenesis

The mode of development of the lesions is unknown. Haemorrhage from the haemangiomata in the bladder wall occurs intermittently and results in varying degrees of blood loss. Deaths are due to haemorrhagic anaemia.

Clinical Findings

Acute cases are manifested by the passage of large quantities of blood, often as clots, in the urine. Acute haemorrhagic anaemia develops and the animal becomes weak and recumbent and may die after an illness lasting 1 to 2 weeks. Subacute cases are characterized by intermittent, mild clinical haematuria or persistent subclinical haematuria. In these cases there is a gradual loss of condition over several months and eventually clinical evidence of anaemia. On rectal examination acute cases may show nothing but subacute cases usually evidence marked thickening of the bladder wall. Secondary bacterial infection of the bladder may lead to the development of cystitis and pyelonephritis.

Clinical Pathology

In the absence of gross haematuria, a urine sample should be centrifuged and the deposit examined for erythrocytes. Repeated examinations may be necessary. Non-specific anaemia and leucopenia are detectable by haematological examination.

Necropsy Findings

Haemorrhages in the bladder mucosa are typical of the disease. In the later stages, there are raised pedunculated tumours which are friable and bleed easily and these are accompanied by fibrotic thickening with scarring and distortion of the bladder wall. The tumours probably arise from transitional epithelium and often show evidence of malignancy, metastasis to regional lymph nodes and lungs having been observed. In uncomplicated cases, the remainder of the urinary tract is usually unaffected although lesions have been observed in ureters and the renal pelvis. The severity of the haemorrhage is not necessarily related to the extent of the lesions and animals may bleed to death when only minor lesions are present.

Diagnosis

It is necessary to determine by microscopic examination that the redness of the urine is due to the presence of erythrocytes and not to the presence of free haemoglobin. Other causes of haematuria in cattle are few. Cystitis and pyelonephritis are usually accompanied by fever, frequent urination and the presence of pus and debris in the urine. Bacteriological examination of the urine will reveal the presence of infection.

Treatment

Blood transfusion is necessary in acute cases and haematinic mixture should be provided in chronic cases. Little can be done to cause regression of the bladder lesions and affected animals are best disposed of.

Control

A general improvement in nutrition is often followed by a decrease in the number of animals affected. A specific recommendation is to apply gypsum (200 to 300 lb. per acre) to the pasture as a fertilizer, a measure which is reputed to delay the onset of the disease.

REFERENCES

(1) Smith, B. L. & Beatson, N. S. (1970). *N.Z. vet. J.*, *18*, 115.
(2) Rosenberger, G. (1963). *Proc. 17th Wld vet. Congr.*, Hanover, *2*, 1167.
(3) Price, J. M. & Pamukcu, A. M. (1968). *Cancer Res.*, *28*, 2247.
(4) Pamukcu, A. M. *et al.* (1971). *Cancer Res.*, *30*, 902.
(5) Pamukcu, A. M. *et al.* (1967). *Cancer Res.*, *27*, 917.
(6) Harbutt, P. R. & Leaver, D. D. (1969). *Aust. vet. J.*, *45*, 473.
(7) Pamukcu, A. M. *et al.* (1970). *Cancer Res.*, *30*, 2671.
(8) Olson, C. *et al.* (1959). *Amer. J. Path.*, *35*, 672.
(9) Pamukcu, A. M. *et al.* (1967). *Cancer Res.*, *27*, 2197.
(10) Bryan, G. T. *et al.* (1963). *Ann. N.Y. Acad. Sci.*, *108*, 924.
(11) Pamukcu, A. M. (1963). *Ann. N.Y. Acad. Sci.*, *108*, 938.
(12) Tokarnia, C. H. *et al.* (1969). *Pesquisa agropec. bras.*, *4*, 209.

Enzootic Posthitis

(*Pizzle Rot, Sheath Rot, Balanoposthitis*)

This enzootic inflammation of the prepuce and penis of principally castrated male sheep is caused by a diphtheroid organism which produces lesions which themselves become severe only in certain circumstances of management and urinary composition.

Incidence

Enzootic posthitis occurs in epizootic proportions in wethers in conditions of excellent pasture growth especially when legumes are plentiful. The incidence in affected flocks may be as high as 40 per cent and in some areas the disease is so common that it is not possible to maintain bands of wethers. Many deaths occur because of uraemia and secondary bacterial infections and all affected sheep show a severe set-back in growth rate and wool production. Young rams are sometimes affected and are subsequently incapable of mating.

Aetiology

Although the disease fluctuates in its incidence depending upon climate and feed conditions it was considered, for many years, to be non-infectious. The two factors considered to be most important were a high alkalinity of the urine causing irritation of the preputial and surrounding skin and a high intake of oestrogens in pasture causing swelling and congestion of the prepuce. Factors of lesser, and largely unknown, importance were considered to be continued wetness of the area around the prepuce due to removal of preputial hairs at shearing, a high calcium, low phosphorus diet and the ingestion of large quantities of alkaline water. In spite of the finding that the disease is caused by an unidentified diphtheroid organism the above factors appear to be of major importance as predisposing causes because their removal has such a beneficial effect on the occurrence of posthitis (1).

The causative organism can be recovered from lesions and from clinically normal prepuces and has also been found in the lesions of vulvitis in ewes and posthitis in bulls (2, 3). Implantation of the organism on a scarified prepuce in the presence of urine is capable of causing the external ulceration which is characteristic of the disease. The organism is capable of hydrolysing urea and proliferates more rapidly in high concentrations of urea which probably accounts for its pathogenicity in this situation. It has been suggested that the exact cytotoxic agent may be the ammonia produced by the bacteria rather than any destructive capacity of the bacteria itself (4). Factors likely to increase the urinary concentration of urea include the provision of a high-protein diet such as would be available on lush, improved pasture, the circumstance in which the disease occurs most commonly.

In Australia enzootic posthitis occurs most commonly in Merino sheep, particularly wethers over 3 years of age and young rams, but in a severe outbreak young wethers and old rams may also be affected. The high incidence in castrates and young rams is probably related to the close adherence of the preputial and penile skins which separate in mature entire animals.

An ulcerative vulvitis occurs in ewes in the same flocks in which posthitis occurs in wethers and is thought to be a venereal extension of that disease. The causative bacteria is transmissible to the prepuce of male cattle and an ulcerative posthitis occurs naturally in bulls and is thought to be caused by the agent of ovine posthitis (5, 6). There appears to be no counterpart to ovine vulvitis in cows.

The causative bacteria persists for 3 to 6 months in the laboratory at room temperature but details of its persistence in the normal ovine environment are not available.

Occurrence and Transmission

Enzootic posthitis occurs most extensively on lush, improved pasture with a high legume content and reaches its highest incidence in autumn in summer rainfall areas and in spring where the major rainfall is in winter. In the early stages the progress of the disease can be halted or reversed by starvation for several days.

Transmission of the causative organism could occur in a number of ways. Infection at dipping or shearing seems not to be important but flies are considered to be probable mechanical vectors and contact with infected soil and herbage is a likely method of spread. Transmission to ewes appears to occur venereally from infected rams (6). Although the natural disease in cattle is usually benign they may act as vectors of infection for sheep on the same farm.

Pathogenesis

It is generally believed that the initial lesion in the wether (the external lesion) is caused by ammonia produced from urea in the urine by the causative bacteria. This lesion may be maintained in a static condition for a long period but, if satisfactory conditions of high urea content of the urine and continued wetting of the wool around the prepuce are maintained, the lesion proceeds to invade the interior of the prepuce producing the 'internal lesion'. A similar pathogenesis is postulated for vulvar lesions.

Clinical Findings

The primary lesion is a small scab on the skin dorsal to the preputial orifice (the external lesion) and this may persist for long periods without the appearance of any clinical signs. The scab is thick, coherent and tenacious. If extension to the interior of the prepuce occurs (the internal lesion) ulceration and scabbing of the preputial opening appear and the sheep may show restlessness, kicking at the belly and dribbling of the urine as in urethral obstruction. Swelling of the prepuce occurs commonly and the area is often infested by blowfly maggots. The development of pus and fibrous tissue adhesions may interfere with urination and protrusion of the penis, and permanent impairment of function in rams.

Some deaths occur due to obstructive uraemia, toxaemia and septicaemia. During an outbreak many sheep may be affected without showing clinical signs and are detected only when they are subjected to a physical examination. Others recover spontaneously when feed conditions deteriorate.

In ewes the lesions are confined to the lips of the vulva and consist of ulcers and scabs. They may cause an increased susceptibility to blowfly-strike. The lesions in bulls are similar to the external lesions which occur in wethers but rarely there may be invasion of the interior of the prepuce. The external lesions occur at any point around the urethral orifice and may encircle it (6). Their severity varies from local excoriation to marked ulceration with exudation and oedema. There is a tendency for the lesions to persist for several months without treatment and with highly alkaline urine (3, 7).

Clinical Pathology

Isolation of the causative diphtheroid bacterium may be necessary if there is doubt as to the identity of the disease (2).

Diagnosis

The occurrence of other forms of enzootic posthitis in cattle and sheep seems likely but ulcerative dermatosis of sheep, caused by a virus, is the only common one. Obstructive urolithiasis in wethers may superficially resemble posthitis but there is no preputial lesion.

Treatment

In bad outbreaks the sheep can be removed on to dry pasture and their feed intake restricted to that required for subsistence only. They should be inspected at regular intervals, the wool shorn from around the prepuce and affected animals treated individually. Weekly application of a 10 per cent copper sulphate ointment is recommended for external lesions and when the interior of the prepuce is involved, it should be irrigated twice weekly with a 5 per cent solution of copper sulphate. Cetrimide (20 per cent in alcohol or water with or without 0·25 per cent acid fuchsin) or alcohol alone (90 per cent) are about as effective as copper sulphate preparations. Penicillin topically or parenterally, may effect a temporary response. Thiabendazole by the mouth appears to have a beneficial effect on the lesions but does not eliminate them (8). In severe cases the only satisfactory treatment is surgical, antibiotics effecting no response and testosterone implants producing a good weight gain without affecting the lesions (9). Surgical treatment may be necessary if the prepuce is obstructed. The recommended procedure is to open the sheath by inserting one blade of a pair of scissors into the external preputial orifice and cutting the prepuce back as far as the end of the urethral process; extension beyond this leads to trauma of the penis. Badly affected rams should be disposed of as they are unlikely to be of value for breeding.

Control

The principal control measures are restriction of the diet to reduce the urea content of the urine, removal of the wool around the prepuce or vulva to avoid a local accumulation of urine, segregation of affected sheep and disinfection of the preputial area. The latter measure may be necessary only if the causative bacteria is present in the environment but it is likely to be a ubiquitous organism. As a preventive measure it is carried out on three occasions over a period of a year commencing at 6 months of age. In wethers the antiseptic is infused into the prepuce and smeared over the skin around the prepuce. In ewes it is swabbed on to the vulva and surrounding skin (6).

Subcutaneous implantation with testosterone propionate is highly effective as a preventive and a treatment especially against the internal lesion, but response in affected animals is improved by the simultaneous application of one of the local treatments listed above. At the dose rate used there is no appreciable deterioration in the quality of the carcase and there is a marked increase in the rate of gain. A slight disadvantage is that there is an increase in the growth of horn. A single implantation of 60 to 90 mg. is effective for 3 months and although the treatments can be repeated four times a year, it is more economical to time them to coincide with periods of maximum incidence which will vary from district to district. Three implantations in autumn, winter and spring provide an effective control programme in most areas (9). The tablets are implanted subcutaneously, pre-

ferably at the base of the ear, using preloaded tubes to avoid undue contact to the operator.

REVIEW LITERATURE

Dent, C. H. R. (1971). Ulcerative vulvitis and posthitis in Australian sheep and cattle. *Vet. Bull.*, *41*, 719.

REFERENCES

(1) Johnstone, I. L. (1963). *Aust. vet. J.*, *39*, 371.
(2) Southcott, W. H. (1965). *Aust. vet. J.*, *41*, 193.
(3) Nielsen, I. (1972). *Aust. vet. J.*, *48*, 39.
(4) Brook, A. H. *et al.* (1965). *Aust. vet. J.*, *42*, 9.
(5) Bassett, C. R. (1963–64). *Vict. vet. Proc.*, p. 38.
(6) Southcott, W. H. (1965). *Aust. vet. J.*, *41*, 225.
(7) Parsonson, I. M. & Clark, B. L. (1972). *Aust. vet. J.*, *48*, 125.
(8) Southcott, W. H. (1968). *Aust. vet. J.*, *44*, 526.
(9) Swan, R. A. (1971). *Vet. Rec.*, *88*, 304.
(10) Southcott, W. H. (1962). *Aust. vet. J.*, *38*, 33.

DISEASES CHARACTERIZED BY NERVOUS SYSTEM INVOLVEMENT

Polioencephalomalacia

(*Cerebrocortical Necrosis, Forage Poisoning*)

This disease occurs sporadically in cattle, sheep and pigs. It is characterized clinically by a syndrome indicative of increased intracranial pressure and at necropsy by cerebral oedema and symmetrical necrosis of the cerebral cortex.

Incidence

Polioencephalomalacia appears to be occurring with increased frequency; at least it is being recognized more often. The disease occurs in most countries, principally in cattle and sheep, and to a lesser extent in pigs. Accurate morbidity and mortality figures are not available but up to 25 per cent of groups of feeder cattle or lambs may be affected. The reported mortality rates vary between 90 per cent for feedlot cattle and 50 per cent for cattle at pasture.

Aetiology

The cause of the disease is incompletely understood although it seems reasonably sure that acute conditioned thiamine deficiency is the cause in most cases (1). High thiaminase levels are found almost constantly in the rumen (4); fungi which occur on stored feeds have high thiaminase activity (2); the disease has been produced by feeding an anti-thiamine analogue (3). However, there are contrary arguments. Lambs given a thiamine deficient diet from 2 days of age die or need euthanasia 18 to 36 days later and although there are nervous signs there are no lesions suggestive of polioencephalomalacia (10). Also for logistic reasons direct fungal inactivation of thiamine seems unlikely (3) and it may be necessary to define other causes, for example factors affecting the ruminal bacterial metabolism of thiamine (5). A high content of thiaminase in plants has been suggested (6) but has not been identified except in bracken and equisetum, plants not normally associated with polioencephalomalacia.

One factor which could affect thiamine production by rumen microflora is cobalt deficiency which has been related to an outbreak of polioencephalomalacia (7). The disease has been produced by feeding amprolium, a cocciostatic drug (23), and there is a field report associating the disease with the feeding of pellets containing considerable quantities of gypsum (calcium sulphate). From a consideration of the pathology, it seems probable that the causative agent produces an initial oedema of the cerebrum, and the similarity of the lesions to those of salt poisoning in pigs suggests that the aetiology may be the same in some reported cases of polioencephalomalacia. Other toxins, particularly enterotoxins such as those produced by *Cl. perfringens* and organic mercury compounds, have also been suggested as causes and it seems probable that a number of agents are capable of causing the disease (8). The disease occurs in cattle and sheep, particularly in young cattle up to 2 years of age, although this distribution may be a reflection of the number exposed rather than of age susceptibility. The age groups most commonly affected are calves about 6 months of age and lambs 2 to 4 months old. Adult cattle are affected rarely (9).

Occurrence

The disease occurs most commonly and in its most acute form in feedlot cattle (10) and lambs. A very high incidence (up to 16 per cent) is recorded on the heavy molasses diets used for fattening cattle in Cuba (11, 12, 22). Less severe outbreaks of a milder form of the disease occur at pasture, usually 5 to 10 days after a change from poor to good pasture. In some instances there is a history of temporary deprivation of water on a diet containing 1 to 2 per cent salt, and in others the salt has been provided in bulk at intervals of 3 to 4 days rather than being added to the diet daily. Deprivation of water may occur when the animals are watered by hand or when water troughs are frozen over during very cold weather. In still other outbreaks, water and salt intake do not seem to be abnormal but there is often a history of sudden change in management. Outbreaks also occur after shearing, only the yearling sheep being affected.

Pathogenesis

In early acute cases, there is severe cerebral oedema with repulsion of the cerebellum into the foramen magnum and flattening of cerebral cortical gyri. This probably accounts for the syndrome of increased intracranial pressure observed in the early stages. If the pressure is maintained for a sufficiently long period, there is probably interference with normal blood supply to the compressed parts of the brain. This may be the explanation for the superficial laminar necrosis of the cerebral cortex seen in subacute cases. It is this cortical necrosis which is responsible for the residual blindness and imbecility of recovered animals.

Clinical Findings

In acute cases in cattle there is a sudden onset of blindness, muscle tremor, particularly of the head, frothy salivation, opisthotonus and, in some animals, convulsions. Initially these signs may occur in episodes with periods of normality between, but subsequently the syndrome is constant, the animal goes down, nystagmus appears, there is coma, mild tetany and an occasional clonic convulsion. Papilloedema may be present. The temperature remains normal. Death usually occurs 24 to 48 hours later but may be delayed for a week or more. In less severe cases, affected animals show the same general signs with the addition of head-pressing, but do not go down. Recovery is more common in this group but the survivors are often blind or stupid.

Sheep usually begin to wander aimlessly, sometimes in circles, or stand motionless and are blind but within a few hours become recumbent with opisthotonus, extension of the limbs, hyperaesthesia, nystagmus and periodic tonic-clonic convulsions. Hoggets affected at shearing time may show blindness and head-pressing, but if fed and watered, usually recover within a few days. Occasional animals show unilateral localizing signs including circling and spasmodic deviation of the head.

Clinical Pathology

Valuable information is obtained by detection of the high blood pyruvate levels which occur after glucose administration and fall after treatment with thiamine, and the low blood transketolase activity, both of which are diagnostic of thiamine deficiency (1, 13). Urine levels of pyruvate are also raised (14). Pyruvate kinase levels are significantly raised, an important diagnostic feature (15). Serum potassium levels are depressed in some calves in the latter stages of the disease (16). Differentiation from thrombo-embolic meningoencephalitis with which polioencephalomalacia is likely to be confused, because of the common occurrence of both diseases in feedlots can be made on the basis of cerebrospinal fluid cell counts. In polioencephalomalacia the cell counts are low, less than 100 per cmm., and are mostly lymphocytes; in the other the cell count is high (over 200 per cmm.) and they are mostly neutrophils (17).

Necropsy Findings

Cerebral oedema with compression and yellow discolouration of dorsal cortical gyri is evident and the cerebellum is pushed back into the foramen magnum with distortion of its posterior aspect. In recovered animals, there is macroscopic decortication about the motor area and over the occipital lobes. Histologically the lesions are restricted to the grey matter and are necrotic in type. Microscopic lesions may also occur in the cerebellar cortex. Subnormal levels of thiamine are detectable in liver and cerebral cortex (13).

Diagnosis

Many diseases of the nervous system are characterized by clinical syndromes indistinguishable from that of polioencephalomalacia. Acute lead poisoning, thrombo-embolic meningoencephalitis, enterotoxaemia caused by *Cl. perfringens* Type D, hypomagnesaemic tetany, hypovitaminosis A, and arsenic and mercury poisonings are some of the diseases which are clinically similar and can be expected to occur in calves under the same circumstances as polioencephalomalacia. The resemblance between these diseases and polioencephalomalacia is strong and one must be guided by the possibility of access to the poisons and assay of faeces, urine and blood, and the management practices followed. Nitrofurazone and furazolidone are commonly administered to calves and if overdosed may produce neurological signs of tremor, ataxia, loss of vision and convulsions (18, 19).

In sheep, enterotoxaemia caused by *Cl. perfringens* Type D causes an almost identical syndrome and occurs under the same management conditions as polioencephalomalacia. The glycosuria in the former disease may be of value in the ante-mortem diagnosis but necropsy examination is usually necessary to confirm the diagnosis. Another disease in sheep which may be confused with polioencephalomalacia is focal symmetrical encephalomalacia. Pregnancy toxaemia of ewes also bears a strong clinical similarity to these diseases.

Encephalitides and meningitides of both species, including listeriosis and thromboembolic meningoencephalitis usually present a more acute syndrome with more severe signs of brain irritation but they need to be considered in the differential diagnosis. They are usually accompanied by fever and, in some diseases, by other specific signs (20). Local space-occupying lesions occur only sporadically and are usually accompanied by localizing signs.

Treatment

On the basis of present knowledge the important treatment to be administered is thiamine in large doses but it may be relatively ineffective in advanced cases. Its efficiency in early cases is reported in many situations. The recommended dose is high (6 to 10 mg. per kg. intravenously).

Ancillary treatment should be directed at decompression of the brain, and the intravenous injection of hypertonic solutions and the administration of diuretics are indicated. Water intake should be restricted to small amounts at frequent intervals. Early cases may derive some benefit from the administration of corticosteroids, which have been partially effective in the prevention of cerebral oedema caused by the administration of triethyl tin (21).

Control

Satisfactory control measures are difficult to recommend because of the uncertain aetiology of the disease. It is safe to recommend that water should be freely available at all times and salt fed continuously rather than intermittently. When cases occur, abrupt changes in diet and management are often followed by cessation of the outbreak. In the circumstances the prophylactic administration of thiamine or a thiamine-rich feed may be of value and the cobalt status of the group should be ensured.

REVIEW LITERATURE

Loew, F. M., Radostits, O. M. & Dunlop, R. H. (1969). Polioencephalomalacia (cerebrocortical necrosis). *Canad. vet. J.*, *10*, 54.
Markson, L. M. & Terlecki, S. (1968). The aetiology of cerebrocortical necrosis. *Brit. vet. J.*, *124*, 309.

REFERENCES

(1) Pill, A. H. *et al.* (1966). *Vet. Rec.*, 78, 737.
(2) Davies, E. T. *et al.* (1968). *Vet. Rec.*, 83, 681.
(3) Loew, F. M. *et al.* (1972). *Vet. Rec.*, 90, 657.
(4) Edwin, E. E. & Jackman, R. (1970). *Nature (Lond.)*, 228, 772.

(5) Loew, F. M. *et al.* (1970). *Canad. vet. J.*, *11*, 57.
(6) Edwin, E. E. *et al.* (1968). *Vet. Rec.*, *83*, 176, 417.
(7) Hartley, W. J. (1962). *N.Z. vet. J.*, *10*, 118.
(8) Howell, J. McC. (1961). *Vet. Rec.*, *73*, 1165.
(9) Harris, A. H. (1962). *Vet. Rec.*, *74*, 370.
(10) Weide, K. D. *et al.* (1964). *Proc. 68th ann. gen. Mtg U.S. Live Stock sanit. Ass.*, 469.
(11) Verdura, T. & Zamora, I. (1970). *Rev. cub. Cienc. agric.*, *4*, 209.
(12) Geerken, C. M. & Figueroa, V. (1971). *Rev. cub. Cienc. agric.*, *5*, 205.
(13) Pill, A. H. (1967). *Vet. Rec.*, *81*, 178.
(14) Markson, L. M. *et al.* (1966). *Vet. Rec.*, *79*, 578.
(15) Edwin, E. E. (1970). *Vet. Rec.*, *87*, 396.
(16) Clegg, F. G. (1966). *Vet. Rec.*, *78*, 505.
(17) Howard, J. & Fawcett, K. (1966). *Iowa St. Univ. Vet.*, *28*, 101.
(18) Gardner, K. E. & Wittorff, W. E. (1955). *J. Anim. Sci.*, *14*, 1204.
(19) Gray, W. V. (1962). *Vet. Rec.*, *74*, 628.
(20) Little, P. B. & Sorenson, D. K. (1969). *J. Amer. vet. med. Ass.*, *155*, 1892.
(21) Taylor, J. M. (1964). *Nature* (*Lond.*), *204*, 891.
(22) Preston, T. R. (1972). *Wld Anim. Rev.*, *1*, 24.
(23) Markson, L. M. *et al.* (1972). *Brit. vet. J.*, *128*, 488.

Focal Symmetrical Encephalomalacia of Lambs

The disease has been recorded at a low level of incidence in lambs in New Zealand (1), Britain (2, 3) and South Africa (4). The cause is unknown although it has been suggested that the disease is a sequel to enterotoxaemia caused by *Cl. perfringens* Type D and vaccination against enterotoxaemia is commonly associated with termination of an outbreak (4). Lambs of 2 weeks to 6 months of age have been affected and manifest apathy, aimless wandering, circling, head-pressing and blindness. Inco-ordination and posterior paralysis have also been observed. More severe cases manifest lateral recumbency, opisthotonus, paddling convulsions, muscle tremor, particularly of the facial muscles, nystagmus and hyperaesthesia (4). Most affected animals become recumbent and die and a proportion of lambs are found dead without manifesting previous illness. More commonly the course is of 3 to 14 days duration.

At necropsy there are focal, symmetrical, haemorrhagic softenings in the internal capsule, basal ganglia and cerebellar penduncles. Infective agents have not been isolated and the strict symmetry of the lesions suggests an initial functional disturbance.

REFERENCES

(1) Hartley, W. J. (1956). *N.Z. vet. J.*, *4*, 129.
(2) Robertson, J. M. & Wilson, A. L. (1958). *Vet. Rec.*, *70*, 1201.
(3) Barlow, R. M. (1958). *Vet. Rec.*, *70*, 884.
(4) Pienaar, J. G. & Thornton, D. J. (1964). *J. S. Afr. vet. med. Ass.*, *35*, 351.

Neuronopathy and Pseudolipidosis of Calves

This disease has been recorded in Aberdeen Angus (1) and Friesian (4) calves. Clinically it is characterized by ataxia, muscle tremor and failure to grow. Signs appear at 1 to 15 months of age and the disease progresses over a period of 3 to 4 months. Affected calves are somewhat stunted. The first positive sign is a swaying of the hindquarters especially after exercise or excitement. A fine head tremor develops and is accompanied by aggressiveness and a tendency to attack. Slow vertical head nodding is also a feature. Ataxia increases and the movements of the limbs are jerky, inco-ordinated, exaggerated and misplaced, and the animal falls easily. The terminal stage is either one of failure to grow, with ataxia evident during movement, or complete paralysis necessitating destruction of the animal. There are no constant macroscopic findings at necropsy although there may be mild hydrocephalus (2). Histologically there is gross abnormality of nerve cells throughout the brain without apparent damage to the axons. Vacuolation of the larger nerve cell bodies is a characteristic finding. Similar lesions are present in the reticulo-endothelial cells of the lymph nodes and pancreatic exocrine cells (2). The cause of the disease is unknown but conditioning by an inherited factor has been suggested and suspected carrier animals should not be used for breeding. The inherited defect is probably one of glycoprotein metabolism (3).

REFERENCES

(1) Whittem, J. H. & Walker, D. (1957). *J. Path. Bact.*, *74*, 281.
(2) Jolly, R. D. (1970). *N.Z. vet. J.*, *18*, 228.
(3) Jolly, R. D. (1971). *J. Path.*, *103*, 113.
(4) Donnelley, W. J. C. *et al.* (1972). *Vet. Rec.*, *91*, 225.

Arthrogryposis and Hydranencephaly

Two congenital abnormalities of newborn calves, arthrogryposis (permanent joint contracture) and hydranencephaly (a compensatory replacement by fluid of missing cerebral cortical tissue in contradistinction to atrophy of brain tissue caused by fluid pressure as in hydrocephalus) have been reported as occurring in outbreak proportions in the same herds at the same time. Both conditions may also occur in the same animal (1, 2, 3). The two conditions appear to be varying degrees of the one disease and their variations may reflect the age at which damage to the developing nervous system occurs. Calves with uncomplicated hydranencephaly are born normally but are blind and imbecile; those with arthrogryposis frequently cause foetal dystocia because of severe joint contracture which may be in flexion or extension and affect one or more limbs. Wry-neck may also be present and there is severe muscle atrophy.

At necropsy, the cerebral hemispheres are almost entirely replaced by fluid in the calves with hydranencephaly. In the calves with arthrogryposis, there is severe muscle degeneration and fixation of the joints by contracted tendons, without abnormality of the joint surfaces. There is a complete absence of motor horn cells in the spinal cord in this latter group. The cause of the disease is unknown but an unidentified virus has been suggested in Australia (4) and has almost certainly caused the extensive outbreaks reported in Israel (5). Ephemeral fever and bluetongue have been eliminated as causes in the respective countries. The disease has been produced experimentally in guinea pigs by exposure to high environmental temperatures (6) but this seems an unlikely cause in practical circumstances.

Congenital arthrogryposis without cranial abnormalities has been observed in pigs born to sows which had ingested burley tobacco stalks between the 10th and 30th day of pregnancy (7).

REFERENCES

(1) Blood, D. C. (1956). *Aust. vet. J.*, *32*, 125.
(2) Whittem, J. H. (1957). *J. Path. Bact.*, *73*, 375.
(3) Bonner, R. B. *et al.* (1961). *Aust. vet. J.*, *37*, 160 (corresp.).
(4) Young, J. S. (1969). *Aust. vet. J.*, *45*, 574.
(5) Markusfield, O. & Mayer, E. (1971). *Refuah. vet.*, *28*, 51.
(6) Edwards, M. J. (1971). *J. Path.*, *104*, 221.
(7) Crowe, M. W. & Pike, H. T. (1973). *J. Amer. vet. med. Ass.*, *162*, 453.

'Barkers' and 'Wanderers' in Thoroughbred Foals

(Neonatal Maladjustment Syndrome)

This series of abnormalities appears to occur only in Britain (1) and only in thoroughbred horses. Cases occur after easy parturitions and may reach an incidence of 1 to 2 per cent. It seems probable that only foals which are assisted at birth are affected and it has been suggested that too early severance of the cord may deprive the foal of large quantities of blood in the placental vascular bed and precipitate the disease. By the same token oxygen deprivation due to any cause is likely to cause the disease and it has been classified as a pulmonary dysfunction (2). A very similar syndrome has been described in hunter foals and is ascribed to hypoglycaemia because of rapid response to oral administration of colostrum (3). A similar hypoxic disease occurs in human infants and has been produced experimentally in laboratory animals.

Clinically there are three stages of the disease, affected foals in each stage being known as 'barkers', 'dummies' or 'wanderers'. Foals that show the 'barker' syndrome pass through the other stages during recovery but some may begin as 'dummies' or 'wanderers' and these progress to recovery. In the first stage, about 50 per cent die but, in the other stages, improvement or recovery is the rule. The disease always commences during the first day of life, sometimes as early as 10 to 30 minutes after birth, but usually after an hour or two.

The barking stage may be ushered in by prodromal signs of weakness, aimless movements and blindness. The characteristic signs in this stage are a barking sound emitted during severe clonic convulsions in which the foal paddles wildly, champs the jaws, shows clonic contractions of the head and neck and often bruises itself extensively about the head by banging it on the floor. Nystagmus is also present and sweating may be profuse. A period of coma follows such a convulsive episode but the foal can be aroused and subsequent, less severe convulsions may occur. The foal is unable to stand or suck and is blind. Affected foals may die during this stage or remain in a coma for hours or days and then pass into the 'dummy' stage.

The 'dummy' and 'wandering' stages are manifested by blindness and failure to respond to most external stimuli. The sucking reflex is absent, the foal shows no fear and there is no excitement or abnormal movement. The foal can walk and wanders about aimlessly, bumping into fixed objects. Most such foals go on to recover completely in from 3 to 10 days.

At necropsy, there is extensive consolidation of the upper parts of both lungs and an absence of central nervous system changes. It is suggested that acute cerebral anoxia may cause the clinical signs which appear.

In the acute stage, sedation is necessary to prevent excessive injury and, in the chronic stage, the foal must be fed by nasal tube, preferably 4 or 5 times a day, until it can learn to drink from a dish or suck from the mare.

REFERENCES

(1) Mahaffey, L. W. & Rossdale, P. D. (1957). *Vet. Rec.*, *69*, 1277.
(2) Rossdale, P. D. (1969). *Res. vet. Sci.*, *10*, 279.
(3) Smith, G. A. (1968). *Vet. Rec.*, *83*, 588.

Shaker Foal Syndrome

This naturally occurring syndrome can be produced experimentally by the intravenous injection of *Clostridium botulinum* type A toxin. There is difficulty in assuming that the disease is a form of botulism in that there is a very strict limitation in the age group affected—3 to 8 weeks of age. The disease occurs sporadically in the U.S.A. (1) and the U.K. (2) where it has been known for many years. It occurs rarely and never more than one or two cases per farm in a year. Either sex and both standardbreds and thoroughbreds are affected.

Clinically there is a sudden onset of severe muscular weakness and prostration, with the foal going down and being unable to rise. If it is held up there is a gross muscle tremor which is not evident when the foal is lying down. Prostrate foals are bright and alert and respond to pinching. They go through periods of rising, followed by onset of the tremor and recumbency and complete prostration.

During this latter period there is a complete cessation of peristalsis, dilation of the pupils with a sluggish response to light. The temperature varies from being slightly elevated to slightly depressed. Death occurs about 72 hours after the onset of signs and is due to respiratory failure.

There is no significant clinico-pathological change although extreme acidosis has been recorded terminally. At necropsy examination the colon is tightly contracted and contains small amounts of dry, hard faecal material. The liver is enlarged and unevenly mottled. The pericardial sac contains excessive clear yellow fluid with fibrin flakes. There are no lesions in the nervous system. There are some similarities to grass sickness.

An heroic treatment schedule of 2 mg. neostigmin every 2 hours (plus mineral oil, steroids, antibiotics and tube feeding) for 4 to 7 days is recorded as curing 2 of 2 cases thus treated (1).

REFERENCES

(1) Rooney, J. E. & Prickett, M. E. (1967). *Mod. vet. Pract.*, *48*, 44.
(2) Rossdale, P. D. & Mullen, P. A. (1969). *Vet. Rec.*, *85*, 702.

Myoclonia Congenita

This congenital disease of the nervous system of piglets has been recorded in most countries. Signs may be present at birth or, more usually, may be delayed until the pigs become active at 2 or 3 days of age. Muscle tremor varying from fibrillary twitching to violent trembling of the head, trunk and limbs is observed when the piglets stand. They have difficulty in sucking and may die of starvation. Surviving piglets improve gradually, the tremor being visible only on exercise in the late stages and disappearing completely in from 2 weeks to 2 months. The incidence in an affected litter is usually about 40 per cent.

Swine fever virus infection, or vaccination with attenuated swine fever virus in early pregnancy (1) is the most important cause of the disease. In natural infections the strains of virus isolated are always of low pathogenicity (2). Infection with swine fever virus is not the only cause; some cases occur in its absence. Histologically the lesions observed are those of spinal hypomyelinogenesis or cerebellar hypoplasia or both (1, 3).

REFERENCES

(1) Harding, J. D. J. *et al.* (1966). *Vet. Rec.*, *79*, 388.
(2) Done, J. T. (1969). *Brit. vet. J.*, *125*, 349.
(3) Emerson, J. L. & Delez, A. L. (1965). *J. Amer. vet. med. Ass.*, *147*, 47.

Hypomyelinogenesis Congenita

This congenital disease has been recorded in lambs in the U.K. (1, 2) and Canada (3) and in calves in the U.S.A. (4). Congenital hypomyelinogenesis also occurs extensively as a lesion in myotonia congenita of piglets and is discussed under that heading (p. 929). Affected lambs manifest severe muscle tremor affecting the whole body and head. The tremor disappears when the lambs are asleep. The gait is erratic and inco-ordinated and the lambs tend to hop or jump with the hindlegs, but they follow the ewe, and suck and grow well. Defaecation, urination and the voice are unaffected. Many lambs recover spontaneously but severely affected lambs may die of starvation within the first few days of life, or nervous signs, including intermittent head-shaking and mild, coarse muscle tremor with ataxia of the hind-legs, may persist for as long as 5 months. These lambs appear normal at rest and grow normally if carefully nursed but appear to be more susceptible than usual to intercurrent disease. The disease has occurred in outbreak form with an incidence as high as 13 per cent (5).

A similar, and possibly identical, disease known as 'border disease' also occurs in the U.K. (6). It is dealt with elsewhere under the title of 'Hairy Shaker' disease. There seems to be little doubt among English workers that hypomyelinogenesis and 'hairy shakers' are the same disease. For this edition at least we have decided to keep a foot in both camps.

Both diseases resemble congenital enzootic ataxia but liver copper levels are normal and histological examination shows absence of myelin but no defect of the nerve fibre. The causative agent has not been isolated but both hypomyelinogenesis congenita and 'border disease' have been reproduced by the injection into pregnant ewes of tissues from affected lambs (7, 8). A closely related syndrome has been produced by injection of mucosal disease virus into pregnant ewes (9).

Affected calves are well formed, alert and have normal eyes but are unable to stand or achieve normal postures from birth. Persistent general tremor is evident at all times, is more pronounced on stimulation and may be accompanied by brief periods of spastic rigidity and moderate opisthotonus and occasionally nystagmus. At necropsy there is a marked deficiency of myelin particularly in the cerebellum and brain-stem. Although the cause of the disease has not been determined, an inherited factor does not appear to be responsible (4).

REFERENCES

(1) Markson, L. M. *et al.* (1959). *Vet. Rec., 71*, 269.
(2) Hughes, L. E. *et al.* (1959). *Vet. Rec., 71*, 313.
(3) Darcel, C. leQ. *et al.* (1961). *Canad. J. comp. Med., 25*, 132.
(4) Young, S. (1962). *Cornell Vet., 52*, 84.
(5) Barr, M. (1964). *Vet. Rec., 76*, 815.
(6) Barlow, R. M. & Dickinson, A. G. (1965). *Res. vet. Sci., 6*, 230.
(7) Shaw, J. G. *et al.* (1967). *Vet. Rec., 81*, 115.
(8) Dickinson, A. G. & Barlow, R. M. (1967). *Vet. Rec., 81*, 114.
(9) Acland, H. M. *et al.* (1972). *Aust. vet. J., 48*, 70.

Enzootic Inco-ordination

(*'Wobbles'*, *Foal Ataxia*, *Equine Sensory Ataxia*)

Enzootic inco-ordination is a disease of young horses affecting the cervical spinal cord and vertebrae and characterized clinically by inco-ordination.

Incidence

Details of incidence are not available but the disease occurs sporadically in most countries, and is of some importance in that affected horses are useless for further work.

Aetiology

The cause of the disease is unknown. There is a tendency for it to be familial (1) but inheritance of a defect or susceptibility has not been satisfactorily proven. The current view is that the spinal cord is damaged by pressure usually in the cervical region, exerted by vertebrae which are rendered excessively mobile by disease in the intervertebral discs and ligaments (2, 3). It is possible that the primary cause of such lesions may be a nutritional deficiency. Most cases are first observed in sucklings and yearlings but clinical signs may appear for the first time in horses up to 2 years of age. Often the horses affected in a group are those in best condition.

Occurrence

The disease occurs in young thoroughbreds, trotting and saddle horses but no association has been noted between the occurrence of the disease and any management or nutritional factor.

Pathogenesis

Osteoarthritic lesions of intervertebral joints, narrowing of the spinal canal and degenerative lesions of the spinal cord are present (4).

Continued contusion of the cervical spinal cord is accepted as the basic lesion, the contusion occurring by overflexion of the neck and momentary dorsal displacement of the vertebral body, or because of fleeting protrusion of the capsule of the lateral spinal joint into the spinal canal (2). It is suggested that the occurrence of the abnormality is related to the length of neck, longer necked horses being more susceptible because of greater bending and retroflexing force (7). Serious exacerbations occur from time to time, often associated with falls or other violent movements. The clinical picture then is one of gradual deterioration in co-ordination of movement, which may go undetected in horses which are not under restraint, until the more serious errors occur.

The specific degenerative lesion of this disease, due to pressure from subluxation of vertebral bodies, may be primarily due to venous occlusion (5). The abnormalities observed are more readily explained as both motor and sensory rather than a purely sensory ataxia (5, 6).

Clinical Findings

Males are more commonly affected and overall the incidence is very low.

Although a history of sudden onset is often obtained it is usually found that there were mild signs previously and that a fall, violent activity or casting have precipitated a more severe disturbance. The onset is insidious, the first signs being a slight inco-ordination of leg movements. This may be apparent in mild cases only when the horse is being ridden. Neck movements are restricted and pain may be elicited on sudden movement of, or pressure over, the cervical vertebrae but there is no cutaneous hypersensitivity in the usual sense.

The defect of gait is difficult to describe. There may be insufficient or excessive flexion or extention or excessive abduction. There is usually a degree of weakness. While moving, there is clumsiness when the horse is turned sharply, and pulling up sharply at a fast gait causes knuckling over at the fetlocks. During walking there may be lurching and swaying, particularly of the hindquarters, and the horse often has difficulty maintaining a normal posture for urination and grazing. The forelimbs may be more seriously involved than the hind and one of a pair may be more affected than the other. The signs are most marked when walking and often disappear at the trot. There is some difference of opinion about the effect of blind-folding on the gait (5, 6) but the consensus is that it has no effect. Dragging of the toes, often inter-mittently, is an early sign in many cases and there may be difficulty in getting up after the horse has rolled or been cast. After the initial appearance of signs, there may be progression of the disease for several weeks, followed by a long period during which the signs remain static. Recovery does not occur but death is unusual unless the animal has a severe accident.

Clinical Pathology

No laboratory examinations have diagnostic value. Blood levels of calcium and phosphorus are within normal limits. Radiographic examination offers some assistance in differentiation.

Necropsy Findings

In 30 to 50 per cent of cases, there are projec-tions of vertebrae or intervertebral discs into the spinal canal and some evidence of compression of the cord. Areas of malacia are present in the spinal cord and there is symmetrical degeneration of ascending and descending spinal cord tracts. Inflammation of the articular processes of both thoracic and cervical vertebrae may be present with involvement of the spinal nerves. Severe inflammation of peripheral nerves may also be present in early cases. Slight atrophy of cervical muscles is sometimes evident.

Diagnosis

Traumatic injury to the spinal cord causes a sudden onset of paralysis often followed by gradual improvement. Pressure on the spinal cord due to space-occupying lesions in the vertebral canal may cause almost identical signs (5). Spinal meningitis or myelitis usually develops slowly; meningitis is accompanied by rigidity and hyperaesthesia of the neck and myelitis by some signs of encephalitis. Inco-ordination during moderate exercise is a prominent sign in iliac thrombosis but usually only one leg is affected and there are circulatory signs on palpation of the affected limb. In tropical countries, cerebrospinal nematodiasis is a more common cause of an almost identical syndrome. A fatal, inherited ataxia of foals in the Oldenburg

breed is much more severe and develops to the stage of recumbency and finally complete paralysis.

Treatment

Treatment is unlikely to be of value and is not usually undertaken.

Control

Because of the possible inherited nature of the disease, a corrective breeding programme may be advisable.

REFERENCES

(1) Dimock, W. W. (1950). *J. Hered.*, *41*, 319.
(2) Dahme, E. & Schebitz, H. (1970). *Zbl. vet. Med.*, *17A*, 120.
(3) Rooney, J. R. (1963). *Cornell Vet.*, *53*, 411.
(4) Pohlenz, J. & Schulz, L. C. (1966). *Dtsch. tierärztl. Wschr.*, *73*, 533.
(5) Fraser, H. & Palmer, A. C. (1967). *Vet. Rec.*, *80*, 338.
(6) Steel, J. D. *et al.* (1959). *Aust. vet. J.*, *35*, 442.
(7) Rooney, J. R. (1972). *Mod. vet. Pract.*, *53*, 42.

DISEASES CHARACTERIZED BY INVOLVEMENT OF THE MUSCULO-SKELETAL SYSTEM

Sporadic Lymphangitis
(*Bigleg, Weed*)

This is a non-contagious disease of horses characterized by acute fever, lymphangitis and severe swelling of one or both hind-legs. The disease commences abruptly with fever (40·5 to 41°C or 105 to 106°F), shivering and a rapid pulse rate and respiration. Pain is severe and the horse is usually quite distressed. There is severe pain on palpation of the affected leg and lameness may be so severe that the horse may refuse to put its foot to the ground. The limb is swollen and hot, the swelling commencing at the top of the leg and extending down to the coronet. There is cording of the lymphatics on the medial aspect of the leg and palpable enlargement of the lymph nodes. Anorexia, thirst and patchy sweating may also be in evidence and constipation is usual. The acute stage lasts for 2 to 3 days but the swelling persists for 7 to 10 days. Occasionally abscesses develop in the lymph nodes and vessels. There is a tendency for the disease to recur and cause chronic fibrotic thickening of the lower part of the limb.

Sporadic lymphangitis usually occurs in horses fed highly nutritious rations with restricted exercise for a number of days. It is usually associated with superficial wounds and ulcers on the lower parts of the limbs, and the disease is thought to develop as a lymphadenitis of the deep inguinal nodes as a result of these wounds. The affected lymph nodes obstruct lymphatic and venous drainage and, because of lack of stimulation of these by exercise, lymphangitis develops, causing lymphatic obstruction oedema and, in some cases, cellulitis (1).

Affected horses require energetic treatment. Penicillin or other antibiotic should be administered parenterally to control the infection. A sedative to ease the pain, and vigorous hot fomentation and massage of the leg to remove the oedema fluid are also advised. The administration of a laxative and a diuretic has long been a standard practice. Hot fomentations, with upward massage of the limb, should be applied frequently and the leg bandaged tightly in the intervals. The efficiency with which this part of the treatment is carried out will determine largely the speed of recovery. Exercise should be encouraged as soon as the horse can put its foot to the ground.

Prevention of the disease necessitates prompt and careful treatment of all wounds of the lower limbs. Provision of daily exercise, restriction of the diet during prolonged rest periods and dry standing in the stable also help to prevent the disease.

REFERENCE

(1) Tufvesson, G. (1952). *Nord. Vet.-Med.*, **4**, 529, 729, 817, 1046.

Porcine Stress Syndrome

(Herztod, Fatal Syncope, Shock-Heart Failure Syndrome)

This is a disease of pigs which has existed for a long time under the name of Herztod, but has come to be very much more important in recent times largely because of the development and popularization of Landrace and Pietrain pigs. It is much more common in the latter and is recorded as a rarity in Large White pigs (1). It is now one of the most serious diseases of pigs in Europe.

Clinically the most common occurrence is death after exercise, especially the driving of fat pigs, but also in boars during mating or sows during parturition. When affected pigs are observed alive the first sign observed is a rapid tremor of the tail, followed by dyspnoea to the point of mouth breathing. The body temperature rises very high and there are irregularly shaped areas of skin blanching and erythema. Finally the pig becomes reluctant to move, collapses and dies, and rigor mortis sets in very rapidly. At post mortem examination there is diffuse and severe degeneration of skeletal muscle (7). There is also an increase in

pericardial fluid but no fibrin is present. Another common observation is the appearance of the disease during anaesthesia, especially with halothane, death usually occurring suddenly but preceded by a period of severe hyperthermia, muscular rigidity and apnoea and the appearance of extrasystoles in the electrocardiogram. The disease has many similarities to malignant hyperthermia in man, a fatal hyperthermia occurring during halothane anaesthesia.

The cause is incompletely understood but appears to be a familial susceptibility to acidosis (2), due to excessive lactic acid production in these heavily muscled breeds of pigs during periods of stress. The stress may be in the form of physical exercise (2, 3), sudden sharp rises in environmental temperature or halothane anaesthesia. It is suggested that during the stress oxidative phosphorylation in muscle becomes uncoupled, resulting in anaerobic glycolysis and coagulation necrosis of the muscle and excessive heat production, causing in turn the very high temperatures observed. There is a concurrent fall in plasma pH and a larger than normal increase in serum inorganic phosphate and plasma potassium (1). The acidity is due to elevation of plasma lactate from the damaged muscle.

In unstressed Pietrain pigs the plasma levels of creatine phosphokinase activity are well above normal and it may be possible to identify highly susceptible pigs by this means (4, 5). Serum aldolase levels are similarly elevated but potassium levels are not (6). Lactate dehydrogenase levels are also raised significantly but of the three enzymes creatine phosphokinase is the most sensitive indicator (5). Death is due to respiratory or cardiac failure due to failure of activity of relevant muscle masses.

An allied disability of breeds and families of pigs susceptible to this disease is their predisposition to produce pale, watery pork (pale, soft exudative post mortem degeneration). This is thought to be due to a rapid glycolysis and adenosine triphosphate breakdown soon after death (4). It seems apparent that the three recognized conditions of acute stress syndrome, malignant hyperthermia and pale soft exudative post mortem degeneration are manifestations of the same myopathy which can be elicited by muscular exercise, or the use of anaesthetic agents or by death (5).

The whole subject is an interesting and exciting one, partly because it marks the outer limit of selection for muscle production in an animal and partly because of its comparative interest for studies in diseases of muscle in man. The subject is by no means closed (5).

REVIEW LITERATURE

Hoorens, J. & Oyaert, W. (1970). *Vlaams diergeneesk. Tijdschr.*, *39*, 246.

REFERENCES

(1) Allen, W. M. *et al.* (1970). *Vet. Rec.*, *87*, 64.
(2) Hadlow, W. J. (1959). *Lab. Invest.*, *8*, 1478.
(3) Goodwin, R. F. W. (1958). *Vet. Rec.*, *70*, 885.
(4) Patterson, D. S. P. & Allen, W. M. (1972). *Brit. vet. J.*, *128*, 101.
(5) Berman, M. C. *et al.* (1971). *S. Afr. med. J.*, *45*, 580, 590, 1208.
(6) Allen, W. M. (1970). *Vet. Rec.*, *87*, 410.
(7) Topel, D. G. *et al.* (1968). *Mod. vet. Pract.*, *49*, 40.

Myofibrillar Hypoplasia

(*Splayleg*)

In this disease of pigs a definitive diagnosis is made on the deficiency of myofibrils as seen histologically. Grossly the muscles have the appearance of foetal muscle and clinically affected pigs display the 'splayleg' syndrome from birth (1). In affected muscle there is an abnormal distribution of potassium and a polysaccharide outside the myofibrils, marked abnormality of muscle fibre cell membranes and plasma enzyme activity (LDH and CPK are raised). Basically the affected muscle is immature. It is probable that the defect is inherited but it has been pointed out that an identical clinical syndrome can be produced in normal newborn pigs by forcing them to stand on a very slippery surface (2).

The histopathological change in this case is interstitial muscular oedema without myofibril immaturity.

Clinically the pigs affected with congenital myofibrillar hypoplasia have varying degrees of difficulty in standing and walking, the legs tend to splay out sideways or forwards; as a result the piglets are likely to be crushed or have difficulty gaining access to their source of nourishment. It has been suggested that the use of farrowing crates, with the sows immobilized, could have permitted the preservation of pigs which would otherwise have been destroyed (3). The incidence is usually low, one or two per litter. Hindlegs are most affected but forelegs may be involved. Unless further traumatic damage is incurred the affected pigs are normal in mobility about 10 days later.

The disease is perhaps more common in the Landrace breed and losses in this breed have been heavy (4). Suggestions that the disease is caused by a nutritional deficiency of choline in the sow appears to have been disposed of effectively (5). The disease does occur in males and females although restriction to male pigs has been recorded (6) and the genetic mechanism suggested is a dominant sex-linked character with varying degrees of penetrance.

One of the important aspects of this disease is to point up the developing importance of the syndrome known as 'leg weakness' in intensively housed pigs. In recent years there has been an increasing problem of young pigs who have a grossly swaying gait in the hindquarters, curvature of the hocks, disinclination to stand on the hindlegs, difficulty in rising and eventual posterior paralysis. The defect may be much more marked in one leg than another. It is often difficult to decide whether the pigs are lame or have weak legs. The condition seems to have increased markedly since the introduction of Landrace pigs, the use of very rapidly growing Specific Pathogen Free pigs, very heavy grain feeding and limited-space, controlled environment housing. Whether any or all of these influences have had any effect on the increase in leg weakness is difficult to say but inherited splayleg, inherited porcine stress syndrome, osteodystrophia fibrosa due to high phosphorus feeding immediately suggest themselves as possible contributors. Irreversible damage to bones and joint cartilages may occur during the period of expression of any of these diseases and maintain a persistent leg weakness (7, 8).

REFERENCES

(1) Patterson, D. S. P. & Allen, W. M. (1972). *Brit. vet. J.*, *128*, 101.
(2) Kohler, E. M. *et al.* (1969). *J. Amer. vet. med. Ass.*, *155*, 139.
(3) Thurley, D. C. *et al.* (1967). *Vet. Rec.*, *80*, 302.
(4) Dobson, K. J. (1968). *Aust. vet. J.*, *44*, 26.
(5) Dobson, K. J. (1971). *Aust. vet. J.*, *47*, 587.
(6) Lax, T. (1971). *J. Hered.*, *62*, 250.
(7) Thurley, D. C. (1967). *Dtsch. tierärztl. Wschr.*, *74*, 336.
(8) Vaughan, L. C. (1971). *Vet. Rec.*, *89*, 81.

'Tying-up' Syndrome of Horses

The all embracing terms 'tying-up' or 'set-fast' are used to denote horses which become stiff and sore in their limbs, showing cramped and slow movement without actual lameness. They include also horses which stumble a little when walking and have a general appearance of rigidity, stiffness and gauntness of the abdomen after exercise, a real problem for race-horse trainers. In many cases the problem is one of muscle soreness due to a sudden change from a soft to a hard track, or overwork, especially in horses coming back into work after a rest. It may be due to a trainer demanding too much too soon. If such factors can be eliminated, and a decision reached that the horse's reaction is abnormal, the following possible causes should be considered (1, 2):

Myopathy (*polymyositis*). Most of the following entities are poorly defined, this being no exception. It is characterized by muscle soreness, often to the point where the horse literally will not move, a sudden onset after brisk exercise, and greatly elevated levels of serum enzymes including glutamic oxalate transanimase (SGOT) aldolase and creatine phosphokinase (CPK). It is identical to azoturia except that there is no myoglobinuria, and there is no immediately preceding history of an enforced rest on a full grain ration. There are distinct clinical and epidemiological differences from the enzootic equine myosites of Scandinavia and New Zealand which are described elsewhere; the principal difference is the tendency for this disease to be a characteristic of a particular horse which is inclined to have successive or intermittently repeated attacks (3). These make it an impossible training proposition and of doubtful suitability for other equine occupations. They are understandably significant sources of client dissatisfaction for veterinarians.

The onset of an attack may occur while the horse is being ridden; within a few strides it falters, goes gingerly and then stops. If it can be persuaded to move it does so with reluctance and with short shuffling steps. The pulse rate and temperature are elevated and the horse is obviously in pain. The muscles are not palpably abnormal. Lesser attacks are usually evident when the horse has cooled off after work; the signs are the same but less marked. SGOT levels are often as high as 4,000 SF units, normal horses rarely go above 600 (occasionally to 1,000) SF units after exercise (4). SGOT is a fairly non-specific enzyme although it is largely influenced by skeletal muscle status, serum creatine phosphokinase is a sensitive and reliable indicator of cellular damage, rather than specifically skeletal muscle. Aldolase is fairly specific for muscle injury but lactic dehydrogenase is too non-specific (5). Susceptible horses often have suspiciously high serum enzyme levels at rest. The muscle stiffness passes off in one to three days depending on the severity of the attack. With little justification treatment with a combination of selenium and vitamin E is usual. Spontaneous recovery occurs and the cause is unknown.

Grain or oat sickness. The existence of this entity depends on observations that individual horses on heavy grain diets develop a 'tying-up' syndrome which can be alleviated by reducing the grain intake or by administering 30 to 60 g. magnesium sulphate daily in the feed (2). The characteristic stiffness and restriction of movement are most noticeable 1 or 2 hours after exercise.

Verminous arteritis/iliac thrombosis is a well known disease. The development of weakness and incoordination during fast work, the obvious pain, lack of sweating, diminution of pulse amplitude in the internal iliac arteries on rectal examination and the volar digital arteries, and lack of warmth in the skin of the affected limb are the diagnostic features. There may be an abnormality of gait while walking and failure of the superficial veins to distend normally.

Spondylopathy. The early stages or mild forms of enzootic incoordination due to repeated contusion of the cervical spinal cord may resemble 'tying-up' and is described elsewhere. There are in addition other poorly defined syndromes caused by damage to the spinal cord and pressure to or irritation of dorsal spinal nerve roots (2). Causes of such pressure include vertebral dislocation, fracture or osteoarthritis, or abscess or haematoma. The stiffness and pain which result can be relieved by anti-inflammatory and pain-killing agents.

Neuritis of the cauda equina. This is characterized by paralysis of the tail, loss of tone of the anal sphincter, distension of the rectal ampulla, paralysis of the bladder and cutaneous anaesthesia of the tail, perineum, caudal upper parts of the hind legs (6). There is an associated weakness and incoordination of gait in the hindlegs and it has been suggested that the defect may have an aetiological relationship with the 'wind-sucking' which occurs in some horses (2). There is a non-suppurative inflammation of nerve trunks of the cauda equina.

Degenerative arthritis. Mild cases of osteodystrophia fibrosa still occur but knowledge of the disease has resulted in its virtual elimination by dietary management. A number of cases of degenerative arthritis still occur (2). They represent a problem dealt with in surgical textbooks; they are mentioned here only as additions to the list of diagnostic possibilities.

REFERENCES

(1) Steel, J. D. & Maclean, J. G. (1967–68). *Vict. Vet. Proc.*, 26, 24.
(2) Steel, J. D. (1969). *Aust. vet. J.*, 45, 162.
(3) Cornelius, C. E. *et al.* (1963). *J. Amer. vet. med. Ass.*, 142, 639.
(4) Hansen, M. A. (1970). *Nord. Vet.-Med.*, 22, 617.
(5) Gerber, H. (1969). *Equine vet. J.*, 1, 129.
(6) Milne, F. J. & Carbonell, P. L. (1970). *Equine vet. J.*, 2, 179.

'Acorn' Calves

A non-inherited condition has been described in the United States and Australia (1) which bears some resemblance to inherited dwarfism. The disease occurs on poor range country and is thought to be due to a maternal nutritional deficiency during the middle third of pregnancy. The specific dietary factors involved have not been determined although supplementary feeding during pregnancy eliminates the condition. Osseous development of the head is abnormal with either a shortened or long, narrow head. Shortening of the shafts of the long bones of the limbs is accompanied by bending of the joints, and calves nurse and stand with difficulty. Inco-ordination, arching of the back and a tendency to bloat, which may cause death, also occur. The dentition is normal. Muscle spasticity, wry neck, circling, falling backwards and goose-stepping occur rarely. Most of the calves are born alive and, in badly affected herds, as many as 15 per cent of calves may be affected. The condition derives its name from the common occurrence of acorns in the diet of affected herds, although the acorns are not thought to have any aetiological significance.

REFERENCE

(1) Barry, M. R. & Murphy, W. J. B. (1964). *Aust. vet. J.*, *40*, 195.

DISEASES CHARACTERIZED BY INVOLVEMENT OF THE SKIN

Pityriasis Rosea

This skin disease of pigs resembles ringworm closely but skin scrapings do not reveal the presence of fungal hyphae or spores, and cultures for fungal growth are usually negative. Treatment with standard preparations used for ringworm is usually ineffective although spontaneous recovery may occur.

The disease occurs in sucking pigs (1) and young pigs in the 10- to 14-weeks age group. Up to 50 per cent of each litter may be affected and in large groups of feeder pigs there may be only individual pigs or the majority of the group with lesions. The disease is usually innocuous although digestive disturbances, particularly anorexia and, to a lesser extent, diarrhoea and vomiting may accompany the appearance of lesions and affected pigs lose some body weight. There is no fever.

Lesions occur most commonly on the ventral abdomen but may spread to the rest of the body. They commence as small, red nodules which enlarge to flat plaques and become covered with thin, dry, brown scales. The lesions appear to enlarge centrifugally leaving a centre of normal appearance surrounded by a narrow zone of elevated, erythematous skin covered by typical scales. Individual lesions are generally circular except that they often coalesce to produce a large, irregular lesion. There is little irritation and the skin lesions, although obvious, are superficial. There is no loss of bristles.

The cause is unknown although there is strong evidence of familial susceptibility, either through inheritance by vertical transmission of an infectious agent (2, 3). Transmission experiments have been unsuccessful and the disease has been observed in SPF pigs produced by Caesarean section (4). By analogy with a similar condition affecting man, it may be a viral infection. Treatment appears to be completely ineffective but in general consists of the local application of a salve containing 5 per cent salicylic acid or iodized mineral oil. Affected pigs should be isolated from the group. Spontaneous recovery occurs in 6 to 8 weeks in most instances.

REFERENCES

(1) Thompson, R. (1960). *Canad. vet. J.*, *1*, 449.
(2) Wellman, G. (1963). *Berl. Münch. tierärztl. Wschr.*, 107.
(3) Corcoran, C. J. (1964). *Vet. Rec.*, *76*, 1407.
(4) McDermid, K. A. (1964). *Canad. vet. J.*, *5*, 95.

Anhidrosis

(Non-Sweating Syndrome, Puff Disease, Dry Coat)

Anhidrosis is a disease characterized by absence of sweating, occurring mainly in horses, and less commonly in cattle.

Incidence

The disease occurs most commonly in horses in countries with hot, humid climates including India, Indonesia, Ceylon, Burma, Malaysia, Australia, Puerto Rico and Trinidad. A similar condition has been described in cattle (1). Indigenous horses may be affected but the major problem is in racehorses imported into tropical areas from temperate climates. Similarly in cattle, the indigenous animals, particularly zebus and their crosses, are unaffected and stock imported for breeding purposes present the major difficulty. High-producing dairy cows are more susceptible than other types. Affected animals rarely die of the disease but are seriously incapacitated and may have to be returned to cooler climates if they are to function efficiently.

Aetiology

The disease is basically a failure in adaptation to a hot climate. Work done in horses suggests that although blockage of sweat gland ducts occurs this is a secondary lesion and that the basic disturbance is one of insensitivity of sweat glands to adrenaline, the sweat glands having been conditioned by persistent high blood adrenaline levels caused by exposure to consistently high environmental temperatures (2). In cattle the capacity of animals reared in temperate climates to adapt themselves to tropical conditions appears to be quite strongly inherited. This may or may not be the case in horses.

Pathogenesis

The failure of the sweating mechanism results in reduction of heat loss from the body and a rise in body temperature, particularly on exercise. Respiration is stimulated by the need for heat dissipation by other routes and the resulting dyspnoea may be so severe that the animal is unable to function efficiently.

Clinical Findings

In the early stages in horses, excessive sweating and dyspnoea after exercise are observed. The skin area over which sweating can be observed is gradually reduced over a period of weeks until sweating can be observed only under the mane. In addition, the skin becomes dry and scurfy and loses its elasticity. Dyspnoea may become extreme, and the animals continually seek the shade. Death from heart failure may occur if exercise is forced. High body temperatures are observed after exercise, sometimes reaching 41·5 to 42°C (107 to 108°F) and persist for long periods. At this stage, the disease is analogous to heat stroke. If animals are returned to cool climates, the condition gradually disappears.

Clinical Pathology

Blood chloride levels are low and blood adrenaline levels are high but these observations are unlikely to be used in clinical diagnosis.

Necropsy Findings

There are no characteristic lesions at necropsy.

Treatment and Control

Treatment is empirical because of the doubtful aetiology of the disease. An adequate salt intake should be maintained and in severe cases, intravenous injections of physiological saline are recommended. The ration should contain adequate green feed. The feeding of iodinated casein (containing 0·72 per cent 1-thyroxine) is claimed to cure the disease in horses when given in daily doses of 10 to 15 g. for 4 to 8 days (3) and good results are reported after the use of thyroid gland extract (50 g. daily for 20 days) (4). The daily administration orally of 1,000 to 3,000 units of vitamin E is also reported to be effective (5). Removal of affected animals to cooler climates is often necessary, although air conditioning of stables and maintenance of horses in higher country where they can be returned after a day's racing may enable susceptible horses to be kept locally (1).

REFERENCES

(1) Stewart, C. M. (1956). *Irish vet. J.*, *10*, 189, 208.
(2) Evans, C. L. (1966). *Brit. vet. J.*, *122*, 117.
(3) Maqsood, M. (1956). *Vet. Rec.*, *68*, 474.
(4) Correa, J. E. & Calderin, G. G. (1966). *J. Amer. vet. med. Ass.*, *149*, 1556.
(5) Marsh, J. H. (1961). *Vet. Rec.*, *73*, 1124.

Index

Page numbers in italic type indicate principal references